Handbuch der experimentellen Pharmakologie
Handbook of Experimental Pharmacology

Heffter-Heubner New Series

XXXIX

Antihypertensive Agents

Contributers

M. E. Conolly · J. Conway · D. Ganten · R. Gaunt · F. Gross
H. Jurevics · O. Krayer · V. A. W. Kreye · J. B. Lüth · R. A. Maxwell
E. Meilman · J. C. Melby · J. A. Oates · C. C. Porter · B. N. C. Prichard
M. J. Rand · G. Schapel · D. G. Shand · E. Schlittler · H. Schmitt
C. A. Stone · M. L. Torchiana · W. B. Wastila

Editor

Franz Gross

With 120 Figures

Springer-Verlag Berlin · Heidelberg · New York 1977

Franz Gross, Professor Dr., Pharmakologisches Institut der Universität,
Im Neuenheimer Feld 366, D-6900 Heidelberg

ISBN 3-540-07594-1 Springer-Verlag Berlin · Heidelberg · New York
ISBN 0-387-07594-1 Springer-Verlag New York · Heidelberg · Berlin

Type setting, printing and binding: Brühlsche Universitätsdruckerei, Lahn-Gießen. 2122/3130-543210

Preface

Between 1950 and 1960, remarkable advances were made in the development of antihypertensive drugs, but since then, progress has been less rapid. This does not mean that no new drugs have been introduced: on the contrary, their number has increased sharply; but since the advent of the beta-adrenergic blockers no new pharmacodynamic principle has been discovered that could be applied widely as an antihypertensive. This has not been for want of efforts, because many attempts have been made to find new ways and means of influencing blood-pressure regulation or the mechanisms involved in the pathogenesis of hypertension. However, the results of these endeavors have mostly been disappointing. Even though high blood pressure can be treated more satisfactorily today than many other diseases, the success achieved in combating one of man's most frequent ailments should not induce complacency, but rather stimulate research towards further improvements.

The present standstill affords an opportunity to review the field of antihypertensive agents, for it is unlikely that fundamentally new drugs will appear in the near future. Although greater knowledge has been gained of the mechanisms of blood-pressure regulation and of the pathogenesis of hypertension, these advances have had no direct consequences in the search for new therapeutics. Antihypertensive drugs are still found by standard screening methods, which are little discriminating and give no information about the possible therapeutic usefulness of a new substance. Various drugs that looked promising in experiments on animals have turned out to be valueless in man, and some of the most widely used antihypertensives have been discovered by clinicians, e.g., the diuretics of the benzothiadiazine type or the beta-adrenergic blockers. It is admittedly not clear why certain drugs that reduce peripheral vascular resistance, either directly by acting on arteriolar smooth muscle or by interfering with the sympathetic innervation of the vascular wall, are inactive as antihypertensives. Theoretically, alpha-adrenergic blocking drugs should be more effective than beta-adrenergic blockers in reducing total peripheral resistance and lowering blood pressure. However, most attempts to use alpha-adrenergic blockers as antihypertensives proved unavailing, and the same holds true for various direct vasodilators that interfere with intracellular calcium release or inhibit phosphodiesterase activity. Attempts to reduce the formation of pressor substances by suppressing or competing with the enzymes involved in the biosynthesis of catecholamines (dopa-decarboxylase, dopamine-beta-hydroxylase) have failed, and it is doubtful whether further efforts in this direction will meet with more success. All these experiences indicate that so far the pathophysiologic approach to the search for antihypertensives has been unproductive, and that almost all the drugs used today have been found by trial and error.

Contributing an article to a handbook and editing a volume have become a laborious undertaking, and it is only a genuine dedication to the subject that can induce an author to accept the task. The editor wishes to express his sincere appreciation and thanks to all contributors to this manual for their excellent cooperation and their continuous efforts to keep their chapters abreast of the latest developments. Special thanks are due to all concerned for the patience with with which they have awaited the appearance of the volume. The editor assumes full responsibility for the undue delay in completing the manuscript and begs the authors' forgiveness for any inconvenience they have had to bear. He hopes that that the volume will reflect due credit upon all those who have contributed to it, and that readers will find in it a useful source of information and reference.

Heidelberg, August 1977 F. Gross

Table of Contents

Chapter 4

The Pharmacology of Rauwolfia Alkaloids. M. J. RAND and HELGA JUREVICS. With 5 Figures

Chapter 5

Adrenergic Neuron Blocking Drugs. R. A. MAXWELL and W. B. WASTILA. With 40 Figures

Chapter 7

The Pharmacology of Clonidine and Related Products. H. SCHMITT. With 29 Figures

Chapter 8

Drugs Acting on Arteriolar Smooth Muscle (Vasodilator Drugs). F. GROSS. The Section "III. Nitroprusside" was written by V. A. W. V. A. W. KREYE and F.GROSS. With 8 Figures

Chapter 9

Antihypertensive Effect of Diuretics. J. CONWAY. With 5 Figures

Chapter 10

The Pathophysiology of Adrenal Inhibitors with Respect to their Antihypertensive Activity
R. GAUNT and J. C. MELBY. With 18 Figures

Chapter 11

Interference with the Renin-Angiotensin System and Their Effects on High Blood Pressure.
D. GANTEN and F. GROSS. With 6 Figures

List of Contributors

M. E. CONOLLY, The Royal Postgraduate Medical School, London/Great Britain

J. CONWAY, Imperial Chemical Industry, Pharmaceutical Division, Mereside Aloerly Park, Maccesfiled, Cheshire SK 10, 4 TG/Great Britain

D. GANTEN, Pharmakologisches Institut der Universität, Im Neuenheimer Feld 366, 6900 Heidelberg/FRG

R. GAUNT, Club House Estates of Countryside, 2673 Pebble Beach Drive, Clearwater, Florida 33519/USA

F. GROSS, Pharmakologisches Institut der Universität, Im Neuenheimer Feld 366, 6900 Heidelberg/FRG

HELGA JUREVICS, Department of Pharmacology, University of Melbourne, Parkville, Victoria 3052/Australia

O. KRAYER, 3940 East Timrod Street 202, Tuscon, Arizona 85711/USA

A. W. KREYE, Physiologisches Institut der Universität, Im Neuenheimer Feld 426, 6900 Heidelberg/FRG

J. B. LÜTH, Pharmakologisches Institut der Universität, Im Neuenheimer Feld 366, 6900 Heidelberg/FRG

R. A. MAXWELL, Pharmacology Department, The Wellcome Research Laboratories, Burroughs Wellcome & Co. Inc. 3030 Cornwallis Road, Research Triangle Park, NC 27709/USA

E. MEILMAN, New Hyde Park, N. Y. 11040/USA

J. C. MELBY, Section of Endocrinology and Metabolism, Department of Medicine, Boston University, School of Medicine, Boston, Mass. 02118/USA

J. A. OATES, Department of Medicine and Pharmacology, Vanderbildt University, School of Medicine, Nashville, Tenn. 37203/USA

C. C. PORTER, Merck Institute for Therapeutic Research, West Point, Pennsylvania 19486/USA

B. N. C. PRICHARD, Medical Unit, Pharmacology and Therapeutics, University College Hospital, Medical School, University Street, London, WC1E 6JJ/Great Britain

M. J. RAND, Head of the Department of Pharmacology, University of Melbourne, Parkville 3052, Victoria/Australia

G. SCHAPEL, Department of Clinical Pharmacology, The Queen Elizabeth Hospital Woodville, 5011/South Australia

D. G. SHAND, The Royal Postgraduate Medical School, London/Great Britain

E. SCHLITTLER, Fürfelder Str. 20, 4125 Riehen/Switzerland

H. SCHMITT, Départment de Pharmacologie, Faculté de Medecine, Paris Broussais Hôtel-Dieu 15, Rue de l'Ecole de Médecine, Paris VIe/France

A. STONE, Merck Institute for Therapeutic Research, West Point, Pennsylvania 19486/USA

M. L. TORCHIANA, Merck Institute for Therapeutic Research, West Point, Pennsylvania 19486/USA

W. B. WASTILA, Pharmacology Department, The Wellcome Research, Laboratories, Burroughs Wellcome & Co. Inc. 3030 Cornwallis Road, Research Triangle Park, NC 27709/USA

Chapter 1

Antihypertensive Drugs

F. Gross

With 1 Figure

I. Introduction

Drugs may be classified according to their chemical structure, their pharmacology, or their therapeutic use, but none of these groupings is completely satisfactory and avoids either overlapping between, or forced attaching to, the various categories. The most debated classification is the one according to therapeutic application, since it may comprise not only substances which vary widely with respect to their chemical structures, but also drugs that differ fundamentally in their pharmacodynamic profiles. The volume on antihypertensive drugs is no exception to this rule and presents quite a few of the problems inherent in an arrangement compiling drugs which are used to lower high blood pressure.

In the treatment of hypertension, drugs are applied that interfere at various sites with the efferent sympathetic system, that occupy α- or β-adrenergic receptors, that have a direct effect on arteriolar smooth muscle, that may stimulate afferent parasympathetic activity, or that influence renal handling of water, sodium and potassium. The pharmacology of various of these classes of drugs has already been described or will be included in other volumes of the Handbook. Hence, chapters such as those dealing with the use of ganglionic blockers, of α- or β-adrenergic blocking drugs, of vasodilators, of diuretics or saluretics, of veratrum alkaloids, do not aim at completeness at all, but consider only the possible application of these drugs in antihypertensive therapy. The main purpose of the present volume is to provide the information necessary for rational and effective drug treatment of high blood pressure. For this reason, drugs which interfere with the renin-angiotensin system have actually been included, but are not extensively reviewed. Despite the interest they may have in the analysis of pathophysiologic mechanisms of hypertension and a few of them also as diagnostic tools, it is doubtful whether they will ever be of significance for the treatment of hypertension. Prostaglandins have been left out completely, although some of them, such as PGA_2 or PGE_2, as well as various of their derivatives have vasodilating activities which might come to be of some practical interest. It remains doubtful, however, that prostaglandins will ever be used in the treatment of hypertension. A chapter on α-sympathicolytics was originally planned, but had to be dropped for technical reasons. In view of the fact that, with some rare exceptions, these drugs are of minor significance as therapeutics for high blood pressure, such an omission was thought to be justifiable.

The title of the book refers to antihypertensive agents and not to hypotensive drugs. The lowering of blood pressure is a pharmacologic effect, elicited by numerous compounds, of which only a few are suitable for the treatment of hypertension. Onset, degree, and duration of the blood pressure lowering effect, the mode of action, the occurrence of side effects and adverse reactions are only some features that eventually determine if a hypotensive drug becomes an antihypertensive agent.

Various reviews on antihypertensive drugs have been published during recent years but none of them may claim to be complete. One of the earlier ones is that of A. F. GREEN (1962) which gives a good survey on what was known until then, but leaves out completely vasodilators such as hydralazine and dihydralazine which at that time had been on the market for 10 years. However, they had never found their way into Britain. The monograph Antihypertensive Agents edited by E. SCHLITTLER was published in 1967; it contains a lot of useful information but does not mention sodium nitroprusside or diazoxide which were already available at that time. In the yearly edited volumes on Drug Research in 1962 SCHLITTLER, DRUEY and MARXER and in 1968 SCHIER amd MARXER have reviewed antihypertensive agents mainly from the chemical point of view, and the same holds true for the review by WILHELM and DE STEVENS (1976). The most recent volume has been edited by ENGELHARDT (1976).

II. Requirements for an Antihypertensive Agent

From a clinical point of view, an antihypertensive should correspond to the following requirements (GROSS, 1974):

1. Induce a decrease in blood pressure that is of slow onset, not too pronounced, and similar in supine and standing positions.
2. Have a duration of action of 12 to 24 h.
3. Be active when taken by mouth.
4. Produce no negative inotropic effect on the heart, and no tachycardia.
5. Cause no tolerance.
6. Cause no adverse reactions or side-effects or only mild ones, and no reduction of physical capacity or mental alertness.
7. Be suitable for long-term treatment.

Today, none of the available drugs meets with all these demands. Whereas intensity and duration of action, absorption when given by mouth, or lack of tolerance are satisfactory with several drugs, none of them is free from side-effects. One of the major obstacles to the effective control of high blood pressure is the fact that many patients feel better without than with drug treatment. This is not only the case with drugs that affect the mood, such as reserpine, which may induce or unmask a depressive state, but also with other centrally acting agents which produce drowsiness and fatigue, loss of libido in man, postural hypotension, or the peripherally acting vasodilators which increase heart rate and cardiac output. The search for new drugs has therefore to be directed to better tolerated rather than to more effective agents.

Remarkable progress has been made in the treatment of high blood pressure since about 1950, when ganglionic blocking drugs became available (Fig. 1). However, it is obvious that during recent years no major contributions have been made, and that the speed of advance has remarkably slowed down since 1968 when the β-adrenergic blockers became accepted in the treatment of hypertension.

In looking on the success which has been achieved, one should also keep in mind that: 1) lowering of high blood pressure is in most cases only a symptomatic treatment. So far no causal therapy exists of primary hypertension, and the same holds true for most cases of secondary hypertension. 2) With a few exceptions, various types of hypertension that differ fundamentally in their pathogenesis are treated with the same drugs by trial and error.

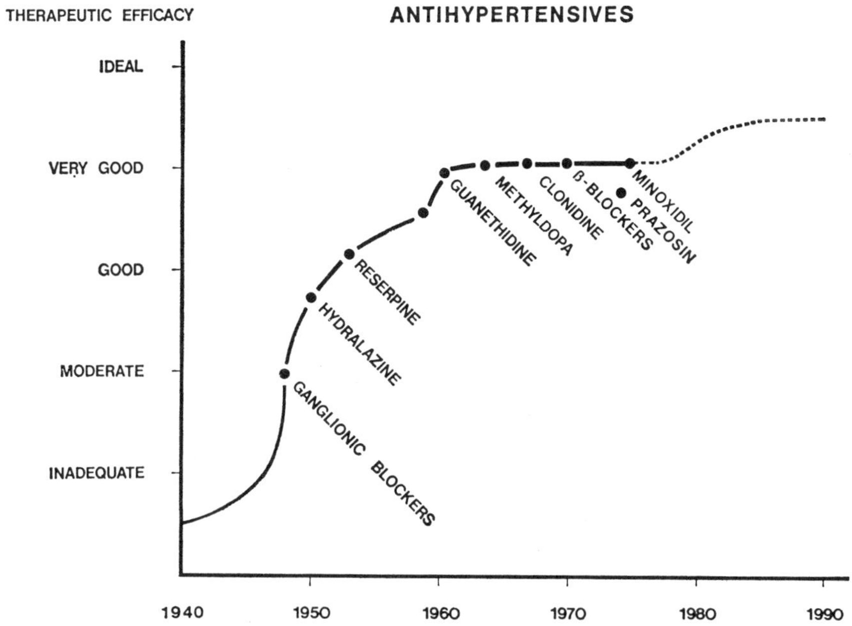

Fig. 1. Introduction of various antihypertensive drugs. Ordinate: Therapeutic assessment A Abscissae: Years

To a major degree this unsatisfactory situation depends on the fact that high blood pressure is not a nosologic entity, and is often an accompanying symptom of an underlying primary disease. Further differentiation of the diagnosis "hypertension" may help in the development of more specifically acting drugs. However, by far the largest share of patients suffering from high blood pressure has to be attributed to primary or essential hypertension, a disease that still retains the enigma of its pathogenesis and has no identifiable underlying mechanism comparable to those of the various forms of secondary hypertension. Primary hypertension depends on hereditary factors, age, and environmental conditions including socioeconomic features which are beyond fundamental alteration by drug treatment. Therefore we may hardly expect antihypertensives which act *specifically* against primary hypertension.

Attempts have been made to subdivide the total group of essential hypertension and about 20% of it has been separated according to a reduced response to various procedures that stimulate the renin-angiotensin system, such as physical exercise, saluretics or sodium restriction, and vasodilators. It soon became evident, however, that patients with suppressed renin response do not form a homogenous group. Age and duration as well as the severity of the disease are determining factors for the activity of the renin-angiotensin system (SCHALEKAMP et al., 1970, 1971, 1974) and for this reason the search for a common pathogenic factor in suppressed renin response would be in vain. Nevertheless, various steroids with sodium-retaining activity have been charged with being responsible for the reduced renin response such as 18-hydroxydesoxycorticosterone (18 OH-DOC) (MELBY et al., 1971; DALE and MELBY, 1973) or 16-β-hydroxy-dihydroepiandrosterone (16-β-OH-DHEA) (SENNET et al., 1975), but the weak mineralocorticoid activity of these steroids makes it improbable that they play a role in the pathogenesis of a group of patients with essential hypertension. Quite recently claims made for 16-β-OH-DHEA have been withdrawn (LIDDLE, 1976).

Despite the inappropriate concept to look for a mineralocorticoid as a responsible factor for the reduced responsiveness of the renin-angiotensin system, it has to be accepted that administration of a diuretic or an aldosterone antagonist for several weeks not only resulted in negative fluid and sodium balance, reduction of intravascular volume, loss of body weight and decrease in blood pressure, but also restored the responsiveness of the renin-angiotensin system (SPARK and MELBY, 1971; CAREY et al., 1972; VAUGHAN et al., 1973). The effective diuretic therapy in patients with reduced renin response indicates a quantitative rather than a qualitative deviation within the whole group of patients with essential hypertension; an observation that is of some significance for the selection of the therapeutic agent, but does not permit a pathogenetic subdivision.

Other efforts have been made to separate groups of patients with essential hypertension according to their response to certain drugs. The plasma renin activity (PRA) has been used as a parameter to predict the effectiveness of β-adrenergic blocking drugs (BÜHLER et al., 1972, 1973). According to the original claim, patients with essential hypertension in whom a high or normal PRA was determined should respond well to β-adrenergic blocking drugs whereas patients with a suppressed PRA would react with no or only a negligible lowering of their blood pressure. This simplified concept of a connection between the activity of the renin-angiotensin system and the blood pressure-lowering effect of β-adrenergic blocking drugs is based on the erroneous assumption that the renin-angiotensin system is of pathogenetic significance in a certain percentage of patients with essential hypertension. This, however, is not the case, although it is in no way excluded that primary essential hypertension may induce renal lesions with the consequence that the hypertension becomes renin dependent. The hypothesis of a relationship between PRA and the blood pressure-lowering effect of β-adrenergic blockers has aroused quite some interest, but only a few investigators have confirmed the original findings, whereas the majority found no such relationship (STOKES et al., 1974; BRAVO et al., 1975; MORGAN et al., 1975). In more recent studies it was observed that in patients with essential hypertension and a low PRA, higher doses of β-adrenergic blockers were necessary than in patients with normal or high PRA (KAPLAN, 1975; SHAND et al., 1975; HOLLIFIELD et al., 1976). Recently the role of renin in the therapy of hypertension has been reviewed by GUTHRIE et al. (1976).

III. Combinations of Antihypertensive Drugs

Since a specific treatment of high blood pressure is possible only in exceptional cases and since various types of antihypertensive drugs are available which differ with respect to their mechanisms of action, the combined use of drugs is a widely accepted practice in the treatment of high blood pressure. Whereas fixed drug combinations are regarded with increasing suspicion and are only reluctantly accepted by clinicians, pharmacologists, and health authorities, combinations have their established place in the treatment of high blood pressure and at least nobody denies the usefulness of giving two or even three drugs together. Of course, an individual combination according to the needs of the patient would be preferable but two or three drugs in one formula may be of practical advantage both for convenience and to obtain a better compliance with the prescription. On the other hand, a stepwise procedure is recommendable and in most patients, even those with severe hypertension, treatment should be started with a single drug (KOCH-WESER, 1973, 1974). Until recently these have been mostly saluretics, in some countries also reserpine. Today, the latter is only rarely used as drug of first choice and the saluretics have to increasingly share their role with the β-adrenergic blockers, which have been the most important contribution to the treatment of high blood pressure during recent years. If treatment has been started with a saluretic, *e.g.*, hydrochlorothiazide, a β-adrenergic blocker may be added after 2 to 3 weeks, in a case where blood pressure has not sufficiently responded to monotherapy, and vice versa: a saluretic may enhance the effectiveness of a β-blocker when it was given first. Should blood pressure not have fallen to normal values with such a combination, hydralazine may be added as a third drug.

The composition of combination products may vary from country to country. Most of the combinations contain a diuretic, many of them reserpine, and in some countries such as Germany, Italy, France, or Finland diuretic-reserpine combinations are still the most widely prescribed antihypertensives. In addition to these two components one or several others may have been included into one formula, but not infrequently these ingredients add nothing but the name to the combination and do not at all contribute to the efficient lowering of blood pressure. It is advisable to combine drugs which act at different sites within the system responsible for the regulation of blood pressure. In this respect the simultanous administration of a diuretic, a drug which influences the efferent sympathetic system and a vasodilator corresponds well to the stipulation of multilocal interferences with blood pressure regulation. Similarly the sympathetic innervation of the arterioles may be affected at various sites. However, not all combinations are useful and the selection of the components should be based on their mechanism of action and their pharmacologic profile, but not on preferences of manufacturers for some of their own products.

Besides the improved antihypertensive effect, combining of drugs may be advantageous in abolishing unwanted side effects. This is especially the case for the increase in heart rate and sometimes salt and fluid retention which occur with vasodilators, some of which have to be given together with β-adrenergic antagonists and with diuretics. Such combination may not only result in a better tolerability of the original drug but also enhance its blood pressure-lowering effect. In view of the variable response to vasodilators it is doubtful if fixed combinations may be suitable or if individual dosage of the components mentioned would be preferable.

IV. Trends in Antihypertensive Therapy

As in other fields of therapeutics, treatment varies according to the development of new drugs. The ganglionic blocking drugs which, around 1950, were the first effective antihypertensive agents, have been abandoned today, since more specifically acting sympatholytics have become available. The use of veratrum alkaloids is reserved for a few selected cases only. On the other hand, some older drugs such as hydralazine and dihydralazine have not only been remarkably resistent but have been more widely prescribed recently, partly because it has become possible to abolish the undesirable increase in heart rate by the simultaneous administration of β-adrenergic blockers. Between 1955 and 1965 an ever increasing share was taken by the drugs which interfere with the efferent sympathetic system such as reserpine, α-methyldopa, guanethidine, bethanidine, debrisoquine and clonidin. With the exception of guanethidine, bethanidine, and debrisoquine all these drugs pass the blood-brain barrier and affect mind and mood. The diuretics entered the field in 1959 and have held a significant share since. A new era began when the adrenergic β-blockers were found to lower high blood pressure, because for the first time drugs became available which reduced pressure similarly in the supine and upright position.

During the last 2 years there has been a growing tendency to concentrate antihypertensive treatment on peripherally acting drugs which do not pass the blood-brain barrier and do not affect wakefulness. An increasing number of patients are being treated with diuretics, vasodilators and β-adrenergic blockers (Gross, 1976). Most efforts have been directed toward the development of new vasodilators and β-adrenergic blocking drugs, but whereas a large number of β-blockers have been issued and still more are in an advanced stage of clinical investigation, only a few of the experimentally promising vasodilators have reached the market. Of those diazoxide and prazosine have to be mentioned, although the latter is less a vasodilator than an α-adrenergic antagonist. The most powerful vasodilator, minoxidil, is still in the phase of clinical evalution. Nevertheless, the tendency is evident to make more use of peripherally acting antihypertensives and to limit the administration of drugs that have a complete or partly central site of action. This trend will have repercussions on research in the field of antihypertensives. Although there is no need for further diuretics or β-adrenergic blockers, except one with a prolonged duration of action in the order of 24 h, new types of vasodilators that differ from those available, would be a valuable contribution to therapeutics. This would be especially the case for a drug having a mechanism of action similar to sodium nitroprusside but with a prolonged duration of action, and active when given by mouth. But so far nothing of such a type is in sight.

V. National Preferences of Treatment Schemes

Large differences exist for the preference of certain antihypertensive agents in various countries. Only a few data are available, but from marketing surveys it is evident that the use of antihypertensive drugs varies widely from country to country (Table 1). The reasons for these discrepancies are difficult to analyse but often lack a rational basis. It was already mentioned that in Britain hydralazine is regarded as a weak but dangerous drug, whereas it is widely used in the USA either alone or in combination. Reserpine is put in the same category as hydralazine in the U. K. whereas in Germany or Finland 80% of antihypertensive preparations contain reserpine or extracts of Rauwolfia. In the United States, Rauwolfia preparations are also still largely prescribed and the same is the case for Italy, France, Spain or countries of Latin America. In Britain guanethidine and more recently bethanidine and debrisoquine are widely used, while they have scarcely been administered in Germany or other countries of the European continent, and α-methyldopa which leads the list in Britain is far from being so popular in Germany or Italy (Gross, 1974; O'Brien, 1974; Freis, 1974). To these examples many others could be added, but it is already obvious from those quoted that it is not possible to establish a firm scheme for the treatment of high blood pressure. Medical education, postgraduate courses, continuing education, and experiences of leading specialists have major influences but also drug regulatory agencies or health services may be responsible for preferences or neglect of certain drugs, not only in hypertension but also in other fields. The position held by the drug manufacturer in a given country is of significance and of course also promotional efforts, although the influence of the latter is often overestimated.

Table 1. *Products prescribed (%) in general practice for the treatment of hypertension*

	United Kingdom	Belgium	Germany	Italy	Spain	Japan	Canada	Argentina
Rauwolfia products	6	13	3	5	8	32	5	16
Rauwolfia combinations	6	30	79	56	77	27	20	46
Other antihypertensive agents (guanethidine,								
Other antihypertensive agents (guanethidine, methyldopa)	50	39	6	17	5	13	22	25
Plain diuretic drugs	29	31	2	11	5	27	41	23
Cardiac glycosides	3	1	17	10	2	1	1	—

Analysis of the preferences and dislikes for certain drugs in individual countries should be followed by an analysis of the results of treatment. Is the hypertensive patient more effectively treated in Britain, in the USA or in Germany, three countries in which the leading antihypertensive drugs vary so widely from each other? An answer to this question is not possible for the time being. Reliable epidemiologic data on the results of treatment in various forms of high blood pressure are not available in most of the countries where data on prescriptions are at hand. It seems fair to assume, however, that the overall outcome of drug treatment of hypertension is similar in the various countries and quite independent of the different treatment schemes that are applied. It would be of considerable value to provide better evidence for such an assumption than that now available (GROSS, 1976).

VI. Experimental Hypertension

High blood pressure is one of the few human diseases which can be produced in experimental animals. Various forms of experimental hypertension have been developed and studied mainly with a view to obtaining information on etiology and pathogenesis of primary and secondary hypertension. In addition high blood pressure in experimental animals may be used as a tool for investigating drugs with regard to their antihypertensive activity. However, research on experimental hypertension has contributed little, if anything to the finding of drugs which are used today in the treatment of hypertension in man. All compounds applied as antihypertensives, with the exception of the saluretics, disclose their blood-pressure lowering effect in normotensive as well as in hypertensive animals, at least when suitable experimental conditions are chosen. It has to be admitted that the antihypertensive effect of some drugs such as the diuretics, clonidine or the β-adrenergic blockers were first observed in man, and only later were studied in animal experiments with respect to their blood pressure-lowering activity. It is, however, doubtful if their therapeutic usefulness in hypertension had been detected in the laboratory on the basis of a larger screening programme in rats with different types of experimental or spontaneous hypertension.

Each type of experimental hypertension should correspond to the following requirements:

1. It should be simple to elicit.
2. It should be easily and uniformly reproducible.
3. It should be comparable to some form of the human disease.
4. It should be elicited in small laboratory animals, preferably rats.

Various forms of experimental hypertension have clinical equivalents (Table 2), whereas others, such as adrenal regeneration hypertension have not. In the beginning of research on hypertension the renovascular forms were predominant, first in dogs (Goldblatt et al., 1934; Goldblatt, 1947) and later on also in rabbits (Pickering and Prinzmetal, 1938) and rats (Byrom and Wilson, 1938). Besides renal artery stenosis, wrapping of the kidneys in cellophane or placing a figure-of-eight ligature by means of a thread around the kidney were also used but did not bring any advantage and worked satisfactorily only in unilaterally nephrectomized rats or when both kidneys were wrapped (Page, 1939; Grollman, 1944).

Table 2. *Comparable forms of experimental and clinical hypertension*

Experimental	Clinical
Spontaneous hypertension of rats (SHR)	Essential hypertension (?)
Renal artery stenosis (rat, rabbit dog)	Renal artery stenosis
Renal infarction (rat rabbit)	Renal infarction
Perinephritis (wrapping, figure-of-8-ligature)	
Overdosage of glucocorticoids	Cushing syndrome
Overdosage of mineralocorticoids	Primary aldosteronism (adenoma, hyperplasia) Overproduction of DOC Overdosage of licorice
Overdosage of salt (rat)	Chronic high salt intake
Subtotal nephrectomy (rat)	Various forms of renal damage, Loss of nephrons

Subsequently endocrine hypertension was described, first produced with DOCA and salt (Selye, 1942) and later on also with glucocorticoids, cortisone or cortisol (Knowlton et al., 1952). The differences between mineralocorticoid- and glucocorticoid-induced forms of hypertension are mainly that DOCA hypertension depends on salt supply whereas glucocorticoids produce hypertension without the additional administration of salt. DOCA is still widely used for the induction of sustained hypertension, whereas the glucocorticoids have been abandoned as drugs to elicit high blood pressure in rats. Instead of them adrenal regeneration hypertension, which occurs after subtotal adrenalectomy (Skelton, 1959), has found wider interest and has been intensively investigated both with respect to its pathogenesis and for its possible use as a screening model for antihypertensive drugs.

Decisive progress in research on experimental hypertension was made, when various strains of rats with spontaneous hypertension were bred in several laboratories, mainly in New Zealand (Smirk and Hall, 1958), in Japan (Okamoto and Aoki, 1963) and in the USA (Dahl et al., 1962). High blood pressure in these strains of rat is hereditary, probably of multifactorial origin. It is relatively easy to select from an inbred strain of rats animals which have a higher blood pressure than the majority of animals of the same strain. After breeding for several generations blood pressure in most and later in all animals will be above average. Substrains with more or less pronounced hypertension have been selected and it is possible to maintain them over many generations (OKAMOTO et al., 1972). Various substrains have undergone changes since they left the laboratories or their origin and the rats kept in numerous places all over the world differ in various respect from the original strains. When studying these rats with spontaneous hypertension it is of importance to use nonhypertensive rats of the same stains as controls. Furthermore in some substrains an increased sensitivity of some vascular beds to high blood pressure has been observed, *e.g.*, in the cerebrovascular system. A stroke-prone substrain of the Kyoto strain was bred in which the incidence of stroke and cerebral infarction (OKAMOTO et al., 1974) rose to 80% of the animals and was found to be directly related to the height of pressure. Additional noxious factors such as high salt intake enhance the severity of cerebrovascular damage. It is of special importance that not only the tendency to develop high blood pressure but also the sensitivity of certain vascular beds for pressure induced lesions is of hereditary origin.

Spontaneous hypertensive rats without vascular complications respond well to antihypertensive drugs. In the original Aoki-Okamoto strain, blood pressure was less stable than in the New Zealand strain and was lowered already by general anesthesia. Such a lability of high blood pressure is of special significance when spontaneous hypertensive rats are used for the evaluation of antihypertensive agents.

In this context the various forms of experimental hypertension will not be discussed, but the reader is referred to some review articles (PLUMMER, 1967; GROSS, 1968, 1969; OKAMOTO, 1972).

Experimental hypertension may be subdivided according to the eliciting factors into hereditary, renal, endocrine, neurogenic and dietary forms. Of them the first three are most widely used in the laboratories of drug companies for the testing of antihypertensive agents. However, one has to keep in mind that some drugs according to their mechanism of action influence only special types of experimental hypertension. Diuretics, for example, are active only in mineralocorticoid or plainly salt-induced hypertension, but are inactive in renal hypertension, and β-adrenergic blockers do not have an effect on hypertension of renal or endocrine origin, when administered perorally or parenterally, but diminish blood pressure and sympathetic nerve activity when given into the cerebral ventricles of normotensive cats and rabbits (LEWIS and HAEUSLER, 1975). Despite the numerous attempts that have been made to develop a suitable method for testing antihypertensive drugs in animals, preferably rats, with experimental hypertension, no procedure has been found that could be generally applied to all the antihypertensives in use. There is also no method available that would give a higher degree of probability for detecting a new blood pressure-lowering drug than screening in the normotensive animal or in spontaneous hypertensive rats. It may be expected that future drugs to be used in the treatment of high blood pressure will also be found with the help of standard pharmacologic screening methods. However, when we try to analyse the current situation in the field of antihypertensives, it is obvious that the changes of discovering new drugs by means of conventional testing methods are rapidly dwindling. For the time being, or even for the next 10 years, no fundamentally new type of antihypertensive drug may be anticipated. Of course, there will be new drugs to treat high blood pressure but they hardly will have other than marginal advantages over those already at hand. The possibility is also not to be excluded that a new drug may be found on the basis of clinical observations; however, progress cannot be based on serendipity, but only on systematic research.

References

1. General

Bravo, E. L., Tarazi, R. C., Dustan, H. P., Lewis, J. W.: Dissociation between renin and arterial pressure responses in β-adrenergic blockade in human essential hypertension. Circulation Res. **36/37**, Suppl. I, 241—247 (1975).

Bühler, F. R., Laragh, J. H., Baer, L.: Propranolol inhibition of renin reaction. New Engl. J. Med. **287**, 1209—1214 (1972).

Bühler, F. R., Laragh, J. H., Vaughan, E. D.: Antihypertensive action of propranolol. Amer. J. Cardiol. **32**, 511—522 (1973).

Carey, R. M., Douglas, J. G., Schweikert, J. R.: The syndrome of essential hypertension and suppressed plasma renin activity. Arch. intern. Med. **130**, 849—854 (1972).

Dale, S. L., Melby, J. C.: Isolation and identification of 16, 18 dihydroxy deoxycorticosterone from human adrenal gland incubations. Steroids **21**, 617—632 (1973).

Engelhardt, E. L., ed.: Antihypertensive Agents. Am. Chem. Soc. Symp. Series 27, 1976.

Freis, E. D.: New drugs for hypertension. J. Amer. med. Ass. **229**, 689 (1974).

Green, A. F.: Antihypertensive agents. Advanc. Pharmacol. **1**, 161—225 (1962).

Gross, F.: Drug therapy of hypertension: What we have, what we need, what we expect. Amer. J. Cardiol. **34**, 471—475 (1974).

Gross, F.: Trends in the treatment of high blood pressure. In: Vascular neuroeffector mechanism, pp. 235—243. Basel: Karger 1976.

Guthrie, Jr., G. P., Genest, J., Kuchel, O.: Renin and the therapy of hypertension. Ann. Rev. Pharmacol. Toxicol. **16**, 287—308 (1976).

Hollifield, J. W., Sherman, K., Roger, R. N., Vander Zwagg, Shand, D. G.: Proposed. mechanism of propranolol's antihypertensive effect in essential hypertension. New Engl. J. Med. **295**, 68—74 (1976).

Kaplan, N. M.: The prognostic implications of plasma renin in essential hypertension. J. Amer. med. Ass. **231**, 167—170 (1975).

Koch-Weser, J.: Vasodilation for vasospastic hypertension. New Engl. J. Med. **289**, 213—214 (1973).

Koch-Weser, J.: Vasodilator drugs in the treatment of hypertension. Arch. intern. Med. **133**, 1017—1027 (1974).

Melby, J.C., Dale, S.L., Wilson, T.E.: 18-hydroxy deoxycorticosterone in human hypertension. Circulation Res. **28/29**, Suppl. II, 143—152 (1971).

Morgan, T., Carney, S., Roberts, R.: Changes in plasma renin activity and blood pressure after acute and chronic administration of β-adrenergic receptor blocking drugs. Clin. Sci. molec. Med. **48**, 81s—83s (1975).

O'Brien, W.: The management of essential hypertension. J. Amer. med. Ass. **229**, 693—694 (1974).

Schalekamp, M. A. D. H., Schalekamp-Kuyken, M. P. A., Birkenhäger, W. H.: Abnormal renal haemodynamics and renin suppression in hypertensive patients. Clin. Sci. **38**, 101—110 (1970).

Schalekamp, M. A. D. H., Krauss, X. H., Schalekamp-Kuyken, M. P. A., Kolsters, G., Birkenhäger, W. H.: Studies on the machanism of hypernatriuresis in essential hypertension in relation to measurements of plasma renin concentration, body fluid compartments and renal function. Clin. Sci. **41**, 219—231 (1971).

Schalekamp, M. A. D. H., Birkenhäger, W. H., Kolsters, G., Lever, A. F.: Pathogenetic aspects of low-renin hypertension. In: Distler, A., Wolff, H.-P. (Eds.): Hypertension. Current Problems, pp. 133—142. Symposium Mainz 1973. Stuttgart: Thieme 1974.

Schier, O., Marxer, A.: Antihypertensive agents 1962—1968. Drug Res. **13**, 101—135 (1968).

Schlittler, E., ed.: Antihypertensive Agents. New York-London: Academic Press 1967.

Schlittler, E., Druey, J., Marxer, A.: Antihypertensive agents. Drug Res. **4**, 295—352 (1962).

Sennett, J. A., Brown, R. D., Island, D. P., Yarbo, L. R., Watson, J. T., Slaton, P. E., Hollifield, J. W., Liddle, S. W.: Evidence for a new mineralocorticoid in patients with low-renin essential hypertension. Circulation Res. **36/37**, Suppl. I, 2—9 (1975).

Shand, D., Frisk-Holmberg, M., McDevitt, D., Sherman, K., Hollifield, J.: A dual antihypertensive mechanism for propranolol based on plasma level/response relationships. In: Berglund, G., Hansson, L., Werkö, L. (Eds.): Pathophysiology and management of arterial hypertension, pp. 175—182. Göteborg: Astra 1975.

Spark, R. F., Melby, J. C.: Hypertension and low plasma renin activity: presumptive evidence for mineralocorticoid excess. Ann. intern. Med. **75**, 831—836 (1971).

Stokes, G. S., Weber, M. A., Thornell, I. R.: Beta-blockers and plasma renin activity. Brit. med. J. **1974 I**, 60—62.

Vaughan, E. D. Jr., Laragh, J. H., Gavras, I., Bühler, F. R., Gavras, H., Brunner, H. R., Baer, L.: Volume factor in low and normal renin essential hypertension. Treatment with either spironolactone or chlorthalidone. Amer. J. Cardiol. **32**, 523—532 (1973).
Wilhelm, M. de Stevens, G.: Antihypertensive agents. Drug Res. **20**, 198—259 (1976).

2. Experimental Hypertension

Byrom, F. B., Wilson, C.: A plethysmographic method for measuring systolic blood pressure in the intact rat. J. Physiol. (Lond.) **93**, 101—104 (1938).
Dahl, L. K., Heim, M., Tassinari, L.: Effect of chronic excess salt injection. Evidence that genetic factors play an important role in susceptibility to experimental hypertension. J. exp. Med. **115**, 1173—1190 (1962).
Goldblatt, H.: The renal origin of hypertension. Physiol. Rev. **27**, 120—165 (1947).
Goldblatt, H., Lynch, J., Hanzal, R. F., Summerville, W. W.: Studies on experimental hypertension. I. The production of persistent elevation of systolic blood pressure by means of renal ischaemia. J. exp. Med. **59**, 347—379 (1934).
Grollman, A.: A simplified procedure for inducing chronic renal hypertension in the mammal. Proc. Soc. exp. Biol. (N. Y.) **57**, 102—104 (1944).
Gross, F.: Experimentell renaler Hochdruck und experimenteller Hochdruck mit Nierenveränderungen. In: Schwirgk, H. (Ed.): Handbuch der Inn. Medizin. Nierenkrankheiten. Teil 2, pp. 3—34. Berlin-Heidelberg-New York: Springer 1968.
Gross, F.: Experimentelle Hypertonie. In: Heintz, R., Losse, H. (Eds.): Arterielle Hypertonie. Pathogenese — Klinik — Therapie, pp. 63—89. Stuttgart: Thieme 1969.
Knowlton, A. L., Loeb, E. N., Stoerk, H. C., White, J. P., Hefferman, J. F.: Induction of arterial hypertension in normal and adrenalectomized rats given cortisone acetate. J. exp. Med. **96**, 187—205 (1952).
Lewis, P. J., Haeusler, G.: Central nervous effects of β-blockers in hypertension. In: Berglung, G., Hansson, L., Werkö, L. (Eds.): Pathophysiology and Management of Hypertension, pp. 203—209. Göteborg: Astra 1975.
Okamoto, K.: In: Okamoto, K., (Ed.): Spantaneous hypertension, its pathogenesis and complications. Tokyo: Igaku Shoin Ltd. 1972.
Okamoto, K., Aoki, K.: Development of a strain of spontaneously hypertensive rats. Jap. Circulat. J. (Ni.) **27**, 282—293 (1963).
Okamoto, K., Yamori, Y., Ooshima, A., Park, C., Haebara, H., Matsumoto, M., Tanaka, T., Okuda, T., Hazama, F., Kyogoku, M.: Establishment of the inbred strain of the spontaneously hypertensive rat and genetic factors involved in hypertension. In: Okamoto, K. (Ed.): Spontaneous hypertension, its pathogenesis and complications, pp. 1—8. Tokyo: Igaku Shoin Ltd. 1972.
Okamoto, K., Yamori, Y., Nagaoka, A.: Establishment of the stroke-prone spontaneously hypertensive rat (SHR). Circulation Res. **34**, Suppl. I, 143—154 (1974).
Page, I. H.: The production of persistent arterial hypertension by cellophane perinephritis. J. Amer. med. Ass. **113**, 2046—2048 (1939).
Pickering, G. W., Prinzmetal, M.: Experimental hypertension of renal origin in the rabbit. Clin. Sci. **3**, 357—368 (1938).
Plummer, A. J.: Experimental hypertension in animals and its use in screening for antihypertensive compounds. In: Schlittler, E. (Ed.): Antihypertensive Agents, pp. 68—114. New York-London: Academic Press 1967.
Selye, H.: Production of nephrosclerosis by overdosage with desoxycorticosterone acetate. Canad. med. Ass. J. **47**, 515—519 (1942).
Skelton, F. R.: Adrenal regeneration and adrenal regeneration hypertension. Physiol. Rev. **39**, 162—182 (1955).
Smirk, F. H., Hall, W. H.: Nature (Lond.) **182**, 727—728 (1958).

Chapter 2

The Chemistry of Antihypertensive Agents

E. SCHLITTLER

In accordance with the wishes of the Editor, a chapter on the chemistry of antihypertensive agents precedes the pharmacological chapters. If the author has not succeeded in giving all chemical structures for antihypertensive agents mentioned in subsequent contributions, his only consolation for this failure is the fact that this "Handbuch" is concerned with activity of drugs and not with their chemistry. It is not the chemistry but the biological activity which counts in this field of research.

There are no contributions on the chemistry of saluretics, false adrenergic transmitters, the use of β-blockers in antihypertensive therapy, pathophysiology of adrenal inhibitors, or clinical pharmacology of antihypertensives, partly because the chemistry of these compounds has been dealt with adequately in earlier volumes of this "Handbuch", and partly because subsequent chapters already contain a fair amount of chemistry.

Research on the chemistry of antihypertensives has been enormous during the last 20 years, but it is still true that "until the mysteries of the etiology of essential hypertension are unravelled", treatment of elevated blood pressure must remain empiric and palliative (GIFFORD, 1972). However, today hypertension is called a "controllable disease" (FREIS, 1972).

As it is impossible to mention all chemical compounds for which hypotensive or antihypertensive activity has been claimed, a selection had to be made. Also compounds mentioned only in patents are mostly not considered, as long as their claims have not been substantiated by scientific publications.

Most literature reviews stress either the pharmacodynamic or the clinical problems of antihypertensive agents. However, there are a few reviews which are mainly concerned with the chemical side. Important reviews can be found in "Annual Reports in Medicinal Chemistry"; vol. 1—10 (1965—1975) ed. Amer. chem. Soc. see also SCHIER and MARXER (1969), CARSTENS (1972), and DE STEVENS, WILHELM (1976).

I. Early Antihypertensives

LEROY (1909) stated "no remedy can or will reduce the blood pressure so kindly and so quickly, when given after a proper manner than the thiocyanates". In 1972 the following announcement appeared in the Federal Register: "There is a lack of evidence that the effectiveness of potassium thiocyanate is sufficient to justify its use for the treatment of hypertension and relief of headaches associated with hypertension, in view of known serious hazards associated with such use."

The thiocyanates, the most important drugs used before the "rational" treatment of high blood pressure, were probably first studied by PAULI (1904), but soon dropped and later resumed by WESTPHAL (1926). In general, there was a great divergence of opinion (BARKER, 1936), the majority of investigators claiming that rhodanide treatment had little effect or that the toxic effects of the drug were so common or dangerous that they interfered seriously with its administration (STIEGLITZ, 1932; GOLDRING and CHASIS, 1932; MASSIE et al., 1938; CAVINESS et al., 1941; RUSSEL and STAHL, 1942; PAGE, 1952; HOFFMEISTER and KRÜCK, 1954). Since the introduction of specific antihypertensives the rhodanides have fallen into disrepute, which justifies the doubts expressed in the Federal Register (see above).

The rhodanides were probably the most frequently used, but not the only antihypertensives employed in the first 30 years of this century. GUTMAN (1941) listed more than 100 preparations including, among others, barbiturates, nitrites, liver extracts, misteltoe extracts, and a great number of ill-defined "patent medicines". Bismuth subnitrate was used as an antihypertensive in the years 1927 to 1935 (STIEGLITZ, 1928, 1932; AYMAN, 1932). Intravenous injections of an aqueous solution of *n*-octyl alcohol were claimed to have an antihypertensive effect (AYMAN, 1930; CLERK et al., 1933; RACINE, 1935; PEZZANGARO, 1936).

The use of inorganic and organic azides dates back to early work of WERLE's (1938) and this work has continued up to the present day (WERLE and FRIED, 1951, 1952; ROTH et al., 1956; WERLE and STÜCKER, 1958; BLACK et al., 1954). According to WERLE, the action of sodium azide is peripheral, but its duration, after oral application to humans, is short (BLACK et al., 1954). Organic azides are the subject of recent patent applications (FMC 1966, 1967, 1968, 1969). MATIER et al. (1972) have recently reported on hypotensive sulfamoylazides. (See also: SIVACH et al., 1975.)

Some consideration should also be given to early investigations of guanidines. Whereas it was found (MAJOR and STEPHENSON, 1924; MAJOR, 1925) that intravenous injection of methylguanidine caused an increase of blood pressure in dogs, ALLES (1926) found that arylguanidines, symmetrical diphenylguanidines, and triphenylguanidine caused a fall in blood pressure with an accompanying decrease in heart rate.

For a very interesting and comprehensive review on drug treatment of high blood pressure see a public lecture by PAGE (1966).

II. Adrenergic Neuronal Blockers: Guanethidine and Similar Compounds

The preparation of guanethidine and guanethidine-like compounds was unrelated to the desire to obtain strongly alkaline, highly ionized compounds with effects possibly similar to the quaternary blockers (BOURA et al., 1961). On the contrary, it was the purpose of a CIBA-US team to look for compounds with activity against trypanosomiasis, the African sleeping sickness. Some pertinent information was available in this respect, since KING et al. (1937) demonstrated that guanidino compounds possess some activity in experimental trypanosomiasis. Also for certain diamidoximes, antitrypanosomal activity has been reported (LAMB and WHITE, 1939). Polymethylene imine rings were chosen as a part of these compounds because their derivatives were largely unknown. Thus, a large number of strongly alkaline compounds with a predictable low absorption on oral application was obtained.

The first compound prepared was the amidoxime SU 4029 (Mull et al., 1957; Maxwell et al., 1958; Maxwell and Schneider, 1961).

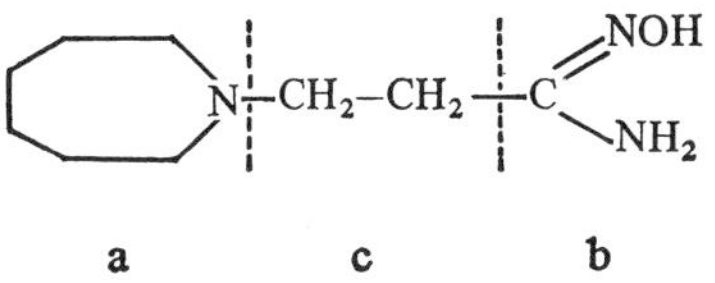

SU 4029: 3-(Hexahydro-1-azepinyl) propionamidoxime

(1)

SU 4029 was completely inactive against trypanosomiasis, but an observant pharmacologist noticed that SU 4029 caused a fall in blood pressure that lasted for several weeks (see Chapter by Maxwell and Wastila in this volume). Clinical trials demonstrated similar activity in man, but the compound was unexplainably pyrogenic. In spite of this undesirable feature, which necessitated immediate with-drawal of SU 4029 from the trials, this provided a valuable lead for continuing research.

A. SU 4029 and Guanethidine

SU 4029 consisted of three parts:

a) the polymethylene imine ring (often called "bridgehead"),
b) the terminal, strongly polar group ("end-group"),
c) the "bridge" between the "end-group" and the polymethylene imine ring.

It was obvious that these three moieties could be manipulated and the following table illustrates how this problem was attacked at an early stage of guanethidine research. The following modifications of the molecular structure were carried out (Mull and Maxwell, 1967):

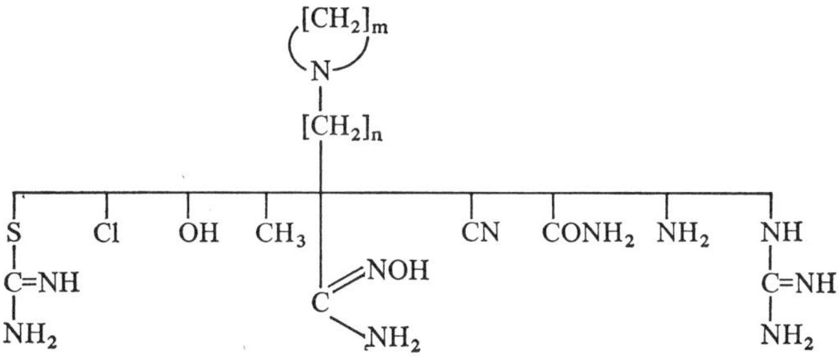

m = 5–7
n = 1–4

The conclusion from these preliminary investigations was the proposal that, among the many compounds with antihypertensive activity, the guanidine SU 5864 should be tested clinically:

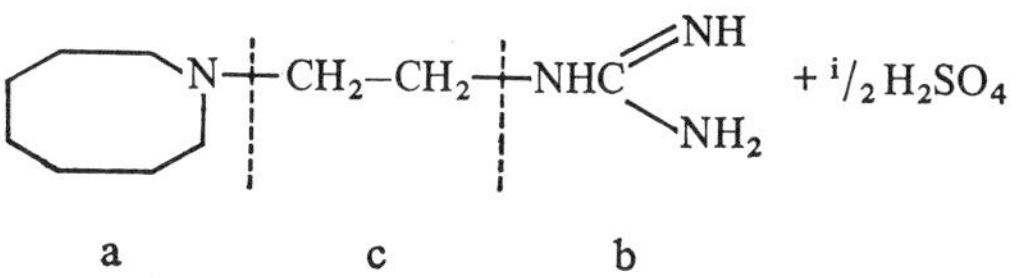

SU 5864: 2-(Hexahydro-1-(2H)-azocinyl)-ethyl-guanidine sulfate (Maxwell et al., 1959; Mull et al., 1960)

(2)

The results of this clinical investigation gave a favorable picture of SU 5864 and it was then given the name guanethidine (ISMELIN) (Octadine or Isobarin in Russia, SPIVAKOVA, 1971; BEGEKA and GROISMAN, 1975). Guanethidine was not as long-acting as 4029, but it possessed strong antihypertensive activity and was free of the pyrogenic effect of SU 4029.

SAH et al. (1966) pointed out that guanethidine should probably be written in a skewed form (3), but its action is not comparable with that of the quaternary "pyrrolizidine analog" (4).

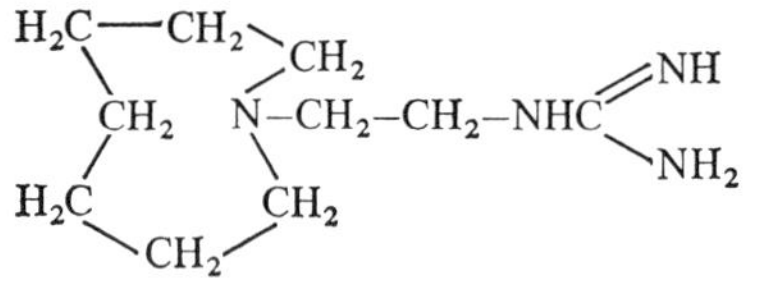

(3)

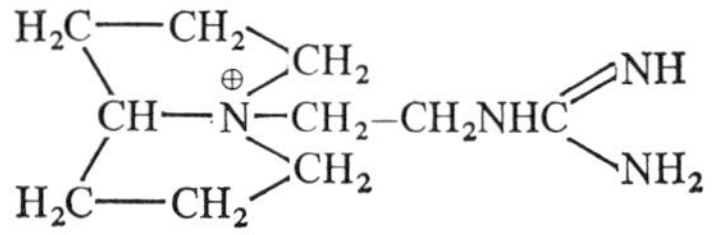

(4)

B. Modification of the Guanethidine Structure

Besides the original inventors of guanethidine, many other groups have participated in this endeavor and today it is almost impossible to survey this field completely. Only the most important compounds will therefore be mentioned below.

The structure of (1) and (2) clearly indicates possibilities for numerous modifications. Few modifications of the "bridge" part (c) have been made; it consists mainly of two or three methylene groups. The polymethylene rings were enlarged and reduced, or bridged by methylene groups or attached to aromatic rings, also additional nitrogen was introduced into the polymethylene imine ring. With some success, the polymethylene imine ring was replaced by a benzene ring, giving compounds like bethanidine (see Chap. 5). Also the strongly polar guanidine or amidoxime end groups were extensively modified. All these modifications were carried out individually, but some changes were made simultaneously. Most structure-activity studies (SAR) were done with the guanidino compounds but, where appropriate, amidoximes will also be mentioned.

a) Large Ring Compounds with Guanidino or Amidoxime Structure

Large rings show decreased activity and in the case of the eleven-membered ring there is also a noticeable increase in toxic side-effects.

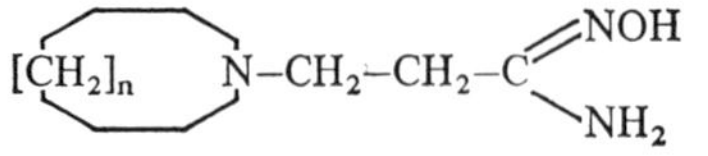

(5)

$n = 6$: very weak (SU 5078)
$n = 5$: very weak (SU 5898)
$n = 4$: very active (SU 4975)
$n = 3$: very active (SU 4852)
$n = 2$: very active (SU 4029)
$n = 1$: very weak (SU 3857)

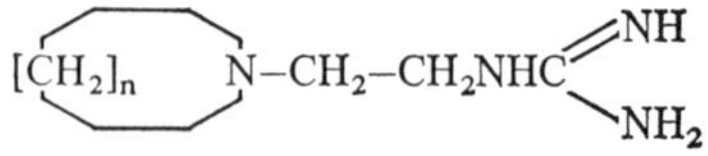

(6)

$n = 5$: weak (SU 6249)
$n = 4$: moderate (SU 6023)
$n = 3$: very active (SU 5864)
$n = 2$: moderate (SU 5690)
$n = 1$: moderate (SU 5954)

b) Eight-membered Rings with Additional Nitrogen or Modified Polar End Groups (e.g. amino guanidines)

Although cardiovascular activity was noted with compound (7), it was not exceptional (MULL et al., 1962).

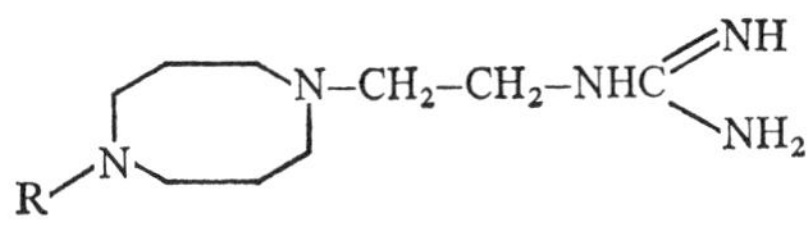

(7) R = CH_3 or C_5H_5

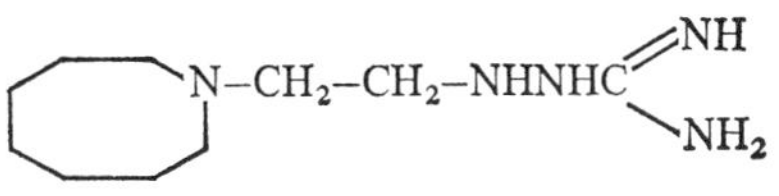

(8) marked hypotensive effect: (BOTTON et al., 1965)

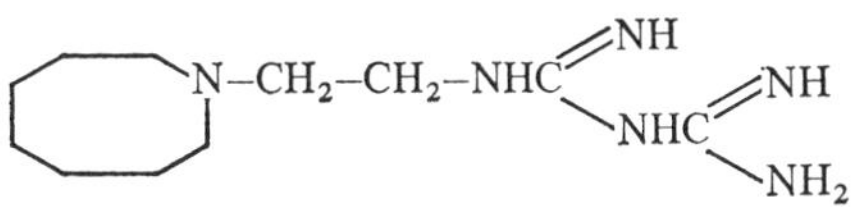

(9) hypotensive: (ROBERTSON, 1963)

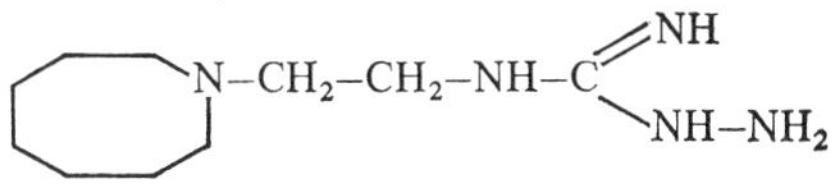

(10) guanethidine-like effect with rapid onset of action: (MULL, 1961)

c) Azepine Rings with End Groups other than Amidoximes

Compound (11) seems to possess only reduced antihypertensive activity; compound (12) is an amidine (BW 1113C60) whose activity was investigated by BOURA et al. (1962).

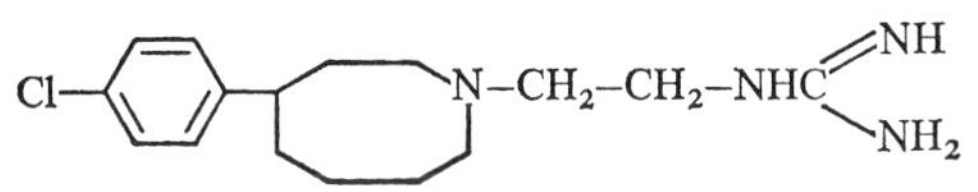

(11) (OZAWA et al., 1965)

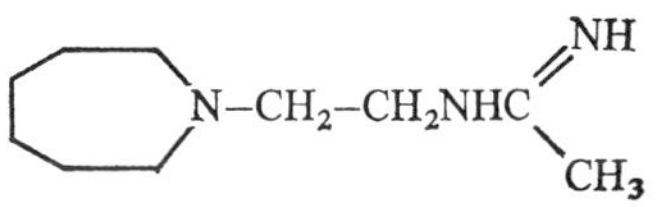

(12)

d) Pyrrolidine, Piperidine, and Piperazine Rings

It was found (WOLLWEBER et al., 1971) that most pyrrolidines with the guanidinoethyl side-chain reacted as ganglionic blockers. According to another investigation (CURWAIN et al., 1971) pyrrolidino ethyl guanidines with a certain number of smaller substituents are active; however, the activity declines with larger substituents. This work indicated that the total number and the distribution of alkyl groups in the pyrrolidine ring is more important than the ring size. Active derivatives are

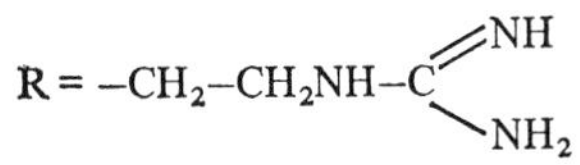

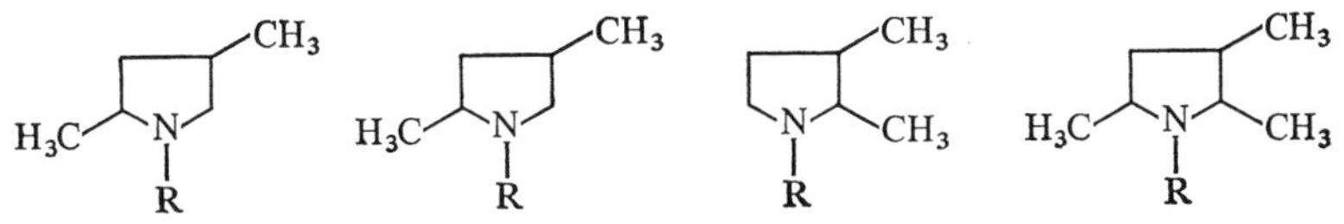

Some piperidines [*e.g.* the pempidine analog (13) were ganglionic blockers, whereas others, like (14) and (15)], were postganglionic adrenergic neuronal blockers.

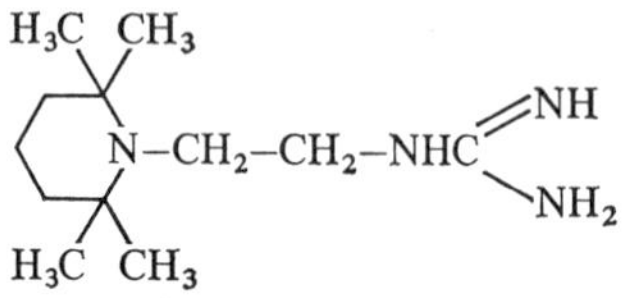

(13)

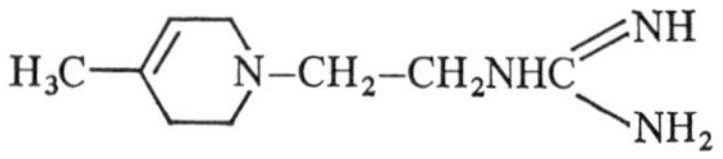

(14) Guanaclin, Cyclazenine, Leron® (KRONEBERG et al., 1967)

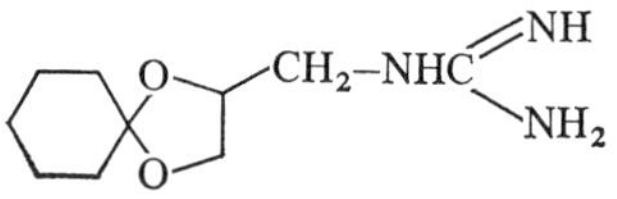

(15)

For some time cyclazenine was a widely used antihypertensive agent, but it had to be recalled from the market in 1971 due to its side-effects.

Piperazine derivatives (16) and (17) had a distinct, but reduced antihypertensive activity. Preliminary clinical trials with (16) were not encouraging.

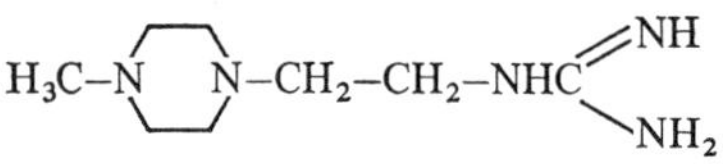

(16) (MULL et al., 1962)

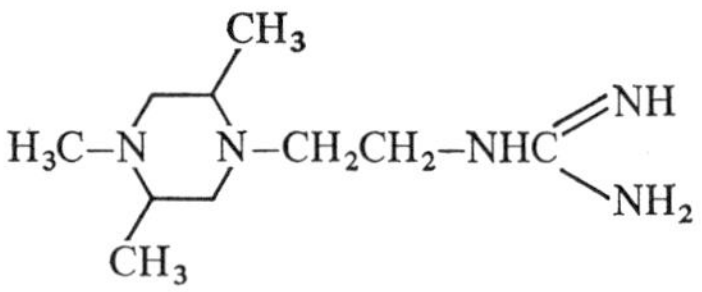

(17) MULL et al. (1962) less active than cpd without methyl in positions 2 and 5

e) Azaspiroalkanes

Several azaspiroalkanes have been synthesized, the most active being (18). It has been tested clinically, but its side-effects were such that it had to be dropped.

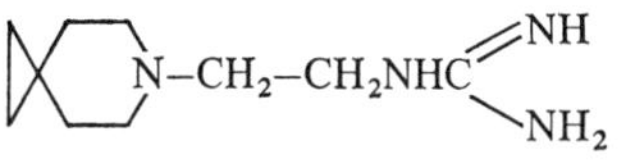

(NAJER et al., 1965)

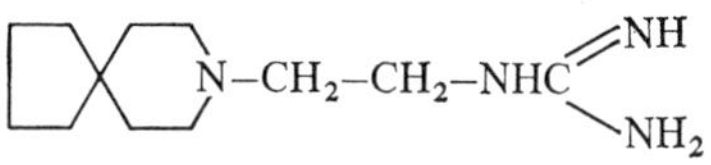

(18) $1^1/_2$–2 x guanethidine (GIUDICELLI et al., 1964)

An oxo spiro compound is guanadrel (19) (U 28.288; CL 1388 R) whose effect appears to be similar to that of guanethidine but with only one third the potency on a weight basis.

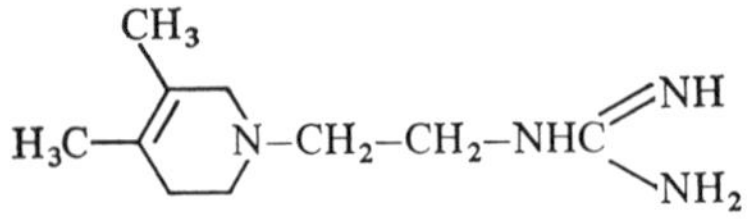

(see also HANSSON et al., 1973)

(19) Guanadrel (BLOOMFIELD and CANGIANO, 1970; PRUSS and HIDALGO, 1972)

f) Bicyclic Compounds

The following two isoquinoline derivatives have been introduced as antihypertensives (20 and 21) and a number of analogs are mentioned in the literature (LAPE et al., 1971)

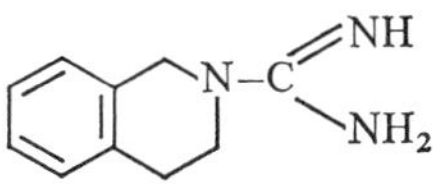

(20) Debrisoquin, Declinax (WENNER et al., 1965)

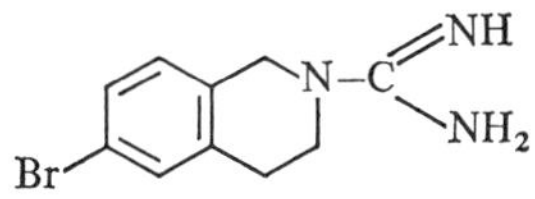

(21) Guanisoquin, (SCRIABINE et al., 1965, 1966)

Three dioxan derivatives, selected from a large number of the synthesized compounds seemed to be interesting, and one has been introduced as guanoxan (22). Compound (23) has a doubly methylated guanidino group like bethanidine. Another dioxan derivative is a spiro compound (24).

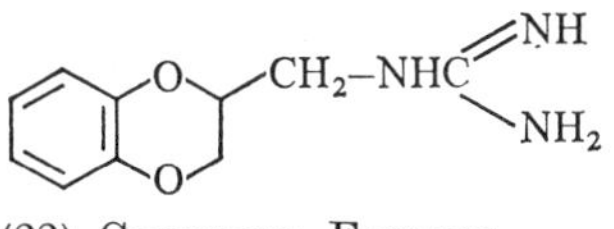

(22) Guanoxan, Encavar (AUGSTEIN et al., 1965; BAINES et al., 1965)

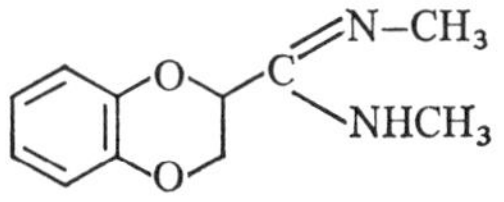

(23) (SCRIABINE et al., 1964)

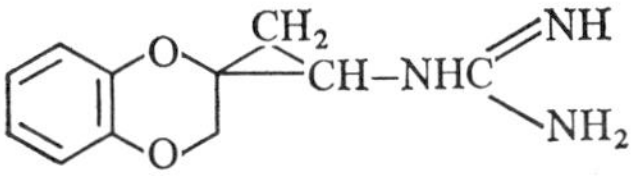

(24) (MONRO et al., 1967)

A later paper (AUGSTEIN et al., 1968) discussed modifications of the heterocyclic ring of guanoxan and general studies of the effect of these changes.

g) Aromatic Guanidino Compounds

Besides guanethidine (2), bethanidine (25) is the most frequently used adrenergic neuronal blocker. Its guanidino group is doubly methylated and for the study of SAR a great number of analogs were made. Most of these compounds have a phenyl group as a bridgehead (a), and one methylene group as "bridge" (c). In general, lengthening of the bridge (c) beyond one CH_2 group (*e.g.* 26) reduced

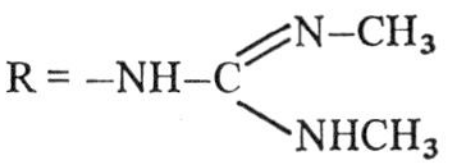

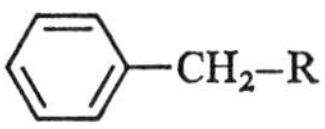

(25) Bethanidine Esbatal (BOURA et al., 1961)

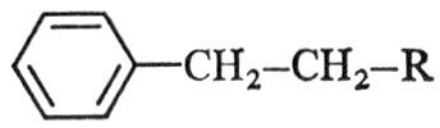

(26) (FIELDEN et al., 1965)

activity. One halogen in position 2 (27) increased activity, whereas the doubly chlorine-substituted compound (28) is mentioned in a patent application of NADOR and KAROLY (1969). Also other substituents like (29) give active compounds.

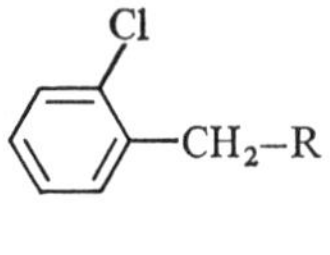

(27)

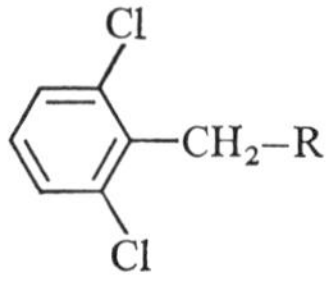

(28)

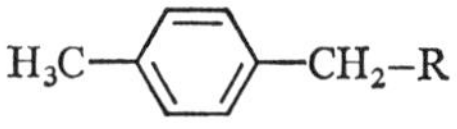

(29)

The observation that a benzene ring can replace the polymethylene imine structure has had a stimulating effect upon research in this group of compounds and besides the therapeutically used bethanidine a large number of experimental derivatives have been prepared. A simple "amphetamine approach" led to compounds like (30) or (31) (FIELDEN et al., 1965) and it is claimed that the (−) isomer of (30) has high adrenergic neuronal blocking action whereas the (+) isomer of (30) antagonizes this effect.

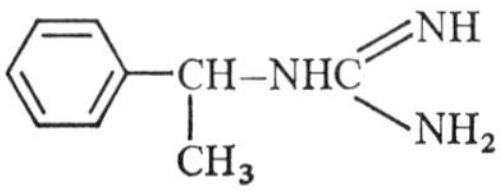

(30)

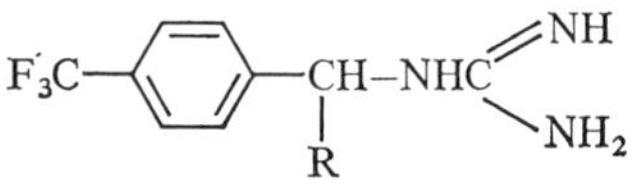

(31) R = H or CH_3
(SHORT et al., 1967)

Two other compounds of interest are (−) β-hydroxyphenethyl guanidine (32) and the two cinnamyl guanidines (cis and trans 33).

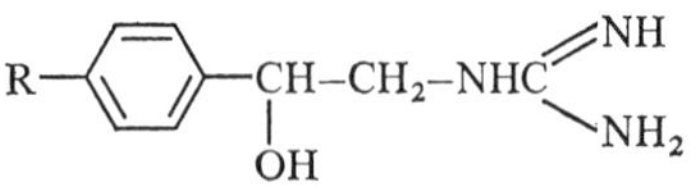

(32) R = H or Cl
(FIELDEN and GREEN, 1967, 1968)

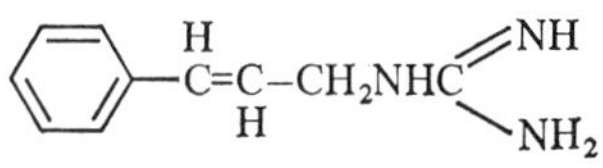

(33) SU 13.686 (cis)
(BARRETT et al., 1965)

Cis-cinnamylguanidine (33), which is considerably more active than the corresponding trans compound, has failed in clinical use in spite of some definite advantages.

Eighty-six aralkylamino guanidines have been prepared by BREAM et al. (1970); the following compounds (34) were found to be the most active:

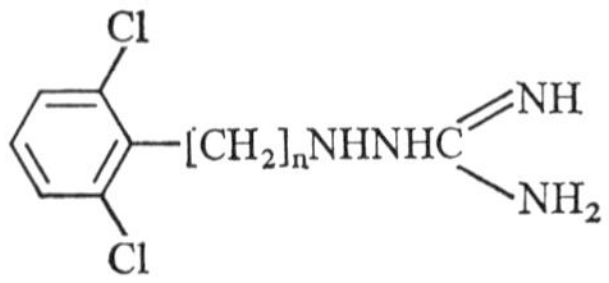

n = 2 and 3

(34)

Even more complex aromatic structures than benzene derivatives can yield active compounds. The antihypertensive properties of a series of 20 indole and azaindole amidoximes have been tested and found to be active, (35) and (36) being the most active ones (BELL et al., 1967; LAPE et al., 1968).

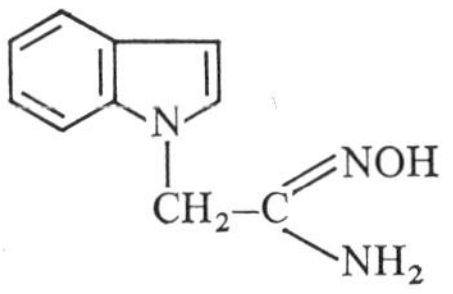

(35) Indole-1-amidoxime

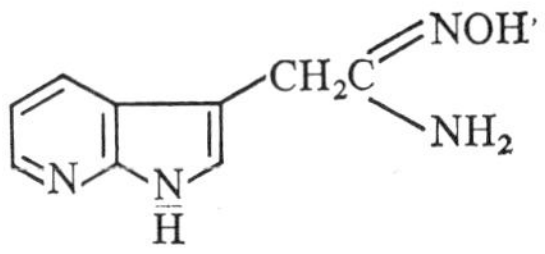

(36) 7-Azaindole-3-acetamidoxime

h) Anilinoguanidines, Phenoxyguanidines and Phenoxyaminoguanidines

The group of anilinoguanidines is small, one of its representatives being (37) (OZAWA and SATO, 1967)

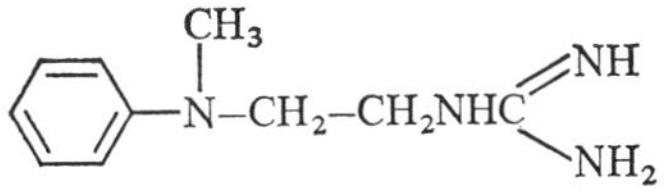

(37) (2-methyl(phenylamino)ethyl guanidine)

The group of phenoxyguanidines and phenoxyaminoguanidines is larger and it is interesting to note that extensive use of *o*—*o'* double substitution of the aromatic ring (as in clonidine) has been made. (38) is claimed to have antihypertensive activity in man similar to guanethidine. Compound (39) is guanoclor.

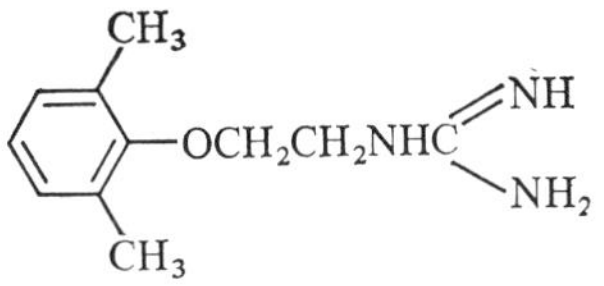

(38) (BARRON et al., 1963a and 1963b)

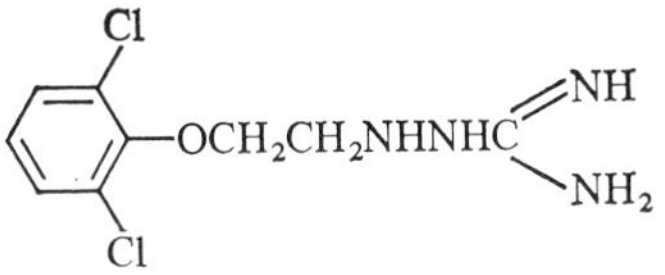

(39) Guanoclor, Vatensol (AUGSTEIN et al., 1965)

The two following isomers of guanoclor show very little antihypertensive activity:

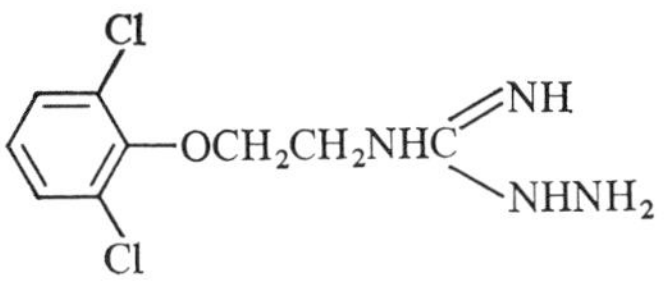

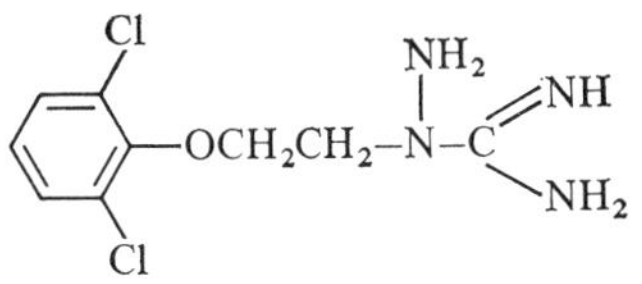

i) Bretylium

Although bretylium (40) (*o*-bromobenzyl ethyldimethylammonium *p*-toluene sulfonate) has the typical structure of a ganglionic blocker, it has adrenergic neuronal blocking effects.

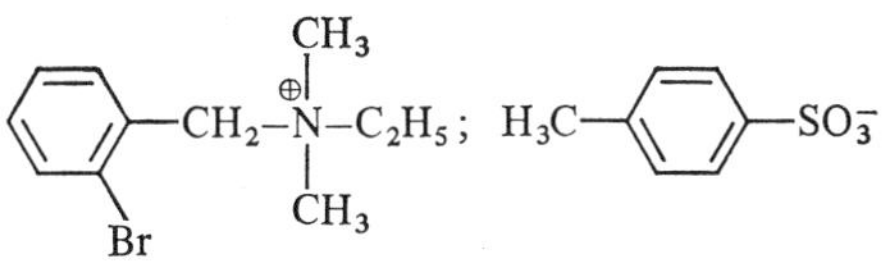

(40) Bretylium, Darenthine

SAR studies of a large number of analogs of bretylium (BOURA et al., 1959a, 1959b, 1959c) mostly concerned changes in the substitution of the aromatic ring. On the basis of activity, specificity and low toxicity, bretylium seemed most promising for therapeutic use and was therefore clinically tested and introduced. The meta and para as well as disubstituted analogs of bretylium failed to show worthwhile activity. Also other alterations of the cationic group of (40) mainly produced less active compounds. Although bretylium plays a lesser role in therapy today, the chemical connection between bretylium and bethanidine is evident.

k) Aliphatic Guanidines

A few aliphatic guanidines have been found to possess antihypertensive activity, provided their "bridgehead" (a) has a certain "bulkiness" (SHORT et al., 1968). This can be illustrated by two amidoximes, (1) being highly active, whereas the di-*n*-propyl compound (41) is inactive.

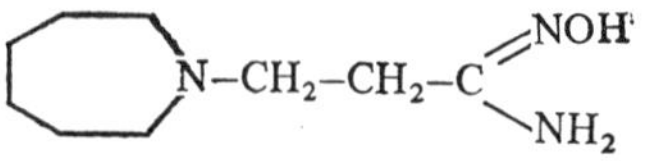

(1) SU 4029: highly active

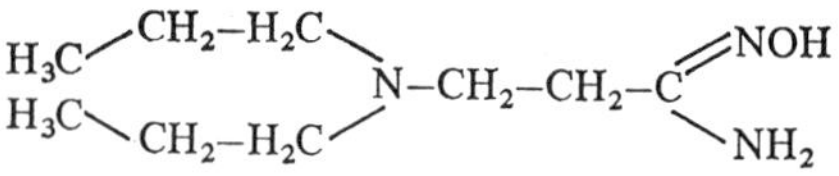

(14) SU 4660: inactive (MAXWELL, 1958)

N-butyl and N-octylguanidines are inactive, whereas tertiary butyl- (42) and to a greater extent tertiary neopentylguanidine (43) show some activity.

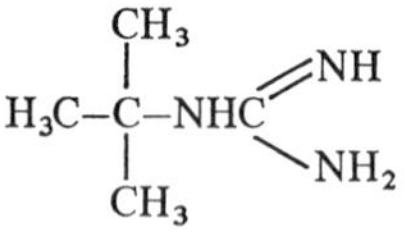

(42)

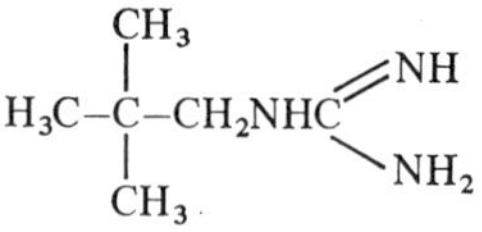

(43)

The failure of 3,3-dimethylbutylguanidine (44) to exhibit activity indicates that branching of the chain beyond the β-carbon atom is not helpful (45).

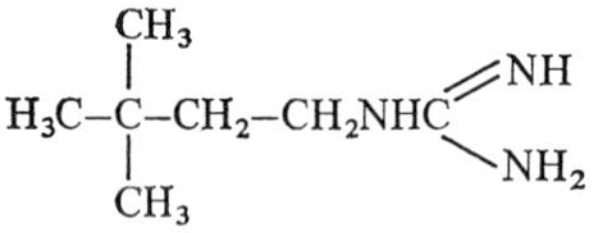

(44) inactive

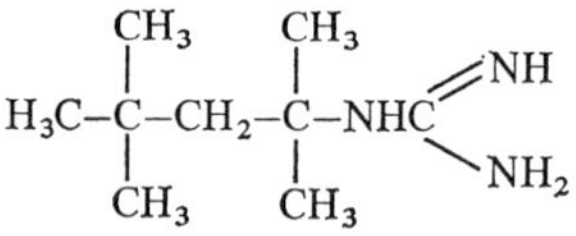

(45) very active (SCHOEPKE et al., 1965)

None of these compounds is used therapeutically. However, the closely related guancydine (46) is presently under clinical study.

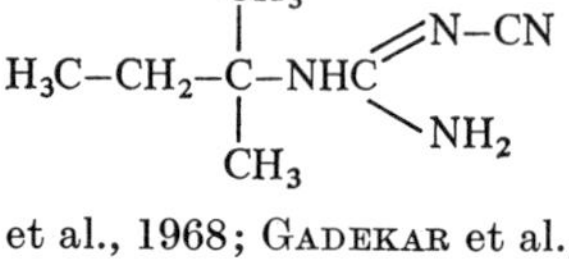

(46) Guancydine (CUMMINGS et al., 1968; GADEKAR et al., 1968; HAMMER et al., 1971)

III. Rauwolfia Alkaloids

Leonhard Rauwolf was a 16th-century German doctor. He registered as a botany student at the University of Montpellier in 1560. Later he undertook a botanical excursion to the Middle East on which he published a book in 1572. He became town-surgeon of Augsburg, Germany, and died a few years later as a military surgeon in Hungary. During the years of his activity he had collected a herbarium, now in the University of Leyden (Rieppel, 1955, 1956; Dannenfeldt, 1968).

Rauwolf never saw the plant called *Rauwolfia*. In the early 18th century it became customary to give names of well-known botanists to newly identified plants, and it was the French botanist Plummier who in his report "Nova Plantarum Americanarum Genera" used the name rauwolfia for the first time (or rauvolfia) for a newly identified apocynaceous plant. It was therefore a plant from Central America and not the Indian species *R. serpentina* Benth. which was first named rauwolfia. However, there were no early observations on the activity and use of rauwolfia, neither in Central America nor in Central Africa, where the species *R. vomitoria* grows abundantly.

In contrast to this lack of early use on two continents, the use of the Indian serpentina root or root extracts as a tranquilizer (sedative) dates back many centuries. In Europe the serpentina root became known fairly early. It was mentioned in Rumphius' "Herbarium Amboinense" (1755) and also in several pharmacopoeias of the late 18th and early 19th centuries. The hypotensive activity of rauwolfia, however, was discovered only recently. It was probably first observed by Sen and Bose (1931) in the early 1930's and later confirmed by Chopra et al. (1941); see also Bhatia (1942) and Mazumdar and Mukherji (1950). The therapeutic use of rauwolfia root for high blood pressure was first reported in a Western journal by Vakil (1949).

About 1890 Greshoff found that *R. serpentina* contained alkaloids and Indian investigators, mostly medical people, were of the opinion that the antihypertensive activity of rauwolfia was due to the presence of alkaloids and assumed that the tranquilizing action was due to some ill-defined "oleo-resins" (Gupta et al., 1944, 1947).

Almost simultaneously Siddiqui and Siddiqui (1931, 1932, 1935, 1939) and van Itallie and Steenhauer (1932) started detailed chemical investigations on the contents of *R. serpentina* roots and isolated the following alkaloids:

Siddiqui and Siddiqui			van Itallie and Steenhauer
colorless	ajmaline	← identical with →	rauwolfine
	ajmalicine		alkaloid B
	ajmalinine		alkaloid A
yellow	serpentine		
	serpentinine		

Most of these alkaloids were tested pharmacologically and some, like ajmaline and serpentine, were found to lower the blood pressure of experimental animals given intravenously. However, it did not occur to anybody that these blood pressure curves looked quite different from those recorded after injection of crude extracts which lowered blood pressure for a much longer time.

It needed the stimulus of Vakil's paper and the isolation of reserpine (Müller et al., 1952) to initiate intense chemical research. One of the most important facts, found soon after the isolation of pure reserpine, was that this alkaloid possessed tranquilizing (sedative) as well as antihypertensive activity.

After reserpine, a large number of rauwolfia alkaloids were isolated from various other rauwolfia species and today about 50 rauwolfia alkaloids are known (Schlittler, 1965). Chemically they are all indole derivatives belonging to a number of structurally different classes. Pharmacologically, some show the typical reserpine activity (reserpinoid alkaloids), some have other activities, and many have no demonstrable activity.

Reserpine has also been isolated in small amounts from other genera of the apocynaceous family (Schlittler, 1965). Whereas all *Rauwolfia* species contain reserpine (albeit in various amounts), deserpidine and rescinnamine (see later) are not broadly distributed. The species with the highest reserpine content is the African *R. vomitoria*, and the best source of deserpidine is *R. canescens* (syn. *R. tetraphylla*). Rescinnamine, besides being isolated from plant material, can be prepared semisynthetically from reserpine.

1. The Reserpinoid Alkaloids

Reserpinoid alkaloids are yohimbine-like bases (47) which have an additional functional group in position 18 and a different stereochemistry in positions 3, 16, and 20. Although about a dozen natural reserpinoid alkaloids are known, only three, reserpine (48), deserpidine (49), and rescinnamine (50), possess typical reserpine-like activity that is strong enough for therapeutic use. Their structures and stereochemistry are as follows:

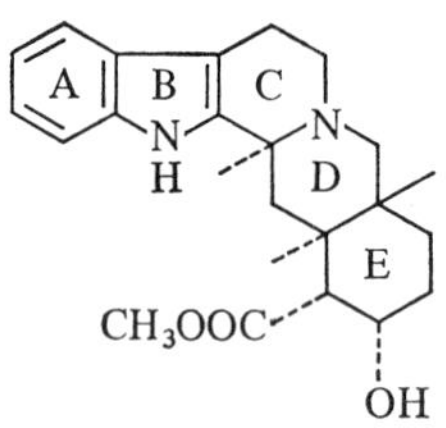

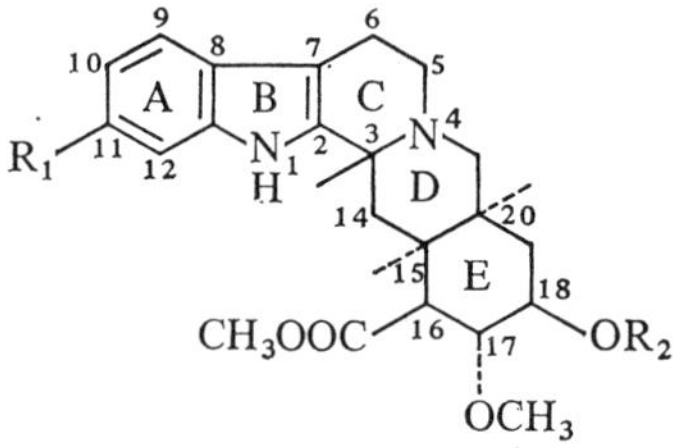

(47) Yohimbine (sympatholytic)

(48) $R_1 = H$; R_2
Deserpidine

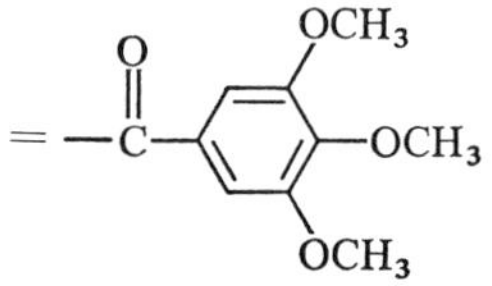

(49) $R_1 = CH_3O$; R_2
Reserpine

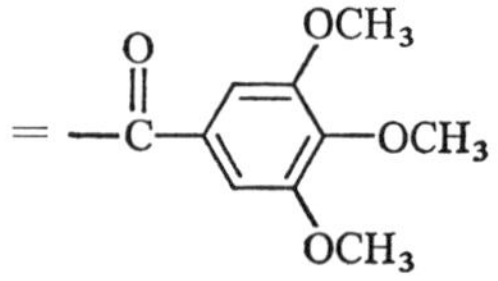

(50) $R_1 = OCH_3$; R_2
Rescinamine

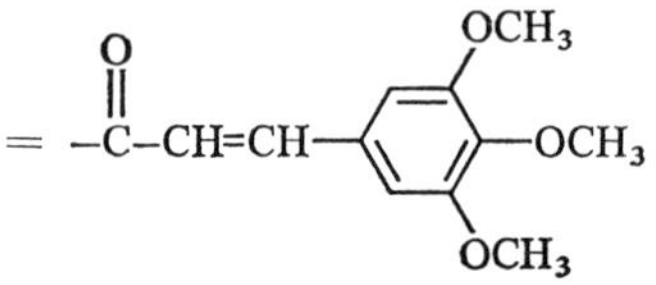

All reserpinoid alkaloids, not only the active ones, have the same stereochemistry as reserpine. Reserpine and deserpidine possess the same qualitative and quantitative activity. Therefore the presence or absence of a methoxyl group in position 11 is of no consequence. Rescinnamine is considerably less active than reserpine and deserpidine, but shows qualitatively the same type of activity.

Once the structure of reserpine was known, the following two questions assumed importance:

1) Can "molecular modification" of the reserpine structure yield derivatives with a higher antihypertensive activity?

2) Can "molecular modification" of the reserpine skeleton yield derivatives which are exclusively antihypertensive?

a) Can Molecular Modification of the Reserpine Structure Yield Derivatives with a Higher Antihypertensive Activity?

The most obvious points of attack for molecular modification are

a) the asymmetric centers in positions 3, 15, 16, 17, 18, and 20;

b) the ester groupings in positions 16 and 18.

a) With the exception of carbon atoms 15, and 20 all other asymmetric centers have been inverted and in no case was antihypertensive activity demonstrable. C-3 is the easiest center for inversion; this actually takes place when reserpine is treated with acids. Even acetic acid treatment for several days is sufficient (McPhillamy et al., 1955; Aldrich et al., 1959). The compound is completely inactive as an antihypertensive; this is explained by the deep-seated change in the shape of the reserpine molecule that takes place as a consequence of the isomerization at C-3.

b) The most amenable possibilities for molecular modifications of the reserpine molecule are the two ester groupings in positions 16 and 18, and it is only natural that such alterations were the first to come under intense scrutiny. Total or partial saponification of reserpine yields the following three compounds:

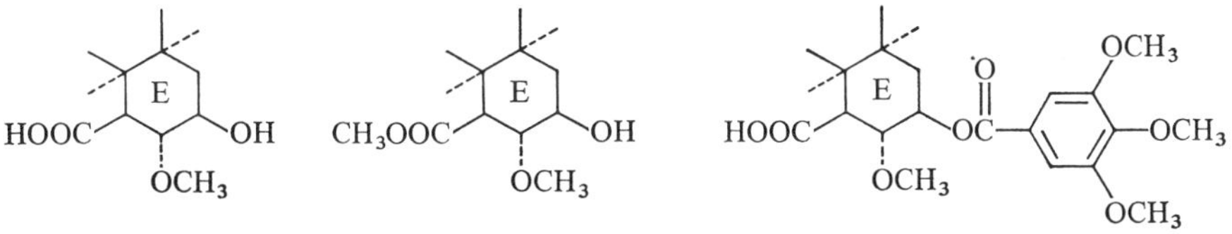

(51) Reserpic acid (52) Methyl reserpate (53) Reserpic acid-18-trimethoxybenzoate

All three compounds are pharmacologically inactive, only simultaneous esterification of both centers 16 and 18 creates activity. This has been done with many alcohols in position 16 and acids in position 18 and, of the hundreds diesters prepared, not a single one was more active than the natural products (Lucas et al., 1959, 1960).

b) Can Molecular Modification Yield Derivatives which are Exclusively Antihypertensive?

In this case too, the ester groups in 16 and 18 were the first places for modification and compounds were indeed found in which the antihypertensive activity was more prominent than sedative and vice-versa. At a therapeutic dose about ten times as high as for reserpine, syrosingopine (54) (Singoserp) shows an exclusively antihypertensive effect. At this dose there is no sign of sedation. If a higher dose is given, the sedative effect reappears.

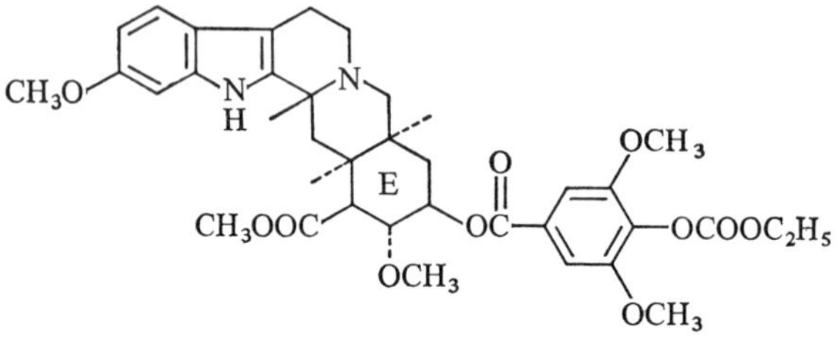

(54) Syrosingopine

A similar case has been reported by PROTIVA and his associates (ERNEST et al., 1965). The methoxyphenoxyacetate of methyl reserpate was exclusively antihypertensive, but its activity was not sufficiently pronounced to justify its therapeutic use.

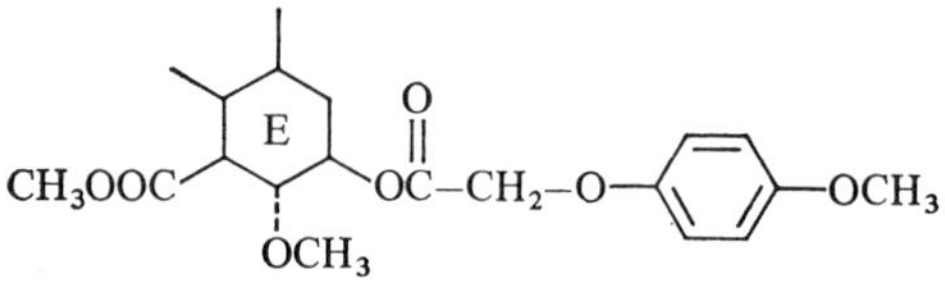

p-Methoxyphenoxyacetate of methyl reserpate

A less obvious point of attack is the two nitrogens of the reserpine molecules. Quaternization of the N_b nitrogen makes all reserpine activity disappear completely. When N_a was substituted by methyl or allyl (HUEBNER, 1954), no reserpine-like action was demonstrable. Strangely enough, when N_a is substituted by a basic side-chain its activity is retained. Compound (55), biétaserpine (BERTHAUX and NEUMAN, 1964; BUZAS and REGNIER, 1960) is claimed to have practically no tranquilizing effect but still a pronounced antihypertensive activity. In hypertensive patients the therapeutic daily dose is about 20 mg compared with 0.25 to 0.5 mg of reserpine.

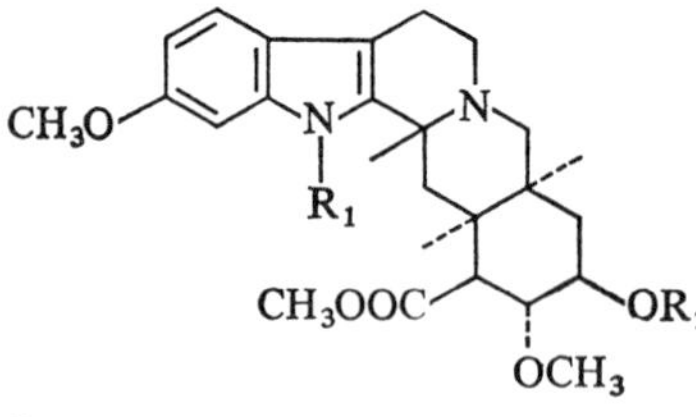

R_1 = methyl or allyl . . . . R_2 = trimethoxybenzoate: inactive
R_1 = $—CH_2—CH_2—N(C_2H_5)_2$ . . . R_2 = trimethoxybenzoate: active (55)

Etherification of the Hydroxyl Group in Position 18: The etherification of the hydroxyl group in position 18 of methyl reserpate has been investigated extensively (ROBISON et al., 1961a, 1961b; POPELAK and LETTENBAUER, 1962), but it has yielded mainly tranquilizing derivatives and therefore will not be considered in this discussion.

2. Reserpine Analogs Obtained by Total Synthesis

The total synthesis by WOODWARD et al. (1956, 1958) and its technical development by a French group under VELLUZ (1959) and a Czech group under PROTIVA not only made reserpine available at roughly the same price as the natural product, but also yielded reserpine analogs not obtainable by molecular modification of natural reserpine. The French and the Czech group, have done a lot of work in this field: substitution in different positions of ring A with alkyl, alkoxy and halogen; substitution in ring C by introducing alkyl groups into the side-chain of tryptamine which served as starting material; replacement of tryptamine by indole-3-propylamine (to yield homoreserpine) or by substituted or unsubstituted β-phenethylamines (to yield isoquinoline derivatives); replacement of the indole nitrogen by sulfur, etc. This research led to countless new derivatives for which a "reserpine-like" activity was often claimed. In most cases, however, it was not stated whether this activity was antihypertensive, tranquilizing or both. The French group found that 10-methoxydeserpidine (56), (Decaserpyl), was exclusively antihypertensive, and 10-chlorodeserpidine (57) exclusively tranquilizing (VELLUZ et al., 1958a; PETERFALVI and JÉQUIER, 1960). Other interesting

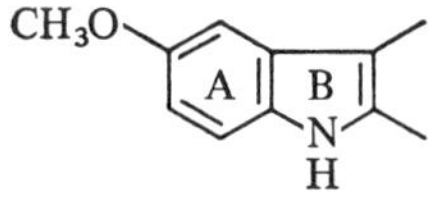

(56)

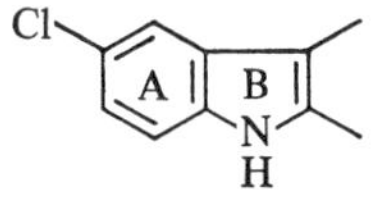

(57)

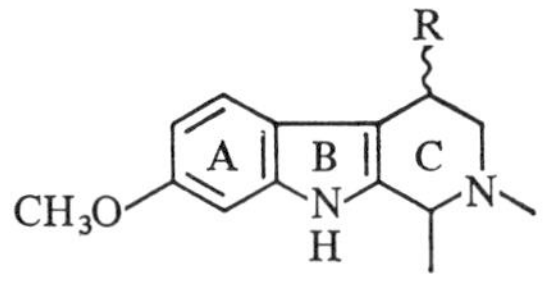

(58)

compounds are the 6-alkylreserpines (VELLUZ et al., 1958b). It is claimed that 6-methylreserpine (58, R=CH_3) is about twice as active as reserpine and the activity of 6-ethylreserpine (58, R=C_2H_5) lasts three times longer than reserpine.

Advantages of 10-methoxydeserpidine over reserpine are also claimed, but the daily dose of (56) for humans is about 30 mg compared with 0.3 to 0.5 mg for reserpine.

The carbethoxysyringoyl ester of 10-methoxy deserpidate (59) has been prepared by several investigators (MULLER and ALLAIS, 1960; ERNEST and

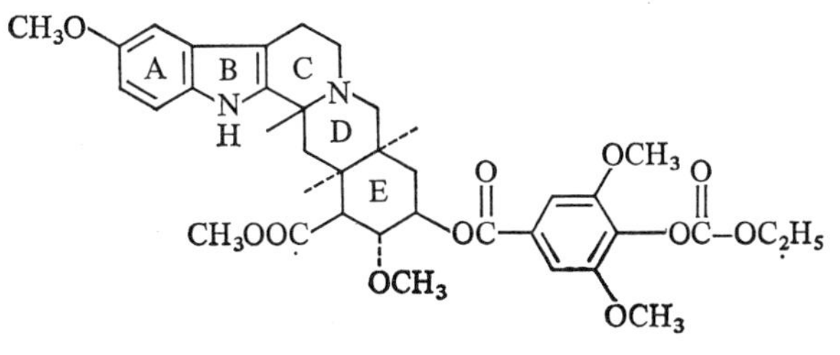

(59) Carbethoxysyringoyl ester of 10-methoxy deserpidate

PROTIVA, 1961), but no pharmacological data are available on this compound. 12-Methylmercapto deserpidine (60) methiopidine (ERNEST and PROTIVA, 1963) was found to possess a considerable antihypertensive effect and was therefore recommended for clinical investigation. The same claims have been made for 12-methoxy deserpidine (61) (VELLUZ et al., 1958c, 1958a).

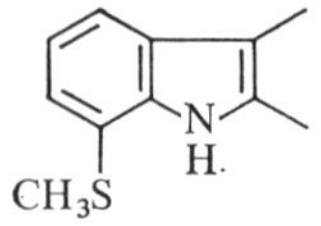

(60) Methiopodine

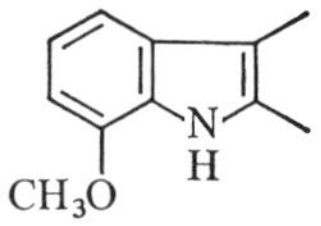

(61) 12-Methoxy deserpidine

A derivative of β-phenethylamine (instead of tryptamine) is 10,11-methylene-dioxy-des-pyrrolo-deserpidine (62) (Mediodespidine, JIRKOVSKY and PROTIVA, 1963) for which considerable antihypertensive, but no tranquilizing effect has been observed in rhesus monkeys (TRCKA et al., 1965; TRCKA and CARLSSON, 1965). So far none of these reserpine analogs obtained by total synthesis has been used as a therapeutic except for synthetic reserpine and deserpidine, Decaserpyl and Biétaserpine.

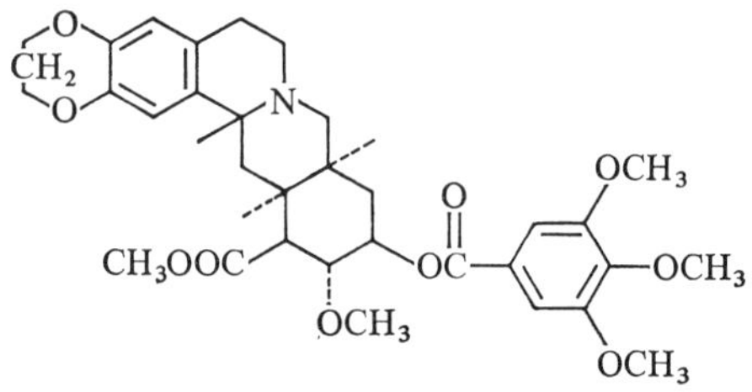

(62) Mediodespidine

3. Synthetic Model Compounds of Reserpine

The synthetic approach to simplified model compounds of reserpine with antihypertensive activity was difficult for several reasons. First and most important, there was not much of an incentive for preparing such compounds because a great number of synthetic substances belonging to chemically different classes have been developed within the last 15 years and have become successful drugs in the treatment of severe hypertension. Secondly, quite minor changes (like inversion at one of the asymmetric C atoms or simple substitution at one of the nitrogens) destroy the antihypertensive activity of reserpine and it would therefore not be expected that model compounds would be active.

If, in spite of this adverse situation, work in the field of model compounds has been intense, it must be assumed that the aim was mostly to obtain tranquilizing derivatives with qualitatively different effects. Unfortunately, in many cases the activity is again described only as "reserpine-like" without any clear definition of what is meant.

Synthetic models can be divided into three classes:

a) tetrahydroharmine derivatives (rings A, B, and C of reserpine),
b) indole derivatives (rings A and B of reserpine),
c) linear derivatives.

For many of these compounds pharmacological information is completely lacking though details are promised in future papers. For obvious reasons, this information has never appeared.

The following list of model compounds is incomplete and is only of illustrative value. Some of the compounds have caused a brief fall in blood pressure which however, was not reserpine-like:

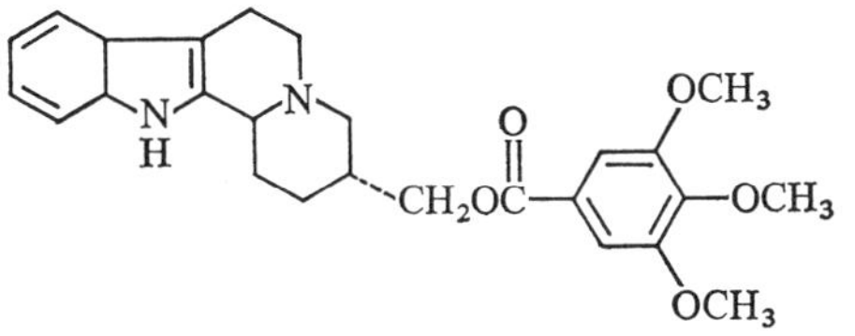

weak reserpine-like activity (DE GROOT and STRATING, 1961)

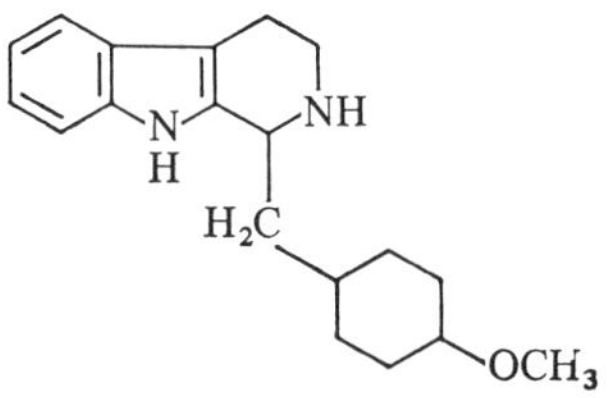

antihypertensive, but not tranquilizing (PROTIVA et al., 1959)

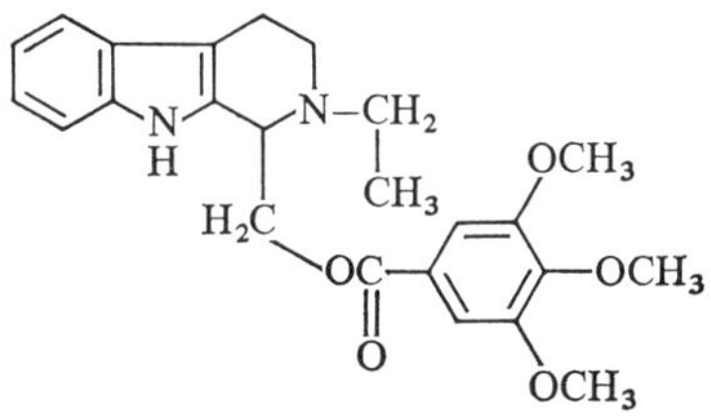

inactive (VEJDELEK et al., 1961)

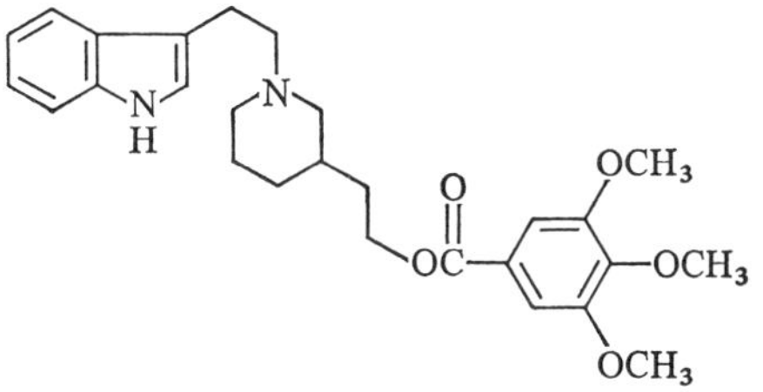

weak antihypertensive and tranquilizing activity (NAJER et al., 1963)

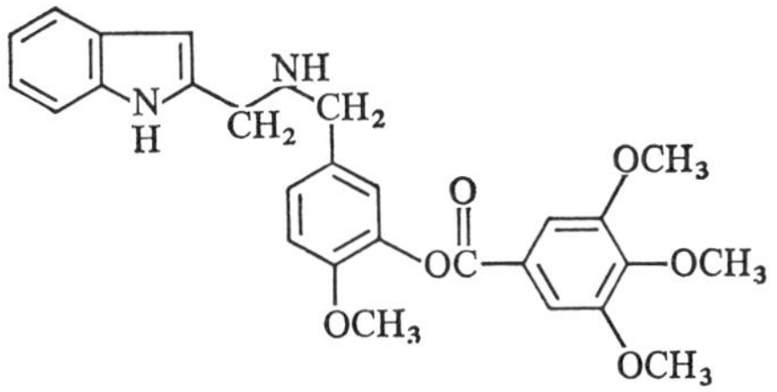

no activity (NOGRADI, 1957b)

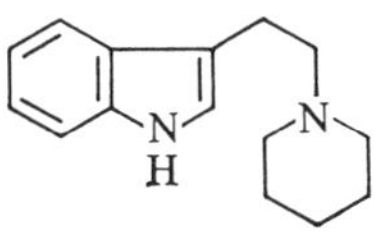

reduced antihypertensive activity, 1/30 tranquiliz. a of reserpine (NOGRADI, 1957a)

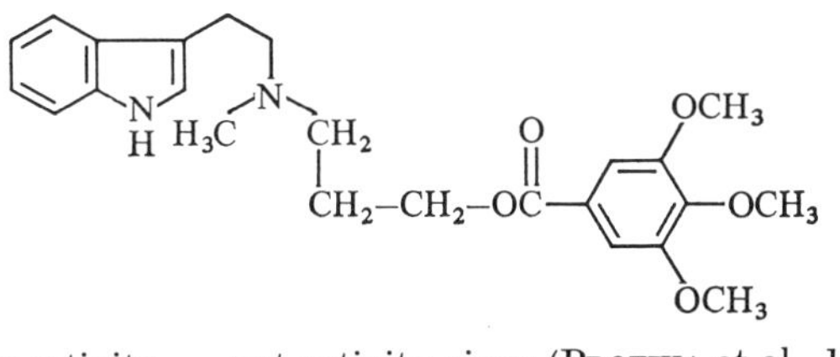

not activity given (PROTIVA et al., 1959b)

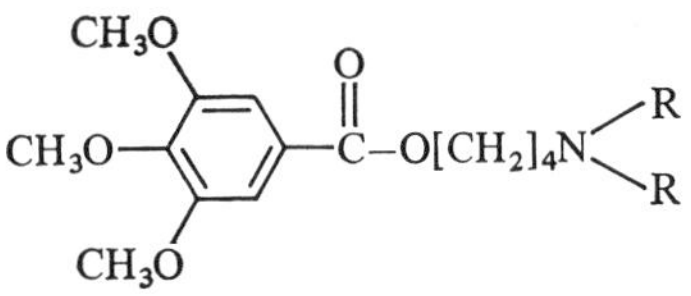

no reserpine activity (VAZAKAS and DOLUISIO, 1964)

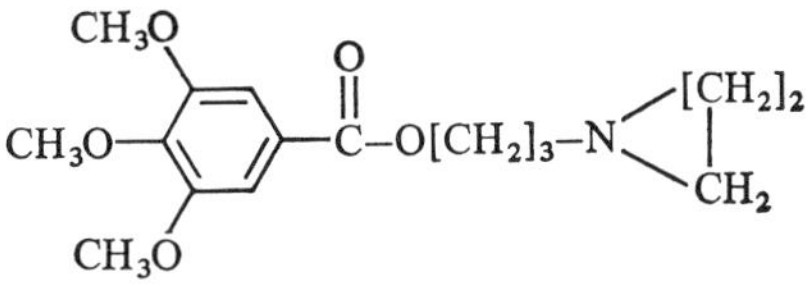

no activity given (DI PACO and TAURO, 1958)

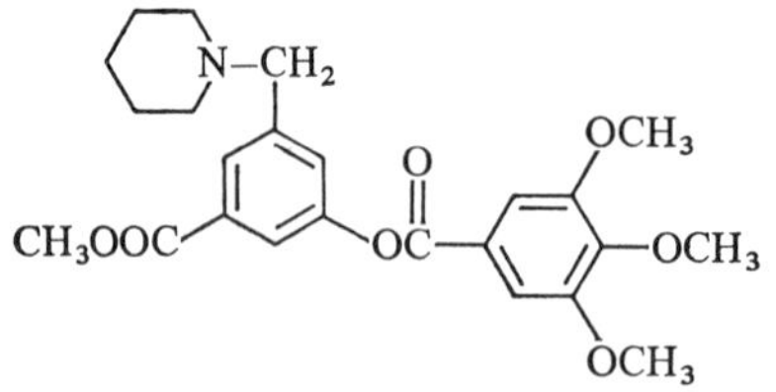

no activity given (TURNER and GEARIEN, 1952)

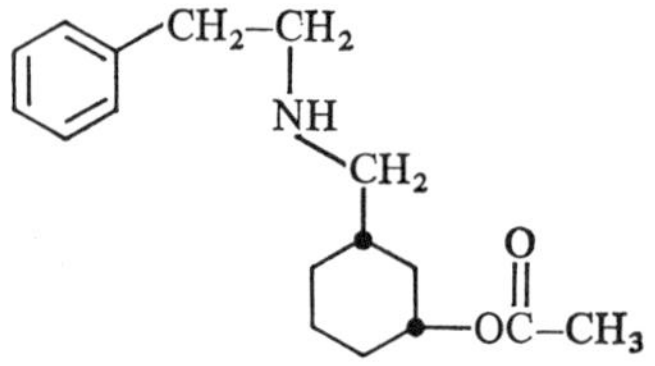

no hypotension, some sedation (LE VINE and GEARIEN, 1961)

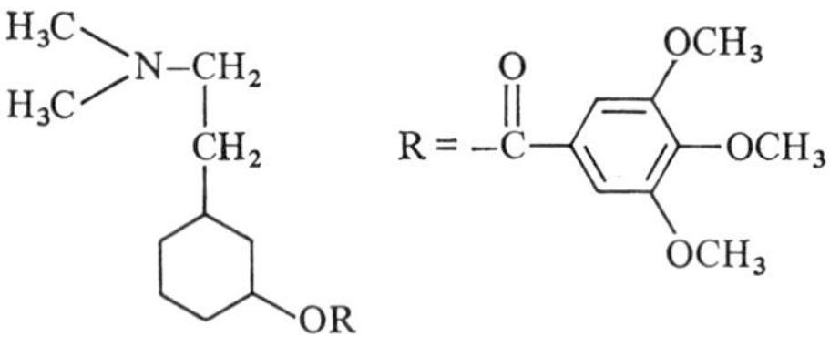

no activity given (PROTIVA et al., 1959)

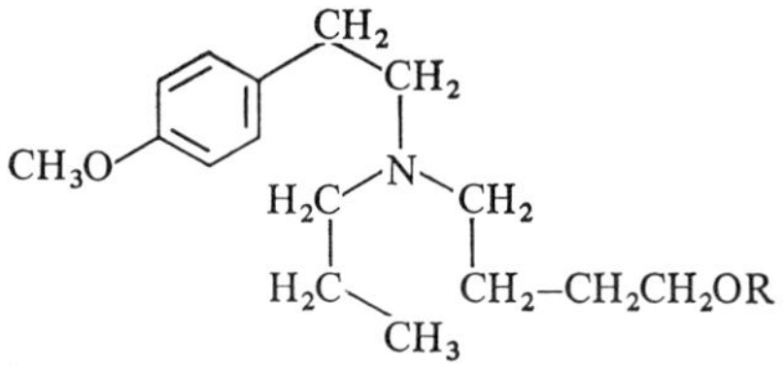

no activity given (KRALT et al., 1961)

In summing up, it should be stated that contrary to experience in other fields, molecular modification of the reserpine molecule has not resulted in any more active substances nor was it possible to separate clearly antihypertensive and tranquilizing action. With high doses of the compounds studied both effects were present.

IV. Ganglionic Blockers

a) Quaternary Ganglionic Blockers

Although in 1914 BURN and DALE had already observed that tetraethylammonium chloride blocks impulse transmission in the ganglia of the autonomous nervous system, research in this field originated from studies with another seemingly doubly quaternized compound, tubocurarine (63). Since the mid-1940's, tubocurarine has been used as a muscle relaxant for patients undergoing surgery. Recently it has been found, however, that tubocurarine contains one tertiary and one quaternary nitrogen (63a) (EVERETT et al., 1970). Thus, all early speculations

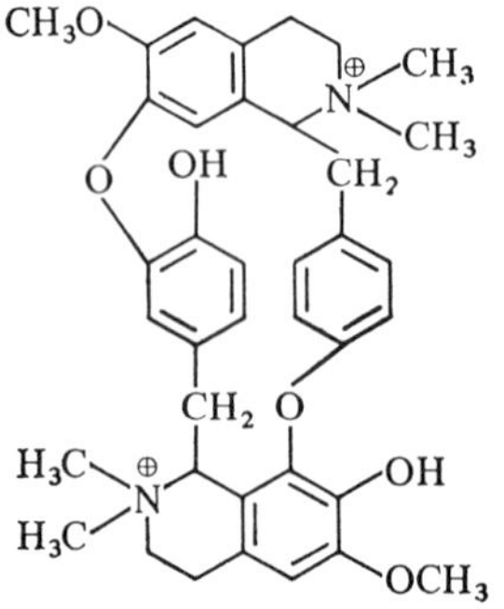

(63) Tubocurarine (old formula)

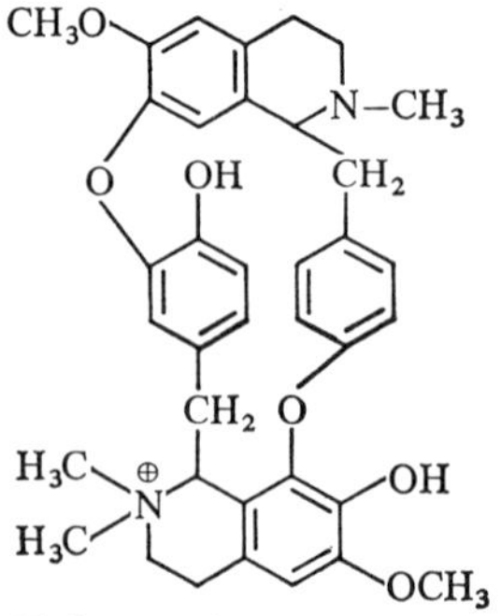

(63a) Tubocurarine (new formula)

on structure activity relations (SAR) between tubocurarine and diquaternary synthetic compounds have to be taken with a grain of salt. Nevertheless, such speculations did lead to active ganglionic blockers.

On the basis of the old hypothesis, BOVET et al. (1947) synthesized a number of polyquaternary compounds, the most important being gallamine triethiodide (**64**) (Flaxedil)

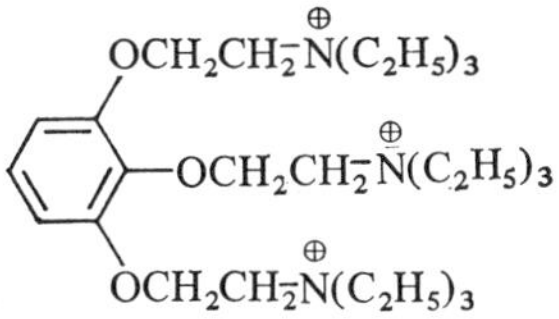

(64) Gallamine ethiodide, Flaxedil

Again postulating the old structure of tubocurarine, BARLOW and ING (1948) and PATON and ZAIMIS (1948, 1949) discovered that diquaternary polymethylenes with ten CH_2 groups (in agreement with the distance of the two nitrogen atoms in tubocurarine) were muscle relaxants (65), whereas with six methylene groups between the two polar centers compound (66) and its analogs possessed predominantly ganglionic blocking activity. Compounds (65) and (66) had already been synthesized by VON BRAUN in 1912 and 1910 respectively, but had never been tested pharmacologically.

$Me_3\overset{+}{N}—(CH_2)_n—\overset{+}{N}—Me_3$

$n = 10$ (65) Decamethonium, inhibitory effect on motor impulses, not introduced

$n = 6$ (66) Hexamethonium, therapeutically used for its ganglionic blocking activity, Vagolysin, Derpressin etc.

The influence of the chain length (n=2—7) on the ganglionic blocking activity has been studied and it has been demonstrated that it reaches a sharp peak, when n=6 (PATON and ZAIMIS, 1948, 1949). Also the nature of the quaternizing alkyl groups is of some importance since (66) with six ethyl groups instead of methyl has lost its ganglionic blocking activity. However, single methyls can be exchanged for ethyls without much loss of activity.

Since quaternary ganglionic blockers were the first antihypertensives to be of therapeutic use, a considerable number of SAR studies were performed in this field. However, for all practical purposes, the use of these compounds has been

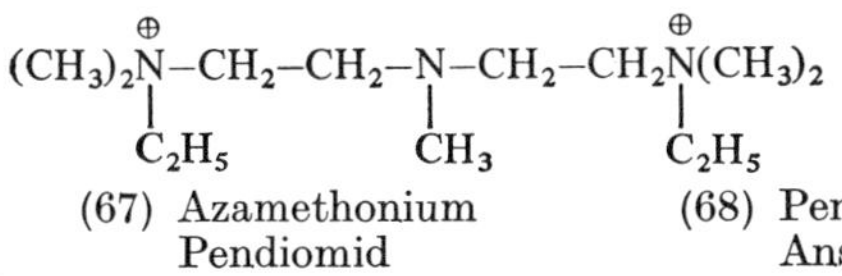

(67) Azamethonium
Pendiomid

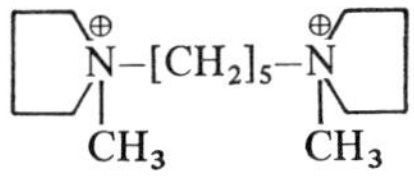

(68) Pentolinium
Ansolysen

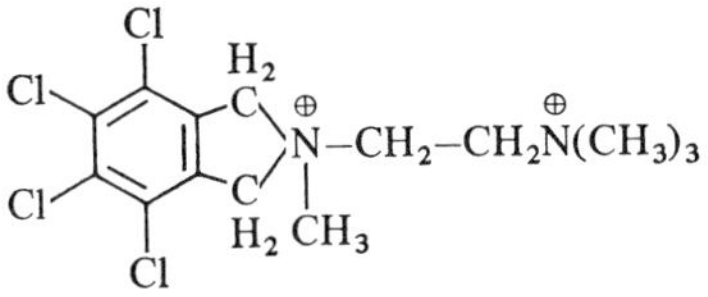

(69) Chlorisondamine
Ecolid

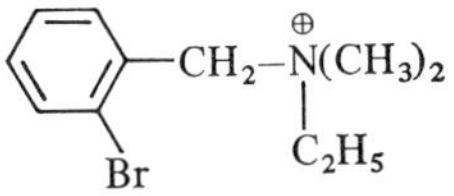

(70) Bretylium
Darenthin

discontinued and it may suffice to quote two important reviews which report such studies and to mention a few of the formerly leading compounds (67—71) (SCHLITTLER et al., 1962; MARXER and SCHIER, 1967).

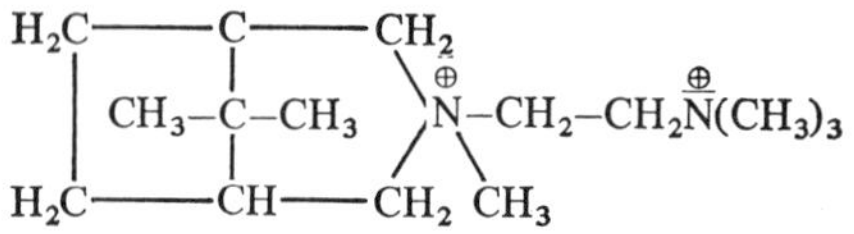

(71) Trimethidinium, Ostensin

Bretylium tosylate is still of theoretical importance (see Adrenergic neuron blockers, p. 163).

b) Non-Quaternary Ganglionic Blockers

Irregular absorption and short activity were two of the many reasons why quaternary ganglionic blockers, although useful at a time, were not a lasting success. When NORTON and PHILLIPS (1953) and PLUMMER et al. (1954) discovered that certain *bis*-tertiary amines also possessed ganglionic blocking activity, research in non-quaternary blockers was intensified. The first non-quaternary agent of clinical importance was mecamylamine (72), 3-methylamino iso-camphane which was claimed to be at least as active hexamethonium. Two research teams, SPINKS and YOUNG (1958) and LEE et al. (1958) discovered the high ganglionic blocking activity of pempidine (73), a compound previously prepared by LEONARD and NOMMENSEN (1949) (see also LEONARD and HAUCK, 1957).

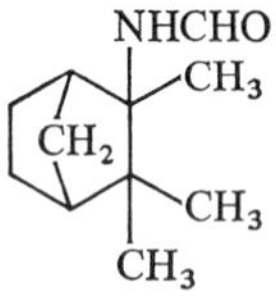

(72) Mecamylamine, Inversine

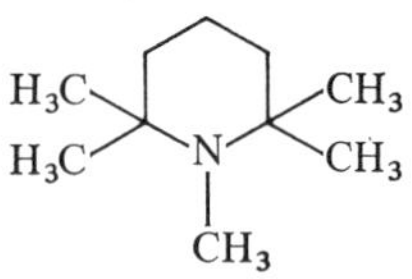

(73) Pempidine, Perolysen

Extensive SAR studies with (72) and (73) have been reported by LEE (1967). A compound of some importance is trimetaphan (74).

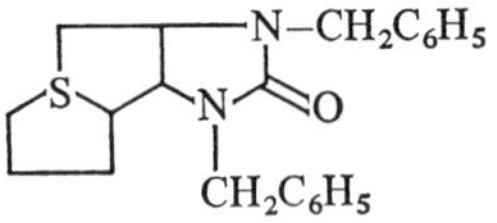

(74) Trimethaphan, Arfonad, RANDALL et al. (1949)

V. Clonidine, ST 155, 2-(2,6-dichlorophenylamino)-2-imidazoline and Analogs

Compounds with an imidazoline ring like naphazoline (75) (Privin), xylomethazoline (76) (Otrivin), oxymethazoline (77) (Nasivin), and tetrahydrazoline (78) (Tyzine) have been used as topical vasoconstrictors for many years, whereas tolazoline (79) (Priscoline), and phentolamine (80) (Regitine) have been employed for their adrenolytic effects. These compounds are substituted amidines, their amidine group being incorporated into an imidazoline complex connected with the rest of the molecule by a CH_2-bridge (EHRHART and RUSCHIG, 1968).

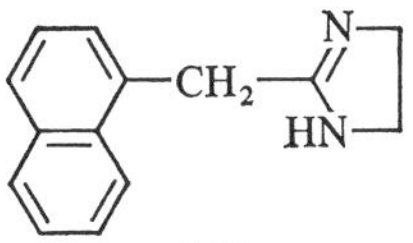

(75)

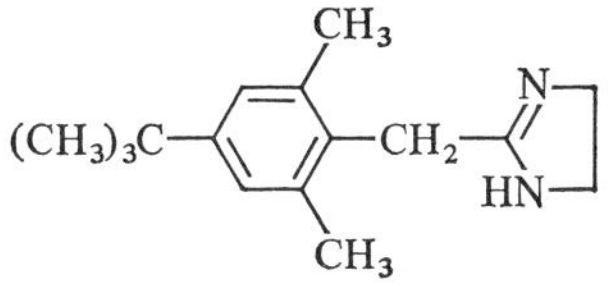

(76)

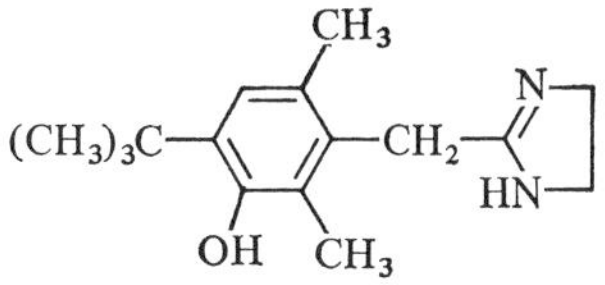

(77)

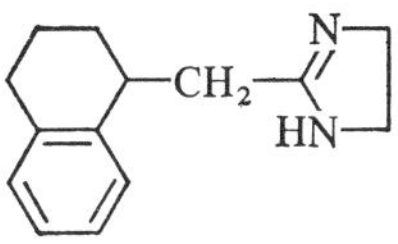

(78)

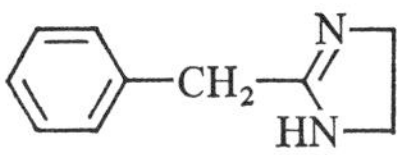

(79)

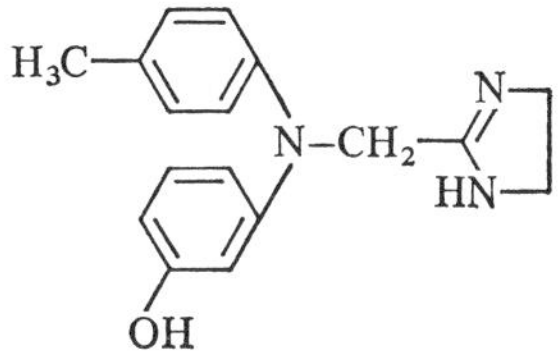

(80)

NAJER et al. (1959, 1960) reported a number of oxazoline analogs (81) and (82). These compounds, in addition to their oxazoline complex, had an NH bridge between the heterocyclic and the benzene ring, the two prototypes being

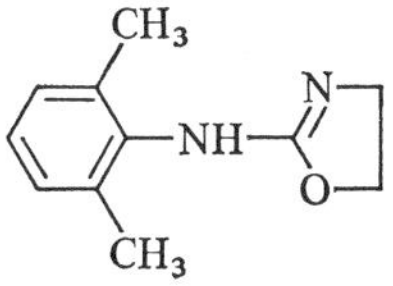

(81)
LD 2855: vasoconstrictor and local anesthetic (GIUDICELLI-NAJER, 1970)

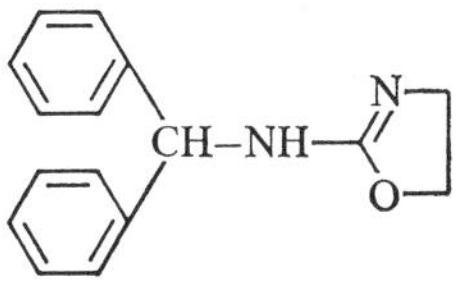

(82)
LD 2849: vasodilator and adrenolytic

Most of the vasoconstrictor LD-compounds had approximately the same activity as compounds (75) to (78) (GIUDICELLI et al., 1959).

NAJER et al. (1961) prepared a number of imidazoline derivatives which differed from (75) to (78) by having the same NH bridge as the compounds discovered two years previously. These compounds were again tested for their vasoconstrictor activity, but were not found to be more active than (75) or (76). The following compounds which are cyclic guanidine derivatives should be mentioned in this connection. LD 3022 had been prepared before by HELGEN et al. (1959):

R = 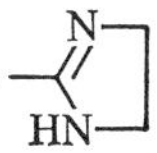

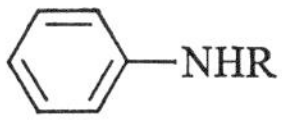

LD 3022

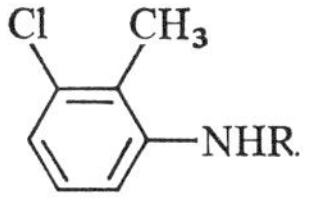

LD 3027

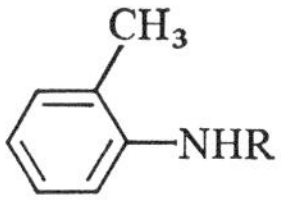

LD 3024

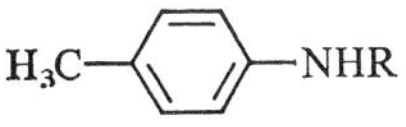

LD 3023

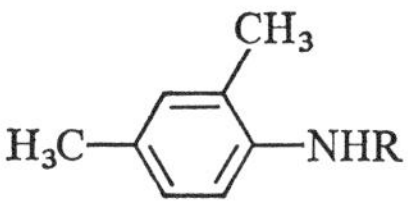

LD 3027

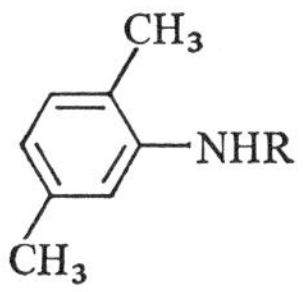

LD 3029

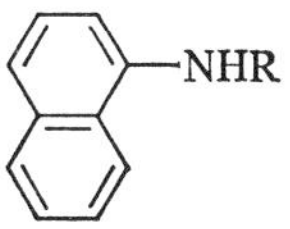

LD 3028

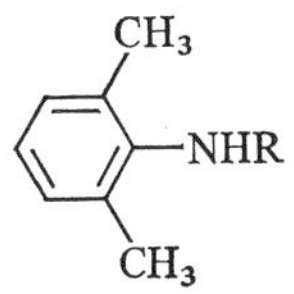

no number

In the same year a patent application was filed by Boehringer-Ingelheim (Germany) for a compound ST 155 (83), later called clonidine (Catapres), which chemically did not differ materially from the above preparations but was unique by having, besides structural elements already present in the LD compounds, an *o,o'* double substitution by chlorine in its aromatic ring.

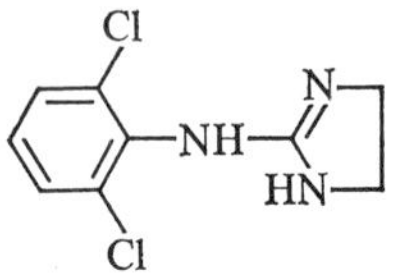

(83)

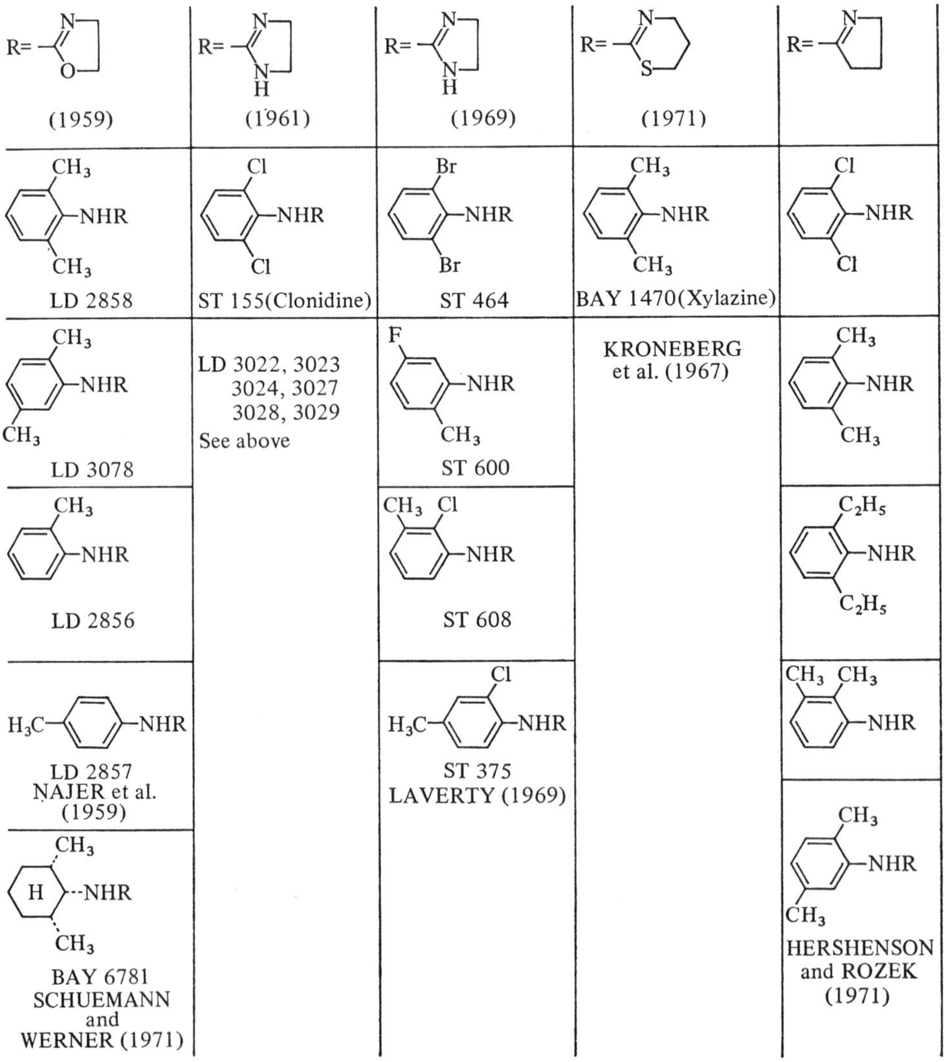

Although clonidine had originally been synthesized and tested as a vasoconstrictor, its blood-pressure-lowering effect was observed incidentally and on detailed investigation revealed a strong antihypertensive activity (HOEFKE and KOBINGER, 1966). By 1966, Boehringer reported that 250 derivatives and analogs of clonidine had been synthesized and tested, but most of them were divulged only in patent applications. None of these compounds was more active than clonidine. A preliminary clinical testing of 20 analogs was also carried out with similar results (GRAUBNER and WOLF, 1966). Additional analogs (all experimental) have been synthesized later by other research teams, some of them are given in the following table.

It can be argued that in (83) the two chlorine substituents in the *o,o'* position of the NH bridge might be responsible for the high activity of clonidine. This may be the result of the NH bridge being forced out of the plane of the benzene ring by the two heavy chlorine atoms, which reduces resonance (see COMER and GOMOLL, 1970). It is also quite possible that the *o,o'*-dichloro substitution reduces free rotation between the aromatic and the heterocyclic complexes and may thus account for the high activity of clonidine, in which case also the corresponding dimethyl derivative should show high antihypertensive activity.

Since clonidine became known, the *o,o'* double substitution of aromatic rings by chlorine, methyl, etc. has become fashionable and in many instances an increase in activity over unsubstituted compounds has been observed. However, it may be pointed out that this information had been exploited before. Compound (76) was synthesized with this fact in mind (HUENI, 1957) and also the anesthetic lidocaine (84) has an analogous substitution by methyl groups (LÖFGREN, 1937; LÖFGREN and ERDTMANN, 1944).

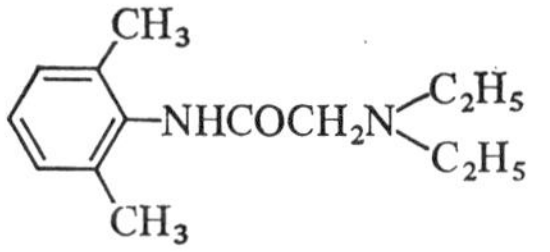

(84) Lidocaine (Xylocaine)

It should be mentioned that doubly substituted "open-ring imidazolines" (actually aminoguanidines) also have antihypertensive activity. Among the compounds prepared, two types (85 and 86) seem to be ineresting:

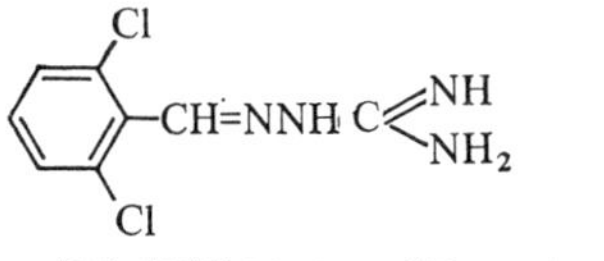

(85) WY 8678 or SD 15.468
BAUM et al. (1970)
SHERMAN et al. (1971)

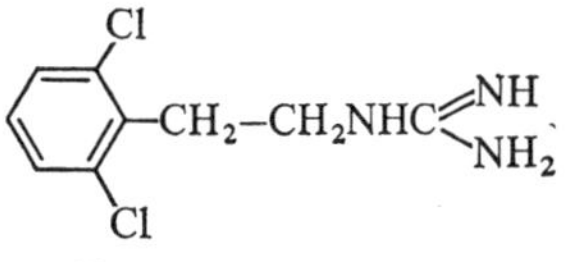

(86) BREAM et al. (1970)

A number of iminohydroxamic acids of the type (87) (R=H or CH_3) have also been found to be antihypertensive (SANDOZ, 1968).

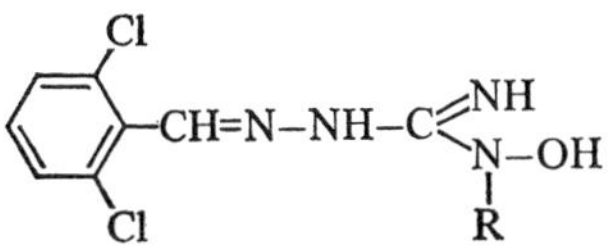

(87) R = H: SAH 43.663

Some heterocyclic and open-ring clonidine analogs have been mentioned only in patents, but it is not planned to give a complete list of such compounds which in many cases have been only superficially investigated for pharmacological activity.

Sandoz 44-549 (88) is a further development of the clonidine structure; it was discussed at the 1972 Congress of Pharmacology in San Francisco.

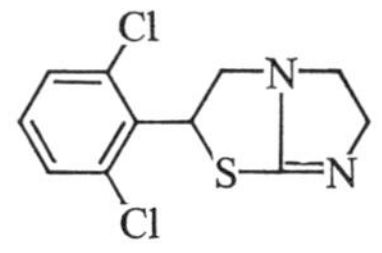

(88) BOYAJI et al. (1972)

Other clonidine-analogs are (89) (COSNIER et al., 1975a, 1975b, 1975c; HOEFKE et al., 1975), (90) (Tiamenidine, KERSTING, 1973; LINDNER and KAISER, 1974) and (91) (Tramazoline, a NH-analog of tetrahydronaphazoline, DELBARRE and SCHMITT, 1975).

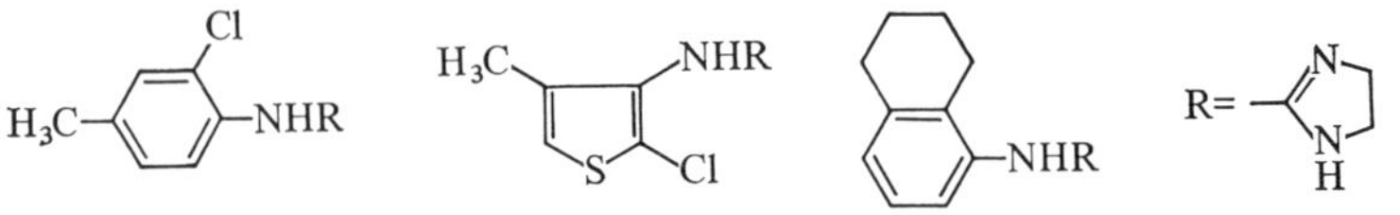

(89) (90) (91)

VI. The Chemistry of the Veratrum Alkaloids

Veratrum alkaloids have been extracted from a number of Liliaceae: from different *Veratrum* species, from *Schoenocaulon (Sabadilla)* and from *Zygadenus*. Also the alkaloids from *Fritillaria* (Liliaceae) belong chemically to this group of alkaloids (see KUPCHAN, 1968). *Fritillaria* grows wild in Turkestan, Iran, Afghanistan and the Western Himalayas. *Veratrum album* is indigenous to Europe, whereas *V. viride* and *Zygadenus venenosus* grow in North America and *Schoenocaulon* in Central and South America (KUPCHAN, 1961). Veratrum extracts have been used for a number of ailments for centuries (DUCHESNE, 1836; BAKER, 1859). KUPCHAN and FLACKE (1967) report that several attempts were made to introduce veratrum extracts into medical practice during the second half of the 19th century, but these attempts were unsuccessful. Purified extracts from *V. viride* and crystalline veratrum alkaloids (protoveratrines) are used clinically for hypertension today.

An excellent review by KUPCHAN and BY (1968) on the chemistry of the veratrum group deals with these problems in great detail. An earlier review by JEGER and PRELOG appeared in 1960.

Veratrum alkaloids are classified in the three following groups:

1) jerveratum alkamines and their glucosides,
2) ceveratum alkamines and their esters,
3) simple steroidal alkaloids (*e.g.* rubijervine and a number recently isolated veratrum bases) which are not discussed here.

a) Jerveratrum Alkamines and Glucosides

Jervine, veratramine and many alkaloids from *Veratrum album* var. *lobelianum:* These alkaloids mostly have 27 carbon atoms and one to three oxygen atoms. There are a number of alkamines whose structures have not been determined yet

(KUPCHAN and BY, 1968). Jerveratrum alkamines also occur in nature as the glucosides veratrosine, pseudojervine and rubijervosine which yield jerveratrum alkamines and D-glucose on hydrolysis. The sugar moiety is attached to position 3 of the steroid molecule. Extracts of *V. californicum* and their alkaloids are said to possess teratogenic activity. These teratogenic agents are veratramine (KEELER and BINNS, 1966, 1967), jervine (KEELER, 1971a), cycloposine (=11-deoxojervine glucoside, KEELER, 1969), cyclopamine (=11-deoxojervine, KEELER 1971a) and muldamine (=veratramine-3β-11α-diol-11-acetate, KEELER, 1971b) (see also KEELER, 1973).

b) Ceveratrum Alkamines and Their Esters

This group contains the principal hypotensive alkaloids. They are known to be ester derivatives of a number of highly hydroxylated ceveratrum alkamines which are all C-nor-D-homosteroids:

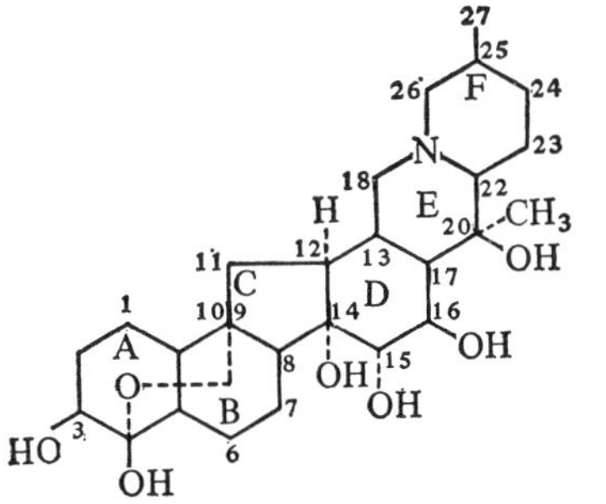

Zygadenine

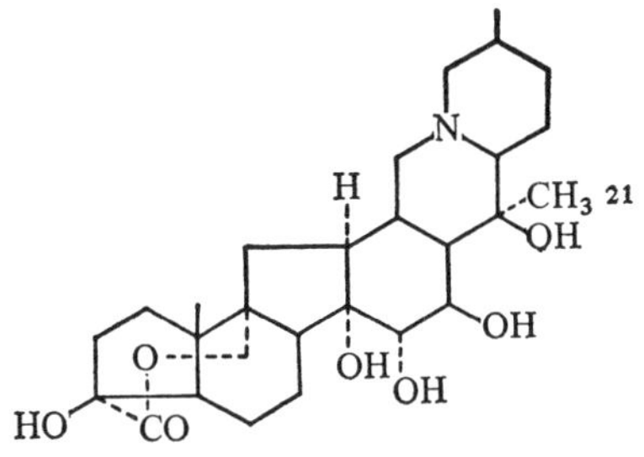

Zygadenylic acid-δ-lactone

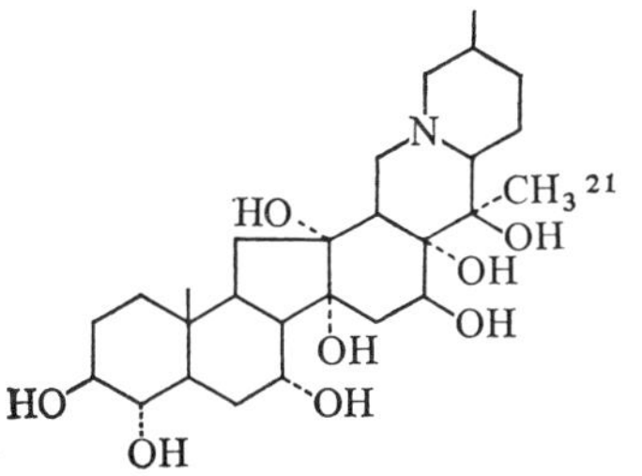

Sabine

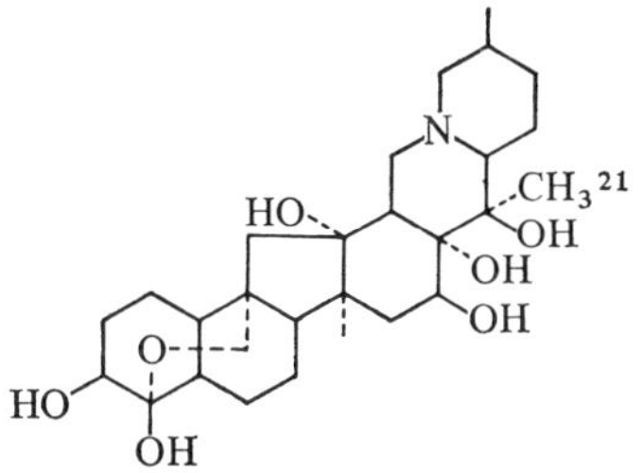

(92) Veracevine

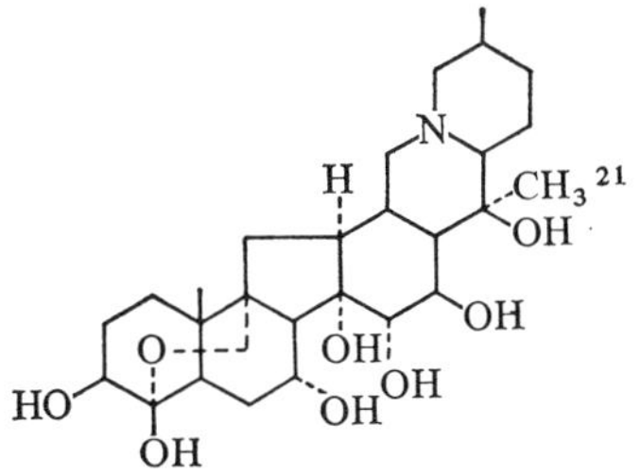

(93) Germine

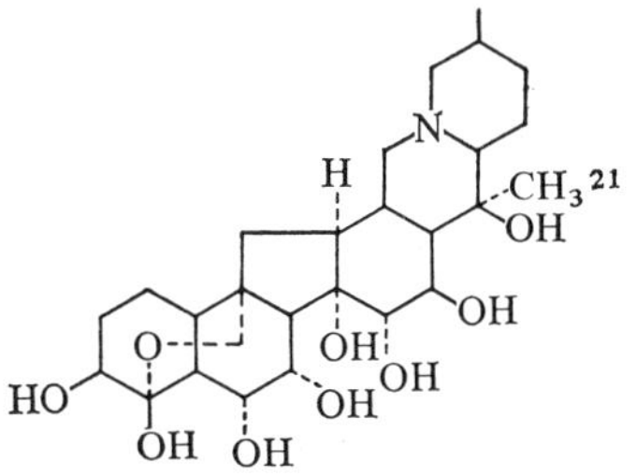

(94) Protoverine

These basic skeletal structures differ in the number, position and stereochemistry of their secondary hydroxyl groups and the acids esterified with these hydroxyls. The tertiary OH groups in position 12, 14, and 17 are never esterified.

The hydroxyl group in 14 is in α-position, *i.e.* opposite to the corresponding hydroxyl in the cardiac glycosides. A feature common to zygadenine, veracevine, germine, and protoverine is the α-ketol hemiketal grouping in rings A and B.

KUPCHAN and FLACKE (1967) give a complete list of all esters of the basic alkamines with different aliphatic and aromatic acids. Furthermore, they report interesting details about SAR in this group of alkaloids. Mostly, the highly esterified alkamines are also highly active, but this statement should not be generalized. Hypotensive action is a function of the proper alkamine, of the number and the nature of the esterifying acids, and of the position of the acyl groups. Only 3-monoesters of veracevine (92) and zygadenine have been found in nature. In spite of their low acylation, 3-veratrolylzygadenine and veratroylveracevine (veratridine) are strongly hypotensive, contrary to observations with more highly esterified, polyhydroxylated alkamines.

For therapeutic purposes, only the esters of germine (93) and of protoverine (94) can be used. The former are contained in the purified extracts from *V. viride* and are essentially germitetrine, germitrine, and neo-germitrine.

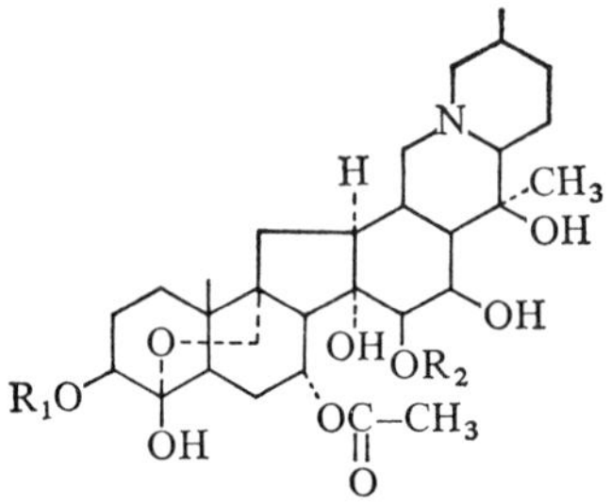

Germine esters

Germitetrine	R_1 = erythro-2-hydroxy-2-methyl-3-acetoxy-butyryl	R_2 = (l)-2-methylbutyryl-
Germitrine	R_1 = (l)-2-methylbutyryl-	R_2 = (d)-2-hydroxy-2-methyl-butyryl-
Neogermitrine	R_1 = acetyl	R_2 = (l)-2-methyl-butyryl-

The ester alkaloids of protoverine, protoveratrin A and B are even more highly esterified. Their structures are as follows:

Protoverine esters

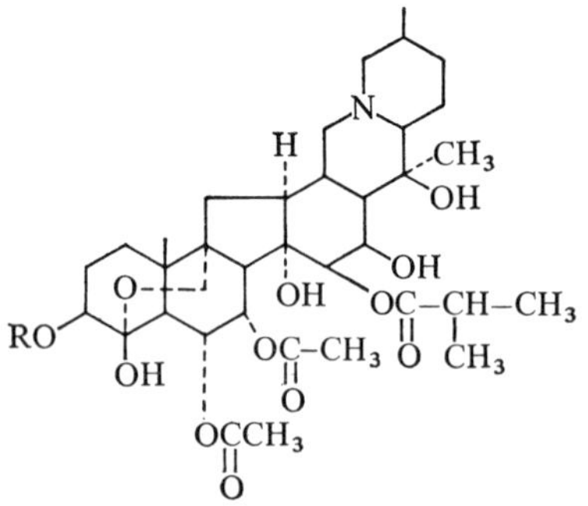

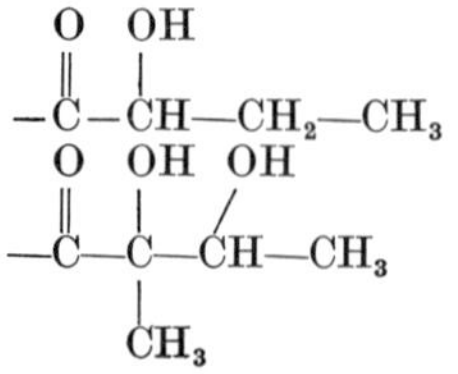

R = –CO–CH(OH)–CH_2–CH_3 = Protoveratrine A

R = –CO–C(OH)(CH_3)–CH(OH)–CH_3 = Protoveratrine B CH_3

Although the differences in the esterifying acids in position 3 are minute (as compared to the identical construction of the rest of the molecule), the two alkaloids differ in their pharmacologic activity.

It is also appropriate to mention cevine which was the subject of much earlier chemical work. However, cevine is not a genuine alkamine but the result of an isomerization. It is readily obtained by treating veracevine (92) with alkali and differs from veracevine only in the steric position of 3-OH (JEGER and PRELOG, 1960; BARTON et al., 1954).

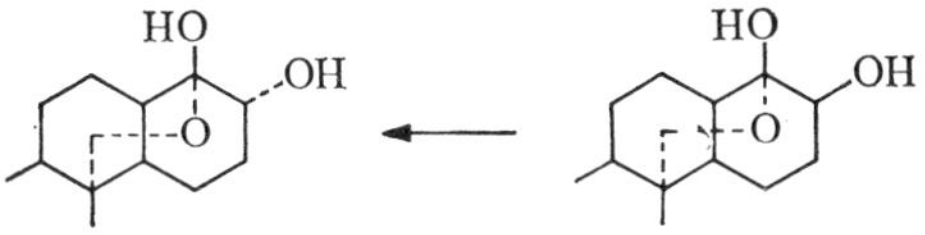

(92) Veracevine Cevine

VII. Compounds Acting Directly on Vascular Smooth Muscles

a) Hydralazine and Derivatives

Hydralazine, 1-Hydrazinophthalazine, Apresoline, originated from the work of a chemist attempting to produce unusual chemical compounds and from the fact that in 1950 very few pyridazines and phthalazines were known, which is quite different from the present situation (DRUEY and RINGIER, 1951). 1-Hydrazinophthalazine was one of the first compounds synthesized. GROSS et al. (1950) drew attention to the antihypertensive effect of 1-hydrazinophthalazine (95). A compound with equal activity with a particularly facile synthesis is dihydralazine (96, Nepresol).

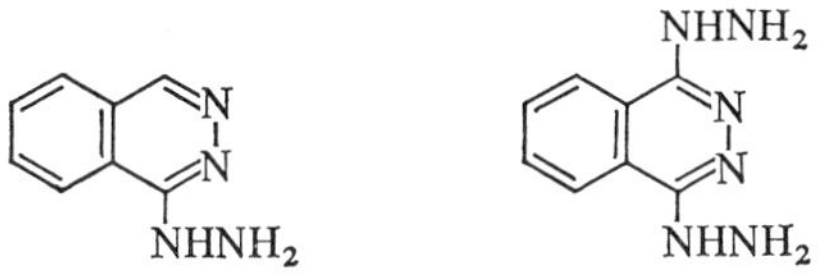

(95) (96)

In the beginning of the 1950's more than 250 analogs of hydralazine were prepared in the laboratories of the original inventors. They found that the specificity of these compounds is quite pronounced and barely half a dozen derivatives proved suitable for clinical testing. This subject has been treated in several reviews (DRUEY and MARXER, 1959; SCHLITTLER et al., 1962; DRUEY and TRIPOD, 1967). Besides (95) and (96), one of the few hydrazinophthalazines introduced into therapy seems to be 1-carbethoxyhydralazine (97) (Binazine or Ecarazin) (KUBISKOWSKI et al., 1965/66; CHRUSCIEL, 1968), which is probably hydrolyzed to (95).

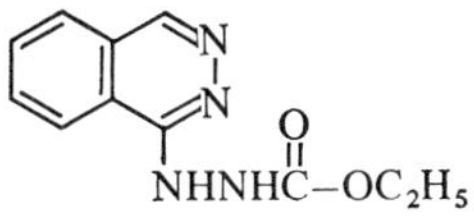

(97)

Compounds which are transformed into hydralazine in the body, *e.g.* Schiff bases (UENO et al., 1972) are also active. The following compounds (98), (99), and (100) are highly active, whereas (101) and (102) show little activity.

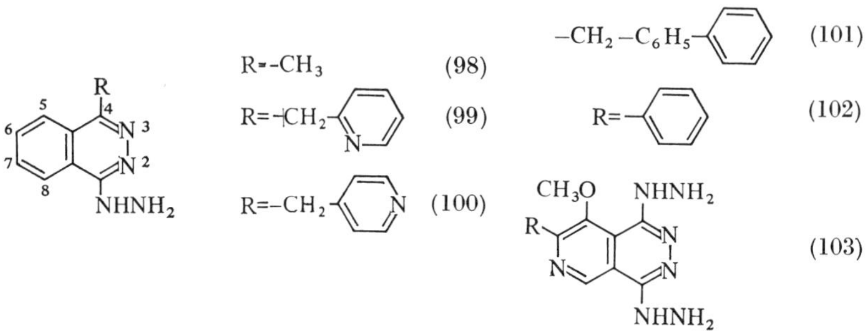

A number of pyridopyridazines, *e.g.* (103) have also been found to be active (UENO et al., 1971). Little work has apparently been done on substitution into the benzene ring of phthalazine and in this connection it is interesting to point out that a trifluoromethyl group in position 7 of dihydralazine had no advantage over the unsubstituted compound (CAVALLERI et al., 1970).

Considerable work has been done in the pyridazine series (DRUEY, 1958) and compound (104) has also been introduced into clinical practice (LIBERMANN and ROUAIX, 1961). Contrary to the experience with the phthalazine (see above), compounds with phenyl in para position to the hydrazino group show good activity.

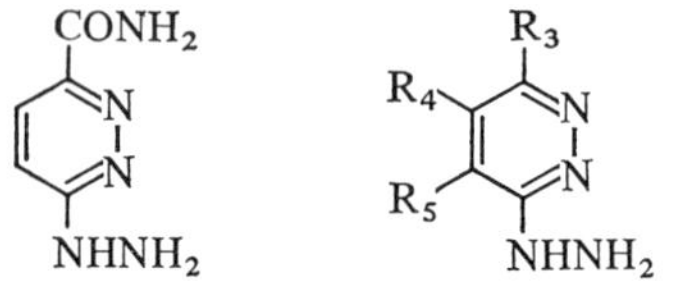

$R_3=R_4=C_6H_5$; $R_5 = H$ $R_4=R_5=H$; $R_3=-C_6H_3(OCH_3)_2$
$R_3=R_5=C_6H_5$; $R_4=H$
(104) good activity

For 3-hydrazino-6-aminopyridazines, see BELLASIO et al. (1969/1971). The following comparison is interesting:

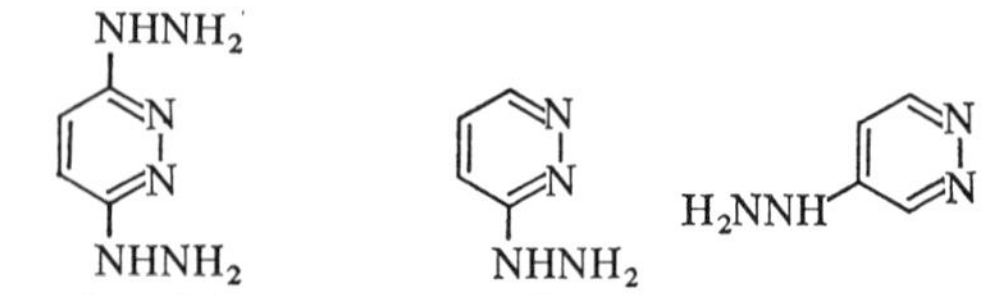

good activity inactive

It has been argued that the antihypertensive activity is closely connected with the hydradizine structure (105), and in agreement with this hypothesis the following basic structures show the highest activity:

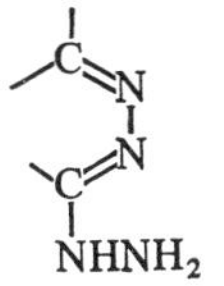

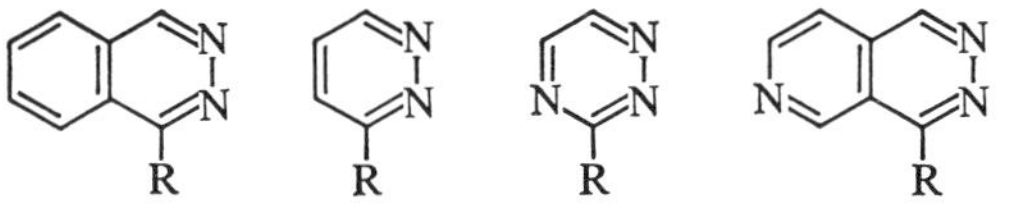

$R = -NHNH_2$

(105) $R = -NHNH_2$

An exception to this rule is the inactivity of (106). In compounds (107) and (108) the hydrazino group has been replaced by sulfur; both compounds are active, albeit at a much higher dose.

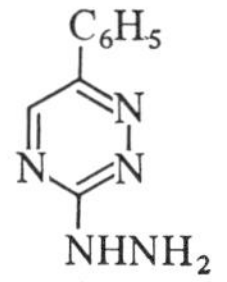

(106)

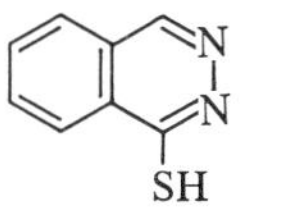

(107)

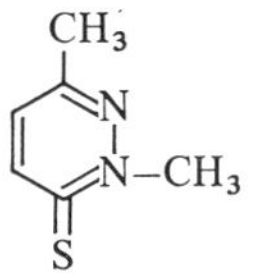

(108)

Hydrazino derivatives of the following heterocyclic structures have been found to be of no value as antihypertensives: pyridine, quinoline, phenanthridine, cinnoline, quinazoline, quinoxaline, phenanthroline, triazole, *sym* triazine.

The most recent review of Schier and Marxer (1969) does not report on hydralazine and its analogs. However, this lead has been actively followed up and in the patent literature a series of new results have been published. Hypotensive activity has been claimed for hydroxyaminophthalazines (109, R=alkyl) (Parsons et al., 1969). Another patent application reports that the hydrazino group has been incorporated into a third ring to give compound (110) (Doebel and Francis, 1969). More recently, among other compounds, hydrazino-4-aminopyridazines were prepared (*e.g.* 111) for which antihypertensive activity is claimed (Anderson et al., 1971; Houlihan and Manning, 1971/1972).

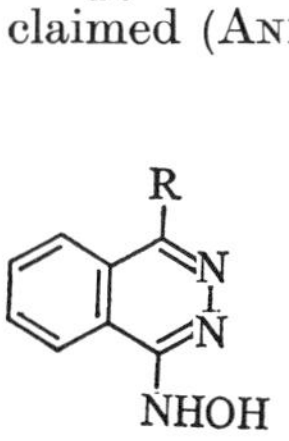

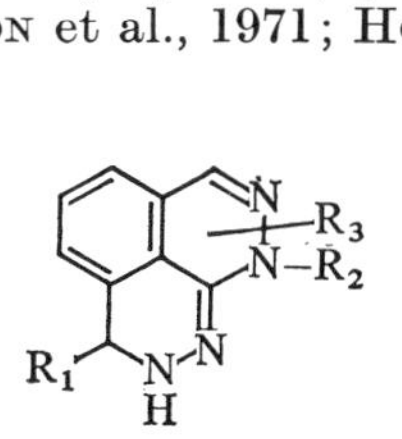

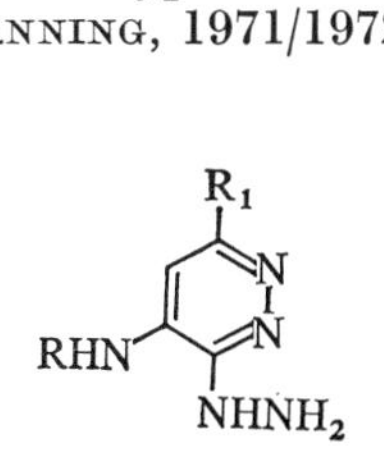

e.g. $R_2 = R_3 = H$; $R_1 = -$ 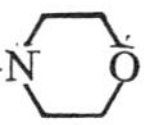 $R_1 = -CH_2{-}CH{=}CH_2$; $R = H, CH_3$ etc.

(109) (110) (111)

However, none of these recent preparations has reached the introductory stage, and for more than 20 years hydralazine and dihydralazine have not had any serious competitor in this specific field of antihypertensives.

b) Diazoxide (2H-1,2,4-Benzothiadiazine-7-chloro-3-methyl-1,1-dioxide)

It was the observation of a group of chemists and pharmacologists of Schering-USA that molecular modification converted the diuretic chlorothiazide (112) into the antihypertensive diazoxide (113) (RUBIN et al., 1961a, 1961b).

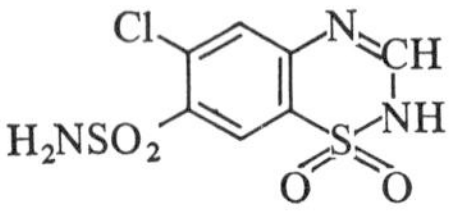

(112)

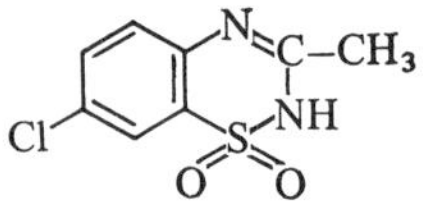

(113)

Diazoxide is the prototype of a number of compounds which have no diuretic activity, but cause an immediate fall in blood pressure in dogs and cats on intravenous injection. Chlorothiazide at 40 mg/kg causes no fall in blood pressure in dogs, whereas diazoxide is hypotensive at 2 to 10 mg. It is therefore reasonable to assume that this is a true separation of the diuretic and the antihypertensive properties, although the latter differs substantially from the properties of saluretics. The type of antihypertensive effect of chlorothiazide and diazoxide is quite different and the two compounds have fundamentally different activity profiles. This is another demonstration of the way in which molecular manipulation can lead to new drugs. Another feature of diazoxide is its hyperglycemic effect, which prevents its general use as an antihypertensive.

In two well-documented publications, TOPLISS and associates (TOPLISS et al., 1963, 1964) reported a large number of analogs; they demonstrated that the transformation from a diuretic into a hypotensive takes place regularly when the sulfamido group is omitted. A similar observation was made with chlorthalidone (114). A corresponding derivative of dihydrochlorothiazide (115) was much weaker than (113):

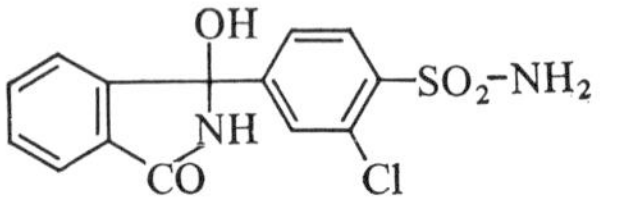

(114)

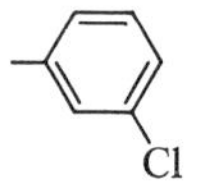

Desulfamyl-(114)

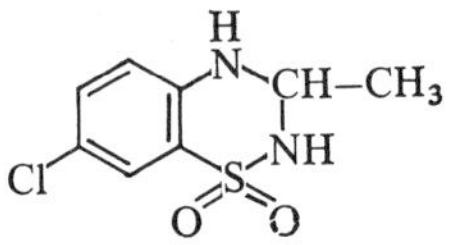

(115)

Analogous observations were made with quinethazone (116)

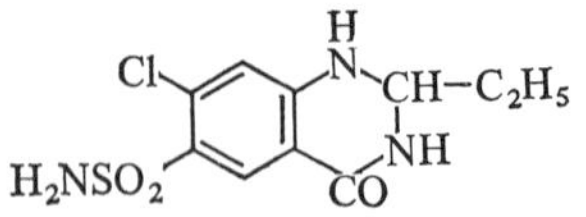

(116) diuretic

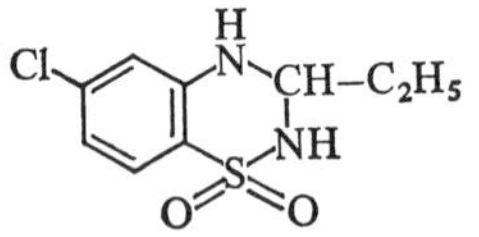

Desulfamyl-(116) hypotensive

RAFFA and MONZANI (1963) reported on an early synthesis of diazoxide which differed from the approach of the Schering chemists, and a group of Lilly chemists (BIERBAUM et al., 1963) has also worked in this field.

TOPLISS and YUDIS (1972) recently reported on the correlation of antihypertensive activity with structure in a series of 2-H-1,2,4-benzothiadiazine-1,1-dioxides using the "substituent constant approach".

c) U 10.858, PDP, Minoxidil

The origin of U 10.858 is somewhat ambiguous. Two pharmaceutical companies were interested in aminopyrimidines and aminotriazines (melamines) like

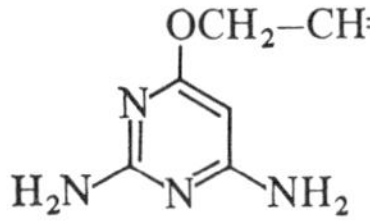

SKF 11.197

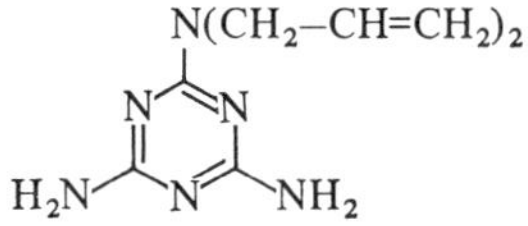

U 7720, DAM

SKF 11.197 lowered the blood pressure in anesthetized dogs, cats, and rabbits (EHRREICH et al., 1967, 1969). The lowered blood pressure was ascribed to direct smooth muscle relaxation.

U 7720 was apparently first described by FREYBURGER et al. (1965). An excellent metabolic study by ZINS (1965, 1968) demonstrated that the formation of the metabolite B (U 20.388) was responsible for the slow onset of action, whereas the other two metabolites A and C were pharmacologically inactive.

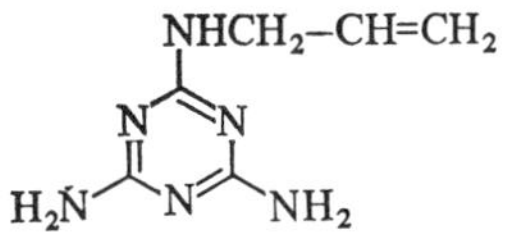

Metabolite A

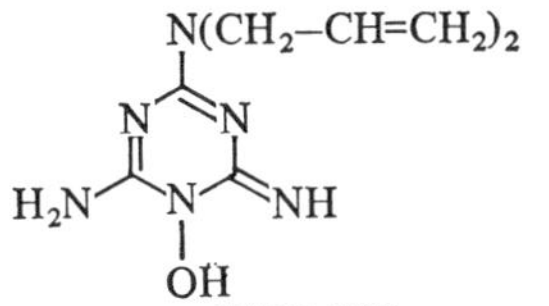

U 20.388
Metabolite B

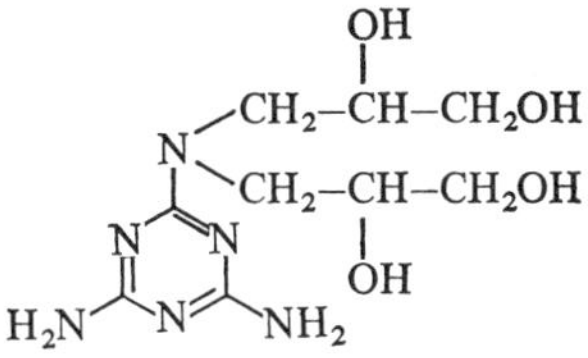

Metabolite C

A number of analogs of B were synthesized, but it was ultimately found that the corresponding pyrimidine derivatives were more active. The following piperidino pyrimidine (U 10.858, PDP) (117) was the most suitable compound for therapy and has been widely studied in clinical trials. Apparently the corresponding hydroxylamine derivative of SKF 11.197 has not been investigated.

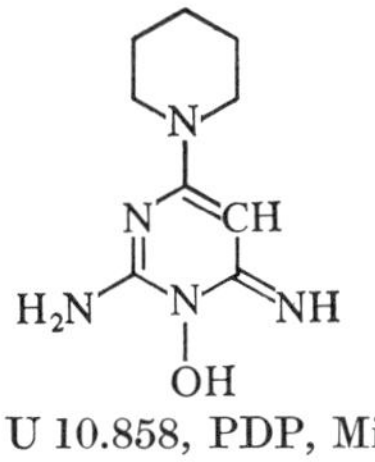

(117) U 10.858, PDP, Minoxidil

d) Guancydine, Verapamil, and Prazosin

For *guancydine* (118) see adrenergic neuron blocking agents (CUMMINGS et al., 1968). GADEKAR et al. (1968) have pointed out that the guanethidine analog (119) is pharmacologically inactive.

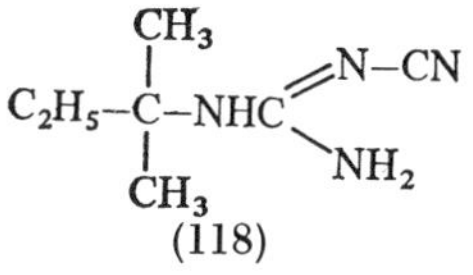

(118)

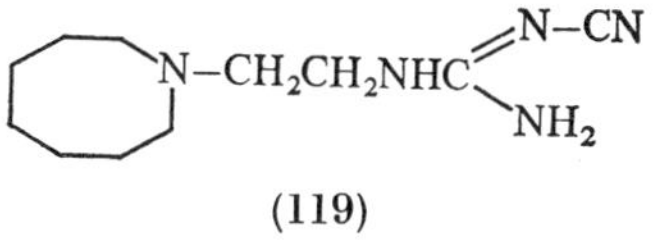

(119)

Verapamil is mostly used as a coronary dilator (APPEL, 1962).

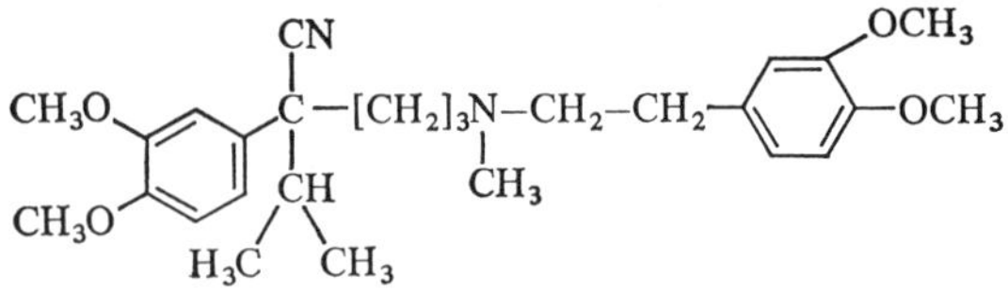

(120)

Prazosine (121) has the following structure:

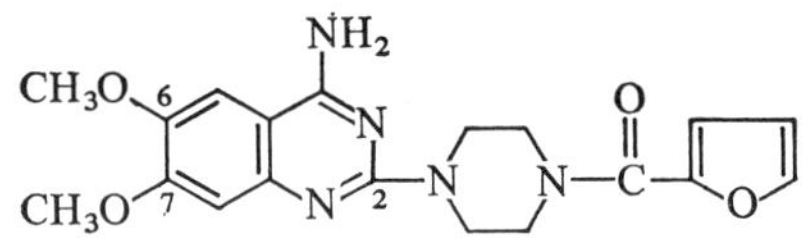

(121)

HESS et al. (1968) demonstrated that dimethylamino-, diethylamino-, diallylamino-, ethylallylamino-, N-methylpiperazino substitution at position 2, and 6,7-dimethoxy substitution in the aromatic ring were optimal for antihypertensive activity.

e) Sodium Nitroprusside, Disodium Nitrosyl Pentacyano Ferrate $Na_2[Fe(CN)_5NO]$

It was HERMANN (1886/87) who first found the hypotensive activity of sodium nitroprusside on injection. Many publications commenting on the activity of sodium nitroprusside have appeared since (JOHNSON, 1929; PAGE, 1956; PAGE et al., 1955; SAUNDERS and HIMWICH, 1950). The rapid hypotensive effect of sodium nitroprusside used intravenously is due to the intact molecule; however, it decomposes fairly rapidly on oral application and its decomposition products are claimed to be responsible for its oral activity, which is rather low. Hydrocyanic acid is thought to be such a decomposition product (HILL, 1942; MAHAFFEY, 1942). Other authors (CASSINELLI, 1958) assume that the liberated cyanogen $(CN)_2$ is converted to $(SCN)_2$ by liver rhodanase and that the rhodanide ion is responsible for the weak peroral activity of sodium nitroprusside (see also PAGE, 1952; WILSON et al., 1971).

The chemistry of sodium nitroprusside does not lend itself to easy molecular modification. In spite of these shortcomings a few interesting observations have been made with "modified nitroprussides". The replacement of the nitroso group by an amino group leads to inactivity although JUNG and PETSCH (1967) disagree with this fact. The two sodium atoms have also been replaced by other elements. According to CAUJOLLE (1968), the toxicity of such compounds is reduced and their activity is extended (PHAM-HUU-CHANH, 1969). A number of additional analogs of sodium nitroprusside has been made, but not tested pharmacologically (KAHN et al., 1968; AYERS, 1969).

KREYE et al. (1973) restudied the vasodilator and antihypertensive effect of sodium nitroprusside. To achieve the powerful vasodilating effect, the whole complex of sodium nitroprusside with its typical configuration must be present. Even with seemingly similar compounds, the vasodilator effect is reduced. However, the following molybdenum (HIEBER et al., 1948) and ruthenium (MANCHOT and DÜSING, 1933) derivatives were fairly active:

$$K_4[Mo(CN)_5NO],\ Na_2[Ru(CN)_5NO]\,.$$

VIII. The α-Adrenolytics (α-Adrenergic Receptor Blocking Agents)

α-adrenergic blocking agents are characterized by their ability to reduce the increase in blood pressure produced in animals by catecholamines and to "reverse" the pressor effect of epinephrine. It was hoped that α-adrenolytics would be active antihypertensives in man by preventing the contraction of the smooth muscles of the vascular walls elicited by epinephrine and nor-epinephrine. To date, these expectations have not been fulfilled.

In spite of the fact that BARGER et al. as early as 1906 observed a blood-pressure-lowering effect of ergotoxine, the beginning of the "α-adrenolytic era" was the work carried out at the Pasteur Institute in Paris in the early 1930's. FOURNEAU and BOVET (1933a, b) reported on a number of compounds which were pharmacologically hypotensive, the best known examples being prosympal (122) and piperoxan (123) (F 883 and 933) (see also FOURNEAU et al., 1933; WERNER and BARRETT, 1967).

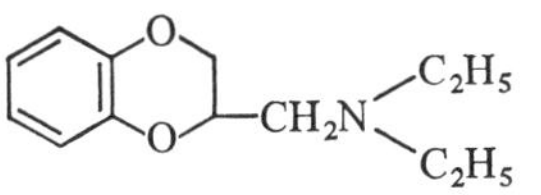

(122) (F 883)

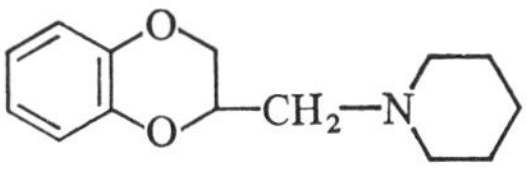

(123) (F 933)

Development in this field was rapid and soon afterwards a few additional compounds were synthesized which, at least pharmacologically, seemed to be more advantageous, such as dibenamine (124), phenoxybenzamine (125) (Dibenzyline), and phentolamine (126) (Regitine).

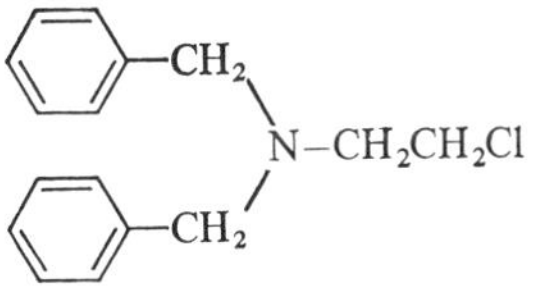

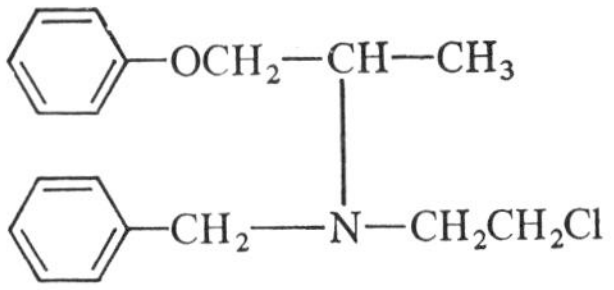

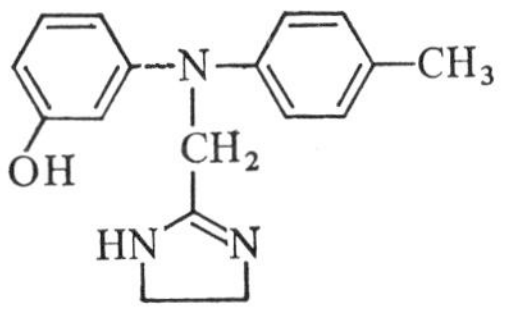

(124) (125) (126)

Expectations for the use of such compounds as antihypertensives were not fulfilled; however, a number of clinically useful drugs were developed. Their main application is as peripheral vasodilators and as diagnostic aids. Phentolamine is excellent for diagnosis of suspected cases of phaeochromocytoma. Much chemical and pharmacological research has been done in this field, although the results have been disappointing in terms of human therapy.

Phenylpiperazines: Special attention has been given to derivatives of phenylpiperazines (WERNER and BARRETT, 1967; SCHIER and MARXER, 1969). MULL et al. (1965) prepared an extensive series of phenylpiperazines differing from previous preparations by having an alkoxy group attached to the aralkyl moiety linked to the phenylpiperazine (*e.g.* 127) (CHRISTENSEN and HALEY, 1966).

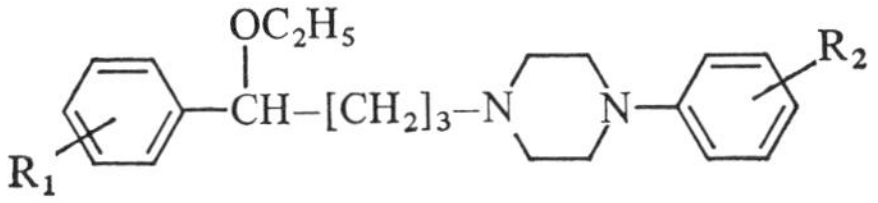

(127)

The phenylpiperazine moiety has also been linked to heterocycles and has yielded compounds with interesting activities (128). Another compound of interest originated from the laboratory of ARYA et al. (1967) (129):

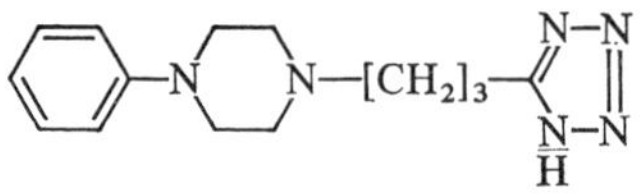

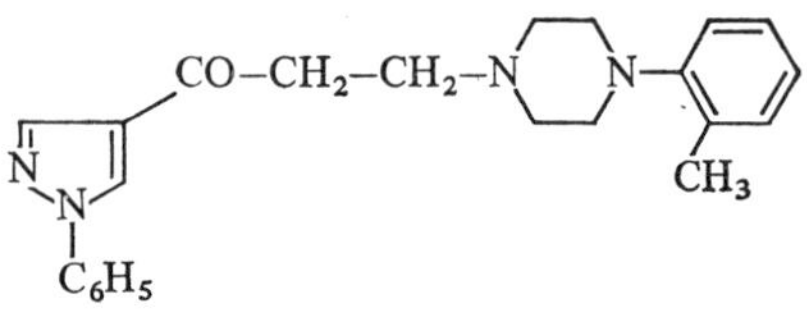

(128) (Rodriguez et al., 1965) 129)

An α-adrenolytic with a completely different structure is azapetine (Ilidar) (130)

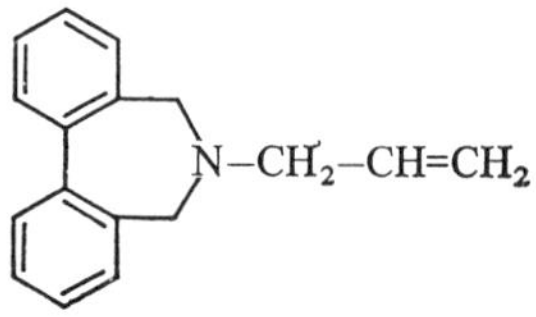

(130)

a) Imidazolines

Another group of pharmacologically interesting compounds are substituted imidazolines, already discussed in connection with the chemistry of clonidine (see p. 33) Tolazoline (79) was of particular interest as a potent adrenolytic and vasodilator, but it is not used as an antihypertensive.

Miscellaneous Compounds. A recently discovered α-adrenolytic is indoramine (131) (Wy 21.901,131). Wy 21.901 was selected from a wide variety of modifications and a number of pharmacological and clinical evaluations have been published (ARCHIBALD et al., 1971)

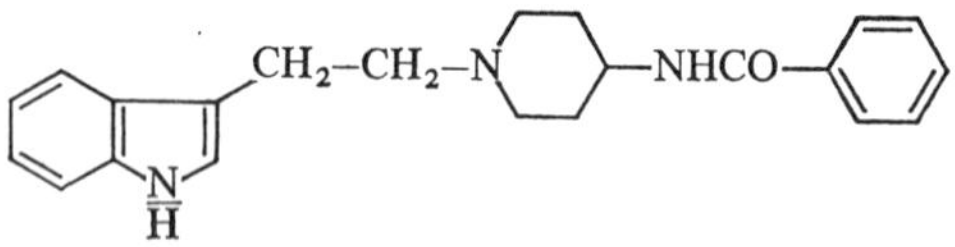

(131)

b) Ergot Alkaloids

Early interest in ergot alkaloids was largely stimulated by their oxytocic and adrenergic blocking activity, investigated by BARGER and DALE (BARGER, 1931; HOFMANN, 1964; STOLL and HOFMANN, 1965, 1970). Drugs of considerable therapeutic value have been found among the ergot alkaloids, some of which are being used for their α-adrenolytic effect.

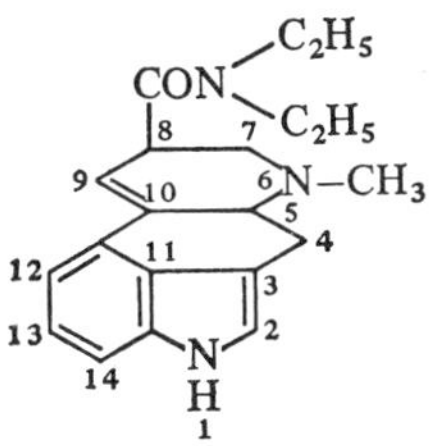

(132) LSD

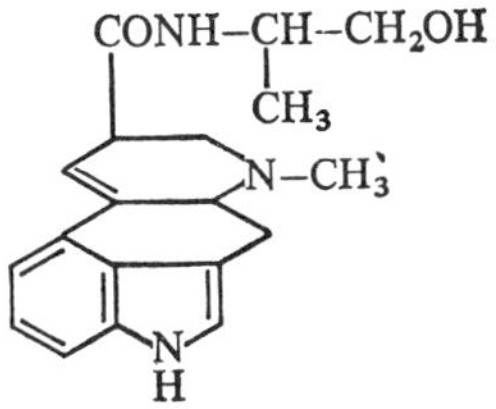

(133) = Ergometrine

BARGERS "ergotoxine" was found to be a mixture of (134), (135), and (136). By hydrogenation of the 9 to 10 double bond of "ergotoxine", "dihydroergotoxine" is obtained which is marketed as an antihypertensive under the trade name Redergam in Russia (VEDERNIKOV, 1963). A more refined technique is the individual hydrogenation of (134), (135), and (136) and recombining the dihydro compounds (as methanesulfonates) in stochiometric amounts. This combination, under the name of Hydergine formerly had an important place in the therapy of high blood pressure. For this purpose, it is obsolete today, but it has found many other clinical uses.

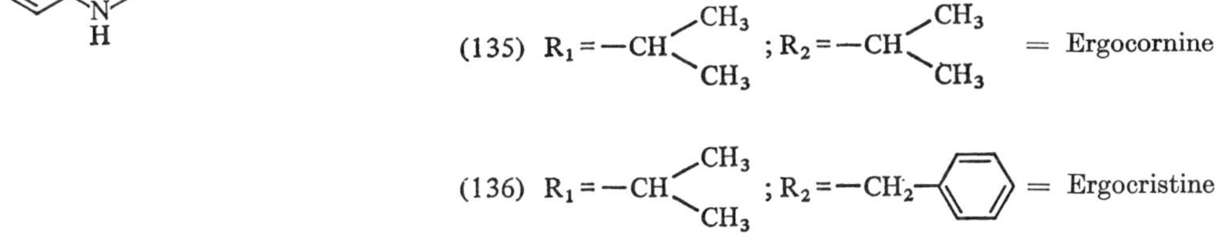

Research in this field was always hampered by the difficulty in obtaining lysergic acid from ergot of rye. Some 14 years ago an Italian group succeeded in growing a specific ergot species in submerged culture and was able to obtain lysergic acid derivatives without having to depend on products from ergot of rye. Such products became readily available as starting material for semisynthetic derivatives. BERNARDI (1969) reviewed recent work in this field. The same group also originated a new vasodilating and α-receptor-blocking ergoline derivative called nicergoline 137, 1,6-dimethyl-8β-(5-bromonicotinoyloxymethyl)-10α-methoxy ergoline (ARCARI et al., 1968, 1972).

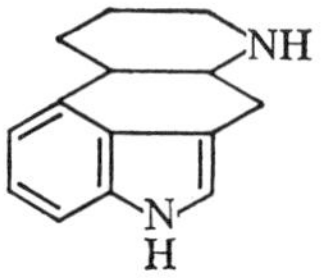

Ergoline

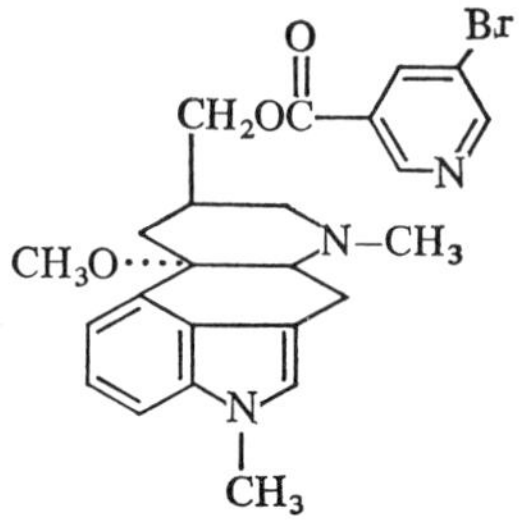

(137)

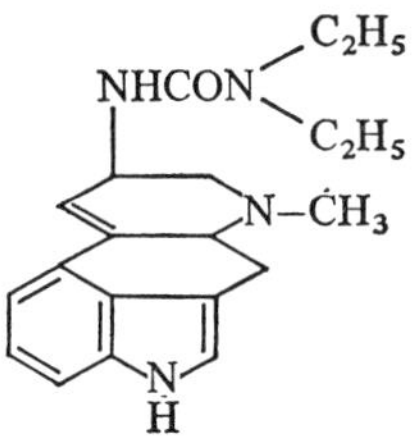

(138)

A Czech group studied the two ergoline ureas Lysenyl (138) and Mesenyl. Lysenyl (138) was introduced as an antimigraine preparation (VOTAVA et al., 1966; SEMONSKY et al., 1968; ZIKAN and SEMONSKY, 1968).

IX. Fusaric Acid

Fusaric acid (139, *n*-butylpicolinic acid, formerly called fusarinic acid) was isolated from Fusarium oxysporum Nees (YABUTA et al., 1935) and from Gibberella fujikuroi (TAMARI and KAJI, 1954; see also PLATTNER et al., 1954).

At the time of its isolation fusaric acid was found to be weakly bacteriostatic, it inhibited the growth of Micrococcus pyogenes, var. aureus, Salmonella typhosa, and E. coli in dilutions of 1:2.000.

It was later found (HIDAKA et al., 1969) that fusaric acid has a hypotensive effect. SUDA et al. (1969) and NAGATSU et al. (1971) made the observation that fusaric acid was an adrenal tyrosine hydroxylase and dopamine β-hydroxylase inhibitor.

During the last few years a number of chemical, pharmacological, and clinical publications concerning its antihypertensive activity have appeared. The best known compounds are fusaric acid itself (139) its amide (140, Sch. 10.595, bupicomide; KORDUBA et al., 1971/73; VELASCO et al., 1974/75), and its dimethylamide. An Abbott patent (JONES and SOMANI, 1974) claims that also the racemic hexahydrofusaric acid (141) is an antihypertensive.

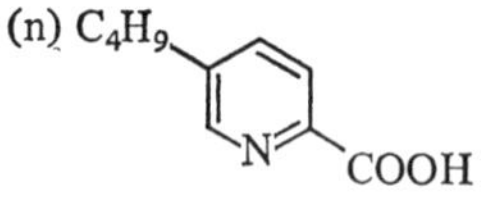

(139)

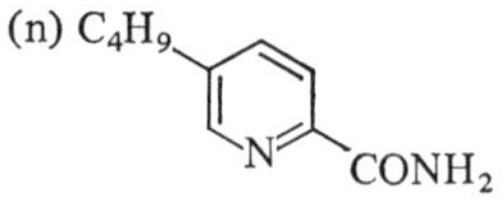

(140)

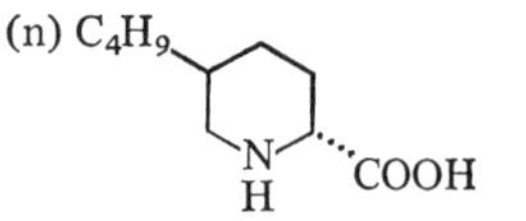

(141)

Since (140) is only active *in vivo* (and not *in vitro*), it may be assumed that the amide is hydrolyzed to fusaric acid in the body (KORDUBA et al., 1971; SYMCHOWICZ and STAUB, 1974). Fusaric acid is also used as the calcium salt (TERASAWA and KAMEYAMA, 1973), whereas salts with heavy metals, described in the literature, are not used therapeutically.

Further modifications of fusaric acid tested pharmacologically are (142), (143), and (144):

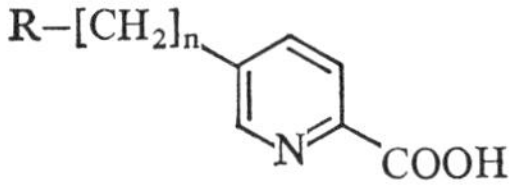

$n = 2$–6
R = Cl,Br,F,CH(Cl)CH_3 = (142)
UMEZAWA et al., 1973
ISHII et al., 1975

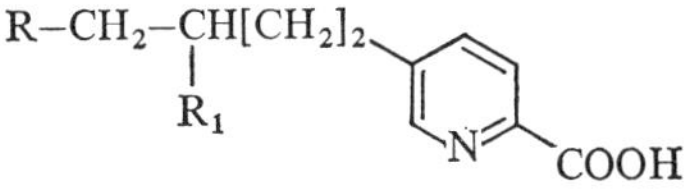

R = H; R_1 = Cl,Br,I = (143)
Japan. Kokei 74–36–681
R = Cl; R_1 = H = (149); ISHII et al. (1975)
R = R_1 = Br (HIDAKA and TAKEYA, 1972)

HIDAKA et al. (1975) claim that the bromine derivatives are usually more active than the chlorine containing compounds. Other, pharmacologically active modifications of fusaric acid are (145) (YP-279, HIDAKA et al., 1974) and (146) (phenopicolinic acid, NAKAMURA et al., 1975).

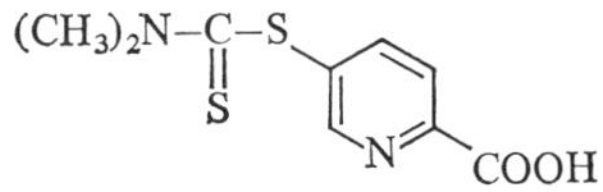

(145)

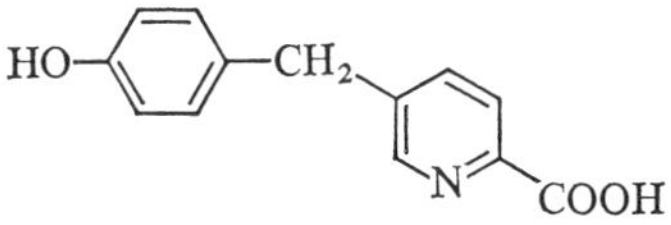

(146)

Very recently a new and interesting synthesis of fusaric acid analogs has been published (WARAWA, 1975).

References

ALDRICH, P. E., DIASSI, P. A., DICKEL, D. F., DYLION, C. M., HANCE, P. D., HUEBNER, C. F., KORZUN, B., KUEHNE, M. E., LIU, L. H., MCPHILLAMY, H. B., ROBB, E. W., ROYCHAUDHURI, D. K., SCHLITTLER, E., ST. ANDRE, A. F., VAN TAMELEN, E. E., WEISENBORN, F. L., WENKERT, E., WINTERSTEINER, O.: The stereochemistry of reserpine, deserpidine and related alkaloids. J. Amer. chem. Soc. **81**, 2481—2494 (1959).

ALLES, G. A.: Comparative physiological action of some derivates of guanidine. J. Pharmacol. exp. Ther. **28**, 251—276 (1926).

ANDERSON, P. L., HOULIHAN, W. J., MANNING, R. E.: Antihypertensive hydrazinopyridazines. Chem. Abstr. **73**, 120,655w (1971).

APPEL, W.: α-Isopropyl-α[(N-methyl-N-homoveratryl)γ-aminopropyl]-3,4-dimethoxyphenyl-acetonitril, sein Nachweis im biologischen Material und sein Verhalten im Blut. Arzneimittel-Forsch. **12**, 562—566 (1962).

ARCARI, G., BERNARDI, L., BOSISIO, G., CODA, S., FREGNAN, G. B., GLÄSSER, A. H.: 10-Methoxyergoline derivatives as α-adrenergic blocking agents. Experientia (Basel) **28**, 819—820 (1972).

ARCARI, G., DORIGOTTI, L., FREGNAN, G. B., GLÄSSER, A. H.: Vasodilating and α-receptor blocking activity of a new ergoline derivative. Brit. J. Pharmacol. **34**, 700P (1968).

ARCHER, S., WYLIE, D. W., HARRIS, L. S., LEWIS, T. R., SCHULENBERG, J. W., BELL, M. R., KULLNIG, R. K., ARNOLD, A.: 1-(Indolalkyl)-4-arylpiperazines a new class of tranquilizers. J. Amer. chem. Soc. **84**, 1306—1307 (1962).

ARCHIBALD, J. L., ALPS, B. J., CAVALLA, J. F., JACKSON, J. L.: Synthesis and hypotensive activity of benzamidopiperidyl ethylindole. J. med. Chem. **14**, 1054—1059 (1971).

ARYA, V. P., GREWAL, R. S., DAVID, J., KAUL, C. L.: 1-(5-Methyl-1-phenyl-4-pyrazolyl)-3-(4-((o-tolyl)piperazinyl)-1-propanone, a new synthetic antihypertensive agent. Experientia (Basel) **23**, 514—515 (1967).

AUGSTEIN, J., GREEN, S. M., KATRITZKY, A. R., MONRO, A. M.: The synthesis, proof of structure, and biological activity of some monosubstituted aminoguanidines. J. med. Chem. **8**, 395—397 (1965a).

AUGSTEIN, J., GREEN, S. M., MONRO, A. M., POTTER, G. W. H., WORTHING, C. R., WRIGLEY, T. I.: Adrenergic neurone blocking agents derived from 1,4 benzodioxan. J. Med. Chem. **8**, 446—456 (1965b); see also MONRO, A. M.: A new synthesis of guanidines. Chem. Ind. (Lond.) **1964**, 1806.

Augstein, J., Monro, A. M., Potter, G. W. H., Scholfield, P.: Adrenergic neurone blocking agents III: Heterocyclic analogs of guanoxan. J. med. Chem. **11**, 844—848 (1968).

Ayers, J. B., Waggoner, W. H.: Synthesis and properties of a series of pentacyanoferrates. J. inorg. nuclear. Chem. **31**, 2045—2051 (1969); Chem. Abstr. **71**, 66.787j (1969).

Ayman, D.: Potassium thiocyanate in the treatment of essential hypertension (its practicability). J. Amer. med. Ass. **96**, 1852—1857 (1931).

Ayman, D.: Bismuth subnitrate in the treatment of essential hypertension. J. Amer. med. Ass. **98**, 545—548 (1932).

Baines, M. W., Cobb, D. B., Eden, R. J., Fielden, R., Gardner, J. N., Roe, A. M., Tertiuk, W., Willey, G. L.: The synthesis and pharmacology of some stubstituted 1,3 benzdioxoles and 1,4-benzdioxans. J. med. Chem. **8**, 81—90 (1965).

Baker, P. D.: Sth. Med. Surg. **15**, 579 (1859).

Barger, G.: Ergot and Ergotism. London-Edinburgh: Gurney and Jackson 1931.

Barger, G., Carr, F. H.: The alkaloids of ergot. J. chem. Soc. **91**, 337—353 (1907).

Barker, M.: The blood cyanates in the treatment of hypertension. J. Amer. med. Ass. **106**, 762—767 (1936).

Barlow, R. B., Ing, H. R.: Curare like action of polymethylene bis-quaternary ammonium salts. Nature (Lond.) **161**, 718 (1948).

Barlow, R. B., Ing, H. R.: Curare-like action of polymethylene bis-quaternary ammonium salts. Brit. J. Pharmacol. **3**, 298—304 (1948).

Barrett, W. E., Mull, R. P., Plummer, A. J.: Hypotensive activity of cis-cinnamyl guanidine sulfate. Experientia (Basel) **21**, 506 (1965).

Barron, D. I., Bavin, P. M. G., Durant, G. J., Natoff, I. L., Spickett, R. G., Vallance, D. K.: Potential antihypertensive agents: Some guanidine derivatives. J. med. Chem. **6**, 705—711 (1963).

Barron, D. I., Natoff, I. L., Vallance, D. K.: Pharmacology of N-[2-(2,6-xylyloxy)ethyl]-guanidine sulfate: An adrenergic neurone blocking agent. Brit. J. Pharmacol. **25**, 534—544 (1965).

Barton, D. H. R., Jeger, O., Prelog, V., Woodward, R. B.: The constitution of cevine and some related alkaloids. Experientia (Basel) **10**, 81—90 (1954).

Baum, T., Shropshire, A. T., Rowles, G., Van Pelt, R., Fernandez, S. P., Eckfeld, D. K., Gluckman, M. I.: General pharmacologic actions of the antihypertensive agent 2,6-dichlorobenzylidene aminoguanidine acetate, WY 8678. J. Pharmacol. exp. Ther. **171**, 276—287 (1970).

Begeka, A. D., Groisman, S. D.: Effect of different doses of sympatholytic isobarin on the evacuative function of the stomach in dogs: Fiziol. Zh. (Kiev) **21**, 649—653 (1975). (Chem. Abstr. **83**, 188405b (1975).

Bell, M. R., Hoppe, J. O., Lape, H. E., Wood, D., Arnold, A., Selberis, W. H.: Antihypertensive activity of 7-azaindole-3-acetamidoxime and indole-1-acetamidoxime. Experientia (Basel) **23**, 298—299 (1967).

Bellasio, E., Carpi, C., Maffii, G., Testa, E.: 3-Hydrazino-6-aminopyridazines. Chem. Abstr. **75**, 151.820s (1971).

Bellasio, E., Parravicini, F., Testa, E.: 3-Hydrazinopyridazines containing basic groups in 6-position and possessing hypotensive activity. Farmaco, Ed. sci. **24**, 919—929 (1969); Chem. Abstr. **72**, 121.471z (1970).

Bernardi, L.: Recent developments in the chemistry of ergot alkaloids. Chimica Industria **51**, 563—569 (1969).

Berthaux, P., Neuman, M.: Etude pharmacologique et clinique d'un nouvel hypotenseur réserpinique: DL 152 ou Biétaserpine. Arzneimittel-Forsch. **14**, 1040—1045 (1964).

Bhatia, B. B.: On the use of Rauwolfia serpentina in high blood pressure. J. Indian med. Ass. **11**, 262—265 (1942).

Bierbaum, B. A., Traverso, J. J., Whitehead, C. W.: Hypotensive 1,2,4-benzothiadiazines. J. med. Chem. **6**, 272—275 (1963).

Black, M. M., Zweifach, B. W., Speer, F. D.: Comparison of hypotensive action of sodium azide in normotensive and hypertensive patients. Proc. Soc. exp. Biol. (N. Y.) **85**, 11—16 (1954).

Bloomfield, D. K., Cangiano, J. L.: Guanadrel and guanethidine in hypertension. Clin. Pharmacol. Ther. **11**, 200—204 (1970).

Boehringer-Ingelheim: U.S. Pat. 3.190.802 (German prior. 10/9/1961). Chem. Abstr. **64**, 2096 (1966).

Botton, I., Kinnard, W. J., Buckley, J. P.: Hypotensive activity of β-heptyleneiminoethyl-amino guanidine sulfate. J. Pharmacol. exp. Ther. **152**, 243—250 (1966).

Boura, A. L. A., Copp, F. C., Green, A. F.: New adrenergic compounds. Nature (Lond.) **184**, BA 70, (1959).

BOURA, A. L. A., COPP, F. C., GREEN, A. F.: Amidines as adrenergic neurone blocking agents. Nature (Lond.) **195**, 1213—1214 (1962).
BOURA, A. L. A., COPP, F. C., GREEN, A. F., HODSON, H. F., RUFFEL, G. K., SIM, M. F., WALTON, E.: Adrenergic neurone blocking agents related to choline 2,6-xylyl ether bromide (T.M.10), bretylium, and guanethidine. Nature (Lond.) **191**, 1312—1313 (1961).
BOURA, A. L. A., GREEN, A. F.: The actions of bretylium: Adrenergic neurone blocking and other effects. Brit. J. Pharmacol. **14**, 536—548 (1959).
BOVET, D., DEPIERRE, F., DE LESTRANGE, Y.: Propriétés curarisantes des éthers phénoliques à fonctions ammonium quaternaires. C. R. Acad. Sci. (Paris) **225**, 74—76 (1947).
BOYAJY, L. D., MANNING, R., MCINTOSH, R. E., SCHÄFER, F., HERZIG, M., SCHAAF, J., TRAPOLD, J. H.: Cardiovascular effects of 2-(2,6-dichlorophenyl)-5,6-dihydroimidazo-(2,1-b-thiazole)-hydrobromide. 166th ACS Meeting, Chicago, August 1973, Abstracts Medi-22.
BREAM, J. B., PICARD, C. W., WHITE, T. G., LAUENER, H.: Aralkylaminoguanidines and related compounds. J. med. Chem. **13**, 1051—1057 (1970).
BURN, J. H., DALE, H. H.: The action of certain quaternary ammonium bases. J. Pharmacol. exp. Ther. **6**, 417—438 (1914).
BUZAS, A., REGNIER, G.: Aminoalcoyl-1-réserpines. C. R. Acad. Sci. (Paris) **250**, 1340—1342 (1960).
CARSTENS, E.: Blutdrucksenkende Pharmaka. Pharmazie **27**, 675—682 (1972).
CASSINELLI, C. M.: Therapeutic applications of the hypotensive action of Na-nitroprusside. Chem. Abstr. **52**, 2283 (1958).
CAUJOLLE, F., CHANH, P. H., LECOINTE, P.: Pharmacology of the nitrosopentocyano ferrate of cobalt. Arch. int. Pharmacodyn. **172**, 487—495 (1968).
CAVALLERI, B., BELLASIO, E., SARDI, A.: Synthesis of 6-trifluoromethyl-1,4-dihydrazinophthalazine. J. med. Chem. **13**, 148—149 (1970).
CAVINESS, V. S., UMPHLET, T. L., PEASLEY, E. D., BELL, T. A., SATTERSFIELD, G. H.: Potassium rhodanide treatment of hypertension. N. C. med. J. **2**, 283—288 (1941).
CHOPRA, R. N., CHAKRAVARTI, M.: A preliminary note on the pharmacology of the alkaloids of R. serpentina. Indian J. Med. Res. **29**, 763—768 (1941).
CHRISTENSEN, H. D., HALEY, T. J.: Comparison of the effect of phentolamine and SU 12.080 on femoral blood flow in the anesthetized cat. Arch. int. Pharmacodyn. **164**, 84—90 (1966).
CHRUSCIEL, M.: Chronic toxicity of carbethoxyphthalazino hydrazine and its influence on the excretion of 5-hydroxyindoleacetic acid and the activity of 5-HTP-decarboxylase in white rats. Brit. J. Pharmacol. **32**, 104—112 (1968).
CLERK, A., PARIS, R., STERNE, J.: Action of octyl alcohol on the arterial pressure and surface tension of the blood of an animal. Compt. rend. soc. biol. **111**, 774—776 (1932). Federal Register **37**, No. 97, p. 10.015 (1972).
COMER, W. T., GOMOLL, A. W.: In: BURGER, A. (Ed.): Medicinal Chemistry, p. 1046. (3rd Ed. New York-London-Sidney-Toronto: Wiley Interscience 1970.
COSNIER, D., DUCHENE-MARULLAZ, P., GRIMAL, J., RISPAT, G., STREICHENBERGER, G.: Pharmacological properties of 2-(2-chloro-p-toluidino)-2-imidazolin enitrate (Tolonidine) I: Action on blood pressure and heart rate. Arzneimittel-Forsch. **25**, 1557—1561 (1975a).
COSNIER, D., HACHE, J., LABRID, C., STREICHENBERGER, G.: Pharmacological properties of 2-(2-chloro-p-toluidino)-2-imidazoline nitrate, III: Action on the secretions of the digestive tract and on the central nervous system, acute toxicity. Arzneimittel-Forsch. **25**, 1926—1933 (1975c).
COSNIER, D., LABRID, C., RISPAT, G., STREICHENBERGER, G.: Pharmacological properties of 2-(2-chloro-p-toluidino)-2-imidazoline nitrate (Tolonidine), a new antihypertensive agent, II: Action on cardiac contraction, circulatory parameters and diuresis. Arzneimittel-Forsch. **25**, 1802–1806 (1975b).
CUMMINGS, J. R., WELTER, A. N., GRACE, J. L., LIPCHUCK, L. M.: Cardiovascular actions of guancydine in normotensive and hypertensive animals. J. Pharmacol. exp. Ther. **161**, 88—97 (1968).
CURWAIN, B. P., FAKE, C. S., GORDON, J. L., MEHTA, M. D., MILLER, D., POYSER, R. H., WATTS, E. A.: Synthesis and antihypertensive properties of some N-(guanidinoalkyl)pyrrolidines. J. med. Chem. **14**, 737—742 (1971).
DANNENFELDT, K. H.: Leonard Rauwolf (a biography), 321 pp. Cambridge Mass.: Harvard University Press 1968.
DELBARRE, B., SCHMITT, H.: Sedative effects of α-sympathomimetic drugs and their antagonism by adrenergic and cholinergic blocking drugs. Europ. J. Pharmacol. **13**, 356—363 (1975).
DE STEVENS, G., WILHELM, M.: Antihypertensive agents. In: JUCKER, E. (Ed.): Progress in Drug Research, Vol. 20, pp. 197—259. Basel-Stuttgart: Birkhäuser 1976.
DOEBEL, K. J., FRANCIS, J. E.: 1,2,8,9-Tetraazaphenalenes. Chem. Abstr. **70**, 106.567a (1969).
DRUEY, J.: Pyridazines in the synthesis of drugs. Angew. Chem. **70**, 5—13 (1958).

DRUEY, J., MARXER, A.: Hypotensive hydrazinophthalazines and related compounds. J. med. Chem. 1, 1—21 (1959).
DRUEY, J., RINGIER, B. H.: Hydrazine derivatives of phthalazines and pyridazines. Helv. chim. Acta **34**, 195—210 (1951).
DRUEY, J., TRIPOD, J.: Hydralazines. In: SCHLITTLER, E. (Ed.): Antihypertensive Agents, pp. 223—262. New York-London: Academic Press 1967.
DUCHESNE, E. A.: Répertoire des plantes utiles et des plantes vénéneuses du globe, p. 35. Paris 1836.
EHRHART, G., RUSCHIG, H.: Arzneimittel, 2.te Aufl., Vol. 2, p. 150, 1972. Weinheim, Germany: Verlag Chemie
EHRREICH, S. J., HERINGSLAKE, J. E., WARREN, F. R., WEINSTOCK, J., TEDESCHI, R. E.: Pharmacological effects of an unusual hypotensive agent (SKF 11.197). Effects on the cardiovascular system. Arch. int. Pharmacodyn. **179**, 284—302 (1969).
ERNEST, I., JILEK, J. O., VEJDELEK, Z. J., PROTIVA, M.: Über einige neue (—)-Methylreserpatester. Coll. Czech. Chem. Commun. **24**, 266—273 (1964).
ERNEST, J., PROTIVA, M.: (±)Methyl-O-(O-carbethoxysyringoyl)-10-methoxydeserpidate. Coll. Czech. Chem. Commun. **26**, 1137—1144 (1961).
ERNEST, I., PROTIVA, M.: Synthese des racem. 12-Methylmercaptodeserpidins. Coll. Czech. Chem. Commun. **28**, 3106—3112 (1963).
EVERETT, A. J., LOWE, L. A., WILKINSON, S.: Revision of the structures of (+)-tubocurarine chloride and (+)-chondrocurine. Chem. Commun. **1970**, 1020—1021.
FIELDEN, R., GREEN, A. L.: A comparative study of the noradrenaline-depleting and sympathetic blocking actions of guanethidine and (—)-β-hydroxyphenethylguanidine. Brit. J. Pharmacol. **30**, 155—165 (1967).
FIELDEN, R., GREEN, A. L.: Optical isomers of β-hydroxyphenethylguanidine: Effects on heart noradrenaline and sympathetic blockade. Brit. J. Pharmacol. **32**, 350—359 (1968).
FIELDEN, R., GREEN, A. L., WILLEY, G. L.: Adrenergic neurone blocking activity of some aralkylguanidines. Brit. J. Pharmacol. **24**, 395—407 (1965).
FOURNEAU, E., BOVET, D.: Recherches sur l'action sympatholytique d'un nouveau dérivé du dioxane. Arch. int. Pharmacodyn. **46**, 178—191 (1933a).
FOURNEAU, E., BOVET, D.: Sympatholytic action of a new derivative of dioxan. Compt. rend. soc. biol. **113**, 388—390 (1933b).
FOURNEAU, E., MADERNI, P., DE LESTRANGE, Y.: Heterocyclic bases derived from coumarans and benzodioxan. J. Pharmacol. Chim. **18**, 185—191 (1933).
FREIS, E. D.: Hypertension: A controllable disease. Clin. Pharmacol. Ther. **13**, 627—632 (1972).
FREYBURGER, W. A., WEEKS, J. R., DUCHARME, D. W.: Cardiovascular actions of the hypotensive agent N,N-diallylmelamine (U 7720) Arch. exp. Path. Pharm. **251**, 39—47 (1965).
GADEKAR, S. M., NIBI, S., COHEN, E.: Hypotensive activity of some cyanoguanidines. J. med. Chem. **11**, 811—814 (1968).
GIFFORD, R. W.: Hypotensive Drugs. In: MODELL, W. (Ed.): Drugs of Choice 1970—1971. St. Louis, Mo.: C. V. Mosby.
GIUDICELLI, R., BEAUVALLET, M., CHABRIER, P., NAJER, H.: Sur l'action vasculaire de quelques amino-2-oxazolines. C. R. Acad. Sci. (Paris) **247**, 891, 2494—2497 (1959).
GIUDICELLI, R., NAJER, H., LEFÈVRE, F.: Relations between structure and activity in the N-(β-guanidinoethyl)azaspiroalkane series. C. R. Acad. Sci. (Paris) **260**, 2944—2947 (1965).
GIUDICELLI, R., NAJER, H., SARRET, M., PROUTEAU, M.: The pharmacologic activity in the N(β-guanidinoethyl)azaspiroalkane series. C. R. Acad. Sci. (Paris) **259**, 1596—1598 (1964).
GIUDICELLI, R., SCHMITT, H.: Propriétés antihypertensives et mécanisme d'action de la (diméthyl-2,6-phenylamino)-2-oxazoline-1,3. J. Pharmacol. **1**, 339—358 (1970).
GOLDRING, W., CHASIS, H.: Thiocyanate therapy in hypertension I: Observations on its toxic effects. Arch. intern. Med. **49**, 321—329 (1932).
GRAUBNER, W., WOLF, M.: Kritische Betrachtungen zum Wirkungsmechanismus des 2-(2,6-dichlorophenylamino)-2-imidazolinhydrochlorids. Arzneimittel-Forsch. **16**, 1055—1058 (1966).
GRESHOFF, M.: Übersicht der alkaloidhaltigen Apocynaceen in Niederländ. Indien. Chem. Ber. **23**, 3543 (1890).
GROOT, S. DE, STRATING, J.: Reserpine analogs I. Rec. Trav. chim. Pays-Bas **80**, 121—133 (1961).
GROSS, F., DRUEY, J., MEIER, R.: A new group of antihypertensive substances with a special mode of action. Experientia (Basel) **6**, 19—21 (1950).
GUPTA, J. C., GHOSH, S., DUTTA, A. T., KAHALI, B. S.: A note on the hypnotic principle of R. serpentina. J. Amer. pharm. Ass. **36**, 416 (1947).
GUPTA, J. C., KAHALI, B. S., DUTT, A.: The hypnotic effect of a resin fraction isolated from the root of R. serpentina Benth., obtained from Dehra-Dun. Indian J. med. Res. **32**, 183—188 (1944).

GUTMAN, J.: Modern Drug Encyclopedia and Therapeutic Guide, 1941, 138—139.
HAMMER, J., ULRYCH, M., FREIS, E.: Hemodynamic and therapeutic effects of guancydine in hypertension. Clin. Pharmacol. Ther. **12**, 78—90 (1971).
HANSSON, L., PASCUAL, A., JULIUS, S.: Comparison of guanadrel and guanethidine. Clin. Pharmacol. Ther. **14**, 204—208 (1973).
HARTMANN, M., ISLER, H.: Chemische Konstitution und pharmakologische Wirksamkeit von in 2-Stellung substituierten Imidazolinen. Naunyn-Schmiedebergs Arch. exp. Path. Pharmak. **192**, 141—154 (1939).
HEISE, A., KRONEBERG, G., SCHLOSSMANN, K.: α-Sympathomimetische Eigenschaften als Ursache der blutdrucksteigernden und blutdrucksenkenden Wirkung von BAY 1470 (2-(2-,6-xylidino)-5,6-dihydro-4H-1,3-thiazinhydrochlorid). Naunyn-Schmiedebergs Arch. Pharmak. **268**, 348—360 (1971).
HELGEN, L., STOUTLAND, O., AGRE, C. L.: Pyrolysis of N-phenylthiocarbamyl ethylenediamine and related materials. J. Org. Chem. **24**, 884—886 (1959).
HERMANN: Arch. f. Physiol. **39**, 419 (1886); Thesis, Univ. Königsberg 1887, p. 34.
HERSHENSON, F. M., ROZEK, L. F.: Synthesis and antihypertensive activity of 2-arylamino-1-azacycloalkenes. J. med. Chem. **14**, 907—909 (1971).
HESS, H. J., CRONIN, T. H., SCRIABINE, A.: Antihypertensive 2-Amino-4(3H)-quinazolinones. J. med. Chem. **11**, 130—136 (1968).
HIDAKA, H., HARA, F., HASHIZUME, V., YANO, M.: Selective inhibition of dopamine β-hydroxylase in the peripheral tissues by 5-dimethyldithio-carbamylpicolinic acid, its effect on stress-induced ulcer, ethanol-induced sleep and blood pressure. J. Pharmacol. exp. Ther. **191**, 384—392 (1974).
HIDAKA, H., NAGATSU, T., TAKEYA, K., TAKEUCHI, T., SUDA, H., KOJIRI, K., MATSUZAKI, M., UMEZAWA, H.: Fusaric acid, a new hypotensive agent produced by fungi. J. Antibiot. (Tokyo) **22**, 228—230 (1969); Chem. Abstr. **71**, 29.127y (1969).
HIDAKA, H., TAKEYA, K.: Blood pressure decreased by halobutylpicolinic acid, an inhibitory of dopamine β-hydroxylase Nature (Lond.) **239**, 334—335 (1972).
HIEBER, W., NAST, R., PROESCHEL, E.: Inorganic compounds of nitric oxide VI: The nitrosylcyano nickel complex. Z. anorg. Chem. **256**, 145—158 (1948).
HILL, H. E.: A contribution to the toxicity of sodium nitroprusside, the decomposition and determination of sodium nitroprusside. Aust. J. chem. Inst. **9**, 82—93 (1942).
HOEFKE, W., KOBINGER, W., WALLAND, A.: Relationship between activity and structure in the derivatives of clonidine: Arzneimittel-Forsch. **25**, 786—793 (1975).
HOFFMEISTER, W., KRUECK, F.: Mechanism of action of potassium rhodanide as explanation for the blood pressure lowering effect in hypertension. Klin. Wschr. **32**, 106—110 (1954).
HOFMANN, A.: Die Mutterkornalkaloide. Encke, Stuttgart 1964.
HOULIHAN, W. J., MANNING, R. E.: Secondary aminopyridazines as central nervous stimulants and as antihypertensives. Chem. Abstr. **75**, 49.118g (1971).
HOULIHAN, W. J., MANNING, R. E.: Pharmacologically active tertiary aminopyridazine derivatives. Chem. Abstr. **77**, 152.207a (1972).
HUEBNER, C. F.: Rauwolfia Alkaloids XIII: Derivatives of reserpine. J. Amer. chem. Soc. **76**, 5792 (1954).
HUENI, A.: Verfahren zur Herstellung eines neuen Imidazolins. A.P. 2.868.802. Chem. Abstr. **53**, 10.253 (1959).
ISHII, Y., FUJII, Y., MIMURA, C., UMEZAWA, H.: Pharmacological action of FD-008, a new dopamine β-hydroxylase inhibitor. Arzneimittel-Forsch. **25**, 55—59 (1975).
ISHII, Y., HOMMA, M., YOSHIKAWA, A., UMEZAWA, H.: Pharmacological action of FD-008, a new dopamine β-hydroxylase inhibitor. Arzneimittel-Forsch. **25**, 181—185 (1975); see also ISHII, Y., FUJII, Y., UMEZAWA, H.: Jap. J. Pharmacol. **23**, Suppl., 53, Abstr. 76 (1973).
ITALLIE, L. VAN, STEENHAUER, A. J.: R. serpentina Benth. Arch. Pharm. **270**, 313—322 (1932).
JEGER, O., PRELOG, V.: Steroid alkaloids: Veratrum group. In: MANSKE, R. H. F. (Ed.): The Alkaloids, Vol. VII, pp. 363—417. New York-London: Academic Press 1960.
JIRKOVSKY, I., PROTIVA, M.: Synthese des racem. 10,11-Methylendioxydespyrrolodeserpidins. Coll. Czech. Chem. Commun. **28**, 2577—2581 (1962).
JOHNSON, C. C.: The actions and toxicity of sodium nitroprusside. Arch. int. Pharmacodyn. **35**, 480—496 (1929).
JONES, P. H., SOMANI, P., Antihypertensive. U.S. Pat. 3840663 (3/23/1973 and 10/8/1974).
JUNG, F., PETSCH, G.: On the hypotensive activity of pentacyano ferrates, especially sodium nitroprusside. Acta biol. med. Germ. **19**, 781—783 (1967).
KAHN, M. M., AHMAD, N.: Nitroprusside complexes of divalent cobalt, nickel, cadmium, zinc, copper, mangan, iron and trivalent titanium. Z. Anorgan. Allgem. Chem. **354**, 301—306 (1967). Chem. Abstr. **68**, 16598 (1968).
KEELER, R. F.: Teratogenic compounds of V. californicum VII: The structure of the glycosidic alkaloid cycloposine. Steroids **13**, 579—588 (1969).

Keeler, R. F.: Teratogenic compounds of V. californicum XI: Gestational chronology and compound specifity in rabbits. Proc. Soc. exp. Biol. (N. Y.) **136**, 1174—1179 (1971a).
Keeler, R. F.: Teratogenic compounds of V. californicum XIII: Structure of muldamine. Steroids **18**, 741—752 (1971b).
Keeler, R. F.: Teratogenic compounds of V. californicum XIV: Limb deformations produced by cyclopamine. Proc. Soc. exp. Biol. (N. Y.) **142**, 1287—1291 (1973).
Keeler, R. F., Binns, W.: Possible teratogenic effects of veratramine. Proc. Soc. exp. Biol. (N. Y.) **123**, 921—923 (1966).
Keeler, R. F., Binns, W.: Teratogenic compounds from V. californicum III: Malformations of veratramine-induced type from ingestio nof plant or roots. Proc. Soc. exp. Biol. (N. Y.) **126**, 452—454 (1967).
Kersting, F.: Klinische Prüfung, Phase I: Arzneimittel-Forsch. **23**, 1657 —1659 (1973).
King, H., Lourie, E. M., Yorke, W.: New trypanocidal substances. Lancet **1937 II**, 1360—1363.
Korduba, C. A., Veals, J., Wohl, A., Symchowicz, S., Tabachnick, I. I. A.: Sch. 10.595, an effective dopamine β-hydroxylase inhibitor and a new hypotensive agent. Pharmacologist **13**, 192, abstr. 010 (1971); J. Pharmacol. exp. Ther. **184**, 671—677 (1973).
Kralt, T., Asma, W. J., Moed, H. D.: Reserpine analogues III: Alkoxy-β-phenylethylamine derivatives. Rec. Trav. chim Pays-Bas **80**, 431—445 (1961).
Kreye, V. A. W., Bechtel, H., Hoebel, M.: Studies on sodium nitroprusside II: Structure-Activity-Relationships (in press).
Kroneberg, G., Oberdorf, A., Hoffmeister, F., Wirth, W.: Zur Pharmakologie von BAY 1470, eines Hemmstoffs adrenergischer und cholinergischer Neurone. Naunyn-Schmiedebergs Arch. Pharmak. exp. Path. **256**, 257—280 (1967).
Kroneberg, G., Schlossmann, K., Stoepel, K.: Pharmacology of N-(2-guanidinoethyl)-4-methyl-1,2,3,6-tetrahydropyridine, a new antihypertensive agent. Arzneimittel-Forsch. **17**, 199—207 (1967).
Kubikowski, P., Majcherczyk, J., Szymanska, J.: New hydrazinophthalazine derivatives of hypotensive activity. Acta physiol. pol. **16**, 289—296 (1965); Chem. Abstr. **64**, 5638 (1966).
Kupchan, S. M.: Hypotensive veratrum ester alkaloids. J. pharm. Sci. **50**, 273—287 (1961).
Kupchan, S. M., By, A. W.: The chemistry of the veratrum group. In: Manske, R. H. F. (Ed.): The Alkaloids, Vol. X, pp. 193—285. New York-London: Academic Press 1968.
Kupchan, S. M., Flacke, W. E.: Hypotensive veratrum alkaloids. In: Schlittler, E. (Ed.): Antihypertensive Agents, pp. 429—458. New York-London: Academic Press 1967.
Lamb, I. D., White, A. C.: Some amidines and amidoximes with trypanocidal activity. J. chem. Soc. **1939**, 1253—1257.
Lape, H. E., Fort, D., Frering, R., Skulan, T.: Antihypertensive activity of a dihydroisoquinoline carboxamidoxime. Pharmacologist **13**, 191 (1971).
Lape, H. E., Hoppe, J. O., Bell, M. R., Wood, D., Selberis, W. H., Arnold, A.: The antihypertensive properties of a series of indole and azaindole amidoximes with particular reference to 7-azaindole-3-acetamidoxime and indole-1-acetamidoxime. Arch. int. Pharmacodyn. **171**, 394—414 (1968).
Laverty, R.: A comparison of the behavioural effects of some hypotensive imidazoline derivatives. Europ. J. Pharmacol. **9**, 163—169 (1969).
Lee, G. E.: Non-quaternary blockers. In: Schlittler, E. (Ed.): Antihypertensive Agents, pp. 295—329. New York-London: Academic Press 1967.
Lee, G. E., Wragg, W. R., Corne, S. J., Edge, N. D., Reading, H. W.: 1:2:2:6:6-Pentamethylpiperidine, a new hypotensive agent. Nature (Lond.) **181**, 1717—1719 (1958).
Leonard, N. J., Hauck, F. P.: Unsaturated amines X: The mercuric acetate route to substituted piperidines, Δ^2-tetrahydropyridines and Δ^2-tetrahydroanabasines. J. Amer. chem. Soc. **79**, 5279—5292 (1957).
Leonard, N. J., Nommensen, E. W.: Studies on the mechanism of the von Braun reaction. J. Amer. chem. Soc. **71**, 2808—2813 (1949).
Leroy, B. R.: The thiocyanates in solution, the natural physiological solvent of the body. N. Y. med. J. **1909**, 802—805.
Le Vine, P. B., Gearien, J. E.: Stereospecific synthesis of a reserpine analog. J. Organ. Chem. **26**, 4060—4062 (1961).
Libermann, D., Rouaix, A.: Hydrazine derivatives of some heterocyclic compounds. Bull. Soc. chim. Fr. **1959**, 1793—1798.
Lindner, E., Kaiser, J.: Tiamenidine (Hoechst 440), a new antihypertensive substance. Arch. int. Pharmacodyn. **211**, 305—325 (1974).
Löfgren, N., Erdtman, H.: A new group of compounds acting as local anesthetics. Svensk Kem. Tid. **49**, 163—174 (1937).
Lucas, R. A., Kiesel, R. J., Ceglowski, M. J.: Rauwolfia Alkaloids XXXII: Further studies on the synthesis and activity of reserpine analogs. J. Amer. chem. Soc. **82**, 493—495 (1960).

LUCAS, R. A., KUEHNE, M. E., CEGLOWSKI, M. J., DZIEMIAN, R. L., MCPHILLAMY, H. B.: Rauwolfia Alkaloids XXXI: The synthesis and activity of some reserpine analogs. J. Amer. chem. Soc. **81**, 1928—1932 (1959).
MAHAFFEY, L. W.: Toxicity of sodium nitroprusside for guinea pigs. Aust. J. chem. Inst. **9**, 93—94 (1942).
MAJOR, R. H.: Possible relationship between guanidine and high blood pressure. Amer. J. med. Sci. **170**, 228—232 (1925).
MAJOR, R. H., STEPHENSON, W.: The effects of methylguanidines. Bull. Johns Hopk. Hosp. **35**, 140—141 (1924).
MANCHOT, W., DÜSING, J.: Studies of the similarity of ruthenium to iron: Sodium nitrosopenta cyano ruthenite. Z. anorg. Chem. **212**, 109—112 (1933).
MARXER, A., SCHIER, O.: Quaternary ganglionic blockers. In: SCHLITTLER, E. (Ed.): Antihypertensive Agents, pp. 279—294. New York-London: Academic Press 1967.
MASSIE, E., ETHERIDGE, C. B., O'HARE, J. P.: Thiocyanate therapy in vascular hypertension. New Engl. J. Med. **219**, 736—740 (1938).
MATIER, W. L., COMER, W. T., DEITCHMAN, D.: Sulfamoyl azides: Hydrolysis rate and hypotensive activity. J. med. Chem. **15**, 538—541 (1972); see also Chem. Abstr. **75**, 150.893f (1971).
MAXWELL, R. A., PLUMMER, A. J., DANIEL, A. I., SCHNEIDER, F., POVALSKI, H.: Concerning the mechanisms of the cardiovascular actions of hexahydro-1-azepine propionamidoxime. J. Pharmacol. exp. Ther. **124**, 127—134 (1958b).
MAXWELL, R. A., MULL, R. P., PLUMMER, A. J.: (2-(Octahydro-1-azocinyl)-ethyl)guanidine sulfate (SU 5864), a new synthetic antihypertensive agent. Experientia (Basel) **15**, 267 (1959).
MAXWELL, R. A., ROSS, S. D., PLUMMER, A. J.: Pharmacology of hexahydro-1-azepine propionamidoxime (SU 4029). J. Pharmacol. exp. Ther. **123**, 128—139 (1958a).
MAXWELL, R. A., SCHNEIDER, F. L.: Some actions of hexahydro-1-azepine propionamidoxime ·HCl (SU 4029) in certain autonomic pathways. J. Pharmacol. exp. Ther. **134**, 347—355 (1961).
MAZUMDAR, D. C., MUKHERJI, K. L.: Rauwolfia in hypertension. J. Indian med. Ass. **19**, 362—367 (1950).
MCPHILLAMY, H. B., HUEBNER, C. F., SCHLITTLER, E., ST. ANDRE, A. F., ULSHAFER, P. R.: Rauwolfia Alkaloids XIX: The constitution of deserpidine and reserpine. J. Amer. chem. Soc. **77**, 4335—4343 (1955).
MULL, R. P.: Belgian Patent 611653 (1962). Aminoguanidines. Chem. Abstr. **57**, 16414 (1962).
MULL, R. P., EGBERT, M. E., DAPERO, M. R.: Guanidines with antihypertensive activity I. J. Org. Chem. **25**, 1953—1956 (1960).
MULL, R. P., MAXWELL, R. A.: Guanethidine and related adrenergic neurone blocking agents. In: SCHLITTLER, E. (Ed.): Antihypertensive Agents, p. 131. New York-London: Academic Press 1967.
MULL, R. P., MAXWELL, R. A., PLUMMER, A. J.: Antihypertensive activity of hexahydro-1-azepine propionamidoxime. Nature (Lond.) **180**, 1200—1201 (1957).
MULL, R. P., MIZZONI, R. H., DAPERO, M. R., EGBERT, M. E.: Guanidines with antihypertensive activity II. J. med. Chem. **5**, 944—949 (1962).
MÜLLER, J. M., SCHLITTLER, E., BEIN, H. J.: Reserpin, der sedative Wirkstoff aus R. serpentina Benth. Experientia (Basel) **8**, 338 (1952).
MULLER, G., ALLAIS, A.: Sur quelques analogues synthétiques de la réserpine et de la déserpidine. Naturwissenschaften **47**, 82 (1960).
MONRO, A. M., POTTER, G. W. H., SEWELL, M. J.: Adrenergic neurone blocking agents II: Some dioxane-substituted derivatives of guanoxan. J. med. Chem. **10**, 880—883 (1967).
NADOR, K.: Benzylguanidines. Hungarian Pat. 155717 (Gedeon Richter) Chem. Abstr. **70**, 114811r (1969).
NAGATSU, I., MITSUTAMI, K., UMEZAWA, H., MATSUZAKI, M., TAKEUCHI, T.: Adrenal tyrosine hydroxylase and dopamine β-hydroxylase in spontaneous hypertensive rats. Nature (Lond.) **230**, 381—382 (1971).
NAJER, H., CHABRIER, P., GIUDICELLI, R.: Sur quelques amino-2-oxazolines N-substituées douées d'activité vasculaire. Bull. Soc. chim. Fr. **1959**, 352—359.
NAJER, H., GIUDICELLI, R.: Sur quelques amino-2-oxazolines N-substituées douées d'activité vasculaire (2° mémoire). Bull. Soc. chim. Fr. **1960**, 1650—1652.
NAJER, H., GIUDICELLI, R., LOISEAU, J., MENIN, J.: Le (triméthoxy-3''-4''-5''-benzoate de β-hydroxyéthyl)-3'-pipéridino-N-ethyl)-3-méthoxy-6-indole. Bull. Soc. chim. Fr. **1963**, 2831—2840.
NAJER, H., GIUDICELLI, R., SETTE, J.: Une nouvelle synthèse des arylamino-2-imidazolines. Bull. Soc. chim. Fr. **1961**, 2114—2126.
NAJER, H., GIUDICELLI, R., SETTE, J.: Guanidines with antihypertensive activity IV: N-(β-guanidinoethyl)azaspiroalkanes. Bull. Soc. chim. Fr. **1964**, 2572—2581.

NAJER, H., GIUDICELLI, R., SETTE, J., MENIN, J.: Guanidines with antihypertensive activity V: N-(β-guanidinoethyl)azaspiroalkanes. Bull. Soc. chim. Fr. **1965**, 204—208.

NAKAMURA, T., YASUDA, H., OBAYASHI, A., TANABE, O., MATSUMURA, S., UEDA, F., OHATA, K.: Antihypertensive and fungal dopamine β-hydroxylase inhibitor. J. Antibiot. (Tokyo) **28**, 477 (1975). Chem. Abstr. **83**, 75.176j (1975).

NOGRADI, T.: Untersuchungen über Rauwolfia-Alkaloid-Modelle I: Tryptamin- und Gramin-derivate. Mh. Chem. **88**, 768—777 (1957a).

NOGRADI, T.: Untersuchung über Rauwolfia-Alkaloid-Modelle II: 2-substituierte Indole, Tetrahydrocarbolin- und Hexahydroyohimbanderivate. Mh. Chem. **88**, 1087—1094 (1957b).

NORTON, S., PHILLIPS, A. P.: A new type of autonomic blocking agent. Nature (Lond.) **172**, 867 (1953).

OZAWA, H., GOMI, Y., OTSUKI, I.: Pharmacological studies of guanethidine dervatives III: Yakugaku Zasshi **85**, 112—119 (1965); Chem. Abstr. **62**, 15314 (1965).

OZAWA, H., SATO, S.: The adrenergic neurone blocking action of 2-(methylphenylamino)ethyl-guanidine sulfate: Chem. Pharm. Bull. (Tokyo) **14**, 1291—1297 (1966); **15**, 840—844 (1967).

PACO, G. DI, TAURO, C. S.: On some new esters and amides of 3,4,5-trimethoxy benzoic acid with potential reserpine activity. Farmaco, Ed. sci. **13**, 64—74 (1958).

PAGE, I. H.: The nature of treatment of hypertension. Trans. Amer. ther. Soc. **48**, 56—70 (1947).

PAGE, I. H.: Humoral and vasomotor controls of blood vessels. Bull. N. Y. Acad. Med. **28**, 131—144 (1952).

PAGE, I. H.: Drug treatment in hypertension. A public lecture given at the Symposium on antihypertensive therapy, principles and practice (GROSS, F. Ed.), pp. 602—614. Berlin-Heidelberg-New York: Springer 1966.

PAGE, I. H., CORCORAN, A., DUSTAN, P. H., KOPPANY, T.: Cardiovascular actions of sodium nitroprusside in animals and hypertensive patients. Circulation **11**, 188—198 (1955).

PARSONS, D. G., TURNER, A. F., MURRAY, B. G.: Substituted 1-aminophthalazines. Chem. Abstr. **70**, 57872k (1969); see also (Vantorex Ltd.) New substituted phthalazines. Chem. Abstr. **68**, 49632a (1968).

PATON, W. D. M., ZAIMIS, E. J.: The pharmacological actions of the polymethylene bistrimethyl-ammonium salts. Nature (Lond.) **161**, 718—719 (1948); Brit. J. Pharmacol. **4**, 381—400 (1949).

PAULI, W.: Zur Kenntnis der Rhodantherapie. Zbl. ges. Ther. **22**, 19 (1904).

PETERFALVI, M., JEQUIER, R.: La 10-méthoxy déserpidine: étude pharmacologique. Arch. int. Pharmacodyn. **124**, 237—254 (1960).

PEZZANGARO, F.: Treatment of arterial hypertension by intravenous injection of octyl alcohol. C. R. Soc. Biol. (Paris) **119**, 1331—1333 (1935).

PHAM-HUU-CHANH, LECOINTE, P., DONNAT, L.: Pharmacology of barium nitrosyl pentacyano ferrate. Arzneimittel-Forsch. **19**, 1836—1842 (1969).

PLATTNER, P. A., KELLER, W., BOLLER, A.: Welkstoffe und Antibiotika. Konstitution und Synthese der Fusarinsäure. Synthese von 5-Äthyl- und 5-n-Hexylpyridin-2-carbonsäure. Helv. chim. Acta **37**, 1379—1392 (1954).

PLUMMER, A. J., SCHNEIDER, J. A., BARRETT, W. E.: A series of tris (dialkylaminoalkyl) amines with ganglionic blocking activity. Arch. int. Pharmacodyn. **97**, 1—12 (1954).

POPELAK, A., LETTENBAUER, G.: Über die Verätherung der Yohimbanalkaloide mit Diazomethan. Arch. Pharm. **295**, 427—430 (1962).

PROTIVA, M., JILEK, J. O., HACH, V., ADLEROVA, E., MICHAJLYSZYN, V.: Einfache Reserpinmodelle mit dem Cyclohexanring E. Coll. Czech. Chem. Commun. **24**, 83—92 (1959a).

PROTIVA, M., VEJDELEK, Z. J., JILEK, J. O., MACEK, K.: Einige weitere Derivate des Tryptamins und 1,2,3,4-Tetrahydronorharmans. Coll. Czech. Chem. Commun. **24**, 3978—3987 (1959b).

PRUSS, T. P., HIDALGO, J.: Cardiovascular profile of the antihypertensive agent guanadrel. Proc. Soc. exp. Ther. **139**, 600—603 (1972).

RAFFA, L., MONZANI, A., DI BELLA, M.: 1,2,4-Benzothiadiazine derivatives XVIII: The chlorination of 3-oxodihydrobenzo-1,2-thiadiazine-1,1-dioxide. Farmaco, Ed. sci. **17**, 234—243 (1962); Chem. Abstr. **58**, 3435 (1963).

RACINE, M.: A propos des traitements récents de l'hypertension artérielle. J. Prat. (Paris) **49**, 753—756 (1935).

RIEPPEL, F. W.: Leonhard Rauwolf. Ein Beitrag zu seiner Biographie. Dtsch. med. Wschr. **80**, 653—655 (1955).

RIEPPEL, F. W.: Zur Frühgeschichte der Rauwolfia. Sudhoffs Arch. Gesch. Med. **40**, 231—239 (1956).

ROBERTSON, J. E.: Biguanides French Patent 1.320.255 (1963); Chem. Abstr. **59**, 10.010 (1963).

ROBISON, M. M., LUCAS, R. A., MCPHILLAMY, H. B., BARRETT, W., PLUMMER, A. J.: Rauwolfia Alkaloids XXXV: Potent, fast acting sedatives from methylreserpate. Experientia (Basel) **17**, 14 (1961a).

ROBISON, M. M., LUCAS, R. A., McPHILLAMY, H. B., DZIEMIAN, R. L., HSU, I., KIESEL, R. J.: Rauwolfia Alkaloids XXXVI: Non-hypotensive sedatives derived from methylreserpate. J. Amer. chem. Soc. **83**, 2694—2700 (1965b).
RODRIGUEZ, R., HONG, E., VIDRIO, H., PARDO, E. G.: Pharmacology of a group of phenylpiperazine tetrazole derivatives with adrenergic blocking actions. J. Pharmacol. exp. Ther. **148**, 54—65 (1965).
ROTH, F. E., SCHURR, J., MOUTIS, E., GOVIER, W. M.: Comparative hypotensive effect and toxicity of sodium azide and selected organic azides. Arch. int. Pharmacodyn. **108**, 473—480 (1956).
RUBIN, A. A., ROTH, F. E., WINBURY, M. M.: A non-diuretic benzothiadiazine with antihypertensive properties. Nature (Lond.) **192**, 176—177 (1961).
RUBIN, A. A., ROTH, F. E., WINBURY, M. M., TOPLISS, J. G., SHERLOCK, M. H., SPERBER, N., BLACK, J.: A new class of antihypertensive agents. Science **133**, 2067 (1961).
RUSSEL, W. O., STAHL, W. C.: Fatal poisoning from potassium rhodanide treatment of hypertension. J. Amer. med. Ass. **119**, 1177—1181 (1942).
SAH, H. J., SAH, P. P. T., PEOPLES, S. A.: The new antihypertensive agent guanethidine: a review. Discovery and development, chemical structure, physical properties, and pharmacological actions. Arzneimittel-Forsch. **16**, 53—58 (1966).
SANDOZ: Belg. Pat. 737.553 (U.S. priority 8/16 and 26/1968).
SAUNDERS, J. P., HIMWICH, W. A.: Properties of the transsulfurase responsible for conversion of cyanide to thiocyanate. Amer. J. Physiol. **163**, 404—409 (1950).
SCHIER, O., MARXER, A.: Antihypertensive agents 1962—1968. In: JUCKER, E. (Ed.): Progress in Drug Research, Vol. 13, pp. 101—135. Basel-Stuttgart: Birkhäuser 1969.
SCHLITTLER, E.: Rauwolfia alkaloids with special reference to the chemistry of reserpine. In: MANSKE, R. H. F. (Ed.): The Alkaloids, Vol. 8, pp. 287—334. New York: Academic Press 1965.
SCHLITTLER, E., DRUEY, J., MARXER, A.: Antihypertensive agents. In: JUCKER, E. (Ed.): Progress in Drug Research, Vol. **4**, pp. 295—351. Basel-Stuttgart: Birkhäuser 1962.
SCHOEPKE, H. G., BRONDYK, H. D., WIEMELER, L. H., SCHMIDT, J. L.: Cardiovascular pharmacology of tertiary octylguanidine (B.P. 1184). Arch. int. Pharmacodyn. **153**, 185—204 (1965).
SCHUEMANN, H. J., WERNER, U.: Hemmung der Hormonfreisetzung aus dem Nebennierenmark durch BAY 6781, eine antihypertensive Substanz. Naunyn-Schmiedebergs Arch. Pharmak. **268**, 71—82 (1971).
SCRIABINE, A., BOOHER, K. D., PEREIRA, J. N., McSHANE, W. K., CONSTANTINE, J. W., KOCH, R. C., MIKNIUS, S.: Pharmacological studies with guanisoquin. J. Pharmacol. exp. Ther. **147**, 277—287 (1965).
SCRIABINE, A., BOOHER, K. D., PEREIRA, J. N., McSHANE, W. K., KOCH, R. C.: Some pharmacological actions of N,N′-dimethyl-1,2,3,4-tetrahydroisoquinoline-2-carboxamidine HCl (P-4746). Arch. int. Pharmacodyn. **164**, 435—443 (1966).
SEMONSKY, M., ZIKAN, V., VOTOVA, Z., PODVALOVA, I., PONEC, K.: N(D-6-Methyl-8-isoergolenyl)-N,N-diethylurea acid maleate (LYSENYL-Spofa, a new antiserotonine drug). Čs. Farm. **17**, 296—305 (1968). C. A. **70**, 1976e (1969).
SEN, G., BOSE, K. C.: Rauwolfia serpentina: A new Indian drug for insanity and high blood pressure. Indian med. World **2**, 194—201 (1931).
SHERMAN, G. P.: Bradycardia effects of the antihypertensive agent 2,6-dichlorobenzylidene aminoguanidine acetate (WY 8678) in the dog. Pharmacologist **13**, 192 (abstr. 005) (1971).
SHORT, J. H., DARBY, T. D.: Sympathetic nervous system blocking agents III: Derivatives of benzylguanidines. J. med. Chem. **10**, 833—840 (1967).
SHORT, J. H., OURS, C. W., RANUS, W. J.: Sympathetic nervous system blocking agents V: Derivatives of isobutyl-, tert. butyl-, and neopentyl-guanidine. J. med. Chem. **11**, 1129—1135 (1968).
SIDDIQUI, S.: A note on the alkaloids of R. serpentina Benth. J. Indian chem. Soc. **16**, 421—422 (1939).
SIDDIQUI, S., SIDDIQUI, R. H.: Chemical examination of the roots of R. serpentina Benth. J. Indian. chem. Soc. **8**, 667—680 (1931).
SIDDIQUI, S., SIDDIQUI, R. H.: Alkaloids of Rauwolfia serpentina Benth. Part. I. J. Indian chem. Soc. **9**, 539—544 (1932).
SIDDIQUI, S., SIDDIQUI, R. H.: The alkaloids of R. serpentina Benth. Part II: Studies in the ajmaline series. J. Indian chem. Soc. **12**, 37—47 (1935).
SIVACH, T. A., KAPITONENKO, T. A.: Hypotensive properties of 3-azidocyclohexanone semicarbazone. Chem. Abstr. **83**, 71780d (1975).
SONN, A.: Imidazolines. U.S. Pat. 2.161.938 (Chem. Abstr. **33**, 7316 (1939).
SPIVAKOVA, R. P.: Pharmacological properties of a number of sympatholytics, derivatives of guanidine. Farmakol. i Toksikol **34**, 650—653 (1971). [Chem. Abstr. **76**, 108017u (1972)].

Spinks, A., Young, E. H. P.: Polyalkylpiperidines: A new series of ganglionic blocking agents. Nature (Lond.) **181**, 1397—1398 (1958).

Stieglitz, E. J.: Bismuth subnitrate in the therapy of hypertension. J. Pharmacol. exp. Ther. **32**, 23—35 (1928).

Stieglitz, E. J.: Therapeutic results with bismuth subnitrate in hypertensive arterial disease. J. Pharmacol. exp. Ther. **46**, 343—356 (1932).

Stoll, A., Hofmann, A.: Die Alkaloide der Ergotoxingruppe: Ergocristin, Ergokryptin und Ergocornin. Helv. chim. Acta **26**, 1570—1601 (1943).

Stoll, A., Hofmann, A.: The ergot alkaloids. In: Manske, R. H. F. (Ed.). The Alkaloids, Chemistry and Physiology, Vol. VIII, pp. 725—783. New York-London: Academic Press 1965.

Stoll, A., Hofmann, A.: The chemistry of the ergot alkaloids. In: Pelletier, S. W. (Ed.): Chemistry of the Alkaloids, pp. 267—300. New York: Van Nostrand Reinhold 1970.

Suda, H., Takeuchi, T., Nagatsu, T., Matsuzaki, U., Matsumoto, I., Umezawa, H.: Inhibition of dopamine β-hydroxylase by 5-alkylpicolinic acids and their hypotensive effects. Chem. pharm. Bull. **17**, 2377—2380 (1969).

Symchowicz, S., Staub, M.: Disposition of Sch. 10595 in animals and man. J. Pharmacol. exp. Ther. **191**, 324—330 (1974).

Tamari, K., Kaji, J.: The mechanism of the growth inhibiting action of fusarinic acid on plants: Chem. Abstr. **48**, 8330 (1954).

Terasawa, F., Kameyama, M.: Clinical trial of a new hypotensive agent, fusaric acid (5-butylpicolinic acid). Chem. Abstr. **79**, 27527 (1973).

Topliss, J. G., Konzelman, L. M., Shapiro, E. P., Sperber, N., Roth, F. E.: Antihypertensive agents II: 3 Substituted 2H 1,2,4 benzothiadiazine-1,1 dioxides. J. med. Chem. **7**, 269—273 (1964).

Topliss, J. G., Sherlock, M. H., Reimann, H., Konzelman, L. M., Shapiro, E. P., Pettersen, B. W., Schneider, H., Sperber, N.: Antihypertensive agents I: Non diuretic 2H-1,2,4-benzothiadiazine-1,1-dioxides. J. med. Chem. **6**, 122—127 (1963).

Topliss, J. G., Yudis, M. D.: Correlation of antihypertensive activity with structure in a series of 2H-1,2,4 benzothiadiazine-1,1-dioxides using the substituent constant approach. J. med. Chem. **15**, 394—400, 400—403 (1972).

Trcka, V., Dlabac, A., Vanecek, M.: Mediodespidine, hypotensive reserpoid without sedative effect I: Comparison of sedative and hypotensive activity in monkeys. Life Sci. **4**, 2257—2261 (1956a).

Trcka, V., Carlsson, A.: Part II: Effect on monoamine levels in mouse organs. Life Sci. **4**, 2263—2267 (1965b).

Turner, F. A., Gearien, J. E.: Synthesis of reserpine analogs. J. org. Chem. **24**, 1952—1955 (1959).

Ueno, K., Ishikawa, F., Miyazaki, S.: Pyrido (3-4d) pyridazine derivatives. Chem. Abstr. **75**, 140874—140876 (1971).

Ueno, K., Miyazaki, S., Akashi, A.: Hypotensive 1-(alkylidenehydrazino)-phthalazines. Chem. Abstr. **77**, 5504s (1972).

Umezawa, H., Takeuchi, T., Miyano, K., Hamano, H., Tanaka, W.: Antihypertensive 5(ω-haloalkyl)picolinic acids. Ger. Offen. 2305758 (Chem. Abstr. **79**, 115.444w (1973).

Urech, E., Marxer, A., Miescher, K.: 2-Aminoalkyl-imidazoline. Helv. chim. Acta **33**, 1386—1407 (1950).

Vakil, R. J.: A clinical trial of R. serpentina in essential hypertension. Brit. Heart J. **11**, 350—355 (1949).

Vazakas, A. J., Doluisio, J. T.: Synthesis and pharmacology of some basic esters of 3,4,5-trimethoxybenzoic acid. J. pharm. Sci. **53**, 165—169 (1964).

Vedernikov, Y. P.: Effects of Redergam on vascular responses to sciatic nerve stimuli. (Russ.). Chem. Abstr. **61**, 12505 (1964).

Vedernikov, Y. P.: Pharmacology of Redergam and assays of its analgesic activity in animal and clinical tests. Farmakol. i Toksikol. **26**, 431—434 (1963) (Russ.). Chem. Abstr. **60**, 2234 (1964).

Vejdelek, Z. D., Trcka, V., Protiva, M.: Chemistry of 1,2,3,4-Tetrahydronorharman-1-carboxylic acid and derivatives. J. Med. Pharm. Chem. **3**, 427—440 (1961).

Velasco, M., Gilbert, C. A., Rutledge, C. O., McNay, J. L.: Bupicomide: Clin. Pharmacol. Ther. **18**, 145—153 (1975).

Velasco, M., McNay, J. L.: Clin. Pharmacol. Ther. **15**, 222 (1974).

Velluz, L.: Réserpines de synthèse. Ann. pharm. franç. **17**, 15—25 (1959); Prod. pharm. **14**, 607—609 (1959).

Velluz, L., Muller, G., Allais, A.: 6-Alcoyl réserpines. C. R. Acad. Sci. (Paris) **247**, 1746—1748 (1958b).

VELLUZ, L., MULLER, G., ALLAIS, A.: Deserpidine derivatives. French pat. 1.180.514 (1959); Chem. Abstr. **55**, 9450 (1961).

VELLUZ, L., PETERFALVI, M., JEQUIER, R.: Un clivage des effects réserpiques. C. R. Acad. Sci. (Paris) **247**, 1905—1907 (1958a).

VOTAVA, Z., PODVALOVA, I., VOJTECHOVSKY, M.: Unterschiede in der pharmakologischen Wirkung von halluzinogenen und nicht halluzinogenen Lysergsäurederivaten (LSD-25, Deseryl, Lysenyl und Mesenyl). Arzneimittel-Forsch. **16**, 220—222 (1966).

WARAWA, E. J.: Synthesis of 3-alkyl-2,6-dicyanopyridines by a unique rearrangement. Preparation of fusaric acid analogs. J. org. Chem. **40**, 2092—2095 (1975).

WENNER, W.: 1,2,3,4-Tetrahydroisoquinoline derivatives with antihypertensive properties. J. med. Chem. **8**, 125—126 (1965).

WERLE, E., FRIED, R.: Zur Kenntnis der biologischen Wirkung organischer Azide. Biochem. Z. **322**, 507—512 (1952).

WERLE, E., FRIED, R.: Über das Azid-entgiftende Ferment tierischer Gewebe. Biochem. Z. **321**, 500—507 (1951).

WERLE, E., FRIED, R.: Monoamidoxydase und Azidabbau durch tierische Gewebe. Biochem. Z. **323**, 14—20 (1952).

WERLE, E., MENNICKEN, G.: Über die Inaktivierung von Tryptamin und Tyramin durch tierische Gewebe. Biochem. Z. **296**, 99—104 (1938).

WERLE, E., STÜCKER, F.: Zur Pharmakologie der Azide. Arzneimittel-Forsch. **8**, 28—31 (1958).

WERNER, L. H., BARRETT, W. E.: Adrenergic blocking agents. In: SCHLITTLER, E. (Ed.): Antihypertensive Agents, pp. 331—392. New York-London: Academic Press 1967.

WESTPHAL, K.: Über die Rhodantherapie des genuinen arteriellen Hochdrucks. Münch. med. Wschr. **73**, 1187 (1926).

WESTPHAL, K., BLUM, R.: Die Rhodantherapie des genuinen arteriellen Hochdrucks und ihre Bedeutung. Dtsch. Arch. klin. Med. **152**, 331—353 (1926).

WILSON, J., VESEY, C. J., COLE, P. V.: Nitroprusside revisited. Brit. med. J. **1971 IV**, 116.

WOLLWEBER, H., WILMS, H., HILTMANN, R., STOEPEL, K., KRONEBERG, G.: Guanidinoalkylazacycloalkanes: Chemical structure and antihypertensive activity. Arzneimittel-Forsch. **21**, 2089—2100 (1971).

WOODWARD, R. B., BADER, F. E., BICKEL, H., FREY, A. J., KIERSTEAD, R. W.: The total synthesis of reserpine. J. Amer. chem. Soc. **78**, 2023—2025, 2657 (1956); Tetrahedron **2**, 1—57 (1958).

WYLIE, D. W., ARCHER, S.: Structure-activity relationships of 1-[(3-indolyl)-alkyl]-4-aryl piperazines, a new series of tranquilizers. J. med. Pharm. Chem. **5**, 932—943 (1962).

YABUTA, T., KAMBE, K., HAYASHI, T.: Fusarinic acid, a new product of the bakanae fungus. Chem. Abstr. **29**, 1132 (1935).

ZIKAN, V., SEMONSKY, M.: Mutterkornalkaloide, Mitt. 31: Ein Beitrag zur Herstellung von N(D-6-Methyl-8-isoergolenyl)N,N′-diäthylharnstoff. Pharmazie **23**, 147—148 (1968).

ZINS, G. R.: The in vivo production of a potent, long-acting hypotensive metabolite from diallylmelamine. J. Pharmacol. exp. Ther. **150**, 109—117 (1965).

ZINS, G. R., EMMERT, D. E., WALK, R. A.: Hypotensive metabolite production and sequential metabolism of N,N-diallylmelamine in rats, dogs, and man. J. Pharmacol. exp. Ther. **159**, 194—205 (1968).

ZWIETEN, P. A. VAN: A new antihypertensive compound, 44—549. Pharmacology **13**, 352 (1975).

Chapter 3

Ganglion-Blocking Drugs in Antihypertensive Therapy

V. A. W. KREYE

I. Introduction

Ganglion-blocking agents are not only among the most powerful blood pressure-lowering drugs but were also the first substances to be found capable of inducing a therapeutically significant antihypertensive effect. As early as 1914/15, BURN and DALE described blockade of impulse transmission in autonomic ganglia by quaternary ammonium bases. But not until 32 years later, on the basis of their own studies with tetraethylammonium (TEA), did ACHESON and MOE (1946) and ACHESON and PERREIRA (1946) propose its use in the treatment of hypertension.

Subsequently, the bisquaternary ammonium compounds were introduced (BARLOW and ING, 1948; PATON and ZAIMIS, 1948, 1949) of which hexamethonium, azamethonium, and later pentolinium have been used in the management of high blood pressure. In the following decade, nonquaternary ammonium compounds and triethyl-sulfonium salts with ganglion-blocking activity were developed, which had the advantage of being better absorbed from the intestinal tract than the bisquaternary compounds.

However, side-effects, which in part were quite unpleasant or even dangerous, limited the use of ganglion-blocking drugs in most countries. Hence, when selective inhibitors of adrenergic transmission were developed, especially guanethidine (MAXWELL et al., 1960), ganglion-blocking drugs were less and less used as antihypertensives and today have been nearly abandoned. A limited field of application is still "controlled hypotension" in neurosurgery as well as in otorhinolaryngology or in ophthalmology, but the drugs used for that purpose have other pharmacokinetics than those applied in the treatment of hypertension. Various reviews on ganglion-blocking agents have been published in the past; therefore we shall restrict ourselves to those aspects of ganglion-blocking agents that are of significance for antihypertensive therapy. More detailed pharmacologic surveys are given in the reviews of AVIADO (1971), GREEN (1962), LEE (1967), MASON (1967), MOE (1950), NADOR (1960), TRENDELENBURG (1961), KHARKEVICH (1967), and VOLLE and KOELLE (1970).

II. Characteristics of Individual Drugs, Generic and Brand Names, Routes of Administration, and Dosages

A. General Remarks

Ganglion-blocking agents may be grouped as quaternary ammonium compounds and nonquaternary compounds, the latter group comprising secondary and tertiary amines and triethyl-sulfonium salts. The rationale for such a classification

Table 1. *Ganglion-blocking agents formerly used in antihypertensive therapy and for induction of "controlled hypotension"*[a]

Compound	Mode of administration	Single doses	Max. daily doses	Form and size of preparations	Brand names	Remarks
A. *Quaternary ganglion blockers*						
1. Tetraethylammonium chloride	i.v. i.m.	0.1–0.5 g 1–2 g		flask with 20 ml of 10% solution	Etamon	
2. Hexamethonium bromide	s.c., i.m., i.v. orally	0.01 –0.1 g 0.125–0.750 g	 2–5 g	flask with 25 ml of 10% solution, tablets	Vegolysen	
3. Pentamethonium bromide	parenterally	0.02–0.1 g			Penthonium	
4. Azamethonium bromide	parenterally orally	as hexamethonium		solution tablets	Pendiomid	
5. Pentolinium tartrate	s.c., i.m.	0.001–0.0035 g	0.0025–0.02–0.1 g	flask with 10 ml of sol. 0.5 w/v	Ansolysen	
	orally	0.01–0.02 g	0.1–1.0 g	tablets 0.01 and 0.04 g		
6. Trimethidinium methosulfate	orally	0.02 g	0.3–0.4 g	tablets 0.02 and 0.04 g	Ostensin	
7. Chlorisondamine chloride	orally	0.01–0.05 g	0.02–0.250 g	tablets 0.01, 0.025 and 0.05 g	Ecolid	
	i.v.	0.001–0.0025 g		ampoules 0.005 g in 1 ml		
8. Phenacyl homatropinium chloride	s.c., i.m. i.v.	0.001–0.015 g 0.2% solution by drip		solution	Trophenium	Short duration of action. Used for controlled hypotension
B. *Nonquaternary ganglion blockers*						
1. Mecamylamine hydrochloride	orally	0.0025–0.02 g	0.005–0.05 g	tablets 0.0025 and 0.01 g	Inversine	
2. Pempidine tartrate	orally	0.0025–0.025 g	0.005–0.08 g	tablets 0.001 and 0.005 g	Perolysen	
3. Trimetaphan camphorsulfonate	i.v.	0.1% solution by drip; 40–60 drops/min		vials with 0.25 g of powder	Arfonad	Short duration of action. Used for controlled hypotension

[a] Only a selection of brand names has been given in this list. Note that dosages of ganglionic blockers dispensed as different salts and/or with different brand names may differ from those given in this list. Also, the higher doses listed under the headings "Single doses" and "Max. daily doses" are not valid for initial treatments, but should only be administered after tolerance to ganglionic blockers has developed. Not all of the compounds listed were available in all countries. Several of the drugs listed are no longer sold.

is the different pharmacokinetics (see below) of these two groups of drugs, the most important difference being the good absorption from the gastrointestinal tract of the nonquaternary as compared to the quaternary compounds.

Special features of individual ganglion-blocking drugs will be described below. Brand names and dosages are listed in Table 1.

B. Quaternary Ganglionic Blockers

1. Tetraethylammonium (TEA), a monoquaternary ammonium compound, was the first ganglion-blocking drug used as an antihypertensive agent. The compound is more toxic than most of its successors because of various pharmacologic effects unrelated to its ganglioplegic activity. Its action is of short duration. It blocks both sympathetic and parasympathetic ganglia but in high doses may also cause inhibition of neuromuscular transmission. Its direct vasoconstrictor effect may interfere with the vasodilation induced by ganglionic blockade. TEA causes release of catecholamines from the adrenal medulla and potentiates postganglionic sympathetic nerve stimulation due to release of catecholamines (THOENEN et al., 1967). In view of these effects, the drug is contraindicated in cases of hypertension due to pheochromocytoma, but a provocative dose of TEA may be successfully used as a diagnostic tool in this condition. TEA has been dispensed as a chloride and a bromide and must be administered parenterally.

2. Hexamethonium, a bisquaternary ammonium salt, was synthetized by BARLOW and ING (1948) and studied by PATON and ZAIMIS (1949, 1951). Subsequently for some time it became the most frequently used ganglion-blocking drug. Untoward side-reactions with hexamethonium can be explained by nonselective blockade of the autonomous nervous system. Since the salts of hexamethonium are almost completely ionized in aequous solutions, absorption from the gastrointestinal tract is poor (5 to 15%) and irregular. Hexamethonium has been dispensed as a chloride (Bistrium Chloride, Hestrium Chloride, Chlor-Hexavict, Hexone Chloride, Esomide Chloride, Hiohex Chloride, Methium Chloride, Depressin, Meton), a bromide (Vegolysen, Vegolysin, Esametina, Gangliostat, Simpatoblock), an iodide (Hexathide), an acid tartrate, a bitartrate, and a benzensulfonate.

3. Pentamethonium has a preponderant action on parasympathetic ganglia and therefore is less suitable as an antihypertensive. It has been dispensed as a bromide (Penthonium, Lytensium) and an iodide. Pentamethonium bromide has been given parenterally.

4. Azamethonium bromide (Azamethone, Pendiomid, Pentamin) has a somewhat shorter duration of action but otherwise is very similar to hexamethonium both qualitatively and quantitatively. However, after development of tolerance to methonium compounds, it is less effective than hexamethonium. It may be administered either orally or patenterally.

5. Pentolinium tartrate is four times as active as the aforementioned methonium derivatives, irrespective of whether it is given by mouth or parenterally. Compared to hexamethonium, its duration of action is prolonged by about 50%. Pentolinium (Ansolysen, Pentilium) should not be given intravenously, since slow and inconstant dissociation of the salt may result in unpredictable effects. For that reason the drug is inappropriate to induce controlled hypotension in surgery because the full response may be obtained only several hours after the injection.

6. **Trimethidinium** methosulfate (Ostensin, Camphidonium) differs from other quaternary ganglion-blocking agents in so far as it acts not only on peripheral autonomic ganglia, but also to some degree on the central nervous system. It is more active than hexamethonium and has a longer duration of action. Therefore, the oral route should be used in preference to the i.v. route.

7. **Chlorisondamine** chloride (Ecolid) is 8 times as potent as hexamethonium and has a longer duration of action. Since its absorption from the gastrointestinal tract is inconstant, oral administration should be started with low doses and then gradually increased until the desired blood pressure-lowering effect is obtained.

8. **Phenacyl Homatropinium** chloride (phenactropinium chloride; Trophenium) is a quaternized derivative of homatropine that has no atropine-like activity but a ganglion-blocking activity of very short duration. Therefore, the compound has been recommended for controlled hypotension in surgery.

C. Nonquaternary Ganglionic Blockers

1. **Mecamylamine,** a secondary amine, is almost completely absorbed from the gastrointestinal tract and therefore became the most frequently used orally administered ganglion-blocking drug to treat severe hypertension. Unlike the quaternary amines, mecamylamine freely passes cellular barriers in the body. Therefore, central nervous system (CNS) side-effects that cannot be explained by autonomic ganglion-blockade may be seen with this drug, *e.g.* malaise, extrapyramidal motor, or psychotic symptoms. Abrupt withdrawal of the drug should be avoided since this may result in a rapid rise of blood pressure. Although equipotent to hexamethonium, much smaller oral doses of mecamylamine are necessary because of its good absorption from the gastrointestinal tract. Mecamylamine is dispensed as a hydrochloride (Mevasine, Inversine, Revertina, Mekamine, Versamine).

2. **Pempidine** was one of the latest ganglionic blockers to be developed for the treatment of hypertension (Lee et al., 1958; Spinks and Young, 1958). As a tertiary amine, it resembles mecamylamine in many respects, *e.g.*, good absorption from the intestinal tract, diffusion of cellular barriers, enhanced renal elimination in acidified urine. Serious side-effects that cannot be attributed to autonomous ganglion-blockade have not been reported. Pempidine is dispensed as a tartrate (Perolysen, Tenormal) for oral use.

3. **Trimethaphan Camphorsulfonate** (trimethaphan camsylate; Arfonad), a sulfonium compound, was studied by Randall et al. (1949) together with other triethylsulfonium salts with ganglion-blocking activity. It has a very short duration of action and may be used for controlled hypotension in surgery. The best way of administration is by constant infusion.

III. Pharmacokinetics

A. Methonium Compounds

At the time when ganglion-blocking agents were in use as antihypertensives, neither the theoretical basis of modern pharmacokinetics nor the methods necessary to measure small concentrations of most drugs in the blood were available. Based on studies of acute toxicity and comparing the LD_{50}-values after oral or intravenous administration, Dollery (1964) calculated a gastrointestinal absorption of 5% for hexamethonium and of 4% for pentolinium. Studying urinary recovery in man, Milne and Oleesky (1951) found about 3 to 15% of orally applied hexamethonium in the urine, but 74 to 104% of the drug when applied parenterally. Similar results were presented by HARINGTON (1953), who also pointed out that hexamethonium was better absorbed when taken on an empty stomach and that absorption of the drug showed great inter- and intraindividual variations. Doubt has been cast on HARINGTON'S statement that, of the various hexamethonium salts, the bromide is absorbed best and the bitartrate worst, since all these compounds should be completely ionized in the gastrointestinal tract (DOLLERY, 1964). In rabbits, urinary recovery of pentolinium was found to range from 59 to 91% after parenteral administration, but only 19 to 23% after oral intake (MASON and WIEN, 1955). Since the quaternary ammonium compounds are totally ionized in the gastrointestinal tract, their low absorption after oral intake is not surprising. In fact, they are even better absorbed than should be expected theoretically, and processes other than diffusive absorption may play a role (LEVINE and PELIKAN, 1961).

Obviously, the methonium compounds do not pass cellular barriers (except for the placental barrier; YOUNG, 1953), and therefore their volume of distribution is that of the extracellular space (PATON and ZAIMIS, 1952).

Elimination of the methonium compounds is mainly by renal excretion of the unchanged drug but some may occur via the feces. They are excreted by glomerular filtration without any tubular reabsorption (PATON and ZAIMIS, 1952). Since YOUNG et al. (1951) found the clearances of hexamethonium and pentamethonium to be somewhat higher than that of inulin, he assumed that some degree of tubular secretion may be involved.

B. Mecamylamine and Pempidine

The reason for the introduction of the nonquaternary ganglion-blockers into human therapy was their good absorption from the gastrointestinal tract when given by mouth. Based on toxicity studies, DOLLERY (1964) calculated an intestinal absorption of 50% for mecamylamine and of 63% for pempidine, but more direct studies by HARINGTON et al. (1958) and MUGGLETON and READING (1959) suggested complete absorption. Both drugs have a high pK_a and are therefore highly ionized in the gut; however, due to good lipid-solubility the non-ionized fraction is highly diffusible. With their high pK_a, absorption of these drugs from the stomach is poor; in fact, pH-dependent secretion into gastric pouches of animals has been reported for mecamylamine (ZAWOISKI et al., 1958).

Both pempidine and mecamylamine pass cellular and blood-brain barriers freely, resulting in higher tissue than plasma levels and accounting for some side-effects not known with the methonium compounds. However, the intracellular storage of these drugs helps to maintain their prolonged and steady effect (MASON, 1967).

Elimination of mecamylamine and pempidine is predominantly by renal excretion of the unchanged drug. A strong pH-dependence of the renal excretion of these drugs, especially of mecamylamine, has been reported by several authors (BAER et al., 1956; HARINGTON et al., 1958; SCRIBNER et al., 1959); the higher the pH value of the urine, the lower is the amount of the drugs excreted, and vice versa.

An unexpected finding was made when pempidine was given together with the diuretic chlorothiazide to patients: the renal clearance of the drug was reduced and the plasma level increased two-to threefold that of normal, as a consequence of enhanced protein binding in the presence of chlorothiazide (DOLLERY et al., 1961).

C. Other Drugs

Little information is available on the pharmacokinetics of other ganglion-blocking agents, but mention has to be made of the rapid metabolism of phenacyl homatropinium chloride and trimetaphan camphorsulfonate which makes these two drugs suitable for "controlled hypotension" in surgery by constant i.v. infusion.

IV. Mode of Action

A. Principles of Ganglionic Transmission

In analogy to the neuromuscular blocking agents, which include both membrane-stabilizing drugs such as tubocurarine and membrane-depolarizing drugs such as suxamethonium, transmission in autonomic ganglia can be blocked either by drugs that prevent acetylcholine-induced depolarization or by drugs that induce persistent depolarization of the postsynaptic membrane. The former group is represented by drugs such as hexamethonium, whereas to the latter belong substances such as nicotine, lobeline, tetramethylammonium (TMA), or dimethylphenylpiperazinium (DMPP). The term "ganglion-blocking drugs" has been reserved, however, for those drugs that prevent acetylcholine-induced depolarization.

The following mechanism of autonomic ganglionic transmission is generally accepted: Acetylcholine is released from intraneuronal presynaptic storage sites as a result of the presynaptic electrical nerve impulses. The released acetylcholine passes the synaptic cleft and attaches to postsynaptic cholinergic receptors, thereby eliciting a localized depolarization that subsequently initiates an action-potential in the postsynaptic fiber. Since postsynaptic cholinergic receptors of the ganglia can also be stimulated by nicotine, they are called "nicotine receptors."

B. Drug-Induced Ganglionic Blockade

Ganglion-blocking drugs interfere with acetylcholine by attaching themselves to the nicotine receptors and thereby preventing acetylcholine from binding to them. By definition, ganglion-blocking drugs (1) do not interfere with the release of acetylcholine from presynaptic storage sites, (2) have no depolarizing activity at the postsynaptic membrane, and (3) do not render the postsynaptic membrane inexcitable, since their blocking effect can be overcome by potassium which depolarizes the postsynaptic membrane (ACHESON and PEREIRA, 1946). The interference of ganglion-blocking drugs with acetylcholine is of the competitive type, and an increase of acetylcholine in the synaptic cleft by applying inhibitors of acetylcholine-esterase (neostigmine, diisopropyl-fluorophosphate) abolishes the ganglionic blockade induced by TEA (REARDON et al., 1947; ZAIMIS, 1955). Similar results were obtained by close intra-arterial injections of large amounts of acetylcholine or nicotine to the autonomic ganglia, a procedure by which the ganglionic block elicited by hexamethonium is reversed (PATON and ZAIMIS, 1952).

Experimentally, receptors that are not blocked by ganglion-blocking drugs have been found in autonomic ganglia. They consist of cholinergic receptors of the muscarinic type which can be blocked by atropine (AMBACHE et al., 1956; SCHAUMANN, 1957; VOLLE, 1963), and of adrenergic receptors, which inhibit ganglionic transmission, and which can be either blocked or not by α-adrenergic blockers (DE GROAT and VOLLE, 1966). The role of these ganglionic receptors in the physiologic process of ganglionic transmission is uncertain.

C. Nonselective Interference with Sympathetic and Parasympathetic Transmission

No major differences are known to exist in the mode of transmission in sympathetic and parasympathetic ganglia. Therefore, all attempts to synthesize ganglion-blocking drugs that selectively interfere with sympathetic transmission have yielded unsatisfactory results. Comparing the effect of ganglion-blocking drugs on sympathetic and parasympathetic ganglia in the cat's heart, PERRY and WILSON (1956) found no differential effects of TEA, hexamethonium, and azamethonium, but pentamethonium had a tenfold higher blocking activity on parasympathetic than on sympathetic transmission. FLORIDA et al. (1960) reported that the superior cervical ganglion of the cat was slightly more susceptible to the blocking action of hexamethonium than the ciliary ganglion. The same drug had a stronger blocking effect on DMPP-induced blood pressure increases than on DMPP-induced bladder stimulation (GARRETT, 1963). However, no ganglion-blocking drug became available for therapeutic purposes that selectively depressed sympathetic ganglionic transmisson. The later developed drugs like mecamylamine and pempidine produced less severe side-effects due to parasympathetic ganglion blockade as a consequence of their more reliable absorption, which reduced the danger of overdosage, rather than because of selective sympathetic blockade.

D. Effects on the Cardiovascular System

The most important although temporary contribution of the ganglion-blocking agents to therapeutics is the marked lowering of blood pressure both in normo- and in hypertensive subjects. As an experimental tool in the investigation of the cardiovascular system, they have greatly improved the knowledge of the distribution of the blood to the various parts of the organism. For a detailed survey of the cardiovascular effects of ganglion-blocking drugs, the reader is referred to the reviews of MASON (1967) and AVIADO (1971), and only a selection of the pertinent findings will be given here.

The hypotensive activity of the ganglion-blocking drugs must be regarded as the sum of two cardiovascular effects: a decrease in cardiac output and a decrease in total peripheral resistance. It has not been established with certainty which of these two effects plays the predominant role. Cardiac output has been found to be decreased in man, dogs, and rats after hexamethonium and pentolinium (BRINK et al., 1963; CROSLEY et al., 1956; CRUMPTON et al., 1954; MOYER et al., 1952; SMITH et al., 1955). This is not the result of a negative inotropic effect, and some of the ganglionic blockers were even found to increase cardiac force in isolated heart preparations (PATEL et al., 1962). It is now generally accepted that reduced cardiac output after ganglionic blockade is the consequence of pooling of blood in the capacitance vessels resulting in a reduction of venous return (FREIS et al., 1953; TRAPPOLD, 1957; WERKO et al., 1951).

For the same reason cardiac output may increase in patients with congestive heart failure (FREIS et al., 1953) because the decrease in venous return, like a venesection, lowers the pressure load to the heart and improves cardiac filling. In addition, due to the reduced total peripheral resistance, a more complete emptying of the left ventricle may result, and the failing heart may recover. These effects have provided the basis for the treatment of congestive heart failure by ganglion-blocking agents.

Since the sympathetic nervous system regulates vascular tone and since ganglionic blockade interferes with the transmission of sympathetic impulses, total peripheral resistance is diminished (Van Bergen, 1955; Freis et al., 1953; Grob et al., 1953; Rakita and Sancetta, 1953; Smith et al., 1955; Varnauskas, 1955). Principally, vascular beds that have a high sympathetic tone (*e.g.*, limb vessels) dilate to a greater extent than those under little sympathetic tone (*e.g.*, cardiac and cerebral vessels). Together with the decreased cardiac output, this effect of ganglionic blockade should lead to a serious diminution of blood supply to vital organs. However, due to autoregulatory vascular mechanisms that are not under sympathetic control, a complex redistribution of cardiac output occurs. Aviado (1971) has applied the data available on blood flow to individual vascular beds after ganglionic blockade with hexamethonium to "the hypothetical man of Bazett" (*i.e.*, a model on blood distribution in the human organism proposed by Bazett, 1956). During treatment with ganglion-blocking drugs . . . "the outcome is favourable to the myocardium and the brain (increase in allocation to +8 and +23%, respectively). The kidneys suffer (by a reduction in allocation to −14%) since the extremities and splanchnic beds still receive the same percentages of cardiac output . . . After the autonomic nervous system is blocked, the local regulatory mechanisms ... come into play . . . Without these nonautonomic mechanisms, cerebral and coronary insufficiency . . . would be more frequently encountered. . . ." The reduced allocation of blood flow to the kidneys, although well documented (Aas and Blegen, 1949; Crosley et al., 1956; Mackinnon, 1952; Moyer et al., 1952), seems to be transient, since renal plasma flow and glomerular filtration may return to normal values during prolonged administration of ganglionic blockers (Freis et al., 1953; Mackinnon, 1952; Morris et al., 1953).

A prominent feature of the blood pressure-lowering ganglion-blocking drugs is that the effect is highly dependent on posture. In the supine position, the blood pressure may be lowered only slightly or not at all, but in an upright position the pressure may fall considerably, and postural hypotension and fainting may be evoked. This effect is explained by the blockade of sympathetic reflex mechanisms which normally would increase the vascular tone of the lower parts of the body; after ganglionic blockade blood is pooled in the lower limbs. Thus, venous return and consequently cardiac output are decreased with a resultant drop in blood pressure. Postural hypotension may cause untoward side-effects. On the other hand, postural hypotension has been claimed to be a favorable feature of antihypertensive therapy with ganglion-blocking agents: During the day when the hypertensive patient's blood pressure is highest, the patient is on his legs, and ganglionic blockade exerts its best antihypertensive effects. Thus, posture reinforces the effect of the drug, and relatively low doses of the ganglion-blocking agents may be necessary to control the patient's blood pressure (Smirk, 1956).

E. Tolerance to Antihypertensive Activity

The development of tolerance to the antihypertensive effect of ganglion-blocking drugs during a time-course of one to two months may make a progressive increase in dosage necessary. As opposed to hexamethonium, pentolinium, or mecamylamine, tolerance to chlorisondamine, pempidine, and trimethidinium seems to be less significant (Smirk, 1960) or absent (Freis and Wilson, 1955). Cross tolerance has been reported to occur among the various quaternary amines (Smirk, 1952), but no cross tolerance between mecamylamine and quaternary amines was observed (Freis and Wilson, 1955). The phenomenon of tolerance to ganglion-blocking drugs is not well understood, but the following two explanations are the most plausible-ones: Denervation supersensitivity of the vascular bed to catecholamines may result from ganglionic blockade (BOURA and GREEN, 1962; EMMELIN, 1959) corresponding to the supersensitivity seen after preganglionic nerve section or after the administration of drugs that selectively interfere with sympathetic neuronal transmission such as bretylium, guanethidine, or reserpine. The other explanation is based on the assumption that neuronal pathways that are not affected by ganglion-blocking drugs (*e.g.*, muscarinic receptors in sympathetic ganglia) (VOLLE, 1963) may progressively take over sympathetic transmission when the nicotinic receptors are occupied by ganglion-blocking drugs (PAGE and McCUBBIN, 1959).

Experimentally, tolerance to the cardiovascular effects of ganglion-blocking drugs can be induced within a few hours (BLACKMAN and LAVERTY, 1961; HAAS and GOLDBLATT, 1959, 1960; MAXWELL et al., 1958; ZAIMIS, 1956), and an increased sensitivity to pressure agents can already be elicited by doses that are too low to produce ganglionic blockade (MANTEGAZZA et al., 1958; MAWJI and LOCKETT, 1963). However, these findings are probably unrelated to the slowly developing tolerance that interferes with the treatment of hypertensive patients by ganglion-blocking drugs (MASON, 1967).

F. Pharmacologic Effects Unrelated to Ganglionic Blockade

Ganglion-blocking drugs may have numerous pharmacologic effects unrelated to their selective activity on autonomic ganglia. TEA specifically blocks potassium conductance in nerve fibers (BERGMANN and STÄMPFLI, 1966) and may increase the release of catecholamines from postganglionic sympathetic fibers (THOENEN et al., 1967). Both effects make the drug unsuitable for therapeutic use. TEA, mecamylamine, and chlorisondamine potentiate the contractile responses of isolated arterial strips to various vasoconstrictor drugs (KELKAR et al., 1964; LUM and RASHLEIGH, 1961). Mecamylamine, when given for a prolonged period (VIDRIO and PARDO, 1963, 1967), and pempidine in high doses (CORNE and EDGE, 1958), may produce hypertensive effects in experimental animals. Trimethaphan camphorsulfonate liberates histamine from cellular storage sites with the danger of untoward side-effects (VOLLE and KOELLE, 1970), and phenacyl homatropinium chloride possesses anticholinesterase activity (ref. LEWIS, 1964).

V. Side-Effects

A. General Remarks

From the viewpoint of antihypertensive drug therapy, only the reduction of pathologically elevated blood pressure is desired, and almost all other drug-induced effects are unwanted and may be considered as side-effects. Side-effects of ganglionic blockers either may be linked intimately to their main effect, *i.e.*, blockade of sympathetic and parasympathetic nervous transmission, or may be unrelated to autonomic ganglionic blockade. The former proved to be of considerably greater significance than the latter. Table 2 summarizes the various side-effects observed during treatment with ganglionic blockers.

Table 2. *Causes and types of side-effects due to treatment with ganglion-blocking drugs*

Cause of side-effects	Type of side-effects
1. Ganglionic blockade	
1.1. Blockade of sympathetic transmission	Postural hypotension with peripheral circulatory collapse and fainting; anginal pain; aggravation of renal insufficiency in malignant hypertensives (fatal uremia) dyspnea, radiologic lung changes, fatal pneumonitis with fibrinous edema; aggravation of hypertension after too rapid withdrawal of ganglionic blockers
1.2. Blockade of parasympathetic transmission	Decreased gastric motility and acidity, constipation, paralytic ileus, urinary retention, strangury, mydrasis, blurring of vision, xerostomia, anhydrosis, impotence
2. Others (unrelated to ganglionic blockade), *e.g.* blockade of neuromuscular junction; various effects on CNS centers (non-quaternary ganglionic blockers); catecholamine release from cellular storage sites (TEA); histamine liberation from mast cells (trimethaphan camphorsulfonate)	Muscular weakness; CNS side-effects, *e.g.*, tremor, confusion, seizures, mania, depression (mecamylamine, pempidine); hypertensive crisis, especially in patients with pheochromocytoma (TEA); allergy-like symptoms (trimethaphan camphorsulfonate)

B. Side-Effects Due to Blockade of the Autonomic Nervous System

Although postural hypotension occasionally has been considered to be a valuable feature of ganglion-blocking drugs since it may reinforce their antihypertensive effect during the day (SMIRK, 1956), it may be extremely disturbing and even dangerous for the patient. Peripheral circulatory collapse with fainting may be encountered especially when the patient changes from the recumbent or sitting position to the upright position. Severe attacks of postural hypotension were more frequent in the early years of treatment with ganglion-blocking drugs, when hexamethonium with its inconsistent intestinal absorption was the ganglion-blocking drug of choice. Muscular activity, by increasing venous return, counteracts to some degree postural hypotension. If severe hypotension persists after ganglionic blockade, sympathomimetic drugs may be given, but only in doses lower than usual because of the supersensitivity of the peripheral vascular beds to vasoconstrictors.

Anginal pain in patients with coronary insufficiency and fatal uremia in patients with malignant hypertension may be elicited by ganglion-blocking drugs, but these side-effects may also be seen with other antihypertensives.

Dyspnea associated with radiologic changes in both lungs, sometimes leading to fatal pneumonitis with organized fibrinous edema found on post-mortem examination, has been reported after prolonged treatment with TEA (MCLEMORE et al., 1951), hexamethonium (AVIADO, 1960; MORRISON, 1953; PERRY et al., 1957), and pentolinium (HILDEEN et al., 1958). The combination of attacks due to left ventricular failure and intermittent hypotension during ganglionic blockade has been proposed as the cause of these pulmonary complications (DONIACH et al., 1954).

During treatment with ganglion-blocking drugs, all possible effects of parasympathetic blockade may be encountered, *i.e.*, decreased gastric motility and reduced gastric acidity, constipation, paralytic ileus, urinary retention, mydriasis, blurring of vision, xerostomia, and anhydrosis. During the course of treatment with increasing doses of ganglion-blocking drugs, these side-effects tend to become more severe since the parasympathetic nervous system does not, in contrast to the sympathetic system, develop tolerance. Nevertheless, patients may cope better with these side-effects than with those resulting from blockade of sympathetic transmission. Laxatives and/or parasympathomimetic drugs should be given to treat constipation.

PATON (1954) attributed the effects and side-effects of pharmacologic ganglionic blockade to a "slightly artificial and distinctly frivolous 'hexamethonium man'", the description of whom will be quoted here because of its comprehensiveness:

> "He is a pink complexioned person, except when he has stood for a long time, when he may get pale and faint. His handshake is warm and dry. He is a placid and relaxed companion; for instance he may laugh, but he can't cry because the tears cannot come. Your rudest story will not make him blush, and the most unpleasant circumstances will fail to make him turn pale. His collars and socks stay very clean and sweet. He wears corsets and may, if you meet him out, be rather fidgety (corsets to compress his splanchnic vascular pool, fidgety to keep the venous return going from his legs). He dislikes speaking much unless helped with something to moisten his dry mouth and throat. He is long-sighted and easily blinded by bright light. The redness of his eye-balls may suggest irregular habits and in fact his head is rather weak. But he always behaves like a gentleman and never belches nor hiccups. He tends to get cold and keeps well wrapped up. But his health is good; he does not have chilblains and those diseases of modern civilization, hypertension and peptic ulcer, pass him by. He is thin because his appetite is modest; he never feels hunger pains and his stomach never rumbles. He gets rather constipated so that his intake of liquid paraffin is high. As old age comes he will suffer from retention of urine and impotence, but frequency, precipitancy, and strangury will not worry him. One is uncertain how he will end, but perhaps if he is not careful, by eating less and less and getting colder and colder, he will sink in a symptomless, hypoglycaemic coma and die as was proposed for the universe, a sort of entropy death."

Paton called his "hexamethonium man" a caricature, but altogether, the unpleasant and serious side-effects of ganglionic blockade have often rendered the treatment with ganglion-blocking drugs a "heroic" one (NADOR, 1960). PAGE (1966) stated that "the side-effects ... were often fearful to behold and even worse to experience." It has been because of these side-effects and not because of ineffectiveness as antihypertensives that ganglion-blocking drugs almost immediately disappeared from treatment regimens when antihypertensive agents selectively interfering with sympathetic transmission became available.

C. Side-Effects Unrelated to Ganglionic Blockade

In very high doses, ganglion-blocking drugs may exert some blocking activity at the neuromuscular junction, and muscular weakness may result. CNS side-effects have been reported to occur with the nonquaternary amines mecamylamine and pempidine, which can pass the blood-brain barrier, *e.g.*, tremor, confusion, mania, and depression. Other drug actions unrelated to ganglionic blockade and giving rise to side-effects have been mentioned previously (IV. F.) or are given in Table 2.

VI. Present Role of Ganglion-Blocking Drugs

In the 1950s and at the beginning of the 1960s antihypertensive drugs became available that selectively interfere with sympathetic transmission (*e.g.*, reserpine, guanethidine, α-methyl-dopa) or reduce blood pressure by mechanisms not fully understood but with relatively few side-effects (*e.g.*, diuretics, hydralazines). This led to a rapid decline of the use of the ganglion-blocking drugs in the treatment of high blood pressure, and today, they have no place in the long-term treatment of hypertension. However, they are still among the drugs advocated to treat hypertensive crises, *e.g.*, trimethaphan (Breslin, 1969; Freis, 1969; Greenfell, 1971; Moser, 1969; Moukheibir, 1970; Sheps, 1971; Finnerty, 1973; Bathia and Frohlich, 1973; Dranov et al., 1974; Stinson et al., 1975) and pentolinium (Bulpitt and Dollery, 1971; Vaamonde et al., 1971). Together with other drugs such as diazoxide, hydralazine, sodium nitroprusside, reserpine, methyldopa and phentolamine, both trimethaphan and pentolinium have been included recently in an AMA-statement on drugs suitable for the treatment of malignant hypertension and hypertensive emergencies (AMA Committee, 1974). Ganglion-blocking drugs have been applied successfully to reduce bleeding from esophageal varices in portal hypertension (Cincotti and Huener, 1971).

In selected cases of acute pulmonary edema, pooling of blood in the lower part of the body may be achieved by ganglion-blocking drugs (Chandrasekhar and Cugell, 1972; Dykes and Fuller, 1969; Saev et al., 1966). In left ventricular failure that no longer responds to glycosides, ganglion-blocking drugs are still worth considering, since both the reduction of venous return and the decrease in peripheral resistance induced by ganglionic blockade may improve cardiac function. In patients with acute myocardial infarction, the reduction of ventricular afterload by administration of trimethaphan has been found to protect the jeopardized ischemic myocardium; the observed "infarct size" was 24% less than that predicted (Shell and Sobel, 1974).

In dissecting aneurysm of the aorta, "induced hypotension" for a period of several days or weeks before surgery greatly improves the patient's chances of survival. Since side-effects in this severe condition may be disregarded, ganglion-blocking drugs are still used because of their potent hypotensive effect (Attar et al., 1971; Aronsta et al., 1970; Brest, 1971; Faidutti and Hahn, 1969; Heinrich, 1972; Lindsay and Hurst, 1971, 1972; Thompson et al., 1969; Wheat et al., 1969). The most important present-day application of a ganglion-blocking drug is probably the induction of "controlled hypotension" by trimethaphan camphorsulfonate to prevent oozing of blood in ophthalmologic, otorhinologic, and plastic surgery and in surgery of the brain and prostate (Cote et al., 1968; Dietzel et al., 1971; Deacock, 1971; Harrison, 1971; Hoffmann et al., 1970; Macrae, 1971; Pietrobono et al., 1968; Porto et al., 1970; Spierdijk and de Ruiter, 1971; Suriani, 1968; Urquhart-Hay et al., 1969; Zervas and Hedley-Whyte, 1972). For controlled hypotension, trimethaphan is highly suitable because of its immediate onset of action on infusion and its rapid inactivation in the body; these features permit a rapid regulation of the blood pressure by simply changing the speed of infusion.

In contrast to the minor role ganglion-blocking drugs play at present in most countries, more than one hundred reports on their clinical application in the treatment of various disorders exploiting their ganglioplegic effects both in the sympathetic and parasympathetic system have been published in the USSR and other Eastern countries since 1967.

References

Aas, K., Blegen, E.: The effect of tetraethylammonium bromide on the kidneys. Lancet **1949 I**, 999.

Acheson, G. H., Moe, G. K.: The action of tetraethylammonium on the mammalian circulation. J. Pharmacol. exp. Ther. **87**, 220 (1946).

Acheson, G. H., Pereira, S. A.: The blocking effect of tetraethylammonium ion on the superior cervical ganglion of the cat. J. Pharmacol. exp. Ther. **87**, 273 (1946).

AMA Committee: The treatment of malignant hypertension and hypertensive emergencies. J. Amer. med. Ass. **228**, 1673 (1974).

AMBACHE, N., PERRY, W. L. M., ROBERTSON, P. A.: The effect of muscarine on perfused superior cervical ganglia of cats. Brit. J. Pharmacol. **11**, 442 (1956).
ARONSTA, E. M., GOMEZ, A. C., O'CONNELL, T. J. JR., GEIGER, J. P.: Recent surgical and pharmacologic experience with acute dissecting and traumatic aneurysms. J. thorac. cardiovasc. Surg. **59**, 231 (1970).
ATTAR, S., FARDIN, R., AYELLA, R., MCLAUGHLIN, J. S.: Medical vs. surgical treatment of acute dissecting aneurysms. Arch. Surg. **103**, 568 (1971).
AVIADO, D. M.: Pharmacology of pulmonary circulation. Pharmacol. Rev. **12**, 159 (1960).
AVIADO, D. M.: Ganglionic stimulant and blocking drugs. In: DIPALMA, J. P. (Ed.): Drill's Pharmacology in Medicine, pp. 708—731. New York: MacGraw-Hill 1971.
BAER, J. E., PAULSON, S. F., RUSSO, H. F., BEYER, K. H.: Elimination of 3-methylamino-isocamphane hydrochloride (mecamylamine). J. Pharmacol. exp. Ther. **116**, 2 (1956).
BARLOW, R. B., ING, H. R.: Curare-like action of polymethylene bis-quaternary ammonium salts. Nature (Lond.) **161**, 718 (1948).
BAZETT, H. C.: The circulation. In: Medical Physiology, p. 221. St Louis: Mesby 1956.
BERGEN, VAN F. H.: Hexamethonium induced hypotension. Minn. Med. **38**, 573 (1955).
BERGMAN, C., STÄMPFLI, R.: Difference de perméabilité des fibres nerveuses myélinisées sensorielles et motrices à l'ion potassium. Helv. physiol. pharmacol. Acta **24**, 247 (1966).
BHATIA, S. K., FROHLICH, E. D.: Hemodynamic comparison of agents useful in hypertensive emergencies. Amer. Heart J. **85**, 367 (1973).
BLACKMANN, J. G., LAVERTY, R.: Peripheral actions of hexamethonium in relation to the decreasing effects of repeated doses on the blood pressure of anaesthetized rats. Brit. J. Pharmacol. **17**, 124 (1961).
BOURA, A. L. A., GREEN, A. F.: Comparison of bretylium and guanethidine: tolerance, and effects on adrenergic nerve function and responses to sympathomimetic amines. Brit. J. Pharmacol. **19**, 13 (1962).
BRESLIN, D. J.: Hypertensive crisis. Med. Clin. N. Amer. **53**, 351 (1969).
BREST, A. N.: Dissecting aortic aneurysm. Cardiovasc. Clin. **3**, 151 (1971).
BRINK, R. V., ROSAS, R., BLAQUIER, P., BOHAR, D. F.: Action of pentolinium on cardiac output and other haemodynamic parameters in rats. Proc. Soc. exp. Biol. (N. Y.) **113**, 652 (1963).
BURN, J. H., DALE, H. H.: The action of certain quaternary ammonium bases. J. Pharmacol. exp. Ther. **6**, 417 (1914/15).
BULPITT, C. J., DOLLERY, C. T.: The drug treatment of hypertension. Practitioner **207**, 4 (1971).
CHANDRASEKHAR, A. J., CUGELL, D. W.: Pulmonary edema. Mod. Treat. **9**, 77 (1972).
CINCOTTI, J., HUEMER, R.: Reduction of portal hypertension by ganglionic blockade. Amer. I. dig. Dis. **16**, 517 (1971).
CORNE, S. J., EDGE, N. D.: Pharmacological properties of pempidine (1:2:2:6:6-pentamethyl piperidine), a new ganglion blocking compound. Brit. J. Pharmacol. **13**, 339 (1958).
COTE, M., GRIGNON, J. L., VILAIN, R.: Hypotension controlée et chirurgie plastique. Ann. Chir. Plast. **13**, 211 (1968).
CROSLEY, A. P., BROWN, J. F., TUCHMANN, H., CRUMPTON, C. W., HUSON, J. H., ROWE, G. G.: The acute hemodynamic and metabolic response of hypertensive patients to pentolinium tartrate. Circulation **14**, 584 (1956).
CRUMPTON, C. W., ROWE, G. G., O'BRIEN, G., MURPHEY, Q. R.: The effect of hexamethonium bromide upon coronary flow, cardiac work and cardiac efficiency in normotensive and renal hypertensive dogs. Circulation Res. **2**, 79 (1954).
DEACOCK, A. R.: Aspects of anaesthesia for middle ear surgery and blood loss during stapedectomy. Proc. roy. Soc. Med. **64**, 1226 (1971).
DEGROAT, W. C., VOLLE, R. L.: The actions of the catecholamines on transmission in the superior cervical ganglion of the cat. J. Pharmacol. exp. Ther. **154**, 1 (1966).
DIETZEL, W., GRUNDLACH, K., WIEDEMANN, K.: Untersuchungen zu einem Anaesthesieverfahren bei intrakraniellen Eingriffen. Z. Prakt. Anaesth. Wiederbeleb. **6**, 417 (1971).
DOLLERY, C. T.: Absorption, distribution and excretion of the drugs used to treat hypertension. In: BINNS, T. B. (Ed.): Absorption and Excretion of Drugs, pp. 159—164. Edinburgh-London: Livingstone 1964.
DOLLERY, C. T., EMSLIE-SMITH, D., MUGGLETON, D. F.: Action of chlorothiazide on the distribution, excretion and hypotensive effect of pempidine in man. Brit. J. Pharmacol. **17**, 488 (1961).
DONIACH, I., MORRISON, B., STEINER, R. E.: Lung changes during hexamethonium for hypertension. Brit. Heart J. **16**, 101 (1954).
DRANOV, J., SKYLER, J. S., GUNNELLS, J. C.: Malignant hypertension. Current modes of therapy. Arch. intern. Med. **133**, 791 (1974).
DYKES, M. H., FULLER, J. E.: Post-transfusion pulmonary edema in surgical patients: etiology, and therapeutic use of trimethaphan camphorsulfonate (Arfonad). Anesthesiology **30**, 101 (1969).

Emmelin, N.: Supersensitivity due to prolonged administration of ganglion blocking compounds. Brit. J. Pharmacol. **14**, 229 (1959).
Faidutti, B., Hahn, C.: Les dissections de l'aorte thoracique (27 observations). J. Chir. (Paris) **98**, 503 (1969).
Finnerty, F. A., Jr.: Hypertensive emergencies. In: J. H. Laragh (Ed.): Hypertension Manual. New York: Yorke Medical Books, Dun-Donnelley Publishing Corp. 1973.
Florida, F. A., de Cato, J., Ranirez, L., Pardo, E. G.: Effects of several blocking agents on the sympathetic and parasympathetic postganglionic action potentials. J. Pharmacol. exp. Ther. **129**, 433 (1960).
Freis, E. D.: Hypertensive crisis. J. Amer. med. Ass. **208**, 338 (1969).
Freis, E. D., Rose, J. C., Partenope, E. A., Higgins, T. F., Kelly, R. T., Schnaper, H. W., Johnson, R. L.: The hemodynamic effects of hypotensive drugs in man. III. Hexamethonium. J. clin. Invest. **32**, 1285 (1953).
Freis, E. D., Wilson, I. M.: Effects of mecamylamine in hypertensive patients. Circulation **12**, 707 (1955).
Garrett, J.: Selective blockade of sympathetic or parasympathetic ganglia. Arch. int. Pharmacodyn. **144**, 381 (1963).
Greenfell, R. F.: Treatment of hypertensive crisis. Chest **59**, 212 (1971).
Green, A. F.: Antihypertensive drugs: In: Garattini, S., Shore, P. S. (Eds.): Advances in Pharmacology, Vol. 1; p. 161. New York-London: Academic Press 1962.
Grob, D., Searborough, W. R., Kahus, A. A. Jr., Langford, H. G.: Further observations on the effects of autonomic blocking agents in patients with hypertension. Circulation 8, 352 (1953).
Haas, E., Goldblatt, H.: Effects of an antihypertensive drug, pentolinium. Amer. J. Physiol. **196**, 768 (1959).
Haas, E., Goldblatt, H.: Effects of various ganglionblocking agents on blood pressure and on the activity of pressor agents. Amer. J. Physiol. **198**, 1023 (1960).
Harington, M.: The absorption and excretion of hexamethonium salts. Clin. Sci. **12**, 185 (1953).
Harington, M., Kinkcaid-Smith, P., Milne, M. D.: Pharmacology and clinical use of pempidine in the treatment of hypertension. Lancet **1958 II**, 6.
Harrison, G. G.: Some recent advances in anesthesia of interest to ophthalmic surgeons. S. Afr. med. J. **45**, 400 (1971).
Heinrich, F.: Therapy of dissecting aneurysm of the aorta. Minerva Med. **63**, 1819 (1972).
Hildeen, T., Krogsgaard, A. R., Vimtrop, B.: Fatal pulmonary changes during the medical treatment of maligant hypertension. Lancet **1958 II**, 330.
Hoffmann, J., Szabo, G., Endroedi, J., Soos, K.: Über einige Fragen der chirurgischen Therapie der Trigeminusneuralgie. Dtsch. Stomat. **20**, 174 (1970).
Kelkar, V. V., Gulati, O. D., Gokhale, S. D.: Effect of ganglion blocking drugs on the responses of the rabbit aortic strip to adrenaline, noradrenaline and other vasoactive substances. Arch. int. Pharmacodyn. **149**, 209—222 (1964).
Kharkevich, D. A.: Ganglion-blocking and ganglion-stimulating agents. Oxford: Pergamon Press 1967.
Lee, G. E.: Non-quaternary blockers. In: Schlittler, E. (Ed.): Antihypertensive Agents, p. 295. New York-London: Academic Press 1967.
Lee, G. E., Wragg, W. R., Corne, S. J., Edge, N. D., Reading, H. W.: 1:2:2:6:6-Pentamethylpiperidine. A new hypotensive drug. Nature (Lond.) **181**, 1717 (1958).
Lewis, J. J.: An introduction to pharmacology. Edinburgh-London: E. and S. Livingstone Ltd. 1964.
Levine, R. M., Pelikan, E. W.: The influence of experimental procedures and dose on the intestinal absorption of an onium compound, benzomethamine. J. Pharmacol. exp. Ther. **131**, 319 (1961).
Lindsay, J. Jr., Hurst, J. W.: Dissecting aneurysm of the aorta. J. Amer. med. Ass. **217**, 1533 (1971).
Lindsay, J. Jr., Hurst, J. W.: Management of dissecting aneurysm of the aorta. Postgrad. Med. **51**, 62 (1972).
Lum, B. K., Rashleigh, P. L.: Potentiation of vasoactive drugs by ganglionic blocking agents. J. Pharmacol. exp. Ther. **132**, 13—18 (1961).
Mackinnon, J.: Effects of hypotension producing drugs on the renal circulation. Lancet **1952 II**, 12.
Macrae, W. R.: Induced hypotension for middle ear surgery. Proc. roy. Soc. Med. **64**, 1223 (1971).
Mantegazza, P., Tyler, C., Zaimis, E.: The peripheral action of hexamethonium and of pentolinium. Brit. J. Pharmacol. **13**, 480 (1958).

MASON, D. F. J.: Ganglion-blocking drugs. In: ROOT, W. S., HOFMANN, F. G. (Eds.): Physiological Pharmacology III. The nervous system. Part C, p. 363. New York-London 1967.
MASON, D. F. J., WIEN, R.: The actions of heterocyclic bisquaternary compounds especially of a pyrrolidinium series. Brit. J. Pharmacol. **10**, 124 (1955).
MAWJI, S., LOCKETT, M.: Pressor effects of adrenaline, noradrenaline and reflex vasoconstriction sensitized by low concentrations of ganglion blocking drugs. J. Pharm. Pharmacol. **15**, 45 (1963).
MAXWELL, R. A., PLUMMER, A. J., ROSS, S. D., SCHNEIDER, F.: Factors affecting the blood pressure response of mammals to the ganglion blocking agent chlorisondamine cloride. J. Pharmacol. exp. Ther. **123**, 288 (1958).
MAXWELL, R. A., PLUMMER, A. J., SCHNEIDER, R., POVALSKI, H., DANIELS, A. I.: Pharmacology of (2- (octahydro-1-azocinyl)-ethyl) guanidine sulfate. J. Pharmacol. exp. Ther. **128**, 22—29 (1960).
McLEMORE, G. A., GREEN, H. O., LIDE, T. N.: Respiratory complications from tetraethylammonium ion: report of two deaths. Circulation **4**, 47 (1951).
MILNE, G. F., OLEESKY, S.: Excretion of the methonium compounds. Lancet **1951 I**, 889.
MOE, G. K., FREYBURGER, W. A.: Ganglionic blocking agents. Pharmacol. Rev. **2**, 61 (1950).
MORRIS, G. C., MOYER, J. H., SYNDER, H. B., HAYNES, B. W.: Vascular dynamics in controlled hypotension. Ann. Surg. **138**, 706 (1953).
MORRISON, B.: Parenteral hexamethonium in hypertension. Brit. med. J. **1953 I**, 1291.
MOSER, M.: Treatment of "hypertensive encephalopathy" (accelerated hypertension). II. Amer. Heart J. **77**, 704 (1969).
MOUKHEIBIR, N.: Hypertensive emergencies and their management. Med. Liban. J. **23**, 219 (1970).
MOYER, J. H., HUGGINS, R. A., HANDLEY, C. A., MILLS, L. C.: Effect of hexamethonium chloride on cardiovascular and renal hemodynamics and on electrolyte excretion. J. Pharmacol. exp. Ther. **106**, 157 (1952).
MUGGLETON, D. F., READING, H. W.: Absorption, metabolism and elimination of pempidine in the rat. Brit. J. Pharmacol. **14**, 202 (1959).
NADOR, K.: Ganglienblocker. In: JUCKER, E. (Ed.): Progress in Drug Reserch, Vol. 2, p. 297. Basel: Birkhäuser 1960.
PAGE, I. H.: Drug treatment of hypertensions. In: GROSS, F. (Ed.): Antihypertensive Therapy. Principles andPractice, p. 602. Berlin-Heidelberg- New York: Springer 1966.
PAGE, I. H., McCUBBIN, J. W.: Buffer reflexes, tolerance to ganglionplegics and their relationship to enhanced pressor responsiveness. Amer. J. Physiol. **197**, 217 (1959).
PATEL, D. G., GULATI, O. D., GOKHALI, S. D.: Cardiac actions of ganglion blocking and certain other drugs. Arch. int. Pharmacodyn. **137**, 348 (1962).
PATON, W. D. M.: Transmission and block in autonomic ganglia. Pharmacol. Rev. **6**, 59 (1954).
PATON, W. D. M., ZAIMIS, E. J.: Curare-like action of polymethylene bisquaternary ammonium salts. Nature (Lond.) **161**, 718 (1948).
PATON, W. D. M., ZAIMIS, E. J.: The pharmacological actions of polymethylene bis-trimethylammonium salts. Brit. J. Pharmacol. **4**, 381 (1949).
PATON, W. D. M., ZAIMIS, E. J.: Paralysis of autonomic ganglia by methonium salts. Brit. J. Pharmacol. **6**, 155 (1951).
PATON, W. D. M., ZAIMIS, E. J.: The methonium compounds. Pharmacol. Rev. **4**, 219 (1952).
PERRY, H. M., O'NEAL, R. M., THOMAS, W. A.: Pulmonary disease following chronic chemical ganglionic blockade. A clinical and pathologic study. Amer. J. Med. **22**, 37 (1957).
PERRY, W. L. M., WILSON, C. W. M.: The relative effects of ganglion blocking compounds on the sympathetic and parasympathetic ganglia supplying the cat heart. Brit. J. Pharmacol. **11**, 81 (1956).
PIETROBONO, P., TIBALDESCHI, C. C., SCOTTI, A.: Reduction of bleeding in laminectomy operations for disk hernia by association of fluothane and camphosulfonate of trimethaphan. Acta anaesth. (Padova, **19**, 557 (1968).
PORTO, A. J., VIEIRA, J. L., FERREIRA, A. A., KATAYAMA, M., DE COSTA, A.: Controlled hypotension with trimethaphan. Rev. bras. Anest. **20**, 462 (1970).
RAKITA, L., SANCETTA, S. M.: Acute hemodynamic effects of hexamethonium in normotensive man. Circulation Res. **1**, 499 (1953).
RANDALL, L. D., PETERSON, W. G., LEHMAN, G.: The ganglionic blocking action of thiophanium derivatives. J. Pharmacol. exp. Ther. **97**, 48 (1949).
REARDON, M. J., MARZONI, F. A., HENDRIX, J. P.: The effect of neostigmine on the actions of tetraethylammonium in dogs and man. Fred. Proc. **6**, 364 (1947).
SAEV, S. K., DIMITROV, D. I., DRAGOICHEV, C. Z., TENEV, K. A.: Emergency treatment of heartrate disturbances and pulmonary oedema. Acta anaesth. scand. **23** (suppl.), 266 (1966).
SCHAUMANN, W.: Resistenz einiger Wirkungen peripherer Vagusreizung gegenüber Ganglienblockern. Arch. exp. Path. Pharmakol. **231**, 738 (1957).

Shell, W. E., Sobel, B. E.: Protection of jeopardized ischemic myocardium by reduction of ventricular afterload. New Engl. Med. **291**, 481 (1974).
Sheps, S. G.: Hypertensive crisis. Postgrad. Med. **49**, 95 (1971).
Scribner, B. H., Crawford, M. A., Dempster, W. J.: Urinary excretion by nonionic diffusion. Amer. J. Physiol. **196**, 1135 (1959).
Smirk, F. H.: Hypotensive actions of hexamethonium bromide and some of its homologues, their use in high blood pressure. Lancet **1952 II**, 1002.
Smirk, F. H.: Principles and details of hypotensive therapy. In: Harington, M. (Ed.): Hypotensive Drugs, p. 109. New York: Macmillan, Pergamon 1956.
Smirk, F. H.: Advances in the treatment of hypertension. Practitioner **185**, 471 (1960).
Smith, J. R., Agrest, A., Hoobler, S. W.: The effect of acute and chronic administration of pentolinium tartrate on the blood pressure and cardiac output of hypertensive patients. Circulation **12**, 777 (1955).
Spierdijk, H., de Ruiter, H. J.: Decreased blood loss in prostate procedures by using continued controlled hypotension. Ned. T. Geneesk. **115**, 226 (1971).
Spinks, A., Young, E. H.: Polyalkylpiperidines: A new series of ganglion-blocking agents. Nature (Lond.) **181**, 1397 (1958).
Stinson, E. B., Holloway, E. L., Derby, G., Oyer, P. E., Hollingsworth, J., Griep, R. B., Harrison, D. C.: Comparative hemodynamic responses to chlorpromazine, nitroprusside, nitroglycerin, and trimethaphan immediately after open-heart operations. Circulation **51/52**, Suppl. I, 26 (1975).
Suriani, U.: Anaesthesiological technics of operative ischemia. Notes on otorhinolaryngological surgery, eye surgery, and surgery of the nervous system. Riv. Oto-neurio-oftal. **43**, 269 (1968).
Thoenen, H., Haefely, H., Staehelin, H.: Potentiation by tetraethylammonium of the response of the cat spleen to postganglionic sympathetic nerve stimulation. J. Pharmacol. exp. Ther. **157**, 532 (1967).
Thompson, A. E., Spracklens, F. H., Besterman, E. M., Bromley, L. L.: Recognition and management of dissecting aneurysms of the aorta. Brit. med. J. **1969 IV**, 134.
Trappold, J. H.: Role of venous return in the cardiovascular response following injection of ganglion-blocking agents. Circulation Res. **5**, 444 (1957).
Trendelenburg, U.: Pharmacology of autonomic ganglia. Ann. Pharmacol. **1**, 219 (1961).
Urquhart-Hay, D., Marshall, N. G., Marsland, J. M.: Comparison of epidural and hypotensive anaesthesia in open prostatectomy: Series 2. N. Z. med. J. **70**, 223 (1969).
Vaamonde, C. A., David, N. J., Palmer, R. F.: Hypertensive emergencies. Med. Clin. N. Amer. **55**, 325 (1971).
Varnauskas, E.: Studies in hypertensive cardiovascular disease with special reference to cardiac function. Scand. J. clin. Lab. Invest. **7**, Suppl. 17, 1 (1955).
Vidrio, H., Pardo, E. G.: Development of hypertension during chronic mecamylamine administration in dogs. Life Sci. **1**, 22 (1963).
Vidrio, H., Pardo, F. G.: Increased sympathetic vasoconstrictor tone in dogs treated chronically with mecamylamine. J. Pharmacol. exp. Ther. **157**, 42 (1967).
Volle, R. L.: Pharmacology of the autonomic nervous system. Ann. Rev. Pharmacol. **8**, 129 (1963).
Volle, R. L., Koelle, G. B.: Ganglionic stimulating and blocking agents. In: Goodmann, L. S., Gilman, A. (Eds.): The Pharmacological Basis of Therapeutics, p. 585. London-Toronto: Macmillan Comp. 1970.
Werko, L., Frisk, A. R., Wade, G., Eliasch, H.: Effect of hexamethonium in arterial hypertension. Lancet **1951 II**, 470.
Wheat, M. W. Jr., Harris, P. D., Malm, J. R., Kaiser, G., Bowman, F. O. Jr., Palmer, R. F.: Acute dissecting aneurysm of the aorta. Treatment of results in 64 patients. J. thorac. cardiovasc. Surg. **58**, 344 (1969).
Young, I. M.: The placental transfer of hexamethonium bromide and the origin of ammiotic fluid in the rabbit. J. Physiol. (Lond.) **122**, 93 (1953).
Young, I. M., de Wardener, H. E., Miles, B. E.: Mechanism of renal excretion of methonium compounds. Brit. med. J. **1951 II**, 1500.
Zaimis, E.: The interruption of ganglion transmission and its problems. J. Pharm. Pharmacol. **7**, 497—511 (1955).
Zaimis, E. J.: A possible explanation for the development of "tolerance" to ganglion blocking substances. In: Harington, M. (Ed.): Hypotensive Drugs, p. 85. New York: Macmillan, Pergamon 1956.
Zawoiski, E. J., Baer, J. E., Braunschweig, L. W., Paulson, S. F., Shermer, A., Beyer, K. H.: Gastrointestinal secretion and absorption of 3-methylaminoisocamphane hydrochloride (mecamylamine). J. Pharmacol. exp. Ther. **122**, 442 (1958).
Zervas, N. T., Hedley-Whyte, J.: Successful treatment of cerebral herniation in five patients. New Engl. J. Med. **286**, 1075 (1972).

Chapter 4

The Pharmacology of Rauwolfia Alkaloids

M. J. RAND and HELGA JUREVICS

With 5 Figures

I. Introduction and History

Preparations derived from species of *Rauwolfia*, a plant genus belonging to the Apocynaceae family, have been used for the treatment of a great variety of diseases in the folk medicine of the regions in which they are found. The species *R. serpentina* is a climbing or twining shrub occurring in the Indian sub-continent and S.E. Asia. The root of this plant has been used since ancient times in both India and the Malay peninsula as an antidote to the stings and bites of insects and poisonous reptiles. It has also been used to reduce fever, as a stimulant to uterine contractions, for insomnia, and particularly for the treatment of insanity.

The earliest reference in Western literature in regard to the curative properties of *Rauwolfia* was as early as 1563 (see BEIN, 1956). Although their use in hypertension was recorded by Indian workers in 1918, enthusiasm regarding their usefulness was aroused only after VAKIL (1949) published, in the British Heart Journal, his findings on the use of *Rauwolfia* extracts in the treatment of hypertension and these were confirmed by WILKINS and JUDSON (1953). *Rauwolfia* preparations were also introduced in psychiatry, in the treatment of schizophrenia, following reports that confirmed the value of the folk medicine. It was rapidly established that they were of worth in reducing aggression so that patients required less restraint and seclusion and the psychiatric wards were more manageable; it was also noted that the blood pressure and pulse rate were lowered (KLINE, 1954).

By the end of the 1960's, reserpine had almost passed out of psychiatric use, having been displaced by more efficacious drugs (LUBY, 1968). However, reserpine still holds a place in antihypertensive therapy (FREIS, 1971).

The development of effective antihypertensive agents has aimed primarily at symptomatic relief since the aetiological factors involved in primary, essential or idiopathic hypertension are still unknown. By 1930, well over a hundred so-called hypertensive remedies had been reported. These included certain natural products such as mistletoe, watermelon seeds, hawthorn, cannabis and veratrum. However, simple sedative measures were considered the most effective therapy (EVANS and LOUGHNAN, 1939). During the 1940's, the drastic measure of radical surgical sympathetic ganglionectomy for the treatment of severe hypertension was brought to a high state of development. The ganglion blocking drugs tetraethylammonium and hexamethonium were used as prognostic aids, the reasoning being that if "chemical ganglionectomy" was successful in lowering the blood pressure temporarily, then surgical ganglionectomy should produce a lasting beneficial effect. In the early 1950's, hexamethonium was introduced for the treatment of severe hypertension which was successful although it produced various unwanted side effects (RESTALL and SMIRK, 1950; CAMPBELL and ROBERTSON, 1950; SMIRK and ALSTAD, 1951). Also in the early 1950's *Rauwolfia serpentina* preparations, and the main active alkaloid (reserpine) were introduced for the treatment of less severe forms of hypertension and rapidly became popular, the peak years of popularity being 1955 and 1956. The initial enthusiasm for the use of reserpine was, however, dampened by its side effects, in particular severe depression resulting in some cases of suicide. The combination of reserpine with the ganglion blocking drug pentolinium resulted in a better control of hypertension and the doses of each drug could be lowered so that side effects were less severe (SMIRK et al., 1954; DOYLE et al., 1955). The thiazide diuretics were introduced in the late 1950's. These had only weak antihypertensive properties in their own right, but in combination with reserpine and other antihypertensive agents they provided an enhanced effectiveness in the lowering of high blood pressure (HOLLANDER and WILKINS, 1957; FREIS et al., 1958) and thus allowed for a reduction in the dose of reserpine. The selective adrenergic neurone blocking drugs, bretylium and guanethidine, replaced the formerly used ganglion blocking drugs in the routine management of patients with severe forms of hypertension (FROLICH and FREIS, 1959). The therapeutic management of hypertension was further advanced by the introduction of methyldopa which forms a false adrenergic transmitter (see Chapter 6). By the early 1960's a choice of effective and fairly well tolerated antihypertensive agents were available for controlling blood pressure. Despite the introduction of newer antihypertensive drugs, reserpine, in combination with diuretics, is still used, particularly in the treatment of mild hypertension.

Reserpine, as well as being a clinically useful drug for the management of hypertension and formerly as a tranquillizer in schizophrenia, has also proved to be a useful tool in biological research. It releases serotonin and catecholamines from stores of these amines and depletes their content in the tissues. Consequently, it has been used to study the role of these substances and their interaction with drugs in the brain and peripheral tissues and has proved of value in the elucidation of physiological and pharmacological mechanisms.

The study of the alkaloid composition of *R. serpentina* was initiated in the 1930's, and the major active constituent, reserpine, was isolated in 1952. An account of the early work in this field with the subsequent isolation, characterization and synthesis of the active alkaloids of *Rauwolfia* is reviewed by SCHLITTLER in Chapter 2.

Some 6,000 papers have been published on the chemistry, pharmacology and clinical aspects of reserpine and other *Rauwolfia* alkaloids. There are numerous comprehensive reviews dealing with the botany and pharmacognosy of *Rauwolfia* (WOODSON et al., 1957; YOUNGKEN, 1957), the chemistry and structure-activity relationships of *Rauwolfia* alkaloids (LUCAS, 1963; SCHLITTLER, 1965), and on the pharmacology of reserpine and other alkaloids from *Rauwolfia* (VAKIL, 1955; BEIN, 1956; BRODIE et al., 1961; LEWIS, 1963; SCHLITTLER and BEIN, 1967).

The majority of the papers dealing with reserpine published during the past several years have been concerned with its use as a tool in the evaluation of the actions of other drugs. In reviewing this literature, a certain amount of selection has been inevitable. Furthermore, our attention has been confined largely to reserpine, since this appears to be by far the most useful and most widely used of the *Rauwolfia* alkaloids and may be taken as the archetype for its congeners.

II. Absorption, Metabolism, and Distribution of Reserpine

In rats, injected ^{14}C-reserpine is rapidly eliminated from the blood and maximal concentrations are attained in all tissues, with the exception of fat tissue, within one hour. Fat tissues accumulate reserpine slowly, the maximal level being reached between 4 and 6 h. After 24 h, some radioactivity is detectable in the liver and in fat tissue but not in the brain or other tissues (SHEPPARD et al., 1955). Essentially the same results are obtained with randomly labelled ^{3}H-reserpine as with the specifically labelled ^{14}C-reserpine (SHEPPARD et al., 1958). The highest concentration in the brain is reached about 20 min after intraperitoneal injection (SHEPPARD et al., 1958; MUELLER and SHIDEMAN, 1968b).

The effects of reserpine do not correlate well with tissue levels. Thus, ^{14}C-reserpine is present at the maximal level in the brain at a time when rats and guinea-pigs still appear normal (SHEPPARD et al., 1957). Moreover, the pharmacological effects of reserpine are still manifested in rabbits at a time when reserpine can no longer be detected in the brain when assayed biochemically (HESS et al., 1956). However, when labelled reserpine is used, radioactivity is present in mouse brain for 5 days (MAGGIOLO and HALEY, 1964) and in rat brain for 12 h (MANARA and GARATTINI, 1967). ALPERS and SHORE (1969) using ^{3}H-reserpine of high specific activity in rats found that the biological half-life in the heart and spleen is approximately 18 h and is about 4 h in the liver. They also noted that unlabelled reserpine given 18 h after the labelled compound is unable to displace ^{3}H-reserpine from the tissues, indicating that the reserpine given initially is firmly bound. WAGNER and STITZEL (1972) found that the converse also held: pretreating with unlabelled reserpine or tetrabenazine reduced the retention of ^{3}H-reserpine in heart, and there was a corresponding increase in the reserpine metabolite ^{3}H-TMBA (3,4,5-trimethoxybenzoic acid).

Evidence that reserpine is bound to adrenergic neurones is provided by the observation of MANARA et al. (1972) that pretreatment of rats with 6-hydroxydopamine reduces the binding of ^{3}H-reserpine in the heart. At the sub-cellular level, reserpine accumulates not only at the sites of catecholamine storage, where it exerts its main effects, but also in mitochondria (STJÄRNE et al., 1969; WAGNER and STITZEL, 1972) and in the membrane of the sarcoplasmic reticulum (BALZER et al., 1968b). The subcellular distribution of ^{3}H-reserpine runs closely parallel to the distribution of total lipid in cardiac subcellular fractions (WAGNER and STITZEL, 1969).

Reserpine crosses the placenta and can affect the newborn if given during pregnancy: the babies often display severe nasal congestion (FINNERTY, 1956), presumably because of loss of vasomotor tone to mucosal blood vessels (see Section VI 6).

Reserpine is metabolized by the liver and intestine, but the contribution of other tissues has not been fully elucidated. The main metabolic event is hydrolysis to methylreserpate and TMBA (Fig. 1).

There are marked species differences in routes of metabolism of reserpine (SHEPPARD et al., 1955). Thus, rat liver has the greatest ability for the oxidation of the 4-methoxy carbon of the 3,4,5-trimethoxybenzoic acid moiety of reserpine to carbon dioxide, but pigeon and rabbit livers are devoid of this activity. Guinea-pig liver has the greatest ability for hydrolysing reserpine to TMBA and methylreserpate; mouse, rabbit and rat livers have fair ability to hydrolyse reserpine, but dog and pigeon livers have practically none. In mouse liver, reserpine is hydrolyzed by an esterase of the microsomal fraction, but may require initial oxidation by a mixed-function oxidase (STITZEL et al., 1972). Reserpine metabolism by microsomal fractions *in vitro* is inhibited by SKF 525-A, hexobarbital, aniline and pethidine (STITZEL et al., 1972).

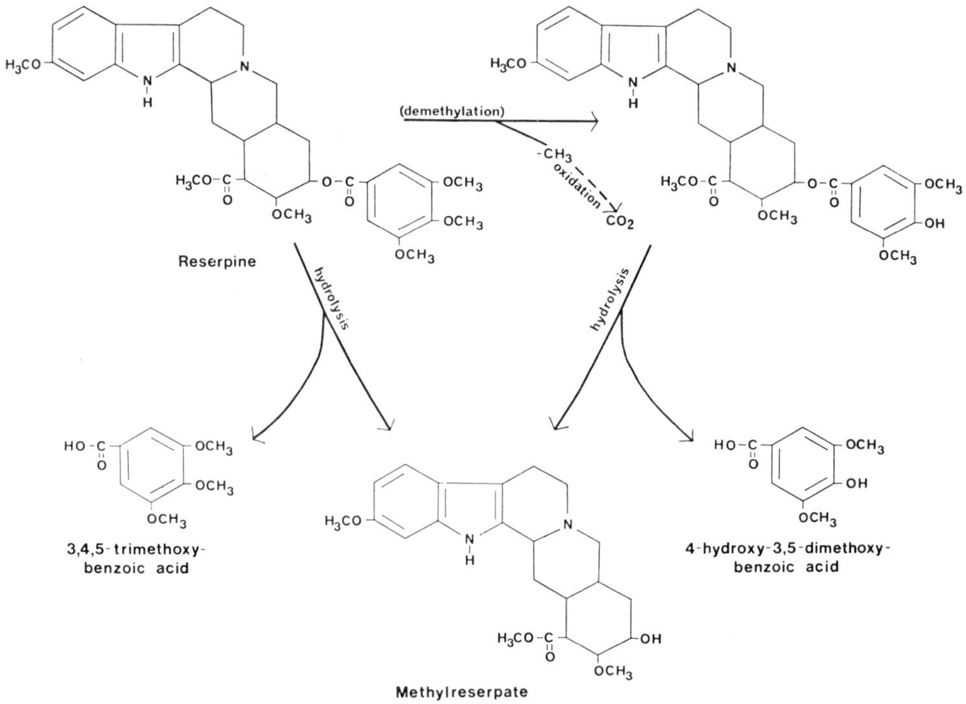

Fig. 1. Metabolism of Reserpine.

The metabolites of reserpine are devoid of pharmacological activity and are excreted by way of the lung, kidney and gut (SHEPPARD and TSEIN, 1955). It has not been established whether the species differences in metabolism of reserpine are responsible for the species differences in pharmacological effects. However, the more pronounced effect of reserpine in infant than in adult rats is probably due to a lower rate of metabolism of reserpine in the infants (MUELLER and SHIDEMAN, 1968b).

III. Effects of Reserpine on Levels of Catecholamines and Serotonin in Tissues

A. Sympathetically Innervated Tissues

Reserpine treatment of animals results in depletion of catecholamines from the sympathetic ganglia, heart, blood vessels, spleen, iris and other tissues with an adrenergic innervation (BERTLER et al., 1956; HOLZBAUER and VOGT, 1956; CARLSSON and HILLARP, 1956; PAASONEN and KRAYER, 1957, 1958; MUSCHOLL and VOGT, 1958; BURN and RAND, 1957, 1958b,d, 1959b; WAUD et al., 1958; MUSCHOLL, 1959; SJÖSTRAND, 1962; SCHAEPDRYVER, 1960; DAHLSTRÖM, 1967; BERKOWITZ et al., 1971). The depleting action of reserpine is produced by small doses. It takes some hours to develop fully, but is then long lasting. Although a circadian cycle has been reported for the depletion of noradrenaline from the brain, there is no such rhythm in the depletion of noradrenaline from the heart and salivary gland of the rat (BLACK et al., 1969; WALKER et al., 1971).

Reserpine is much less effective in reducing cardiac catecholamine stores when given *in vitro* (CERVONI et al., 1966; KUBO et al., 1970).

It has been reported that reserpine, even in high doses, does not cause depletion of catecholamines from tissues of the toad (NAYLER, 1963; BOYD et al., 1964); however, when the body temperature of the toad is raised, reserpine becomes effective in causing almost complete loss of cardiac catecholamines (CHANG and RAND, 1971).

In addition to the findings with animals, reserpine treatment reduces the content of noradrenaline in atrial appendages of human patients (CHIDSEY et al., 1963).

B. Tissue Chromaffin Cells

The depletion of catecholamines from sympathetically innervated tissues by reserpine is generally attributed to loss of transmitter from adrenergic nerve terminals, however, part of the depletion may be from chromaffin-staining cells in various tissues that are reduced in number by reserpine treatment (BURN et al., 1959).

Recently, VAN ORDEN et al. (1970) presented evidence for two morphologically distinct stores of noradrenaline in rat autonomic ganglia: the stores are differentially affected by catecholamine-depleting drugs. One storage site, in "chromaffin" cells, is resistant to depletion by reserpine or α-methyl-*m*-tyrosine but responds to α-methyl-*p*-tyrosine. The other type of noradrenaline store is in clusters of small granular vesicles within the perikarya of ganglionic adrenergic neurones, in the small dendrite-like processes and in the nerve fibres throughout the ganglion. This latter type of noradrenaline storage site is easily depleted by reserpine, α-methyl-*m*-tyrosine and α-methyl-*p*-tyrosine.

C. Adrenal Medullary Amines

Reserpine depletes the adrenaline and noradrenaline content of the adrenal medulla of cat, rabbit, rat and dog (HOLZBAUER and VOGT, 1956; CARLSSON and HILLARP, 1956; PARRATT and WEST, 1957; KRONEBERG and SCHÜMANN, 1957a, b, 1958; SCHÜMANN, 1958; COUPLAND, 1958, 1959; SCHAEPDRYVER and PREZIOSI, 1959; SCHAEPDRYVER, 1960). It was reported that noradrenaline is selectively depleted from adrenal glands of mouse (ERÄNKÖ and HOPSU, 1958) and cat (STJÄRNE and SCHAPIRO, 1959) but this does not occur in rats (COUPLAND, 1958; CALLINGHAM and MANN, 1962). The rate of depletion of adrenal stores is slower than that of amine stores in brain or other peripheral tissues (CALLINGHAM and MANN, 1962), and higher doses of reserpine are required (CARLSSON et al., 1957a; LEE, 1967). The relative insensitivity of the adrenal medulla to depletion arises from the slower turn-over rate of medullary amines than of amines in other tissues.

Role of the Splanchnic Nerves in Depletion of Adrenal Amines

HOLZBAUER and VOGT (1956) and MUSCHOLL and VOGT (1958) found that reserpine does not cause depletion of the catecholamine content of the denervated adrenal gland in the cat. In the rabbit, splanchnic nerve section confers only partial protection against the catecholamine-depleting action of reserpine (KROneberg and Schümann, 1957a), but spinal section at T1 prevents the depleting action (Taketomo et al., 1957; Brodie et al., 1957a). In the mouse, splanchnicectomy prevents the selective release of noradrenaline (Eränkö and Hopsu, 1958). Furthermore, reserpine-induced depletion of catecholamines from the adrenal medulla is inhibited by prior treatment with hemicholinium which inhibits synthesis of acetylcholine (Stitzel et al., 1965) and causes transmission failure at cholinergic junctions, suggesting that there is considerable traffic in the splanchnic nerves to the adrenal medulla. The effects of high doses of reserpine in destroying the integrity of the adrenal granular membrane in the rabbit is prevented by the ganglion blocking drug chlorisondamine (Viveros et al., 1969). These observations suggest a permissive role of the adrenal innervation for the depleting action of reserpine, or possibly that the action is exerted in the central nervous system and that depletion is due to a massive rate of splanchnic nerve excitation. Splanchnic nerve stimulation would increase the turn-over rate of medullary amines, and so facilitate the depleting action of reserpine.

However, in the rat, depletion of adrenal catecholamines by reserpine is not affected by splanchnic nerve section (Mirkin, 1958; Callingham and Mann, 1962) or by spinal section at C6 (Kroneberg and Schümann, 1957b). It was suggested that reserpine may act centrally in small doses to cause depletion of the adrenal catecholamines, but large doses have a more direct peripheral action which overshadows any central effect; most studies in the rat have been concerned with the latter effect (Callingham and Mann, 1962).

D. Peripheral Serotonin

Reserpine depletes serotonin from the intestinal tract, stomach, platelets, kidney, lung and spleen in a number of animal species (Brodie et al., 1955; Pletscher et al., 1955, 1956; Erspamer, 1956; Hardisty et al., 1956; Sanyal and West, 1958; Garattini et al., 1960a; Kim and Shore, 1963; Thompson and Campbell, 1967). The literature on the depletion of serotonin from enterochromaffin cells has been recently reviewed by Thompson (1971).

Serotonin with a ^{14}C-label which has been taken up by the vas deferens, presumably in the sympathetic nerves, is released by reserpine (Thoa et al., 1969).

E. Central Nervous System

Reserpine depletes the brain of its contents of noradrenaline (Holzbauer and Vogt, 1956) and serotonin (Pletscher et al., 1956; Hess et al., 1956; Kärki and Paasonen, 1959). The depletion of these two amines from rabbit brain follows parallel time courses and amounts to 90% in 4 h (Brodie et al., 1957a). Reserpine also depletes the rabbit and sheep brain of dopamine, the depletion of dopamine occuring more rapidly than that of noradrenaline (Bertler, 1961). In pigeons, reserpine causes depletion of the serotonin content of brain most rapidly, then dopamine and finally noradrenaline (Juorio and Vogt, 1967). Not only are there inter-species differences, but there are differences within a species, thus reserpine causes a more pronounced depletion of brain catecholamines in infant than in adult rats (Kulkarni and Shideman, 1966). Further observations on the depletion of amines from the central nervous system are dealt with in the section concerned with the functional effects of the depletion (Section VII).

The effects of reserpine on the levels in brain of catecholamines (noradrenaline and dopamine) and serotonin, as well as histamine and acetylcholine are summarized in Table 1.

Table 1. Effect of reserpine on brain amine content. (See page 85 for footnotes)

Amine	Species	Area of brain	Reserpine Route	Reserpine Dose	Reserpine Time	Control µg/g tissue	Reserpine treated µg/g tissue	Change	Ref.
Noradrenaline	Cat	Whole brain	i. a.	0.08 mg/kg	5 h	0.30	0.08	—73%	Zwieten et al., 1966.
		Hypothalamus	i. p.	0.4 mg/kg	18 h	1.40	0.20 to 0.86	—85 to —39%	Holzbauer and Vogt, 1956.
		Hypothalamus	i. p.	2.0 mg/kg	2 h	3.3	1.6	—52%	Laverty and Sharman, 1965.
	Mouse	Whole brain	i. p.	1.0 mg/kg	$23^1/_2$ h	0.50	0.20	—60%	Carlsson and Lindqvist, 1966.
		Whole brain	i. p.	3.0 mg/kg	24 h	0.41	0.04	—90%	Carlsson and Lindqvist, 1967.
	Pigeon	Hypothalamus	i. m.	1.0 mg/kg	4 h	1.42	0.62	—56%	Juorio and Vogt, 1967.
	Rabbit	Whole brain	i. v.	1.0 mg/kg	$23^3/_4$ h	0.27	0.01	—96%	Carlsson and Lindqvist, 1966.
		Telencephalon	i. v.	2.0 mg/kg/day	2 days	0.316	0.055	—83%	Meter and Karczmar, 1971.
		Hippocampus	i. v.	2.0 mg/kg/day	2 days	0.468	0.060	—87%	Meter and Karczmar, 1971.
		Cerebellum	i. v.	2.0 mg/kg/day	2 days	0.233	0.082	—65%	Meter and Karczmar, 1971.
		Midbrain	i. v.	2.0 mg/kg/day	2 days	0.348	0.038	—89%	Meter and Karczmar, 1971.
		Medulla-Pons	i. v.	2.0 kg/mg/day	2 days	0.496	0.082	—84%	Meter and Karczmar, 1971.
		Brain stem	i. v.	1.0 mg/kg	24 h	0.56	0.14	—75%	Quinn et al., 1959.
	Rat	Whole brain	i. v.	0.9 mg/kg	1 h	—	—	—71%	Brodie et al., 1966.
		Whole brain	i. cv.	0.25 mg/kg	4 h	0.306	0.088	—71%	Jobe et al., 1973.
		Brain stem	i. p.	2.0 mg/kg	3 h	0.54	0.06	—89%	Pirch et al., 1967.
		Caudate nucleus	i. p.	5.0 mg/kg	4 h	1.27(1)	1.02(1)	—20%	Walker et al., 1971.
						0.90(2)	0.72(2)	—20%	
		Hypothalamus	i. p.	5.0 mg/kg	4 h	1.78(1)	1.13(1)	—37%	Walker et al., 1971.
						1.06(2)	0.69(2)	—35%	
	Sheep	Corpus striatum	s. c.	2—4 mg/kg	13 h	1.0	0.0	—100%	Bertler, 1961.
Dopamine	Cat	Whole brain	i. a.	0.08 mg/kg	5 h	0.50	0.16	—68%	Zwieten et al., 1966
		Caudate nucleus	i. p.	2.0 mg/kg	2 h	4.90	<1.0	>—76%	Laverty and Sharman, 1965.
	Mouse	Whole brain	i. p.	1.0 mg/kg	$23^1/_2$ h	1.10	0.55	—51%	Carlsson and Lindqvist, 1966.
		Whole brain	i. p.	3.0 mg/kg	24 h	0.76	0.08	—89%	Carlsson and Lindqvist, 1967.
	Pigeon	Nucleus basalis-anterior part	i. m.	1.0 mg/kg	4 h	3.33	0.10	—97%	Jurio and Vogt, 1967.
	Rabbit	Whole brain	i. v.	1.0 mg/kg	$23^3/_4$ h	0.33	0.06	—82%	Carlsson and Lindqvist, 1966.
	Rat	Whole brain	i. v.	0.9 mg/kg	1 h	—	—	—78%	Brodie et al., 1966.
		Whole brain	i. cv.	0.25 mg	4 h	0.953	0.518	—45%	Jobe et al., 1973.
		Telencephalon	i. p.	2.0 mg/kg	3 h	1.12	0.08	—93%	Pirch et al., 1967.
	Sheep	Corpus striatum	s. c.	2—4 mg/kg	13 h	5.6	0.0	—100%	Bertler, 1961

Table 1. (continued)

Amine	Species	Area of brain	Reserpine Route	Reserpine Dose	Reserpine Time	Control μ/g tissue	Reserpine treated μ/g tissue	Change	Ref.
Serotonin	Cat	Thalamus	i. p.	2.0 mg/kg	2 h	0.98	0.35	—64%	LAVERTY and SHARMAN, 1965.
	Dog	Hypothalamus	i. p.	5.0 mg/kg	22 h	0.443	< 0.031	> —93%	PAASONEN and VOGT, 1956.
		Caudate nucleus	i. p.	5.0 mg/kg	22 h	0.150	0.016	—89%	PAASONEN and VOGT, 1956.
		Area postrema	i. p.	5.0 mg/kg	22 h	0.858	< 0.107	> —88%	PAASONEN and VOGT, 1956.
	Mouse	Whole brain	i. p.	1.0 mg/kg	$23^1/_2$ h	0.55	0.30	—44%	CARLSSON and LINDQVIST, 1966.
		Whole brain	i. p.	3.0 mg/kg	24 h	0.47	0.10	—98%	CARLSSON and LINDQVIST, 1967.
	Pigeon	Cerebral cortex	i. m.	1.0 mg/kg	4 b	0.88	0.33	—63%	JUORIO and VOGT, 1967.
	Rabbit	Whole brain	i. v.	1.0 mg/kg	$23^3/_4$ h	0.38	0.03	—92%	CARLSSON and LINDQVIST, 1966.
		Brain stem	i. v.	1.0 mg/kg	24 h	0.74	0.40	—46%	QUINN et al., 1959.
		Brain stem	i. v.	2.0 mg/kg	6 h	0.88	0.09	—90%	BRODIE et al., 1966.
	Rat	Whole brain	i. p.	2.0 mg/kg	3 h	0.71	0.16	—77%	PIRCH et al., 1967.
		Whole brain	i. v.	0.9 mg/kg	1 h	0.51	0.16	—70%	BRODIE et al., 1966.
		Pineal gland	i. p.	1.0 mg/kg/day	3 days	62.0	27.0	—56%	SNYDER and AXELROD, 1965.
	Sheep	Corpus striatum	s. c.	2—4 mg/kg	13 h	0.6	0.1	—83%	BERTLER, 1961.
Histamine	Cat	Anterior hypophysis	i. p.	0.5 to 10 mg/kg	18 h	2.40	1.70	N. S.	ADAM and HYE, 1966.
		Posterior hypophysis	i. p.	0.5 to 10 mg/kg	18 h	1.70	2.30	N. S.	ADAM and HYE, 1966.
		Hypopyseal stalk	i. p.	0.5 to 10 mg/kg	18 h	5.20	4.50	N. S.	ADAM and HYE, 1966.
		Hypothalamus-corpora mammallaria	i. p.	0.5 to 10 mg/kg	18 h	1.15	0.40	—65%	ADAM and HYE, 1966.
		Vertical hypothalamus	i. p.	0.5 to 10 mg/kg	18 h	0.80	0.27	—66%	ADAM and HYE, 1966.
		Dorsal hypothalamus	i. p.	0.5 to 10 mg/kg	18 h	4.80	0.20	—96%	ADAM and HYE, 1966.
		Preoptic nucleus	i. p.	0.5 to 10 mg/kg	18 h	0.43	0.19	—56%	ADAM and HYE, 1966.
		Medial thalamus	i. p.	0.5 to 10 mg/kg	18 h	0.25	0.16	—36%	ADAM and HYE, 1966.

Table 1 (continued)

Amine	Species	Area of brain	Reserpine Route	Reserpine Dose	Reserpine Time	Control µg/g tissue	Reserpine treated µg/g tissue	Change	Ref.
	Rat	Whole brain	i. p.	5.0 mg/kg	16 h	0.056	—	N. S.	MEDINA et al., 1970.
Acetylcholine	Dog	Cerebral cortex	i. v.	5.0 mg/kg	20 m	1.30	2.07	+59%	MALHOTRA and MEHTA, 1966.
		Hypothalamus	i. v.	0.5 mg/kg	1 h	4.81	6.01	+25%	MALHOTRA and DAS, 1962.
		Hypothalamus	i. v.	0.5 mg/kg	3 h	3.39	4.25	+25%	MALHOTRA and PUNDLIK, 1959.
		Hippocampus	i. v.	5.0 mg/kg	3 h	3.06	2.22	—27%	MALHOTRA and MEHTA, 1966.
		Temporal Lobe	i. v.	5.0 mg/kg	3 h	2.43	2.85	+17%	MALHOTRA and MEHTA, 1966.
		Frontal Lobe	i. v.	5.0 mg/kg	3 h	1.69	2.36	+40%	MALHOTRA and MEHTA, 1966.
		Cerebellum	i. v.	5.0 mg/kg	3 h	1.00	1.28	+28%	MALHOTRA and MEHTA, 1966.
	Rat	Brain stem	i. p.	1.0 mg/kg	30 m	3.0	7.5	+150%	MALPICA et al., 1970.

i. a. = intra-arterial.
i. cv. = intracerebroventricular.
i. m. = intramuscular.
i. p. = intraperitoneal.
i. v. = intravenous.
s. c. = subcutaneous.
— = value not given in original paper.
N.S. = no significant difference.
(1) = noradrenaline levels at end of dark period.
(2) = noradrenaline levels at end of light period.

IV. Effects of Reserpine on Uptake, Storage, Synthesis and Catabolism of Catecholamines and Serotonin

Of all the drugs which are known to affect adrenergic mechanisms, none has been as long or as extensively studied as reserpine. Despite this, its precise mode of action in depleting transmitter stores has not been completely clarified. Adrenergic neurones possess a number of special mechanisms for handling their transmitter substance: they synthesize, store and release noradrenaline, and they inactivate part of the released noradrenaline by transporting it back into the neurone. Similar mechanisms exist for dopaminergic and tryptaminergic neurones in the central nervous system. The effects of reserpine on the various transmitter mechanisms are considered in the following sections.

A. Effect of Reserpine on Uptake of Amines

Noradrenaline. The re-uptake of noradrenaline released by nerve impulses is considered to be the major means for termination of transmitter action. Several studies have indicated that up to 95% of released noradrenaline may be re-incorporated into adrenergic nerves (Brown, 1965; Gillespie, 1966).

Exogenous noradrenaline is taken up by the adrenergic axons in sympathetically innervated tissues, *in vivo* and *in vitro*. In tissues of reserpine-pretreated animals, the uptake of exogenous noradrenaline has been demonstrated with histochemical methods (Hamberger et al., 1964; Malmfors, 1967; Gillespie et al., 1970), with radioisotopic techniques (Weiner and Trendelenburg, 1962; Iversen et al., 1965) and by bioassay (Pennefather and Rand, 1960).

Although uptake occurs, the retention of exogenous catecholamines by a number of adrenergically innervated tissues both *in vivo* and *in vitro* after reserpine pretreatment of the animal is less than that of tissues from untreated animals (Muscholl, 1960; Axelrod et al., 1961a, b, 1962a; Hertting et al., 1961; Dengler et al., 1961, 1962; Weiner and Trendelenburg, 1962; Potter and Axelrod, 1963; Lindmar and Muscholl, 1964; Kuntzman and Jacobson, 1964; Cervoni et al., 1970; Trendelenburg and Draskóczy, 1970). The impairment of retention of exogenous noradrenaline caused by reserpine has been equated with failure of the adrenergic neurones to accumulate endogenous noradrenaline.

The processes involved in the storage, uptake and retention of noradrenaline in peripheral adrenergic axon varicosities are illustrated diagrammatically in Fig. 2. Similar processes are thought to operate in central adrenergic axon terminals and in chromaffin cells. Uptake and retention involve two components. One component is located at the cell membrane and is concerned with the uptake of extracellular noradrenaline (and other structurally related amines) into the cytoplasm: this process is not affected by reserpine (Kopin et al., 1962; Lindmar and Muscholl, 1964; Hamberger et al., 1964; Carlsson and Waldeck, 1965b; Carlsson, 1966; Hamberger, 1967; Herr and Costa, 1969). A second, intraneuronal uptake process occurs from the cytoplasm into subcellular storage particles: this process is ATP-dependent, and is impaired by reserpine in isolated adrenal storage granules and in nerve storage vesicles (Kirshner, 1962; Euler and Lishajko, 1963; Carlsson et al., 1963b; Stjärne, 1964; Carlsson, 1965a; Dahlström et al., 1965; Euler, 1966; Giachetti and Shore, 1966; Lundborg and Stitzel, 1967a, b).

IVERSEN et al. (1965) showed that in perfused rat hearts there are two components in the plot of rate of uptake against time. In hearts from reserpine-treated rats, the initial uptake of the amine is the same as in normal hearts, but the second component of uptake is absent and little of the amine can be found in subcellular particles.

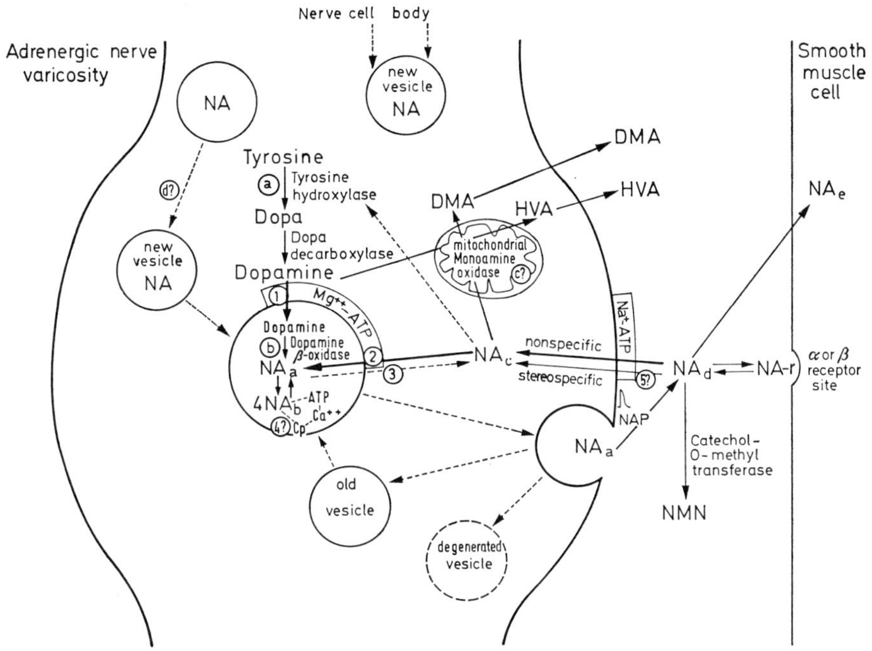

Fig. 2. Interaction of reserpine with components of the adrenergic nerve varicosity. NA_a Mobile pool of noradrenaline within storage granule. NA_b Bound pool of noradrenaline, possibly in association with calcium, ATP and protein. NA_c Mobile pool of noradrenaline in nerve cytoplasm. NA_d Noradrenaline in region of receptor. NA-r Noradrenaline-receptor complex. NA_e Extraneuronal uptake of noradrenaline by smooth muscle cell. NAP Nerve action potential (excitation—secretion coupling). Cp Proteins (chromagranins) associated with storage vesicles and may function in binding noradrenaline. DMA 3,4-Dihydroxymandelic acid, metabolite of intraneuronal noradrenaline. HVA Homovanillic acid, metabolite of dopamine. NMN Normetanephrine, metabolite of extraneuronal noradrenaline. **1—5** Sites of direct effect of reserpine. 1 and 2 Inactivation of Mg^{++} ATP dependent uptake of dopamine and noradrenaline by storage granula (Section IV A 2). 3 Inhibition of spontaneous release of noradrenaline from storage granula (Section IV C). 4 ? Dissassociation of noradrenaline from bound complex (Section IV B). 5 ? Inhibition of Na^+-ATP dependent, optically specific uptake of noradrenaline by the neuronal membrane (Section IV A 1). **a** to **d** Sites of indirect effect of reserpine. **a** and **b** Delayed increase in activity of tyrosine hydroxylase and dopamine-β-oxidase (dopamine-β-hydroxylase) (Section IV D 1). c ? Increase in activity of monoamine oxidase (Section IV E). d ? Stimulation of synthesis of new storage vesicles (Section IV F).

There is, therefore, clear evidence that reserpine impairs the intracellular binding and storage of noradrenaline. However, there is accumulation of catecholamines in reserpine-treated tissues when a monoamine oxidase inhibitor is administered prior to administration of catecholamines (FUXE and HILLARP, 1964; HAMBERGER et al., 1964; CARLSSON, 1965a, 1966; MALMFORS, 1965; NORBERG, 1965; HÄGGENDAL and HAMBERGER, 1967; GARCIA and KIRPEKAR, 1973). Presumably, the noradrenaline taken up intraneuronally, being protected from destruction by monoamine oxidase, presents a higher concentration gradient for uptake into the storage vesicles.

Other amines. The accumulation of serotonin by slices of the corpus striatum and hypothalamus is inhibited by reserpine to a greater extent than that of catecholamines (SHASKAN and SNYDER, 1970). The accumulation of dopamine by these tissues is affected less by reserpine than that of noradrenaline (DORRIS and SHORE, 1971). Thus it appears that there are differences in the effects of reserpine on tryptaminergic, dopaminergic and noradrenergic neurones.

1. Uptake of Amines across Neuronal Membranes

The reserpine-resistant uptake mechanism for noradrenaline and related amines is present in all parts of noradrenergic neurones, that is, in the cell body, the conducting axon and the axon terminals (FUXE and HILLARP, 1964).

The membrane uptake mechanism has the properties of a transport system. It exhibits Na^+ dependency (IVERSEN and KRAVITZ, 1966; BOGDANSKI and BRODIE, 1966, 1969; BOGDANSKI et al., 1968; GILLIS and PATON, 1967; SUGRUE and SHORE, 1969), the Na^+ electrochemical gradient across the axonal membrane being maintained by the Na^+ -K^+ ATPase system (SKOU, 1965). The inactivation of the Na^+ -K^+ ATPase *in vitro*, either by ouabain (DENGLER et al., 1961; GIACHETTI and SHORE, 1966; PATON, 1971) or by omission of K^+ (GILLIS and PATON, 1967; BOGDANSKI and BRODIE, 1969), results in a decrease of amine uptake. The tricyclic antidepressants and cocaine also act on the reserpine-resistant membrane uptake mechanism to inhibit uptake of exogenous catecholamines (HAMBERGER, 1967; BERTI and SHORE, 1967a; MAXWELL et al., 1969).

Although reserpine does not significantly affect the axonal membrane transport of amines, it potentiates the inhibitory effects of ouabain or low Na^+ concentration on the uptake of amines by rabbit heart slices (BERTI and SHORE, 1967b; SUGRUE and SHORE, 1971). These effects have been attributed to a Na^+-dependent, optically specific, reserpine-sensitive amine uptake mechanism which is separate and distinct from the main, relatively non-specific, reserpine-resistant membrane amine uptake system. Tetrabenazine but not guanethidine shares this action of reserpine (SUGRUE and SHORE, 1971). Since the intraneuronal concentration of sodium is low, it has been proposed that the Na^+-dependent reserpine-sensitive amine uptake system may operate both at the axonal membrane and at the membrane of the intraneuronal storage granule and may be associated with a functional or "available" noradrenaline pool (SUGRUE and SHORE, 1969, 1971). The rate of release of ^{3}H-noradrenaline from spleen slices taken from reserpine-treated cats is not altered by reduction of the Na^+-concentration of the medium (GARCIA and KIRPEKAR, 1973).

2. Uptake of Amines by Nerve Vesicles and Adrenal Granules

The uptake and storage of noradrenaline and other amines by intraneuronal storage vesicles are inhibited not only by reserpine but by a number of other drugs, including prenylamine, desmethylimipramine and other tricyclic antidepressants, tetrabenazine, chlorpromazine and other phenothiazines, haloperidol and other butyrophenones, some indirectly acting sympathomimetic amines, uncouplers of oxidative phosphorylation, metabolic inhibitors, EDTA, some α-receptor antagonists and some β-receptor antagonists (KIRSHNER, 1962; CARLSSON et al., 1963b; EULER and LISHAJKO, 1968; TAUGNER and HASSELBACH, 1966; PHILIPPU et al., 1965, 1967, 1969; BURGER et al., 1968, 1969).

The reserpine-sensitive uptake of catecholamines into isolated granules at 37° C is stimulated by Mg^{++} and ATP (KIRSHNER, 1962; CARLSSON et al., 1963b). This uptake process is dependent on active metabolism since at 4° C reserpine has no effect on splenic nerve vesicles (POTTER, 1966; EULER, 1966; STJÄRNE, 1966) or adrenal chromaffin granules (HILLARP, 1959). At this temperature, the catecholamine content is retained for a considerable length of time and there is only passive diffusion of the amines, even in the presence of reserpine.

Isolated chromaffin granules also take up ATP, although to a considerably lesser extent than amines, and ATP uptake is only partially inhibibited by reserpine (CARLSSON et al., 1963b). It has been suggested that reserpine inhibits the ATP-dependent amine-transport process (KIRSHNER, 1962; CARLSSON et al., 1962; EULER and LISHAJKO, 1965). In accord with this, it has been found that reserpine reduces the ATPase activity of storage granules and vesicles isolated from the adrenal medulla, splenic nerve, sympathetic ganglia and hypothalamus (TAUGNER and HASSELBACH, 1966; PHILIPPU et al., 1967, 1969; BURGER et al., 1968, 1969).

The inhibition by reserpine of noradrenaline uptake by splenic nerve granules can be overcome when the concentration of noradrenaline is raised to 10^{-4}M or higher (EULER and LISHAJKO, 1967). Although this was attributed to a non-specific uptake, it may explain the reversal by monoamine oxidase inhibitors of the reserpine-induced inhibition of uptake mechanisms and depletion of catecholamine stores.

Isolated amine-storing vesicles from the hypothalamus of the pig take up noradrenaline by two different mechanisms (PHILIPPU et al., 1968). The first type of uptake is independent of temperature and occurs in the absence of ATP and Mg^{++}, so it is attributed to a passive transport of the amine through the membrane. The second type is temperature sensitive and dependent on ATP and Mg^{++}, and is considered to be due to active transport. Reserpine (and prenylamine) inhibits both the active and passive transport of noradrenaline into these vesicles (PHILIPPU et al., 1969). However, the passive transport which occurs in the presence of high amounts of noradrenaline is inhibited only at 37° C; at 0° C reserpine does not influence the diffusion of the amine.

B. Effect of Reserpine on Amine Storage Mechanisms

Noradrenaline. Combined electron microscopy and autoradiography have provided evidence that exogenous ^{3}H-noradrenaline is stored in intraneuronal vesicles (WOLFE et al., 1962). Electron micrographs of adrenergic axons show three morphological types of intraneuronal vesicles (RICHARDSON, 1962, 1964; BONDAREFF, 1965; GRILLO, 1966; VAN ORDEN et al., 1966): (1) agranular vesicles, 300 to 600 Å in diameter; (2) small granular vesicles which are the same size as the agranular type but contain an electron-dense core of variable size; (3) large granular vesicles, 600 to 1200 Å in diameter which are more sparsely distributed throughout the axon and occur most commonly in nerve terminals in autonomic ganglia and more sparsely in adrenergic terminals. Reserpine produces changes in the ultrastructure of adrenergic terminals in peripheral tissues (RICHARDSON, 1964; BURNSTOCK et al., 1970) and in the central nervous system (ROBERTIS, 1964); in particular, the proportion of granulated vesicles is decreased (PELLEGRINO DE IRALDI and ROBERTIS, 1963; WALKER et al., 1971).

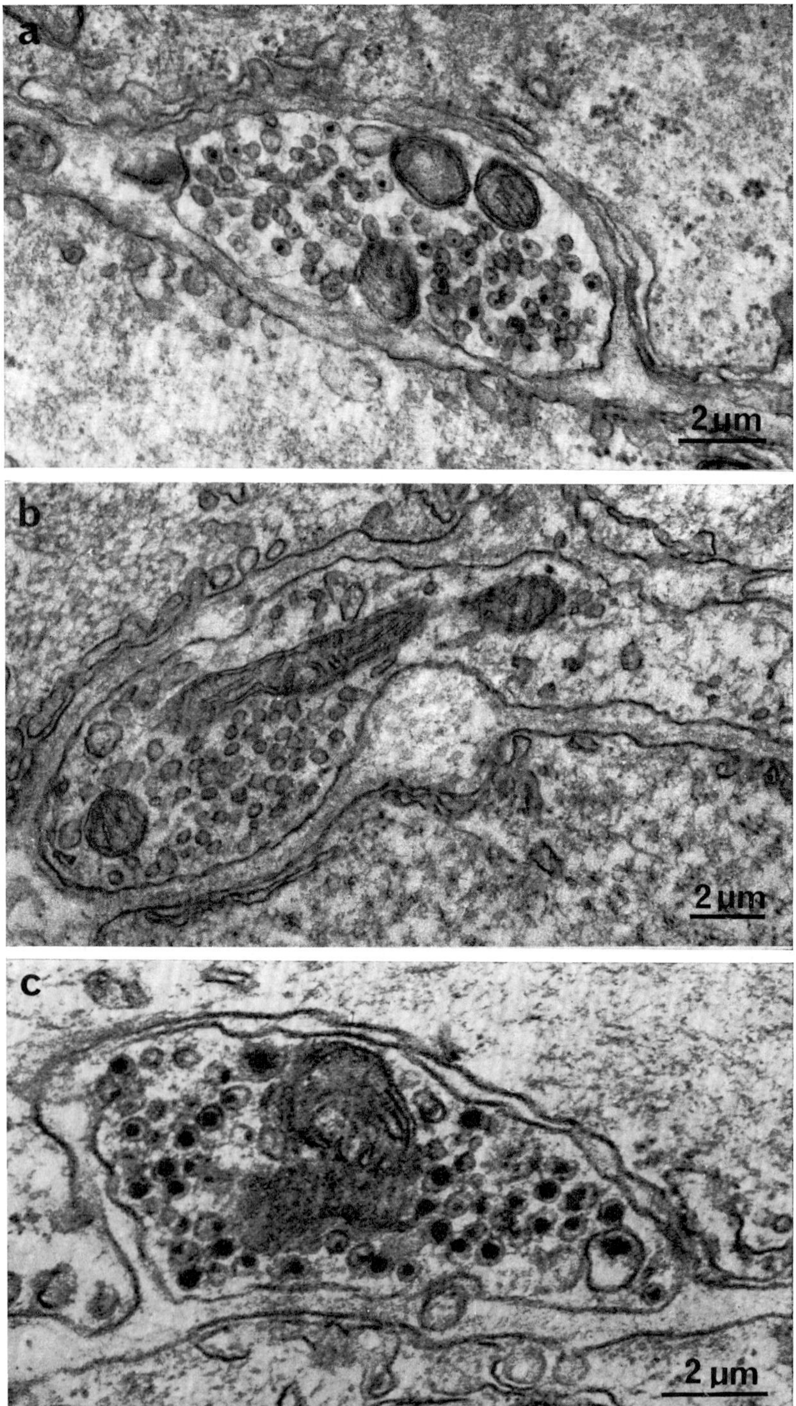
a
2 µm
b
2 µm
c
2 µm

The small granular vesicles are thought to be the important storage sites for noradrenaline (POTTER, 1967; BURNSTOCK et al., 1970), as shown in Fig. 3. The large granular type may represent a precursor of the synaptic vesicles in transit from the site of synthesis in the cell bodies in ganglia along the fibres to the axon terminals (GEFFEN and OSTBERG, 1969; BONDAREFF, 1965; TAFURI, 1964). Evidence in support of somatofugal transport of granular vesicles containing noradrenaline has been obtained from studies of the effects of reserpine on ligated nerves. In doubly ligated nerves it has been shown that endogenous noradrenaline (DAHLSTRÖM and HÄGGENDAL, 1966a, b), granular vesicles (MAYOR and KAPELLER, 1967), radioactive noradrenaline and protein (LIVETT et al., 1968) accumulate above the proximal but not the distal ligature. Also the granules which accumulate proximal to a constriction are significantly larger and more completely granulated than those in the terminals (GEFFEN and OSTBERG, 1969). Reserpine depletes the noradrenaline (DAHLSTRÖM, 1967) and the granular contents of the vesicles (MAYOR and KAPELLER, 1967) accumulated above the ligature. After reserpine treatment, recovery of the noradrenaline content (DAHLSTRÖM et al., 1965) and of granular vesicles (HASSLER and BAK, 1966) occurs first in the cell body and later in the nerve terminals in unconstricted nerves. In doubly ligated nerves, recovery occurs only above the proximal ligature and the rate is faster the closer the ligature is placed to the cell bodies (DAHLSTRÖM, 1967).

Among the reasons why large granular vesicles are thought to differ qualitatively from the smaller type is that they are less affected by reserpine (BONDAREFF, 1965; HÖKFELT, 1966; CLEMENTI et al., 1966). However, VAN ORDEN et al. (1966), in experiments on depletion of granular vesicles in the vas deferens with reserpine and with nerve stimulation, could not detect a differential effect on the two types of granular vesicles. Similar results were obtained in ligated splenic nerves of cats with reserpine (GEFFEN and OSTBERG, 1969).

The form in which catecholamines are complexed within storage particles is not clear. The occurrence of catecholamines and adenine nucleotides in an approximately 4 : 1 molar ratio in chromaffin granules has led to the suggestion that these two substances are associated in a nondiffusible complex (HILLARP, 1958a). Similar proportionate amounts of catecholamines and adenine nucleotides are released from chromaffin granules both *in vitro* and *in vivo* by a wide variety of stimuli (CARLSSON and HILLARP, 1956; SCHÜMANN, 1958; KIRPEKAR et al., 1958). Reserpine releases ATP as well as noradrenaline from isolated nerve vesicles, but the ratio of released noradrenaline to released ATP is higher than is the ratio within the vesicles (STJÄRNE, 1964). Although ATP-amine complexes in concentrated solutions are weak (WEINER and JARDETZKY, 1964), low concentrations of calcium which are equivalent to the ion content of chromaffin granules (SMITH, 1968) have been found to enhance the aggregation of noradrenaline plus ATP in aqueous solutions (BERNEIS et al., 1969, 1970). Small amounts of reserpine (0.3 μM) cause phase separation of the ATP-noradrenaline complex (BERNEIS et al., 1970). Whether this has any bearing on the *in vivo* depletion of catecholamines is not known. The breakdown of RNA by granular RNAase has been suggested as the

---

Fig. 3. Electronmicrographs showing profiles of adrenergic neurone terminal varicosities. (a) Varicosity in vas deferens from untreated rat. Note preponderance of small vesicles with variably sized granular cores. (b) Varicosity in rat vas deferens, 18 h after intraperitoneal injection with reserpine (5 mg/kg). Note the loss of granular cores from the vesicles. (c) Varicosity of mouse vas deferens, 30 min after intravenous injection of 6-hydroxydopamine. Note that the granular cores of the vesicles are particularly well defined. (The authors are grateful to Professor G. Burnstock for providing these illustrations).

primary event in the release of catecholamines and ATP from adrenal granules (SCHÜMANN, 1966). It has not been established, apparently, whether the activity of this enzyme is affected by reserpine. The effects of reserpine (and other psychotropic drugs) on catecholamine storage mechanisms have been related to their physicochemical property of lowering surface tension (PALM et al., 1970). However, this does not explain the unique properties of reserpine, nor does it help in identifying the molecular basis of the effect of reserpine.

Serotonin. Blood platelets are subcellular particles derived from megakaryocytes and contain structures analogous to storage granules. The accumulation of serotonin by platelets is blocked by reserpine (BRODIE et al., 1957b; PLETSCHER et al., 1967). Reserpine has no effect on the uptake of ^{14}C-serotonin by perfused lungs of the rat. However, the lungs, unlike the brain and blood platelets, do not store serotonin but metabolize it rapidly (JUNOD, 1972).

The binding of serotonin to a ganglioside *in vitro* is prevented by reserpine (GIELEN, 1966). However, it is not established whether a ganglioside forms a part of the serotonin storage complex.

C. Effect of Reserpine on Retention of Amines by Isolated Storage Particles

High concentrations of reserpine (5×10^{-4}M and higher) increase the rate of loss of catecholamines from isolated bovine splenic nerve vesicles whereas a concentration of 10^{-4}M has no effect (EULER and LISHAJKO, 1961a). Similarly, reserpine in concentrations of approximately 10^{-4}M has no effect on the release of catecholamines from the perfused adrenal gland (EULER et al., 1964) or from adrenal slices although it decreases their rate of O_2 consumption (DRASKÓCZY et al., 1963). The rate of spontaneous release of noradrenaline is greater than that of adrenaline in bovine adrenal medullary granules at 37° C (OKA et al., 1966); this difference remains in the presence of 10^{-5}M of reserpine but with 10^{-4}M there are equal rates of release of both amines.

In low concentrations (between 10^{-8} and 10^{-5}M), reserpine strongly inhibits the spontaneous release of noradrenaline (EULER and LISHAJKO, 1961b, 1966; WEIL-MALHERBE and POSNER, 1963; EULER et al., 1964). Thus after partial depletion, the retention of noradrenaline has been reported to be even greater in the presence of reserpine than in its absence as a result of the retarded release (EULER and LISHAJKO, 1963). The inhibitory effect of reserpine on the spontaneous release of catecholamines from isolated granules or adrenal slices is temperature sensitive. At temperatures of 0 to 4° C, the spontaneous release is very slow and is not influenced by reserpine, whereas at 37° C, the spontaneous release rate is very rapid and is sensitive to reserpine (HILLARP, 1958b; KIRSHNER, 1962). The inhibitory effect of reserpine on the release of catecholamines from adrenal medullary granules has also been reported to show marked variations among different species of animals and these could not be correlated with the spontaneous rates of release (STJÄRNE and SCHAPIRO, 1959; EULER and LISHAJKO, 1961b).

D. Effect of Reserpine on the Synthesis of Catecholamines and Serotonin

Three enzymes are required in the synthesis of noradrenaline and four in the synthesis of adrenaline from their dietary precursor, tyrosine. The first and rate-limiting step requires tyrosine hydroxylase for the *meta*-hydroxylation of tyrosine to dopa (NAGATSU et al., 1964; LEVITT et al., 1965). Dopa is converted to dopamine by dopa decarboxylase (LOVENBERG et al., 1962). Both dopa and dopa decarboxylase are found in the soluble portion in subcellular fractions of adrenergic nerves (LOVENBERG et al., 1962; POTTER and AXELROD, 1963). Synthesis of noradrenaline from dopamine takes place within the storage vesicles (KIRSHNER, 1962) and is catalyzed by dopamine β-hydroxylase (LEVIN et al., 1960), an enzyme which is associated with the storage granule (KIRSHNER, 1962). In the adrenal medulla and other chromaffin cells noradrenaline is converted to adrenaline within the storage granule by the enzyme phenylethanolamine-N-methyltransferase (AXELROD, 1962a, b).

Although reserpine has not been demonstrated to have a direct action on the individual enzymes involved in the synthesis of catecholamines (GLOWINSKI et al., 1966; RUTLEDGE and WEINER, 1967), it nervertheless exerts a profound inhibitory effect in organized tissues and in particle-containing homogenates on the synthesis of noradrenaline (STJÄRNE and LISHAJKO, 1966; STJÄRNE et al., 1967; RUTLEDGE and WEINER, 1967; ROTH and STONE, 1968) and at the same time increases the metabolites of both endogenous and administered noradrenaline (KOPIN et al., 1962; KOPIN and GORDON, 1962, 1963; RUTLEDGE and WEINER, 1967).

BERTLER (1961) suggested that reserpine inhibits the synthesis of noradrenaline by inhibiting the uptake of the immediate precursor, dopamine, into the storage vesicles which contain the enzyme dopamine-β-hydroxylase. Evidence in support of this proposal has been obtained mainly from studies with radioactive precursors of noradrenaline. Thus, the formation of ^{14}C-noradrenaline from ^{14}C-dopamine by intact chromaffin granules is inhibited by reserpine, but the synthesis by lysed granules is not affected (KIRSHNER, 1962). A similar difference is observed in the activities of particulate and non-particulate homogenates of the adrenal medulla after pretreatment of the donor animal with reserpine (KIRSHNER et al., 1963). Reserpine inhibits the formation of noradrenaline from dopamine by isolated splenic nerve granules (STJÄRNE and LISHAJKO, 1966) and by splenic nerve homogenates (ROTH and STONE, 1968), bot does not affect the formation of dopamine from tyrosine (STJÄRNE and LISHAJKO, 1966). However, in perfused hearts and adrenal medullary slices from reserpine-treated rabbits, the amounts of both ^{3}H-noradrenaline and ^{3}H-dopamine formed from ^{3}H-tyrosine are markedly reduced (WEINER and RUTLEDGE, 1966; RUTLEDGE and WEINER, 1967). In splenic nerve homogenates incubated with tyrosine, reserpine prevents the accumulation of dopamine, but after inhibition of monoamine oxidase with pargyline there is accumulation of dopamine. Thus the reduction by reserpine of the noradrenaline formed from tyrosine in intact tissues can be readily explained by an inhibition of uptake of the precursor amine, dopamine, into the storage granules as originally proposed by BERTLER (1961).

Brain Amines. It has been reported that reserpine does not affect the formation of dopamine in the brain of rabbit, pig and mouse (ROSENGREN, 1960). Reserpine treatment of rats leads to an increase in brain levels of tyrosine and tryptophan (TAGLIAMONTE et al., 1971), suggesting impairment of synthesis of amines derived from these amino acids. The turn-over rate of dopamine in the striatum of rats is depressed by reserpine (BESSON et al., 1971), but the turn-over rate of serotonin is increased (TOZER et al., 1966; BARKAI et al., 1972).

Effects of Reserpine on the Activity of Enzymes Concerned in Catecholamine Synthesis

After the administration of reserpine, tyrosine hydroxylase activity is increased in the adrenal gland, brain, and sympathetic ganglia of a number of animals

(THOENEN et al., 1969a, b; MUELLER et al., 1969a, b; AXELROD et al., 1970; BHAGAT et al., 1971; MOLINOFF et al., 1972). Although the effect of reserpine on tyrosine hydroxylase activity is dose-related, there is no relationship between the increase in enzyme activity and the decrease in endogenous catecholamines (MUELLER et al., 1969b). Ganglionic blockade (BHAGAT et al., 1971), inhibition of protein synthesis or decentralization (THOENEN et al., 1969a; MUELLER et al., 1969b; AXELROD et al., 1970) prior to the administration of reserpine abolishes its effect in increasing tyrosine hydroxylase activity, suggesting that the increase may be a compensatory mechanism to overcome the inhibition of catecholamine synthesis (BESSON et al., 1971). Actinomycin D inhibits the reserpine-induced increase in tyrosine hydroxylase activity in rat stellate ganglia (MOLINOFF et al., 1972), suggesting that the increase is due to induction of enzyme synthesis. It has also been suggested that the small, reserpine-resistant amine pools in various tissues may in part reflect a maintenance of the levels of catecholamines by an induction of tyrosine hydroxylase (BERKOWITZ et al., 1971).

In adrenergic nerve terminals, free (axoplasmic) noradrenaline exerts a feedback inhibitory effect on the activity of tyrosine hydroxylase. BOADLE-BIBER and ROTH (1972) showed that reserpine pretreatment of guinea-pigs which produces a 50% depletion of the noradrenaline content of the vas deferens results in inhibition of the formation of dopa from ^{14}C-tyrosine, presumably because of an increase in axoplasmic noradrenaline; however, when there is 95% depletion of noradrenaline the conversion of ^{14}C-tyrosine is as in control tissues. The reserpine-induced increase in tyrosine hydroxylase activity of sympathetic ganglia is counteracted by administration of dopa or monoamine oxidase inhibitors (MOLINOFF et al., 1972): in this case the increased enzyme activity associated with increased neuronal activity is offset by the inhibitory effect of increased intraneuronal noradrenaline.

Reserpine has a dose-dependent effect on dopamine-β-hydroxylase activity of rabbit adrenal glands (VIVEROS et al., 1969). After 5 mg/kg there is a marked fall in dopamine-β-hydroxylase along with depletion of catecholamines. After 1 mg/kg, there is still almost complete depletion of adrenal catecholamines but only a slight decrease in enzyme activity. Low doses of reserpine (0.25 mg/kg) produce considerable depletion of catecholamines but there is no fall in dopamine-β-hydroxylase activity; in fact, after 5 days, the enzyme level starts to rise and is twice normal in 8 days. In these studies, dopamine-β-hydroxylase activity was used as a marker for membranes of storage granules. The findings suggest that destruction of granules occurs with higher doses of reserpine, but with low doses the integrity of the granule is not destroyed although amine storage capacity is deranged. The decrease in enzyme activity produced by the larger doses of reserpine is prevented by prior treatment with the ganglionic blocking agent, chlorisondamine, suggesting that neuronal traffic is a necessary adjunct to the effect.

An increase in phenylethanolamine-*N*-methyl transferase activity has been reported in rat adrenal glands after reserpine (BHAGAT et al., 1971). The increase in activity of this enzyme does not appear to be neuronally mediated since ganglionic blockade with chlorisondamine fails to antagonize the reserpine-induced increase in activity.

In hypophysectomised rats, in which the activities of both tyrosine hydroxylase and phenylethanolamine-N-methyl transferase are decreased, ACTH restores the activities of both enzymes but reserpine increases only that of tyrosine hydroxylase (BHAGAT et al., 1971).

E. Effect of Reserpine on Catabolism of Catecholamines and Serotonin

The two enzymes involved in the degradation of catecholamines are monoamine oxidase and catechol-O-methyl transferase. It is generally accepted that extraneuronal catecholamines are metabolized largely by catechol-O-methyl transferase whereas the intraneuronal unbound amines are metabolized by monoamine oxidase.

In rat submaxillary gland reserpine pretreatment causes a reduction in catechol-O-methyl transferase activity (MARSDEN et al., 1971), and the maximal effect on activity coincides in time with the maximal effect of reserpine on the noradrenaline level in this tissue (JONASON, 1969).

Reserpine causes an increase in monoamine oxidase activity of mitochondria and microsomes in several tissues (IZUMI et al., 1967, 1969; YOUDIN and SANDLER, 1968), but a small reduction of activity has been observed in rat submaxillary gland (MARSDEN et al., 1971).

In reserpine-pretreated animals, there is an increase in the deaminated product of noradrenaline and a decrease in the O-methylated product, normetanephrine, in adrenergically innervated tissues (KOPIN and GORDON, 1962, 1963; RUTLEDGE and WEINER, 1967) and in the brain (HÄGGENDAL, 1963; GLOWINSKI and AXELROD, 1965; GLOWINSKI et al., 1966). The effect has been attributed to the impaired uptake of noradrenaline into the storage vesicles by reserpine which results in a greater exposure of the amine to intraneuronal catabolizing enzymes (KOPIN and GORDON, 1962, 1963). It has also been suggested that the increased deamination may result from activation of mitochondrial monoamine oxidase or from facilitated penetration of noradrenaline into the mitochondria (IZUMI et al., 1969).

Increased amounts of catabolic products of dopamine are formed from ^{3}H-dopamine in hearts of reserpine-treated animals (RUTLEDGE and WEINER, 1967) and from tyrosine in splenic nerve homogenates in the presence of reserpine (ROTH and STONE, 1968). The increased rate of catabolism is attributed to the inhibition of dopamine uptake and accumulation in the storage vesicles.

The rate of metabolism of serotonin by brain synaptosomes is increased (BOGDANSKI et al., 1968).

Interaction between Reserpine and Monoamine Oxidase Inhibitors

The tissue contents of amines that have been depleted by reserpine treatment are generally restored by administration of a monoamine oxidase inhibitor, and the behavioural effects of reserpine are also reversed (SHORE, 1962). The extent of repletion of amines must depend on the intensities of the effects of reserpine in impairing accumulation of amines, on the degree of inhibition of monoamine oxidase, and on the rates of synthesis and utilization of the amine. Monoamine oxidase inhibitors do not restore the noradrenaline content of the heart of reserpinized mice (CARLSSON and WALDECK, 1967), probably because of the high turn-over rate of cardiac noradrenaline.

In animals pretreated with a monoamine oxidase inhibitor, the amine-depleting action of reserpine is abolished and there is increased behavioural activity rather than depression (PLETSCHER et al., 1956; HOLTZ et al., 1957; CARLSSON et al., 1957a; CHESSIN et al., 1957; SPECTOR et al., 1960, 1963; STEIN and RAY, 1960; CHEN and BOHNER, 1961; CARLSSON, 1961; GREEN and ERICKSON, 1962).

The ability of tissues of reserpine-treated animals to accumulate exogenous noradrenaline is restored by monoamine oxidase inhibitors; in fact, in certain tissues the levels of noradrenaline in the tissue may even exceed that in control tissues (FUXE and HILLARP, 1964; HAMBERGER et al., 1964; CARLSSON, 1965a, 1966; MALMFORS, 1965; NORBERG, 1965; HAMBERGER and MASUOKA, 1965; GLOWINSKI et al., 1966; HÄGGENDAL and HAMBERGER, 1967; KRELL and PATIL, 1972). Similarly, the ability to accumulate serotonin is restored (CARLSSON, 1965b, 1966; BOGDANSKI et al., 1968).

The accumulation of amines that possess an α-methyl group, and are thereby not substrates for monoamine oxidase, is not affected by reserpine treatment in brain tissue (HAMBERGER et al., 1964; CARLSSON et al., 1965).

The antagonism by monoamine oxidase inhibitors of the amine-depleting effect of reserpine has been attributed to prevention of destruction of the released amine. It was suggested that the amine remained in the tissues in a free form (SHORE and BRODIE, 1957b), however, noradrenaline is in fact located in appreciable amounts in the particulate fraction of homogenates (STITZEL and LUNDBORG, 1967), where it is presumably bound. The blockade of monoamine oxidase will alter the equilibrium between free and bound noradrenaline by a mass action effect, as suggested by RAND and TRINKER (1966). However, there is some evidence suggesting that monoamine oxidase inhibitors may interfere directly with the action of reserpine on the storage sites (SCHANBERG and GIARMAN, 1962).

F. Recovery of Amine Stores After Reserpine Treatment

The effects of reserpine on stores of monoamines, and the consequences of these effects for behaviour and autonomic control mechanisms, persist for a considerable time after the drug has been completely eliminated. Consequently, BRODIE and BEAVAN (1963) described reserpine as a "hit-and-run" drug.

The recovery of catecholamine content, as well as the content of other biogenic amines, depends on at least three factors: (i) the disappearance of reserpine from the tissues; (ii) the restoration of amine storage capacity, either by generation of new storage vesicles or by the return of function to previously existing vesicles; (iii) the rates of synthesis of the amines (see Fig. 2). There is no conclusive evidence that a single factor predominates in the recovery of biogenic amine stores; in fact, there is interaction between the factors since the rate of synthesis of noradrenaline is dependent on the binding capacity of the storage vesicle for dopamine. It is difficult to construct a comprehensive review of the recovery of amine contents since there are many methodological differences between the various studies. Thus, a variety of species and tissues have been examined, reserpine has been administered at various doses and for varying periods of time, the methods of analysis have differed, and the times at which analyses have been performed have been chosen arbitrarily.

After the initial depletion of catecholamines by a single injection of reserpine, the tissue concentrations recover slowly, complete return taking several weeks (CARLSSON, 1965a; CARLSSON et al., 1957a). Total recovery of noradrenaline content in the brain, heart and skeletal muscle has been reported to occur in 4 to 5 weeks in the rat and 7 weeks in the rabbit after injection of 10 mg/kg of reserpine (DAHLSTRÖM and HÄGGENDAL, 1966a, b). However, according to CORRODI et al.

(1971) the noradrenaline content of rat heart returns to normal after 12 days. Other investigators have found that 2 to 3 weeks are required for the recovery of catecholamine stores after reserpine in the rabbit (CARLSSON et al., 1957a), rat (PAASONEN and KRAYER, 1958) and dog (WAUD et al., 1958).

The rate of recovery of noradrenaline in adrenergic nerves is most rapid in the first two weeks (HÄGGENDAL and DAHLSTRÖM, 1970). During recovery from reserpine-induced depletion, the amount of noradrenaline accumulating above a ligature on the sciatic nerve exceeds that in control ligated nerves, the overshoot occuring between the second and sixth days (DAHLSTRÖM and HÄGGENDAL, 1969). This overshoot suggests stimulation of synthesis of noradrenaline.

The onset of recovery of endogenous noradrenaline levels after a single dose of reserpine occurs after 24 to 36 h, and corresponds to the restoration of capacity to take up and retain exogenous ^{3}H-noradrenaline (HÄGGENDAL and DAHLSTRÖM, 1970).

Large differences in the rates of recovery of amine content in various monoamine terminal systems of the brain have been reported (FUXE, 1965). In pigeon brain the serotonin content completely recovers by 19 days after reserpine while recovery of noradrenaline content is still not complete (JUORIO and VOGT, 1967). However, BERTLER (1961) found that the recovery of dopamine content paralleled that of noradrenaline in the brains of sheep and rabbits.

Several factors are known to affect the rate of repletion of catecholamines after reserpine. Fasting of rats pretreated with reserpine retards the recovery of the cardiac noradrenaline content (MUELLER and SHIDEMAN, 1968a). Daily injections of sodium phenobarbital for 4 days prior to reserpine results in a less complete depletion and an earlier repletion of cardiac noradrenaline (MUELLER and SHIDEMAN, 1968a). It has not been established whether this effect of phenobarbital is due to induction of an increase in the activity of the liver microsomal enzyme system which metabolizes reserpine (SHEPPARD and TSIEN, 1955), but it seems likely. Daily injections of SKF 525-A, a known inhibitor of hepatic microsomal drug-metabolizing enzymes, retards the repletion of cardiac noradrenaline in the rat (MUELLER and SHIDEMAN, 1968c), but this effect does not appear to be associated with prolongation of the action of reserpine by inhibition of its metabolism. Actinomycin D, an inhibitor of RNA-mediated protein synthesis, delays restoration to normal values of serotonin levels in mouse kidneys (SARTORELLI and MAGUS, 1965) and noradrenaline levels in rat hearts (MUELLER and SHIDEMAN, 1968c) after reserpine depletion of the amines. However, actinomycin D does not affect repletion of catecholamines in the rat adrenal gland after reserpine (MUELLER and SHIDEMAN, 1968c).

The age of the animal also appears to influence recovery from the effects of reserpine. Thus in infant rats (11 days old) there was a more pronounced depletion and a longer time was required to replenish brain catecholamines than in adult rats (KULKARNI and SHIDEMAN, 1966; MUELLER and SHIDEMAN, 1968b). The change with age may be attributed to a lesser ability of infant rats to metabolize reserpine (MUELLER and SHIDEMAN, 1968b).

The return of catecholamine content after depletion by reserpine has been attributed to the return of storage function of existing vesicles in the nerve terminals (ANDÉN and HENNING, 1966; CARLSSON, 1966; ALPERS and SHORE, 1969), or to the synthesis of new storage vesicles (DAHLSTRÖM and HÄGGENDAL, 1966a, b; DAHLSTRÖM, 1970). After a single dose of reserpine which depletes amines within 2 h from both the cell bodies and terminals of adrenergic fibres (DAHLSTRÖM et al., 1965), recovery occurs in the cell bodies long before the amine can be found in the nerve terminals (DAHLSTRÖM and FUXE, 1965; DAHLSTRÖM et al., 1965; NORBERG

1965; DAHLSTRÖM, 1967). Within the cell body, noradrenaline fluorescence appears first in the perinuclear zone (DAHLSTRÖM, 1970). After a dose of 10 mg/kg of reserpine in the rat, the first sign of noradrenaline fluorescence appears in 10 h and in 15 h it is present throughout all the cell bodies and small amounts are in the proximal portions of axons, the axonal transport rate being about 5 mm/h (DAHLSTRÖM, 1967). About 24 h must elapse before fluorescence is detectable in terminal axons (NORBERG, 1965).

Two actions of reserpine must be taken into account to explain the relationship between amine uptake, accumulation and the return of adrenergic function after reserpine (SUGRUE and SHORE, 1971; NORN and SHORE, 1971). One action is the short-lasting blockade of an intraneuronal catecholamine carrier system; the other is a prolonged inactivation of the vesicular storage mechanism. Evidence for the two actions advanced by NORN and SHORE (1971) was that there are two components of reserpine binding: a reversible phase occurring within 18 h of reserpine administration, and an irreversible binding occuring after 30 h. The suggestion was offered that the reversible phase is associated with temporary inhibition of an intraneuronal amine carrier system and the irreversible phase is associated with a permanent alteration of the amine storage mechanism. Because of the permanent inactivation of the storage vesicles, synthesis of new vesicles would be essential for the return of endogenous catecholamine levels to normal values, whereas the temporary reversible phase would account for the relatively fast recovery of adrenergic neurone function.

After depletion of adrenal catecholamines by reserpine, the catecholamine stores are repleted in 5 to 14 days (TAKETOMO et al., 1957; KRONEBERG and SCHÜMANN, 1957a; MUSCHOLL and VOGT, 1958; COUPLAND, 1959; CALLINGHAM and MANN, 1958, 1962). During repletion, there is a considerable overshoot of the noradrenaline content (250% of control) after 7 days followed by a return to the control value in 21 days (CALLINGHAM and MANN, 1962). The ability of adrenal storage granules to accumulate labelled catecholamine returns after reserpine treatment well before the normal levels are restored (LUNDBORG, 1963).

V. Effect of Reserpine on Other Neurotransmitters and Autacoids

Although the main effects of reserpine are due to its actions on adrenergic and serotoninergic mechanisms, it does have effects on other transmitters and autocoids which should not be overlooked.

A. Acetylcholine

In peripheral tissues, treatment with reserpine leads to increases in the acetylcholine content of ileum and heart in the dog (MALHOTRA and PUNDLIK, 1959; MALHOTRA and DAS, 1962) and of heart and blood in the rat (MALPICA et al., 1970). Atria from reserpine-treated rabbits are more responsive to the inhibitory and to a non-nicotinic excitatory action of acetylcholine and vagus nerve stimulation than are those from control rabbits (BURN and RAND, 1958c). Reserpine does not alter skeletal neuromuscular transmission, or the stores of acetylcholine, or the amount of acetylcholine released (LEDDA and BALDI, 1965; BIANCHI and BEANI, 1966). However, the dose of tubocurarine required to induce muscle paralysis in rabbits is increased after pretreatment with reserpine, suggesting an altered excitability of the end plate (CARRIER et al., 1969).

In the brain, treatment with reserpine leads to an increase in acetylcholine content in the dog (MALHOTRA and PUNDLIK, 1959; MALHOTRA and DAS, 1962; MALHOTRA and MEHTA, 1966), the rat (GIARMAN and PEPEU, 1962; MALPICA et al., 1970) and the cat (MALHOTRA and PRASAD, 1968). The effects of reserpine appear to be localized to certain regions since in the dog there is an increase in the acetylcholine content of the hypothalamus, but a decrease in that of the hippocampus (MALHOTRA and PUNDLIK, 1959). These changes in cholinergic systems may be related to the change in electrical activity of the hippocampus produced by reserpi.ne (KILLAM and KILLAM, 1967).

The mechanisms by which reserpine increases tissue levels of acetylcholine have not been elucidated. However, MANDELL and KNAPP (1971) showed that reserpine pretreatment of chicks results in an increase in activity of choline acetyltransferase in the optic lobe.

The effects of reserpine on brain cholinergic systems may prove to be of greater importance than was previously recognized in the light of new evidence about cholinergic-adrenergic interactions. Thus, METER and KARCZMAR (1967, 1971) showed that the block of recruitment produced by inhibition of cholinesterase does not occur after reserpine treatment, but the effect of the anticholinesterase is restored by administration of dopa and a monoamine oxidase inhibitor. Further, the effects of intraventricular choline in dogs are modified by pretreatment with reserpine (SRIMAL et al., 1969). It has been suggested that there may be a relationship between free catecholamines or their metabolites and the increased levels of acetylcholine produced by reserpine since tyramine has a similar, but less pronounced effect to that of reserpine (MALPICA et al., 1970).

An interaction between adrenergic and cholinergic mechanisms has long been recognized in ganglionic transmission. In 1939, MARRAZZI found that adrenaline impaired transmission in the cervical ganglion of the cat. However, catecholamines have also been reported to enhance transmission in some circumstances (MARRAZZI, 1939; BÜLBRING, 1944; MATTHEWS, 1956). It might be expected that reserpine, by altering tissue catecholamine levels, would have effects on ganglionic transmission. COSTA et al. (1961) reported that ganglionic transmission is enhanced in cats and rabbits pretreated with reserpine, but enhancement of ganglionic transmission in animals treated with reserpine is not a constant finding (REINERT, 1963; WEIR and MCLENNAN, 1963; HONG et al., 1965; VOLLE, 1966).

B. Histamine

Histamine is present in parts of the brain that are known to contain other monoamines. ADAM (1961) showed that the regional distribution of histamine in the dog brain follows closely the pattern described for noradrenaline (VOGT, 1954) and serotonin (AMIN et al., 1954). The distribution of histamine in various tissues of the dog is similar to that of noradrenaline after administration of tritiated amines (RYAN and BRODY, 1970). Although mast cells have been suggested as a possible storage site for histamine associated with neural tissues (THORP, 1961), evidence has also been presented for the existence of non-mast cell histamine (GREEN, 1970; RYAN and BRODY, 1970) and, in fact, for the existence of histaminergic sympathetic nerves. In neural tissue, the highest concentrations of histamine have been found in the subcellular fraction containing microsomes and soluble material (EULER, 1958) whereas mast cell histamine is found in the mitochondrial fraction (HAGEN et al., 1959).

After reserpine treatment of dogs, there is an increase in histamine concentrations in splenic, renal, splanchnic, sciatic and phrenic nerves, and in the lung and skin, although reserpine decreases the catecholamine contents of those tissues (Ryan and Brody, 1970). The histamine depletor 48/80 does not reduce the histamine concentration in the autonomic nerves.

Reserpine does not affect the histamine content of mast cells *in vivo* (Parratt and West, 1957). However, neoplastic mast cells exposed to reserpine *in vitro* exhibit ultrastructural changes with swelling of cytoplasmic granules and are significantly depleted of their histamine content (Mannaioni et al., 1968), although reserpine injected intraperitoneally into mice bearing a similar strain of neoplast mast cells does not release histamine from them (Day and Green, 1962). Pretreatment of rat peritoneal mast cells *in vitro* with colchicine, a mitotic inhibitor, decreases the histamine-releasing action of reserpine (Gillespie et al., 1968).

Reserpine treatment of rats decreases the histamine content of the gastric mucosa (Haverbach and Wirtschafter, 1962; Kim and Shore, 1963; Moran and Westerholm, 1963; Shore and Busfield, 1964) but not of the lung, heart and arteries (Johnson, 1970; Howland and Spector, 1972). Pretreatment of rats with the monoamine oxidase inhibitor, pheniprazine, does not prevent the reserpine-induced depletion of histamine from the stomach (Kim and Shore, 1963). Rosengren and Svensson (1969) reported that histamine-forming capacity is increased in the gastric mucosa and decreased in the lung after reserpine treatment of rats. Similar effects on the histamine-forming capacity of the lung and gastric mucosa have been observed after the administration of cortisone (Schayer, 1956) or subcutaneous injection of adrenaline; however, demedullation of the adrenals does not abolish these effects of reserpine (Rosengren and Svensson, 1969). Since reserpine releases adreno-corticosteroids (see Section VIII A 1) it may have an indirect effect on tissue histamine. The effect of reserpine on gastric histamine may be related to its ulcerogenic action which is considered in Section VIII D 1.

Treatment of rats with reserpine does not alter the histamine content of the whole brain (Medina et al., 1969). However, reserpine treatment of cats results in reduction of the histamine content of the hypothalamus and medial thalmus but not of the hypophysial stalk or the anterior and posterior lobe of the hypophysis (Adam and Hye, 1966). Lack of depletion in the hypophysis may be related to the finding that reserpine, *in vivo*, does not release histamine from mast cells, and these comprise the histamine-containing cells of the hypophysis (Adam and Hye, 1966).

The accumulation and retention of ^{3}H-histamine injected into the lateral ventricles of the rat is unaffected by reserpine pretreatment (Snyder et al., 1966). Similarly, reserpine treatment of rats does not affect the catabolism and tissue uptake of circulating ^{3}H-histamine, but alters the kinetics of the subsequent decline of ^{3}H-histamine levels in some tissues (Johnson, 1970).

C. Tryptamine

Tryptamine occurs in mammalian tissue (Hess et al., 1959; Björklund and Falck, 1969) and is formed by decarboxylation of tryptophan (Weissbach et al., 1959). Tryptamine is hydroxylated *in vivo* by liver microsomes to form 6-hydroxytryptamine which appears in the urine (Jepson et al., 1962; Lemberger et al., 1971). Brain slices take up 6-hydroxytryptamine into tryptaminergic neurones where it is believed to replace serotonin (Hökfelt, 1969).

Reserpine decreases tissue levels of ^{14}C-tryptamine and increases its polar acidic metabolites in lung, kidney, ileum and plasma (Lemberger et al., 1971). The increase in acid metabolites would be expected if the amine were being released from intracellular storage sites, and made available for enzymatic degradation by monoamine oxidase.

The findings that certain derivatives of tryptamine have hallucinogenic properties (SZARA, 1956) and that animal tissues are capable of synthesizing N-methylated derivates of tryptamine (AXELROD, 1962b; MORGAN and MANDELL, 1969) have led to the proposal that endogenous tryptamine may play some role in psychotic behaviour (SZARA, 1956; LEMBERGER et al., 1971). The effect of reserpine on endogenous tryptamine may be of some significance for its antipsychotic activity.

VI. Effects of Reserpine on Function of Peripheral Tissues

Animals treated with reserpine display a number of signs indicative of impairment of autonomic control. Typically these include bradycardia, hypotension with peripheral vasodilatation, miosis, relaxation of the nictitating membrane and diarrhoea.

The reduction in sympathetic activity produced by reserpine is generally attributed to the depletion of catecholamines from stores in peripheral adrenergic nerves rather than to the effects of reserpine in the central nervous system (SULSER and BASS, 1968). One reason for this belief is that the reserpine analogue, syrosingopine, depletes noradrenaline from peripheral stores and reduces sympathetic activity in doses that do not cause sedation or an appreciable decrease of brain catecholamines (ORLANS et al., 1960). It does not follow, however, that the actions of reserpine on autonomic function are exerted *only* peripherally: in fact, the view that the autonomic nervous system acts autonomously (as is suggested, albeit erroneously, by its name) has all but disappeared from the thinking of physiologically orientated pharmacologists. There is, however, impairment of peripheral adrenergic function after reserpine treatment.

A. Effect of Reserpine on Adrenergic Mechanisms

1. Responses to Sympathetic Nerve Stimultation

The administration of reserpine results in reduction of responses of effector organs to stimulation of post-ganglionic adrenergic nerves even though the effector organ remains responsive to noradrenaline (BURN and RAND, 1958d; MUSCHOLL and VOGT, 1958; TRENDELENBURG and GRAVENSTEIN, 1958; KRAYER et al., 1962). The loss of peripheral adrenergic transmission has a latency period for onset and occurs some time after the appearance of the usual signs of the reserpine syndrome such as sedation, bradycardia, decrease in blood pressure and relaxation of the nictitating membrane.

The degree of impairment of responses to sympathetic nerve stimulation depends on the extent of depletion of transmitter stores. In dogs, the positive chronotropic response to cardioaccelerator nerve stimulation is completely abolished by reserpine pretreatment only after the catecholamine content of the heart has decreased from 2.5 to 3.0 μg/g to less than 0.3 μg/g (GAFFNEY et al., 1963). In cats, the decrease in responses of the nictitating membrane to sympathetic nerve stimulation is greater with increasing doses of reserpine (TRENDELENBURG, 1961; FLEMING and TRENDELENBURG, 1961). A significant decrease in response of the nictitating membrane and atrium occurs only when the noradrenaline content of these tissues is reduced to 50% of normal and responses to maximal stimulation are still present after depletion of more than 90% of the noradrenaline store (LEE, 1967).

The loss of responses to splanchnic nerve stimulation occurs 8 to 25 h after administration of reserpine in dogs, when the medullary amine stores are considerably depleted (BIANCHI and FARGIER, 1962). As in other tissues, the loss of responses due to catecholamine release produced by splanchnic nerve stimulation is only complete when the adrenal stores have been depleted by at least 90% (LEE, 1967).

The vas deferens from reserpine-treated animals exhibits a reduction in both the frequency and amplitude of spontaneous potentials in the muscle cells (BURNSTOCK and HOLMAN, 1962; BELL, 1969) indicating decreased transmitter release, and contractions in response to stimulation of the hypogastric nerve are reduced (HUKOVÍC, 1961; BURNSTOCK and HOLMAN, 1962; BHARGAVA et al., 1965; BELL, 1969; VAN ORDEN et al., 1967). However, after 99% depletion of catecholamines from guinea-pig vas deferens, contractile responses to hypogastric nerve stimulation were reduced to only 60% of control (WAKADE and KRUSZ, 1972).

A different kind of effect of reserpine on responses of the guinea-pig isolated vas deferens to hypogastric nerve stimulation has been reported by VON EULER (1969, 1970). *In vitro*, reserpine and methoserpidine produce a rapid decrease in responses to stimulation which is rapidly reversible after washing the preparation providing that the exposure time is only a few minutes. This effect of reserpine is probably due to impairment of transmitter release since responses to noradrenaline are not affected. The effects of *in vitro* reserpine on responses to sympathetic nerve stimulation have also been noted in rabbit isolated atria: again there is a reduction in response to stimulation but not to noradrenaline (TODA et al., 1970) and there is a decreased release of noradrenaline from rabbit heart in response to nerve stimulation (KUBO et al., 1970).

Loss of adrenergic transmission after reserpine treatment is not a constant finding. Thus, after reserpine treatment adrenergic nerve stimulation still produces a positive inotropic response in guinea-pig atria (TRENDELENBURG, 1965; BARNETT and BENFORADO, 1966; BLINKS, 1966) and chick hearts (BOLTON, 1967) but the response is abolished in rabbit (HUKOVIĆ, 1959a; TRENDELENBURG, 1965) and kitten (BLINKS, 1966) atria. Activation of liver phosphorylase in rabbits by splanchnic nerve stimulation is not blocked by previous injection of reserpine (SHIMAZU and AMAKAWA, 1968). It has been suggested that there are species differences in reserpine-releasable pools of catecholamines (TRENDELENBURG, 1965).

Reserpine treatment may not only result in the loss of responses to sympathetic stimulation mediated by noradrenaline release, but the response may be replaced by one which is due to acetylcholine release. This has been demonstrated in isolated rabbit colon (GILLESPIE and MACKENNA, 1961) isolated rabbit atria (HUKOVIĆ, 1959b), nictitating membrane, spleen and uterus of the cat (BURN and RAND, 1960b), the cat isolated spleen (BRANDON and RAND, 1961) and the rabbit ear, isolated (BURN and RAND, 1960b) and *in situ* (HOLTON and RAND, 1962). These findings may be explained by an admixture of cholinergic fibres running with the adrenergic fibres in the sympathetic nerve trunk, or by the presence of a cholinergic mechanism in the adrenergic nerves as suggested by BURN and RAND (1959c, 1962, 1965). It has been reported that there is no cholinergic component in the response of the nictitating membrane of the reserpinized cat (MIRKIN and CERVONI, 1962).

2. Responses to Indirectly Acting Sympathomimetic Amines

The pressor response to tyramine in cats and dogs is greatly reduced or abolished after treatment with reserpine (CARLSSON et al., 1957a; BURN and RAND, 1958d; MAXWELL et al., 1959; SCHMITT and SCHMITT, 1960; LOUIS and DOYLE,

1966) as are responses of the cat spleen and nictitating membrane, dog hind leg blood vessels and rabbit ear vessels (BURN and RAND, 1958d). Reserpine treatment also reduces the actions of a number of other sympathomimetics, including phenethylamine, ephedrine, amphetamine, phenylethanolamine, methamphetamine, mephentermine and phenylpropylmethylamine (BURN and RAND, 1958d, 1959a). In the dog heart-lung preparation, reserpine pretreatment decreases the response to ephedrine (INNES and KRAYER, 1958), phenylpropanolamine (LIEBMAN, 1961) and dopamine (BEJRABLAYA et al., 1958) and abolishes responses to tyramine and dexamphetamine (LIEBMAN, 1961). Reserpine has been used as a tool to classify a range of sympathomimetic amines into those acting directly on receptors, those acting only by releasing noradrenaline from stores and those having dual actions. Observations have been made on the blood pressure and nictitating membrane in reserpine-pretreated cats (TRENDELENBURG et al., 1962) and on the rate of beating of atria from reserpine-pretreated guinea-pigs (TRENDELENBURG et al., 1963). The effects of reserpine on indirectly acting sympathomimetic amines has been reviewed by MUSCHOLL (1966).

The extent of the decrease in the response to an indirectly acting sympathomimetic amine is proportional to the dose of reserpine (FLEMING and TRENDELENBURG, 1961; TRENDELENBURG, 1961; LIEBMAN, 1961; WAUD, 1961; MUSKUS, 1962; LIEBMAN et al., 1962; CLARKE, 1967). In guinea-pig isolated atria, the response to tyramine begins to decrease only after reserpine is given in a dose sufficient to cause depletion of atrial noradrenaline by 50% or more (CROUT et al., 1962).

Raunescine and syrosingopine are less potent than reserpine in reducing responses of guinea-pig atria (MUSKUS, 1962) and dog heart-lung preparation (LIEBMAN et al., 1962) when donor animals are pretreated with these alkaloids, but deserpidine is more potent (LIEBMAN et al., 1962).

In man, low doses of reserpine which exert effects on the cardiovascular system do not cause loss of the vasoconstrictor action of ephedrine or amphetamine (WHELAN and SKINNER, 1963), but high doses abolish the adipokinetic action of amphetamine in adipose tissue (PINTER and PATTEE, 1968).

There are residual responses to tyramine in atria from several animal species after reserpine. These findings have led to the suggestion that there are two or more pools of noradrenaline in compartments with different sensitivities to the depleting action of reserpine and the releasing action of tyramine (TRENDELENBURG, 1961; CROUT et al., 1962). Responses of isolated aortas from rats and guinea-pigs are not affected by pretreatment of the donor animals with reserpine although the responses of aortas from pretreated rabbits are considerably reduced: the degree of depletion of noradrenaline from rat and guinea-pig tissue was as great as that from rabbit tissue (MALING et al., 1971).

3. Nicotinic Drugs

The stimulant actions of nicotine and of acetylcholine in the presence of atropine on isolated atria are abolished by pretreatment of donor rabbits with reserpine (BURN and RAND, 1958a, c). Pretreatment of donor guinea-pigs does not abolish these nicotinic effects in isolated atria according to BARNETT and BENFORADO (1966), but LINDMAR (1962) and BHAGAT (1966) noted that responses to nicotine and DMPP are considerably reduced.

Reserpine pretreatment considerably reduces the pilomotor responses to nicotine and acetylcholine in the cat's tail, the contraction of the cat's isolated nictitating membrane in response to nicotine, the vasconstrictor effect of nicotine in the perfused rabbit ear (BURN et al., 1959), the contractions produced by acetylcholine and nicotine in isolated spleen strips from rabbits (MACMILLAN and RAND, 1962) and cats (BRANDON and RAND, 1961) and the inhibitory effect of nicotine on the rabbit isolated colon (GILLESPIE and MACKENNA, 1961).

Pretreatment with large doses of reserpine decreases the pressor response to carbachol in atropinized cats (CARLSSON et al., 1957a) and to acetylcholine in atropinized dogs (SCHAEPDRYVER, 1960; GARDIER et al., 1963), but small doses, producing only partial depletion of tissue catecholamine, have no effect (SCHAEPDRYVER, 1960).

4. Recovery of Adrenergic Function After Reserpine

The return of sympathetic nerve function after reserpine is associated with partial recovery of noradrenergic uptake mechanisms into storage vesicles (ANDÉN et al., 1964; STJÄRNE, 1964; IVERSEN et al., 1965; ANDÉN and HENNING, 1966; CARLSSON, 1966; ALPERS and SHORE, 1969). *In vivo* and *in vitro* studies indicate that 48 h after reserpine, adrenergically innervated tissues are capable of accumulating noradrenaline even though endogenous catecholamine levels remain depressed (IVERSEN et al., 1965; SUGRUE and SHORE, 1971).

DAHLSTRÖM and HÄGGENDAL (1966a, b) proposed that functional recovery in adrenergic neurones is associated with the transfer of newly synthesized granules in the cell body to the nerve terminal. This proposal was largely based on the findings that functional recovery returns within 24 to 72 h and that 18 h after a single dose of reserpine, the first granules formed in the cell body and not affected by reserpine had reached the mid-part of the sciatic nerve. As further evidence for this proposal, HÄGGENDAL and DAHLSTRÖM (1970, 1972) reported that recovery of the ability of adrenergically innervated tissues to take up and store ^{3}H-noradrenaline after reserpine is impaired by axotomy and ganglionectomy.

Effect of Noradrenaline, Its Precursors and Their Analogues. The main observations on restoration of responses to sympathetic nerve stimulation and tyramine after treatment with noradrenaline, noradrenaline precursors and noradrenaline analogues are summarized in Table 2.

The failure of adrenergic transmission produced by reserpine has been reported to be reversed by the administration of noradrenaline or its precursors dopamine and dopa. Thus, restoration of the response to sympathetic nerve stimulation has been demonstrated for cat nictitating membrane (BURN and RAND, 1960a; TRENDELENBURG and PFEFFER, 1964), iris (BURN and RAND, 1960a), uterus and spleen (BURN and RAND, 1960a; PENNEFATHER and RAND, 1960), rabbit ileum (GILLESPIE and MACKENNA, 1961) and guinea-pig vas deferens (HUKOVIĆ, 1961). Infusions of the α-methyl derivatives of dopa, dopamine and noradrenaline are also capable of restoring responses to sympathetic nerve stimulation (DAY and RAND, 1964). The depression of the frequency-response curve to sympathetic nerve stimulation in isolated perfused mesenteric and intestinal blood vessels from dogs treated with low doses of reserpine for 12 months is also reversed by noradrenaline (CLARKE et al., 1970).

It has been reported that responses to sympathetic nerve stimulation are not restored by noradrenaline in atria from guinea-pigs, rabbits and cats (FURCHGOTT et al., 1963; TRENDELENBURG, 1965) and in the dog heart *in situ* (GAFFNEY et al., 1963). Inhibition of monoamine oxidase does not affect the failure of noradrenaline to restore responses in rabbit atria (TODA et al., 1970).

According to BURN and RAND (1960a), dopamine and dopa are more effective than noradrenaline in restoring responses. In reserpinized rabbits, dopamine infusions, but not noradrenaline infusions, restore vasoconstrictor responses in the

Table 2. Effect of noradrenaline, its precursors, and their analogues on adrenergic function after reserpine

Species	Tissue or system	Stimulating agent or procedure	Effective agents for restoring response after reserpine	Ineffective agents for restoring response after reserpine	Ref.
Cat	Atria	Sympathetic nerve stimulation		noradrenaline dopamine	FURCHGOTT and GARCIA, 1968.
		or Tyramine	noradrenaline dopamine		
	Iris	Sympathetic nerve stimulation or Tyramine	adrenaline noradrenaline dopamine (—)-dopa		BURN and RAND, 1960a.
	Nictitating membrane	Sympathetic nerve stimulation or Tyramine	noradrenaline dopamine (—)-dopa		BURN and RAND, 1960a.
			α-methyl-noradrenaline α-methyl-dopamine α-methyl-dopa		DAY and RAND, 1964.
	Spleen	Sympathetic nerve stimulation or Tyramine	noradrenaline		BURN and RAND, 1960a.
	Uterus	Sympathetic nerve stimulation	noradrenaline adrenaline dopamine		BURN and RAND, 1960a. PENNEFATHER and RAND, 1960.
	Blood pressure	Tyramine	noradrenaline dopamine	adrenaline	BURN and RAND, 1960a.
			dopa (—)-α-methyl-dopa		DAY and RAND, 1964.
			(—)-α-methyl-dopa	(+)-α-methyl-dopa	KRONEBERG and STOEPEL, 1963.
Dog	Heart	Sympathetic nerve stimulation		noradrenaline dopamine	GAFFNEY et al., 1963.
	Blood vessels (mesenteric and intestinal)	Sympathetic nerve stimulation	noradrenaline		CLARKE et al., 1970.

Table 2 (continued)

Species	Tissue or system	Stimulating agent or procedure	Effective agents for restoring response after reserpine	Ineffective agents for restoring response after reserpine	Ref.
Guinea-pig	Atria	Sympathetic nerve stimulation		noradrenaline	TRENDELENBURG, 1965.
		Tyramine	noradrenaline α-methyl-noradrenaline α-methyl-dopa (slight)	dopamine[a] dopa[a] tyrosine	FURCHGOTT and GARCIA, 1968.
	Vas deferens	Sympathetic nerve stimulation	noradrenaline		HUKOVIĆ, 1961.
			dopamine α-methyl-noradrenaline α-methyl-dopamine	dopa α-methyl-dopa	DAY and RAND, 1964.
Rabbit	Aortic strip	Tyramine	noradrenaline		FURCHGOTT et al., 1963.
	Atria	Sympathetic nerve stimulation		noradrenaline noradrenaline plus MAO Inhibitor	TRENDELENBURG, 1965. TODA et al., 1970.
		Tyramine	noradrenaline		TRENDELENBURG, 1965.
	Ear blood vessels	Sympathetic nerve stimulation	dopamine	noradrenaline	HOLTON and RAND, 1960a.
		Nicotine	noradrenaline		BURN and RAND, 1960a.
	Colon	Sympathetic nerve stimulation	adrenaline noradrenaline dopamine dopa	tyrosine	GILLESPIE and MACKENNA, 1961.
	Ileum	Sympathetic nerve stimulation	adrenaline noradrenaline dopa	tyrosine	GILLESPIE and MACKENNA, 1961.
			dopamine α-methyl-noradrenaline α-methyl-dopamine α-methyl-dopa		DAY and RAND, 1964.

Table 2 (continued)

Species	Tissue or system	Stimulating agent or procedure	Effective agents for restoring response after reserpine	Ineffective agents for restoring response after reserpine	Ref.
Rat	Atria	Tyramine	adrenaline noradrenaline α-methyl-noradrenaline α-methyl-dopamine α-methyl-norphenyl-ephrine (metaraminol)	dopamine[a] epinine[a] phenylephrine[a] norphenylephrine[a] synephrine[b] norsynephrine[b] isoprenaline	MURNAGHAN, 1968.
	Blood pressure	Tyramine	noradrenaline dopamine (—)-dopa phenylalanine (±)-meta-tyrosine	adrenaline tyrosine	BURN and RAND, 1960a.
			α-methyl-noradrenaline α-methyl-dopamine α-methyl-dopa		DAY and RAND, 1964.

[a] Restoration of response in presence of MAO Inhibitor.
[b] Slight restoration of response in presence of MAO Inhibitor.

ear to sympathetic nerve stimulation (Holton and Rand, 1962). However, in the isolated vas deferens from reserpinized guinea-pigs, responses were restored after incubation with noradrenaline, dopamine or their α-methylated analogues, but not after incubation with dopa or methyldopa (Day and Rand, 1964). These observations suggest either that the amino acids do not enter the adrenergic nerves, or that the activity of dopa decarboxylase is inadequate to form sufficient of the amines. Furthermore, infusion of dopa into reserpinized cats fails to increase the noradrenaline content of the tissues if the cat is eviscerated (Pennefather and Rand, 1960), suggesting that the conversion of dopa to dopamine occurs in tissues which are excluded from the circulation by the evisceration procedure; of these, the liver is probably the critical one.

Responses to tyramine in reserpinized animals can be restored by infusions of noradrenaline (Bejrablaya et al., 1958; Burn and Rand, 1958d, 1960a; Gaffney et al., 1962), precursors of noradrenaline (Burn and Rand, 1960a) or their α-methyl analogues (Kroneberg and Stoepel, 1963; Day and Rand, 1964).

Treatment of isolated atria from reserpinized guinea-pigs, rabbits and cats with noradrenaline restores the positive inotropic and chronotropic responses to tyramine, but not the responses to sympathetic nerve stimulation (Furchgott et al., 1963; Trendelenburg, 1965; Toda et al., 1970). When radiolabelled noradrenaline is used, tyramine causes an efflux of radio-activity (Axelrod et al., 1962b).

Inhibition of monoamine oxidase increases the capability of dopamine to restore the inotropic and chronotropic responses of rabbit atria to tyramine and other indirectly acting sympathomimetic amines (Furchgott and Garcia, 1968; Murnaghan, 1968), but not to sympathetic nerve stimulation (Toda et al., 1970).

The effect of dopamine in restoring responses to tyramine is reduced by disulfiram, an inhibitor of dopamine-β-hydroxylase (Musacchio et al., 1966; Murnaghan, 1968).

5. Sympathomimetic Responses to Reserpine

Although reserpine can deplete tissues of nearly all their catecholamine content, there are few signs of increased sympathetic activity in response to released catecholamines. Reserpine gradually lowers blood pressure without causing an initial pressor response in most animals and in man (Plummer et al., 1954; McQueen et al., 1955; Bein, 1956).

Kopin and Gordon (1962, 1963) showed that the reserpine-induced depletion of catecholamines is accompanied by the release of inactive deaminated metabolites. Thus the appearance of active catecholamines at the site of action is minimal. However, a primary hypertensive response to reserpine has been observed in spinal animals (Jongh and Proosdij-Hartzema, 1958; Schneider and Rinehardt, 1956; Maxwell et al., 1957; Schmitt and Schmitt, 1960), and in animals pretreated with ganglion blocking drugs (Maxwell et al., 1956; Domino and Rech, 1957; Beck et al., 1957). Both these procedures result in considerable enhancement of pressor responses to noradrenaline and adrenaline. The pressor response to reserpine in a pithed rat, which is also sensitive to pressor effects of catecholamines, is shown in Fig. 4. Furthermore, denervated tissues which are supersensitive to noradrenaline respond to administration of reserpine, indicating the release of noradrenaline (from other tissues): thus, reserpine causes contraction of the denervated nictitating membrane (Maxwell et al., 1957) and vasoconstriction in the denervated ear of the rabbit (McQueen et al., 1955).

Reserpine given intravenously to rabbits raises the plasma adrenaline concentration (MUSCHOLL and VOGT, 1957). This effect may explain the hyperglycaemic action of reserpine in rats (TAKETOMO et al., 1957) and in rabbits which is blocked by ergot alkaloids but is not abolished by splanchnic nerve sections (KUSCHKE and FRANTZ, 1955).

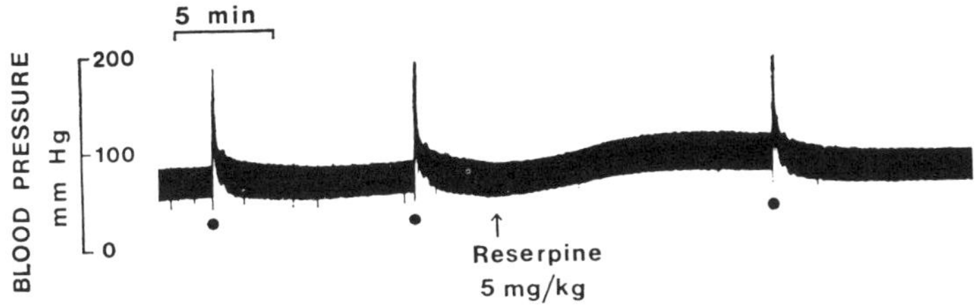

Fig. 4. Pressor response to reserpine injected intravenously in pithed rat. The black dots indicate the pressor response to sympathetic stimulation

The acute administration of reserpine to dog heart-lung preparations markedly increases the rate of beating (PLUMMER et al., 1954; KRAYER and FUENTES, 1958), but only if cardiac noradrenaline stores are intact (PAASONEN and KRAYER, 1958; WAUD et al., 1958; LIEBMAN et al., 1962). Similarly, BRIMIJOIN and TRENDELENBURG (1971) found that the increase in heart rate produced by acutely administered reserpine depends on the release of physiologically significant amounts of noradrenaline and is partly counteracted by a rate-lowering effect which appears to be exerted directly by reserpine on the pacemaker.

Pretreatment of animals with a monoamine oxidase inhibitor results in a pressor response to a subsequent dose of reserpine (PLETSCHER et al., 1956; CHESSIN et al., 1957; GARATTINI et al., 1960b; BONACCORSI, 1968; CASHIN, 1972), presumably because intraneuronal deamination of released noradrenaline is inhibited and more free noradrenaline is liberated. In animals whose cardiac amine stores are loaded with the false transmitter metaraminol (which is not a substrate for monoamine oxidase or catechol-O-methyl transferase), pretreatment with a tricyclic antidepressant to block re-uptake of released amine results in an enhanced release by reserpine or tetrabenazine (CARLSSON and WALDECK, 1965a, 1968; MURAD and SHORE, 1966).

In animals pretreated with amphetamine, tyramine or other indirectly acting sympathomimetic amines, injection of reserpine produces a pressor response (SCHMITT and SCHMITT, 1957, 1959, 1960; BONACCORSI, 1968; CASHIN, 1972). This effect is probably due to "labilization" of the noradrenaline store by the indirectly acting sympathomimetic amine. If a tricyclic antidepressant is given before amphetamine the pressor response to reserpine is prevented (SCHMITT and SCHMITT, 1966), presumably because the access of amphetamine to the noradrenaline store was blocked (BONACCORSI, 1968).

Reserpine has been reported to have pressor effects in hypertensive rats and rabbits (JONGH and PROOSDIJ-HARTZEMA, 1958).

Acute Effects of Reserpine. Although pretreatment with reserpine abolishes the response to indirectly acting sympathomimetic amines when these are administered some 12 to 24 h later, the responses are enhanced when the amines are given immediately after reserpine (SCHMITT and SCHMITT, 1960; NASMYTH, 1962; SCHMITT et al., 1962). The pressor response of the cat to *iso*-monomethylnicotinium bromide (a weak nicotinic stimulant) is markedly enhanced when it is given soon after a low dose of reserpine which itself has no action (EULER and PERSSON, 1970). These effects are probably due to labilization of the noradrenaline stores by reserpine, resulting in facilitated release.

6. Antihypertensive and Peripheral Side Effects of Reserpine

The antihypertensive action of reserpine is often attributed to the loss of vasomotor and cardiac sympathetic tone consequent to the depletion of noradrenaline from the peripheral adrenergic nerves subserving cardiovascular control (GREEN, 1962). However, depletion of noradrenaline from cardiovascular control centres in the hypothalamus and medulla, and from neurones in the lateral horns of the spinal cord which make synaptic connection with thoracico-lumbar sympathetic preganglionic neurones, could also be responsible for the fall in blood pressure. Evidence indicating that loss of peripheral function is not responsible for the effects of reserpine in man is provided by the observations of WHELAN and SKINNER (1963) that sympathetic reflex activity and vascoconstrictor responses to ephedrine and amphetamine are not impaired by treatment with reserpine that results in prolonged peripheral vasodilatation.

Reserpine-treated rats which have been subjected to a procedure for producing renal hypertension (removal of one kidney, clipping of the remaining renal artery) fail to become hypertensive. The isolated perfused hind-quarters of these rats exhibit a lesser increase in the vasoconstrictor action of noradrenaline than do those of untreated hypertensive rats (McQUEEN, 1961). The effect of reserpine was interpreted as prevention of the development of hypertrophy of blood vessels, and hence of reactivity, in response to the hypertension. Reserpine treatment also prevents the rise in blood pressure in rats made hypertensive by clipping one renal artery and leaving the other kidney intact and, as a consequence, fewer renal lesions develop in the untouched kidney (McQUEEN and HODGE, 1961).

The hypotensive action of reserpine is greater in hypertensive patients than in normotensive subjects although the incidence of side effects does not differ between the two groups (McQUEEN et al., 1955). The same finding has been made with animals. The hypotensive effect of reserpine in rats made hypertensive by wrapping the kidney is very much greater than in normotensive rats; furthermore, the threshold antihypertensive dose is ten times less and the slope of the dose effect curve is much steeper in the hypertensive rats (FLÜCKIGER, 1969). Rats made hypertensive with DOCA-salt treatment also give a greater hypotensive response to reserpine than do normotensive rats (GARRETT et al., 1967).

Many of the side effects of reserpine can be attributed to impairment or imbalance of autonomic function. Nasal stuffiness, which is the most common side effect with an incidence of 39% (SIGG, 1968), is probably due to loss of sympathetic vasoconstrictor tone in mucosal blood vessels. There is also conspicuous conjunctival injection (SMIRK and DOYLE, 1954) which is probably due to the same effect. However, dryness of the oral mucosa which is reported by about 3.5% of patients is more likely to be due to a central inhibition of cholinergic secretory tone.

Miosis, which has a reported incidence of 2.5%, is unlikely to be due to imbalance of autonomic tone since the sympathetic innervation of the dilator pupillae plays only a minor role in governing the pupillary aperture. It may be due to increased parasympathetic tone to the constrictor pupillae arising from facilitation of the pupillary light reflex. In animals, the dopamine-containing neurones of the retina are depleted of their amine content by reserpine (MALMFORS, 1963; HÄGGENDAL and MALMFORS, 1963) and this may explain the heightening of the reflex response to light of blepharospasm which occurs in reserpinized animals. Ptosis, which is induced in rats by reserpine, appears to be due to peripheral failure of sympathetic nerve function since it is reversed by an infusion of noradrenaline which can restore responses to nerve stimulation by re-loading the peripheral transmitter stores, but it does not enter the brain (TEDESCHI et al., 1967).

Gastro-intestinal side effects of reserpine include constipation, diarrhoea, abdominal cramps, nausea, vomiting and ulcer formation. Loss of sympathetic control of intestinal function would predictably lead to diarrhoea and abdominal cramps, but it is difficult to attribute the other effects to this. On the other hand, it has been suggested that diarrhoea and abdominal cramps could be caused by serotonin liberated by reserpine (GROSS, personal communication). The ulcerogenic action of reserpine is discussed more fully elsewhere in this review (Section VIII D 1).

Weight gain which commonly occurs in patients treated with reserpine is probably due largely to fluid retention (PERERA, 1955) consequent on the fall in arterial blood pressure: the fluid retention reflects the role of the kidney in long-term arterial pressure regulation (GUYTON, 1971).

Asthmatic attacks and dyspnoea due to reserpine treatment occur in a small proportion of patients (DOYLE et al., 1955; FERGUSON, 1955). Loss of sympathetic bronchodilator nerve function probably explains this effect. Reserpinized guinea-pigs are more sensitive to the bronchoconstrictor effect of histamine than normal guinea-pigs (MCCULLOCH et al., 1967).

B. Effects of Reserpine on Cardiac and Smooth Muscle Function

1. Cardiac Muscle

a) Contractility

Reserpine *in vitro* depresses contractility of frog ventricular strips (NAYLER, 1963) and rabbit atria (TODA et al., 1970), although cardiac noradrenaline content is only slightly reduced by *in vitro* reserpine (CERVONI et al., 1966).

There is a depression of contractility of papillary muscle from reserpine-pretreated cats (LEE and SHIDEMAN, 1959a, b). It has been suggested that endogenous noradrenaline stores were important for the maintenance of normal contractility. PENEFSKY and KAHN (1971) reported that papillary muscle from reserpine-pretreated cats and puppies exhibit decreased tension and velocity in all phases of contraction and relaxation to about 40% of the control values. Furthermore, reserpine pretreatment abolishes the "staircase effect" in cardiac muscle (PENNA et al., 1965). According to WHITRINGTON and ZAIMIS (1961) the heart of the reserpinized cat is in failure.

However, other investigators have reported that reserpine does not change the contractile force of cat heart (TANZ and MARCUS, 1966; SPILKER and CERVONI, 1969) or of cat papillary muscle (CAIROLI et al., 1962). Moreover, no differences have been reported between the frequency-force curves of papillary muscle from normal and reserpine-pretreated cat (FURCHGOTT et al., 1959; KOCH-WESER, 1965; SPANN et al., 1966; SPILKER and CERVONI, 1969) and rabbit atria (TODA et al., 1970). Post-stimulation and post-quiescent potentiation have also been reported not to differ among normal, denervated and reserpine-pretreated atria and ventricles from cats (SPILKER and CERVONI, 1969); these findings suggest that endogenous stores of noradrenaline are not necessary for the production of such changes in the contractile force of cardiac tissue.

The impaired myocardial function observed in dogs treated with low doses of reserpine (25 µg/kg/per day for 4 days) by WILCKEN et al. (1967) was attributed to a direct depressant effect on cardiac contraction since an equal reduction in cardiac catecholamines produced by denervation (DONALD and SHEPHERD, 1964) does not appear to impair myocardial function.

BOLTON (1967) reported that ventricular strips from 6-week old chicks pretreated with reserpine have a greater basal force of contraction and contractile amplitudes in response to field stimulation than do strips from untreated chicks. The increased basal force of contraction in strips from reserpinized chicks is not abolished by doses of β-receptor blocking drugs and by adrenergic neurone blocking drugs which abolish the effects of nerve stimulation in strips from control chicks. It was concluded that the increased basal force of contraction is due to a direct action of reserpine on the cardiac muscle cell. JUREVICS and CARRIER (1973) also observed that reserpine pretreatment resulted in an increase in force of contraction in isolated rabbit atria, and showed that this effect was due to increased sensitivity to the inotropic action of calcium in the medium.

b) Heart Rate

Pretreatment of rabbits with reserpine results in a decrease of the rate of beating of the isolated atria (BURN and RAND, 1958a; AZARNOFF and BURN, 1961; TODA et al., 1970), but pretreatment of guinea-pigs does not affect the rate of their isolated atria (TRENDELENBURG et al., 1963). Reserpine pretreatment leads to a decrease in the heart rate in the spinal cat (FLEMING and TRENDELENBURG, 1961) and in the dog heart-lung preparation (WAUD et al., 1958; INNES and KRAYER, 1958; INNES et al., 1958; ALPER and SCHMIER, 1962). Addition of large doses of reserpine to the dog heart-lung preparation decreases the rate (KRAYER and FUENTES, 1958), although small doses increase the rate by releasing catecholamines. *In vitro*, reserpine reduces the rate of beating of heart preparations (TRIPOD and MEIER, 1954b).

c) Electrical Activity

INNES and KRAYER (1958) observed that the addition of reserpine to the circulation blood in the heart-lung preparation of the dog caused marked shortening of A-V propagation time and a reduction of the functional refractory period of A-V transmission as well as an increase in heart rate. These effects were similar to those produced by a constant infusion of adrenaline. In dogs treated with reserpine 2 to 3 days previously to deplete catecholamine stores, reserpine did not shorten the A-V propagation time or the functional refractory period, but prolonged their duration. The effects of reserpine are also exhibited by raunescine, isoraunescine, deserpidine, and rescinnamine (INNES et al., 1958), but in preparations from dogs pretreated with reserpine all these alkaloids and also ajmaline, serpentine, aricine and α-yohimbine produce slowing and prolongation of A-V conduction and functional refractory period.

Application of reserpine to rabbit pacemaker and atrial tissues prolongs the action potential duration, reduces the size of the overshoot, slows the heart rate and decreases the slope of diastolic depolarization in the pacemaker cells, from which it was concluded that reserpine has direct depressant effects on the cell membrane (TODA, 1960). However, the effects of quinidine and propranolol in depressing the excitability of cat pupillary muscle, and in reducing Na^+ and K^+ exchanges in this tissue, are delayed by pretreatment with reserpine (CHOI et al., 1972).

The duration of repolarization is prolonged in atrial muscle and ventricular strips from reserpine-treated rabbits (MISU et al., 1965). On the other hand, reserpine pretreatment of cats has no effect on the electrophysiological parameters of the heart (SPILKER and CERVONI, 1969).

d) Responses to Cardiotonic Agents

Cardiac Glycosides. Reserpine pretreatment of dogs increases the amount of acetylstrophanthidin required to produce ventricular arrhythmias (ROBERTS et al., 1963), decreases the sensitivity of the chronically digitalized dog to countershock (TEN EICK et al., 1967), and decreases the lethality of digoxin (TAKAGI et al., 1965). In cats pretreated with reserpine, significantly higher doses af acetylstrophanthidin, digitoxin, ouabain and deslanoside are required to induce arrhythmias (LEVILL and ROBERTS, 1967). These studies suggest that catecholamines may be involved in some of the toxic effects of cardiac glycosides, and this view is supported by findings with β-receptor antagonists (see, for example, RAPER and WALE, 1968).

The positive inotropic action of cardiac glycosides is also reduced by reserpine treatment, and numerous studies on the relationship between the cardiac actions of ouabain and endogenous catecholamine stores have been reviewed by TANZ (1967). It has been reported that a minimal ventricular catecholamine content of 8.5% of normal is required for ouabain to exert its maximum positive inotropic effect in cats (TANZ et al., 1968). However, it was pointed out that because reserpine modifies ouabain-induced cardiac responses and also depletes catecholamines, it does not necessarily follow that these two actions of reserpine are causally related. In fact, the ability of the heart to take up digoxin is reduced by reserpine pretreatment of dogs (MARCUS et al., 1966).

Other Cardiotonic Drugs (Excluding Sympathomimetics). The stimulant action of various other agents on the heart has been studied after reserpine pretreatment of donor animals to determine if their action is mediated through the release of catecholamines. Thus, the cardiac responses to nicotine in rabbit atria are abolished by reserpine pretreatment while the response to histamine is unaffected (BURN and RAND, 1958a). Similar findings have also been reported in guinea-pig and cat hearts (TRENDELENBURG, 1960). However, species differences were noted in the effect of reserpine on the stimulant response to serotonin: hearts from reserpinized cats and guinea-pigs remain responsive whereas the response is lost in hearts from rabbits pretreated with reserpine (TRENDELENBURG, 1960).

The positive inotropic effect of the purine compounds adenosine and inosine is reported to be dependent on endogenous catecholamine stores while that of the pyrimidine nucleosides uridine and cytidine is still present after reserpine treatment of rabbits (BUCKLEY, 1970).

2. Smooth Muscle

Reserpine *in vitro* reduces the action of many agonist drugs on smooth muscle (TRIPOD and MEIER, 1954a, b) and causes direct relaxation of horse carotid artery strips and relaxes artery strips contracted by acetylcholine, noradrenaline, adrenaline, histamine, serotonin, $BaCl_2$ and KCl (KIRPEKAR and LEWIS, 1958). However, pretreatment of animals with reserpine over a longer period produces a different pattern of change in vascular reactivity (TRIPOD et al., 1960).

In reserpine-pretreated dogs, vascular resistance is reduced in the perfused hindquarters (BAUM, 1963) and perfused hind leg (MOHAMMED et al., 1968).

However, isolated perfused lateral branches of the femoral artery from normal and reserpine-treated dogs do not differ in intrinsic resistance (CARRIER et al., 1967).

Reserpine pretreatment of rabbits increases conducted spontaneous electromechanical activity in spike-generating vascular smooth muscle (HUGHES and VANE, 1967; SOMLYO et al., 1969). However, the size of the spontaneous spike potentials in the taenia coli is reduced after pretreatment of guinea-pigs with reserpine (DAVIS, 1970).

C. Reserpine-Induced Supersensitivity

An increased sensitivity of vascular smooth muscle to noradrenaline after reserpine treatment of dogs and rabbits was described by BURN and RAND (1958b, d) and has since been confirmed by others working with dog and rabbit vascular preparations (MACMILLAN et al., 1962; TAKENAKA, 1963; BAUM, 1963; FURCHGOTT et al., 1963; CARRIER and HOLLAND, 1965; HUDGINS and FLEMING, 1966; CARRIER and SHIBATA, 1967). In addition, increased sensitivity to noradrenaline after reserpine treatment has been observed in other smooth muscle preparations such as cat spleen and iris (BURN and RAND, 1959b), cat nictitating membrane (TRENDELENBURG and WEINER, 1962), guinea-pig and rat vas deferens (WESTFALL, 1970a, b; POLLOCK et al., 1972), and in cardiac muscle preparations (WESTFALL and FLEMING, 1968a, b).

The effects of reserpine on the sensitivity of various tissues to noradrenaline depend on the experimental procedure. Thus chronic reserpine treatment of the cat produces an increased sensitivity of the nictitating membrane to noradrenaline *in situ*, but not when the membrane is isolated from the cat (BURN et al., 1959; TSAI et al., 1968). There is increased sensitivity of the cat spleen *in situ*, but no supersensitivity to noradrenaline could be demonstrated in isolated spleen strips from cats after reserpine treatment (GREEN and FLEMING, 1968). There are similar differences in responses of the guinea-pig heart *in situ* and isolated (WESTFALL and FLEMING, 1968a).

Various mechanisms have been postulated to account for the sensitivity changes induced by reserpine pretreatment. BURN and RAND (1959b) suggested that fewer receptors were occupied by endogenously released noradrenaline, hence more were available to mediate responses to exogenous noradrenaline. However, short-term treatment with large doses of reserpine which greatly reduce noradrenaline stores does not result in supersensitivity (FLEMING and TRENDELENBURG, 1961; TRENDELENBURG and WEINER, 1962). To explain the faster increase in response to noradrenaline of isolated arteries in dogs after reserpine treatment, CARRIER and HOLLAND (1965) suggested that reserpine increases the effective receptor area on the effector organ. However, supersensitivity does not appear to result from a change in the affinity of the receptor for drugs (GREEN and FLEMING, 1967; TAYLOR and GREEN, 1971). Another explanation for supersensivity to noradrenaline is that neuronal uptake is impaired: such an explanation appears to account satisfactorily for supersensitivity induced by denervation or cocaine, but it is not tenable in the case of reserpine since uptake is not impaired although storage is (see Section IV A and B), and the noradrenaline taken up by adrenergic neurones is rapidly attacked by intraneuronal monoamine oxidase. Recent findings indicate that the role of catechol-O-methyl transferase, but not that of monoamine oxidase, in terminating the action of noradrenaline is increased in vascular tissue after reserpine pretreatment (KALSNER and NICKERSON, 1969).

The most satisfactory explanations for reserpine-induced supersensitivity take into account the fact that it is not specific for noradrenaline. In the rat, the vasoconstrictor action of naphazoline and the vasodilator action of isoprenaline on the perfused hind legs are enhanced after pretreatment with reserpine (SABELLI, 1960), but neither of these drugs is taken up by adrenergic neurones. Supersensitivity after reserpine treatment of rabbits is "relatively non-specific" in that the aortic strips are supersensitive to noradrenaline, acetylcholine and potassium chloride, but not to histamine, serotonin or angiotensin (HUDGINS and FLEMING, 1966). There are also non-specific sensitivity changes in dog and guinea-pig hearts (WESTFALL and FLEMING, 1968a, b) after reserpine. The "non-specific" sensitization to several different agonists after reserpine pretreatment has been attributed to prolonged interruption of the action of the transmitter at the effector cell (see reviews by EMMELIN, 1961, and TRENDELENBURG, 1963, 1966), rather than to a direct action of reserpine on the muscle cell. The development of non-specific supersensitivity in most tissues after reserpine is slow in onset and shows no apparent correlation with catecholamine depletion (FLEMING and TRENDELENBURG, 1961; TRENDELENBURG and WEINER, 1962).

The nature of the change in muscle cells which is responsible for reserpine-induced supersensitivity may be concerned with calcium transport or binding. The supersensitivity of aortic strips from reserpine-treated rabbits to acetylcholine and potassium is entirely dependent on the presence of external calcium, but the supersensitivity to noradrenaline and isoprenaline is demonstrable in calcium-free media (CARRIER and JUREVICS, 1973). Reserpine decreases the calcium content of vascular tissue of young but not old rabbits, and the decrease can be correlated with the development of supersensitivity (CARRIER and SHIBATA, 1967). Less extracellular calcium is required for contractile responses to noradrenaline in isolated artery preparations from reserpinized dogs and rabbits than in control arteries (PEGRAM and CARRIER, 1969; GARRETT and CARRIER, 1971), and the binding affinity for calcium is increased (HUDGINS and HARRIS, 1970; GARRET and CARRIER, 1971; CARRIER and JUREVICS, 1973). The sensitivity of phosphorylase to activation by adrenaline and calcium is increased after reserpine treatment in rabbits (McNEILL, 1969).

Little is known about supersensitivity to transmitters in the central nervous system. However, reserpine treatment of rats increases the sensitivity of brain stem neurones to the excitatory action of iontophoretically applied noradrenaline, but does not modify the inhibitory responses to noradrenaline (BOAKES et al., 1971, 1972).

VII. Effects of Reserpine on Central Nervous Function

The effects of reserpine on the function of the central nervous system are generally thought to be closely linked to changes it produces in the brain levels of the monoamines noradrenaline, dopamine and serotonin.

A. The Sedative and Tranquillizing Activity of Reserpine

A distinction between sedation and tranquillization is largely a matter of definitions. One may regard a drug that allays such symptoms as anxiety, anger and fear without producing somnolence as a tranquillizer. *Rauwolfia* preparations have been known to have such an effect long before they were introduced into modern therapeutics, and the effect is also exerted by reserpine.

The sedative (behavioural depressant) action of reserpine in animals was at first attributed to its effects on brain serotonin, and in particular to an increase in the concentration of "free" serotonin rather than to depletion of stores (BRODIE and SHORE, 1957; BRODIE et al., 1957a, b; SHORE and BRODIE, 1957a, b). Part of the evidence was that morphine, which causes excitement in cats, depletes only noradrenaline whereas reserpine depletes both amines (HOLZBAUER and VOGT, 1956). However, later work showed that the sedative effect of reserpine does not correlate well with its effect on the level of any one amine in the brain (HÄGGENDAL and LINDQVIST, 1964). The best correlation between the sedative action of reserpine and effects on monoamines is with the loss of ability of the brain to accumulate monoamines (BRODIE et al., 1966; GLOWINSKI et al., 1966). There is still fairly recent support for the view that the reserpine-induced behavioural syndrome is mediated through serotonin, the impaired binding of this amine resulting in an increase in that interacting with receptors (BRODIE et al., 1966). However, the bulk of the evidence suggests that the sedative effect of reserpine is due to depletion of catecholamines. Thus PAASONEN and DEWS (1958) observed that raunescine, a *Rauwolfia* alkaloid with a reserpine-like central effect, reduces brain levels of noradrenaline to a greater extent than those of serotonin and argued that the typical reserpine-like central effects are due more to depletion of noradrenaline than of serotonin.

Much of the evidence for the role of particular amines in the functional effects of reserpine on the central nervous system has been obtained from experiments in which the interactions between reserpine and other drugs have been observed.

One complicating factor in the study of the effect of reserpine on the relationship between behaviour and amine levels is the existence of a circadian cycle in the endogenous noradrenaline content of rat brain (FRIEDMAN and WALKER, 1968; REIS et al., 1968; WALKER et al., 1971). A circadian cycle in the rate of depletion of noradrenaline by reserpine has been reported in rat brain (BLACK et al., 1969). It seems possible that some of the conflicting interpretations for the role of individual monoamines in the reserpine-induced syndrome, as deduced from studies of the antagonistic action of monoamine precursors and the use of agents which selectively protect individual monoamine stores, may be reflected in the diurnal variation of endogenous levels of monoamines.

Agents with weak or short-lasting reserpine-like activity confer some protection against the effect of reserpine. Thus, pretreatment of animals with prenylamine (CARLSSON and LINDQVIST, 1966) or tetrabenazine (QUINN et al., 1959) protects against the effects of reserpine, presumably by competition with reserpine for receptor sites. Support for the role of serotonin in reserpine-induced sedation was provided by experiments with tetrabenazine (QUINN et al., 1959). Rabbits pretreated with tetrabenazine and then with reserpine behave essentially as if they had received tetrabenazine alone and recovered from sedation much sooner than those treated only with reserpine. The brain serotonin level at the time of behavioural recovery in rabbits treated with tetrabenazine plus reserpine is normal, but it is still low in the reserpine-treated group. There are no corresponding differences in the noradrenaline content of the brain. However, it has been reported that tetrabenazine does not selectively protect brain amines from depletion in rabbits or mice (CARLSSON and LINDQVIST, 1966).

In rats, *para*-chlorophenylalanine depletes the brain of its serotonin content but does not produce sedation. Moreover, reserpine still has a sedative action in rats pretreated with *para*-chlorophenylalanine (KOE and WEISSMAN, 1966).

In mice, metatyrosine (*meta*-hydroxyphenylalanine) causes a marked but short-lasting depletion of brain noradrenaline and dopamine, but does not affect brain serotonin. There is increased activity following metatyrosine injection. Treatment with metatyrosine provides protection against the catecholamine-depleting action of reserpine and prevents the behaviour syndrome but there is still depletion of serotonin (CARLSSON and LINDQVIST, 1967). In mice pretreated with protriptyline, metatyrosine protects only against the dopamine-depleting action of reserpine, and in such mice the behaviour syndrome is prevented. It was concluded that depletion of brain catecholamines, in particular dopamine, is responsible for the gross behavioural action of reserpine.

One experimental method that has been used to identify the tranquillizer activity of a drug is to determine whether it has selective activity on conditioned avoidance responses. In fact, reserpine blocks conditioned avoidance responses in doses which do not interfere with escape behaviour or bar pressing to obtain food (COOK and CATANIA, 1964). Many other studies on the effects of reserpine in disrupting conditioned avoidance responses have been reviewed by HERZ (1960) and DEWS and MORSE (1961).

There is evidence that the effect of reserpine on conditioned avoidance responses may be due to depletion of catecholamines. Thus, HANSON (1965, 1966, 1967) showed that amphetamine restores conditioned avoidance in reserpine-treated rats, but this effect of amphetamine is blocked by α-methyl-m-tyrosine, although doses of dopa which are themselves too low to reverse the effect of reserpine overcome the block of amphetamine-reversal produced by α-methyl-m-tyrosine. However, experiments of this type are difficult to interpret since the effect of a particular drug given alone may be modified by interaction with other drugs.

Self-Stimulation. Rats with electrodes implanted in various subcortical areas of the brain will engage in repeated self-stimulation. This behaviour is depressed by reserpine (STEIN, 1964). Reserpine pretreatment abolishes the facilitating action of nicotine on self-stimulation (PRADHAN and BOWLING, 1971). It has been suggested that the reinforcement of self-stimulation involves the release of noradrenaline (STEIN, 1964) or serotonin (STARK et al., 1964; MARGULES, 1969).

B. Extrapyramidal Effects of Reserpine

In some patients the prolonged administration of reserpine has been reported to induce extrapyramidal symptoms indistinguishable from those seen in idiopathic and postencephalitic Parkinsonism. The findings that reserpine depletes extrapyramidal centres of dopamine and that the striatal dopamine is reduced in brains of patients with Parkinsonism (EHRINGER and HORNYKIEWICZ, 1960) led to the hypothesis that deficiency of the striatal dopaminergic mechanisms is responsible for the major symptoms of Parkinsonism. Experimental evidence has accumulated to suggest that dopamine acts as a neurotransmitter to mediate inhibition in a nigrostriatal pathway and that acetylcholine functions as an excitatory transmitter between the substantia nigra, pallidum and striatum. In Parkinsonism it is believed that an imbalance exists between the dopaminergic and cholinergic pathways in the direction of cholinergic dominance (see reviews by KLAWANS, 1958; CALNE, 1970; WEISS and CHASE, 1971; BROGDEN et al., 1971). Brain levels of noradrenaline and serotonin are also reduced in Parkinsonism, as after reserpine treatment, but these probably have no significance for the extrapyramidal symptoms since it has been reported that brain noradrenaline levels of patients with Parkinsonism are elevated after treatment with monoamine oxidase inhibitors whereas dopamine levels are unaffected (CALNE, 1970). This is in accord with clinical findings that monoamine oxidase inhibitors confer no benefit in idiopathic Parkinsonism.

The extrapyramidal effects of reserpine are thought to be due to depletion of dopamine from the striatum (see reviews on the role of brain dopamine by HORNYKIEWICZ, 1966, and BERTLER and ROSENGREN, 1959). However, poor results were originally reported with *l*-dopa in the treatment of reserpine-induced extrapyramidal disorders in man (McGEER et al., 1961), although at the time of that report the doses of *l*-dopa tested experimentally in parkinsonian patients generally were lower than in recent years and were of little benefit. Later, larger doses of *l*-dopa and long periods of treatment were found to be effective in the treatment of idiopathic Parkinsonism (see, for example, COTZIAS et al., 1969) and it has been suggested that *l*-dopa can in fact ameliorate the symptoms in reserpine-induced Parkinsonism (DUVOISIN, 1968). It is to be expected that it should since dopa reverses the central effects of reserpine in animals (see Section VII F). Dopa abolishes the tremor produced by reserpine in monkeys with lesions of the lateral cerebellar nuclei (LAROCHELLE et al., 1971).

The akinesia, muscle rigidity, tremor and hunchback posture produced by reserpine treatment in experimental animals are thought to be due to disturbed extrapyramidal function.

Reserpine produces an increase of α-motoneurone and a decrease of γ-fibre activity in rats (STEG, 1964); these effects are of supraspinal origin and are reversed by administration of dopa (ROOS and STEG, 1964). The rigidity and changes in α-motoneurone and γ-fibre activity in rats produced by reserpine are also abolished by amantadine (JURNA et al., 1972): this agent acts by inhibiting dopamine uptake into synaptosomes from rat basal ganglia (HEIMANS et al., 1972), and would thereby facilitate dopaminergic transmission.

In experimental animals, tremor, which is supposedly related to parkinsonian tremor, is induced with tremorine or with *Harmala* alkaloids. There have been a number of studies on the interaction between these effects and reserpine. AGARWAL and BOSE (1967) found that pretreatment of mice with reserpine (or pargyline) reduces the effect of tremorine but increases that of harmaline. Depletion of the catecholamine content of the brain by α-methyl-*m*-tyrosine does not induce tremor or modify the tremor produced by these drugs, from which it was concluded that changes in the catecholamine levels in the brain produced by reserpine are not responsible for its effects on responses to harmaline or tremorine. ZETLER (1957) found that reserpine antagonizes harmine-induced tremor in mice when the two drugs are given together. BOWMAN and OSUIDE (1968) noted that acute administration of reserpine or tetrabenazine depresses the tremor responses to tremorine and harmine whereas chronic treatment potentiates the tremor responses. Akinesia produced by tremorine and harmine is slightly augmented by an acute dose of reserpine whereas chronic treatment does not alter the akinesia. They concluded that changes in catecholamine levels are not directly involved in the tremor and akinesia produced by tremorine and harmine but can influence the responses.

Coordinated but stereotyped behaviour like that produced by amphetamine has been observed in rats 7 to 21 h following an injection of reserpine (RANDRUP et al., 1963; SHIØRRING and RANDRUP, 1968). Similar stereotyped behaviour characterized by locomotion, rearing, sniffing and gnawing is also produced by oxotremorine and other cholinergic drugs such as arecoline and physostigmine in reserpine-sedated rats (KRÜGER and RANDRUP, 1968; AMBANI and WOERT, 1972). Antiparkinsonian drugs of the centrally active anticholinergic type, such as hyoscine, benactyzine, benzhexol, benztropine and caramiphen, abolish completely the stereotyped behaviour in reserpine-treated rats (KRÜGER and RANDRUP, 1968). Benztropine reduces tremors induced by physostigmine in reserpine-pretreated and chlorpromazine-pretreated rats, whereas dopa is effective only in reserpine-pretreated rats (AMBANI and WOERT, 1972). These observations may be related to the effects of reserpine on brain acetylcholine (see Section V A).

C. Effect of Reserpine on Body Temperature

Although the body temperature is the resultant between heat production and heat loss which involve peripheral mechanisms, the regulation of body temperature is due to the activity of central control mechanisms involving catecholamines and serotonin. The effects of reserpine on the body temperature are mainly exerted through its effects on these amines in the central nervous system.

A single injection of reserpine produces a fall in body temperature in the rabbit (BEIN, 1953), monkey (PLUMMER et al., 1954), pigeon (HOFFMAN, 1958a), rat (HOFFMAN, 1958b; TAYLOR and FREGLY, 1962) and mouse (DANDIYA et al., 1960). In rabbits, there is a biphasic temperature response with a rise in the first 30 min followed by a gradual fall which is significant at 3.5 h (SHELLENBERGER and ELDER, 1967). A similar biphasic temperature change is produced by an injection of reserpine into the lateral ventricle of the rabbit (COOPER et al., 1967; BANERJEE et al., 1968). Conversely, intraventricular injection of reserpine in the cat produces an initial fall of body temperature followed by a rise (BANERJEE et al., 1968). After the initial temperature response to reserpine in the cat and rabbit, intraventricular noradrenaline produces a rise in temperature in the rabbit and a fall in the cat (BANERJEE et al., 1968) which parallels the effects of noradrenaline in untreated rabbits (COOPER et al., 1965) and cats (FELDBERG and MYERS, 1965). Similarly, injection of serotonin intraventricularly in untreated (FELDBERG and MYERS, 1963, 1964) or reserpine-treated cats (BANERJEE et al., 1968) produces hyperthermia which is blocked by noradrenaline and adrenaline (FELDBERG and MYERS, 1963, 1964). It has been suggested that the initial temperature effects of reserpine in the rabbit and cat are not due to a direct action but to noradrenaline released from adrenergic nerve endings in hypothalamic temperature-regulating centres (BANERJEE et al., 1968). Pretreatment of rabbits with α-methyl-*m*-tyrosine modifies the usual biphasic temperature response to reserpine, the initial rise in temperature being unaffected while the fall is blocked, suggesting that serotonin is the causative agent in mediating the initial hyperthermic response (SHELLENBERGER and ELDER, 1967).

The administration of imipramine-like drugs before reserpine enhances and prolongs the hyperthermic response to reserpine in rats and prevents the succeeding hypothermia (see Section VII G 1). This is not due to their anticholinergic activity since the administration of atropine-like drugs to reserpine-treated hypothermic rats induces an increase in body temperature (ASKEW, 1963; JORI and GARATTINI, 1965; BERNARDI et al., 1966; REWERSKI and JORI, 1968), which is prevented or reduced by spinal transection (BERNARDI et al., 1968).

Reserpine increases the rate at which rats cool when exposed to low environmental temperature due to impaired vasoconstriction, although piloerection is exhibited and there is a hunched posture (HOFFMAN, 1958a); the failure of the reserpine-treated rat to maintain its body temperature is not attributed to the lack of muscular work. However, impaired free fatty acid and glucose metabolism (GILGEN et al., 1962; MUELLER and MCDONALD, 1968), a decrease in oxygen consumption (LETTAU et al., 1964) and a decrease in insulin levels (MUELLER and MCDONALD, 1968) have been reported in cold-exposed reserpine-treated rats. Physiological doses of thyroxine return the cooling rates of reserpine-treated rats to that of untreated animals but TSH is without effect (TAYLOR and FREGLY, 1962). Survival is significantly increased by pretreatment with hydrocortisone but not with ACTH, suggesting that the adrenal cortex has a decreased responsiveness to ACTH in the cold-exposed reserpine-treated rats (LETTAU et al., 1964). An inadequate mobilization of calorigenic substrate has been proposed as a factor in the production of the hypothermia (MUELLER and MCDONALD, 1968).

D. Electrical Activity of the Brain

It would be expected that a drug having such profound effects on brain function as reserpine would produce marked changes in electroencephalographic activity. However, the effects are slight and their interpretation is difficult, since the relationships between amine levels and electrical activity in particular parts of the brain are not well understood.

The effects of reserpine treatment on electroencephalographic activity in man have been reviewed by FINK (1968). There is decreased α-rhythm activity, an increase in abundance of slow wave patterns and enhancement of bursts and seizure activity.

The effects of reserpine on electroencephalographic activity in animals have been reviewed by LEWIS (1963) and JONVET (1968) and its effect on the reticular formation have been reviewed by KILLAM (1962, 1968). Reserpine pretreatment increases arousal thresholds and abolishes the electroencephalic accompaniment of arousal in cats (KEY and BRADLEY, 1960), and it reduces the cortical potentials evoked by stimulation of the dorsal hippocampus in rabbits (MONNIER and GRABER, 1962). The time course of the changes produced by reserpine in the electrocorticogram of rats is related to changes in brain amines (PIRCH et al., 1967; BROOKS and GERSHON, 1972; BROOKS et al., 1972).

Sleep. Reserpine treatment results in an increase in the time spent in paradoxical (rapid eye movement) sleep in man (HARTMANN, 1966). The alterations in sleep pattern may be associated with the bizarre and disturbing dreams that occasionally occur as a side effect of reserpine treatment (MCQUEEN et al., 1955), and may be related to increased availability of extraneuronal serotonin.

E. Effects of Reserpine on Reflexes and Centrally Maintained Autonomic Nervous Tone

1. Somatic Reflex Activity

The flexor reflex is depressed in spinal cats by reserpine in the presence of a monoamine oxidase inhibitor (ENGBERG et al., 1968). The effect is probably on the central portions of the reflex pathway since reserpine does not modify the behaviour of sensory receptors, at least, in the skin of cats (IGGO and MUIR, 1969). The depressant effect of reserpine on the flexor reflex is partially reversed by the serotonin antagonist methysergide, suggesting that it may be due to excess of free serotonin (ENGBERG et al., 1968).

Reserpine pretreatment of cats prevents the development of decerebrate rigidity (HERMAN and BARNES, 1967; BARNES and POMPEIANO, 1971) and blocks tension responses of the gastrocnemius-soleus to stimulation of the ipsilateral VIIIth nerve (BARNES and POMPEIANO, 1971).

Blepharospasm in response to light is facilitated by reserpine treatment. Blepharospasm is the result of somatic muscle contraction, whereas the reserpine-induced effect of ptosis occurs in the dark and is due to failure of adrenergic transmission to smooth muscle (TEDESCHI et al., 1967).

2. Autonomic Reflexes

WHELAN and SKINNER (1963) reported that reserpine treatment in man exerting a prolonged vasodilator action does not interfere with sympathetic reflex activity. However, MASON and BRAUNWALD (1964) found that long term reserpine therapy does result in a decrease of reflex vasoconstriction elicited by cold stimulation. Nevertheless, since hypotensive episodes in man are rare with small doses of reserpine, it is likely that cardiovascular reflexes are not greatly impaired.

In dogs, reserpine reduces cardiovascular reflexes (SCHAEPDRYVER, 1960) and abolishes the reflex vasodilatation elicited by an intravenous injection of noradrenaline in perfused hind quarters (BECK and BRODY, 1961) and hind leg (MOHAMMED et al., 1968).

The rise in plasma free fatty acid elicited by anxiety-provoking electric shocks is abolished by reserpine (KHAN et al., 1964). However the cardiovascular concomitants of a conditioned withdrawal reflex are not abolished, although the conditioned withdrawal is abolished (GANTT, 1960); the latter finding may be related to the specific tranquillizing activity of reserpine.

The loss of circulatory reflexes to carotid body and sinus stimulation produced by reserpine in experimental animals can be largely explained in terms of peripheral failure of adrenergic transmission. However, injection into the vertebral arteries of cats of small doses of reserpine which do not deplete peripheral catecholamines leads to loss of chemoreceptor reflexes in parallel with a decrease in central catecholamines (ZWIETEN et al., 1966).

In acute experiments injection of reserpine is reported to modify cardiovascular reflexes (BEIN, 1953, 1955; MCQUEEN et al., 1955). This is probably due to central effects of reserpine and is probably attributable to the release of amines during the acute phase of depletion.

3. Activity in Autonomic Nerves After Reserpine

a) Sympathetic Nerves

Electrical activity in the sympathetic nerves to the heart in the cat is reduced by reserpine (BEIN, 1955) but there is no change or possibly a slight increase in activity in cervical sympathetic nerves (IGGO and VOGT, 1960; SCHMIDT et al., 1968). There is a decrease in splanchnic nerve activity in dogs and cats (DONTAS, 1956; MCCUBBIN and PAGE, 1958); however, this finding is apparently at variance with data regarding the role of the splanchnic nerves in the amine-depleting action of reserpine in the adrenal medulla (see Section III C).

Neuronal activity facilitates the reserpine-induced depletion of noradrenaline from adrenergic neurones in the spinal cord since there is greater depletion above than below a spinal transection (ANDÉN et al., 1966, 1967). Most of the spinal adrenergic nerves are concerned with sympathetic activity. There is no difference in the serotonin-depleting action above and below the spinal transection. GLOVER and MCCULLOCH (1970) also provided evidence that reserpine has a greater effect when activity is present since it is less effective in impairing responses to sympathetic nerve stimulation in pithed rats than in those with an intact central nervous system.

b) Parasympathetic Nerves

The effects of miosis, lacrimation and salivation produced by reserpine are due to central stimulation of the parasympathetic centres concerned with these functions since section of the efferent parasympathetic nerves abolishes the effects (BOGDANSKI et al., 1961).

F. Recovery from the Central Actions of Reserpine

There are many reports that there is recovery from the sedative action of reserpine within 48 h while brain amine content remains low. These observations have led to the suggestion of a dissociation of brain monoamine content and sedation (Bertler, 1961; Brodie and Costa, 1962; Carlsson et al., 1963a).

After a single dose of reserpine or after the cessation of chronic reserpine treatment, recovery from the effects, as assessed in various behavioural tests, occurs in 1 to 8 days. Recovery of spontaneous locomotor activity in the rat occurs within 1 day when measured in an enclosed chamber by means of photocells (Magus et al., 1964) and in open field exploration (Faith et al., 1968), but in 3 days when measured in a circular alley (Pirch et al., 1967).

Recovery from ptosis (Rubin et al., 1957), from abnormal tone and hunched posture (Faith et al., 1968) and of electro-corticogram activity (Pirch et al., 1967) are complete or nearly complete 2 days after reserpine. Recovery of the conditioned avoidance response does not occur until more than 8 days after reserpine (Rech, 1964; Levison and Freedman, 1967; Faith et al., 1968). It has been suggested that the different durations of action reflect differences in neurochemical effects of the reserpine in the brain (Faith et al., 1968).

Effects of Amino Acid Precursors of Catecholamines and Serotonin on Recovery. An indication of the relative roles of the catecholamine and serotonin contents of brain as determinants of behaviour has been obtained with the use of precursors of these amines. The precursor of noradrenaline, dopa (the *dl*-form was used), reverses reserpine-induced ptosis and sedation in mice and rabbits, whereas 5-hydroxytryptophan, the precursor of serotonin, does not antagonize these effects; a combination of both amino acids was found to be more effective than dopa alone (Carlsson et al., 1957b). The store of catecholamines in the brain is repleted by injections of dopa (Carlsson et al., 1957b; Blaschko and Chruściel, 1960). The findings that dopa reverses the central effects of reserpine, and that 5-hydroxytryptophan does not, have been confirmed (Holtz et al., 1957; Everett and Toman, 1959; McGeer et al., 1963; Wada et al., 1963; Graeff et al., 1965; Butcher et al., 1972). However, the reversal of some effects of reserpine by 5-hydroxytryptophan has been reported (Chen and Bohner, 1961).

Although administration of the amino acid precursor of noradrenaline or serotonin raises the level of the particular amine in the brain, it has been suggested that this does not provide definitive evidence of the role of that amine in normal tissues since the distribution of an amine in the brain after a large dose of its amino acid precursor may not correspond to the normal distribution of that amine (McGeer et al., 1963; Bertler et al., 1966). A further complication arises from the finding that brain noradrenaline is released by 5-hydroxytryptophan when that substance is given in doses that cause excitation (Brodie et al., 1966); on the other hand, dopa partially protects serotonin stores in the brain from depletion by reserpine (Butcher et al., 1972).

Specific effects of reserpine that are reversed by dopa include gastric secretion (Kim and Shore, 1963), conditioned avoidance (Hanson, 1967; Seiden and Peterson, 1968), motoneurone activity (Roos and Steg, 1964): reversal of responses to sympathetic nerve stimulation is discussed elsewhere (Section VI A 4).

In man, dopa is reported to counteract the psychological effects of reserpine (Degkwitz et al., 1960), and the extrapyramidal symptoms (see Section VII B). The reversal of reserpine-induced catatonia in mice by dopa is directly correlated with brain dopamine levels (Horst et al., 1973).

However, it has been reported that dopa alone causes little change in behaviour and fails to reverse reserpine-induced miosis, relaxation of the nictitating membrane and diarrhoea, whereas dopa given after a monoamine oxidase inhibitor produces a state of intense excitation which is associated with an increase in the level of noradrenaline in the brain (REIS et al., 1970). There are other reports that the reversal of the behavioural effects of reserpine by dopa is enhanced by additional treatment with a monoamine oxidase inhibitor (CARLSSON et al., 1957b; BLASCHKO and CHRUŚCIEL, 1960; CHEN and BOHNER, 1961). Methyldopa, which forms the false transmitters α-methyldopamine and α-methylnoradrenaline that are not attacked by monoamine oxidase, reverses reserpine-induced sedation (DAY and RAND, 1963b), although in normal rats it produces sedation.

G. Interaction Between Reserpine and Other Centrally Acting Drugs

1. Tricyclic Antidepressant Drugs

The behavioural depressant effects of reserpine in animals are abolished by subsequent administration of drugs of the imipramine type (tricyclic antidepressants). This was observed with imipramine itself (DOMENJOZ and THEOBALD, 1959) and with a number of its congeners (GILLETTE et al., 1961; SULSER et al., 1964; SIGG et al., 1965; JORI et al., 1966). The reversal of reserpine-induced behavioural depression forms the basis of a screening test for antidepressant activity (SULSER et al., 1961). In rats, the most potent amongst a series of clinically useful antidepressants has been found to be desipramine, followed by imipramine and then by dibenzepine, nortriptyline and amitriptyline with about one-tenth the potency of desipramine (STILLE et al., 1965).

Depression may develop in hypotensive patients treated with *Rauwolfia* preparations (QUETSCH et al., 1959), reserpine (KLEIN, 1968) or methoserpidine (BERLIN, 1965). Desipramine reverses the depressant action of reserpine in patients (PÖLDINGER, 1963).

The hypothermic effect of reserpine in rats and mice, which is due to actions exerted in the central nervous system (see Section VII C), is also abolished by subsequent administration of tricyclic antidepressants (COSTA et al., 1960; GARATTINI et al., 1962; ASKEW, 1963; BOISSIER et al., 1966; JORI et al., 1966; GARATTINI and JORI, 1967). The tricyclic antidepressants are active in this respect if they are injected into the cerebral ventricles of reserpinized animals (BERNARDI et al., 1966). In general, it is easier to reverse the hypothermic than the sedative effects of reserpine with tricyclic antidepressants.

The effect of tricyclic antidepressants in reversing the sedative and hypothermic effects of reserpine is attributed to their action in blocking the re-uptake of released amines across the axonal membranes. The amounts of transmitter amines released in reserpinized animals are too low to be effective, but after blockade of re-uptake they remain longer and in higher concentrations at their sites of action in synaptic clefts and thereby become effective as transmitters. The small amounts that are released are generated by continued synthesis since inhibition of synthesis as a result of treatment with α-methyl-*m*-tyrosine abolishes the effect of antidepressants in reversing the sedative action of reserpine (SULSER et al., 1964).

In animals pretreated with tricyclic antidepressant drugs, reserpine produces increased behavioural activity instead of sedation (SULSER et al., 1964). Again, this effect is due to blockade of re-uptake of released amines across the axonal membrane. As a consequence, the amounts of noradrenaline and its metabolites released into perfusates from a push-pull cannula inserted into the rat hypothalamus are increased, the relative proportion of free plus O-methylated noradrenaline being greater and that of deaminated metabolites being lower than in controls (SULSER et al., 1969). Tricyclic antidepressants, unlike monoamine oxidase inhibitors, do not prevent the depletion of catecholamines and serotonin from the brain although they decrease the rate of depletion (COSTA et al., 1960; GARATTINI et al., 1962; PLETSCHER and GEY, 1962; BARTONICEK, 1965; MANARA et al., 1966).

The interactions between reserpine and tricyclic antidepressant drugs on peripheral tissues appear to differ from those occurring in the central nervous system. Thus, desipramine does not affect the failure of responses to sympathetic nerve stimulation induced by reserpine in pithed rats (GLOVER and MCCULLOCH, 1970). However, when desipramine is given before pithing it delays the effect of reserpine in decreasing responses to sympathetic stimulation. MANARA et al. (1966) showed that desipramine-pretreatment slows the rate of depletion of noradrenaline from the heart by reserpine. Desipramine decreases the turnover rate of noradrenaline in the heart and elevates the endogeneous level (NEFF and COSTA, 1967); however this may not explain its effect in slowing the rate of depletion by reserpine since in the brain the turnover rate of noradrenaline is increased by desipramine (NEFF and COSTA, 1967), but the rate of depletion by reserpine is slowed as in the heart.

The findings suggest that the interaction between reserpine and tricyclic antidepressants is confined to their actions in the central nervous system. This conclusion could explain the observations that imipramine and desipramine inhibit the effect of reserpine in releasing catecholamines from the adrenal medulla (ZBINDEN, 1962; SHORE and BUSFIELD, 1964) since there is evidence that centrally mediated splanchnic nerve activity is involved in the release of medullary amines by reserpine (see Section III C).

Reserpine produces narrowing of the palpebral fissure either by producing ptosis, which is due to loss of peripheral adrenergic transmission to smooth muscle, or to blepharospasm, which is due to a reflex involving motoneurones and striated muscle, or to both (TEDESCHI et al., 1967). There have been many reports that tricyclic antidepressants antagonize the effect of reserpine on the palpebral fissure (RUBIN et al., 1957; COSTA et al., 1960; CHEN and BOHNER, 1961; MAXWELL and PALMER, 1961; GARATTINI et al., 1962; HALLIWELL et al., 1964; SULSER et al., 1964; ACETO and HARRIS, 1965; COTILLO and BONACCORSI, 1972). The effect has been variously referred to as reversal of ptosis and reversal of blepharospasm. It would appear highly likely that what has been observed in all cases is reversal of blepharospasm which has resulted from an interaction of the drugs on the reflex pathways in the brain.

Other Drugs Related to the Tricyclic Antidepressants. Certain antihistamines antagonize the behavioural depressant action of reserpine (SIGG et al., 1965; GARATTINI and JORI, 1967). This effect is not related to specific antihistamine activity but probably to blockade of catecholamine uptake as occurs with the tricyclic antidepressants (GARATTINI and JORI, 1967; ISAAC and GOTH, 1965; CARLSSON and LINDQVIST, 1969).

The amine-depleting action of reserpine is reduced by chlorpromazine (GEY and PLETSCHER, 1964), which also has uptake blocking activity.

2. Amphetamines

Pretreatment with reserpine confers protection against the enhanced toxicity of amphetamine in grouped mice (LASAGNA and MCCANN, 1957; BURN and HOBBS, 1958). This effect may be allied to the tranquillizing action of reserpine which is associated with catecholamine depletion, or to the hypothalamic action of reserpine.

The central stimulant actions of amphetamine and methamphetamine are, however, still present in reserpinized rats and mice (BRODIE and SHORE, 1957; ROSSUM et al., 1962; SMITH, 1963) and monkeys (COLE and GLEES, 1957). Put another way, amphetamine antagonizes the central depressant action of reserpine. The increase in motor activity and social interaction produced in rats by amphetamine is enhanced after reserpine treatment (MORPURGO and THEOBALD, 1966). However, these effects are variable and occur only in those animals that suffer marked loss of weight as a result of reserpine treatment (FIBIGER et al., 1972).

It is thought that amphetamine accelerates the release of newly formed noradrenaline and even though the store is small, the response to amphetamine remains as long as synthesis is not impaired (WEISSMAN et al., 1966; DINGELL et al., 1967; HANSON, 1967; SULSER et al., 1968). This explanation raises the question of why the peripheral sympathomimetic effects of amphetamines are abolished by reserpine pretreatment. One possible reason for the difference is that the rate of synthesis of noradrenaline is greater in central than in peripheral adrenergic neurones, another is that residual stores of catecholamines are larger in central adrenergic neurones. Another factor that has to be taken into account is the time course of the action of reserpine, which may differ in different tissues. In the first two hours after the administration of reserpine, the peripheral sympathomimetic effect of amphetamine is enhanced and is only lost after 12 or more hours (SCHMITT and SCHMITT, 1960).

3. Lysergide

The interaction of reserpine and lysergide (LSD-25) on behaviour has been studied in both experimental animals and humans. The effect of reserpine in prolonging hexobarbital sleeping time is antagonized by lysergide (SHORE et al., 1955) and by 2-bromolysergide (SALMOIRAGHI et al., 1956), but reserpine enhances the effect of lysergide in impairing the performance of hungry rats climbing a rope to obtain food (WINTER and FLATAKER, 1956). The timing of the two drugs is evidently an important factor in determining their interaction. It was reported that reserpine given acutely enhances the effects of lysergide but after chronic pretreatment with reserpine the effects of lysergide are reduced or abolished (ISBELL and LOGAN, 1957). However, it has also been reported that pretreatment with reserpine enhances and prolongs the effects of lysergide (APPEL and FREEDMAN, 1964; RESNICK et al., 1965). The doses of the drugs must also be taken into account. Thus, in rats pretreated with reserpine, low doses of lysergide or methysergide reverse the blepharospasm and sedation, but high doses of lysergide produce convulsions, aggressive and hostile behaviour and vocalization (VOTAVA et al., 1967).

In man, treatment with reserpine alters the subjective effect of lysergide in that it was reported to evoke unpleasant and unusual hallucinations described as a hissing sound in the back of the head culminating to an expanding flash of light (ISBELL and LOGAN, 1957). The side effects of tremor and nausea produced by reserpine are enhanced by lysergide.

Lysergide elevates brain serotonin levels (FREEDMAN, 1961, 1963; FREEDMAN and GIARMAN, 1962; VOTAVA et al., 1967) and reduces the levels of noradrenaline and dopamine (VOTAVA et al., 1967). After depletion of brain amines by reserpine treatment, it has been reported that lysergide does not increase serotonin levels, nor does it produce an additional decrease in catecholamine levels (VOTAVA et al.,

1967); however, there are other findings that lysergide does increase serotonin levels (APPEL and FREEDMAN, 1964).

4. Convulsants

Severe reactions to electroconvulsive therapy have been reported in patients undergoing treatment with reserpine (FOSTER and GAYLE, 1955) and it is now generally recognized that such therapy is contraindicated (GONZALEZ and IMAHARA, 1964).

In rats, low doses of reserpine facilitate electroshock seizures whereas high doses inhibit the seizures (KOSLOW and ROTH, 1971). Reserpine facilitates drug-induced convulsions in mice (CHEN et al., 1954) and causes loss of the anticonvulsant effectiveness of diphenylhydantoin and acetazolamide (GRAY et al., 1963). The anticonvulsant effect of acetazolamide can, however, be produced by raising the dose even if a very large dose of reserpine has been given (KOSLOW and ROTH, 1971). The reserpine-induced effect of facilitation of seizures provoked by leptazol is abolished by methamphetamine (KOBINGER, 1958).

The lowering of the extensor seizure threshold by reserpine in mice has been ascribed to a depletion of brain biogenic amines (CHEN et al., 1968). The reduction by reserpine of the threshold for electroshock-induced convulsion in mice correlates with the reduction of brain levels of catecholamines and serotonin (AZZARO et al., 1972). Injection of reserpine into the cerebral ventricles intensifies audiogenic seizures at a time when noradrenaline levels are markedly reduced but dopamine levels are only moderately lowered, suggesting that noradrenaline exerts an inhibitory effect to limit the spread of seizure discharge (JOBE et al., 1973). However, low doses of reserpine, which did not produce a significant depletion of brain amines, still antagonized the anticonvulsant action of acetazolamide (GRAY and RAUH, 1967).

The effects of convulsants are thought to be due to blockade of the action of inhibitory amino acid transmitters in the central nervous system. It is of interest, therefore, to note that the brain concentrations of glutamic acid, glutamine, aspartic acid and γ-aminobutyric acid in the cat are decreased after treatment with reserpine and the turnover rates were increased 3-fold (BERL and FRIGYESI, 1969).

The convulsant activity and lethality of digitoxigenin in rats and mice is reduced by pretreatment with reserpine, syrosingopine or tetrabenazine in doses which deplete brain stores of biogenic amines (LAGE and SPRATT, 1967; BUTTERBAUGH and SPRATT, 1970). However these drugs are of a different type to those generally recognized as convulsants (picrotoxin, leptazol, strychnine) and their mode of action is probably different.

VIII. Endocrinological, Metabolic and Structural Effects of Reserpine

A. Effects of Reserpine on Endocrine Systems

1. Pituitary-Adrenal Axis

Reserpine evokes in experimental animals a biochemical picture strikingly similar to the classical responses to stress (BEIN, 1956; WELLS et al., 1956). Thus, there is a fall in adrenal ascorbic acid, a rise in plasma corticosterone, an increase in liver tryptophan pyrrolase activity, an increase in the weight of the adrenal glands and an excessive mobilization of free fatty acids from fat depots (KRUGER et al., 1960b; MAICKEL et al., 1961; MONTANARI and STOCKHAM, 1962b; CHATTERJEE, 1965; TAYLOR, 1972). The toxicity of reserpine in rats is greatly increased by adrenalectomy (GAUNT et al., 1954; MONTANARI and STOCKHAM, 1962a). This effect is probably due to the loss of the protective action of corticosteroids against the stress imposed by reserpine.

Reserpine depletes CRF from the median eminence of the hypothalamus (BHATTACHARYA and MARKS, 1969) and ACTH from the anterior pituitary (MAHFOUZ and EZZ, 1958; KITAY et al., 1959; SAFFRAN and VOGT, 1960; MAICKEL et al., 1961; BHATTACHARYA and MARKS, 1969). The ACTH depletion occurs only with doses of reserpine that lower the brain amine stores by 50% or more, and the failure of rats to respond to stressful stimuli after such large doses of reserpine has been attributed to an exhaustion of pituitary ACTH stores (WESTERMANN et al., 1962). Small doses of reserpine induce a smaller loss of ACTH and the animals are thus able to respond to cold-exposure by an elevation of corticosterone (MAICKEL et al., 1961; WESTERMANN et al., 1962). Ascorbic acid in high doses has been reported to reduce the hyperactivity of the pituitary corticotrophins evoked by reserpine (CHATTERJEE, 1965; BARDHAN and CHATTERJEE, 1969).

It has been suggested that the effect of reserpine in releasing ACTH is due to changes in serotonin in neuronal pathways concerned with anterior pituitary release, since α-methyl-*m*-tyrosine, which selectively depletes noradrenaline stores, does not induce ACTH release (WESTERMANN et al., 1962).

2. Thyroid

A single injection of reserpine inhibits release of thyroxine from the thyroid in the rabbit (HARRISON, 1961) and reserpine is of benefit in the treatment of thyrotoxicosis and protects against "thyroid storm" (HARRISON, 1964). However, there are still conflicting views as to the role of the autonomic nervous system in mediating the symptoms of hyperthyroidism, thus the manner by which reserpine exerts its normalizing effect in thyrotoxicosis is not clearly understood. It is not certain to what extent an excessive adrenergic influence on the cardiac pacemaker (BREWSTER et al., 1956), a deficient cholinergic (vagal) influence (HOFFMANN et al., 1947) or a direct action of thyroxine (CAIROLI and CROUT, 1967) contribute to the tachycardia of thyrotoxicosis.

There is a proportionately greater fall in heart rate after reserpine in thyroxine-treated animals than in euthyroid animals (CAIROLI and CROUT, 1967). The bradycardia induced by reserpine is reversed by atropine in both euthyroid and thyroxine-treated animals (BRAY, 1964; BOGDANSKY et al., 1961) suggesting that there is an increase in parasympathetic activity as well as a decrease in adrenergic activity after reserpine. However, it has been reported that neither bilateral vagotomy nor atropine abolishes reserpine-induced bradycardia in the intact animal (RAAB et al., 1961; TANZ and MARCUS, 1966). It has also been suggested that reserpine may induce a greater activity of efferent vagal impulses in thyroxine-treated animals than in normal animals by an action mediated in the central nervous system (CAIROLI and CROUT, 1967).

3. Reproductive Hormones

Hypothalamic and pineal mechanisms mediated by catecholamines, serotonin and melatonin are generally believed to be concerned in the secretion of gonadotropins although it is not possible to correlate precisely changes in specific amines with endocrinological actions of reserpine.

Administration of reserpine to experimental animals inhibits gonadotropin secretion and ovarian oestrogen production. This is manifested as effects on oestrous (CRANSTON, 1958), ovulation (PURSHOTTAM, 1962; HOPKINS and PINCUS, 1963; BROWN, 1966), vaginal histology (BENSON, 1958), milk secretion (MEITES et al., 1959), pituitary histology (PASTEELS, 1961), implantation (MAYER et al., 1960) and egg transport (BENNETT and KENDLE, 1967).

Reserpine delays development in puberty (KHAZAN et al., 1960), but this does not appear to be a result of depletion of brain catecholamines (WEINER and GANONG, 1971). Reserpine blocks spontaneous ovulation when administered before the critical period (BARRACLOUGH and SAWYER, 1957; FRANCE, 1970), possibly by a direct effect of reserpine on the ovary (PURSHOTTAM, 1962; HOPKINS and PINCUS, 1963; FRANCE, 1970). However, reserpine treatment of rats prevents the fall in pituitary FSH content normally occurring between the age of 34 and 39 days (BROWN, 1971).

Intraperitoneal administration of reserpine (COPPOLA et al., 1965) and implantation of reserpine into the median eminence of rabbits and rats (KANEMATSU and SAWYER, 1963; MAANEN and SMELIK, 1968) induces pseudopregnancy whereas implantation into the pituitary (KANEMATSU and SAWYER, 1963) has no effect.

Reserpine lowers pituitary prolactin content and induces lactation (KANEMATSU et al., 1963). This effect of reserpine may be due to a depression of prolactin-inhibiting factor of the hypothalamus, thus removing the hypothalamic inhibition to pituitary prolactin release (RATNER et al., 1965). The mammotropic and lactogenic effects of fifteen reserpine analogues have been reported by BEN-DAVID et al. (1968).

Melatonin. No references to the effect of reserpine on the melatonin content of the pineal gland have been found. However, SNYDER and AXELROD (1965) reported that reserpine abolishes the circadian rhythm in the serotonin content of the pineal gland and this amine is a precursor of melatonin. Thus, in reserpinized rats the content of serotonin during the day is decreased and at night it is increased, in relation to levels in control rats, and the level remains constant through the 24 h period. Sympathetic denervation has the same effect as reserpine, hence the effect of reserpine may be due to failure of adrenergic transmission, or to disruption elsewhere in the retinal-pineal reflex.

B. Electrolyte Metabolism

Reserpine treatment of animals alters the electrolyte metabolism in a variety of tissues. There is loss of myocardial potassium accompanied by cardiac decompensation in rats treated with reserpine (TROQUET et al., 1966). Vascular tissues from dogs, rabbits and rats treated with reserpine have less calcium (CARRIER and SHIBATA, 1967), sodium and potassium (CARRIER et al., 1967) than do control tissues. However, the calcium loss is transient, the maximum loss occurring at 2 to 4 h after reserpine following which the levels return to control or above control by 24 h (GARRETT et al., 1970), and it occurs only with relatively high doses of reserpine (GARRETT and CARRIER, 1971). In guinea-pig vas deferens, reserpine treatment produces an elevation in the magnesium content but no change in calcium, sodium or potassium (WESTFALL, 1970b).

Reserpine produces a transient decrease in the calcium content of brain tissue which parallels the depletion of brain monoamines (RADOUCO-THOMAS et al., 1971). Intraventricular injection of reserpine in the cat results in increases in the potassium, magnesium and calcium concentrations of cerebral spinal fluid without affecting the blood pressure or heart rate (MELVILLE and JOHNSON, 1970). However, reserpine abolishes both the increase in spinal fluid potassium concentration and the tachycardia induced by high doses of noradrenaline, but does not modify the associated pressor responses (MELVILLE and JOHNSON, 1970).

Reserpine *in vitro* has a marked effect on ^{45}Caefflux from both stimulated and quiescent frog ventricular strips (NAYLER, 1963) and inhibits the calcium-induced increase in ATPase activity and rate of ^{45}Ca uptake by the sarcoplasmic reticulum vesicles of rabbit skeletal muscle (BALZER et al., 1968a). In aortic strips from reserpine-treated rabbits there is a delay in ^{45}Ca efflux (HUDGINS and HARRIS, 1970) and a retention of tissue calcium content during soaking in a calcium-free solution (HUDGINS and HARRIS, 1970; GARRETT and CARRIER, 1971).

C. Tissue Metabolism

1. Cardiac Mitochondria

Some of the circulatory effects of reserpine in the cat were attributed by ZAIMIS (1961) to a damaging action on the myocardium which was manifested as widespread and degenerative changes, but TANZ and MARCUS (1966) were unable to confirm her findings. However, reserpine does produce changes which are detectable by electron microscopy. Thus, WILCKEN et al. (1967) reported that heart mitochondria from reserpine-treated dogs are fragmented and the cristae are lost. In the hearts of reserpine-treated rats and mice, the mitochondria are swollen and distorted in shape, the cristae are deranged and electron-dense material is accumulated (SUN et al., 1968; BURNSTOCK et al., 1970; PALM et al., 1970). These effects of reserpine do not appear to be a direct result of depletion of cardiac catecholamines, since there are no ultrastructural changes in cardiac mitochondria after surgical denervation of the dog heart (POTTER et al., 1965). Furthermore, IWAYAMA et al. (1973) demonstrated that the administration of low doses of reserpine for seven days to guinea-pigs does not affect cardiac mitochondria, although the same treatment produces maximal depletion of noradrenaline from the heart (CROUT et al., 1962); however, large doses of reserpine produce characteristic alterations in the ultrastructure of mitochondria, as illustrated in Fig. 5.

There are functional changes in mitochondrial activity accompanying the structural changes. Oxidative phosphorylation is uncoupled by reserpine, *in vivo* and *in vitro*, in cardiac mitochondria of cats and guinea-pigs (SCHWARTZ and LEE, 1960), and there are multiple defects in oxidative metabolism of lipids and carbohydrates by cardiac mitochondria from reserpine-treated mice (SUN et al., 1968). The Mg^{++}-activated ATPase of rat heart mitochondria is inhibited by reserpine, 50% inhibition being produced by about 5×10^{-5} M; however, the same effect is also produced by prenylamine, chlorpromazine and propranolol (PALM et al., 1970).

2. Cyclic-AMP System

Reserpine increases brain glycogen concentrations (HUTCHINS and ROGERS, 1970); however, the relationship between brain glycogen and catecholamines is unknown. Reserpine *in vitro* inhibits phosphodiesterase (HONDA and IMMURA, 1968) and enhances the adenylcyclase activity of the pineal gland (WEISS and COSTA, 1967). The behavioural effects of dibutyryl-cyclic-AMP injected into the lateral ventricles of the rat are not altered by pretreatment with reserpine (GESSA et al., 1970).

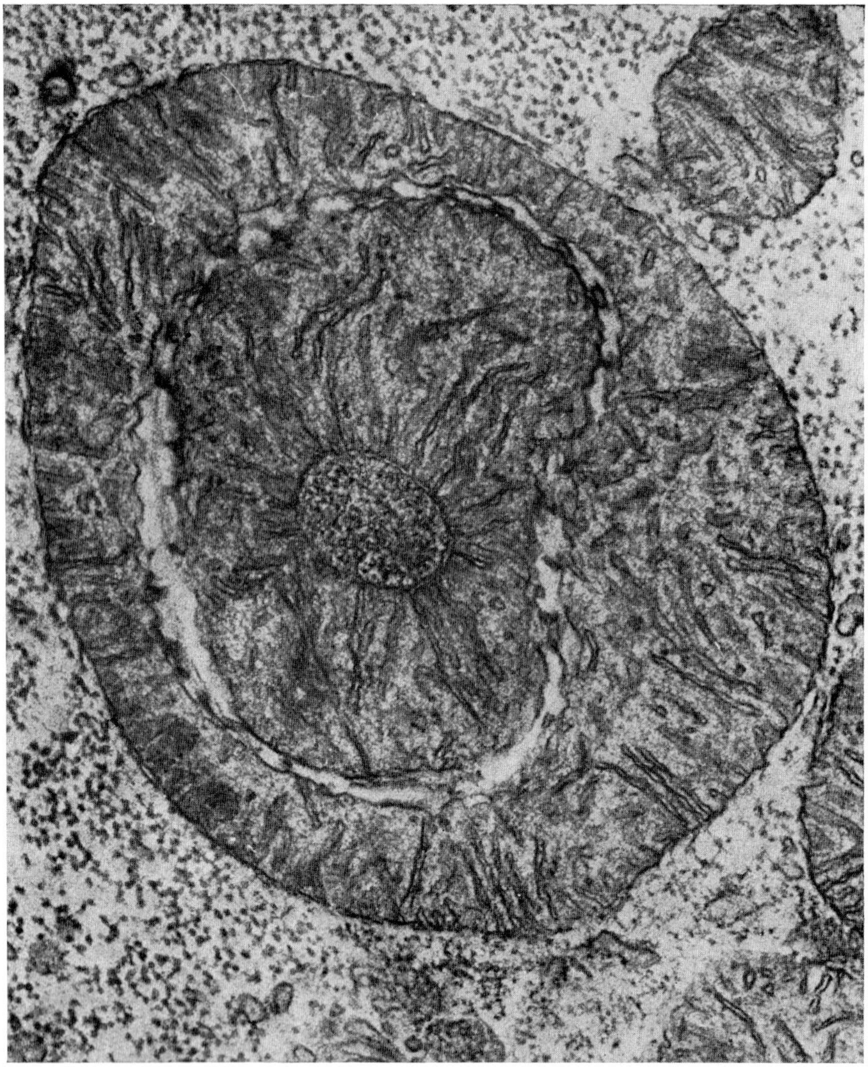

Fig. 5. Electronmicrograph through a mitochondria in the right atrium of a guinea-pig treated with reserpine (5 mg/kg) 18 h before sacrifice and removal of tissue. Note characteristic infoldings and disordered arrangement of cristae (× 61,000). (Reproduced by permission from T. IWAYAMA, W. W. FLEMING and G. BURNSTOCK: *J. Pharmacol. exp. Ther.* **184**, 95—105 1973).

D. Structural Effects

1. Ulcerogenic Action

A tendency for formation of peptic ulcers is a recognized hazard of clinical reserpine treatment (KLEIN, 1968). In patients treated with reserpine, the volume and acidity of gastric secretions are increased (HAVERBACK et al., 1955), and gastric lesions occur (HAVERBACK et al., 1965; HUSSAR and BRUNO, 1956; WOFFORD and CUMMINS, 1956).

Reserpine produces haemorrhagic lesions or ulceration of gastric mucosa and stimulates gastric secretion in rats (BENDITT and WONG, 1956; KIM and SHORE, 1963), mice (BLACKMAN et al., 1959), hamsters (BRODIE and HANSON, 1960), cats (GAITONDE et al., 1960; EMÅS, 1965), dogs (BARRETT et al., 1955) and pigs (MUGGENBURG et al., 1966).

The damage to the gastric mucosa is confined to the glandular portion of the stomach. The effect is apparent within a few hours of administration of a single dose of reserpine and the lesions are partially healed in 72 h (BRODIE et al., 1963). The increase in gastric secretion occurs after a delay of up to 60 min and persists for more than 12 hours (EMÅS, 1965). Age, sex and environmental conditions influence the effect of reserpine in producing gastric lesions in rats (REILLY et al., 1969).

Reserpine decreases the histamine and serotonin contents of the stomach wall by about 30% (HAVERBACK and WIRTSCHAFTER, 1962; KIM and SHORE, 1963). Insulin also stimulates gastric secretions, causes mucosal lesions and lowers gastric histamine but does not affect gastric serotonin (KIM and SHORE, 1963). A monoamine oxidase inhibitor (pheniprazine) inhibits all the effects of reserpine on the stomach except the decrease in histamine content but does not modify the effects of insulin, from which it was concluded that the lesions are produced by the excessive secretion but that a high local concentration of free serotonin exerts a protective action (KIM and SHORE, 1963).

A large part of the effects of reserpine on the gastric mucosa involves a vagal mechanism since anticholinergic drugs and vagotomy confer protection against the production of lesions (BLACKMAN et al., 1959) and there is a smaller increase in secretions after atropine (BARRETT et al., 1965; EMÅS, 1965), chlorisondamine (KIM and SHORE, 1963) and vagotomy (KIM and SHORE, 1963; EMÅS, 1965). Vagal integrity is not obligatory for the stimulatory effect of reserpine on gastric secretions since it occurs in the vagally denervated Heidenhain pouch of the dog (BARRETT et al., 1955) and after vagotomy in the rat (KIM and SHORE, 1963) and cat (EMÅS, 1965). However, the vagus is necessary for the optimal stimulatory effect of reserpine on gastric secretion (EMÅS, 1965).

The effect of reserpine on gastric secretion does not involve the sympathetic nerves to the stomach (EMÅS, 1965).

2. Anti-Toxic Actions of Reserpine

Reserpine pretreatment of mice confers protection against the hepatotoxic effect of carbon tetrachloride (CLOWER et al., 1967); it is not clear whether the toxicity of carbon tetrachloride involves the autonomic nervous system (CALVERT and BRODY, 1960).

Reserpine protects against the production of lenticular opacities by morphine in mice (SMITH et al., 1966).

The death rate and the incidence of atrial thrombosis in mice induced by a high-fat, low-protein, choline-deficient diet are much reduced by reserpine treatment (CLOWER et al., 1967).

The survival time of leukaemic mice is prolonged by treatment with reserpine (GOLDIN et al., 1957), and other *Rauwolfia* alkaloids and related drugs (KRUGER et al., 1960a).

Reserpine pretreatment protects mice against the lethal effect of X-irradiation, the maximal protective effect being with administration 12 to 18 h before irradiation (LANGENDORFF, 1957).

3. Anti-Atheroma Action

Reserpine lessens the degree of atheromatous lesion formation and lowers the associated high levels of cholesterol in rats (SMITH and ROSSI, 1962). In rabbits, reserpine lessens the atherosclerotic process and reduces the calcium content of aortic tissue (CARRIER et al., 1968; WHITTINGTON-COLEMAN et al., 1968) without lowering the serum cholesterol (WHITTINGTON-COLEMAN et al., 1968). Reserpine as an additive in feed has been shown to reduce the damage of environmental stress to the cardiovascular system and thus lessen the mortality rate in chickens and turkeys (RINGER, 1959, 1960). At 2·5 ppm in the diet of turkeys, reserpine delays the onset of aneurism induced by feeding β-aminopropionitrile, and also lowers the blood pressure and heart rate (KRISTA et al., 1963). Reserpine has also been shown to be effective in the treatment of dissecting aneurisms in humans (WHEAT et al., 1965). Although the beneficial effects of reserpine in atherosclerosis and in the treatment of dissecting aneurisms have been proposed to stem from its hypotensive action (see DEMING, 1966), similar beneficial effects of reserpine have been found in both normotensive and hypertensive rats (SMITH and ROSSI, 1962). It has been suggested that reserpine exerts a direct action on vascular tissue to lessen the atherosclerotic processes (WHITTINGTON-COLEMAN et al., 1968).

References

ACETO, M., HARRIS, L. S.: Effects of various agents on reserpine-induced blepharoptosis. Toxicol. appl. Pharmacol. **7**, 329—336 (1965).

ADAM, H. M.: Histamine in the central nervous system and hypophysis of the dog. In: KETY, S.S., ELKES, J. (Eds.): Regional Neurochemistry, pp. 293—306. London: Pergamon Press 1961.

ADAM, H. M., HYE, H. K. A.: Concentration of histamine in different parts of brain and hypophysis of cat and its modification by drugs. Brit. J. Pharmacol. **28**, 137—152 (1966).

AGARWAL, S. L., BOSE, D.: A study of the role of brain catecholamines in drug induced tremor. Brit. J. Pharmacol. **30**, 349—353 (1967).

ALPER, M. H., SCHMIER, J.: Modification by guanethidine of the chronotropic action of sympathomimetic amines in the heart-lung preparation of the dog pretreated with reserpine. J. Pharmacol. exp. Ther. **137**, 235—241 (1962).

ALPERS, H. S., SHORE, P. A.: Specific binding of reserpine-association with norepinephrine depletion. Biochem. Pharmacol. **18**, 1363—1372 (1969).

AMBANI, L. M., WOERT VAN M. H.: Modification of the tremorigenic activity of physostigmine. Brit. J. Pharmacol. **46**, 344—347 (1972).

AMIN, A. H., CRAWFORD, T. B., GADDUM, J. H.: The distribution of substance P and 5-hydroxytryptamine in the central nervous system of the dog. J. Physiol. (Lond.) **126**, 596—618 (1954).

ANDÉN, N. E., FUXE, K., HÖKFELT, T.: The importance of nerve impulse flow for the depletion of the monoamines from central neurones by some drugs. J. Pharm. Pharmacol. **18**, 630—632 (1966).

ANDÉN, N. E., FUXE, K., HÖKFELT, T.: Effect of some drugs on central monoamine nerve terminals lacking nerve impulse flow. Europ. J. Pharmacol. **1**, 226—232 (1967).

ANDÉN, N. E., HENNING, M.: Adrenergic nerve function, noradrenaline level and noradrenaline uptake in cat nictitating membrane after reserpine treatment. Acta physiol. scand. **67**, 498—504 (1966).

ANDÉN, N. E., MAGNUSSON, T., WALDECK, B.: Correlation between noradrenaline uptake and adrenergic nerve function after reserpine treatment. Life Sci. **3**, 19—25 (1964).

APPEL, J. B., FREEDMAN, D. X.: Chemically-induced alterations in the behavioural effects of LSD-25. Biochem. Pharmacol. **13**, 861—869 (1964).

ASKEW, B. M.: A simple screening procedure for imipramine-like antidepressant agents. Life Sci. **10**, 725—730 (1963).

AXELROD, J.: Purification and properties of phenyl-ethanolamine-*N*-methyl transferase. J. biol. Chem. **237**, 1657—1660 (1962a).

AXELROD, J.: The enzymatic-*N*-methylation of serotonin and other amines. J. Pharmacol. exp. Ther. **138**, 28—33 (1962b).

AXELROD, J., GORDON, E., HERTTING, G., KOPIN, I. J., POTTER, L. T.: On the mechanism of tachyphylaxis to tyramine in the isolated rat heart. Brit. J. Pharmacol. **19**, 56—63 (1962b).
AXELROD, J., HERTTING, G., PATRICK, R. W.: Inhibition of H^3-norepinephrine release by monoamine oxidase inhibitors. J. Pharmacol. exp. Ther. **134**, 325—328 (1961a).
AXELROD, J., HERTTING, G., POTTER, L.: Effect of drugs on the uptake and release of ^3H-norepinephrine in the rat heart. Nature (Lond.) **194**, 297 (1962a).
AXELROD, J., MUELLER, R. A., THOENEN, H.: Neuronal and hormonal control of tyrosine hydroxylase and phenylethanolamine *N*-methyltransferase activity. In: SCHÜMANN, M. J., KRONEBERG, G. (Eds.): New Aspects of Storage and Release Mechanisms of Catecholamines, pp. 212—219. Berlin-Heidelberg-New York: Springer 1970.
AXELROD, J., WHITBY, L. G., HERTTING, G.: Effect of psychotropic drugs on the uptake of ^3H-norepinephrine by tissues. Science **133**, 383—384 (1961b).
AZARNOFF, D. L., BURN, J. H.: Effect of noradrenaline on the action of nicotine and tyramine on isolated atria. Brit. J. Pharmacol. **16**, 335—343 (1961).
AZZARO, A. J., WENGER, G. R., CRAIG, C. R., STITZEL, R. E.: Reserpine-induced alterations in brain amines and their relationship to changes in the incidence of minimal electroshock seizures in mice. J. Pharmacol. exp. Ther. **180**, 558—568 (1972).
BALZER, H., MAKINOSE, M., FIEHN, W., HASSELBACH, W.: The binding of calcium transport inhibitors reserpine, chlorpromazine and prenylamine to the lipid of the membranes of the sarcoplasmic reticulum. Naunyn-Schmiedeberg's Arch. exp. Path. Pharmak. **260**, 456—473 (1968b).
BALZER, H., MAKINOSE, M., HASSELBACH, W.: The inhibition of the sarcoplasmic calcium pump by prenylamine, reserpine, chlorpromazine and imipramine. Naunyn-Schmiedeberg's Arch. exp. Path. Pharm. **260**, 444—455 (1968a).
BANERJEE, U., BURKS, T. F., FELDBERG, W., GOODRICH, C. A.: Temperature effects of reserpine injected into the cerebral ventricles in rabbits and cats. J. Physiol. (Lond.) **197**, 221—231 (1968).
BARDHAN, N. R., CHATTERJEE, A.: Failure of ascorbic acid in the prevention of adrenal hypertrophy and ovarian inhibition in reserpinized rats. Acta anat. (Basel) **73**, 278—280 (1969).
BARKAI, A., GLUSMAN, M., RAPPORT, M. M.: Serotonin turnover in the intact cat brain. J. Pharmacol. exp. Ther. **181**, 28—35 (1972).
BARNES, C. D., POMPEIANO, O.: The interaction of brain stem adrenergic systems and VIIIth nerve stimulation on the spinal cord. Neuropharmacology **10**, 437—446 (1971).
BARNETT, A., BENFORADO, J. M.: The nicotinic effects of choline esters and of nicotine in guinea pig atria. J. Pharmacol. exp. Ther. **152**, 29—36 (1966).
BARRACLOUGH, C. A., SAWYER, C. H.: Blockage of the release of pituitary ovulating hormone in the rat by chlorpromazine and reserpine: possible mechanisms of action. Endocrinology **61**, 341—351 (1957).
BARRETT, W. E., PLUMMER, A. J., EARL, A. E., ROGIE, B.: Effect of reserpine on gastric secretion of the dog. J. Pharmacol. exp. Ther. **113**, 3 (1955).
BARTONICEK, V.: Failure of imipramine to influence serotonin and catecholamine levels in specific neurons of rat brain. Med. Pharmac. Exp. **12**, 395—398 (1965).
BAUM, T.: Vascular reactivity of reserpine-pretreated dogs. J. Pharmacol. exp. Ther. **141**, 30—35 (1963).
BECK, L., BRODY, M. J.: The physiology of vasodilatation. Angiology **12**, 202—222 (1961).
BECK, L., YBARRA-FALCON, L., DOMINO, E. F.: Hemodynamic responses to reserpine in unanesthetized dogs immobilized with neuromuscular blocking agents. J. Pharmacol. exp. Ther. **119**, 133 (1957).
BEIN, H. J.: Zur Pharmakologie des Reserpin, eines neuen Alkaloids aus Rauwolfia Serpentina Benth. Experientia (Basel) **9**, 107—110 (1953).
BEIN, H. J.: Significance of selected central mechanisms for the analysis of the action of reserpine. Ann. N. Y. Acad. Sci. **61**, 4—16 (1955).
BEIN, H. J.: The pharmacology of rauwolfia. Pharmacol. Rev. **8**, 435—483 (1956).
BEJRABLAYA, D., BURN, J. H., WALKER, J. M.: The action of sympathomimetic amines on heart rate in relation to the effect of reserpine. Brit. J. Pharmacol. **13**, 461—466 (1958).
BELL, C.: The pharmacological nature of the response of the reserpinized guinea-pig vas deferens to postganglionic nerve stimulation. Brit. J. Pharmacol. **37**, 52—56 (1969).
BEN-DAVID, M., KHAZEN, K., KHAZAN, N., SULMAN, F. G.: Correlation between depressant and mammotropic effects in fifteen reserpine analogues. Arch. int. Pharmacodyn **171**, 274—284 (1968).
BENDITT, E. P., WONG, R. L.: The release of enterochromaffin cell substance by reserpine. Amer. J. Path. **32**, 638 (1956).
BENNETT, J. P., KENDLE, K. E.: The effect of reserpine upon the rate of transport in the Fallopian tube of the mouse. J. Reprod. Fertil. **13**, 345—348 (1967).

BENSON, G. K.: Effect of reserpine on mammary gland involution and on other organs in the rat. Proc. Soc. exp. Biol. (N. Y.) **99**, 550—553 (1958).
BERKOWITZ, B. A., TARVER, J. H., SPECTOR, S.: Norepinephrine in blood vessels: concentration, binding, uptake and depletion. J. Pharmacol. exp. Ther. **117**, 119—126 (1971).
BERL, S., FRIGYESI, T. L.: Effect of reserpine on the turnover of glutamate, glutamine, aspartate and GABA labeled with 1—^{14}C acetate in caudate nucleus, thalamus and sensorimotor cortex (cat). Brain Res. **14**, 683—695 (1969).
BERLIN, R.: Depression after methoserpidine. Lancet **1965** II, 497.
BERNARDI, D., JORI, A., MORSELLI, P., VALZELLI, L., GARATTINI, S.: Further effects of imipramine and its desmethyl derivative on the hypothermia induced by reserpine. J. Pharm. Pharmacol. **18**, 278—282 (1966).
BERNARDI, D., PAGLIALUNGA, S., JORI, A.: Peripheral and central components in the hyperthermic effects of desipramine in reserpinized rats. J. Pharm. Pharmacol. **20**, 204—209 (1968).
BERNEIS, K. H., PLETSCHER, A., DA PRADA, M.: Metal dependent aggregation of biogenic amines: A possible explanation for their storage and release. Nature (Lond.) **224**, 281—283 (1969).
BERNEIS, K. H., PLETSCHER, A., DA PRADA, M.: Phase separation in solutions of noradrenaline and adenosine triphosphate: influence of bivalent cations and drugs. Brit. J. Pharmacol. **39**, 382—389 (1970).
BERTI, F., SHORE, P. A.: A kinetic analysis of drugs that inhibit the adrenergic neuronal membrane amine pump. Biochem. Pharmacol. **16**, 2091—2094 (1967a).
BERTI, F., SHORE, P. A.: Interaction of reserpine and ouabain on amine concentrating mechanisms in the adrenergic neurone. Biochem. Pharmacol. **16**, 2271—2274 (1967b).
BERTLER, Å.: Affect of reserpine on the storage of catecholamines in brain and other tissues. Acta physiol. scand. **51**, 75—83 (1961).
BERTLER, Å., CARLSSON, A., ROSENGREN, E.: Release by reserpine of catecholamines from rabbits' hearts. Naturwissenschaften **43**, 521 (1956).
BERTLER, Å., FALCK, B., OWMAN, C., ROSENGREN, E.: The localization of monoaminergic blood-brain barrier mechanisms. Pharmacol. Rev. **18**, 369—385 (1966).
BERTLER, Å., ROSENGREN, E.: Occurrence and distribution of catechol amines in brain. Acta physiol. scand. **47**, 350—361 (1969).
BESSON, M. J., CHERAMY, A., GLOWINSKI, J.: Effects of some psychotropic drugs on dopamine synthesis in the rat striatum. J. Pharmacol. exp. Ther. **177**, 196—205 (1971).
BHAGAT, B.: Response of isolated guinea-pig atria to various ganglion-stimulating agents. J. Pharmacol. exp. Ther. **154**, 264—270 (1966).
BHAGAT, B., BURKE, W. J., DAVIS, J. W.: Effect of reserpine on the activity of adrenal enzymes involved in the synthesis of adrenaline. Brit. J. Pharmacol. **43**, 819—827 (1971).
BHARGAVA, K. P., KAR, K., PARMAR, S. S.: Independent cholinergic and adrenergic mechanisms in the guinea-pig isolated vas deferens preparation. Brit. J. Pharmacol. **24**, 641—650 (1965).
BHATTACHARYA, A. N., MARKS, B. H.: Reserpine- and chlorpromazine-induced changes in hypothalamo-hypophyseal-adrenal system in rats in the presence and absence of hypothermia. J. Pharmacol. exp. Ther. **165**, 108—116 (1969).
BIANCHI, C., BEANI, L.: Reserpine and the neuromuscular junction. J. Pharm. Pharmacol. **18**, 757—758 (1966).
BIANCHI, M. DE, FARGIER, M. C.: Etude dans le temps de l'effect de la reserpine sur la médullosurrénale. C. R. Soc. Biol. (Paris) **156**, 1797—1802 (1962).
BJÖRKLUND, A., FALK, B.: Histochemical characterization of a tryptamine-like substance stored in cells of the mammalian adenohypophysis. Acta physiol. scand. **77**, 475—489 (1969).
BLACK, I. B., PARKER, L., AXELROD, J.: A daily rhythm in the rate of depletion of brain norepinephrine by reserpine. Biochem. Pharmacol. **18**, 2688—2691 (1969).
BLACKMAN, J. G., CAMPION, D. S., FASTIER, F. N.: Mechanism of action of reserpine in producing gastric hemorrhage and erosion in the mouse. Brit. J. Pharmacol. **14**, 112—116 (1959).
BLASCHKO, H., CHRUŚCIEL, T. L.: The decarboxylation of amino acids related to tyrosine and the awakening action in reserpine-treated mice. J. Physiol. (Lond.) **151**, 272—284 (1960).
BLINKS, J. R.: Field stimulation as a means of effecting the graded release of autonomic transmitters in isolated heart muscle. J. Pharmacol. exp. Ther. **151**, 221—235 (1966).
BOADLE-BIBER, M. C., ROTH, R. H.: Effect of drugs on the synthesis of noradrenaline in guinea-pig vas deferens. Brit. J. Pharmacol. **46**, 696—707 (1972).
BOAKES, R. J., BRADLEY, P. B., CANDY, J. M.: Supersensitivity of central noradrenaline receptors after reserpine. Brit. J. Pharmacol. **43**, 443P—444P (1971).
BOAKES, R. J., BRADLEY, P. B., CANDY, J. M.: A neuronal basis for the altering action of (+)-amphetamine. Brit. J. Pharmacol. **45**, 391—403 (1972).

BOGDANSKI, D. F., BRODIE, B. B.: Role of sodium and potassium ion in storage of norepinephrine by sympathetic nerve endings. Life Sci. **5**, 1563—1569 (1966).

BOGDANSKI, D. F., BRODIE, B. B.: The effects of inorganic ions on the storage and uptake of H^3-norepinephrine by rat heart slices. J. Pharmacol. exp. Ther. **165**, 181—189 (1969).

BOGDANSKI, D. F., SULSER, F., BRODIE, B. B.: Comparative action of reserpine, tetrabenazine, and chlorpromazine on central parasympathetic activity: Effects on pupillary size and lacrimation in rabbit and on salivation in dog. J. Pharmacol. exp. Ther. **132**, 176—182 (1961).

BOGDANSKI, D. F., TISSARI, A., BRODIE, B. B.: The effects of inorganic ions on uptake, storage and metabolism of biogenic amines in nerve endings. Pp. 17—26. In: Psychopharmacology: A review of progress 1957—1967. Washington, Public Health Service Publication No. 1836 (1968).

BOISSIER, J.-R., FICHELLE-PAGNY, J., SIMON, P.: Activité antirésèrpine chez la sqauris de l'imipramine, de l'amitriptyline et de leur dérivés monodesméthylés. Therapie **21**, 109—117 (1966).

BOLTON, T. B.: Intramural nerves in the ventricular myocardium of the domestic fowl and other animals. Brit. J. Pharmacol. **31**, 253—268 (1967).

BONACCORSI, A.: Studies on the hypertensive response elicited by reserpine or tetrabenazine in rats treated with amphetamine-like drugs. Europ. J. Pharmacol. **3**, 97—105 (1968).

BONDAREFF, W.: Submicroscopic morphology of granular vesicles in sympathetic nerves of rat pineal body. Z. Zellforsch. **67**, 211—218 (1965).

BOWMAN, W. C., OSUIDE, G.: Interaction between the effects of tremorine and harmine and of other drugs in chicks. Europ. J. Pharmacol. **3**, 106—111 (1968).

BOYD, H., BURNSTOCK, G., ROGERS, D.: Innervation of the large intestine of the toad (*Bufo marinus*). Brit. J. Pharmacol. **23**, 151—163 (1964).

BRANDON, K. W., RAND, M. J.: Acetylcholine and the sympathetic innervation of the spleen. J. Physiol. (Lond.) **157**, 18—32 (1961).

BRAY, G. A.: Studies on the interactions of thyroid hormone and catecholamines. J. clin. Invest. **43**, 285—294 (1964).

BREWSTER, W. R., ISAACS, J. P., OSGOOD, P. F., KING, T. L.: The hemodynamic and metabolic interrelationships in the activity of epinephrine, norepinephrine and the thyroid hormones. Circulation **13**, 1—20 (1956).

BRIMIJOIN, S., TRENDELENBURG, U.: Reserpine-induced release of norepinephrine from isolated spontaneously beating guinea-pig atria. J. Pharmacol. exp. Ther. **176**, 149—159 (1971).

BRODIE, B. B., BEAVAN, M. A.: Neurochemical transducer systems. Med. exp. (Basel) **8**, 320—351 (1963).

BRODIE, B. B., COMER, M. S., COSTA, E., DLABAC, A.: The role of brain serotonin in the mechanism of a central action of reserpine. J. Pharmacol. exp. Ther. **152**, 340—349 (1966).

BRODIE, B. B., COSTA, E.: Some current views on brain monoamines. Psychopharmacol. Bull. **2**, 1—25 (1962).

BRODIE, B. B., OLIN, J. S., KUNTZMAN, R. B., SHORE, P. A.: Possible interrelationship between release of brain norepinephrine and serotonin by reserpine. Science **125**, 1293—1294 (1957a).

BRODIE, B. B., PLETSCHER, A., SHORE, P. A.: Evidence that serotonin has a role in brain function. Science **122**, 968 (1955).

BRODIE, B. B., SHORE, P. A.: A concept for the role of serotonin and norepinephrine as chemical mediators in the brain. Ann. N. Y. Acad. Sci. **66**, 631—642 (1957).

BRODIE, B. B., SULSER, F., COSTA, E.: Psychotherapeutic drugs. Ann. Rev. Med. **12**, 349—368 (1961).

BRODIE, B. B., TOMICH, E. G., KUNTZMAN, R., SHORE, P. A.: On the mechanism of action of reserpine: Effect of reserpine on capacity of tissues to bind serotonin. J. Pharmacol. exp. Ther. **119**, 461—467 (1957b).

BRODIE, D. A., HANSON, H. M.: A study of the factors involved in the production of gastric ulcers by the restraint technique. Gastroenterology **38**, 353—360 (1960).

BRODIE, D. A., HANSON, H. M., SINES, J. O., ADER, R.: A symposium on current research on gastric ulcers. J. Neuropsychiat. **4**, 388—408 (1963).

BROGDEN, R. N., SPEIGHT, T. M., AVERY, G. S.: Levodopa: A review of its pharmacological properties and therapeutic uses with particular reference to parkinsonism. Drugs **2**, 262—400 (1971).

BROOKS, D. C., GERSHON, M. D.: An analysis of the effect of reserpine upon ponto-geniculo-occipital wave activity in the cat. Neuropharmacology **11**, 499—510 (1972).

BROOKS, D. C., GERSHON, M. D., SIMON, R. P.: Brain stem serotonin depletion and ponto-geniculo-occipital wave activity in the cat treated with reserpine. Neuropharmacology **11**, 511—520 (1972).

BROWN, G. L.: The release and fate of the transmitter liberated by adrenergic nerves. Proc. roy. Soc. B **162**, 1—19 (1965).
BROWN, P. S.: The effect of reserpine, 5-hydroxytryptamine and other drugs on induced ovulation in immature mice. J. Endocr. **35**, 161—168 (1966).
BROWN, P. S.: Pituitary follicle-stimulating hormone in immature female rats treated with drugs that inhibit the synthesis or antagonise the actions of catecholamines and 5-hydroxytryptamine. Neuroendocrinology **7**, 183—192 (1971).
BUCKLEY, N. M.: Role of endogenous norepinephrine in cardiac inotropic effects of nucleosides Arch. int. Pharmacodyn **188**, 92—104 (1970).
BÜLBRING, E.: The action of adrenaline on transmission in the superior cervical ganglion. J. Physiol. (Lond.) **103**, 55—67 (1944).
BURGER, A., PHILIPPU, A., SCHÜMANN, H. J.: Untersuchungen zur Bedeutung einer ATPase aus Milznervengranula. Naunyn-Schmiedeberg's Arch. exp. Path. Pharmak. **260**, 101—102 (1968).
BURGER, A., PHILIPPU, A., SCHÜMANN, H. J.: ATP-Spaltung und Aminaufnahme durch Milznervengranula. Naunyn-Schmiedeberg's Arch. exp. Path. Pharmak. **262**, 208—220 (1969).
BURN, J. H., HOBBS, R.: A test for tranquillizing drugs. Arch. int. Pharmacodyn. **113**, 290—295 (1958).
BURN, J. H., LEACH, E. H., RAND, M. J., THOMPSON, J. W.: Peripheral effects of nicotine and acetylcholine resembling those of sympathetic stimulation. J. Physiol. (Lond.) **148**, 332—352 (1959).
BURN, J. H., RAND, M. J.: Reserpine and noradrenaline in artery walls. Lancet **1957** II, 1097.
BURN, J. H., RAND, M. J.: Action of nicotine on the heart. Brit. med. J. **1958** a I, 137—139.
BURN, J. H., RAND, M. J.: Noradrenaline in artery walls and its dispersal by reserpine. Brit. med. J. **1958** b I, 903—908.
BURN, J. H., RAND, M. J.: Excitatory action of the vagus in the isolated atria in relation to adrenaline. J. Physiol. (Lond.) **142**, 173—186 (1958c).
BURN, J. H., RAND, M. J.: The action of sympathomimetic amines in animals treated with reserpine. J. Physiol. (Lond.) **144**, 314—336 (1958d).
BURN, J. H., RAND, M. J.: Fall of blood pressure after a noradrenaline infusion and its treatment by pressor agents. Brit. med. J. **1959** a I, 394—397.
BURN, J. H., RAND, M. J.: The cause of the supersensitivity of smooth muscle to noradrenaline. J. Physiol. (Lond.) **147**, 135—143 (1959b).
BURN, J. H., RAND, M. J.: Sympathetic postganglionic mechanism. Nature (Lond.) **184**, 163—165 (1959c).
BURN, J. H., RAND, M. J.: The effect of precursors of noradrenaline on the response to tyramine and sympathetic stimulation. Brit. J. Pharmacol. **15**, 47—55 (1960a).
BURN, J. H., RAND, M. J.: Sympathetic postganglionic cholinergic fibres. Brit. J. Pharmacol. **15**, 56—66 (1960b).
BURN, J. H., RAND, M. J.: A new interpretation of the adrenergic nerve fibres. Advanc. Pharmacol. **1**, 1—30 (1962).
BURN, J. H., RAND, M. J.: Acetylcholine in adrenergic transmission. Ann. Rev. Pharmacol. **5**, 163—182 (1965).
BURNSTOCK, G., GANNON, B., IWAYAMA, T.: Sympathetic innervation of vascular smooth muscle in normal and hypertensive animals. Circulat. Res. **27**, Suppl. 2, 5—23 (1970).
BURNSTOCK, G., HOLMAN, M. E.: Effect of denervation and of reserpine treatment on transmission at sympathetic nerve endings. J. Physiol. (Lond.) **160**, 461—469 (1962).
BUTCHER, L. L., RHODES, D. L., YUWILER, A.: Behavioural and biochemical effects of preferentially protecting monoamines in the brain against the action of reserpine. Europ. J. Pharmacol. 18, 204—212 (1972).
BUTTERBAUGH, G. G., SPRATT, J. L.: The possible role of brain monoamines in the acute toxicity of digitoxigenin. (Protective effects of Serpasil, Singoserp, and tetrabenazine.) J. Pharmacol. exp. Ther. **175**, 121—130 (1970).
CAIROLI, V. J., CROUT, J. R.: Role of the autonomic nervous system in the resting tachycardia of experimental hyperthyroidism. J. Pharmacol. exp. Ther. **158**, 55—65 (1967).
CAIROLI, V. J., REILLY, J. F., ROBERTS, J.: Effect of reserpine pretreatment on the response of isolated papillary muscle to ephedrine. Brit. J. Pharmacol. **18**, 588—594 (1962).
CALLINGHAM, B. A., MANN, M.: Adrenaline and noradrenaline, replacement of, in the innervated and denervated adrenal gland of the rat, following depletion with reserpine. Nature (Lond.) **182**, 1020—1021 (1958).
CALLINGHAM, B. A., MANN, M.: Depletion and replacement of the adrenaline and noradrenaline contents of the rat adrenal gland, following treatment with reserpine. Brit. J. Pharmacol. **18**, 138—149 (1962).
CALNE, D. B.: Parkinsonism: Physiology, pharmacology and treatment. London: Arnold 1970.

CALVERT, D. N., BRODY, T. M.: Role of the sympathetic nervous system in CCl_4 hepatotoxicity. Amer. J. Physiol. **198**, 669—676 (1960).
CAMPBELL, A., ROBERTSON, E.: Treatment of severe hypertension with hexamethonium bromide. Brit. med. J. **1950** II, 804—806.
CARLSSON, A.: Brain monoamines and psychotropic drugs. Neuropsychopharmacol. **2**, 417—421 (1961).
CARLSSON, A.: Pharmacological depletion of catecholamine stores. Pharmacol. Rev. **18**, 541—549 (1965a).
CARLSSON, A.: Drugs which block the storage of 5-hydroxytryptamine and related amines. In: ERSPAMER, V. (Ed.): Handbuch der Exp. Pharmakol., Vol. 19, pp. 529—592. Berlin-Heidelberg-New York: Springer 1965b.
CARLSSON, A.: Physiological and pharmacological release of monoamines in the central nervous system. In: VON EULER, U. S., ROSELL, S., UVNÄS, B. (Eds.): Mechanisms of Release of Biogenic Amines, pp. 331—346. Oxford: Pergamon Press 1966.
CARLSSON, A., DAHLSTRÖM, A., FUXE, K., HILLARP, N.-Å.: Failure of reserpine to deplete noradrenaline neurons of α-methylnoradrenaline formed from α-methyldopa. Acta pharmacol. (Kbh.) **22**, 270—276 (1965).
CARLSSON, A., HILLARP, N.-Å.: Release of adenosine triphosphate along with adrenaline and noradrenaline following stimulation of adrenal medulla. Acta physiol. scand. **37**, 235—239 (1956).
CARLSSON, A., HILLARP, N.-Å., WALDECK, B.: A Mg^{++}-ATP dependent storage mechanism in the amine granules of the adrenal medulla. Med. exp. (Basel) **6**, 47—53 (1962).
CARLSSON, A., HILLARP, N.-Å., WALDECK, B.: Analysis of the Mg^{++}-ATP dependent storage mechanisms in the amine granules of the adrenal medulla. Acta physiol. scand. **59**, Suppl. 215, 1—38 (1963)b.
CARLSSON, A., JONASSON, J., ROSENGREN, E.: Time correlation between the effects of reserpine on behaviour and storage mechanism for arylalkyamines. Acta physiol. scand. **59**, 474—477 (1963a).
CARLSSON, A., LINDQVIST, M.: The interference of tetrabenazine, benzquinamide and prenylamine with the action of reserpine. Acta pharmacol. (Kbh.) **24**, 112—120 (1966).
CARLSSON, A., LINDQVIST, M.: Metatyrosine as a tool for selective protection of catecholamine stores against reserpine. Europ. J. Pharmacol. **2**, 187—192 (1967).
CARLSSON, A., LINDQVIST, M.: Central and peripheral monoaminergic membrane-pump blockade by some addictive analgesics and antihistamines. J. Pharm. Pharmacol. **21**, 460—464 (1969).
CARLSSON, A., LINDQVIST, M., MAGNUSSON, T.: 3,4-Dihydroxy-phenylalanine and 5-hydroxytryptophan as reserpine antagonists. Nature (Lond.) **180**, 1200 (1957b).
CARLSSON, A., ROSENGREN, E., BERTLER, A., NILSSON, J.: Effect of reserpine on the metabolism of catecholamines. In: GARATTINI, S., GHETTI, V. (Eds.): Psychotropic Drugs, Vol. 6, pp. 363—372. Amsterdam: Elsevier 1957a.
CARLSSON, A., WALDECK, B.: Rapid release of H^3-metaraminol induced by combined treatment with protriptyline and reserpine. J. Pharm. Pharmacol. **17**, 327—328 (1965a).
CARLSSON, A., WALDECK, B.: Mechanism of amine transport in the cell membranes of the adrenergic nerves. Acta pharmacol. (Kbh.) **22**, 293—300 (1965b).
CARLSSON, A., WALDECK, B.: The accumulation of H^3-noradrenaline in the adrenergic nerve fibers of reserpine-treated mice. J. Pharm. Pharmacol. **19**, 182—190 (1967).
CARLSSON, A., WALDECK, B.: Different mechanisms of drug-induced release of noradrenaline and its congeners α-methylnoradrenaline and metarminol. Europ. J. Pharmacol. **4**, 165—168 (1968).
CARRIER, G. O., PEGRAM, B. L., CARRIER, O., Jr.: Antagonistic effects of reserpine on d-tubocurarine action on motor function of rabbits. Europ. J. Pharmacol. **6**, 125—128 (1969).
CARRIER, O., Jr., CLOWER, B. R., WHITTINGTON, P. J.: Inhibition of cholesterol-induced vascular lesions by dietary reserpine. J. Atheroscler. Res. 8, 229—236 (1968).
CARRIER, O., Jr., DOUGLAS, B. H., GARRETT, L., WHITTINGTON, P. J.: The effect of reserpine on vascular tissue sodium and potassium content. J. Pharmacol. exp. Ther. **158**, 494—503 (1967).
CARRIER, O., Jr., HOLLAND, W. C.: Supersensitivity in perfused isolated arteries after reserpine. J. Pharmacol. exp. Ther. **149**, 212—218 (1965).
CARRIER, O., Jr., JUREVICS, H. A.: The role of calcium in "nonspecific" supersensitivity of vascular muscle. J. Pharmacol. exp. Ther. **184**, 81—94 (1973).
CARRIERE, O., JR., SHIBATA, S.: A possible role for tissue calcium in reserpine supersensitivity. J. Pharmacol. exp. Ther. **155**, 42—49 (1967).
CARRIER, O., Jr., WHITTINGTON-COLEMAN, P. J., MATHENY, J., SHIBATA, S.: Tissue calcium losses following reserpine administration in rabbits. Arch. int. Pharmacodyn. **187**, 97—105 (1970).

CASHIN, C. H.: Effect of sympathomimetic drugs in eliciting hypertensive response to reserpine in the rat, after pretreatment with monoamineoxidase inhibitors. Brit. J. Pharmacol. **44**, 203—209 (1972).

CERVONI, P., KIRPEKAR, S. M., SCHWAB, A.: The effect of drugs on uptake and release of catecholamines in the isolated left atrium of the guinea pig. J. Pharmacol. exp. Ther. **151**, 196—206 (1966).

CERVONI, P., REIT, E., MCCULLOUGH, J.: Studies on the decentralized nictitating membrane of the cat. II. Uptake and retention of norepinephrine and epinephrine. J. Pharmacol. exp. Ther. **175**, 649—663 (1970).

CHANG, P., RAND, M. J.: Temperature dependence of catecholamine depletion by reserpine in the heart of the toad (*Bufo marinus*). Brit. J. Pharmacol. **42**, 371—374 (1971).

CHATTERJEE, A.: Effect of reserpine on adrenal cortical activity in rats. Endokrinologie **48**, 265—268 (1965).

CHEN, G., BOHNER, B.: The anti-reserpine effects of certain centrally-acting agents. J. Pharmacol. exp. Ther. **131**, 179—184 (1961).

CHEN, G., ENSOR, C. R., BOHNER, B.: A facilitation of reserpine on the central nervous system. Proc. Soc. exp. Biol. (N. Y.) **86**, 507—510 (1954).

CHEN, G., ENSOR, C. R., BOHNER, B.: Studies of drug effects on electrically induced extensor seizures and clinical implications. Arch. int. Pharmacodyn. **172**, 183—218 (1968).

CHESSIN, M., KRAMER, E. R., SCOTT, C. C.: Modification of the pharmacology of reserpine and serotonin by iproniazid. J. Pharmacol. exp. Ther. **119**, 453—460 (1957).

CHIDSEY, C. A., BRAUNWALD, E. MORROW, A. G., MASON, D. T.: Myocardial norepinephrine concentration in man. New Engl. J. Med. **269**, 653—658 (1963).

CHOI, S. J., ROBERTS, J., KELLIHER, G. J.: Modification of the action of propranolol and quinidine on Na^{22}- and K^{42}-exchange by reserpine. Europ. J. Pharmacol. **20**, 22—33 (1972).

CLARKE, D. E.: The effect of differing reserpine pretreatments on the cardiovascular response to tyramine. J. Pharm. Pharmacol. **19**, 474—475 (1967).

CLARKE, D. E., ADAMS, H. R., BUCKLEY, J. P.: Chronic reserpine treatment on adrenergic neuronal and receptor function in the isolated perfused mesenteric blood vessels of the dog. Europ. J. Pharmacol. **12**, 378—381 (1970).

CLEMENTI, F., MANTEGAZZA, P., BOTTURI, M.: Pharmacologic and morphologic study on the nature of the dense-core granules present in the presynaptic endings of sympathetic ganglia. Int. J. Neuropharmacol. **5**, 281—285 (1966).

CLOWER, B. R., CARRIER, O., Jr., BALL, C. R.: The protective action of reserpine against diet-induced atrial thrombosis. Europ. J. Pharmacol. **2**, 131—135 (1967).

CLOWER, B. R., DOUGLAS, B. H., CARRIER, O., Jr.: Protection by reserpine of carbon tetrachloride-induced hepatic necrosis. Europ. J. Pharmacol. **2**, 276—280 (1968).

COLE, J., GLEES, P.: Reserpine and its antagonists methyl-phenidate (Ritalin) and amphetamine in monkeys. 2nd Intern. Cong. Psychiat. Zürich, 1957, **2**, 398—403 (1957).

COOK, L., CATANIA, A. C.: Effects of drugs on avoidance and escape behaviour. Fed. Proc. **23**, 818—835 (1964).

COOPER, K. E., CRANSTON, W. I., HONOUR, A. J.: Effects of intraventricular and intrahypothalamic injection of noradrenaline and 5-HT on body temperature in conscious rabbits. J. Physiol. (Lond.) **181**, 852—864 (1965).

COOPER, K. E., CRANSTON, W. I., HONOUR, A. J.: Observations on the site and mode of action of pyrogens in the rabbit brain. J. Physiol. (Lond.) **191**, 325—337 (1967).

COPPOLA, J. A., LEONARDI, R. G., LIPPMAN, W., PERRINE, J. W., RINGLER, I.: Induction of pseudopregnancy in rats by depletors of endogenous catecholamines. Endocrinology **77**, 485—490 (1965).

CORRODI, H., MASUOKA, D. T., CLARK, W. G.: Effect of 6-hydroxydopamine on rat heart noradrenaline. Europ. J. Pharmacol. **15**, 160—163 (1971).

COSTA, E., GARATTINI, S., VALZELLI, L.: Interactions between reserpine, chlorpromazine, and imipramine. Experientia (Basel) **16**, 461—463 (1960).

COSTA, E., REVZIN, A. M., KUNTZMAN, R., SPECTOR, S., BRODIE, B. B.: Role for ganglionic norepinephrine in sympathetic synaptic transmission. Science **133**, 1822—1823 (1961).

COTILLO, P., BONACCORSI, A.: Observations on the interactions between desipramine and reserpine on adrenergic transmission in the rat. J. Pharm. Pharmacol. **24**, 103—107 (1972).

COTZIAS, G. C., PAPAVASILIOU, P. S., GELLENE, R.: Modifications of Parkinsonism-chronic treatment with *l*-dopa. New Engl. J. Med. **280**, 337—345 (1969).

COUPLAND, R. E.: Strain sensitivity of albino rats to reserpine. Nature (Lond.) **181**, 930—931 (1958).

COUPLAND, R. E.: The catecholamine content of the adrenal medulla of the rat following reserpine-induced depletion. J. Endocr. **18**, 154—161 (1959).

CRANSTON, E.M.: Effect of tranquilizers and other agents on sexual cycle of mice. Proc. Soc. exp. Biol. (N.Y.) **98**, 320—322 (1958).
CROUT, J.R., MUSKUS, A.J., TRENDELENBURG, U.: Effect of tyramine on isolated guinea pig atria in relation to their noradrenaline stores. Brit. J. Pharmacol. **18**, 660—611 (1962).
DAHLSTRÖM, A.: The effect of reserpine and tetrabenazine on the accumulation of noradrenaline in the rat sciatic nerve after ligation. Acta physiol. scand. **69**, 167—179 (1967).
DAHLSTRÖM, A.: The effects of drugs on axonal transport of amine storage granules. In: SCHÜMANN, H.J., KRONEBERG, G. (Eds.): New Aspects of Storage and Release of Catecholamines, pp. 20—36. Bayer Symposium II. Berlin-Heidelberg-New York: Springer 1970.
DAHLSTRÖM, A., FUXE, K.: Evidence for the existence of monoamine neurons in the central nervous system. II. Experimentally induced changes in the intraneuronal amine levels of bulb-spinal neuron systems. Acta physiol. scand. **64**, Suppl. 247, 1—36 (1965).
DAHLSTRÖM, A., FUXE, K., HILLARP, N.-Å.: The site of action of reserpine. Acta pharmacol. (Kbh.) **22**, 277—292 (1965).
DAHLSTRÖM, A., HÄGGENDAL, J.: Studies on the transport and lifespan of amine storage granules in a peripheral adrenergic neurone system. Acta physiol. scand. **67**, 278—288 (1966a).
DAHLSTRÖM, A., HÄGGENDAL, J.: Recovery of noradrenaline levels after reserpine compared with the life span of amine storage granules in rat and rabbit. J. Pharm. Pharmacol. **18**, 750—752 (1966b).
DAHLSTRÖM, A., HÄGGENDAL, J.: Recovery of noradrenaline in adrenergic axons of rat sciatic nerves after reserpine treatment. J. Pharm. Pharmacol. **21**, 633—638 (1969).
DANDIYA, P.C., JOHNSON, G., SELLERS, E.A.: Influence of variation in environmental temperature on the acute toxicity of reserpine and chlorpromazine in mice. Canad. J. Biochem. **38**, 591—596 (1960).
DAVIS, W.G.: The effects of beta adrenoceptor blocking agents on the membrane potential and spike generation in the smooth muscle of guinea-pig taenia coli. Brit. J. Pharmacol. **38**, 12—19 (1970).
DAY, M., GREEN, J.P.: The uptake of amino acids and the synthesis of amines by neoplastic mast cells in culture. J. Physiol. (Lond.) **164**, 210—226 (1962).
DAY, M.D., RAND, M.J.: A hypothesis for the mode of action of α-methyldopa in relieving hypertension. J. Pharm. Pharmacol. **15**, 221—224 (1963a).
DAY, M.D., RAND, M.J.: Awakening from reserpine sedation by α-methyl dopa. J. Pharm. Pharmacol. **15**, 631—632 (1963b).
DAY, M.D., RAND, M.J.: A possible mechanism of action for α-methyldopa (Aldomet). Int. J. Neuropharmacol. **3**, 173—175 (1964).
DEGKWITZ, R., FROWEIN, R., KULENKAMPFF, C., MOHS, U.: Über die Wirkungen des *l*-Dopa beim Menschen und deren Beeinflussung durch Reserpin, Chlorpromazin, iproniazid and Vitamin B_6. Klin. Wschr. **38**, 120—123 (1960).
DEMING, Q.B.: Experimental atherosclerosis and hypertension. In: GROSS, F. (Ed.): Antihypertensive therapy: Principles and practice, pp. 111—124. Berlin-Heidelberg-New York: Springer 1966.
DENGLER, H.J., MICHAELSON, I.A., SPIEGEL, H.E., TITUS, E.: The uptake of labeled norepinephrine by isolated brain and other tissues of the cat. Int. J. Neuropharmacol. **1**, 23—38 (1962).
DENGLER, H.J., SPIEGEL, H.E., TITUS, E.O.: Effects of drugs on uptake of isotopic norepinephrine by cat tissues. Nature (Lond.) **191**, 816—817 (1961).
DEWS, P.B., MORSE, W.H.: Behavioural pharmacology. Ann. Rev. Pharmacol. **1**, 145—174 (1961).
DINGELL, J.V., OWENS, M.L., NORVICH, M.R., SULSER, F.: On the role of norepinephrine biosynthesis in the central action of amphetamine. Life Sci. **6**, 1155—1162 (1967).
DOMENJOZ, R., THEOBALD, W.: Zur Pharmakologie de Tofranil (N-(3-dimethylaminopropyl)-iminodibenzyl-hydrochlorid). Arch. int. Pharmacodyn. **120**, 450—489 (1959).
DOMINO, E.F., RECH, R.H.: Observations on the initial hypertensive response to reserpine. J. Pharmacol. exp. Ther. **121**, 171—182 (1957).
DONALD, D.E., SHEPHERD, J.T.: Initial cardiovascular adjustment to exercise in dogs with chronic cardiac denervation. Amer. J. Physiol. **207**, 1325—1329 (1964).
DONTAS, A.S.: The hypotensive property of hydralazine and reserpine. J. Pharmacol. exp. Ther. **116**, 17 (1956).
DORRIS, R.L., SHORE, P.A.: Amine uptake and storage mechanisms in the corpus striatum of rat and rabbit. J. Pharmacol. exp. Ther. **179**, 15—19 (1971).
DOYLE, A.E., MCQUEEN, E.G., SMIRK, F.H.: Treatment of hypertension with reserpine, with reserpine in combination with pentapyrrolidinium, and with reserpine in combination with veratrum alkaloids. Circulation **11**, 170—181 (1955).

Draskóczy, P. R., Burack, W. R., Weiner, N.: Catecholamine release from adrenal slices and rate of respiration. J. Pharmacol. exp. Ther. **141**, 58—64 (1963).

Duvoisin, R. C.: Neurological reactions to psychotropic drugs. Pp. 561—573 In: Psychopharmacology. A review of progress: 1957—1967. Washington: Public Health Service Publication No. 1836 (1968).

Ehringer, H., Hornykiewicz, O.: Verteilung von Noradrenalin und Dopamin (3-hydroxytyramin) im Gehirn des Menschen und ihr Verhalten bei Erkrankungen des extrapyramidalen Systems. Klin. Wschr. **38**, 1236—1239 (1960).

Emås, S.: On the mechanism for the stimulating action of reserpine on acid secretion in gastric fistula cats. Acta physiol. scand. **64**, 224—237 (1965).

Emmelin, N.: Supersensitivity following "pharmacological denervation". Pharmacol. Rev. **13**, 17—37 (1961).

Engberg, I., Lundberg, A., Ryall, R. W.: The effect of reserpine on transmission in the spinal cord. Acta physiol. scand. **72**, 115—122 (1968).

Eränkö, O., Hopsu, V.: Effect of reserpine on the histochemistry and content of adrenaline and noradrenaline in the adrenal medulla of the rat and the mouse. Endocrinology **62**, 15—23 (1958).

Erspamer, V.: Observations on the 5-hydroxytryptamine (Enteramine) release caused by reserpine in the rat. Experientia (Basel) **12**, 63—64 (1956).

Euler, U. S. von: The presence of the adrenergic neurotransmitter in intraaxonal structures. Acta physiol. scand. **43**, 155—166 (1958).

Euler, U. S. von: Catecholamines in nerve and organ granules. In: von Euler, U. S., Rosell, S., Uvnäs, B. (Eds.): Mechanisms of Release of Biogenic Amines, pp. 211—222. Oxford: Pergamon Press 1966.

Euler, U. S. von: Acute neuromuscular transmission failure in vas deferens after reserpine. Acta physiol. scand. **76**, 255—256 (1969).

Euler, U. S. von: Effect of some metabolic factors and drugs on uptake and release of catecholamines *in vitro* and *in vivo*. In: Schümann, H. J., Kroneberg, G. (Eds.): New Aspects of Storage and Release Mechanisms of Catecholamines, pp. 144—158. Berlin-Heidelberg-New York: Springer 1970.

Euler, U. S. von, Lishajko, F.: Noradrenaline release from isolated nerve granules. Acta physiol. scand. **51**, 193—203 (1961a).

Euler, U. S. von, Lishajko, F.: Effect of reserpine on the release of catecholamines from isolated nerve and chromaffin cell granules. Acta physiol. scand. **52**, 137—145 (1961b).

Euler, U. S. von, Lishajko, F.: Effect of reserpine on the uptake of catecholamines in isolated nerve storage granules. Int. J. Neuropharmacol. **2**, 127—134 (1963).

Euler, U. S. von, Lishajko, F.: Effects of drugs on the storage granules of adrenergic nerves. Proc. 2nd. int. Pharmac. Meeting, Prague, August 1963, Vol. 3, 245—259. Oxford: Pergamon Press 1965.

Euler, U. S. von, Lishajko, F.: Inhibitory action of adrenergic blocking agents on catecholamine release and uptake in isolated nerve granules. Acta physiol. scand. **68**, 257—262 (1966).

Euler, U. S. von, Lishajko, F.: Mechanism of drug-induced catecholamine release from adrenergic nerve granules. Circulat. Res. **21**, Suppl. 3, 63—69 (1967).

Euler, U. S. von, Lishajko, F.: Inhibitory action of adrenergic blocking agents on re-uptake and net uptake of noradrenaline in nerve granules. Acta physiol. scand. **74**, 501—506 (1968).

Euler, U. S. von, Persson, N.-Å.: Potentiation of adrenergic cardiovascular effects of two quaternary nicotine analogues by reserpine. Acta physiol. scand. **78**, 459—464 (1970).

Euler, U. S. von, Stjärne, L., Lishajko, F.: Effect of reserpine, segontin and phenoxybenzamine on the catecholamines and ATP of isolated nerve and adrenomedullary storage granules. Life Sci. **3**, 35—40 (1964).

Evans, W., Loughnan, O.: The drug treatment of hyperpiesia. Brit. Heart J. **1939** I, 199—228.

Everett, G. M., Toman, J. E. P.: Mode of action of Rauwolfia alkaloids and motor activity. Recent Advanc. Biol. Psychiat. **1**, 75—81 (1959).

Faith, M. E., Young, L. D., Grabarits, F., Harvey, J. A.: Differences in the duration of reserpine action in the rat depending on the measure employed. Int. J. Neuropharmacol. **7**, 575—585 (1968).

Feldberg, W., Myers, R. D.: A new concept of temperature by amines in the hypothalamus. Nature (Lond.) **200**, 1325 (1963).

Feldberg, W., Myers, R. D.: Effects of temperature of amines injected into the cerebral ventricles. A new concept of temperature regulation. J. Physiol. (Lond.) **173**, 226—237 (1964).

Feldberg, W., Myers, R. D.: Changes in temperature produced by microinjections of amines into the anterior hypothalamus of cats. J. Physiol. (Lond.) **177**, 239—245 (1965).

FERGUSON, R. S.: Reserpine and Rauwolfia in psychoneuroses. Brit. med. J. **1955** II, 1563.
FIBIGER, H. C., TRIMBACH, C., CAMPELL, B. A.: Enhanced stimulant properties of (+)-amphetamine after chronic reserpine treatment in the rat: Mediation by hypophagia and weight loss. Neuropharmacology **11**, 57—67 (1972).
FINK, M.: EEG classification of psychoactive compounds in man: a review and theory of behavioural associations. Pp. 497—507 In: Psychopharmacology. A Review of Progress: 1957—1967. Washington, Public Health Service Publication No. 1836 (1968).
FINNERTY, F. A.: Reserpine and the newborn infant. J. Amer. med. Ass. **160**, 997 (1956).
FLEMING, W. W., TRENDELENBURG, U.: The development of supersensitivity to norepinephrine after pretreatment with reserpine. J. Pharmacol. exp. Ther. **133**, 41—51 (1961).
FLÜCKIGER, E.: Pharmakologie der Antihypertonika. In: SARRE, H. (Ed.): Hypertonie: Pathogenese, Klinik and Therapie, pp. 235—249. Stuttgart: Schattauer 1969.
FOSTER, M. N., GAYLE, R. F.: Dangers in combining reserpine (Serpasil) with electroconvulsive therapy. J. Amer. med. Ass. **159**, 1520—1522 (1955).
FRANCE, E. S.: Reversal by pargyline of reserpine block of induced ovulation — direct ovarian effects. Neuroendocrinology **6**, 77—89 (1970).
FREEDMAN, D. X.: Effect of LSD-25 on brain serotonin. J. Pharmacol. exp. Ther. **134**, 160—166 (1961).
FREEDMAN, D. X.: Psychotomimetic drugs and brain biogenic amines. Amer. J. Psychiat. **119**, 843—850 (1963).
FREEDMAN, D. X., GIARMAN, N. J.: LSD-25 and the status and level of brain serotonin. Ann. N. Y. Acad. Sci. **96**, 98—106 (1962).
FREIS, E. D.: Effectiveness of drug therapy in hypertention: present status. Circulat. Res. **28**, Suppl. 2, 70—75 (1971).
FREIS, E. D., WANKO, A., WILSON, I. M., PARRISH, A. E.: Treatment of essential hypertension with chlorothiazide (diuril); its use alone and combined with other antihypertensive agents. J. Amer. med. Ass. **166**, 137—140 (1958).
FRIEDMAN, A. H., WALKER, C. A.: Circadian rhythms in rat mid-brain and caudate nucleus biogenic amine levels. J. Physiol. (Lond.) **197**, 77—85 (1968).
FROHLICH, E. D., FREIS, E. D.: Clinical trial of guanethidine, a new type of antihypertensive agent. Med. Ann. D. C. **28**, 419—422 (1959).
FURCHGOTT, R. F., GARCIA, P. S.: Effects of inhibition of monoamine oxidase in the actions and interactions of norepinephrine, tyramine and other drugs on guinea-pig left atrium. J. Pharmacol. exp. Ther. **163**, 98—122 (1968).
FURCHGOTT, R. F., GUBAREFF, T. de, GROSSMAN, A.: Release of autonomic mediators in cardiac tissue by suprathreshold stimulation. Science **129**, 328—329 (1959).
FURCHGOTT, R. F., KIRPEKAR, S. M., RIEKER, M., SCHWAB, A.: Actions and interactions of norepinephrine, tyramine and cocaine on aortic strips of rabbit and left atria of guinea pig and cat. J. Pharmacol. exp. Ther. **142**, 39—58 (1963).
FUXE, K.: Evidence for the existence of monoamine neurons in the central nervous system. IV. The distribution of monoamine nerve terminals in the central nervous system. Acta physiol. scand. **64**, Suppl. 247, 37—85 (1965).
FUXE, K., HILLARP, N.-Å.: Uptake of *l*-dopa and noradrenaline by central catecholamine neurons. Life Sci. **3**, 1403—1406 (1964).
GAFFNEY, T. E., CHIDSEY, C. A., BRAUNWALD, E.: Study of the relationship between the neurotransmitter store and adrenergic nerve block induced by reserpine and guanethidine. Circulat. Res. **12**, 264—269 (1963).
GAFFNEY, T. E., MORROW, D. H., CHIDSEY, C. A.: The role of myocardial catecholamines in the response to tyramine. J. Pharmacol. exp. Ther. **137**, 301—305 (1962).
GAITONDE, B. B., SATOSKAR, R. S., MANDREKAR, S. S.: The effect of reserpine on acid gastric secretion in anaesthetized cat. Arch. int. Pharmacodyn. **127**, 118—127 (1960).
GANTT, W. H.: Cardiovascular component of the conditional reflex to pain, food and other stimuli. Physiol. Rev. Suppl. **40**, 266—291 (1960).
GARATTINI, S., FRESIA, P., MORTARI, A., PALMA, V.: The pressor effect of reserpine after monoamine-oxidase inhibitors. Med. exp. (Basel) **2**, 252—259 (1960b).
GARATTINI, S., GIACHETTI, A., JORI, A., PIERI, L., VALZELLI, L.: Effect of imipramine, amitriptyline and their monomethyl derivatives on reserpine activity. J. Pharm. Pharmacol. **14**, 509—514 (1962).
GARATTINI, S., JORI, A.: Interactions between imipramine-like drugs and reserpine on body temperature. In: GARATTINI, S., DUKES, N. M. G. (Eds.): First Intern. Symp. on Antidepressant Drugs, p. 179—193. Amsterdam: Exerpta Medica Foundation 1967.
GARATTINI, S., KATO, R., VALZELLI, L.: Effect of reserpine analogues on tissue serotonin. Experientia (Basel) **16**, 120 (1960a).
GARCIA, A. G., KIRPEKAR, S. M.: Release of noradrenaline from the cat spleen by sodium deprivation. Brit. J. Pharmacol. **47**, 729—747 (1973).

GARDIER, R. W., JAMES, E. A., JOHNSON, P. C., RICHARDS, A. B., ROESCH, R. P.: Vasodepression induced by acetylcholine in the atropinized dog. Brit. J. Pharmacol. **20**, 579—585 (1963).
GARRETT, R. L., CARRIER, O., Jr.: Alteration of extracellular calcium dependence in vascular tissue by reserpine. Europ. J. Pharmacol. **13**, 306—311 (1971).
GARRETT, R. L., CARRIER, O., Jr.: DOUGLAS, B. H.: Effects of reserpine on blood pressure and vascular electrolytes in hypertension. Europ. J. Pharmacol. **2**, 236—238 (1967).
GAUNT, R., RENZI, A. A., ANTONCHAK, N., MILLER, G. J., GILMAN, M.: Endocrine aspects of the pharmacology of reserpine. Ann. N. Y. Acad. Sci. **59**, 22—35 (1954).
GEFFEN, L. B., OSTBERG, A.: Distribution of granular vesicles in normal and constricted sympathetic neurons. J. Physiol. (Lond.) **204**, 583—592 (1969).
GESSA, G. L., KRISHNA, G., FORN, J., TAGLIAMONTE, A., BRODIE, B. B.: Behavioural and vegetative effects produced by dibutyryl cyclic AMP injected into different areas of the brain. In: GREENGARD, P., COSTA, E. (Eds.): Role of cyclic AMP in cell function. Advances in biochemical psychopharmacology, Vol. 3, pp. 371—381. New York: Raven Press 1970.
GEY, K. F., PLETSCHER, A.: Effects of chlorpromazine on the metabolism of *dl*-2-C^{14}-dopa in the rat. J. Pharmacol. exp. Ther. **145**, 337—343 (1964).
GIACHETTI, A., SHORE, P. A.: Studies *in vitro* of amine-uptake mechanisms in heart. Biochem. Pharmacol. **15**, 607—614 (1966).
GIARMAN, N. J., PEPEU, G.: Drug-induced changes in brain acetylcholine. Brit. J. Pharmacol. **19**, 226—234 (1962).
GIELEN, W. Z.: Über die Funktion von Gangliosiden. Ein Serotonin- und Ca^{+2}-Receptor. Z. Naturforsch. **21**, 1007—1008 (1966).
GILGEN, A., MAICHEL, R. P., NIKODIJEVIC, O., BRODIE, B. B.: Essential role of catecholamines in the mobilization of free fatty acids and glucose after exposure to cold. Life Sci. **1**, 709—715 (1962).
GILLESPIE, E., LEVINE, R. J., MALAWISTA, S. E.: Histamine release from rat peritoneal mast cells: Inhibition by colchicine and potentiation by deuterium oxide. J. Pharmacol. exp. Ther. **164**, 158—165 (1968).
GILLESPIE, J. S.: Tissue binding of noradrenaline. Proc. roy. Soc. B **116**, 1—10 (1966).
GILLESPIE, J. S., HAMILTON, D. N. H., HOSIE, R. J. A.: The extraneuronal uptake and localization of noradrenaline in the cat spleen and the effect on this of some drugs, of cold and of denervation. J. Physiol. (Lond.) **206**, 563—590 (1970).
GILLESPIE, J. S., MACKENNA, B. R.: The inhibitory action of the sympathetic nerves on the smooth muscle of the rabbit gut, its reversal by reserpine and restoration by catecholamines and by dopa. J. Physiol. (Lond.) **156**, 17—34 (1961).
GILLETTE, J. R., DINGELL, J.-V., SULSER, F., KUNTZMAN, R., BRODIE, B. B.: Isolation from rat brain of a metabolite product, desmethylimipramine, that mediates the antidepressant activity of imipramine. Experientia (Basel) **17**, 417—418 (1961).
GILLIS, C. N., PATON, D. M.: Cation dependence of sympathetic transmitter retention by slices of rat ventricle. Brit. J. Pharmacol. **29**, 309—318 (1967).
GLOVER, A. B., MCCULLOCH, M. W.: Interactions between reserpine and desmethylimipramine. Europ. J. Pharmacol. **11**, 163—168 (1970).
GLOWINSKI, J., AXELROD, J.: Effect of drugs on the uptake, release and metabolism of H^3-norepinephrine in the rat brain. J. Pharmacol. exp. Ther. **149**, 43—49 (1965).
GLOWINSKI, J., IVERSEN, L. L., AXELROD, J.: Storage and synthesis of norepinephrine in the reserpine-treated rat brain. J. Pharmacol. exp. Ther. **151**, 385—399 (1966).
GOLDIN, A., BURTON, R. M., HUMPHREYS, S. R., VENDETTI, J. M.: Antileukemic action of reserpine. Science **125**, 156—157 (1957).
GONZALEZ, J. R., IMAHARA, J. K.: Electroshock therapy with the phenothiazines and reserpines — a survey and report. Amer. J. Psychiat. **121**, 253—256 (1964).
GRAEFF, F. G., LEME, J. G., ROCHA e SILVA, M.: Role played by catechol and indoleamines in the central actions of reserpine after monoaminoxidase inhibition. Int. J. Neuropharmacol. **4**, 17—26 (1965).
GRAY, W. D., RAUH, C. E.: The anticonvulsant action of inhibitors of carbonic anhydrase: Site and mode of action in rats and mice. J. Pharmacol. exp. Ther. **156**, 383—396 (1967).
GRAY, W. D., RAUH, C. E., SHANAHAN, R. W.: The mechanism of the antagonistic action of reserpine on the anticonvulsant effect of inhibitors of carbonic anhydrase. J. Pharmacol. exp. Ther. **139**, 350—360 (1963).
GREEN, A. F.: Antihypertensive drugs. Advanc. Pharmacol. **1**, 161—225 (1962).
GREEN, H., ERICKSON, R. W.: Further studies with tranylcypromine (monoamine oxidase inhibitor) and its interaction with reserpine in rat brain. Arch. int. Pharmacodyn. **135**, 407—425 (1962).
GREEN, J. P.: Histamine. In: LIJTHE, A. (Ed.): Handbook of Neurochemistry. Vol. 4, pp. 221—250. New York: Plenum Publ. Corp. 1970.

GREEN, R. D., FLEMING, W. W.: Agonist-antagonist interactions in the normal and supersensitive nictitating membrane of the spinal cat. J. Pharmacol. exp. Ther. **156**, 207—214 (1967).

GREEN, R. D., FLEMING, W. W.: Analysis of supersensitivity in the isolated spleen of the cat. J. Pharmacol. exp. Ther. **162**, 254—262 (1968).

GRILLO, M. A.: Electron microscopy of sympathetic tissues. Pharmacol. Rev. **18**, 387—399 (1966).

GUYTON, A. C.: Textbook of Medical Physiology, pp. 301—304. Fourth Edition. Philadelphia: Saunders 1971.

HÄGGENDAL, J.: The presence of 3-*O*-methylated noradrenaline (normetanephrine) in normal brain tissue. Acta physiol. scand. **59**, 261—268 (1963).

HÄGGENDAL, J., DAHLSTRÖM, A.: Uptake and retention of ^{3}H-noradrenaline in adrenergic nerve terminals after reserpine and axotomy. Europ. J. Pharmacol. **10**, 411—415 (1970).

HÄGGENDAL, J., DAHLSTRÖM, A.: The recovery of noradrenaline in adrenergic nerve terminals of the rat after reserpine treatment. J. Pharm. Pharmacol. **23**, 81—89 (1971).

HÄGGENDAL, J., DAHLSTRÖM, A.: The recovery of the capacity for uptake-retention of ^{3}H-noradrenaline in rat adrenergic nerves after reserpine. J. Pharm. Pharmacol. **24**, 565—574 (1972).

HÄGGENDAL, J., HAMBERGER, B.: Quantitative *in vitro* studies on noradrenaline uptake and its inhibition by amphetamine, desipramine and chlorpromazine. Acta physiol. scand. **70**, 277—280 (1967).

HÄGGENDAL, J., LINDQVIST, M.: Disclosure of labile monoamine fractions in brain and their correlation to behaviour. Acta physiol. scand. **60**, 351—357 (1964).

HÄGGENDAL, J., MALMFORS, T.: Evidence of dopamine-containing neurons in the retina of rabbits. Acta physiol. scand. **59**, 295—296 (1963).

HAGEN, R., BARRNETT, R., LEE, F.: Biochemical and electron microscopic study of particles isolated from mastocytoma cells. J. Pharmacol. exp. Ther. **126**, 91—97 (1959).

HALLIWELL, G., QUINTON, R. M., WILLIAMS, F. E., A comparison of imipramine, chlorpromazine and related drugs in various tests involving autonomic function and antagonism of reserpine. Brit. J. Pharmacol. **23**, 330—350 (1964).

HAMBERGER, B.: Reserpine-resistant uptake of catecholamines in isolated tissues of the rat: a histochemical study. Acta physiol. scand. **71**, Suppl. 295, 1—56 (1967).

HAMBERGER, B., MALMFORS, T., NORBERG, K.-A., SACHS, C.: Uptake and accumulation of catecholamines in peripheral adrenergic neurons of reserpinized animals, studied with a histochemical method. Biochem. Pharmacol. **13**, 841—844 (1964).

HAMBERGER, B., MASUOKA, D.: Localization of catecholamine uptake in rat brain slices. Acta pharmacol. (Kbh.) **22**, 363—368 (1965).

HANSON, L. C. F.: The disruption of the conditioned avoidance response following selective depletion of brain catecholamines. Psychopharmacologia (Berl.) **6**, 100—110 (1965).

HANSON, L. C. F.: Evidence that the central action of amphetamine is mediated via catecholamines. Psychopharmacologia (Berl.) **9**, 79—80 (1966).

HANSON, L. C. F.: Evidence that the central action of (+)-amphetamine is mediated via catecholamines. Psychopharmacologia (Berl.) **10**, 289—297 (1967).

HARDISTRY, R. M., INGRAM, G. I. C., STACEY, R. S.: Reserpine and human platelet 5-hydroxytryptamine. Experientia (Basel) **12**, 42 (1956).

HARRISON, T. S.: Some factors influencing thyrotropin release in the rabbit. Endocrinology **68**, 466—478 (1961).

HARRISON, T. S.: Adrenal medullary and thyroid relationships. Physiol. Rev. **44**, 161—185 (1964).

HARTMANN, E.: Reserpine: its effect on the sleep-dream cycle in man. Psychopharmacologia (Berl.) **9**, 242—247 (1966).

HASSLER, R., BAK, I. J.: Submikroskopische Catecholaminspeicher als Angriffspunkte der Psychopharmaka Reserpin und Monoaminohemmer. Nervenarzt **37**, 493—498 (1966).

HAVERBACK, B. J., STEVENSON, T. D., SJOERDSMA, A., TERRY, L. L.: The effects of reserpine and chlorpromazine on gastric secretion. Amer. J. med. Sci. **230**, 601—604 (1955).

HAVERBACK, B. J., WIRTSCHAFTER, S. K.: The gastrointestinal tract and naturally occurring pharmacologically active amines. Advanc. Pharmacol. **1**, 309—347 (1962).

HEIMANS, R. L., RAND, M. J., FENNESSY, M. R.: Effects of amantadine on uptake and release of dopamine by a particulate fraction of rat basal ganglia. J. Pharm. Pharmacol. **24**, 875—879 (1972).

HERMAN, E. H., BARNES, C. D.: Drug modification of the Schiff-Sherrington phenomenon. J. Pharmacol. exp. Ther. **516**, 48—54 (1967).

HERR, B., COSTA, E.: Normal rate of ^{3}H-norepinephrine uptake by isolated iris of rabbits injected with reserpine and pargyline. Int. J. Neuropharmacol. **8**, 463—469 (1969).

HERTTING, G., AXELROD, J., WHITBY, L. G.: Effect of drugs on the uptake and metabolism of H^3-norepinephrine. J. Pharmacol. exp. Ther. **134**, 146—153 (1961).
HERZ, A.: Drugs and conditioned avoidance response. Int. Rev. Neurobiol. **2**, 229—277 (1960).
HESS, S. M.., REDFIELD, B. G., UDENFRIEND, S.: The effect of monoamine oxidase inhibitors and tryptophan on the tryptamine content of animal tissues and urine. J. Pharmacol. exp. Ther. **127**, 178—181 (1959).
HESS, S. M., SHORE, P. A., BRODIE, B. B.: Persistence of reserpine action after the disappearance of drug from brain. J. Pharmacol. exp. Ther. **118**, 84—90 (1956),
HILLARP, N.-Å.: Adenosinephosphate and inorganic phosphate in the adrenaline and noradrenaline containing granules of the adrenal medulla. Acta physiol. scand. **42**, 321—332 (1958a).
HILLARP, N.-Å.: The release of catecholamines from the amine containing granules of the adrenal medulla. Acta physiol. scand. **43**, 292—302 (1958b).
HILLARP, N.-Å.: Further observations on the state of the catecholamines stored in the adrenal medullary granules. Acta physiol. scand. **47**, 271—279 (1959).
HÖKFELT, T.: The effect of reserpine on the intraneuronal vesicles of the rat vas deferens. Experientia (Basel) **22**, 56 (1966).
HÖKFELT, T.: Ultrastructural studies on the uptake and accumulation of monoamines in peripheral and central neurones, p. 70. In: Abstracts of the Fourth International Congress on Pharmacology, Basel (1969).
HOFFMANN, F., HOFFMANN, E. J., TALESNIK, J.: Influence of the thyroid hormone on the effector systems of the mammalian heart. Amer. J. Physiol. **148**, 689—699 (1947).
HOFFMAN, R. A.: Effect of and interaction between tranquilizers, serotonin and lysergic acid diethylamide on the body temperature of pigeons. Amer. J. Physiol. **195**, 751—754 (1958a).
HOFFMAN, R. A.: Temperature response of the rat to action and interaction of chlorpromazine, reserpine and serotonin. Amer. J. Physiol. **195**, 755—758 (1958b).
HOLLANDER, W., WILKINS, R. W.: Chlorothiazide: New type of drug for the treatment of hypertension. Boston med. Quart. **8**, 69—75 (1957).
HOLTON, P., RAND, M. J.: Sympathetic vasodilatation in the rabbit ear. Brit. J. Pharmacol. **19**, 513—526 (1962).
HOLTZ, P., BALZER, H., WESTERMANN, E., WEZLER, E.: Beeinflussung der Evipannarkose durch Reserpin, Iproniazid und biogene Amine. Naunyn-Schmiedeberg's Arch. exp. Path. Pharmak. **231**, 333—348 (1957).
HOLZBAUER, M., VOGT, M.: Depression by reserpine of the noradrenaline concentration in the hypothalamus of the cat. J. Neurochem. **1**, 8—11 (1956).
HONDA, F., IMMURA, H.: Inhibition of cyclic 3′, 5′ nucleotide phosphodiesterase by phenthiazine and reserpine derivatives. Biochim. biophys. Acta (Amst.) **161**, 267—269 (1968).
HONG, E., MENDOZA, P. A., PARDO, E. G.: Influence of previous reserpine administration on the ganglionic action of selected sympathomimetic amines. Life Sci. **4**, 2383—2392 (1965).
HOPKINS, T. F., PINCUS, G.: Effects of reserpine on gonadotropin-induced ovulation in immature rats. Endocrinology **73**, 775—780 (1963).
HORNYKIEWICZ, O.: Dopamine (3-hydroxytyramine) and brain function. Pharmacol. Rev. **18**, 925—964 (1966).
HORST, W. D., POOL, W. R., SPIEGEL, H. E.: Correlation between brain dopamine levels and *l*-dopa activity in anti-parkinson tests. Europ. J. Pharmacol. **21**, 337—342 (1973).
HOWLAND, R. D., SPECTOR, S.: Disposition of histamine in mammalian blood vessels. J. Pharmacol. exp. Ther. **182**, 239—245 (1972).
HUDGINS, P. M., FLEMING, W. W.: A relatively nonspecific supersensitivity in aortic strips resulting from pretreatment with reserpine. J. Pharmacol. exp. Ther. **153**, 70—80 (1966).
HUDGINS, P. M., HARRIS, T. M.: Further studies on the effects of reserpine pretreatment on rabbit aortas: Calcium and histologic studies. J. Pharmacol. exp. Ther. **175**, 609—618 (1970).
HUGHES, J., VANE, J. R.: An analysis of the responses of the isolated portal vein of the rabbit to electrical stimulation and to drugs. Brit. J. Pharmacol. **30**, 46—66 (1967).
HUKOVIĆ, S.: Isolated rabbit atria with sympathetic nerve supply. Brit. J. Pharmacol. **14**, 372—376 (1959a).
HUKOVIĆ, S.: The action of sympathetic blocking agents on isolated and innervated atria and vessels. Brit. J. Pharmacol. **15**, 117—121 (1959b).
HUKOVIĆ, S.: Responses of the isolated sympathetic nerve-ductus deferens preparation of the guinea pig. Brit. J. Pharmacol. **16**, 188—194 (1961).
HUSSAR, E., BRUNO, E.: Acute duodenal ulcer associated with reserpine therapy. Gastroenterology **31**, 500—504 (1956).

HUTCHINS, D.A., ROGERS, K.J.: Physiological and drug-induced changes in the glycogen content of mouse brain. Brit. J. Pharmacol. **39**, 9—25 (1970).

IGGO, A., MUIR, A.R.: The structure and function of a slowly adapting touch corpuscle in hairy skin. J. Physiol. (Lond.) **200**, 763—796 (1969).

IGGO, A., VOGT, M.: Preganglionic sympathetic activity in normal and reserpine-treated cats. J. Physiol. (Lond.) **150**, 114—133 (1960).

INNES, I.R., KRAYER, O.: Studies on veratrum alkaloids. XXVII. The negative chronotropic action of veratramine and reserpine in the heart depleted of catechol amines. J. Pharmacol. exp. Ther. **124**, 245—251 (1958).

INNES, I.R., KRAYER, O., WAUD, D.R.: The action of Rauwolfia alkaloids on the heart rate and on the functional refractory period of atrio-ventricular transmission in the heart-lung preparation of the dog. J. Pharmacol. exp. Ther. **124**, 324—332 (1958).

ISAAC, L., GOTH, A.: Interaction of antihistaminics with norepinephrine uptake: a cocaine-like effect. Life Sci. **4**, 1899—1904 (1965).

ISBELL, H., LOGAN, C.R.: Studies on the diethylamide of lysergic acid (LSD-25). II. Effects of chlorpromazine, azacyclonal and reserpine on the intensity of the LSD reaction. Arch. Neurol. Psychiat. (Chic.) **77**, 350—358 (1957).

IVERSEN, L.L., GLOWINSKY, J., AXELROD, J.: Uptake and storage of H^3-norepinephrine in the reserpine-pretreated rat heart. J. Pharmacol. exp. Ther. **150**, 173—183 (1965).

IVERSEN, L.L., KRAVITZ, E.A.: Sodium dependence of transmitter uptake at adrenergic nerve terminals. Molec. Pharmacol. **2**, 360—362 (1966).

IWAYAMA, T., FLEMING, W.W., BURNSTOCK, G.: Ultrastructure of mitochondria in atrial muscle associated with depression and supersensitivity produced by reserpine. J. Pharmacol. exp. Ther. **184**, 95—105 (1973).

IZUMI, F., OKA, M., YOSHIDA, H., IMAIZUMI, R.: Effect of reserpine on monoamine oxidase activity in guinea pig heart. Life Sci. **6**, 2333—2343 (1967).

IZUMI, F., OKA, M., YOSHIDA, H., IMAIZUMI, R.: Stimulatory effects of reserpine on monoamine oxidase in guinea pig heart. Biochem. Pharmacol. **18**, 1739—1748 (1969).

JEPSON, J.B., ZALTZMAN, P., UDENFRIEND, S.: Microsomal hydroxylation of tryptamine, indole-acetic acid and related compounds to 6-hydroxyderivatives. Biochim. biophys. Acta (Amst.) **62**, 91—102 (1962).

JOBE, P.C., PICCHIONI, A.L., CHIN, L.: Role of brain norepinephrine in audiogenic seizure in the rat. J. Pharmacol. exp. Ther. **184**, 1—10 (1973).

JOHNSON, H.L.: Nonmast-cell histamine kinetics. III. Uptake, metabolism and decline of H^3-histamine in the female rat and effects of endogenous histamine release. J. Pharmacol. exp. Ther. **171**, 88—97 (1970).

JONASON, J.: Effects of reserpine on the noradrenaline content of atrophied rat salivary glands. Acta physiol. scand. **75**, 73—77 (1969).

JONGH, D.K. DE, VAN PROOSDIJ-HARTZEMA, E.G.: Investigations into experimental hypertension. IV. The acute effects of Rauwolfia alkaloids on the blood pressure of rats with experimental renal hypertension. Acta physiol. pharmacol. neerl. **4**, 175—179 (1955).

JONGH, D.K. DE, VAN PROOSDIJ-HARTZEMA, E.G.: Augmentation of blood pressure in rabbits by reserpine. Acta physiol. pharmacol. neerl. **7**, 364—365 (1958).

JONVET, M.: Neuropharmacology of sleep, pp. 523—540. In: Psychopharmacology. A review of progress: 1957—1967. Washington, Public Health Service Publication, No. 1836 (1968).

JORI, A., GARATTINI, S.: Interaction between imipramini-like agents and catecholamine-induced hyperthermia. J. Pharm. Pharmacol. **17**, 480—488 (1965).

JORI, A., PAGLIALUNGA, S., GARATTINI, S.: Adrenergic mediation in the antagonism between desipramine and reserpine. J. Pharm. Pharmacol. **18**, 326—327 (1966).

JUNOD, A.F.: Uptake, metabolism and efflux of ^{14}C-5-hydroxytryptamine in isolated perfused rat lungs. J. Pharmacol. exp. Ther. **183**, 341—355 (1972).

JUORIO, A.V., VOGT, M.: Monoamines and their metabolites in the avian brain. J. Physiol. (Lond.) **189**, 489—518 (1967).

JUREVICS, H.A., CARRIER, O., Jr.: The influence of reserpine on the calcium-induced responses of spontaneously beating isolated rabbit atria. J. Pharmacol. exp. Ther. **184**, 189—197 (1973).

JURNA, I., GROSSMANN, W., NELL, T.: Depression by amantadine of drug-induced rigidity in the rat. Neuropharmacology **11**, 559—564 (1972).

KÄRKI, N.T., PAASONEN, M.K.: Selective depletion of noradrenaline and 5-hydroxytryptamine from rat brain and intestine by Rauwolfia alkaloids. J. Neurochem. **3**, 352—357 (1959).

KALSNER, S., NICKERSON, M.: Effects of reserpine on the disposition of sympathomimetic amines in vascular tissue. Brit. J. Pharmacol. **35**, 394—405 (1969).

KANEMATSU, S., HILLIARD, J., SAWYER, C.H.: Effect of reserpine on pituitary prolactin content and its hypothalamic site of action in the rabbit. Acta endocr. (Kbh.) **44**, 467—474 (1963).

Kanematsu, S., Sawyer, C. H.: Effects of intrahypothalamic implants of reserpine on lactation and pituitary prolactin content in the rabbit. Proc. Soc. exp. Biol. (N.Y.) **113**, 967—970 (1963).

Key, B. J., Bradley, P. B.: The effect of drugs on conditioning and habituation to arousal stimuli in animals. Psychopharmacologia (Berl.) **1**, 450—462 (1960).

Khan, A. U., Forney, R. B., Hughes, F. W.: Plasma free fatty acids in rats after shock as modified by centrally acting drugs. Arch. int. Pharmacodyn **151**, 466—474 (1964).

Khazan, N., Sulman, F., Winnik, H.: Effect of reserpine on pituitary-gonadal axis. Proc. Soc. exp. Biol. (N.Y.) **105**, 201—204 (1960).

Killam, E. K.: Drug action on the brain stem reticular formation. Pharmacol. Rev. **14**, 175—223 (1962).

Killam, E. K.: Pharmacology of the reticular formation, pp. 411—445. In: Psychopharmacology. A review of progress: 1957—1967. Washington, Public Health Service Publication No. 1836 (1968).

Killam, K. F., Killam, E. K.: Rhinencephalic activity during acquisition and performance of conditional behaviour and its modification by pharmacological agents. Progr. Brain Res. **27**, 388—399 (1967).

Kim, K. S., Shore, P. A.: Mechanism of action of reserpine and insulin on gastric amines and gastric acid secretion, and the effect of monoamine oxidase inhibition. J. Pharmacol. exp. Ther. **141**, 321—325 (1963).

Kirpekar, S. M., Goodlad, S. A. J., Lewis, J. J.: Reserpine depletion of adenosine triphosphate from the rat suprarenal medulla. Biochem. Pharmacol. **1**, 232—233 (1958).

Kirpekar, S. M., Lewis, J. J.: Effects of reserpine and hydrallazine on isolated strips of carotid arteries. J. Pharm. Pharmacol. **10**, 255—259 (1958).

Kirshner, N.: Uptake of catecholamines by a particulate fraction of the adrenal medulla. J. biol. Chem. **237**, 2311—2317 (1962).

Kirshner, N., Rorie, M., Kamin, D. L.: Inhibition of dopamine uptake *in vitro* by reserpine administered *in vivo*. J. Pharmacol. exp. Ther. **141**, 285—289 (1963).

Kitay, J. I., Holub, D. A., Jailer, J. W.: "Inhibition" of pituitary ACTH release after administration of reserpine or epinephrine. Endocrinology **65**, 548—554 (1959).

Klawans, H. L.: Pharmacology of parkinsonism: a review. Dis. nerv. Syst. **29**, 805—816 (1968).

Klein, F.: Hypotensive drugs. In: Meyler, L., Herxheimer, A. (Eds.): Side Effects of Drugs, pp. 202—211. Amsterdam: Exerpta Medica Foundation 1968.

Kline, N. S.: The use of *Rauwolfia serpentia* Benth. in neuropsychiatric conditions. Ann. N.Y. Acad. Sci. **59**, 107—132 (1954).

Kobinger, W.: Reversibility of a facilitatory action of reserpine on the central nervous system by methylamphetamine. Experientia (Basel) **14**, 337—338 (1958).

Koch-Weser, J.: Role of norepinephrine release in the interval-strength relationship of heart muscle. J. Pharmacol. exp. Ther. **150**, 184—189 (1965).

Koe, B. K., Weissman, A.: p-Chlorophenylalanine: A specific depletor of brain serotonin. J. Pharmacol. exp. Ther. **154**, 499—516 (1966).

Kopin, I. J., Gordon, E. K.: Metabolism of norepinephrine-H^3 released by tyramine and reserpine. J. Pharmacol. exp. Ther. **138**, 351—359 (1962).

Kopin, I. J., Gordon, E. K.: Metabolism of administered and drug-released norepinephrine-H^3 in the rat. J. Pharmacol. exp. Ther. **140**, 207—216 (1963).

Kopin, I. J., Hertting, G., Gordon, E. K.: Fate of norepinephrine-H^3 in the isolated perfused rat heart. J. Pharmacol. exp. Ther. **138**, 34—40 (1962).

Koslow, S. H., Roth, L. J.: Reserpine and acetazolamide in maximum electroshock seizure in the rat. J. Pharmacol. exp. Ther. **176**, 711—717 (1971).

Krayer, O., Alper, M. H., Paasonen, M. K.: Action of guanethidine and reserpine upon the isolated mammalian heart. J. Pharmacol. exp. Ther. **135**, 164—173 (1962).

Krayer, O., Fuentes, T.: Changes of heart rate caused by direct cardiac action of reserpine. J. Pharmacol. exp. Ther. **123**, 145—152 (1958).

Krell, R. D., Patil, P. N.: Steric aspects of adrenergic drugs. XIX. Influence of various factors on the stereoselectivity of pre-and postjunctional sites to norepinephrine isomers in isolated rat vasa deferentia. J. Pharmacol. exp. Ther. **182**, 101—115 (1972).

Krista, L. M., Burger, R. E., Waibel, P. E.: The influence of various drugs on the growth and beta-aminopropionitrile-induced dissecting aneurysm of turkeys. Poultry Sci. **42**, 522—526 (1963).

Kroneberg, G., Schümann, H. J.: Der Einfluß der *Rauwolfia*-Alkaloide Reserpin, Rescinnamin und Canescin auf den Katecholamin-Gehalt des Nebennierenmarks. Arzneimittel-Forsch. **7**, 279—280 (1957a).

Kroneberg, G., Schümann, H. J.: Die Wirkung des Reserpins auf den Hormongehalt des Nebennierenmarks. Naunyn-Schmiedeberg Arch. exp. Path. Pharmak. **231**, 349—360 (1957b).

KRONEBERG, G., SCHÜMANN, H. J.: Adrenalinsekretion und Adrenalinverarmung der Kaninchennebennieren nach Reserpin. Naunyn-Schmiedeberg Arch. exp. Path. Pharmak. **234**, 133—146 (1958).

KRONEBERG, G., STOEPEL, K.: Der Einfluß von α-methyl-dopa auf die Tyraminwirkung an mit Reserpin vorbehandelten Katzen. Experientia (Basel) **19**, 252—253 (1963).

KRÜGER, J. S., RANDRUP, A.: Pharmacological evidence for a cholinergic mechanism in brain involved in a special stereotyped behaviour of reserpinized rats. Brit. J. Pharmacol. **34**, 217P—218P (1968).

KRUGER, S., ROBINSON, G. A., SCHUELER, F. W.: A study of the antileukemic activity of Rauwolfia alkaloids. Arch. int. Pharmacodyn. **129**, 125—130 (1960a).

KRUGER, S., STANDEFFER, W. C., SCHUELER, F. W.: Some effects of reserpine on normal and leukemic mice. Arch. int. Pharmacodyn. **129**, 395—400 (1960b).

KUBO, T., NISHIO, H., MISU, Y.: The acute partial failure of neuromuscular transmission by reserpine in the isolated perfused rabbit's heart. Jap. J. Pharmacol. **20**, 442—445 (1970).

KULKARNI, A. S., SHIDEMAN, F. E.: Sensitivities of the brains of infant and adult rats to the catecholamine-depleting actions of reserpine and tetrabenazine. J. Pharmacol. exp. Ther. **153**, 428—433 (1966).

KUNTZMAN, R., JACOBSON, M. M.: On the mechanism of heart norepinephrine depletion by tyramine, guanethidine and reserpine. J. Pharmacol. exp. Ther. **144**, 399—404 (1964).

KUSCHKE, H. J., FRANTZ, J.: Über eine hyperglykamische Wirkung von Reserpin. Naunyn-Schmiedeberg Arch. exp. Path. Pharmak. **224**, 269—274 (1955).

LAGE, G. L., SPRATT, J. L.: Antagonism of intravenous digitoxigenin lethality by reserpine pretreatment in the mouse. Proc. Soc. exp. Biol. (N.Y.) **125**, 580—583 (1967).

LANGENDORFF, M., MELCHING, H.-J., LANGENDORFF, H., KOCH, R., JAQUES, R.: Untersuchungen über einen biologischen Strahlenschutz XXI. Mitteilung: Weitere Untersuchungen zur Wirkung zentral-erregender und -dämpfender Pharmaka auf die Strahlenempfindlichkeit des Tieres. Strahlentherapie **104**, No. 3, 1—8 (1957).

LAROCHELLE, L., BÉDARD, P., POIRIER, L. J., SOURKES, T. L.: Correlative neuroanatomical and neuropharmacological study of tremor and catatonia in the monkey. Neuropharmacology **10**, 273—288 (1971).

LASAGNA, L., MCCANN, W. P.: Effect of tranquilizing drugs on amphetamine toxicity in aggregated mice. Science **125**, 1241—1242 (1957).

LEDDA, F., BALDI, V.: The effect of reserpine on mammalian neuro-muscular transmission. Life Sci. **4**, 955—957 (1965).

LEE, F. L.: The relation between norepinephrine content and response to sympathetic nerve stimulation of various organs of cats pretreated with reserpine. J. Pharmacol. exp. Ther. **156**, 137—141 (1967).

LEE, W. C., SHIDEMAN, F. E.: Role of myocardial catecholamines in cardiac contractility. Science **129**, 967—968 (1959a).

LEE, W. C., SHIDEMAN, F. E.: Mechanism of the positive inotropic response to certain ganglionic stimulants. J. Pharmacol. exp. Ther. **126**, 239—249 (1959b).

LEMBERGER, L., AXELROD, J., KOPIN, I. J.: The disposition and metabolism of tryptamine and the *in vivo* formation of 6-hydroxy-tryptamine in the rabbit. J. Pharmacol. exp. Ther. **177**, 169—176 (1971).

LETTAU, H. F., SELLERS, E. A., SCHÖNBAUM, E.: Modification of drug-induced hypothermia. Canad. J. Physiol. Pharmacol. **42**, 745—755 (1964).

LEVILL, B., ROBERTS, J.: The capacity of different digitalis materials to induce ventricular rhythm disturbances in the reserpine-pretreated cat. J. Pharmacol. exp. Ther. **156**, 159—161 (1967).

LEVIN, E. Y., LEVENBERG, B., KAUFMAN, S.: Enzymic conversion of 3,4-dihydroxyphenylethylamine to norepinephrine. J. biol. Chem. **235**, 2080—2086 (1960).

LEVISON, P. K., FREEDMAN, D. X.: Recovery of a discriminated leverpress avoidance performance from the effects of reserpine, chlorpromazine and tetrabenazine. Arch. int. Pharmacodyn. **170**, 31—38 (1967).

LEVITT, M., SPECTOR, S., SJOERDSMA, A., UDENFRIEND, S.: Elucidation of the rate-limiting step in norepinephrine biosynthesis in the perfused guinea-pig heart. J. Pharmacol. exp. Ther. **148**, 1—8 (1965).

LEWIS, J. J.: Rauwolfia Derivatives. In: ROOT, W. S., HOFMANN, F. G. (Eds.): Physiological Pharmacology, pp. 479—536. Vol. I, London: Academic Press 1963.

LIEBMAN, J.: Modification of the chronotropic action of sympathomimetic amines by reserpine in the heart-lung preparation of the dog. J. Pharmacol. exp. Ther. **133**, 63—69 (1961).

LIEBMAN, J., MUSKUS, A. J., WAUD, D. R.: The depletion of norepinephrine stores in the heart of the dog by reserpine-type alkaloids. J. Pharmacol. exp. Ther. **136**, 75—79 (1962).

Lindmar, R.: Die Wirkung von 1,1-Dimethyl-4-Phenyl-Piperazinium-Jodid am isolierten Vorhof im Vergleich zur Tyramin- und Nicotinwirkung. Naunyn-Schmiedeberg Arch. exp. Path. Pharmak. **242**, 458—466 (1962).

Lindmar, R., Muscholl, E.: Die Wirkung von Pharmaka auf die Elimination von Noradrenalin aus der Perfusionsflüssigkeit und die Noradrenalinaufnahme in das isolierte Herz. Naunyn-Schmiedeberg Arch. exp. Path. Pharmak. **247**, 469—492 (1964).

Livett, B. G., Geffen, L. B., Austin, L.: Proximo-distal transport of (^{14}C) noradrenaline and protein in sympathetic nerves. J. Neurochem. **15**, 931—939 (1968).

Louis, W. J., Doyle, A. E.: The pressor response to noradrenaline and tyramine during angiotensin tachyphylaxis in the dog. Clin. Sci. **31**, 247—254 (1966).

Lovenberg, W., Weissbach, H., Udenfriend, S.: Aromatic l-amino acid decarboxylase. J. biol. Chem. **237**, 89—93 (1962).

Luby, E.: Reserpine-like drugs — Clinical efficacy, pp. 1077—1082. In: Psychopharmacology: A review of progress, 1957—1967. Washington, Public Health Service Publication No. 1836 (1968).

Lucas, R. A.: The chemistry and pharmacology of the Rauwolfia alkaloids. Progr. Med. Chem. **3**, 146—186 (1963).

Lundborg, P.: Storage function and amine levels of the adrenal medullary granules at various intervals after reserpine treatment. Experientia (Basel) **19**, 479—480 (1963).

Lundborg, P., Stitzel, R.: Uptake of biogenic amines by two different mechanisms present in adrenergic granules. Brit. J. Pharmacol. **29**, 342—349 (1967a).

Lundborg, P., Stitzel, R.: Effect of reserpine and protriptyline on the subcellular distribution of H^3-metaraminol in the mouse heart. Brit. J. Pharmacol. **30**, 379—384 (1967b).

Maanen, J. H. van, Smelik, P. G.: Induction of pseudopregnancy in rats following local depletion of monoamines in the median eminence of the hypothalamus. Neuroendocrinology **3**, 177—186 (1968).

Macmillan, W. H., Rand, M. J.: The effects in rabbits of thyroidectomy and treatment with triiodothyronine on the sensitivity to noradrenaline and the content of noradrenaline in aorta and spleen. J. Pharm. Pharmacol. **14**, 257—267 (1962).

Macmillan, W. H., Smith, D. J., Jacobson, J. H.: Responses of normal, denervated and reserpine-treated arteries to sympathomimetic amines and nicotine in dogs. Brit. J. Pharmacol. **18**, 39—48 (1962).

Maggiolo, C., Haley, T. J.: Brain concentration of reserpine-H^3 and its metabolites in the mouse. Proc. Soc. exp. Biol. (N.Y.) **115**, 149—151 (1964).

Magus, R. D., Krause, F. W., Riedel, B. E.: Dissociation of reserpine-induced depression of spontaneous motor activity and release of brain serotonin in rats. Biochem. Pharmacol. **13**, 943—947 (1964).

Mahfouz, M., Ezz, E. A.: The effect of reserpine and chlorpromazine on the response of the rat to acute stress. J. Pharmacol. exp. Ther. **123**, 39—42 (1958).

Maickel, R. P., Westermann, E. O., Brodie, B. B.: Effects of reserpine and cold-exposure on pituitary-adrenocortical function in rats. J. Pharmacol. exp. Ther. **134**, 167—175 (1961).

Malhotra, C. L., Das, P. K.: Effect of reserpine on the acetylcholine content of the heart, the ileum and the hypothalamus of the dog. Brit. J. Pharmacol. **18**, 190—193 (1962).

Malhotra, C. L., Mehta, V. L.: The effect of reserpine on the acetylcholine release of the cerebral cortex of dog under different anaesthetics. Brit. J. Pharmacol. **27**, 131—134 (1966).

Malhotra, C. L., Prasad, S.: Effect of some drugs on the acetylcholine release from the cerebral cortex of cat. Indian J. Physiol. Pharmacol. **12**, 103—106 (1968).

Malhotra, C. L., Pundlik, P. G.: The effect of reserpine on the acetylcholine content of different areas of the central nervous system of the dog. Brit. J. Pharmacol. **14**, 46—47 (1959).

Maling, H. M., Fleisch, J. H., Saul, W. F.: Species differences in aortic responses to vasoactive amines: The effects of compound 48/80, cocaine, reserpine and 6-hydroxydopamine. J. Pharmacol. exp. Ther. **176**, 672—683 (1971).

Malmfors, T.: Evidence of adrenergic neurons with synaptic terminals in the retina of rats demonstrated with fluorescence and electron microscopy. Acta physiol. scand. **58**, 99—100 (1963).

Malmfors, T.: Studies on adrenergic nerves. The use of rat and mouse iris for direct observations on their physiology and pharmacology at cellular and subcellular levels. Acta physiol. scand. **64**, Suppl. 248, 1—95 (1965).

Malmfors, T.: Fluorescent histochemical studies on the uptake, storage, and release of catecholamines. Circulat. Res. **21**, Suppl. 3, 25—42 (1967).

Malpica, J. F., Jurupe, H., Campos, H. A.: Actions of reserpine and tyramine on the acetylcholine content of brain stem, heart and blood of the rat. Arch. int. Pharmacodyn. **185**, 13—19 (1970).

MANARA, L., GARATTINI, S.: Time course of ^{3}H-reserpine levels in brains of normal and tetrabenazine-pretreated rats. Europ. J. Pharmacol. **2**, 139—141 (1967).
MANARA, L., MENNINI, T., CARMINATI, P.: Reduced binding of ^{3}H-reserpine to the hearts of 6-hydroxydopamine-pretreated rats. Europ. J. Pharmacol. **17**, 183—185 (1972).
MANARA, L., SESTINI, M. G., ALGERI, S., GARATTINI, S.: On the ability of desipramine to interfere with reserpine-induced noradrenaline release. J. Pharm. Pharmacol. **18**, 194—195 (1966).
MANDELL, A. J., KNAPP, S.: The effects of chronic administration of some cholinergic and adrenergic drugs on the activity of choline acetyltransferase in the optic lobes of the chick brain. Neuropharmacology **10**, 513—516 (1971).
MANNAIONI, P. F., LEDDA, F., BALDI, V., CATINI, C.: Differential release of histamine by 5-hydroxytryptamine, noradrenaline and reserpine from neoplastic mast cells *in vitro*: biological and fluorescence microscope observations. Europ. J. Pharmacol. **3**, 203—211 (1968).
MARCUS, F. I., PAVLOVICH, J., CUCCIA, C.: Inhibition of myocardial uptake of tritiated digoxin by reserpine pretreatment in the dog. Circulation **34**, Suppl. 3, 162—163 (1966).
MARGULES, D. L.: Noradrenergic rather than serotonergic basis of reward in the dorsal tegmentum. J. comp. physiol. Psychol. **67**, 32—35 (1969).
MARRAZZI, A. S.: Electrical studies on the pharmacology of autonomic synapses. II. The action of a sympathomimetic drug (epinephrine) on sympathetic ganglia. J. Pharmacol. exp. Ther. **65**, 395—404 (1939).
MARSDEN, G. A., BROCH, O. J. Jr., GULDBERG, H. C.: Catechol-*O*-Methyl transferase and monoamine oxidase activities of rat submaxillary glands: Effects of ligation, sympathectomy and some drugs. Europ. J. Pharmacol. **15**, 335—342 (1971).
MASON, D. T., BRAUNWALD, E.: Effects of guanethidine, reserpine, and methyldopa on reflex venous and arterial constriction in man. J. Clin. Invest. **43**, 1449—1463 (1964).
MATTHEWS, R. J.: The effects of epinephrine, levarterenol, and *dl*-isoproterenol on transmission in the superior cervical ganglion. J. Pharmacol. exp. Ther. **116**, 433—443 (1956).
MAXWELL, D. R., PALMER, H. T.: Demonstration of antidepressant or stimulant properties of imipramine in experimental animals. Nature (Lond.) **191**, 84—85 (1961).
MAXWELL, R. A., KEENAN, P. D., CHAPLIN, E., ROTH, B., ECKHARDT, S. B.: Molecular features affecting the potency of tricyclic antidepressants and structurally related compounds as inhibitors of the uptake of tritiated norepinephrine by rabbit aortic strips. J. Pharmacol. exp. Ther. **166**, 320—329 (1969).
MAXWELL, R. A., PLUMMER, A. J., OSBORNE, M. W., ROSS, S. D.: Evidence for a peripheral action of reserpine. J. Pharmacol. exp. Ther. **116**, 42 (1956).
MAXWELL, R. A., POVALSKI, H., PLUMMER, A. J.: A differential effect of reserpine on pressor amine activity and its relationship to other agents producing this effect. J. Pharmacol. exp. Ther. **125**, 178—183 (1959).
MAXWELL, R. A., ROSS, S. D., PLUMMER, A. J., SIGG, E. B.: A peripheral action of reserpine. J. Pharmacol. exp. Ther. **119**, 69—77 (1957).
MAYER, G., MEUNIER, J. M., THEVENOT-DULUC, A. J.: Prolongation de la grossesse par retards de nidation obtenus chez la ratte par administration de réserpine. Ann. Endocr. (Paris) **21**, 1—13 (1960).
MAYOR, D., KAPELLER, K.: Fluorescence microscopy and electron microscopy of adrenergic nerves after constriction at two points. J. roy. micr. Soc. **87**, 277—294 (1967).
MCCUBBIN, J. W., PAGE, I. H.: Do ganglion-blocking agents and reserpine affect central vasomotor activity? Circulat. Res. **6**, 816—824 (1958).
MCCULLOCH, M. W., PROCTOR, C., RAND, M. J.: Evidence for an adrenergic homeostatic bronchodilator reflex mechanism. Europ. J. Pharmacol. **2**, 214—223 (1967).
MCGEER, P. L., BOULDING, J. E., GIBSON, W. C., FOULKES, R. G.: Drug-induced extrapyramidal reactions. J. Amer. med. Ass. **177**, 665—670 (1961).
MCGEER, P. L., MCGEER, E. G., WADA, J. A.: Central aromatic amine levels in behaviour. II. Serotonin and catecholamine levels in various cat brain areas following administration of psychoactive drugs or amine precursors. Arch. Neurol. (Chic.) **9**, 81—89 (1963).
MCNEILL, J. H.: Reserpine supersensitivity to catecholamine-induced cardiac phosphorylase activation. Canad. J. Physiol. Pharmacol. **47**, 515—519 (1969).
MCQUEEN, E. G.: The effect of control of blood pressure on vascular reactivity in experimental renal hypertension. Clin. Sci. **21**, 133—140 (1961).
MCQUEEN, E. G., DOYLE, A. E., SMIRK, F. H.: The circulatory effects of reserpine. Circulation **11**, 161—169 (1955).
MCQUEEN, E. G., HODGE, J. V.: Modification of secondary lesions in renal hypertensive rats by control of the blood pressure with reserpine. Quart. J. Med. **30**, 213—230 (1961).
MEDINA, M. A., LANDEZ, J. H., FORSTER, L. L.: Inhibition of tissue histamine formation by decaborane. J. Pharmacol. exp. Ther. **169**, 132—137 (1969).

Meites, J., Nicoll, C. S., Taiwalker, P. K.: Effects of reserpine and serotonin on milk secretion and mammary growth in the rat. Proc. Soc. exp. Biol. (N.Y.) **101**, 563—565 (1959).

Melville, K. I., Johnson, M. C.: Cerebrospinal fluid electrolyte changes during lateral ventricular perfusion with noradrenaline and associated cardiovascular responses. Neuropharmacology **9**, 79—95 (1970).

Meter, W. van, Karczmar, A. G.: Effect of catecholamine depletion on anticholinesterase activity in the central nervous system. Fed. Proc. **26**, 651 (1967).

Meter, W. van, Karczmar, A. G.: An effect of physostigmine on the central nervous system of rabbits related to brain levels of norepinephrine. Neuropharmacology **10**, 379—390 (1971).

Mirkin, B. L.: Catechol amine depletion in the rat's denervated adrenal gland following chronic administration of reserpine. Nature (Lond.) **182**, 113—114 (1958).

Mirkin, B. L., Cervoni, P.: The adrenergic nature of neurohumoral transmission in the cat nictitating membrane following treatment with reserpine. J. Pharmacol. exp. Ther. **138**, 301—308 (1962).

Misu, Y., Tanaka, C., Takaori, S.: Effects of dichloroisoproterenol and phenoxybenzamine on the transmembrane potentials of the isolated rabbits' heart. Jap. J. Pharmacol. **15**, 176—186 (1965).

Mohammed, S., Gaffney, T. E., Yard, A. C., Gomez, H.: Effects of methyldopa, reserpine and guanethidine on hindleg vascular resistance. J. Pharmacol. exp. Ther. **160**, 300—307 (1968).

Molinoff, P. B., Brimijoin, S., Axelrod, J.: Induction of dopamine-β-hydroxylase and tyrosine hydroxylase in rat hearts and sympathetic ganglia. J. Pharmacol. exp. Ther. **182**, 116—129 (1972).

Monnier, M., Graber, S.: Classification electrophysiologique des substances psycholeptiques. (Position du chlordiazepoxide "Librium".) Arch. int. Pharmacodyn. **140**, 206—216 (1962).

Montanari, R., Stockham, M. A.: The effect of imipramine on the reserpine toxicity in adrenalectomized rats. J. Pharm. Pharmacol. **14**, 126—127 (1962a).

Montanari, R., Stockham, M. A.: Effects of single and repeated doses of reserpine on the secretion of adrenocorticotrophic hormone. Brit. J. Pharmacol. **18**, 337—345 (1962b).

Moran, N. C., Westerholm, B.: The influence of reserpine on 5-hydroxyptamine and histamine content of rat mast cells and of some rat tissues. Acta physiol. scand. **58**, 20—29 (1963).

Morgan, M., Mandell, A. J.: Indole (ethyl) amine-N-methyl transferase in the brain. Science **165**, 492—493 (1969).

Morpurgo, C., Theobald, W.: Behavioural reactions to amphetamine in reserpinized rats. Int. J. Neuropharmacol. **5**, 375—377 (1966).

Mueller, P. S., McDonald, R. K.: Observations on hypothermia induced by reserpine and chlorpromazine. Proc. Soc. exp. Biol. (N.Y.) **128**, 826—830 (1968).

Mueller, R. A., Shideman, F. E.: Restoration of cardiac responsiveness to tyramine after reserpine. J. Pharmacol. exp. Ther. **160**, 53—60 (1968a).

Mueller, R. A., Shideman, F. E.: A comparison of the absorption, distribution and metabolism of reserpine in infant and adult rats. J. Pharmacol. exp. Ther. **163**, 91—97 (1968b).

Mueller, R. A., Shideman, F. E.: The prolongation of reserpine-induced cardiac norepinephrine depletion by metabolic inhibitors. Biochem. Pharmacol. **17**, 451—467 (1968c).

Mueller, R. A., Thoenen, H., Axelrod, J.: Compensatory increase in adrenal tyrosine hydroxylase activity after chemical sympathectomy. Science **163**, 468—469 (1969a).

Mueller, R. A., Thoenen, H., Axelrod, J.: Increase in tyrosine hydroxylase activity after reserpine administration. J. Pharmacol. exp. Ther. **169**, 74—79 (1969b).

Muggenberg, A., Kowalczyk, T., Hoekstra, G., Grummer, R. H.: Experimental production of gastric ulcers in swine by reserpine. Amer. J. vet. Res. **27**, 1663—1669 (1966).

Murad, J. E., Shore, P. A.: Association between biochemical and behavioural actions of tricyclic antidepressants. Int. J. Neuropharmacol. **5**, 299—304 (1966).

Murnaghan, M. F.: Restoration of the chronotropic effect of tyramine on rat atria after reserpine. Brit. J. Pharmacol. **34**, 88—98 (1968).

Musacchio, J. M., Bhagat, B., Jackson, D. J., Kopin, I. J.: The effect of disulfiram on the restoration of the response to tyramine by dopamine and α-methyldopa in the reserpine-treated cat. J. Pharmacol. exp. Ther. **152**, 293—297 (1966).

Muscholl, E.: Die Konzentration von Noradrenalin und Adrenalin in den einzelnen Abschnitten des Herzens. Naunyn-Schmiedeberg's Arch. exp. Path. Pharmak. **237**, 350—364 (1959).

Muscholl, E.: Die Hemmung der Noradrenaline-Aufnahme des Herzens durch Reserpin und die Wirkung von Tyramin. Naunyn-Schmiedeberg Arch. exp. Path. Pharmak. **240**, 234—241 (1960).

Muscholl, E.: Indirectly acting sympathomimetic amines. Pharmacol. Rev. **18**, 551—559 (1966).

MUSCHOLL, E., VOGT, M.: The concentration of adrenaline in the plasma of rabbits treated with reserpine. Brit. J. Pharmacol. **12**, 532—535 (1957).

MUSCHOLL, E., VOGT, M.: The action of reserpine on the peripheral sympathetic system. J. Physiol. (Lond.) **141**, 132—155 (1958).

MUSKUS, A. J.: Effect of pretreatment with reserpine and reserpine analogs on the response of isolated guinea-pig atria to tyramine. J. Pharmacol. exp. Ther. **133**, 296—300 (1962).

NAGATSU, T., LEVITT, M., UDENFRIEND, S.: Tyrosine hydroxylase: The initial step in norepinephrine synthesis. J. biol. Chem. **239**, 2910—2917 (1964).

NASMYTH, P. A.: An investigation of the action of tyramine and its interrelationship with the effects of other sympathomimetic amines. Brit. J. Pharmacol. **18**, 65—75 (1962).

NAYLER, W. G.: A direct effect of reserpine on ventricular contractility. J. Pharmacol. exp. Ther. **139**, 222—229 (1963).

NEFF, N. H., COSTA, E.: Effect of tricyclic antidepressants and chlorpromazine on brain catecholamine synthesis, pp. 28—34. In: Antidepressant drugs. Proceedings of 1st Int. Symposium. Int. Congress Series No. 122. Excerpta Medica, Foundation. Amsterdam, New York, London (1967).

NORBERG, K.-A.: Drug-induced changes in monoamine levels in the sympathetic adrenergic ganglion cells and terminals: a histochemical study. Acta physiol. scand. **65**, 221—234 (1965).

NORN, S., SHORE, P. A.: Further studies on the nature of persistent reserpine binding: evidence for reversible and irreversible binding (in heart, spleen, adrenals and small intestine of rats). Biochem. Pharmacol. **20**, 1291—1295 (1971).

OKA, M., OHUCHI, T., YOSHIDA, H., IMAIZUMI, R.: Selective release of noradrenaline and adrenaline from isolated adrenal medullary granules. Life Sci. **5**, 433—438 (1966).

ORLANS, F. B. H., FINGER, K. F., BRODIE, B. B.: Pharmacological consequences of the selective release of peripheral norepinephrine by syrosingopine (SU 3118). J. Pharmacol. exp. Ther. **128**, 131—139 (1960).

PAASONEN, M. K., DEWS, P. B.: Effects of raunescine and isoraunescine on behaviour and on the 5-hydroxytryptamine and noradrenaline contents of brain. Brit. J. Pharmacol. **13**, 84—88 (1958).

PAASONEN, M. K., KRAYER, O.: Effect of reserpine upon the mammalian heart. Fed. Proc. **16**, 326—327 (1957).

PAASONEN, M. K., KRAYER, O.: The release of norepinephrine from the mammalian heart by reserpine. J. Pharmacol. exp. Ther. **123**, 153—160 (1958).

PALM, D., GROBECKER, H., BAK., I. J.: Membrane effects of catecholamine releasing drugs. In: SCHÜMANN, H. J., KRONEBERG, G. (Eds.): New Aspects of Storage and Release Mechanisms of Catecholamines, pp. 188—198. Berlin-Heidelberg-New York: Springer 1970.

PARRATT, J. R., WEST, G. B.: Release of 5-hydroxytryptamine and histamine from tissues of the rat. J. Physiol. (Lond.) **137**, 179—192 (1957).

PASTEELS, J. L.: Comparaison entre l'action des androgénes et de la réserpine sur l'hypophyse et la glande mammaire chez le rat. Ann. endocr. (Paris) **22**, 257—268 (1961).

PATON, D. M.: Effects of Na^+ and K^+ on the uptake of metaraminol by rabbit ventricular slices. Brit. J. Pharmacol. **41**, 65—75 (1971).

PEGRAM, B. L., CARRIER, O., Jr.: Change in calcium dependence of isolated arteries after reserpine. Amer. J. Physiol. **217**, 1736—1741 (1969).

PELLEGRINO de IRALDI, A., de ROBERTIS, E.: Action of reserpine, iproniazid and pyrogallol on nerve endings of the pineal gland. Int. J. Neuropharmacol. **2**, 231—239 (1963).

PENEFSKY, Z. J., KAHN, M.: Inotropic effects of dexamethasone in mammalian heart muscle. Europ. J. Pharmacol. **15**, 259—266 (1971).

PENNA, M., LINARES, F., CÁCERES, L.: Mechanism for cardiac stimulation during hypoxia. Amer. J. Physiol. **208**, 1237—1242 (1965).

PENNEFATHER, J. N., RAND, M. J.: Increase in noradrenaline content of tissues after infusion of noradrenaline, dopamine and *l*-dopa. J. Physiol. (Lond.) **154**, 277—287 (1960).

PERERA, G. A.: Edema and congestive failure related to administration of *Rauwolfia serpentina*. J. Amer. med. Ass. **159**, 439—440 (1955).

PHILIPPU, A., BECKE, H., BURGER, A.: Effect of drugs on the uptake of noradrenaline by isolated hypothalamic vesicles. Europ. J. Pharmacol. **6**, 96—101 (1969).

PHILIPPU, A., BURKAT, U., BECKE, H.: Uptake of norepinephrine by the isolated hypothalamic vesicles. Life Sci. **7**, 1009—1017 (1968).

PHILIPPU, A., PALM, D., SCHÜMANN, H. J.: Effect of segontin and reserpine on isolated medullary granules. Nature (Lond.) **205**, 183 (1965).

PHILIPPU, A., PFEIFFER, R., SCHÜMANN, H. J., LICKFELD, K.: Eigenschaften der Noradrenalin speichernden Granula des sympathischen Ganglion stellatum. Naunyn-Schmiedeberg Arch. exp. Path. Pharmak. **258**, 251—265 (1967).

PINTER, E. J., PATTEE, C. J.: Fat-mobilizing action of amphetamine. J. clin. Invest. **47**, 394—402 (1968).
PIRCH, J. H., RECH, R. H., MOORE, K. E.: Depression and recovery of the electrocorticogram, behaviour and brain amines in rats treated with reserpine. Int. J. Neuropharmacol. **6**, 375—385 (1967).
PLETSCHER, A., BURKARD, W. F., TRANZER, I. P., GEY, K. F.: Two sites of 5-hydroxytryptamine uptake in blood platelets. Life Sci. **6**, 273—288 (1967).
PLETSCHER, A., GEY, K. F.: Action of imipramine and amitriptyline on cerebral monoamines as compared with chlorpromazine. Med. exp. (Basel) **6**, 165—168 (1962).
PLETSCHER, A. SHORE, P. A., BRODIE, B. B.: Serotonin release as a possible mechanism of reserpine action. Science **122**, 374—375 (1955).
PLETSCHER, A., SHORE, P. A., BRODIE, B. B.: Serotonin as a mediator of reserpine action in brain. J. Pharmacol. exp. Ther. **116**, 84—89 (1956).
PLUMMER, A. J., EARL, A., SCHNEIDER, J. A., TRAPOLD, J., BARRET, W.: Pharmacology of Rauwolfia alkaloids, including reserpine. Ann. N. Y. Acad. Sci. **59**, 8—21 (1954).
PÖLDINGER, W.: Combined administration of desipramine and reserpine or tetrabenazine in depressive patients. Psychopharmacologia (Berl.) **4**, 308—310 (1963).
POLLOCK, D., MUIR, T. C., MACDONALD, A., HENDERSON, G.: Morphine-induced changes in the sensitivity of the isolated colon and vas deferens of the rat. Europ. J. Pharmacol. **20**, 321—328 (1972).
POTTER, L. T.: Storage of norepinephrine in sympathetic nerves. Pharmacol. Rev. **18**, 439—451 (1966).
POTTER, L. T.: Role of intraneuronal vesicles in the synthesis, storage and release of noradren aline. Circulat. Res. **21**, Suppl. 3, 13—24 (1967).
POTTER, L. T., AXELROD, J.: Studies on the storage of noradrenaline and the effect of drugs. J. Pharmacol. exp. Ther. **140**, 199—206 (1963).
POTTER, L. T., COOPER, T., WILLMAN, V. L., WOLFE, D. E.: Synthesis, binding, release and metabolism of norepinephrine in normal and transplanted dog hearts. Circulat. Res. **16**, 468—481 (1965).
PRADHAN, S. N., BOWLING, C.: Effects of nicotine on self-stimulation in rats. J. Pharmacol. exp. Ther. **176**, 229—243 (1971).
PURSHOTTAM, N.: Effects of tranquilizers on induced ovulation in mice. Amer. J. Obstet. Gynec. **83**, 1405—1409 (1962).
QUETSCH, R. M., ACHOR, R. W. P., LITIN, E. M., FAUCETT, R. L.: Depressive reactions in hypertensive patients: a comparison of those treated with rauwolfia and those receiving no specific antihypertensive treatment. Circulation **19**, 366—375 (1959).
QUINN, G. P., SHORE, P. A., BRODIE, B. B.: Biochemical and pharmacological studies of Ro I—9569 (tetrabenazine), a non-indole tranquilizing agent with reserpine-like effects. J. Pharmacol. exp. Ther. **127**, 103—109 (1959).
RAAB, W., MARCHET, H., HERRLICH, H. C.: Effect of reserpine and syrosingopine on the rate of contractility of the human heart. Amer. J. Cardiol. **7**, 404—411 (1961).
RADOUCO-THOMAS, S., TESSIER, L., LAJIUNESSEY, N., GARCIN, F.: Role of calcium in the reserpine-induced cerebral monoamines depletion. Int. Z. klin. Pharmakol. Ther. Toxikol. **5**, 5—11 (1971).
RAND, M. J., TRINKER, F. R.: Pharmacological agents affecting the activity and release of catecholamines. Brit. J. Anaesth. **38**, 666—689 (1966).
RANDRUP, A., MUNKVAD, I., UDSEN, P.: Adrenergic mechanisms and amphetamine induced abnormal behaviour. Acta pharmacol. (Kbh.) **20**, 145—157 (1963).
RAPER, C., WALE, J.: Propranolol, MJ 1999 and Ciba 39089-Ba in ouabain and adrenaline induced cardiac arrhythmias. Europ. J. Pharmacol. **4**, 1—12 (1968).
RATNER, A., TALWALKER, P. K., MEITES, J.: Effect of reserpine on prolaction-inhibiting activity of rat hypothalamus. Endocrinology **77**, 315—319 (1965).
RECH, R. H.: Antagonism of reserpine behavioural depression by *d*-amphetamine. J. Pharmacol. exp. Ther. **146**, 369—376 (1964).
REILLY, J. F., AHLSTROM, A. P., WATTS, J. S., CASSIDY, P., LUSKY, L. M.: Influence of age, sex and cold exposure on susceptibility to reserpine-induced gastric lesions. Toxicol. appl. Pharmacol. **15**, 97—105 (1969).
REINERT, H.: Role and origin of noradrenaline in the superior cervical ganglion. J. Physiol. (Lond.) **167**, 18—29 (1963).
REIS, D. J., MOORHEAD, D. T., MERLINO, N.: Dopa-induced excitement in the cat. Its relationship to brain norepinephrine concentrations. Arch. Neurol. (Chic.) **22**, 31—39 (1970).
REIS, D. J., WEINBREN, M., CORVELLI, A.: A circadian rhythm of norepinephrine regionally in cat brain: its relationship to environmental lighting and to regional diurnal variations in brain serotonin. J. Pharmacol. exp. Ther. **164**, 135—145 (1968).

RESNICK, O., KRUS, D.M., RASKIN, M.: Accentuation of the psychological effects of LSD-25 in normal subjects treated with reserpine. Life Sci. **4**, 1433—1437 (1965).

RESTALL, P.A., SMIRK, F.H.: Treatment of high blood pressure with hexamethonium iodide. N. Z. med. J. **49**, 206—209 (1950).

REWERSKI, W., JORI, A.: Effect of desipramine injected intracerebrally in normal or reserpinized rats. J. Pharm. Pharmacol. **20**, 293—296 (1968).

RICHARDSON, K.C.: Fine structure of autonomic nerve endings in smooth muscle of the rat vas deferens. J. Anat. (Lond.) **96**, 427—442 (1962).

RICHARDSON, K.C.: Fine structure of the albino rat iris with special reference to identification of adrenergic and cholinergic nerves and nerve endings in its intrinsic muscles. Amer. J. Anat. **114**, 173—206 (1964).

RINGER, R.K.: The influence of reserpine on early growth, blood pressure and dissecting aneurysms in turkeys, pp. 21—28. In: Proceedings of the conference on the use of the tranquilizing and antihypertensive agent serpasil in animal and poultry production. New Brunswick, N.J.: Rutgers University 1959.

RINGER, R.K.: Aortic rupture, plasma cholesterol and arteriosclerosis following serpasil administration to turkeys, pp. 32—39. In: The second conference on the use of reserpine in poultry production. Summut, N.J.: University of Minnesota, St. Paul, Minn., sponsored by Ciba Pharmaceutical Products, Inc. 1960.

ROBERTIS, E.D.P. de: Histophysiology of synapses and neurosecretion. London: Pergamon Press 1964.

ROBERTS, J., ITO, R., REILLY, J., CAIROLI, V.J.: Influence of reserpine and TM 10 on digitalis-induced ventricular arrhythmia. Circulat. Res. **13**, 149—158 (1963).

ROOS, B.-E., STEG, G.: The effect of L-3,4-dihydroxyphenylalanine and DL-5-hydroxytryptophan on rigidity and tremor induced by reserpine, chlorpromazine, and phenoxybenzamine. Life Sci. **3**, 351—360 (1964).

ROSENGREN, E.: On the role of monoamine oxidase for the inactivation of dopamine in brain. Acta physiol. scand. **49**, 370—375 (1960).

ROSENGREN, E., SVENSSON, S.E.: Histamine formation in rat gastric mucosa and lung after injecting reserpine or adrenaline. Brit. J. Pharmacol. **37**, 659—665 (1969).

ROSSUM, J.M. VAN, SCHOOT, J.B. VAN DER, HURKMANS, J.A.TH.M.: Mechanism of action of cocaine and amphetamine in the brain. Experientia (Basel) **18**, 229—231 (1962).

ROTH, R.A., STONE, C.A.: The action of reserpine on noradrenaline biosynthesis in sympathetic nerve tissue. Biochem. Pharmacol. **17**, 1581—1590 (1968).

RUBIN, B., MALONE, M.H., WAUGH, M.H., BURKE, J.C.: Bioassay of rauwolfia roots and alkaloids. J. Pharmacol. exp. Ther. **120**, 125—136 (1957).

RUTLEDGE, C.O., WEINER, N.: The effect of reserpine upon the synthesis of norepinephrine in isolated rabbit heart. J. Pharmacol. exp. Ther. **157**, 290—302 (1967).

RYAN, M.J., BRODY, M.J.: Distribution of histamine in the canine autonomic nervous system. J. Pharmacol. exp. Ther. **174**, 123—132 (1970).

SABELLI, H.C.: Influence on the effect of vasoconstrictor amines by pretreatment with reserpine. Nature (Lond.) **187**, 784—785 (1960).

SAFFRAN, M., VOGT, M.: Depletion of pituitary cortiocotrophin by reserpine and by a nitrogen mustard. Brit. J. Pharmacol. **15**, 165—169 (1960).

SALMOIRAGHI, G.C., SOLLERO, L., PAGE, I.H.: Blockade by Brom-Lysergic-acid-Diethylamide (BOL) of the potentiating action of serotonin and reserpine on hexobarbital hypnosis. J. Pharmacol. exp. Ther. **117**, 166—168 (1956).

SANYAL, R.K., WEST, G.B.: The relationship of histamine and 5-hydroxytryptamine to anaphylactic shock in different species. J. Physiol. (Lond.) **144**, 525—531 (1958).

SARTORELLI, A.C., MAGUS, R.D.: Interaction of reserpine with polynucleotides. Pharmacologist **7**, 171 (1965).

SCHAEPDRYVER, A.F. de: Hypertensive responses in reserpinized dogs. Arch. int. Pharmacodyn. **124**, 45—52 (1960).

SCHAEPDRYVER, A.F. de, PREZIOSI, P.: Pharmacological depletion of adrenaline and noradrenaline in various organs of mice. Arch. int. Pharmacodyn. **121**, 177—221 (1959).

SCHANBERG, S.M., GIARMAN, N.J.: Drug-induced alterations in the sub-cellular distribution of 5-hydroxytryptamine in rat's brain. Biochem. Pharmacol. **11**, 187—194 (1962).

SCHAYER, R.W.: Formation and binding of histamine in rat tissues *in vitro*. Amer. J. Physiol. **187**, 63—65 (1956).

SCHLITTLER, E.: *Rauwolfia* alkaloids with special reference to the chemistry of reserpine. In: The Alkaloids, Vol. 8. New York: Academic Press 1965.

SCHLITTLER, E., BEIN, H.J.: Rauwolfia Alkaloids, In: SCHLITTLER, E. (Ed.): Antihypertensive Agents, pp. 191—221. New York: Academic Press (1967).

SCHMIDT, G., KÜSEL, H. J., DAL RI, H.: Über die Wirkung von Reserpin auf die sympathisch-motorische Innervation des Auges. Naunyn-Schmiedeberg Arch. exp. Path. Pharmak. **261**, 75—88 (1968).
SCHMITT, H., SCHMITT, H.: Interaction de la réserpine et de quelques amines sympathicomiméthiques. C. R. Soc. Biol. (Paris) **151**, 2030—2032 (1957).
SCHMITT, H., SCHMITT, H.: Sur les effets hypertenseurs de la reserpine apres certains sympathicomimetiques. Arch. int. Pharmacodyn. **120**, 251—262 (1959).
SCHMITT, H., SCHMITT, H.: Modifications des effets des amines sympathicomimétiques sur la pression artérielle et la membrane nictitante par la réserpine. Arch. int. Pharmacodyn. **125**, 30—47 (1960).
SCHMITT, H., SCHMITT, H.: Inhibition de l'hypertension réserpinique postamphétaminique par les substances anti-dépressives du groupe de l'imipramine. C. R. Soc. Biol. (Paris) **160**, 303—306 (1966).
SCHMITT, H., SCHMITT, H., DEPOILLY, F.: Potentiation of the effects of indirect sympathomimetic amines by reserpine and bretylium. Nature (Lond.) **196**, 73 (1962).
SCHNEIDER, J. A., RINEHART, R. K.: Pharmacological interactions of serotonin and reserpine in dogs. J. Pharmacol. exp. Ther. **116**, 51 (1956).
SCHÜMANN, H. J.: Die Wirkung von Insulin und Reserpin auf den Adrenalin- und ATP-Gehalt der chromaffinen Granula des Nebennierenmarks. Naunyn-Schmiedeberg Arch. exp. Path. Pharmak. **233**, 237—249 (1958).
SCHÜMANN, H. J.: Medullary particles. Pharmacol. Rev. **18**, 433—438 (1966).
SCHWARTZ, A., LEE, K. S.: Effect of reserpine on heart mitochondria. Nature (Lond.) **188**, 948—949 (1960).
SEIDEN, L. S., PETERSON, D. D.: Reversal of the reserpine-induced suppression of the conditioned avoidance response by L-dopa: correlation of behavioural and biochemical effects in two strains of mice. J. Pharmacol. exp. Ther. **159**, 422—428 (1968).
SHASKAN, E. G., SNYDER, S. H.: Kinetics of serotonin accumulation into slices of rat brain: relationship to catecholamine uptake. J. Pharmacol. exp. Ther. **175**, 404—418 (1970).
SHELLENBERGER, M. K., ELDER, J. T.: Changes in rabbit core temperature accompanying alterations in brainstem monoamine concentrations. J. Pharmacol. exp. Ther. **158**, 219—226 (1967).
SHEPPARD, H., LUCUS, R. C., TSIEN, W. H.: The metabolism of reserpine-C^{14}. Arch. int. Pharmacodyn. **103**, 256—269 (1955).
SHEPPARD, H., TSIEN, W. H.: Metabolism of reserpine-C^{14}. II. Species differences as studied *in vitro*. Proc. Soc. exp. Biol. (N. Y.) **90**, 437—446 (1955).
SHEPPARD, H., TSIEN, W. H., PLUMMER, A. J., PEETS, E. A., GILETTI, B. U., SHULERT, A. R.: Brain reserpine levels following large and small doses of reserpine-H^3. Proc. Soc. exp. Biol. (N. Y.) **97**, 717—721 (1958).
SHEPPARD, H., TSIEN, W. H., SIGG, E. B., LUCAS, R. H., PLUMMER, A. J.: The metabolism of reserpine-C^{14}. III. C^{14}-concentration vs. time in the brains and other tissues of rats and guinea pigs. Arch. int. Pharmacodyn. **113**, 160—168 (1957).
SHIMAZU, T., AMAKAWA, A.: Regulation of glycogen metabolism in liver by the autonomic nervous system. III. Differential effects of sympathetic stimulation and of catecholamines on liver phosphorylase. Biochim. biophys. Acta (Amst.) **165**, 349—356 (1968).
SHIØRRING, E., RANDRUP, A.: "Paradoxical" stereotyped activity of reserpinized rats. Int. J. Neuropharmacol. **7**, 71—73 (1968).
SHORE, P. A.: Release of serotonin and catecholamines by drugs. Pharmacol. Rev. **14**, 531—550 (1962).
SHORE, P. A., BRODIE, B. B.: LSD-like effects elicited by reserpine in rabbits pretreated with iproniazid. Proc. Soc. exp. Biol. (N. Y.) **94**, 433—435 (1957a).
SHORE, P. A., BRODIE, B. B.: Influence of various drugs on serotonin and norepinephrine in the brain. In: GARATTINI, S., GHETTI, V. (Eds.): Psychotropic Drugs, pp. 423—427. London: Elsevier 1957b.
SHORE, P. A., BUSFIELD, D.: The effect of desmethylimipramine on reserpine-induced release of gastric histamine and adrenal catecholamines. Life Sci. **3**, 361—366 (1964).
SHORE, P. A., SILVER, S. L., BRODIE, B. B.: Interaction of reserpine, serotonin and lysergic acid diethylamide in brain. Science **122**, 284—285 (1955).
SIGG, E. B.: Autonomic side-effects induced by psychotherapeutic agents, pp. 581—588. In: Psychopharmacology. A review of progress: 1957—1967. Washington, Public Health Service Publication No. 1836 (1968).
SIGG, E. B., GYERMEK, L., HILL, R.: Antagonism to reserpine-induced depression by imipramine, related psychoactive drugs and some autonomic agents. Psychopharmacologia (Berl.) **7**, 144—149 (1965).

SJÖSTRAND, N. O.: Effect of reserpine and hypogastric denervation on the noradrenaline content of the vas deferens and the seminal vesicle of the guinea-pig. Acta physiol. scand. **56**, 376—380 (1962).
SKOU, J. C.: Enzymatic basis for active transport of Na^+ and K^+ across cell membrane. Physiol. Rev. **45**, 596—617 (1965).
SMIRK, F. H., ALSTAD, K. S.: Treatment of arterial hypertension by penta- and hexamethonium salts, based on 150 tests on hypertension of various aetiology and 53 patients treated for periods of two to fourteen months. Brit. med. J. **1951** I, 1217—1228.
SMIRK, F. H., DOYLE, A. E.: Hypotensive action of reserpine. Lancet **1954** I, 1096—1097.
SMIRK, F. H., DOYLE, A. E., MCQUEEN, E. G.: Control of blood pressure by combined action of reserpine and pentapyrrolidinium. Lancet **1954** II, 159—161.
SMITH, A. A., KARMIN, M., GAVITT, J. A.: Interaction of catecholamines with levorphanol and morphine in the mouse eye. J. Pharmacol. exp. Ther. **151**, 103—109 (1966).
SMITH, A. D.: Biochemistry of adrenal chromaffin granules. In: CAMPBELL, P. N. (Ed.): The Interaction of Drugs and Subcellular Components on Animal Cells, pp. 239—292. London: Churchill 1968.
SMITH, C. B.: Enhancement by reserpine and α-methyl dopa of the effects of *d*-amphetamine upon the locomotor activity of mice. J. Pharmacol. exp. Ther. **142**, 343—350 (1963).
SMITH, T. H. F., ROSSI, G. V.: The effect of reserpine and mecamylamine on experimental atheromatosis in the normotensive and hypertensive rat. J. Pharmacol. exp. Ther. **135**, 367—373 (1962).
SNYDER, S. H., AXELROD, J.: Circadian rhythm in pineal serotonin: Effect of monoamine oxidase inhibition and reserpine. Science **149**, 542—544 (1965).
SNYDER, S. H., GLOWINSKI, J., AXELROD, J.: The physiological disposition of H^3-histamine in the rat brain. J. Pharmacol. exp. Ther. **153**, 8—14 (1966).
SOMLYO, A. V., VINALL, P., SOMLYO, A. P.: Excitation-contraction coupling and electrical events in two types of vascular smooth muscle. Microvasc. Res. **1**, 354—373 (1969).
SPANN, J. F. Jr., SONNENBLICK, E. H., COOPER, T., CHIDSEY, C. A., WILLMAN, V. L., BRAUNWALD, E.: Cardiac norepinephrine stores and the contractile state of heart muscle. Circulat. Res. **19**, 317—325 (1966).
SPECTOR, S., HIRSCH, C. W., BRODIE, B. B.: Association of behavioural effects of parygyline, a non-hydrazide MAO inhibitor with increase in brain norepinephrine. Int. J. Neuropharmacol. **2**, 81—93 (1963).
SPECTOR, S., SHORE, P. A., BRODIE, B. B.: Biochemical and pharmacological effects of the monoamine oxidase inhibitors iproniazid, 1-phenyl-2-hydrazinopropane (JB 516) and 1-phenyl-3-hydrazinobutane (JB 835). J. Pharmacol. exp. Ther. **128**, 15—21 (1960).
SPILKER, B., CERVONI, P.: Electrical membrane activity and frequency force relations in normal, denervated and reserpine pretreated cat heart muscle. J. Pharmacol. exp. Ther. **168**, 60—69 (1969).
SRIMAL, R. C., JAJU, B. P., SINHA, J. N., DIXIT, K. S., BHARGAVA, K. P.: Analysis of the central vasomotor effects of choline. Europ. J. Pharmacol. **5**, 239—244 (1969).
STARK, P., BOYD, E. S., FULLER, R. W.: A possible role of serotonin in hypothalamic self-stimulation in dogs. J. Pharmacol. exp. Ther. **146**, 147—153 (1964).
STEG, G.: α-Rigidity in reserpinized rats. Experientia (Basel) **20**, 79—80 (1964).
STEIN, L.: Self-stimulation of the brain and the central stimulant action of amphetamine. Fed. Proc. **23**, 836—850 (1964).
STEIN, L., RAY, O. S.: Accelerated recovery from reserpine depression by monoamine oxidase inhibitors. Nature (Lond.) **188**, 1199—1200 (1960).
STILLE, G., LAUENER, H., EICHENBURGER, E.: Ein pharmakologischer Vergleich klinisch gebräuchlicher Antidepressiva unter besonderer Berücksichtigung von Noveril (HF-1927 Wander). Schweiz. med. Wschr. **95**, 366—372 (1965).
STITZEL, R. E., CAMPOS, H. A., SHIDEMAN, F. E.: Effect of hemicholinium on the catecholamine depleting actions of reserpine, morphine and insulin in rabbit tissues. J. Pharmacol. exp. Ther. **149**, 193—198 (1965).
STITZEL, R. E., LUNDBORG, P.: Effect of reserpine and monoamine oxidase inhibition on the uptake and subcellular distribution of H^3-noradrenaline. Brit. J. Pharmacol. **29**, 99—104 (1967).
STITZEL, R. E., WAGNER, L. A., STAWARZ, R. J.: Studies on the microsomal metabolism of ^3H-reserpine. J. Pharmacol. exp. Ther. **182**, 500—506 (1972).
STJÄRNE, L.: Studies of catecholamine uptake storage and release mechanisms. Acta physiol. scand. **62**, Suppl. 228, 1—97 (1964).
STJÄRNE, L.: Storage particles in noradrenergic tissues. Pharmacol. Rev. **18**, 425—432 (1966).
STJÄRNE, L., LAGERCRANTZ, H., HEDQVIST, P.: Subcellular distribution of reserpine in sympathetic nerves and in the adrenal medulla. Abstracts, 4th Int. Congr. Pharmac., Basel, p. 495 (1969).

Stjärne, L., Lishajko, F.: Drug induced inhibition of noradrenaline synthesis *in vitro* in bovine splenic nerve tissue. Brit. J. Pharmacol. **27**, 398—404 (1966).
Stjärne, L., Roth, R. H., Lishajko, F.: Noradrenaline formation from dopamine in isolated subcellular particles from bovine splenic nerve. Biochem. Pharmacol. **16**, 1729—1739 (1967).
Stjärne, L., Schapiro, S.: Effect of reserpine on secretion from the denervated adrenal medulla. Nature (Lond.) **184**, 2023—2024 (1959).
Sugrue, M. F., Shore, P. A.: The mode of sodium dependency of the adrenergic neuron amine carrier. Evidence for a second, sodium-dependent, optically specific and reserpine-sensitive system. J. Pharmacol. exp. Ther. **170**, 239—245 (1969).
Sugrue, M. F., Shore, P. A.: Further evidence for a sodium-dependent, optically specific and reserpine-sensitive amine carrier mechanism at the adrenergic neuron. J. Pharmacol. exp. Ther. **177**, 389—397 (1971).
Sulser, F., Bass, A. D.: Pharmacodynamic and biochemical considerations on the mode of action of reserpine-like drugs, pp. 1065—1075. In: Psychopharmacology: A review of progress: 1957—1967. Washington, Public Health Service Publication No. 1836 (1968).
Sulser, F., Bickel, M. H., Brodie, B. B.: The action of desmethylimipramine in counteracting sedation and cholinergic effects of reserpine-like drugs. J. Pharmacol. exp. Ther. **144**, 321—330 (1964).
Sulser, F., Owens, M. L., Norvich, M. R., Dingel, J. V.: The relative role of storage and synthesis of brain norepinephrine in the psychomotor stimulation evoked by amphetamine or by desipramine and tetrabenazine. Psychopharmacologia (Berl.) **12**, 322—332 (1968).
Sulser, F., Owens, M. L., Strada, S. J., Dingell, J. V.: Modification by desipramine (DMI) of the availability of norepinephrine released by reserpine in the hypothalamus of the rat *in vivo*. J. Pharmacol. exp. Ther. **168**, 272—282 (1969).
Sulser, F., Watts, J., Brodie, B. B.: On the mechanism of antidepressant action of imipramine-like drugs. Ann. N. Y. Acad. Sci. **96**, 279—288 (1961).
Sun, S. C., Sohal, R. S., Colcolough, H. J., Burch, G. E.: Histochemical and electron microscopic studies of the effects of reserpine on the heart muscle of mice. J. Pharmacol. exp. Ther. **161**, 210—221 (1968).
Szara, S.: Dimethytryptamine: Its metabolism in man; the relation of its psychotic effect to the serotonin metabolism. Experientia (Basel) **12**, 441—442 (1956).
Tafuri, W. L.: Ultrastructure of the vesicular component in the intraneural nervous system of the guinea-pig's intestines. Z. Naturforsch. (B) **19**, 622—625 (1964).
Tagliamonte, A., Tagliamonte, P., Perez-Cruet, J., Stern, S., Gessa, G. L.: Effect of psychotropic drugs on tryptophan concentration in the rat brain. J. Pharmacol. exp. Ther. **177**, 475—480 (1971).
Takagi, M., Zanerttini, D., Khalil, E.: Tolerance of reserpinized dogs to digitalis. Amer. J. Cardiol. **15**, 203—205 (1965).
Takenaka, F.: Response of vascular strip preparations to noradrenaline and tyramine. Jap. J. Pharmacol. **13**, 274—281 (1963).
Taketomo, Y., Shore, P. A., Tomich, E. G., Kuntzman, R., Brodie, B. B.: Studies on the mechanism of reserpine-induced epinephrine release and hyperglycaemia. J. Pharmacol. exp. Ther. **119**, 188 (1957).
Tanz, R. D.: Possible relationship between ouabain-induced augmentation and endogenous cardiac catecholamine release. In: Tanz, R. D., Kavaler, F., Roberts, J. (Eds.): Factors influencing myocardial contractility, pp. 563—577. New York: Academic Press 1967.
Tanz, R. D., Coram, W. M., Brining, C., Cavaliere, T.: The inotropic action of ouabain in relation to ventricular norepinephrine content. Arch. int. Pharmacodyn. **173**, 294—305 (1968).
Tanz, R. D., Marcus, S. M.: Influence of endogenous cardiac catecholamine depletion on the force and rate of isolated heart preparations and their response to ouabain. J. Pharmacol. exp. Ther. **151**, 38—45 (1966).
Taugner, G., Hasselbach, W.: Über den Mechanismus der Catecholamin-Speicherung in den "chromaffinen Granula" des Nebennierenmarks. Naunyn-Schmiedeberg's Arch. exp. Path. **255**, 266—286 (1966).
Taylor, A. W.: Free fatty acid levels in exercised and nonexercised reserpinized rats. Amer. J. Physiol. **223**, 319—322 (1972).
Taylor, J., Green, R. D.: Analysis of reserpine-induced supersensitivity in aortic strips of rabbits. J. Pharmacol. exp. Ther. **177**, 127—135 (1971).
Taylor, R. E., Jr., Fregly, M. J.: Effect of reserpine on body temperature regulation of the rat. J. Pharmacol. exp. Ther. **138**, 200—207 (1962).
Tedeschi, D. H., Fowler, P. J., Fugita, T., Miller, R. B.: Mechanisms underlying reserpine-induced ptosis and blepharospasm: Evidence that reserpine decreases central sympathetic outflow in rats. Life Sci. **6**, 515—523 (1967).

TEN EICK, R. E., WYTE, S. R., ROSS, S. M., HOFFMAN, B. F.: Post-countershock arrhythmias in untreated and digitalized dogs. Circulat. Res. **21**, 375—389 (1967).
THOA, N. B., ECCLESTON, D., AXELROD, J.: The accumulation of C^{14}-serotonin in the guinea-pig vas deferens. J. Pharmacol. exp. Ther. **169**, 68—73 (1969).
THOENEN, H., MUELLER, R. A., AXELROD, J.: Transynaptic induction of adrenal tyrosine hydroxylase. J. Pharmacol. exp. Ther. **169**, 249—254 (1969a).
THOENEN, H., MUELLER, R. A., AXELROD, J.: Increased tyrosine hydroxylase activity after drug-induced alteration of sympathetic transmission. Nature (Lond.) **221**, 1264 (1969b).
THOMPSON, J. H.: Serotonin and the alimentary tract. Res. Communications in Chem. Pathol. and Pharmacol. **2**, 687—781 (1971).
THOMPSON, J. H., CAMPBELL, L. B.: The effect of reserpine upon gastrointestinal serotonin in the Sprague-Dawley rat. Experientia (Basel) **23**, 826—827 (1967).
THORP, A.: Histamine and mast cells in nerves. Med. exp. (Basel) **4**, 180—182 (1961).
TODA, N.: Effects of adrenaline, noradrenaline and reserpine on the transmembrane potentials in both pacemaker and non-pacemaker fibers of the rabbit atrium. Jap. J. Pharmacol. **10**, 78—91 (1960).
TODA, N., YAMASAKI, Y., FUJIWARA, M.: Response to sympathetic nerve stimulation and noradrenaline in atria treated with reserpine and in atria from rabbits pretreated with reserpine. Jap. J. Pharmacol. **20**, 517—529 (1970).
TOZER, T. N., NEFF, N. M., BRODIE, B. B.: Application of steady state kinetics to the synthesis rate and turnover time of serotonin in the brain of normal and reserpine-treated rats. J. Pharmacol. exp. Ther. **153**, 177—182 (1966).
TRENDELENBURG, U.: The action of histamine and 5-hydroxytryptamine on isolated mammalian atria. J. Pharmacol. exp. Ther. **130**, 450—460 (1960).
TRENDELENBURG, U.: Modification of the effect of tyramine by various agents and procedure. J. Pharmacol. exp. Ther. **134**, 8—17 (1961).
TRENDELENBURG, U.: Supersensitivity and subsensitivity to sympathomimetic amines. Pharmacol. Rev. **15**, 225—276 (1963).
TRENDELENBURG, U.: The effect of sympathetic nerve stimulation on isolated atria of guinea pigs and rabbits pretreated with reserpine. J. Pharmacol. exp. Ther. **147**, 313—318 (1965).
TRENDELENBURG, U.: Mechanisms of supersensitivity and subsensitivity to sympathomimetic amines. Pharmacol. Rev. **18**, 629—640 (1966).
TRENDELENBURG, U., DRASKÓCZY, P. R.: The effect of intraneuronal inactivation on the transmembranal uptake of *l*- and *d*-norepinephrine. J. Pharmacol. exp. Ther. **175**, 521—522 (1970).
TRENDELENBURG, U., GRAVENSTEIN, J. S.: Effect of reserpine pretreatment on stimulation of the accelerans nerve of the dog. Science. **128**, 901—903 (1958).
TRENDELENBURG, U., MUSKUS, A., FLEMING, W. W., SIERRA, B. G. A. de la: Modification by reserpine of the action of sympathomimetic amines in spinal rats; a classification of sympathomimetic amines. J. Pharmacol. exp. Ther. **138**, 170—180 (1962).
TRENDELENBURG, U., PFEFFER, R. I.: Effect of infusion of sympathomimetic amines on the response of spinal cats to tyramine and to sympathetic stimulation. Naunyn-Schmiedeberg Arch. exp. Path. Pharmak. **248**, 39—53 (1964).
TRENDELENBURG, U., SIERRA, B. G. A. de la, MUSKUS, A.: Modification by reserpine of the response of the atrial pacemaker to sympathomimetic amines. J. Pharmacol. exp. Ther. **141**, 301—309 (1963).
TRENDELENBURG, U., WEINER, N.: Sensitivity of the nictitating membrane after various procedures and agents. J. Pharmacol. exp. Ther. **136**, 152—161 (1962).
TRIPOD, J., MEIER, R.: Wirkung von Serpasil (Reserpin, ein neues Alkaloid von *Rauwolfia serpentina B.*) auf isolierte Kreislauforgane. Arch. int. Pharmacodyn. **97**, 251—266 (1954a).
TRIPOD, J., MEIER, R.: Détermination et classification pharmacodynamique de l'action vasculaire périphérique de l'aprésoline, du néprésol et du serpasil. Arch. int. Pharmacodyn. **99**, 104—125 (1954b).
TRIPOD, J., STUDER, A., WIRZ, E., MEIER, R.: Modifications de la réactivité vasculaire périphérique "in vivo" par quelques hypotenseurs, entre autres la réserpine et l'hydralazine. Arch. int. Pharmacodyn. **126**, 126—139 (1960).
TROQUET, J., CALINET-LAGNEAUX, D., HERMANN-GEDANG, I.: Influence of reserpine on myocardial content of potassium in the rat. Arch. int. Pharmacodyn. **163**, 232—234 (1966).
TSAI, T. H., DENHAM, S., MCGRATH, W. R.: Sensitivity of the isolated nictitating membrane of the cat to norepinephrine and acetylcholine after various procedures and agents. J. Pharmacol. exp. Ther. **164**, 146—157 (1968).
VAKIL, R. J.: Clinical trial of *Rauwolfia serpentina* in essential hypertension. Brit. Heart. J. **11**, 350—355 (1949).
VAKIL, R. J.: Rauwolfia serpentina in the treatment of high blood pressure. Circulation **12**, 220—229 (1955).

VAN ORDEN, L. S., BENSCH, K. G., GIARMAN, N. J.: Histochemical and functional relationships of catecholamines in adrenergic nerve endings. II. Extravesicular norepinephrine. J. Pharmacol. exp. Ther. **155**, 428—439 (1967).
VAN ORDEN, L. S., BLOOM, F. E., BARRNETT, R. J., GIARMAN, N. J.: Hictochemical and functional relationships of catecholamines in adrenergic nerve endings. I. Participation of granular vesicles. J. Pharmacol. exp. Ther. **154**, 185—199 (1966).
VAN ORDEN, L. S., BURKE, J. P., GEYER, M., LODOEN, F. V.: Localization of depletion-sensitive and depletion-resistant norepinephrine storage sites in autonomic ganglia. J. Pharmacol. exp. Ther. **174**, 56—71 (1970).
VIVEROS, O. H., ARQUEROS, L., KIRSHNER, N.: Mechanism of secretion from the adrenal medulla. V. Retention of storage vesicle membranes following release of adrenaline. Molec. Pharmacol. **5**, 342—349 (1969).
VOGT, M.: Concentration of sympathin in different parts of central nervous system under normal conditions and after administration of drugs. J. Physiol. (London) **123**, 451—481 (1954).
VOLLE, R. L.: Modification by drugs of synaptic mechanisms in autonomic ganglia. Pharmacol. Rev. **18**, 839—869 (1966).
VOTAVA, Z., GLISSON, S. M., HIMWICH, H. E.: Behavioural reaction of rats pretreated with reserpine to LSD-25. Int. J. Neuropharmacol. **6**, 543—547 (1967).
WADA, J. A., WRINCH, J., HILL, D., MCGEER, P. L., MCGEER, E. G.: Central aromatic amine levels and behaviour. Arch. Neurol. (Chic.) **9**, 69—80 (1963).
WAGNER, L. A., STITZEL, R. E.: Studies on the subcellular distribution of H^3-reserpine. J. Pharm. Pharmacol. **21**, 875—876 (1969).
WAGNER, L. A., STITZEL, R. E.: The relation between the subcellular distribution of ^3H-reserpine and its proposed site of action. J. Pharm. Pharmacol. **24**, 396—402 (1972).
WAKADE, A. R., KRUSZ, J.: Effect of reserpine, phenoxybenzamine, and cocaine on neuromuscular transmission in the vas deferens of the guinea-pig. J. Pharmacol. exp. Ther. **181**, 310—317 (1972).
WALKER, C. A., SPECIALE, S. G., FRIEDMAN, A. H.: The influence of drug treatment on norepinephrine levels and ultrastructure of the rat hypothalamus and caudate nucleus during a programmed light-dark cycle. Neuropharmacology **10**, 325—334 (1971).
WAUD, D. R.: The influence of reserpine upon the changes in femoral blood flow produced by stimulation of the lumbar sympathetic chain. Experientia (Basel) **17**, 234 (1961).
WAUD, D. R., KOTTEGODA, S. R., KRAYER, O.: Threshold dose and time course of norepinephrine depletion of mammalian heart by reserpine. J. Pharmacol. exp. Ther. **124**, 340—346 (1958).
WEIL-MALHERBE, H., POSNER, H.: The effect of drugs on the release of epinephrine from adreno-medullary particles *in vitro*. J. Pharmacol. exp. Ther. **140**, 93—102 (1963).
WEINER, N., JARDETZKY, O.: Study of catecholamine nucleotide complexes by nuclear magnetic resonance spectroscopy. Naunyn-Schmiedebergs Arch. exp. Path. Pharmak. **248**, 308—318 (1964).
WEINER, N., RUTLEDGE, C. O.: The actions of reserpine on the biosynthesis and storage of catecholamines. In: VON EULER, U. S., ROSELL, U. S., UVNÄS, B. (Eds.): Mechanisms of Release of Biogenic Amines, pp. 307—318. Oxford: Pergamon Press 1966.
WEINER, N., TRENDELENBURG, U.: The effect of cocaine and of pretreatment with reserpine on the uptake of tyramine-2-C^{14} and *dl*-epinephrine-2-C^{14} into heart and spleen. J. Pharmacol. exp. Ther. **137**, 56—61 (1962).
WEINER, R. I., GANONG, W. F.: Effect of the depletion of brain catecholamines on puberty and the estrous cycle in the rat. Neuroendocrinology **8**, 125—135 (1971).
WEIR, M. C. L., MCLENNAN, H.: The action of catecholamines in sympathetic ganglia. Canad. J. Biochem. **41**, 2627—2636 (1963).
WEISS, B., COSTA, E.: Adenyl cyclase activity in rat pineal gland: effects of chronic denervation and norepinephrine. Science **156**, 1750—1752 (1967).
WEISS, J. L., CHASE, T. N.: Levodopa in Parkinsonism. Drugs **2**, 257—261 (1971).
WEISSBACH, H., KING, W., SJOERDSMA, A., UDENFRIEND, S.: Formation of indole-3-acetic acid and tryptamine in animals. J. biol. Chem. **234**, 81—86 (1959).
WEISSMAN, A., KOE, B. K., TENEN, S. S.: Antiamphetamine effects following inhibition of tyrosine hydroxylase. J. Pharmacol. exp. Ther. **151**, 339—352 (1966).
WELLS, H., BRIGGS, F. N., MUNSON, P. L.: The inhibitory effect of reserpine on ACTH secretion in response to stressful stimuli. Endocrinology **59**, 571—579 (1956).
WESTERMANN, E. O., MAICKEL, R. P., BRODIE, B. B.: On the mechanism of pituitary-adrenal stimulation by reserpine. J. Pharmacol. exp. Ther. **138**, 208—217 (1962).
WESTFALL, D. P.: Nonspecific supersensitivity of the guinea-pig vas deferens produced by decentralization and reserpine treatment. Brit. J. Pharmacol. **39**, 110—120 (1970a).

WESTFALL, D. P.: The effect of reserpine treatment and decentralization on the ion distribution in the vas deferens of the guinea pig. Brit. J. Pharmacol. **39**, 121—127 (1970b).

WESTFALL, D. P., FLEMING, W. W.: Sensitivity changes in the dog heart to norepinephrine, calcium and aminophylline resulting from pretreatment with reserpine. J. Pharmacol. exp. Ther. **159**, 98—106 (1968a).

WESTFALL, D. P., FLEMING, W. W.: The sensitivity of the guinea-pig pacemaker to norepinephrine and calcium after pretreatment with reserpine. J. Pharmacol. exp. Ther. **164**, 259—269 (1968a).

WHEAT, M., Jr., PALMER, R. F., BARTLEY, T. D., SELLMAN, R. C.: Treatment of dissecting aneurysms of the aorta without surgery. J. thorac. cardiovasc. Surg. **50**, 364—373 (1965).

WHELAN, R. F., SKINNER, S. L.: Autonomic transmitter mechanisms. Brit. med. Bull. **19**, 120—124 (1963).

WHITRINGTON, P., ZAIMIS, E.: The reserpine-treated cat. Brit. J. Pharmacol. **17**, 380—391 (1961).

WHITTINGTON-COLEMAN, P. J., CARRIER, O., Jr., CLOWER, B. R.: The effects of reserpine on vasopressin-cholesterol-induced atheromatous lesions. J. Pharmacol. exp. Ther. **160**, 32—39 (1968).

WILCKEN, D. E. L., BRENDER, D., SHOREY, C. D., MACDONALD, G. J.: Reserpine: Effect on structure of heart muscle. Science **157**, 1332 (1967).

WILKINS, R. W., JUDSON, W. E.: The use of *Rauwolfia serpentina* in hypotensive agents. New Engl. J. Med. **248**, 48—53 (1953).

WINTER, C. H., FLATAKER, L.: Effects of lysergic acid diethylamide upon performance of trained rats. Proc. Soc. exp. Biol. (N. Y.) **92**, 285—289 (1956).

WOFFORD, J. J., CUMMINS, A. J.: Hemorrhage from duodenal ulcer during the administration of reserpine. New Engl. J. Med. **255**, 1193—1194 (1956).

WOLFE, D., POTTER, L. T., RICHARDSON, K. C., AXELROD, J.: Localizing tritiated norepinephrine in sympathetic axons by electron microscopic autoradiography. Science **138**, 440—442 (1962).

WOODSON, R. E., YOUNGKEN, H. W., SCHLITTLER, E., SCHNEIDER, J. A.: *Rauwolfia:* Botany, Pharmacognosy, Chemistry and Pharmacology. Boston: Little, Brown 1957.

YOUDIN, M. B. H., SANDLER, M.: Activation of monoamine oxidase by reserpine. Europ. J. Pharmacol. **4**, 105—108 (1968).

YOUNGKEN, H. W.: *Rauwolfia serpentina*. Herbalist **23**, 35—43 (1957).

ZAIMIS, E.: Reserpine induced circulatory failure. Nature (Lond.) **192**, 521—523 (1961).

ZBINDEN, G.: Reserpine antagonists and their effects on reserpine induced catecholamine depletion of the adrenal medulla. Int. J. Neuropharmacol. **1**, 435—445 (1962).

ZETLER, G.: Der Harmin-tremor und seine Antagonisten. Naunyn-Schmiedebergs Arch. exp. Path. Pharmak. **231**, 34—54 (1957).

ZWIETEN, P. A. VAN, BERNSHEIMER, H. HORNYKIEVICZ, O.: Zentrale Wirkung des Reserpins auf die Kreislaufreflexe des Carotissinus. Naunyn-Schmiedebergs Arch. exp. Path. Pharmak. **253**, 310—326 (1966).

Chapter 5

Adrenergic Neuron Blocking Drugs

R. A. MAXWELL and W. B. WASTILA

With 40 Figures

I. Introduction to Adrenergic Neuron Blocking Agents

Adrenergic neuron blocking agents have been prominent on the pharmacologic and therapeutic scenes for approximately 15 years. In that time, an extremely large literature has accumulated regarding these agents. The literature has received extensive reviews (GREEN, 1962; BOURA and GREEN, 1965), shorter reviews (MAXWELL, 1962; MULL and MAXWELL, 1967) and extensive textbook treatments (NICKERSON, 1970; MAXWELL, 1971). In addition, several reviews of the chemistry of these agents have appeared (SCHLITTLER et al., 1962; COPP, 1964; MULL and MAXWELL, 1967). The biochemistry of guanethidine has also been reviewed (FURST, 1967b; LUKAS, 1973). The reader is directed to these earlier publications, especially the excellent one by BOURA and GREEN (1965), for full coverage of the literature available up to the time of their appearance.

The authors have decided to stress the more recent work that has not yet been reviewed because 1) it exists and 2) with new knowledge, especially that concerning the "amine pump" in the adrenergic neuron and the biochemistry of the adrenergic neuron in general, it has become possible to rationalize many previously contradictory and disconnected observations related to the mechanisms of action of these drugs. This is especially true in regard to the interactions of the adrenergic neuron blocking agents with other drugs. General acknowledgement of the earlier literature is given in the next three sections (I A–C). In those instances where an understanding of the significance of recent information is dependent upon comprehension of the earlier literature the earlier material has been covered in the detail required.

In reviewing the more recent experimental work one is struck with the very sophisticated knowledge that has been obtained regarding these compounds. On the other hand, one is also struck with the fact that, in the last analysis, we still do not know their intimate mode of action in dissociating the action potential from the release of norepinephrine in the adrenergic nerve terminal. It is hoped that this will be known by the time of the next review.

The authors have devoted significant space at the end of this presentation to a discussion of the "receptor of the amine pump" in the adrenergic neuron since this review emphasizes its central position in the pharmacology of adrenergic neuron blocking agents and in their interrelation with many other adrenergic drugs.

It has not been the author's intent to ignore any significant work in this field, but it seems inevitable that this may happen. If so, the authors give their sincere apologies to the authors whose work they may have overlooked.

A. General Pharmacology

1. Adrenergic Neuron Blockade Defined

The group of agents reviewed in this chapter has in common the capacity to inhibit the transmission of neuronal activity across the junction between sympathetic nerve terminals and effector cells. In this way they superficially resemble the adrenergic blocking agents. In contrast to adrenergic blocking agents, however, adrenergic neuron blocking agents act at the sympathetic nerve terminals to prevent the release of transmitter substance, rather than at the effector cell to inhibit the association of the transmitter with its receptors. The adrenergic neuron blocking agents produce only transient reduction in parasympathetic and motor function *in vivo* and this occurs only with high intravenous doses.

The general pharmacologic evidence defining adrenergic neuron blockade was similar for all the known agents (EXLEY, 1957, 1960; BOURA et al., 1959a, b; BOURA and GREEN, 1959, 1963, 1965; MAXWELL et al., 1960; MCLEAN et al., 1960; LAWRIE et al., 1964; MOE et al., 1964; DAVEY and REINERT, 1965; SCRIABINE et al., 1965). Three important observations were made following the intravenous administration of these drugs in doses which were sufficient to block the response of effector organs to sympathetic nerve stimulation. (1) Preganglionic and postganglionic conduction and ganglionic transmission in sympathetic nerves were only transiently inhibited relative to the duration of neuron blockade. This clearly ruled out the possibility that these drugs dampened the response of effector cells to nerve stimulation by an action on axons and/or ganglia. (2) Sympathetic effector organs were fully responsive to injected catecholamines. Thus, adrenergic blockade, of the type produced by propranolol or phentolamine was not involved in the action of these agents. (3) TM10 and bretylium were demonstrated to prevent the output of norepinephrine from the spleen on stimulation of the splenic nerves. Thus by a combination of direct measurement and inference, the site of action of adrenergic neuron blocking drugs was determined to be at the terminal ramifications of sympathetic nerves where they somehow interfered with the release of norepinephrine.

Almost the complete gamut of the pharmacologic activities of adrenergic neuron blocking agents which can be elicited *in vivo* following acute administration of moderate doses can be understood in terms of their actions at the sympathetic nerve terminal. These agents exert several or all of the following actions at sympathetic nerve terminals (Table 1) which are presented here in outline and discussed in detail in subsequent sections:

a) *Inhibition of the Release by Action Potentials of a Fraction of the Transmitter Stored in the Nerve Terminals*

The term "release" in this review means the passage out of the neuron of an amount of physiologically-active transmitter which is sufficient to be measured or to produce a response in effector cells. The quantity of norepinephrine released usually does not diminish the overall magnitude of the store of norepinephrine since it is normally rapidly replaced by synthesis or by uptake as described in c. This inhibition of the release normally evoked by action potentials is the primary useful effect of these drugs and has lead to the term "adrenergic neuron blockade".

b) *Release of Transmitter from Stores in Nerve Endings*

Release is sufficient following intravenous administration of neuron blocking agents to lead to sympathomimesis in many effector cells. Release is a result of a

Table 1. *Profile of the actions of some adrenergic neuron blocking agents at the sympathetic nerve terminals, in Vivo*

Blocking agent	Block release of norepinephrine by nerve action potentials[a]	Direct, transient release of norepinephrine[b]	Inhibit uptake and/or binding of norepinephrine from extracellular fluid[c]	Deplete norepinephrine stores In heart	In brain	Inhibit release of norepinephrine by other drugs[d]	Ref.
Guanethidine	+	+	+	+	—	+	MAXWELL et al. (1960)
Bretylium	+	+	+[e]	+[e]	—	—	BOURA et al. (1960)
Bethanidine	+	+	+[e]	+[e]	—	+	BOURA and GREEN (1963; 1965)
Debrisoquin	+	+	—	—	—	(±)	MOE et al. (1964)
Guanisoquin	+[f]	+	+	+	—	+	SCRIABINE (1964)
Guanoxan	+[f]	+	+[e]	+	+[e]	+	DAVEY and REINERT (1965)
Guanoclor	+	No data	+	+[e]	+[e]	+	LAWRIE et al. (1964)

[a] + = Phenomenon occurs. — = Phenomenon does not occur.
[b] As judged by occurrence of sympathomimetic effects following administration of the drug.
[c] As judged by an increase in the responsiveness of effectors to norepinephrine injection.
[d] As judged by inhibition of response of effectors to injected tyramine.
[e] Observed only after repeated administration of blocking drug. Not observed following a single dose which produces significant neuronal blockade.
[f] A part of this blockade may be alpha adrenergic blockade in addition to adrenergic neuron blockade. From MULL and MAXWELL (1967).

direct action of the compound at the nerve endings and is presumably independent of electrical activity in the neurons. This action is short compared to the duration of neuron blockade.

c) *Inhibition of the Capacity of the Nerve Terminal to Take up and/or to Bind Transmitter from the Extracellular Fluid Surrounding the Nerve Terminals and Effector Cells*

Uptake and binding into nerve terminals apparently is a primary mechanism terminating the physiological actions of norepinephrine in many adrenergic neuroeffector junctions (Iversen, 1967). The uptake mechanism is operative regardless of whether the norepinephrine reaches the region of the nerve endings as a result of local release or as a consequence of exogenous administration.

d) *Depletion of Norepinephrine Stored within Effector Organs*

Adrenergic neuron blocking drugs may bring about measurable depletion in the content of stored norepinephrine. This depletion is slow and of long duration relative to phenomenon of release. Depletion is probably due in part to release as described in (b), inhibition of uptake as described in (c) and in larger part to "damage" to storage vesicles and the subsequent intraneuronal metabolism of the transmitter.

e) *Inhibition of Drug-Induced Release of Transmitter from Nerve Endings*

Several phenethylamines, typified by tyramine, release norepinephrine from adrenergic nerve terminals. This release is blocked by several adrenergic neuron blocking agents. Blockade of tyramine-induced release is a protracted action.

The exact molecular mechanisms whereby the above-listed five actions are mediated are controversial. The reader is referred to the body of this review for further discussion concerning these mechanisms.

2. Effects Due to Administration *in vivo*

a) *Consequences of Adrenergic Neuron Blockade*

Circulation. Blockade of the sympathetic nervous system leads to hypotension especially in hypertensive man and animals. Neuron blocking agents have considerably greater hypotensive effect when patients or animals are in the erect position than when they are supine (Green, 1962; Maxwell, 1962). The hypotension which occurs during acute treatment is due to a reduction in the capacity of vasoconstrictor nerves to mediate the usual reflex compensations when the erect posture is assumed. As a consequence venous return and cardiac output fall and hypotension results (Fawaz, 1963).

Sympathetic neuron blockade slows the heart rate (Green, 1962). Presumably this is due to suppression of the sympathetic influences on the heart, which leaves the vagal influences unopposed.

Central Nervous System. Adrenergic neuron blocking agents have little central action following systemic administration. Guanethidine, bretylium and bethanidine are charged molecules at physiological pH and do not penetrate into the brain to any great extent (Boura et al., 1960; Boura and Green, 1962; Kuntzman et al., 1962). Guanoxan and guanoclor may penetrate into the brain since both compounds depleted stores of norepinephrine from the hypothalamus during chronic administration (Table 1).

Salivary Glands. Dampening of sympathetic impulses by neuron blocking agents or by surgical removal of the superior cervical ganglion may cause tenderness and pain in the region of the parotid glands (GREEN, 1962). The pain associated with the use of these drugs is presumably secondary to neuron block and not to some toxic action of the drugs.

Alimentary Tract. Guanethidine and bretylium produce loose stools or diarrhea in animals and man. The predominance of the parasympathetic system over the sympathetic system after the blockade of the latter leads to increased gastrointestinal activity. Other factors are probably involved since bethanidine is a potent neuron blocking agent but produces significantly less diarrhea than guanethidine in man (SMIRK, 1963). Diarrhea did not occur following subcutaneous administration of bethanidine to guinea pigs. In contrast, guinea pigs showed diarrhea following injection of guanethidine (BOURA and GREEN, 1963).

Genitourinary System. Adrenergic neuron blocking agents cause failure of ejaculation without loss of potency in man (DOLLERY et al., 1960; GREEN, 1962; PRICHARD et al., 1968). The inhibitory effect on ejaculation is directly attributable to sympathetic blockade.

Bretylium elicits a transient fall in renal clearance values in man, but these subsequently rise to levels greater than control despite the presence of hypotension (DOYLE et al., 1960). Guanethidine produces variable effects on glomerular filtration rate and renal plasma flow in man. These measurements are decreased if the hypotensive action of guanethidine is large (RICHARDSON et al., 1960; PAGE, 1961). Progressive azotemia or oliguria is observed only when renal function has been compromised prior to administration of neuron blockers (MAXWELL, 1962; PAGE, 1961).

Eye. Local instillation of guanethidine in the eyes of rabbits and man leads to miosis and a lowering of intraocular pressure (CASTREN and POHJOLA, 1962; OOSTERHIUS, 1962). It is uncertain whether guanethidine acts by reducing the rate of secretion or by enhancing the rate of outflow of aqueous humor, or both (CASTREN and POHJOLA, 1962).

All neuron blocking agents relax the nictitating membranes of dogs and cats since this membrane is normally held in a retracted state by tonic sympathetic activity. Bethanidine appears to be the most active in this regard. The single oral doses of bethanidine, guanethidine and bretylium required to produce equal relaxation of the cat nictitating membranes were related approximately as 1:7:20, respectively (BOURA and GREEN, 1963).

b) *Consequences of Direct Release of Norepinephrine from Nerve Endings*

All adrenergic neuron blocking agents when administered intravenously produce signs of sympathetic excitation (Table 1), such as tachycardia, hypertension, piloerection, retraction of the nictitating membrane and mydriasis. These actions are brief relative to the duration of sympathetic blockade.

c) *Consequences of Inhibition of the Capacity of Nerve Terminals to Take up Norepinephrine*

Most neuronal blocking agents enhance the response of effector organs to injected norepinephrine (Table 1). This supersensitivity to norepinephrine is generally considered to occur because these drugs inhibit the uptake of norepinephrine by adrenergic nerves. Presumably, inhibition of uptake leads to a greater accumulation of norepinephrine in the vicinity of the effector cells and/or to an increase in its plasma level (see TRENDELENBURG, 1959, 1963, 1966).

d) Consequences of Depletion of Norepinephrine Stored in Effector Organs

Severe depletion of norepinephrine from adrenergic nerve endings in itself may lead to impairment of transmission to effector cells. Such an effect supports the primary adrenergic neuron blocking action of these compounds. Guanethidine and guanisoquin deplete norepinephrine stores in the heart after single injection while the other agents deplete only during repeated administration (Table 1).

e) Consequences of Inhibition of Drug-Induced Release of Norepinephrine from Nerve Endings

Phenethylamines such as tyramine, which appear to act primarily by releasing norepinephrine from adrenergic nerve endings are rendered impotent by most neuron blocking agents (Table 1). Bretylium is frequently reported to be an exception in acute experiments; tyramine action usually is not affected or is enhanced following bretylium.

B. History of Development

There were two main branches in the evolution of adrenergic neuron blocking agents: one led to the quaternary ammonium compounds, as exemplified by bretylium, and one led to guanidine derivatives, as epitomized by guanethidine.

1. Quaternary Ammonium Compounds

Choline 2,6-xylyl ether bromide (Fig. 1), known generically as xylocholine or TM10, was prepared in the early 1950's as part of a systematic study of choline phenyl ethers. It was related to choline p-tolyl ether bromide (TM-6) (Fig. 1) which was an inhibitor of monoamine oxidase (Brown and Hey, 1956; Bain, 1960). Xylocholine was the first compound reported to antagonize the response of effector organs to postganglionic nerve activity without simultaneously antagonizing their response to injected catecholamines (Hey and Willey, 1954; Exley 1957, 1960). Unfortunately, xylocholine had pronounced muscarinic side effects which rendered it useless as a therapeutic agent. A systematic search among substances related to xylocholine was undertaken and an active series of quaternary benzylammonium salts was prepared. The most active member of this series was bretylium tosylate (Boura et al., 1959a; Boura and Green, 1959; Boura et al., 1961; Copp, 1964) (Fig. 1). Bretylium has been of limited therapeutic usefulness due to the rapid development of tolerance to its hypotensive actions in a large number of hypertensive patients.

2. Guanidine Derivatives

The development of guanidine derivatives as neuron blocking agents, especially guanethidine, had its pharmacological origin in experiments with the central nervous stimulant, methylphenidate HCl (Fig. 1). Methylphenidate was discovered to block completely the pressor and cardiac effects of amphetamine in dogs (Maxwell et al., 1957, 1958a). During the course of these experiments it was the practice for purposes of economy to use, in addition to the normal supply of animals, a few dogs from concluded, unrelated studies. In this case the dogs were those which had been given three or four new compounds at a rate of one a week in order to assess the behavioral effects of these agents. A week was allowed to elapse after the administration of the last compound before they were used for

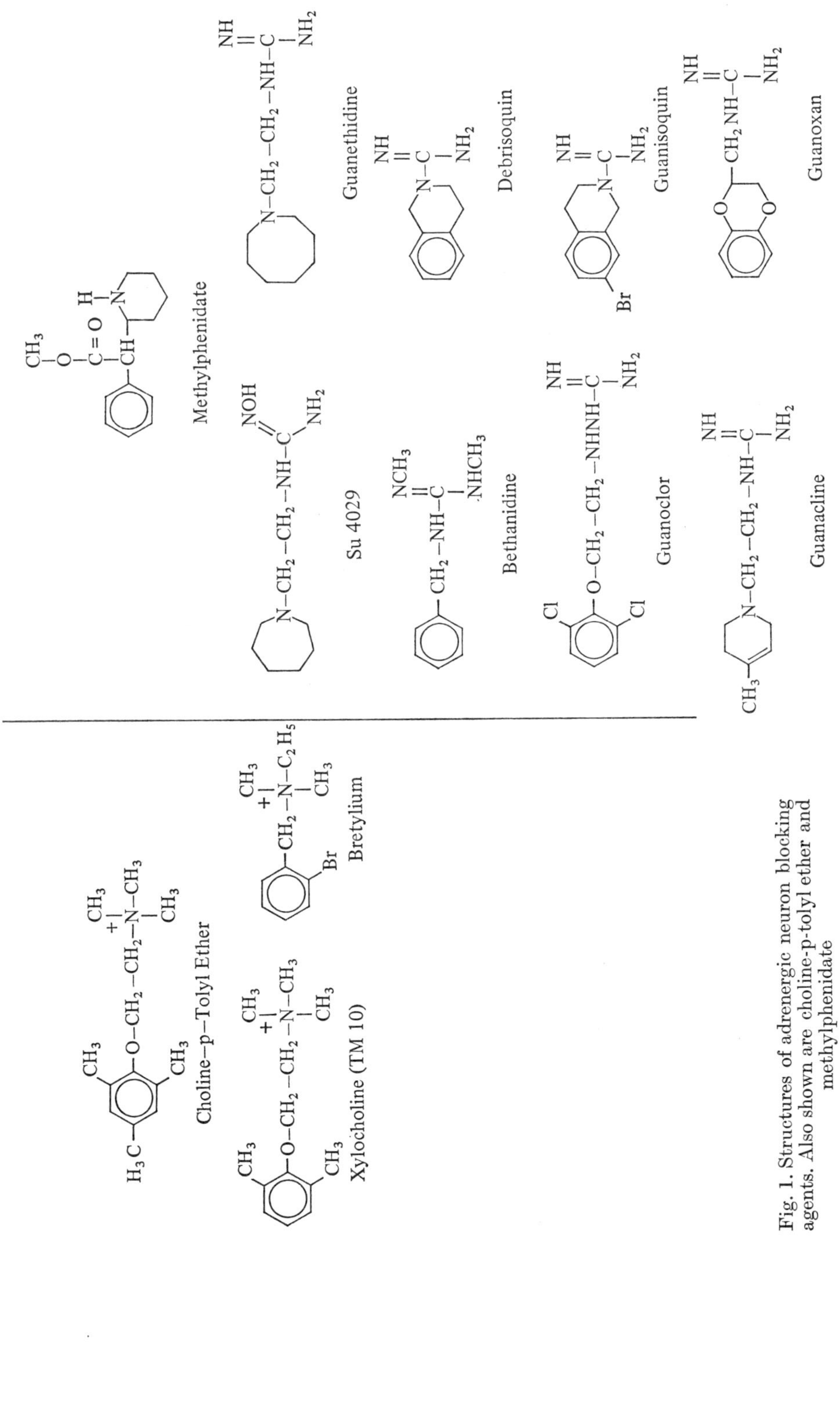

Fig. 1. Structures of adrenergic neuron blocking agents. Also shown are choline-p-tolyl ether and methylphenidate

cardiovascular experimentation. One such dog was given a very large intravenous dose of amphetamine but the amphetamine produced only a negligible increase in blood pressure. The blockade was as complete as if the animal had been given methylphenidate. This was a startling observation since as stated the last compound the dog had received had been administered one week earlier.

Each of the three or four compounds which the animals had received over the previous weeks was given singly to other dogs and a week allowed to elapse. After this time, the dogs were challenged with amphetamine. In a most unlikely manner, it turned out that the compound which had been responsible for the blockade was the one which had been given three weeks earlier! This compound was hexahydro-1 azepinepropionamidoxime HCl (Su-4029) (Fig. 1). It was synthesized originally as part of an antitrypanosomal program (see Chapter 2). Its pharmacology was subsequently described (MAXWELL et al., 1958b; MAXWELL and SCHNEIDER, 1961). The long-lasting blocking effect on amphetamine is shown in Fig. 2.

Su-4029 was subsequently given a trial in man as an antihypertensive agent but was unsuccessful because it produced fever, rash and headache. A systematic study of the capacity of congenors of Su-4029 to block the pressor effects of amphetamine at 24 h following administration was undertaken. Compound Su-5864, which was [2-(octahydro-1-azocinyl)-ethyl]-guanidine sulfate, in addition to blocking amphetamine pressor activity also relaxed the nictitating membranes of the dog, an action not shared by Su-4029. Relaxation of the nictitating membranes was indicative of reduced sympathetic activity in this effector organ. The pharmacology of Su-5864, which had not yet received the generic name of guanethidine, appeared soon thereafter (MAXWELL et al., 1959, 1960). Subsequently, many guanidine derivatives were synthesized and several were developed into potential therapeutic agents such as bethanidine, debrisoquin, guanacline, guanoclor and guanoxan. Not all of them have been successful. For example, VEJLSGAARD et al. (1967) demonstrated that guanoclor was a difficult drug to use for the maintenance treatment of hypertension. In addition, although guanoxan performed fairly well in early studies, there have been reports of impaired liver function in many patients receiving it (MONTUSCHI and LOVEL, 1964; SHEPS et al., 1966; COTTON and MONTUSCHI, 1966). Guanacline has been reported to produce irreversible hypotensive effects in patients and its usefulness may be limited for this reason (see Section VII K).

C. Therapeutic Use in Hypertension

The primary clinical use for adrenergic neuron blocking agents is in the treatment of arterial hypertension. The clinical pharmacology of these agents is reviewed in detail in Chapter 13 of this volume. Also see SANNERSTEDT and CONWAY (1970).

Hemodynamic Effects in Man. When guanethidine was administered intravenously there was a short-lived pressor phase in both normotensive and hypertensive patients (COHN et al., 1963). The effects on heart rate were variable. Peripheral resistance was not changed but there was a substantial reduction in cardiac output (COHN et al., 1963; BREST, 1965). If the patients were tilted, blood pressure and cardiac output were further reduced and systemic resistance fell (VILLARREAL, 1964). Vasoconstrictor reflexes were inhibited (WILSON et al., 1960; TAYLOR et al., 1962; COHN et al., 1963).

Following treatment for approximately one week, blood pressure was moderately lower in patients in the supine position. Tilting enhanced the fall in pressure

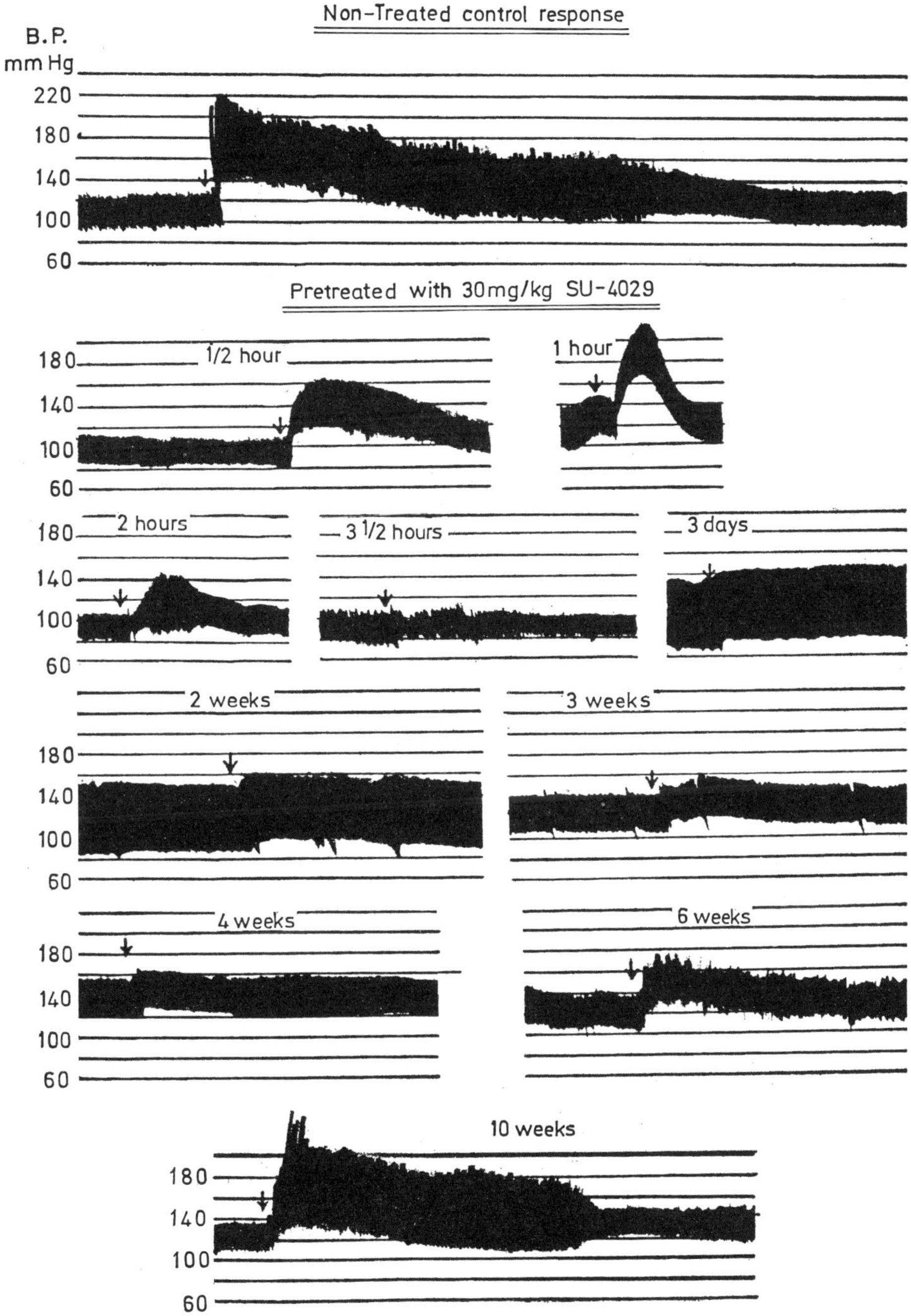

Fig. 2. Time course of inhibition of amphetamine-induced hypertension by Su-4029 in the normotensive anesthetized dog. Time notations refer to time elapsed after a single intravenous injection of Su-4029. Five-tenths mgm./kgm. of amphetamine administered intravenously at arrows. From MAXWELL et. al. (1958)

which was presumably due to reduction in cardiac output since resistance was only moderately lowered. Heart rate was decreased. Pressor reflexes were inhibited (RICHARDSON et al., 1960; SHAPIRO and KRIFCHER, 1964). Guanethidine blocked arterial and venous vasoconstriction evoked by cold immersion of one hand and by leg exercise in normal subjects (MASON and BRAUNWALD, 1964).

In longer-term therapy, cardiac output was not lowered in either the recumbent or standing position and systemic vascular resistance and heart rate were reduced (CHAMBERLAIN and HOWARD, 1964; VILLARREAL et al., 1964).

Clinical trials with bethanidine have shown that the hemodynamic effects in hypertensive patients are similar to those produced by guanethidine treatment (MONTUSCHI and PICKENS, 1962; JOHNSON et al., 1962; SMIRK, 1963; FEWINGS et al., 1964; BATH et al., 1967). PRICHARD et al. (1968) did not show any significant difference between bethanidine and guanethidine in their ability to lower and control blood pressure in hypertensive patients. Both agents produced postural and exercise hypotension. Bethanidine produced a slightly greater fall in blood pressure in standing patients and after erect exercise than did guanethidine. However, GIFFORD (1965) did not find any difference in orthostatic hypotension after bethanidine or guanethidine. Guanethidine produced a greater reduction in heart rate after long-term therapy (PRICHARD et al., 1968). The hemodynamic effects of debrisoquin in man have been reported by several groups of investigators (ABRAMS et al., 1964; LURIA and FREIS, 1965; ONESTI et al., 1966) and have been found to be similar to those observed with guanethidine.

II. Distribution of Neuron Blocking Agents in Tissues Following Their Administration to Animals and Man

KUNTZMAN et al. (1962), SCHANKER and MORRISON (1965), and CHANG et al. (1965) studied the distribution of guanethidine in rats following its intravenous administration. Half of the administered dose disappeared from the animals in the first hour. After two hours the rate of disappearance slowed and declined with a half-life of approximately 7 h (Fig. 3). According to SCHANKER and MORRISON (1965) the kidney and liver had the greatest concentrations during the first 15 min following guanethidine administration; however, these levels declined rapidly, the rate of fall roughly paralleling that of the plasma level. As should be noted in Fig. 4 the plasma level fell precipitately over the first hour and then very slowly over the next 24 h. Heart and skeletal muscle concentrations, on the other hand, rose steadily during the first 30 min and attained levels greater than those of liver, kidney or plasma. Maximal levels were attained in heart and skeletal muscle in one hour with the heart value exceeding that of the skeletal muscle. During the next 2 to 5 h the tissue levels of guanethidine fell slowly, and thereafter even more slowly (Fig. 4). As shown in Table 2, at 2 h following intravenous administration of a moderate dose of guanethidine it was highly concentrated by a number of organs when compared to its content in plasma. The capacity of the rat heart to concentrate guanethidine was demonstrated earlier by BISSON and MUSCHOLL (1962).

SCHANKER and MORRISON (1965) demonstrated that slices of rat heart accumulated guanethidine by two separate processes. One required oxygen and was saturable, suggesting a specialized transport process. The second process was non-specific tissue binding. Additional evidence supporting two types of accumulation has been presented by CHANG et al. (1965) for the rat heart and spleen and by MITCHELL and OATES (1970) for the rat heart.

KUNTZMAN et al. (1970) studied the kinetics of disappearance of ^{14}C-bretylium from the plasma of human subjects given an intramuscular injection of 300 mgs. During the first 24 h after drug administration the plasma level did not decrease as a simple first order function but exhibited a multiphasic decline. The half-life

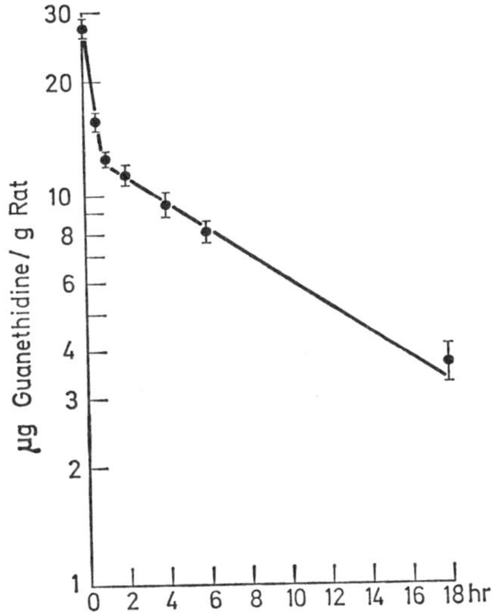

Fig. 3. Concentration of guanethidine in whole body of the rat at various times after intravenous administration (28 mg/kg). Each value is the mean of three to four experiments ± S. E. From SCHANKER and MORRISON (1965)

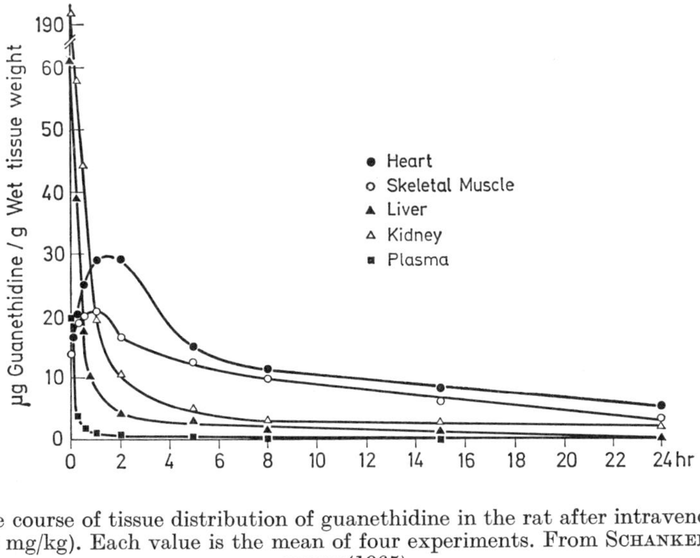

Fig. 4. Time course of tissue distribution of guanethidine in the rat after intravenous administration (28 mg/kg). Each value is the mean of four experiments. From SCHANKER and MORRISON (1965)

Table 2. *Tissue distribution of guanethidine in the rat 2 h after intravenous administration of 7 mg/kg of drug*

Tissue	Concentration of guanethidine[a] (μg/g wet weight)
Heart	10·2 ± 0·1
Lung	5·8 ± 1·8
Intestine	4·9 ± 0·8
Skeletal muscle	3·2 ± 0·7
Spleen	3·1 ± 1·2
Kidney	2·3 ± 0·3
Liver	1·1 ± 0·2
Plasma	0·5 ± 0·1
Brain	< 0·5

[a] Each value is the mean of three experiments ± the range of values. From SHANKER and MORRISON (1965).

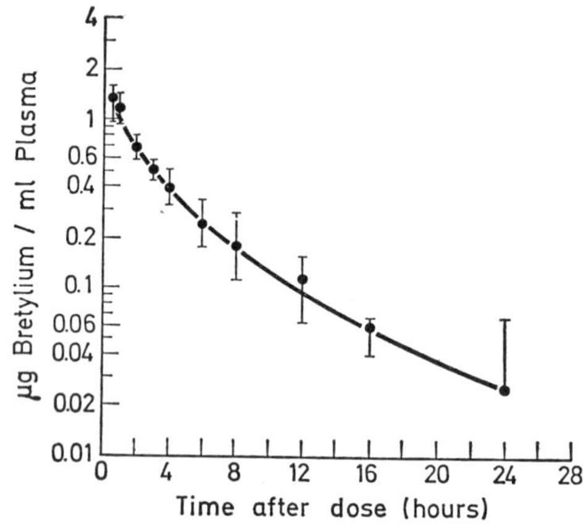

Fig. 5. Rate of decrease of bretylium from plasma in man. Four human volunteers were given an intramuscular dose of 300 mg. of ^{14}C-bretylium tosylate (19.8 μc). Plasma samples obtained 1/2 to 24 h thereafter were assayed for bretylium. The values represent the average and range from the 4 subjects. From KUNTZMAN.et. al. (1970)

increased from 1 to 5.5 h during this period. The plasma level decreased by 90% in 12 h (Fig. 5).

The distribution of bretylium in tissues of the cat following subcutaneous administration is seen in Table 3 (BOURA et al., 1960). The distribution of bethanidine (Table 4) in tissues of the cat at 16 h after its subcutaneous administration (BOURA et al., 1962) resembled that of bretylium at 12 to 18 h after its subcutaneous administration. Several of the major organs accumulated tissue levels far in excess of those in the blood but the concentrations were generally considerably less than those in adrenergic neurons (compare Tables 7 and 8 in Section III A with Tables 3 and 4). In general, organs known to contain high concentrations of catecholamines *i.e.*, those with a dense adrenergic innervation, accumulated the drugs.

Table 3. *The concentration of bretylium in various tissues.* Values for individual cats at intervals after subcutaneous injection of 10 or 50 mg/kg of [^{14}C]-labelled bretylium iodide. Concentrations are expressed as mμmoles/g. wet tissue. 1 mμmole=0·37 μg. bretylium iodide. (a) Other tissue concentrations in this cat were: parotid gland 20 mμmole, ovary 38 mμmole, thyroid 14 mμmole, cervical lymph gland 5 mμmole; (b) and (c) are the concentrations in the cortex and medulla respectively; (d) left ventricle; (e) cerebral and cerebellar cortex and spinal cord

	10 mg/kg							50 mg/kg
	1 h	3 h	3 h	12 h	18 h (a)	18 h	72 h	18 h
Blood	23	15	—	13	28	17	< 1	24
Liver	288	78	201	62	23	27	—	—
Kidney	113	—	—	—	9	13	—	—
Adrenal gland	77	53	—	20	78	110 (b) 164 (c)	< 1	85
Heart (d)	400	131	146	44	22	32	< 1	38
Spleen	205	34	102	235	142	108	25	45
Lung	—	88	—	—	—	—	—	—
Diaphragm	52	—	—	—	45	50	—	—
Area postrema	1	25	—	—	—	20	—	—
C. N. S. (e)	< 1	< 1	—	< 1	—	< 1	—	—
Hypothalamaus	1	3	—	—	—	—	—	—

From Boura et al. (1960).

Table 4. *Concentrations of N-benzyl-N′N″-dimethylguanidine*[a] (*BW* 467C60) *in cat tissues at 16 h after a subcutaneous dose.* Dose: 3 mg/kg of *N′*-[α-^{14}C]benzyl labelled drug. Concentrations are expressed as mμmoles/g wet tissue. Values from two cats

Adrenal	17·5,	53.2	Kidney	1·3,	1·4
Lung	6·7,	16·4	Cerebral cortex	0·3,	0·0
Spleen	14·5,	14·0	Cerebellar cortex	0·4,	0·0
Left ventricle	6·9,	11·8	Hypothalamus	Trace	0·0
Liver	4·5,	6·8	Spinal cord	2·0,	0·0
Diaphragm	5·4,	5·4	Blood	1·3,	1·7
Thyroid	2·8,	2·2	Area postrema	1·9,	—
Pancreas	2·3,	2·2	Pituitary	52·0	—
Parotid	—	6·6	Lymph gland	—	0·8
Renal fat	—	Trace	Cerebrospinal fluid	—	0·0

[a] Bethanidine. From Boura et al. (1962).

The distribution of debrisoquin following i.p. administration in rats is shown in Table 5 (Medina et al., 1969). Debrisoquin was concentrated in several organs, especially heart, as early as 30 min after injection. Tissue levels declined exponentially for about the first 4 h and the half-life during this period in heart, liver, and plasma was approximately 40 min. Thereafter, the rate of decline of debrisoquin in these tissues decreased. The slowing in the rate of disappearance of drug occurred earlier in the spleen. Debrisoquin was detectable in most tissues for as long as 16 h after drug administration. The drug could not be detected in brain at any time. The relationship between dose and concentration in heart and plasma for the 2 h after injection was linear over a 10-fold dose range (Fig. 6). Debrisoquin

Table 5. *Physiological distribution of debrisoquin*[a]

Tissue	Conc of debrisoquin (μg/g wet wt) 30 min	1 h	2 h	3 h	4 h	8 h	16 h
Heart	27·10 ±1·31	18·17 ±1·43	5·66 ±0·41	1·97 ±0·31	0·92 ±0·07	0·32 ±0·07	0·33 ±0·04
Spleen	5·67 ±0·84	3·45 ±0·04	2·62 ±0·17	1·81 ±0·03	1·57 ±0·18	1·06 ±0·21	0·93 ±0·12
Liver	6·62 ±1·69	1·34 ±0·05	1·02 ±0·08	0·48 ±0·02	0·19 ±0·16		
Lung	10·23 ±0·91	5·46 ±0·38	2·02 ±0·15	0·99 ±0·03	0·55 ±0·05	0·30 ±0·05	0·27 ±0·09
Kidney	3·91 ±0·96	1·90 ±0·15	0·84 ±0·04	0·42 ±0·06	0·31 ±0·04	0·16 ±0·04	0·11 ±0·03
Fat	7·31 ±1·49	2·24 ±0·25	0·96 ±0·24	0·61 ±0·06	0·64 ±0·10	0·10 ±0·02	0·11 ±0·03
Muscle	2·52 ±0·73	3·56 ±0·35	1·57 ±0·28	2·07 ±0·08	0·15 ±0·04	0·43 ±0·14	0·27 ±0·12
Plasma	0·76 ±0·25	0·50 ±0·06	0·25 ±0·06	0·22 ±0·01	0·25 ±0·03	0·23 ±0·03	0·15 ±0·11

[a] Rats were treated with debrisoquin (10 mg/kg i. p.) and killed at the times indicated. Each value is the mean ± S. E. M. of 5—13 experiments. From MEDINA et al. (1969).

did not appear to accumulate with successive doses since rats treated for three consecutive days and sacrificed 4 h after the last injection did not show any significant difference in the concentration of the drug in heart, spleen or liver when compared to animals sacrificed 4 h after a single injection (MEDINA et al., 1969).

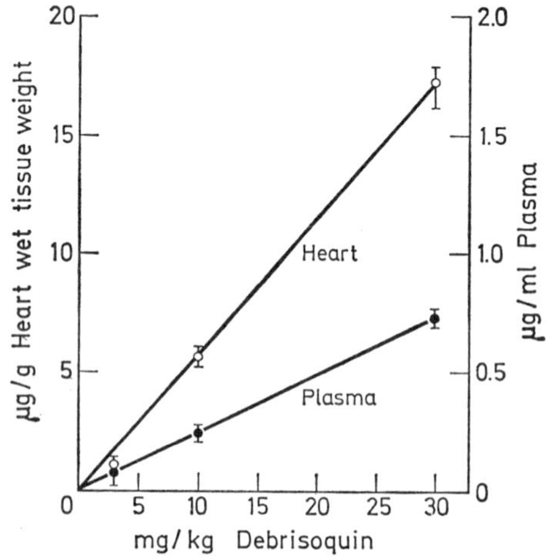

Fig. 6. Concentration of debrisoquin in heart and plasma 2 h after intraperitoneal administration of various doses of the drug. Figures denote mean + S. E. From MEDINA et al. (1969)

III. Interactions of Neuron Blocking Agents with Adrenergic Neurons

A. Retention by Adrenergic Neurons

Considerable evidence was presented in the mid 1960's that guanethidine was taken up and retained in sympathetic nerves by a process involving a high affinity for norepinephrine storage sites. Thus, CHANG et al. (1964), Brodie et al. (1965), CHANG et al. (1965) demonstrated that this specific accumulation could be inhibited or reversed by reserpine treatment (Table 6) while the accumulation in skeletal muscle was not affected. The maximal uptake of guanethidine by this specific process was estimated by CHANG et al. (1965) to be approximately 3 molecules of drug to each molecule of endogenous norepinephrine in the rat heart.

Bretylium (BOURA et al., 1960) and bethanidine (BOURA et al., 1962) were slowly accumulated to very high concentrations by sympathetic ganglia and their postganglionic nerve trunks. Other ganglia and nerve trunks never attained such high concentrations of the drug (Tables 7 and 8).

Table 6. *Depletion of H^3-guanethidine by reserpine from heart.* Rats were given H^3-guanethidine (25 μg/kg i. v.) 1 h before reserpine (2 mg/kg i. p.). Control rats were given H^3-guanethidine only. Animals were killed 5 h after injection of guanethidine. Figures in parentheses indicate number of experiments. In each experiment, the tissues of 3 rats were pooled

	Guanethidine Level in Heart (μg/g ± S. E.)
Controls	0.175 ± 0.013 (4)
Treated with reserpine	0.095 ± 0.010[a] (4)
% Release	45

[a] $P < 0.01$. From CHANG et al. (1965).

B. Mechanism of Uptake into Adrenergic Neurons

MITCHELL and OATES (1970) confirmed the uptake of guanethidine into adrenergic neurons in rat heart as elucidated by SCHANKER and MORRISON (1965) and others (see Section II and IIIA) and in addition presented evidence that the related agents, bethanidine and debrisoquin, were also accumulated against a concentration gradient by an oxygen-requiring, temperature-dependent, saturable uptake system. In the case of the latter two agents, this seemed to be the only significant uptake that occurred. In addition, MITCHELL and OATES (1970) demonstrated by kinetic methods that the uptake of tritiated bethanidine into rat heart slices was competitively inhibited by adrenergic amines: norepinephrine, metaraminol, tyramine; other neuronal blocking agents: guanethidine, bretylium,

Table 7. *The concentration of bretylium in peripheral nervous tissues.* Values for individual cats at intervals following subcutaneous injection of 10,6 or 50 mg/kg of [^{14}C]-labelled bretylium iodide. Concentrations are expressed as mμmoles/g wet tissue. 1 mμmole = 0·37 μg bretylium iodide

Tissue	10 mg/kg					6 mg/kg	50 mg/kg
	3 h	12 h	18 h	18 h	72 h	18 h	18 h
Adrenergic nerves							
Postganglionic cervical sympathetic	42	78	—	700	31	49	696
Hypogastric	—	174	—	—	41	61	421
Gastric	—	99	—	—	—	62	—
Inferior cardiac	22	136	—	—	19	63	196
Cholinergic nerves							
Preganglionic cervical sympathetic	28	29	—	80	8	23	114
Greater splanchnic	14	30	—	—	8	24	37
Vagus	15	19	—	40	2	—	47
Phrenic	11	94	—	40	—	—	—
Sympathetic ganglia							
Superior cervical	197	270	445	890	61	174	965
Middle cervical	—	—	—	610	—	—	—
Stellate	168	315	303	770	16	185	728
Coeliac	158	374	450	950	41	225	634
Superior mesenteric	—	59	258	700	—	—	—
Inferior mesenteric	290	362	—	430	49	152	440
Other ganglia							
Nodose	38	15	41	30	1	6	37
Ciliary	—	64	—	30	—	—	—
Otic	—	7	—	1	—	—	—
Dorsal root	—	16	—	10	—	—	—
Semilunar	—	< 1	—	1	—	—	—

From BOURA et al. (1960).

Table 8. *Concentrations of N-benzyl-N′ N″-dimethylguanidine*[a] (*BW* 467C60) *in nerves and ganglia of cats at* 16 *h after a subcutaneous dose.* Dose: 3 mg/kg of the *N*-[α-^{14} C]benzyl labelled drug. Concentrations are expressed as mμmoles/g. wet tissue. Values from two cats

Sympathetic ganglia		*Adrenergic nerves*	
Superior cervical	43·0, 28·4	Postganglionic superior cervical	33·0, 21·6
Stellate	31·0, 59·3	Hypogastric	46·0, 33·8
Coeliac	31·0, 11·7	Inferior cardiac	40·0, 67·2
Inferior mesenteric	14·5, 43·5	Splenic	30·0, 75·4
		Gastric	— 49·6
		Colonic	— 16·4
Other ganglia		*Other nerves*	
Nodose	— 2·3	Vagus	5·2, 2·6
Ciliary	7·1, 8·6	Preganglionic superior cervical	2·1, 5·7
Dorsal root	1·4, 3·7	Sciatic	2·0, 3·1
Semilunar	3·8, —	Greater splanchnic	9·3, 10·8

[a] Bethanidine. From BOURA et al. (1962).

debrisoquin; and by the tricyclic antidepressant, desmethylimipramine (Fig. 7). GULATI and JAYKAR (1970) observed that the onset of adrenergic neuron blockade in the isolated Finkleman preparation was prevented if the tissue was exposed to guanethidine a) at low temperatures (10° C), b) in the absence of sodium or in the presence of tetrodotoxin or c) in the presence of high concentrations of norepinephrine. Once established, guanethidine blockade was not reversed by these procedures.

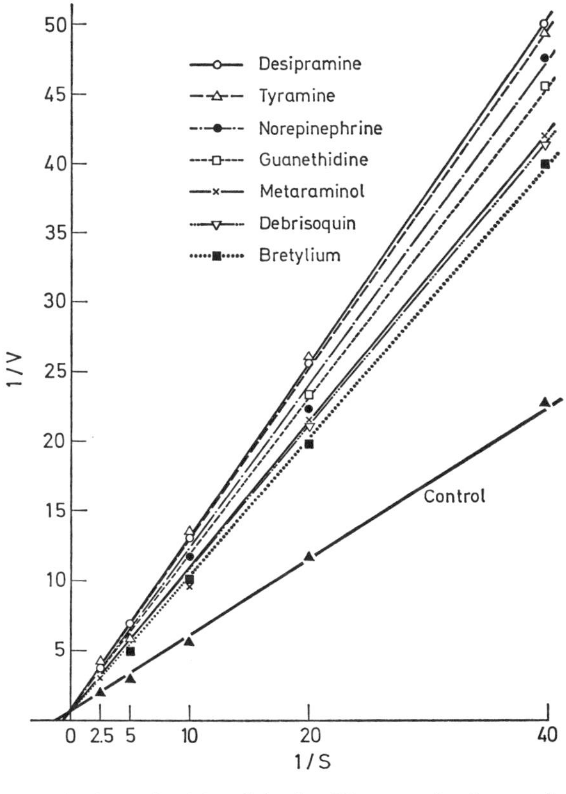

Fig. 7. Double reciprocal plots of tritiated bethanidine uptake by rat heart slices and the effect of drugs on uptake. Velocity (V) is expressed as active uptake of bethanidine by slices during 30-min incubation. Substrate concentration (S) is micrograms of bethanidine per milliliter of medium. Inhibitor concentrations: desipramine, 2×10^{-8}M; debrisoquin, 7×10^{-6}M; metaraminol, 1×10^{-5}M; bretylium, 1×10^{-5}M; norepinephrine, 2×10^{-5}M; guanethidine, 3×10^{-5}M and tyramine, 5×10^{-5}M. Each point is the mean of four (inhibitor) or 16 (control) experiments. From MITCHELL and OATES (1970)

ROSS and GOSZTONYI (1975) studied the uptake of bretylium (N—^{3}H-methyl) iodide in rat atrium *in vitro*. The uptake was saturable with an apparent Km of 3×10^{-6} M. The uptake was inhibited by amphetamine, norepinephrine, desmethylimipramine, cocaine, guanethidine, low sodium and ouabain. GARCÍA and SÁNCHEZ-GARCÍA (1975) using indirect methods studied the uptake of bretylium in reserpine-treated, guinea-pig atria. Cocaine and low sodium greatly reduced the retention of bretylium.

Norepinephrine and related catecholamines are also known to be taken up across adrenergic neuronal membranes by a saturable, energy-dependent, active transport system, the so called "amine pump" (DENGLER et al., 1961; WHITBY et al., 1961; IVERSEN, 1963; LINDMAR and MUSCHOLL, 1964; HILLARP and MALMFORS, 1964; BOGDANSKI and BRODIE, 1966; CARLSSON, 1966; GIACHETTI and SHORE, 1966; IVERSEN and KRAVITZ, 1966; BERTI and SHORE, 1967). This uptake mechanism of the adrenergic neuron membrane was depressed by cold, heat, cardiac glycosides and low Na^+. Tricyclic antidepressants and adrenergic neuron blockers were, likewise, potent competitive inhibitors of this uptake mechanism for norepinephrine and l-metaraminol in adrenergic neuron membranes (HERTTING et al., 1961; BURGEN and IVERSEN, 1965; CARLSSON and WALDECK, 1956a, b; IVERSEN, 1965; BERTI and SHORE, 1967; CALLINGHAM, 1967; MAXWELL et al., 1969).

The competition for the uptake site in adrenergic neurons which is exhibited by the various adrenergic neuron blockers, the adrenergic amines, cocaine, and the tricyclic antidepressants indicated very clearly that the adrenergic neuron blockers are taken up by the same membrane pump that takes up norepinephrine.

Recent kinetic studies reported by HORST and GATTANELL (1970) indicated that debrisoquin inhibited noncompetitively the uptake of tritiated norepinephrine in rat heart. This report would be more convincing if it were based on a larger number of data points and if results obtained with a known competitive inhibitor of uptake were also presented for purposes of comparison.

PRASAD et al. (1973) presented evidence that the onset of neuron blockade produced by guanethidine (3.3×10^{-5} M), debrisoquin (8.4×10^{-4} M), bretylium (5×10^{-4} M) and xylocholine (10^{-3} M) in guinea pig vas deferens was prevented by 3×10^{-3} M norepinephrine and by low temperature (0° C). However, they stated that the onset of neuron blockade by only one of these agents, guanethidine, was inhibited by removal of sodium from the incubation medium. The authors concluded that, since sodium is an absolute requirement for uptake of catecholamines into adrenergic nerve endings, guanethidine must share the uptake mechanism of norepinephrine while debrisoquin, bretylium and xylocholine appear to be transported differently. These experiments are open to question since the figures of the authors indicate that neuron block due to the relatively low concentration of guanethidine (3.3×10^{-5} M) is considerably less than produced by the other agents. In addition with the high concentrations of the other agents (5×10^{-4} M to 10^{-3} M) significant non-neuronal binding would be expected. Such binding of guanidiniums and quaternary bases could easily be temperature-dependent and also readily competed for by norepinephrine but not necessarily affected by sodium concentration. An explanation is needed for the use of widely different degrees of neuron blockade as well as experiments to rule out a smooth muscle depressant effect as a result of non-neuronal binding.

C. Storage in Adrenergic Neurons

MAÎTRE and STAEHELIN (1971) compared the subcellular distribution of tritiated guanethidine with that of tritiated norepinephrine following intravenous injections of these agents into the rat. The microsomal pellet (105,000 × G) obtained from a heart homogenate was subjected to density gradient centrifugation. Tritiated guanethidine was present in the same narrow band of particles as contained the tritiated norepinephrine, thus, demonstrating directly that guanethidine was taken up into the same granules which stored norepinephrine (Fig. 8). In reserpine-pretreated rats the uptake of tritiated guanethidine and norepineph-

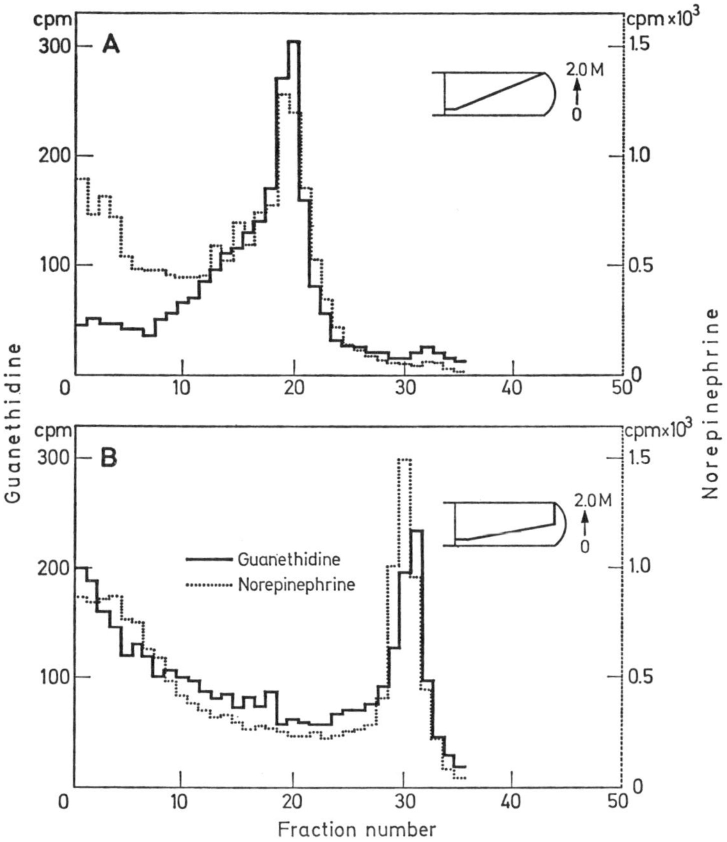

Fig. 8. Subcellular distribution of tritiated guanethidine and tritiated norepinephrine in resuspended highspeed sediment from rat heart. Tritiated norepinephrine (100 μc/rat) or tritiated guanethidine (100 μc/rat) were administered 30 min before removing the hearts. (a) Gradient Type A (0.25—2 M sucrose). (b) Gradient Type B (0.5—1 M sucrose with a layer of 2 M sucrose in the bottom). These gradients are schematically shown in the figure. Solid line: guanethidine. Dotted line: norepinephrine. From MAÎTRE and STAEHELIN (1971)

rine was greatly reduced as compared to untreated controls (Fig. 9). OBIANWU et al. (1968) had found earlier that tritiated guanethidine injected intravenously into mice was preferentially retained in a high speed particulate fraction (100,000 $\times$ G) of the heart known to be high in norepinephrine content. One hour after administration, the ratio *guanethidine in particulate/guanethidine in particulate + supernatant* was 0.56 which indicated a high affinity for the same particulate fraction that stored norepinephrine.

Several drugs, in addition to reserpine, caused a loss of bound tritiated guanethidine and if given before the guanethidine prevented its accumulation. Thus, amphetamine (Fig. 10) given after guanethidine reduced the amount of guanethidine in the rat heart. Amphetamine also prevented guanethidine accumulation when given as a pretreatment (CHANG et al., 1965). These authors interpreted their results to mean that amphetamine directly caused a loss of guanethidine from its specific intracellular binding sites. However, amphetamine appears to have a relatively low affinity for the subcellular particulate fraction which retained norepinephrine and guanethidine (OBIANWU et al., 1968). This low affinity

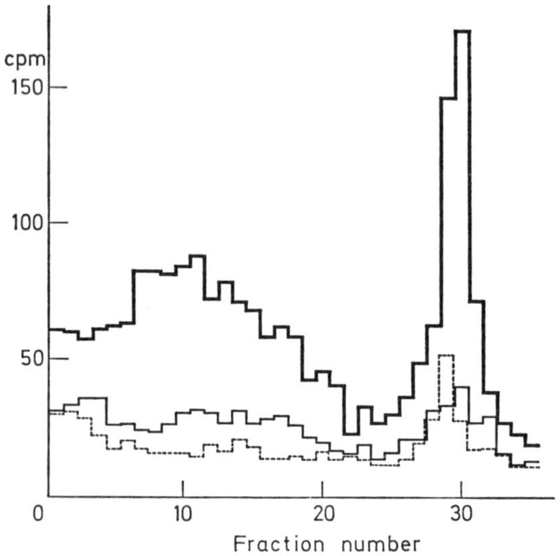

Fig. 9. Reserpine-induced inhibition of uptake of tritiated norepinephrine and tritiated guanethidine in norepinephrine storage granules of the rat heart. Tritiated norepinephrine (100 μc/rat) or tritiated guanethidine (100 μc/rat) were injected intravenously in reserpine treated rats 30 min before removing the hearts. Control rats were similarly injected with tritiated guanethidine. Sucrose density gradient of Type B (0.5—1 M sucrose with a layer of 2 M sucrose in the bottom). Reserpinization (1 mg/kg, subcutaneously) was performed 17 h before injection of the tritiated substances. Heavy Line: Distribution of tritiated guanethidine in non-reserpinized hearts. Light line: Distribution of tritiated guanethidine in reserpinized hearts. Dotted Line: Distribution of tritiated norepinephrine in reserpinized hearts. After MAÎTRE and STAEHELIN (1971)

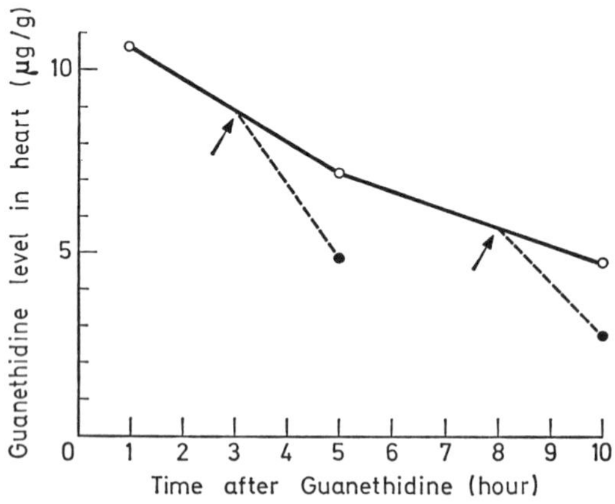

Fig. 10. Decline of guanethidine in heart of rats with and without amphetamine treatment at various times after a single dose of guanethidine. Amphetamine was injected 3 and 8 hours after guanethidine and animals were killed 2 h later. Guanethidine alone (8 mg/kg i.v.), 0———0; decline in guanethidine produced by amphetamine (0.75 mg/kg i. p.), ●——●. Each point is the mean of 4 experiments (12 animals). The difference between control and amphetamine treated rats at 3 and 8 h was significant ($P < 0.05$). From CHANG et al. (1965)

suggests that amphetamine action on guanethidine stores may have another explanation (see Section V D). Methamphetamine, like amphetamine has been demonstrated to prevent the accumulation of guanethidine in rabbit hearts (MATSUMOTO and HORITA, 1963).

Bretylium, although accumulated by adrenergic nerves, appeared not to be retained in the same storage sites as were norepinephrine and guanethidine in rat heart and spleen. COSTA et al. (1964) have reported (in abstract) that reserpine released guanethidine but not bretylium and that, as shown by density gradient centrifugation, the bretylium taken up into the adrenergic nerves was not associated with the norepinephrine containing granules. CHANG et al. (1967a) stated that the particulate to supernatant ratio for bretylium was 0.06 as compared to 0.80 for guanethidine when measured in the rat heart 3 h after administration of tracer doses of these drugs.

Although debrisoquin was initially concentrated to a greater extent in the heart than any other tissue, examination of the subcellular distribution of the drug in this organ (Table 9) did not reveal specific subcellular localization in the microsomal (100,000 × G) fraction. This fraction is commonly associated with amine storage vesicles. The fact that the relative subcellular distribution of debrisoquin in heart was the same after 2 and 5 h indicated that the intracellular binding of the drug was relatively nonspecific (MEDINA et al., 1969).

Table 9. *Subcellular distribution of debrisoquin in rat heart*[a]

	2 h		5 h	
Fraction	(μg ± S. E.)	(%)	(μg ± S. E.)	(%)
1000 *g*	1·246 ± 0·325	34·1	0·672 ± 0·098	50·5
10,000 *g*	0·543 ± 0·241	14·8	0·096 ± 0·010	7·2
100,000 *g*	0·159 ± 0·060	4·3	0·055 ± 0·012	4·1
Supernatant	1·709 ± 0·487	46·7	0·508 ± 0·072	38·2

[a] Hearts from rats given 10 mg/kg debrisoquin i. p. 2 or 5 h before killing were homogenized in 4 vol. of isotonic sucrose. The homogenates were centrifuged for 30 min at the indicated forces. Figures denote amounts of drug found in fractions of 1 g of tissue. Four experiments were performed at each time. From MEDINA et al. (1969).

D. Release from Adrenergic Neurons

Tritiated guanethidine was released from the isolated perfused cat colon into the effluent by stimulation of its sympathetic nerve supply (BOULLIN et al., 1966). This is demonstrated in Fig. 11.

BOULLIN (1966, 1967) demonstrated that extracellular calcium ion was an absolute requirement for the release of tritiated guanethidine from the isolated cat colon during nerve stimulation. In this regard, guanethidine was similar to norepinephrine. If the cation was present, increasing its concentration did not further enhance the efflux of guanethidine or norepinephrine released in response to sympathetic nerve stimulation. The spontaneous efflux of tritiated guanethidine was not changed by alterations in the calcium concentration.

The level of ^{14}C-guanethidine accumulated at steady state in rat ventricle slices was reduced when the calcium ion concentration was raised from 2.2 mM to 10 or 20 mM (BOULLIN, 1966). However, the increases in calcium ion did not affect the initial rate of uptake of guanethidine. It was concluded that excess calcium ion reduced the uptake of guanethidine by an indirect action, possibly by releasing guanethidine from intracellular storage sites in adrenergic nerves.

BOULLIN (1968) reported that zero calcium and 20 mM calcium both enhanced guanethidine efflux from isolated rat heart as compared to 2.2 mM calcium. The high calcium level increased efflux from one compartment by 25% whereas perfusion with zero calcium enhanced efflux by 274%. The kinetics of efflux suggested that the drug was released from different cellular compartments in the presence and absence of calcium. BOULLIN concluded that removal of calcium ions caused release of guanethidine only from non-specific cellular sites and not from the intra-neuronal store and that high calcium enhanced release from the intra-neuronal store.

Bretylium was released from the perfused cat spleen by sympathetic nerve stimulation (FISCHER et al., 1966; KOPIN, 1968).

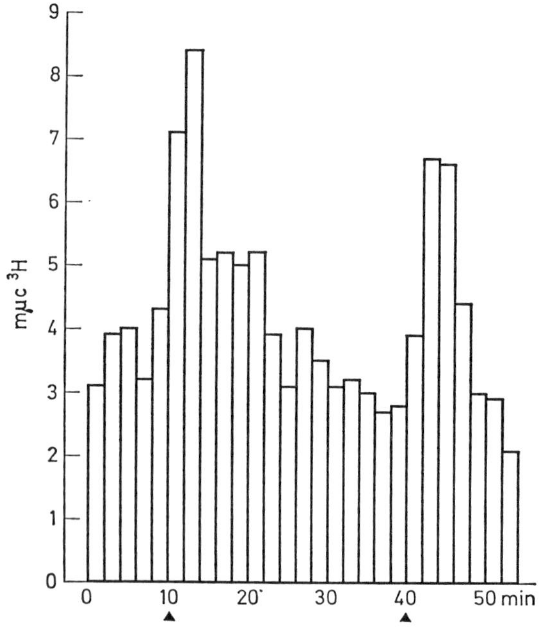

Fig. 11. Release of tritiated guanethidine from the isolated perfused cat colon by nerve stimulation. Sympathetic stimuli were administered after perfusion for 2 h with Krebs solution. Trains of 3000 impulses at 10\sec are shown by the arrows. Each histogram represents tritiated guanethidine output per 2-min collection period. These results are typical of 3 experiments. From BOULLIN et al. (1966)

IV. Interactions of Neuron Blocking Agents with Norepinephrine in Adrenergic Neurons

A. Capacity to Release Norepinephrine from Nerve Endings and Simultaneously to Inhibit the Release of Norepinephrine Elicited by Sympathetic Neuronal Activity

Guanethidine, bretylium and bethanidine blocked adrenergic transmission by inhibiting the release of norepinephrine which occurs as a result of nerve stimulation (BOURA and GREEN, 1959, 1963; MAXWELL et al., 1959, 1960; GILMORE and SIEGEL, 1962; HERTTING et al., 1962; HUKOVIC and MUSCHOLL, 1962;

ABERCROMBIE and DAVIES, 1963). As can be seen in Fig. 12 upon stimulation of the splenic nerves of cats which had previously received tritiated norepinephrine, large amounts of the tritiated norepinephrine were released into venous blood. Both guanethidine and bretylium caused a rise in the tritiated norepinephrine in the splenic outflow following their injection into the splenic artery. Subsequent stimulation of the splenic nerve failed to release tritiated norepinephrine (HERTTING et al., 1962). BOURA and GREEN (1959), HERTTING and WIDHALM (1965), and FISCHER et al. (1966) also demonstrated directly the capacity of bretylium to prevent release of both endogenous and tritiated norepinephrine during stimulation of the sympathetic nerve supply to cat spleen and heart.

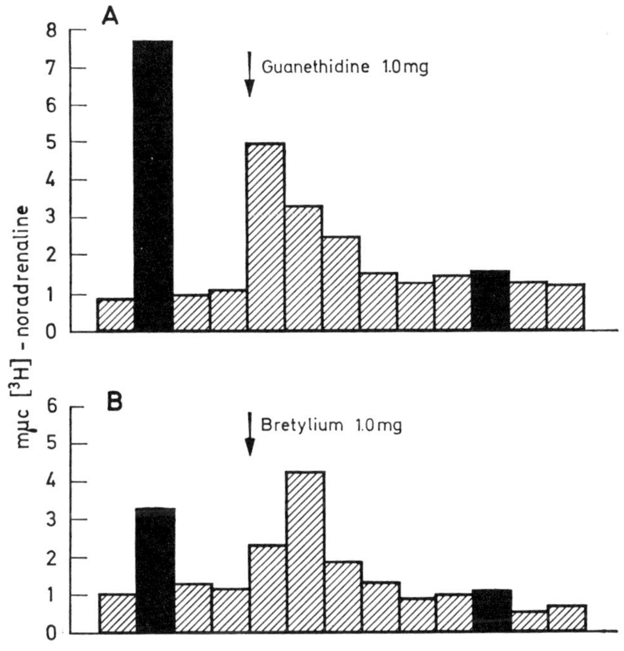

Fig. 12. Effect of guanethidine (A) and bretylium (B) on the release of tritiated norepinephrine in the spleen. Cats were given 200 μc/kg tritiated norepinephrine intravenously. Splenic nerves were stimulated at a frequency of 30/sec for a total of 300 stimuli. Guanethidine (1 mg) or bretylium (1 mg) was injected into the splenic artery. Each column represents tritiated norepinephrine (in mμc) released during a 1-min collection period. Hatched columns represent tritiated norepinephrine measured before stimulation and solid columns for 1 min, during and after stimulation. From HERTTING et al. (1962)

As alluded to earlier (Section I A) there is considerable physiologic evidence that release of norepinephrine by guanethidine and other neuron blocking agents accounts in large part for the transient sympathomimesis produced by these compounds. PLUCHINO et al. (1969) proposed that in the dog heart guanethidine released norepinephrine from both "available" (i.e. tyramine-sensitive) and "bound" (i.e. reserpine-sensitive) functional compartments. ABBS (1966) demonstrated that guanethidine and bretylium increased initially the output of norepinephrine and epinephrine in plasma samples from the splenic vein of adrenalectomized, eviscerated cats but the increase was not sustained. The increase was adequate to account for the initial sympathomimetic effects of the compounds. HARRI-

SON et al. (1963) demonstrated a temporal relationship between the increases in arterial blood pressure, heart rate and ventricular contractile force elicited by guanethidine and the outflow of norepinephrine from the dog heart as determined by the difference in the norepinephrine content of the arterial and the coronary sinus blood. Other investigators have demonstrated release of norepinephrine following guanethidine administration to perfused organs: cat spleen (THOENEN et al., 1966), rat heart (NASH et al., 1964), rat stomach (GOKHALE et al., 1963) and rabbit heart (BUTTERFIELD and RICHARDSON, 1961). NASH et al. (1964) showed that during the first 30 min of perfusion with guanethidine, the rat heart which had been labelled earlier with tritiated norepinephrine, released mainly norepinephrine and normetanephrine and little of the deaminated metabolites.

BURNSTOCK and HOLMAN (1964) measured the effects of bretylium on the smooth muscle-membrane potentials in the isolated guinea-pig vas deferens. After 15 min exposure to bretylium (ca. 3×10^{-5}M) both the miniature spontaneous discharges and the junction potentials in response to hypogastric nerve stimulation were greatly depressed. However, after 40 min exposure the spontaneous discharges showed a great increase over control but the response to nerve stimulation was completely blocked. On the basis that it was likely that the spontaneous discharges were due to release of "packets" or quanta of norepinephrine the authors considered that their data was in accord with the widely accepted hypothesis that bretylium blocked transmission at a prejunctional site. The physiological significance of this bretylium-resistant, spontaneous release shown in Fig. 12 (HERTTING et al., 1962) and shown by the spontaneous discharges in the work of BURNSTOCK and HOLMAN (1964) has not been elaborated on by either set of authors.

HORST and GATTANELL (1970) showed that in the rat debrisoquin (25 mg/kg i.p.) given one hour after tritiated norepinephrine produced within 2 h a 24% reduction (release) in the tritiated norepinephrine and deaminated catechols in heart and also a 20% increase in triated normetanephrine.

B. Effect on the Norepinephrine Content of Adrenergically Innervated Organs and the Adrenal Medulla

1. Organs Other than the Adrenal Gland

SHEPPARD and ZIMMERMAN (1959) were the first to report that guanethidine partially reduced the catecholamine content of the heart and spleen of the rat. CASS et al. (1960) reported that in rabbits and cats, guanethidine completely depleted the norepinephrine stores from heart, spleen and intestine without affecting the catecholamine content in brain. Similar results were found with rat heart, spleen and intestine (CASS and SPRIGGS, 1961) (Fig. 13). Small and transient reductions in the norepinephrine content of the rabbit and cat hypothalamus and rat brain were reported following guanethidine (KRONEBERG and SCHÜMANN, 1962; SANAN and Vogt, 1962; CASS and CALLINGHAM, 1964). These minor effects on brain levels may have been due to reflex stimulation of central noradrenergic fibers. Daily treatment of rats with 10 mg/kg guanethidine for 3 weeks was without effect on brain norepinephrine (CASS and CALLINGHAM, 1964). In contrast to these reports, DES PREZ et al. (1966) found a 72% reduction of brain stem norepinephrine in the rabbit at 16 h following 10 mg/kg intraperitoneal guanethidine. In addition, PFEIFER et al. (1962) observed a 60% decrease in the norepinephrine content of rat brain following a single subcutaneous dose of 5 mg/kg. DAGIRMANJIAN (1963) found that a single dose of 15 mg/kg of guanethidine by the intraperitoneal route did not lower hypothalamic norepinephrine in cats, but, daily injections of 15 mg/kg, subcutaneously, over a 7 day period consistently produced a decrease in hypothalamic norepinephrine. There is no ready explanation for these discrepant results. The failure of most investigators to demonstrate a profound effect of guanethidine on norepinephrine stores in brain is probably attributable to poor penetration of guanethidine into the brain. Such poor penetration has been described for mice and rats (KUNTZMAN et al., 1962; SCHANKER and MORRISON, 1965; FURST, 1967b) (Table 2).

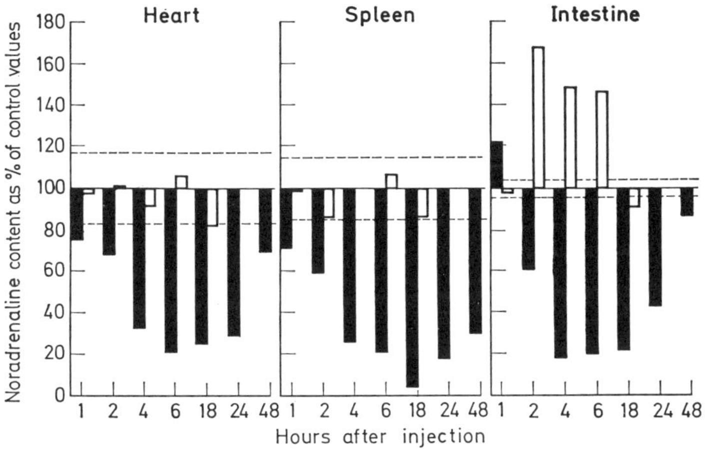

Fig. 13. Norepinephrine content of rat tissues after the subcutaneous injection of guanethidine 15 mg/kg (black columns) or bretylium 15 mg (open columns). The dotted lines represent the standard error of the control levels. From CASS and SPRIGGS (1961)

OSADA and WESTFALL (1969) demonstrated that the recovery of myocardial or renal norepinephrine levels following 90% depletion with guanethidine was similar in both adrenalectomized and sham-operated animals. This indicated that the amines from the adrenal gland were not important in the repletion process. DAILY and WESTFALL (1969) failed to demonstrate that pretreatment of rats with the protein synthesis inhibitor, actinomycin D, influenced the recovery of myocardial norepinephrine following its depletion by guanethidine. The authors concluded that their experiments failed to provide evidence that resynthesis of storage vesicles is a necessary requirement for repletion of norepinephrine stores after guanethidine treatment.

Bretylium was reported not to lower the norepinephrine content of tissues in most studies (Fig. 13) (BRODIE and KUNTZMAN, 1960; CASS and SPRIGGS, 1961; DAVEY and FARMER, 1963; SPRIGGS, 1966). Bretylium, in fact, inhibited guanethidine or reserpine-induced norepinephrine depletion (CALLINGHAM and CASS, 1962; KUNTZMAN et al., 1962). A similar action has been demonstrated with large doses of cocaine (CALLINGHAM and CASS, 1962). BOURA and GREEN (1965) refer to reports that single subcutaneous doses of bretylium did not deplete tissue norepinephrine and to the finding that daily subcutaneous administration for 14 days of 30 mg/kg to the cat caused a marked depletion of the norepinephrine content of the heart, spleen, and superior cervical and stellate ganglia. These authors suggested that doses of bretylium producing prolonged, substantial, adrenergic neuron blockade would over a time course similar to that following sympathectomy, lead to depletion of amines. The implications of this suggestion have never been elaborated on. Presumably in man, where it is unlikely that full sympathetic blockade is achieved, significant depletion probably does not occur. Recent data of Abbs and Robertson (1970), which demonstrated 50% depletion of norepinephrine from the cat spleen following a single 10 mg/kg intravenous dose of bretylium, stand in contrast to the results of Cass and Spriggs (1961) (Fig. 13) as well as others mentioned above. Cass and Spriggs (1961) administered 15 mg/kg by the subcutaneous route. It is most likely that differences in species and route of administration may explain the discrepancy. It seems clear that guanethidine readily depletes norepinephrine from peripheral tissues in doses producing neuron blockade and that bretylium *may* deplete especially if given repeatedly in doses greater than those required for neuronal blockade.

Bethanidine did not lower the pressor amine content of the iris of cats 24 h after subcutaneous administration of single doses of 3 to 30 mg/kg under circumstances where 10 mg/kg guanethidine lowered the pressor amine content (Boura and Green, 1963). Daily subcutaneous administration of 10 mg/kg of bethanidine to cats for 6 months reduced the pressor amine content of the hearts and spleens (Boura et al., 1961). A single intravenous dose of 7.5 mg/kg of bethanidine to the rat reduced the norepinephrine content of the heart by 30% under conditions where a single intravenous dose of 7.5 mg/kg of guanethidine reduced the norepinephrine content by 82% (Costa et al., 1962).

Moe et al. (1964) and Abrams et al. (1965) demonstrated that debrisoquin in a single intraperitoneal dose of 50 mg/kg did not alter the content of endogenous norepinephrine or serotonin in rat heart under experimental conditions in which the norepinephrine-depleting properties of a single dose of guanethidine were quite apparent. The effect of chronic administration of debrisoquin on catecholamine levels in heart has not been reported.

Tomlinson and Mayor (1973) demonstrated that very high concentrations of guanethidine, bretylium and debrisoquin reduced the accumulation of norepinephrine proximal to a constriction applied to cat hypogastric nerves *in vitro*. This reduction was paralleled by a decrease in the accumulation of dense-cored vesicles. The authors concluded that all three drugs exerted a norepinephrine-depleting action upon storage vesicles. The pharmacological significance of these findings is unclear since the concentrations of the drugs employed were in the order of 10^{-1} M and at least 18 h treatment with bretylium and debrisoquin were necessary before an amine depleting action was evident.

2. Adrenal Medulla

a) Catecholamine Content

Cass et al. (1960) found that guanethidine did not lower the catecholamine content of the adrenal glands of rabbit and cat. Kuntzman et al. (1962) also demonstrated that the catecholamines of the adrenal medulla of the rat were resistant to depletion by guanethidine even though the drug entered the adrenal glands. Large doses, however, reduced the level of adrenal catecholamines. Cass and Callingham (1964) observed that chronic treatment with moderate doses of guanethidine or bretylium increased the norepinephrine content of the rat adrenal gland but did not affect the content of epinephrine. This observation suggests that the release of norepinephrine from the adrenal may be inhibited selectively by adrenergic neuron blocking agents.

b) Catecholamine Secretion

ATHOS et al. (1962) reported that direct perfusion of the isolated, denervated, adrenal gland with guanethidine did not affect catecholamine secretion. Guanethidine, given in a single intravenous dose into intact dogs with cannulation of the adrenal vein, did not stimulate catecholamine secretion from the adrenal medulla. ABERCROMBIE and DAVIES (1963) found that guanethidine did not depress the blood pressure response to splanchnic nerve stimulation in the intact cat.

Several investigators found that chemical stimulation of the adrenal medulla was inhibited by guanethidine. Thus, PHILIPPU and SCHÜMANN (1962) reported that guanethidine inhibited the release of catecholamines from perfused bovine adrenal glands which had been evoked by carbachol. JAANUS et al. (1968) demonstrated that guanethidine inhibited acetylcholine-induced catecholamine release from the isolated cat adrenal gland in concentrations similar to those required for hexamethonium and atropine. Guanethidine also inhibited, initially, the medullary catecholamine secretion elicited by nicotinic agents and excess K^+ ion in the intact cat and dog (HAZARD et al., 1964; MIELE, 1966). JAANUS et al. (1968) suggested that guanethidine acted on the chromaffin cell to interfere with the action of acetylcholine on the cell membrane rather than by interfering with the movement of calcium into the cell. The apparent discrepancy in the failure of guanethidine to inhibit neuronally-evoked secretion (Ach-mediated) while it effectively blocked stimulation by cholinergic drugs may be a function of the doses of guanethidine involved. Higher doses may be needed to block effector organ responses evoked by nerve activity than are required to block responses evoked by exogenous mediators. This is true in some adrenergic systems (BEVAN and SU, 1971).

PHILIPPU and SCHÜMANN (1962) and SCHÜMANN and PHILIPPU (1962) reported that guanethidine, like tyramine and related agents, was able in high concentrations ($> 10^{-3}$ M) to release catecholamines from isolated chromaffin granules. WEIL-MALHERBE and POSNER (1963) found that 4×10^{-4} M guanethidine did not release epinephrine from rabbit adrenomedullary particles *in vitro*. CARLSSON et al. (1963) reported that high concentrations of guanethidine (8×10^{-4} M) were only weakly active in inhibiting the uptake of epinephrine into bovine adrenal granules. LUNDBORG and STITZEL (1968), indicated that 10^{-4} and 5×10^{-3} M guanethidine inhibited the bovine granular uptake mechanism. LUNDBORG and STITZEL (1968) made the interesting speculation that very high concentrations may be needed to effect adrenal granular stores (and possibly neuron granule stores as well, Section IV D) and that they may not occur in the adrenal because the adrenal medullary cell membrane, unlike the adrenergic neuron membrane, lacks an effective pump to concentrate guanethidine inside the cell. If this is the case, it would suggest that the guanethidine measured by KUNTZMAN et al. (1962) in the adrenal was largely outside the medullary cells (see 2a above).

C. Effects on Synthesis and Degradation of Norepinephrine in Adrenergic Neurons

1. Synthesis

The information regarding the effects of guanethidine and related agents on the synthesis of norepinephrine is not extensive. Bretylium produces adrenergic neuron blockade without depleting amines. It was and is tacitly assumed that it does not interfere with synthesis. Since guanethidine depleted norepinephrine, the suggestion was made that it might decrease the rate of its synthesis (KUNTZ-

MAN et al., 1962). The authors abandoned this view since they showed (unpublished observations) that although intracisternal injection of guanethidine depleted brain norepinephrine, an increase in the content of catecholamine in these treated brains occurred if monamine oxidase was inhibited. This indicated that synthesis was presumably unimplaired but accumulation did not occur because storage mechanisms were not functional.

Some information is available regarding the effects of guanethidine and related agents on *in vitro* preparations of the enzymes involved in the synthesis of norepinephrine.

a) *Tyrosine Hydroxylase*

Tyrosine hydroxylase activity in homogenates prepared from the guinea pig vas deferens was not affected by bretylium concentrations up to 1.1 mM (POSIVIATA et al. 1971).

b) *Dopa Decarboxylase*

KUNTZMAN et al. (1962, unpublished results) found that guanethidine did not inhibit dopa decarboxylase *in vitro*. Likewise, CHRUSCIEL (1962) reported that this enzyme was not affected by guanethidine. Bretylium did not inhibit dopa decarboxylase (MCCOUBREY, 1962).

c) *Dopamine Beta-Hydroxylase*

Guanethidine and bretylium at concentrations of 10^{-3} M did not inhibit the formation of octopamine (beta-hydroxy tyramine) from tyramine by dopamine beta-hydroxylase isolated from bovine adrenal gland (CREVELING et al., 1962).

Guanoclor inhibited dopamine beta-hydroxylase *in vitro* by 50% at a concentration of 9×10^{-5} M (AUGSTEIN and GREEN, 1964). LAWRIE et al. (1964) showed that guanoclor had a greater inhibitory activity on dopamine beta-hydroxylase than the inhibitor, benzyloxamine. Guanoxan and guanethidine had no effect on the enzyme (Table 10).

Table 10. *Effect of agents on dopamine beta-hydroxylase*

Concentration of compound	Percent inhibition norepinephrine synthesis	
	5×10^{-4}M	1×10^{-4}M
Guanoclor	80.8	41.2
Guanoxan	0	0
Guanethidine	9.1	—
Benzyloxamine	64.4	33.9

After LAWRIE et al. (1964).

LAWRIE et al. (1964) interpreted results from a study with beagle dogs as indicating that guanoclor inhibited dopamine beta-hydroxylase *in vivo*. They found that the norepinephrine in a 24 h urine sample — after 5 months of treatment with guanoclor — was reduced, whereas after guanoxan, which is a more potent adrenergic neuron-blocking and amine-depleting agent than guanoclor, the 24 h urinary norepinephrine was not changed from control. This may be an erroneous interpretation since tyrosine hydroxylase rather than dopamine beta-hydroxylase is rate limiting in the norepinephrine synthetic pathway (UDENFRIEND, 1966). It would be interesting to know if guanoclor inhibits tyrosine hydroxylase.

2. Degradation

a) *Monoamine Oxidase (MAO)*

Guanethidine caused negligible inhibition of MAO of rat heart (CHRUSCIEL, 1962; KUNTZMAN and JACOBSON, 1963a, b), rat brain (KUBIKOWSKI and WYSOKOWSKI, 1963) and rat liver (KADZIELAWA, 1962). Bretylium and bethanidine, on the other hand, had weak inhibiting action on the MAO of the liver of several species and of the rat heart (MCCOUBREY, 1962; DVORNIK et al., 1963; KUNTZMAN and JACOBSON, 1963a, b; MEDINA et al., 1969). MEDINA et al. (1969) presented direct evidence that debrisoquin and its bromo derivative, guanisoquin, inhibited MAO in rabbit liver homogenates (Table 11). Debrisoquin and guanisoquin were the most potent inhibitors among the drugs tested. Debrisoquin has been shown to inhibit MAO in human platelets *in vitro* and *in vivo* (SOLOMON et al., 1969).

Table 11. *Inhibition of rabbit liver MAO by adrenergic neuronal blocking drugs*

Compound	Molar concn producing 50% inhibition
Bethanidine	$5 \cdot 0 \times 10^{-4}$
Bretylium	$8 \cdot 6 \times 10^{-5}$
BW 392C60	$3 \cdot 0 \times 10^{-5}$
Debrisoquin	$2 \cdot 0 \times 10^{-6}$
Guanisoquin	$4 \cdot 4 \times 10^{-7}$

From MEDINA et al. (1969).

FURCHGOTT (1964), FURCHGOTT and SANCHEZ-GARCIA (1966) and FURCHGOTT et al. (1971) demonstrated that bretylium, like classical MAO inhibitors, greatly enhanced the ability of a temporary exposure to norepinephrine to restore the inotropic response of reserpinized guinea pig atria to indirectly acting sympathomimetics such as tyramine. These authors proposed that although bretylium was a relatively weak inhibitor of MAO, it was concentrated in the nerve terminals to such an extent that it effectively inhibited the MAO in these terminals. CLARKE and LEACH (1968) and CLARKE (1970) reported findings with bretylium and bethanidine in rats *in vivo* which were similar to those of FURCHGOTT (1964) and FURCHGOTT and SANCHEZ-GARCIA (1966). Guanethidine, unlike bretylium did not enhance the capacity of norepinephrine to restore responses to tyramine (FURCHGOTT, 1964; FURCHGOTT and SANCHEZ-GARCIA, 1966).

GIACHETTI and SHORE (1967) have shown in rabbit heart slices that 2×10^{-6} M bretylium and debrisoquin, but not guanethidine, markedly increased the accumulation of l-m-octopamine, a MAO substrate, but did not enhance accumulation of l-metaraminol, which is not a substrate for MAO. In these actions bretylium resembled the classical MAO inhibitors iproniazid and pheniprazine (GIACHETTI and SHORE, 1966). CARLSSON and WALDECK (1967) also demonstrated that retention of tritiated norepinephrine by the mouse heart was enhanced by bretylium and certain classical MAO inhibitors.

Similar indirect evidence of MAO inhibition by debrisoquin and several other adrenergic neuron blocking agents is shown in Table 12 (MEDINA et al., 1969). All of the drugs at a concentration of 10^{-4} M greatly inhibited the uptake of metaraminol, indicating that at 10^{-4} M the drugs effectively blocked the membrane amine pump. When heart slices were incubated in media containing the same drugs at a concentration of 1 or 2×10^{-6} M, there was little or no inhibition of uptake of metaraminol, while accumulation of 1-m-octopamine, a substrate for MAO was markedly enhanced. The results suggested that MAO was inhibited by these neuron blocking agents.

MALMFORS and ABRAMS (1970) presented data obtained with fluorescence histochemical methods (see also Section VII B 2) which provided additional support for the idea that debrisoquin and bretylium were reversible, intraneuronal MAO inhibitors and that their effectiveness in adrenergic neurons was the result of accumulation by membrane transport. The nature of the MAO inhibition produced by these drugs differed from that observed with classical MAO inhibitors in being more transient, reversible and localized to sympathetic tissues.

HERTTING et al. (1962) reported that the concentration of endogenous norepinephrine as well as the MAO activity in hearts from bretylium-treated rats, unlike hearts from rats treated with classical MAO inhibitors, were the same as untreated controls. This finding is subject to criticism in that 24 h were allowed to elapse between the injection of bretylium and the subsequent determination of norepinephrine levels and MAO activity. In addition, bretylium is a reversible inhibitor of MAO *in vitro* (WHITE and MAXWELL, unpublished observation) and, therefore, probably dissociated from the enzyme during the *in vitro* assay procedures.

Table 12. *Effect of adrenergic neuronal blocking drugs on amine accumulation by rabbit heart slices*[a]

Drug	Drug concn	Net amine uptake (μg/ml slice water ± S. E.) *l*-Metaraminol	Net amine uptake (μg/ml slice water ± S. E.) *l-m*-Octopamine
None		0·38 ± 0·04	0·20 ± 0·02
Debrisoquin	10^{-6}	0·26 ± 0·02	0·97 ± 0·04
Debrisoquin	10^{-4}	0·04 ± 0·02	0·09 ± 0·02
Bretylium	2×10^{-6}	0·35 ± 0·05	0·57 ± 0·02
Bretylium	10^{-4}	0·10 ± 0·01	0·26 ± 0·02
BW 392C60	10^{-6}	0·34 ± 0·02	1·05 ± 0·09
BW 392C60	10^{-4}	0·10 ± 0·02	0·56 ± 0·02
Bethanidine	2×10^{-6}	0·27 ± 0·01	0·49 ± 0·06
Bethanidine	10^{-4}	0·07 ± 0·01	0·22 ± 0·03
Guanisoquin	10^{-6}	0·28 ± 0·03	0·49 ± 0·05
Guanisoquin	10^{-4}	0·01 ± 0·01	0·07 ± 0·02

[a] Slices were incubated with *l*-metaraminol (0·025 μg/ml) or *l-m*-octopamine (0·2 μg/ml) for 60 min. The blocking drugs were added at the start of the 15-min preincubation period. Net uptake denotes accumulation per ml slice water minus concentration in the medium. From MEDINA et al. (1969).

b) *Catechol O-Methyltransferase (COMT)*

Guanethidine and bretylium did not inhibit COMT of rat and cat liver (ABBS, 1962; HATTORI and SHIBATA, 1971).

D. Effect on the Uptake of Norepinephrine into Adrenergic Nerves, Storage of Norepinephrine in and Release from Intraneuronal Granules, and Disappearance of Norepinephrine from Adrenergic Nerves

LINDMAR and MUSCHOLL (1964) presented strong evidence that two mechanisms existed for concentrating catecholamines within the adrenergic neuron and that guanethidine inhibited both of these mechanisms. The two mechanisms were 1) the transport across the cell membrane and 2) the uptake of norepinephrine into storage sites. These authors found from balance studies with isolated rabbit and rat hearts that 60% of a perfused dose of norepinephrine was recoverable in the perfusate. Essentially all of the norepinephrine removed from the perfusion fluid was recoverable from the heart as norepinephrine. In the presence of guanethidine in the perfusion fluid the removal of norepinephrine was impaired and the net uptake into heart correspondingly decreased (Fig. 14). However, after pretreatment

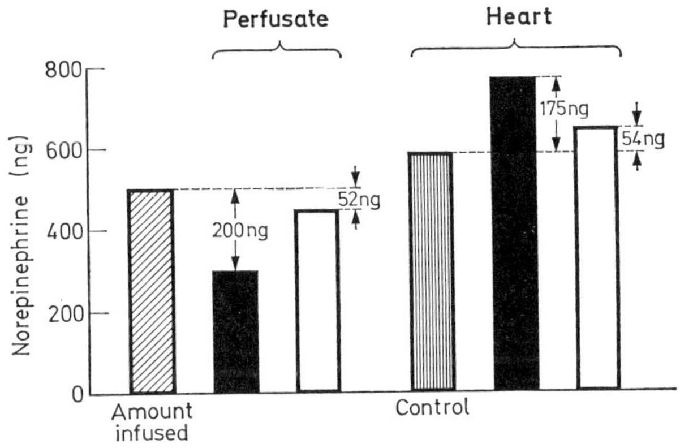

Fig. 14. Effects of guanethidine on the elimination of norepinephrine from the perfusion fluid and on norepinephrine uptake in the isolated rat heart. Norepinephrine (496 ng) was infused for ten minutes. Solid columns represent norepinephrine content in the absence of guanethidine and open columns represent norepinephrine content in the presence of guanethidine (15 μg/ml) in the perfusion fluid. Each column represents the mean of seven experiments. Amount Infused = total amount perfused through the heart; Control = endogenous content of norepinephrine. After LINDMAR and MUSCHOLL (1964)

of animals with guanethidine the removal of norepinephrine from the perfusion fluid was unchanged from control but there was no corresponding net increase of norepinephrine in the heart (Fig. 15). Guanethidine, when added to the perfusion fluid of guanethidine-pretreated hearts increased greatly the norepinephrine in the perfusates. Thus, it was clear that guanethidine (as seen when it was added to the perfusion fluid) prevented entrance of norepinephrine into the nerves of the heart. It also had the capacity (as seen in hearts from pretreated animals) to prevent entrance of norepinephrine into storage sites within the neurons where it could be protected from MAO and the norepinephrine was, therefore, destroyed by MAO and not observable as norepinephrine in the heart. SHORE and GIACHETTI (1966) also presented data in support of a dual action of guanethidine in adrenergic neurons. Low concentrations of guanethidine (5×10^{-6} M) prevented the accumulation of l-m-octopamine, a MAO substrate, by rabbit heart slices but not the accumulation of l-metaraminol, which is not a substrate for MAO. Higher concentrations of guanethidine (10^{-4} M) inhibited the uptake of both l-metaraminol and l-m-octopamine. The data indicated that inhibition of the neuronal membrane pump by a high concentration of guanethidine inhibited the access of both substrates into the neuron. At lower concentrations the pump was not inhibited, thus, l-metaraminol accumulated. m-Octopamine did not accumulate at low concentrations of guanethidine because access to the intraneuronal binding sites was blocked and it was thus degraded by intraneuronal MAO. The inhibition of the l-metaraminol accumulation by 10^{-4} M guanethidine was readily reversed by washing, whereas, the inhibiting action on m-octopamine accumulation was not.

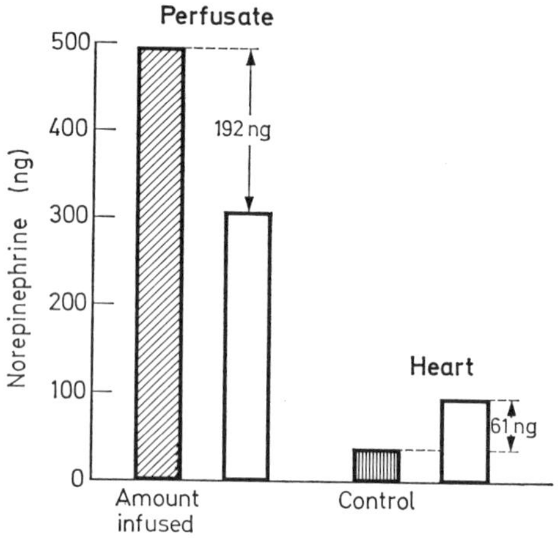

Fig. 15. Effects of guanethidine pretreatment on the elimination of norepinephrine from the perfusion fluid and on norepinephrine uptake in the isolated rat heart. Rats were pretreated with guanethidine (15 mg/kg) 48 and 24 h prior to the experiment. Each column represents the results of five experiments. Amount infused = total amount perfused through heart; Control = endogenous content of norepinephrine. After LINDMAR and MUSCHOLL (1964)

LUNDBORG and STITZEL (1968) also presented evidence for a dual site of action of guanethidine. They studied the effect of guanethidine on the subcellular distribution of tritiated α-methyl-norepinephrine in the heart of mice. α-Methyl-norepinephrine is not a substrate for MAO. Within a half-hour after its injection, guanethidine reduced the uptake of injected α-methyl-norepinephrine by 70%. The remaining 30% was distributed between particulate and supernatant fractions in a manner similar to that in control animals, indicating normal functioning of intraneuronal storage mechanisms. The inhibition, therefore, was at the level of the neuronal membrane pump. Twelve hours after the administration of guanethidine, however, uptake of α-methyl-norepinephrine was increased as compared to the uptake at a half-hour, but the proportion residing in the particulate fraction was reduced as compared to control, indicating that guanethidine had a prolonged effect on intraneuronal binding sites. The authors concluded that guanethidine blocked both of the uptake mechanisms for norepinephrine, but the onset of blockade of the membrane pump was more rapid while the blockade of the granules was more persistent.

Since, as presented in an earlier section (III B) it is clear that guanethidine, as well as other neuron blockers, are substrates for the adrenergic neuron membrane pump (MITCHELL and OATES, 1970) and that norepinephrine and related phenethylamines are also substrates for the same pump, competition between substrates readily explains the inhibitory actions of guanethidine and other blockers on the uptake of norepinephrine into neurons. Furthermore, since it is known (Section III C) that the subcellular distributions of tritiated guanethidine and tritiated norepinephrine in adrenergically innervated tissue (rat heart) are similar and that they are concentrated in the same catecholamine storage granules (OBIANWU et al., 1968; MAÎTRE and STAEHELIN, 1971), the occurrence of an action of guanethidine at this storage granule is not surprising.

CHANG et al. (1965) reported that a direct relationship existed between the amount of guanethidine retained in rat heart and the degree of norepinephrine depletion which occurred in this organ. This was highly suggestive that some form of displacement of norepinephrine by guanethidine was occurring in the storage granules. MAÎTRE and STAEHELIN (1971) compared the amount of guanethidine found in granules with the amount of norepinephrine lost from granules. Thirty minutes after intravenous injection of guanethidine, significant amounts of guanethidine appeared in the granules, whereas no loss of norepinephrine was observed. Between 30 min and 5 h following guanethidine administration, the granules lost an amount of norepinephrine which was greater than the increment of guanethidine taken up during this time. The authors concluded that the norepinephrine depletion was not due to a simple displacement by guanethidine. They further suggested that if displacement was involved it must consist of at least two phases : 1) uptake of guanethidine into stores and 2) subsequent displacement. This would imply, according to the authors, some kind of migration of guanethidine from uptake sites to release sites within the granules.

HIFT and CAMPOS (1962) using hemorrhagic shock as a stress to the heart in dogs, CHANG and CHANG (1965) using long duration of coaxial stimulation of the vas deferens, and CHANG and SU (1967) using cold as a stress to the rat heart reported that these procedures elicited approximately 25 to 50% reduction in total catecholamine content of the organs and similar percentage loss of norepinephrine from the microsomal fraction (ca. 100,000 × G). Depletion from the supernatant fraction was considerably less. STITZEL et al. (1965) on the other hand found that stimulation of the right accelerans nerve of the isolated perfused rabbit heart decreased only the norepinephrine in the soluble fraction. CHANG and CHANG (1965) and CHANG and SU (1967) suggested that the norepinephrine in the particulate fraction was the functional pool of the amine available for release by nerve impulses.

BHAGAT (1964) demonstrated that the first effect of guanethidine was to deplete endogenous norepinephrine from the soluble fraction of a homogenate of rat heart that had been separated into coarse, particulate and soluble fractions by differential centrifugation (Table 13). CHANG et al. (1967a) also found that guanethidine did not cause a significant decrease of endogenous particulate norepinephrine from rat heart within 30 min. Unlike BHAGAT (1964), they did not find depletion of norepinephrine from the supernatant fraction. However, CHANG et al. (1967a) were able to show 20% depletion of tritiated norepinephrine from rat heart particulate fraction at 30 min following guanethidine although as stated above endogenous norepinephrine was not reduced. In the vas deferens, CHANG et al (1967a) found that at 30 min following guanethidine administration, the endogenous amine in the particulate fraction was decreased by approximately 30% whereas the norepinephrine in the supernatant fraction was unchanged. At five hours, both fractions were reduced. SCHÜMANN et al. (1964) found that at 20 h after a low dose of guanethidine (0.3 mg/kg i. m.) a 40% depletion in the catecholamine content of guinea pig heart had occurred. The particulate and supernatant fractions were equally reduced. For discussion of these conflicting results see Section V A.

Table 13. *Effect of guanethidine on the intracellular distribution of noradrenaline in the rat heart.* Rats were killed at different times after the intramuscular injection of 20 mg/kg of guanethidine, and the concentration of cardiac catecholamines in various fractions, separated by centrifugation, were determined. Catecholamine concentrations (means and standard errors) are expressed in terms of noradrenaline. An asterisk indicates that the mean is significantly different ($P < 0.05$) from that of the controls

Time after guan-ethidine (min)	No. of rats	Catechol amine concentration (μg/g of fresh tissue)			
		Coarse fraction	Particulate fraction	Soluble fraction	Whole homogenate
Control	6	0·23 ± 0·026	0·29 ± 0·02	0·29 ± 0·015	0·76 ± 0·05
45	7	0·27 ± 0·024	0·31 ± 0·024	0·20 ± 0·02*	0·70 ± 0·02
60	7	0·24 ± 0·024	0·30 ± 0·02	0·18 ± 0·014*	0·71 ± 0·04
75	9	0·19 ± 0·02	0·26 ± 0·013	0·15 ± 0·014*	0·59 ± 0·045*
90	4	0·16 ± 0·02	0·23 ± 0·03	0·16 ± 0·017*	0·57 ± 0·034*
120	7	0·14 ± 0·014*	0·19 ± 0·01*	0·12 ± 0·012*	0·54 ± 0·025*

From BHAGAT (1964).

It is interesting that MAÎTRE and STAEHELIN (1971) found that whereas tritiated norepinephrine was effectively taken up by isolated bovine splenic nerve granules, no measurable uptake of tritiated guanethidine into these granules was noted with a concentration as high as approximately 10^{-4} M (15.2 μg/ml). Earlier, EULER and LISHAJKO (1964) demonstrated that 10^{-4} M guanethidine did not enhance the release of norepinephrine from isolated bovine splenic nerve granules. It is not understood why isolated storage granules are so insensitive to guanethidine action when *in vivo* they are quite sensitive to its effects. It is quite likely, however, that concentrations of guanethidine greater than 10^{-4} M may be attained in adrenergic neurons as a result of the amine pump and that these high concentrations may exert an effect on the granules (Section II, III B).

KOPIN and GORDON (1963) studied the changes caused by guanethidine in the urinary excretion of tritiated norepinephrine and metabolites in the rat. While there were significant increases in norepinephrine and normetanephrine, the largest increase was in the deaminated catechols. These observations suggest that while some norepinephrine is released intact from the nerve (and therefore accounts for the transient sympathomimesis) considerable amounts of the norepinephrine which is depleted from nerve endings is subject to intraneuronal degradation by MAO prior to its release.

As discussed earlier, bretylium and debrisoquin are taken up into adrenergic nerves in a manner similar to guanethidine but in contrast to guanethidine they do not exhibit specific subcellular localization in amine storage vesicles (Section III B, C). ABBS and ROBERTSON (1970) presented evidence that at 15 min after intravenous administration of 10 mg/kg bretylium, 50% depletion of norepinephrine occurred in the supernatant fraction but not from other subcellular fractions of an homogenate of cat spleen. The depletion was apparent up to 18 h later but disappeared by 7 days. Significant depletion (60%) of norepinephrine from the particulate fraction occurred only after 30 min and continued for 60 min and 18 h after bretylium administration. On the other hand, CHANG et al. (1967a) found that 5 h after intraperitoneal administration of 10 mg/kg to rats, bretylium did not cause any change in the pattern of subcellular distribution of norepinephrine in the rat vas deferens. It seems likely that differences in species, routes of administration and doses may account for these disparate results. It is possible that high doses, especially if given repeatedly to the appropriate species may lead to an interaction of bretylium with amine storage granules. More information is needed.

As pointed out above (Section IV C2), bretylium, debrisoquin and bethanidine, unlike guanethidine have weak, reversible MAO inhibiting activities which can become significant within the adrenergic neuron. It is likely that their intraneuronal MAO inhibiting effect is an important factor in the failure of these agents to deplete norepinephrine from adrenergic nerve endings.

HORST and GATTANELL (1970) reported that low doses (1 mg/kg) of debrisoquin did not significantly alter the accumulation *in vivo* of tritiated norepinephrine by rat heart, but doses of 5 to 50 mg/kg, were effective in inhibiting the accumulation of tritiated norepinephrine. In these studies debrisoquin was nearly as potent as cocaine in preventing the accumulation of norepinephrine.

V. Hypotheses Regarding the Mechanism of Neuron Blockade

A. Subcellular Pool Depletion Hypothesis

The findings of CASS and SPRIGGS (1961), GAFFNEY et al. (1962, 1963), SANAN and VOGT (1962), and SPRIGGS (1966) that following the administration of guanethidine, adrenergic neuron blockade preceded depletion of norepinephrine and waned before recovery of the norepinephrine content, suggested that neuronal blockade was not a direct result of the general depletion of amines. According to CHANG et al. (1967a) and ABBS and ROBERTSON (1970) this did not necessarily mean that the neuron blocking effect of guanethidine and bretylium was unrelated to the storage mechanism of the transmitter amine. They felt as did others (e.g. CARLSSON, 1966; GREEN, 1971) that some small, but necessary, compartment might be depleted. CHANG et al. (1967a) pointed out that guanethidine caused a significant decrease in the tritiated norepinephrine of the particulate subcellular fraction of rat heart and vas deferens within 30 min following its administration. At this time, depletion of total norepinephrine had not yet reached significance. BHAGAT (1964) on the other hand, reported rapid depletion (within 45 min) of only the supernatant norepinephrine in rat heart following guanethidine. Approximately 3 times as long was required for depletion of particulate fractions.

ABBS and DODD (1974) found that 5 mg/kg i.v. guanethidine or a related compound (−)—N-(1-phenylethyl) guanidine (PEG) decreased the norepinephrine content of the high-speed particulate (100,000 × G) and supernatant fractions of splenic homogenates. These changes were temporally correlated with neuron blockade. Dexamphetamine prevented and antagonized neuron blockade produced by both agents. The restoration of nerve function was temporally correlated with a selective repletion of the norepinephrine content of the supernatant fraction. High doses of PEG or guanethidine (15 mg/kg i.v.) selectively depleted norepinephrine in only the supernatant fraction of the spleen. The depletion was temporally correlated with neuron blockade.

ABBS and ROBERTSON (1970) demonstrated rapid depletion (within 15 min) of the supernatant norepinephrine of cat spleen and somewhat less rapid depletion (within 30 min) of particulate norepinephrine following bretylium administration.

ROBERTSON and ABBS (1971) reported that the intravenous administration of 10 mg/kg debrisoquin into cats thirty minutes before splenectomy depleted > 60% of the norepinephrine content of the high speed supernatant fraction (100,00 × G) but did not change the norepinephrine levels in the low-speed particulate (12,000 × G) or high speed particulate (100,000 × G). The authors state that these results, like those obtained with bretylium (ABBS and ROBERTSON, 1970) show that depletion of the norepinephrine of the high-speed supernatant fraction of the cat spleen may be correlated with adrenergic neuron blockade.

ABBS and PYCOCK (1973) studied the effects of intravenous bretylium on the content and subcellular distribution of norepinephrine in the rat heart. They found that bretylium at doses of 2.5 mg/kg, 20 mg/kg and 60 mg/kg was without effect on the norepinephrine content of the rat heart at one hour after administration. Curiously, 10 mg/kg elevated the content by 16% at one hour and reduced it by 11% at 10 h. Changes in the norepinephrine content of several subcellular fractions were associated with onset of adrenergic neuron blockade, however, the only change which occurred at the onset and persisted during blockade was the decrease in the highspeed (100,000 × G) particulate fraction. ABBS and PYCOCK (1973) concluded that the results of their experiments add weight to the earlier suggestions of ABBS and ROBERTSON (1970) that bretylium, and possibly other adrenergic neuron blocking agents bring about blockade by depleting an important small store of norepinephrine which is essential for nerve function.

Since these several workers had differing results with the same and different tissues 1) there may be technical difficulties to overcome or 2) it appears that these early subcellular effects are unrelated to neuron blockade or 3) neuron blocking agents may have different mechanisms of action in different tissues. This latter possibility should be accepted only in the presence of highly persuasive evidence. The possibility that a small but select pool of norepinephrine within the neuron terminal is involved in the mode of action of neuron blocking agents is still a viable idea, but one for which no undisputed, direct evidence exists.

B. Membrane Depolarizing and Stabilizing Hypotheses and Local Anesthetic Action

CHANG et al. (1965) suggested that there was a link between the degree of neuron blockade as measured by appearance of ptosis in the rat, the amount of guanethidine in sympathetic neurons of the rat heart, and the norepinephrine depleted from the rat heart (Fig. 16). These authors considered that their evidence indicated that the blockade of adrenergic neurons and the loss of norepinephrine from nerve endings was a consequence of the same primary action of guanethidine and speculated that this action might be a persistent depolarization of adrenergic terminals. On the other hand, BRODIE et al. (1965) concluded that bretylium, which did not deplete amines and was not taken up into storage vesicles must produce its neuron blockade by some other mechanism.

Some support for the interpretations of CHANG et al. (1965) and BRODIE et al. (1965) comes from the work of KUBO and MISU (1974) who induced neuron blockade with 4×10^{-6} M or 2×10^{-5} M guanethidine in sympathetically-innervated Langendorff preparations and found that wash out of the guanethidine with a high Na (286 mM) solution enhanced,w hile washout with a low Na (86 mM) solution reduced neuron blockade as compared to that seen during washout with normal Na (143 mM). On the other hand while the neuron blockade produced by 1.2×10^{-5} M bretylium was enhanced by washout with high Na (286 mM) it was not reduced by washout with low Na (86 mM) (MISU and KUBO, 1964). These investigators suggested that guanethidine increases the permeability of adrenergic nerve ending membranes to Na thereby leading to adrenergic neuron blockade and that it appeared unlikely that bretylium had the same action as guanethidine.

Evidence that neither guanethidine nor bretylium depolarized sympathetic terminals was presented by CABRERA et al. (1966). These authors used the "collision technique" in cats. With this technique the antidromic impulses which were induced in adrenergic nerve terminals in the heart by injection of drugs into the left atrium, were assessed by their capacity to reduce the amplitude of orthodromic impulses arriving in postganglionic fibers (inferior cardiac nerve). The orthodromic impulses were initiated by electrical stimulation of preganglionic fibers.

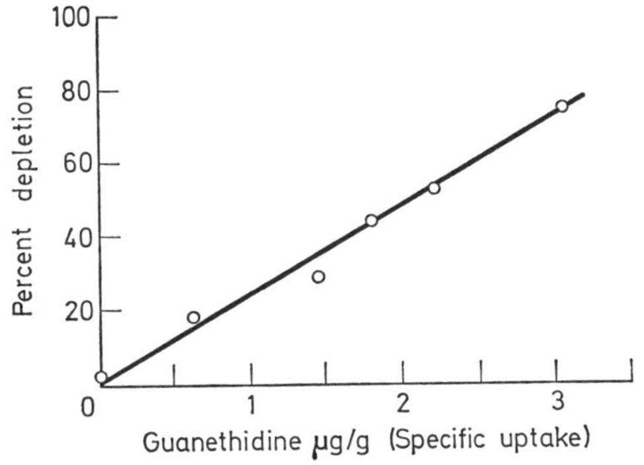

Fig. 16. Depletion of heart norepinephrine 5 h after a single dose of guanethidine as a function of the specific (*i.e.*, neuronal) uptake of drug. The data describe the results of 11 experiments (33 animals) in which the guanethidine uptake and norepinephrine depletion were determined in the same animals. The two points nearest the origin each represent one experiment; the other four points represent the average of 2 or more experiments. The specific uptake of guanethidine was calculated as the difference between uptake of guanethidine in control rats pretreated with various doses of amphetamine. The norepinephrine depletion is calculated as the difference between the norepinephrine level in rats given guanethidine and rats given guanethidine after pretreatment with various doses of amphetamine. From CHANG et al. (1965)

The presence of antidromic impulses indicated that the postganglionic nerve endings had been depolarized. Acetylcholine readily initiated antidromic impulses, but bretylium and guanethidine did not. The failure of these two agents to do so indicated that depolarization of the nerve membrane was not essential for their neuron block. On the contrary, guanethidine and bretylium, like local anesthetics, were strong antagonists of acetylcholine depolarization suggesting that guanethidine and bretylium blocked the sympathetic terminals by stabilizing their membranes. Similar findings were presented by HÄUSLER et al. (1968) using a cat Langendorff preparation with its innervation intact. Guanethidine (2×10^{-7}M) completely blocked the antidromal discharges produced by acetylcholine (0.05 mM), in the postganglionic sympathetic innervation of this preparation. At a concentration of 10^{-6}M, guanethidine blocked the effect of electrical stimulation of sympathetic nerves of the heart after a contact time of 15 to 20 min. The effects of a high concentration of acetylcholine (2.5 mM) were also antagonized by a high concentration (10^{-6}M) of guanethidine. HÄUSLER et al. (1969) presented similar findings for bretylium. On the other hand, DAVEY et al. (1968) reported that at a time when bretylium blocked the acetylcholine-induced liberation of norepinephrine from the cat spleen, acetylcholine still induced antidromic firing in splenic C-fibers. These results seem to contradict those of HÄUSLER et al. (1969). However, HÄUSLER et al. (1969) after confirming these observations in the spleen, attributed the effect to the presence of non-adrenergic C-fibers since some of the fibers were resistant to the destructive action of 6-hydroxydopamine. The evidence of CABRERA et al. (1966) and that of HÄUSLER et al. (1968, 1969) argues strongly against the depolarization hypothesis of BRODIE et al. (1965) and CHANG et al. (1965).

KUBO and MISU (1974) criticized the work of HÄUSLER et al. (1968, 1969) because the stabilizing (local anesthetic-like) effect noted with guanethidine and bretylium was observed when these blocking agents were present in the bath medium. KUBO and MISU (1974) reasoned that once established, neuron blockade is persistent and does not require these presence of the blocking agents in the bath and that a stabilizing effect may in essence be an artifact due to the presence of excessive blocking agents. This reasoning does not seem likely in that the concentrations of blocking agents used by HÄUSLER et al. (1968, 1969) (2×10^{-7} to 10^{-5} M) were at least 1000 times lower than those needed to inhibit the stimulation of sensory endings, e.g., in baroreceptors (8×10^{-3} M to 10^{-2} M), and the time course for onset of neuron blockade was considerably longer than for the onset of baroreceptor blockade. By way of comparison, the local anesthetic agent, tetracaine, blocked adrenergic nerve endings and baroreceptors at the same concentration (10^{-5} M) and with identical rapid time courses.

The idea that bretylium and guanethidine might exert a depressant action on the adrenergic terminals which was analogous to the impairment of conduction in a nerve trunk caused by local anesthetics was first made by BOURA et al. (1960) and BOURA and GREEN (1965) (Section VII G). Bretylium and especially guanethidine (BEIN, 1961) and bethanidine (BOURA and GREEN, 1963) are relatively weak local anesthetic agents but they are taken up and highly concentrated within the adrenergic nerve terminals because they are substrates for the "amine-pump" in the terminal neuronal membrane (see Section III B). In further discussion to this point, HÄUSLER (1971) estimated that guanethidine and bretylium were accumulated within the adrenergic nerve endings as compared to their concentration in the extracellular space by a ratio of 1000 to 3000:1.

BOYD et al. (1961) reported that the differences between the action of bretylium and procaine in several preparations did not support the idea that bretylium blocked sympathetic nerves by producing local anesthesia. RAND and WILSON (1967c) using several isolated preparations showed that in a group of compounds there was no direct relationship between the local anesthetic activity of individual drugs and their potency as adrenergic neuron blocking agents. This study was open to criticism in that there was no evidence that all of the agents studied were taken up and concentrated by the adrenergic terminals. Recently, WILSON (1970) reported that EM 97 (3-cyclohexylamino-n-propylguanidine) which was equipotent with guanethidine as a local anesthetic agent and was taken up into adrenergic nerve endings in rat heart as well as was guanethidine, was virtually inactive as a neuronal blocking agent. FURCHGOTT (1971) and GREEN (1971) pointed out that to speak about the "local anesthetic action" of the adrenergic neuron blocking agents at the nerve terminals might be misleading in that the term connotes an identical mode of action, whereas, the effect of neuron blocking agents may just be analogous but not identical to a true local anesthetic action. The site and mode of action of these agents on a neuronal membrane might be quite different from those of a classical local anesthetic. FURCHGOTT (1971) suggested that it is more likely that these agents produced their blockade of action potentials by acting at "receptor" sites on the inside surface of the membrane of the terminals rather than on the outside. FURCHGOTT (1971) further suggested that, presumably, the high concentration of neuronal blocking agents needed to interrupt norepinephrine release by action potentials would be maintained by reuptake of a significant fraction of the agent which spontaneously leaked out of the terminals. CARLSSON (1966) and GREEN (1971) have suggested that adrenergic neuron blocking agents may exert their blocking effects on a small pool of norepinephrine which is critical to the release mechanism at the adrenergic terminal. A stabilizing action of adrenergic neuron blocking agents on such a pool – whether it was located in some sub-compartment of granules, or in selected granules, or in the neuronal membrane or elsewhere – similar to that demonstrated for the complete terminal by CABRERA et al. (1966) and HÄUSLER et al. (1968, 1969) might be involved. If the "active" site at this pool is capable of recognizing structural differences among blocking agents, then the failure of WILSON (1970) to see neuronal blocking activity in a guanethidine analog (EM97) having equal local anesthetic potency and equal capacity to be taken up by nerve terminals can be understood.

MISU et al. (1976) reported that compound No. 865-123 (4-7-exo-methylene-hexahydroisoindoline-ethyl-guanidine hemisulfate) was a potent neuron blocking agent which lacked local anesthetic activity (in the guinea pig weal test) at concentrations (0.25% to 1%) in which bretylium and guanethidine were active. However, since No. 865-123 is approximately equipotent with guanethidine as a neuron blocking agent but has a much slower onset of action it may well be that considerably more of No. 865-123 needs to be taken up into neurons in order to exert equivalent blockade. It would be very desirable to know the local anesthetic effect of No. 865-123 at concentrations between 1% and 10%.

MITCHELL and OATES (1970) and OATES et al. (1971) have re-emphasized that guanethidine, bretylium and related adrenergic neuron blocking drugs in high concentrations are general inhibitors of nerve and muscle function. Perhaps this is related to their local anesthetic-like actions (Section VII G). Bretylium and guanethidine, administered intravenously to dogs and cats briefly inhibited cholinergic junctions in the sympathetic, parasympathetic and somatic motor outflow (Section VII H). Transient ganglionic blockade was observed as well as transient blockade of the cardiac response to peripheral vagal stimulation (BOURA and GREEN, 1959). Transient paralysis of neuromuscular transmission has been described in several preparations both *in vivo* and *in vitro* (BOURA and GREEN, 1959; DIXIT et al., 1961; CHANG et al., 1967b) (Section VII E). Bethanidine (300 μg/ml, ca. 10^{-3} M) decreased by approximately 10-fold the sensitivity of the guinea-pig isolated ileum preparation to acetylcholine and histamine. Concentrations of 3 to 30 μg/ml (ca. 10^{-5} to 10^{-4} M) inhibited the peristaltic reflex of the guinea-pig isolated ileum and depressed its sensitivity to acetylcholine and to nicotine (BOURA and GREEN, 1963). These blocking actions required high concentrations of the agents *in vitro* and relatively large intravenous doses *in vivo*. *In vivo* these responses were very transient relative to the adrenergic neuron blockade. The brief duration of these effects was undoubtedly due to the rapidly falling plasma level of the compounds which occurs after their intravenous administration and the consequent reduction in concentrations at the various synapses and junctions (see Section II). On the other hand, adrenergic neuron blockade persists because the blocking agents are actively taken up by the amine pump in adrenergic nerves and thereby held in sufficiently high concentrations within the neuron to elicit an effect. Thus, as suggested by earlier work (BOURA et al., 1960; BOURA and GREEN, 1963; SCHANKER and MORRISON, 1965), it can be argued that the selective inhibition of the adrenergic neuron, *in vivo*, results solely from the fact that these agents are substrates for the amine pump in adrenergic neurons and is not because they interrupt a function specific to adrenergic nerve terminals.

C. Cholinergic Link Hypothesis and the Possible Role of Ca-Ion

Burn and Rand (1962) and Burn (1967) speculated that the site of action of neuron blocking agents on the pool of physiologically-releasable norepinephrine was the site of the "cholinergic link" in adrenergic fibers. In other words, guanethidine and bretylium were considered to compete with acetylcholine for the site in the neuron where it was proposed that acetylcholine interacted to release norepinephrine as one step in a series of events initiated by the action potential. Rand and Wilson (1967b), on the basis of structure-activity relationships among adrenergic neuron blockers, nicotine, DMPP and acetylcholine, postulated a receptor that is complementary to the structure of adrenergic neuron blockers.

Hertting and Widhalm (1965) and Fischer et al. (1966) noted that bretylium blocked the neuronally-induced release of norepinephrine from the isolated perfused cat spleen at concentrations that did not affect the release due to acetylcholine. In addition, Hertting and Widhalm (1965) reported that eserine potentiated the effect of injected acetylcholine but not the effects of nerve stimulation. These authors drew the conclusion that it was unlikely that acetylcholine was an intermediate transmitter working at the same site as bretylium as postulated by Burn and Rand (1962). Fischer et al. (1966) drew a somewhat different conclusion; namely, that bretylium acted at a step "proximal" to the cholinergic link. They felt that if bretylium "replaced" intraneuronal acetylcholine it should reduce the amount of acetylcholine "mobilized" during nerve stimulation and as a consequence the amount of norepinephrine relased by the terminals. In this scheme bretylium would not inhibit the release of norepinephrine evoked by exogenous acetylcholine. Davey et al. (1968) reported that the difference in sensitivity to blockade by bretylium of the effects of nerve stimulation and of the sympathomometic effects of acetylcholine did not exist if stimulus frequencies of 10 cps or less were employed. Boura and Green (1965) have drawn attention to the fact that anticholinergic effects of neuron blockers, unlike adrenergic neuron blockade, are rapidly removed by washout in *in vitro* systems.

Some evidence is at hand that neuron blocking agents have the capacity to block acetylcholine selectively in a few systems. Watson (1967) presented evidence that intravenous or intra-arterial guanethidine blocked the afferent discharge produced by acetylcholine in sensory C fibers of the rabbit saphenous nerve without impairing the response to touch or to KCl, whereas, effective doses of lidocaine abolished responses to acetylcholine, KCl and touch. Jaanus et al. (1968) reported that addition of guanethidine to the perfusing solution produced a dose-dependent inhibition of the secretory response of the adrenal medulla of the cat to acetylcholine. This inhibition could be antagonized by increasing the concentration of either acetylcholine or calcium. Thus guanethidine has some "anticholinergic" effects. Their significance to the phenomenon of neuron blockade, however, is obscure. The hypothesis of a "cholinergic active site" for neuron blockade remains highly speculative and awaits convincing substantiation.

Burn and Welsh (1967) reported that after the responses of the rabbit ileum to sympathetic nerve stimulation had been partially blocked by guanethidine, they were restored by raising the extracellular calcium level to 11 mM. These authors suggested that guanethidine and bretylium might produce their blocking action by preventing the access of calcium into the nerve terminal and thereby preventing the release of norepinephrine. They argued that the permeability increase to calcium was normally produced by acetylcholine (the cholinergic link hypothesis) and that guanethidine and bretylium competed with acetylcholine for a common site. KIRPEKAR et al. (1969) reported that exceedingly high calcium (50 mM) in the perfusion fluid restored the norepinephrine release due to splenic nerve stimulation to 50% of normal after it had been greatly reduced by guanethidine treatment. High levels of calcium (5 and 7.5 mM) were without effect in restoring norepinephrine release. From these results, these investigators suggested that guanethidine depressed release of norepinephrine during nerve stimulation by limiting access of calcium to sites in postganglionic sympathetic nerve endings with which the ion must interact to cause liberation of norepinephrine. Since inordinately high concentrations of Ca^{++} were required in the studies of KIRPEKAR et al. (1969) the significance of their finding is problematic.

Much of the force of the argument of BURN and WELSH (1967) has been vitiated by the report of WILSON (1970). In his study, the effects of increasing extracellular calcium on the responses to sympathetic nerve stimulation of three isolated organs were investigated: rabbit ileum, guinea-pig vas deferens and rabbit ear artery. Thus, after partial blockade by guanethidine of the responses of the ileum to sympathetic nerve stimulation, the responses were restored to their original size by a 2- to 4-fold increase in the concentration of Ca^{++} in the bath. However, doubling the Ca^{++} concentration of the bath (from 2.2 to 4.4 mM) increased responses of the ileum to sympathetic stimulation even in the absence of guanethidine. The maximum increase in response of both untreated and guanethidine-treated preparations was obtained with 8.8 mM calcium. In the vas deferens and rabbit ear artery preparations, an increase in extracellular calcium did not antagonize the blocking action of guanethidine. These experiments did not support the theory that guanethidine acted by preventing the access of calcium to its site of action in the sympathetic nerve endings. Similarly, CHANG et al. (1971) working with rat vas deferens and rabbit ileum concluded that the antagonism between calcium and guanethidine was physiologic in nature rather than pharmacologic.

D. Amphetamine Receptor Site Hypothesis

It was reported by WILSON and LONG (1960) that the hypotensive actions of bretylium and guanethidine in man were reduced by simultaneous treatment with dexamphetamine. DAY and RAND (1962) demonstrated that dexamphetamine reversed the adrenergic neuron blocking action of guanethidine in anesthetized cats and dogs. It was suggested by DAY and RAND (1963) that the antagonism between guanethidine and dexamphetamine was competitive and that both drugs interacted with the receptor concerned with the blocking action of guanethidine in sympathetic neuron terminals. CHANG et al. (1965) presented evidence which they interpreted as showing that amphetamine selectively displaced guanethidine from its specific binding sites in adrenergic neurons and suggested that it thereby reversed neuronal blockade. Methamphetamine is also known to prevent accumulation of guanethidine in rabbit hearts (MATSUMOTO and HORITA, 1963).

More recently, GERKENS et al. (1969) demonstrated that cocaine was also effective in reversing the adrenergic neuron blockade in isolated rabbit ileum, ear artery and spleen. Cocaine was effective in a concentration which reduced norepinephrine uptake to the same extent as a concentration of dexamphetamine which also reversed adrenergic neuron blockade in these tissues (Fig. 17). The principal interaction of cocaine with adrenergic neurons is to block the uptake mechanism in the terminals. This result suggested strongly that amphetamine, like cocaine, was antagonizing the effects of guanethidine by inhibiting the uptake of guanethidine. The more rapid recovery from neuronal blockade after amphetamine as compared to after cocaine (Fig. 17) suggests that release of guanethidine by amphetamine may also play a part. KIRPEKAR et al. (1969) demonstrated that cocaine antagonized the guanethidine-induced blockade of the response of the cat nictitating membrane to stimulation of the cervical sympathetic nerve. GERKENS et al. (1969) suggested that the rapid reversal of guanethidine-induced neuronal blockade by compounds which prevented its

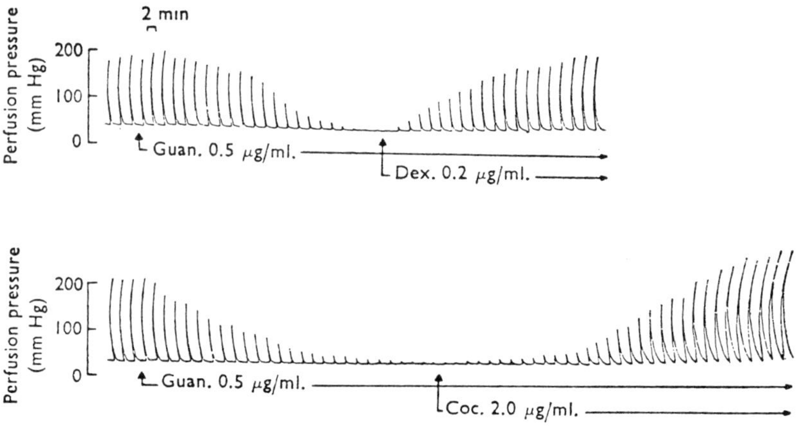

Fig. 17. Isolated rabbit ear artery. The periarterial sympathetic nerves were stimulated for 10 sec every 2 min using 1 msec pulses at a frequency of 15/sec. The records show the effects of dexamphetamine (0.2 μg/ml) and cocaine (2 μg/ml) on the adrenergic neuron blockade produced by guanethidine (0.5 μg/ml). From GERKENS et al. (1969)

uptake indicated that the "pool" of guanethidine involved in neuronal block was in facile steady state with the guanethidine outside the neuron. Alternatively, guanethidine may readily leak out of neurons, only to be taken up again by the neuronal pump in a rapid recycling process. In either case, blockade of the uptake of guanethidine would be expected to result in a net movement of guanethidine away from its site of action and out of the nerve. In direct support of this idea is the report by FLEGIN et al. (1970) that dexamphetamine injection into the guanethidine-pretreated isolated cat spleen produced a "striking increase" in the resting output of guanethidine without releasing norepinephrine. In addition, FLEGIN et al. (1970) reported that in three subjects, given amphetamine 8 days after an injection of tritiated guanethidine, a pronounced increase in the rate of excretion of tritiated guanethidine occurred.

FOLLENFANT and ROBSON (1970) studied the antagonism of adrenergic neuron blockade by amphetamine and dexamphetamine in the rat and guinea pig. These investigators found that in all preparations studied the effect of bretylium was antagonized by amphetamine; in contrast, neuronal blockade produced by bethanidine or guanethidine was antagonized by sympathomimetic amines only in its early stages. The blockade after prolonged exposure to the latter two agents was more resistant to antagonism by amphetamine and dexamphetamine. FOLLENFANT and ROBSON (1970) suggested this change in susceptibility to reversal could be due either to receptor attachment of the guanethidine becoming "firmer" with time so that it is not readily detached by amphetamine or dexamphetamine or to depletion of adrenergic transmitter by guanethidine (Section IV B).

MITCHELL and OATES (1970) concluded on the basis of convincing evidence that desmethylimipramine and related tricyclic antidepressants competitively inhibited uptake of adrenergic neuron blocking agents and thereby prevented their pharmacologic effect on adrenergic neurons (Section III B). Again, implicit in this explanation is the idea that desmethylimipramine interferes with 1) a recycling process for guanethidine or 2) with a steady state relationship between neuronal guanethidine and plasma guanethidine or 3) with both. Desmethylimipramine was first reported to prevent the neuronal blockade due to guanethidine *in vivo* by STONE et al. (1964) and KAUMANN et al. (1965). It has also been reported to antagonize the antihypertensive action of guanethidine in man (LEISHMAN et al., 1963; MITCHELL et al., 1967). SKINNER et al. (1969), MEYER et al. (1970), and FANN et al. (1971a, b) have noted similar troublesome interactions when tricyclic compounds were administered to patients receiving bethanidine and debrisoquin. CARLSSON and WALDECK (1965b) and MITCHELL et al. (1967) in an attempt to explain the reversal of neuron blockade with antidepressant drugs were the first to postulate that desmethylimipramine acted by blocking the uptake of guanethidine into adrenergic neurons.

OBIANWU (1969) has shown in rats that amphetamine potentiated the response of the lower eyelid to sympathetic stimulation. It also antagonized the blocking actions of guanethidine, even in the presence of protriptyline, a potent inhibitor of the neuronal norepinephrine uptake. He concluded from these observations that inhibition of the reuptake of released norepinephrine by amphetamine could not account for potentiation since reuptake was already blocked by protriptyline. Therefore, inhibition of reuptake of released norepinephrine also could not account for the "deblocking" effect of amphetamine. It is likely, however, that the deblocking effect was due to inhibition of the uptake of guanethidine by the protriptyline and amphetamine combined. It is also likely that the facts reported by OBIANWU (1969) are partly explicable on the grounds that protriptyline (as well as other tricyclic compounds) disrupt the metabolism of both amphetamine and guanethidine (see Section VI and VIII for elaboration).

E. MAO Inhibition Hypothesis

GIACHETTI and SHORE (1967) have made the interesting proposal that part of the antihypertensive action of certain adrenergic neuron blocking agents is a consequence of their possessing weak MAO inhibiting activity and of their being concentrated sufficiently into the adrenergic neuron to block intraneuronal MAO. Considerable evidence exists to support a MAO inhibiting effect of some adrenergic neuron blocking agents in adrenergic nerves (Section IV C2). Histochemical studies by MALMFORS and ABRAMS (1970) (Section VII B2) indicated that in the rat iris the MAO-inhibiting and neuron-blocking activities of bretylium and debrisoquin were separable since evidence of MAO inhibition occurred at doses which did not impair the responses of the iris to sympathetic nerve stimulation.

It is possible that bretylium and debrisoquin may have an independent component of antihypertensive action which is the same as that for specific MAO inhibitors such as pargyline, pheniprazine, etc. The short duration of the observable adrenergic neuron blocking effects of debrisoquin contrasted sharply with the capacity of the drug to lower blood pressure of hypertensive rats for periods up to 24 h (MOE et al., 1964; MEDINA et al., 1969). Therefore, it would seem that the initial marked sympatholytic properties of debrisoquin may not be the main or sole mechanism involved in the antihypertensive action of the drug. Presumably MAO inhibition may be involved. The mechanism whereby MAO inhibitors lower blood pressure was suggested by KOPIN (1968) to be the accumulation of the "false transmitter" octopamine (*beta*-hydroxy tyramine) in adrenergic granules in the absence of the normal MAO degradation of endogenous tyramine. Since guanethidine is without MAO-inhibiting action, even in high concentrations (Section IV C2) any mechanism revolving around MAO inhibition seems unlikely to be a reasonable general rationale to explain adrenergic neuron blockade.

F. False Transmitter Hypothesis

The possibility was raised by BOULLIN et al. (1966) that some part of the neuronal blocking action produced by guanethidine might be due to its acting as a "substitute" or false transmitter. As these workers point out, their results with isolated, perfused cat colon showed that guanethidine met the criteria for a false transmitter in that it replaced norepinephrine in its storage sites in sympathetic nerve endings, and on nerve stimulation was released into the region of the adrenergic receptors. FLEGIN et al. (1970) reported that the injection of amphetamine into the isolated cat spleen which had been pretreated with tritiated guanethidine did not cause splenic contraction but produced a striking increase in the resting output of guanethidine without releasing norepinephrine. These authors considered that the lack of splenic response despite the release of large amounts of guanethidine indicated that guanethidine had no post-synaptic agonist properties in this preparation. POLLARD and BECK (1971), working with the perfused dog hind limb, calculated that the sustained vascular dilations resulting from sympathetic nerve stimulation of guanethidine-pretreated preparations could not be due to release of guanethidine from nerves since the dose required to produce dilation exceeded by more than 10,000 times the theoretical amount which could be released from nerve endings. In a recent report covering results in isolated cat spleen, MORGAN et al. (1970) and SHAND et al. (1973) found that the guanethidine released by splenic nerve stimulation was directly proportional to the norepinephrine released during a 3 h period in which the preparation was recovering from the effects of the guanethidine. Furthermore, it was found that the amount of guanethidine released was inversely proportional to the degree of block present. It is, therefore, unlikely that the mechanism of "false neurotransmission" is of importance in explaining the neuronal block produced by guanethidine or other neuronal blockings agents.

Although bretylium is released by adrenergic nerve stimulation (FISCHER et al., 1966), it does not meet the criteria for a false transmitter since it is apparently not stored preferentially at norepinephrine binding sites (KOPIN, 1968).

VI. Absorption, Metabolism and Excretion of Neuron Blocking Agents

A. Guanethidine

Early investigations in man suggested that guanethidine was extensively bound in tissues and that absorption from the gastro-intestinal tract was incomplete. Thus DOLLERY et al. (1960) reported that when guanethidine was given by mouth to patients, 36% was recovered from the urine in 72 h, but following intravenous administration, 72% was recovered in the same time. From 20 to 25% of an orally-administered dose was recovered from the feces. Approximately 40% of an oral dose was unaccounted for. Guanethidine did not appear to be excreted in the bile in man but may have been excreted into the gut in the rat. SCHANKER and MORRISON (1965) reported that 8% of an intravenous dose in the rat was excreted in the feces over an 18 hour period. CALESNICK et al. (1961) showed that after oral administration the absorption of guanethidine was slow and traces of the drug could still be found in the urine and bile 14 days after its administration.

As already reported (Section II), several authors (BISSON and MUSCHOLL, 1962; KUNTZMAN et al., 1962; SCHANKER and MORRISON, 1965) have shown that intravenously-administered guanethidine was initially rapidly removed from the plasma by 1) distribution into tissues, 2) metabolism, 3) concentration into tissues containing adrenergic neurons, and 4) excretion of both the parent compound and metabolites through the kidneys. The subsequent low plasma levels, which declined very slowly thereafter, represented largely the loss of compounds from sites of binding.

The occurrence of metabolites of guanethidine in both man and rats has been reported from the very earliest studies onward. DOLLERY et al. (1960) detected small quantities of three metabolites of guanethidine in rat urine following a subcutaneous dose. Nothing was known of their composition except that they apparently were guanidinium derivatives. BISSON and MUSCHOLL (1962), SCHANKER and MORRISON (1965), FURST (1967a, b, 1968) and RAHN and DAYTON (1969) demonstrated in man, animals and liver homogenates that guanethidine was rapidly and extensively metabolized and they all presented evidence for at least one polar metabolite. The metabolism of guanethidine in liver homogenates required oxygen (FURST, 1967a) and was dependent on nicotinamide-adenine dinucleotide phosphate (ABRAMSON et al., 1969) suggesting involvement of the liver microsomal hydroxylating system. RAHN and DAYTON (1969) indicated that the urine of patients treated with ^{14}C-guanethidine contained more radioactivity than could be accounted for by guanethidine and the one metabolite they described. They suggested that this discrepancy indicated the presence of at least one more metabolite of the drug. MCMARTIN (1969) demonstrated that two partially resolved peaks could be eluted with ammonia from a column of a sulphonic acid ion-exchange resin which had been exposed to large volumes of an acidified radioactive sample. The second peak which was considerably larger than the first, consisted of a single radioactive metabolite (metabolite 1). This metabolite was unstable and was transformed in hot aqueous alkaline solution into a product with changed electrophoretic characteristics. When the column was subsequently eluted with hydrochloric acid solution a mixture of guanethidine and one other major metabolite (metabolite 2) was obtained. These two metabolites and the one transformation product were the only metabolites excreted in significant quantities in the urine of rats that had been treated with guanethidine (MCMARTIN and VINTER, 1969). Subsequently ABRAMSON et al. (1969) working with rabbit and pig liver homogenates, identified metabolite 1 as 2-(6-carboxyhexylamino) ethylguanidine (Fig. 18) on the basis of elemental analysis, infrared spectrum and pH titration curve of the pure compound, and the partial loss of tritium from ring-labelled guanethidine during the formation of this metabolite. This identification was confirmed by synthesis. The compound, 2-(6-carboxyhexylamino) ethylguanidine underwent ring-closure in hot alkaline solution to form 1-(6-carboxyhexyl)-2-iminoimidazolidine (Fig. 18). Metabolite 2 was identical with synthetic guanethidine N-oxide (Fig. 18).

ABRAMSON et al. (1969) pointed out that, although, the presence of the polar guanidine group in guanethidine permitted only a low chloroform/water partition at physiological pH, the drug was metabolized *in vitro* by liver homogenates and was rapidly metabolized *in vivo*. Guanethidine, therefore, provided a clear exception to the rule that only lipid soluble drugs are metabolized by liver microsomes.

MCMARTIN et al. (1970) studied the fate of guanethidine in two hypertensive patients. It was found that 90% of the radioactivity in urine could be accounted for as guanethidine and metabolites 1 and 2 (see Figs. 18 and 19). After intramuscular injection, half of the dose of radioactive guanethidine was eliminated in the urine in the first 2 to 3 days and 2 to 3% in the feces. After this time the dose remaining in the body declined exponentially with a half-life of 9 to 10 days

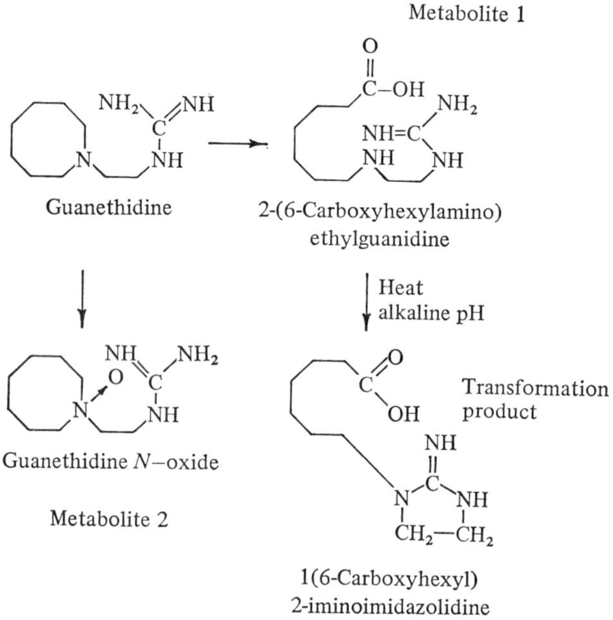

Fig. 18. Scheme illustrating the metabolites of guanethidine isolated from homogenates of rabbit or pig liver and urine from pretreated rats. After MCMARTIN (1969)

(Fig. 20). Hepatic clearance of guanethidine was high. The ratio of metabolites to unchanged guanethidine in the urine was much larger after oral than after intramuscular injection suggesting that a significant amount of drug was metabolized during a single passage through the liver.

MAÎTRE et al. (1971) showed that metabolite 1 and metabolite 2 have approximately 1/30th of the antihypertensive effect of guanethidine in rats made hypertensive by clamping the left renal artery with silver clips (Goldblatt method). Metabolite 2 but not metabolite 1 caused depletion of cardiac norepinephrine stores. Metabolite 2 was only 1/10th to 1/30th as potent as guanethidine in this respect. The transformation product of metabolite 1 was inactive as an antihypertensive agent and as a norepinephrine-depleting agent.

The tricyclic antidepressant compounds, desmethylimipramine, amitriptyline, protriptyline as well as chlorpromazine (Table 14) and several phenethylamines inhibited the metabolism of guanethidine, debrisoquin and guanoxan by an oxygen- and reduced nictinamide adenine nucleotide phosphate-requiring enzyme

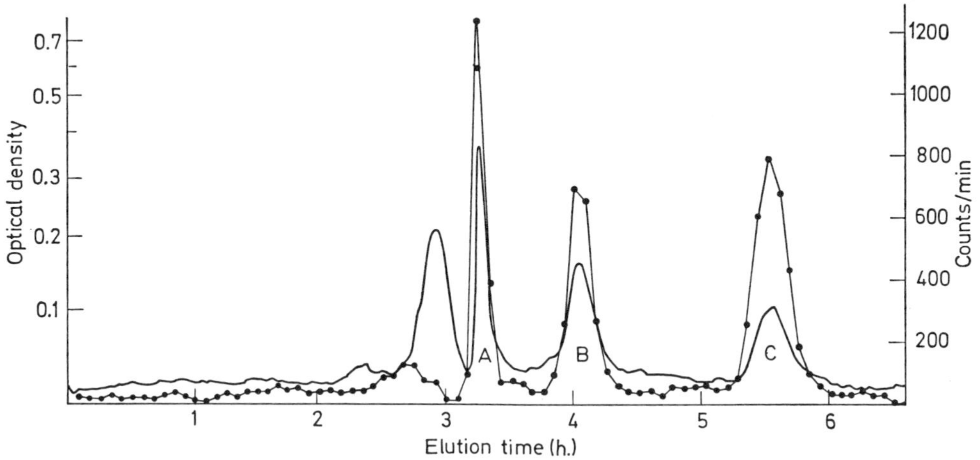

Fig. 19. Chromatography on a series of four 6 × 12 cm CM-cellulose columns of a 1 ml aliquot of human urine excreted 12 to 24 h after an intramuscular injection of 10 mg of tritiated guanethidine sulfate to which excess unlabeled 2-(6-carboxyhexylamino)-ethylguanidine sulfate, guanethidine N-oxide sulfate, and guanethidine sulfate were added. Radioactivity, dots joined by straight lines. Optical density, thick continuous trace. Peaks A, B, and C correspond to 2-(6-carboxyhexyl-amino)-ethylguanidine, guanethidine N-oxide, and guanethidine, respectively. From McMartin et al (1970)

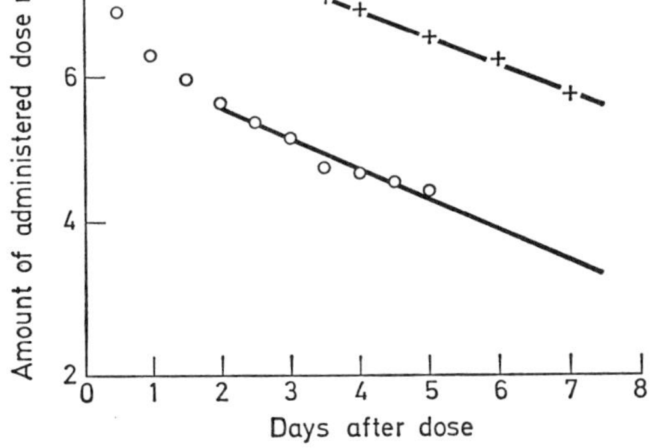

Fig. 20. Semilogarithmic plot of the amount of tritiated guanethidine and its metabolites remaining in the body at different times after a single intramuscular dose given to two hypertensive patients. + ——— + Patient 1, after 15 mg tritiated guanethidine sulfate intramuscularly; 0 ——— 0 Patient 2, after 10 mg tritiated guanethidine sulfate intramuscularly. From McMartin et al. (1970)

system in hepatic microsomes of the rat (MITCHELL et al., 1970). Desmethylimipramine pretreatment increased the cardiac and skeletal muscle contents of guanethidine and bethanidine above control levels. Subsequent experiments showed that even very low doses of desmethylimipramine elevated the concentration of guanethidine and related guanidinium agents in the whole rat (Table 15). The same effect was obtained with SKF-525A, a known inhibitor of the metabolism

Table 14. *Inhibition by desipramine, chlorpromazine, amitriptyline and protriptyline of in vitro metabolism of guanidinium antihypertensive drugs.* Supernatant fraction equivalent to 0.5 g of rat liver was incubated with substrates, co-factors and inhibitors for 30 minutes as described in methods. Values are means ± S. E. of four to nine experiments with at least 12 controls.

Inhibitors	Substrate metabolized *mμmol*		
	Guanethidine[a]	Guanoxan[a]	Debrisoquin[a]
Control	85 ± 6	238 ± 12	168 ± 10
Desipramine, 10^{-5} M	32 ± 9	149 ± 7	74 ± 5
Chlorpromazine, 10^{-5} M	26 ± 4	143 ± 11	22 ± 8
Amitriptyline, 10^{-5} M	40 ± 4	209 ± 4	171 ± 13
Amitriptyline, 10^{-4} M			41 ± 5
Protriptyline, 10^{-5} M	70 ± 6	233 ± 10	168 ± 14
Protriptyline, 10^{-4} M		55 ± 10	68 ± 10

[a] 252 mμmol of guanethidine, 283 mμmol of guanoxan or 571 mμmol of debrisoquin substrate were added to mixture at start of incubation. From MITCHELL et al. (1970).

Table 15. *Effect of desipramine and SKF-525A on the concentration of guanidinium drugs in homogenates of rats with or without their excreta.* Control rats and rats treated with desipramine (DMI) 0.5 h previously or with SKF-525A one hour previously were given guanethidine (15 mg/kg i.p.), bethanidine (15 mg/kg i.p.), guanoxan (50 mg/kg i.p.) or debrisoquin (50 mg/kg i.p.) and homogenized with or without their excreta five hours later. Values are means ± S. E. with number of experiments in parentheses

Treatment	Guanidinium concentration in homogenates				
	Guanethidine (whole rat only)	Guanethidine (whole rat plus excreta)	Bethanidine (whole rat plus excreta)	Guanoxan (whole rat plus excreta)	Debrisoquin (whole rat plus excreta)
	μg/g				
Control	2.7±0.2 (6)	5.7±1.3 (4)	5.8±0.2 (5)	6.1±0.5 (4)	5.8±0.6 (4)
DMI, 1 mg/kg i.p.	7.0±1.4[a](6)				
DMI, 30 mg/kg i.p.	9.0±1.5[a](6)	11.7±1.2[a](4)	19.6±0.2[b](5)	19.2±1.2[b](4)	15.1±3.0[a](4)
SKF-525A, 50 mg/kg i.p.	6.1±1.1[a](6)				

[a] $P < 0.02$ (compared with the levels seen after the guanidinium alone).
[b] $P < 0.005$ (compared with the levels seen after the guanidinium alone). From MITCHELL et al. (1970).

of drugs by liver microsomal enzymes (MITCHELL et al., 1970). The authors pointed out that investigations of drug-drug interactions *in vivo* must be considered in the light of the possibility that one drug might interfere with the metabolism of the other.

WALTER et al. (1975) demonstrated that a steady-state plasma level of guanethidine above 8 ng/ml was always associated with a high degree of sympathetic blockade in man. The level between 5 and 8 ng/ml represented a border zone where some patients had effect and others did not. The relationship between plasma level and sympathetic block was better than the relationship between dose and sympathetic block.

B. Bretylium

Bretylium was pharmacologically effective by the oral, intramuscular, subcutaneous and intravenous routes. It was partially absorbed from the gastrointestinal tract. Since it is a quaternary ammonium salt, it was erratically and poorly absorbed in clinical use (HURLEY et al., 1960). Bretylium was not metabolized in the cat (DUNCOMBE and McCOUBREY, 1960) or in the human or rat (KUNTZMAN et al., 1970). In the cat and rat, 50 to 60% of a parenteral dose was excreted unchanged in the urine in 24 h. A minor amount was passed in the feces in the cat. In the rat, 15% was excreted in the feces in 24 h. In the rat within 5 to 6 days, 63% of a dose was excreted unchanged in the urine and 31% in the feces (KUNTZMAN et al., 1970). Excretion in the bile probably accounted for the bretylium found in rat feces.

C. Bethanidine

Bethanidine was absorbed from the alimentary tract. Comparative studies of bethanidine with guanethidine in man revealed that the drugs were similar in potency. The duration of the hypotensive action of bethanidine was relatively short. The onset of action occurred within 2 h, was maximal in 4 to 5 h and had a total duration of effect between 8 and 12 h (SMIRK, 1963; JOHNSTON et al., 1964; MOSER, 1969).

Studies with ^{14}C-labelled bethanidine in cats demonstrated that approximately half the dose was excreted unchanged in urine within 24 h, and no metabolites were found. Excretion continued for more than seven days (BOURA et al., 1962). In man there appeared to be a highly significant correlation between the proportion of the dose of bethanidine excreted in 24 h and the creatinine clearance indicating that the excretion rate was directly related to glomerular filtration rate (DOYLE and MORLEY, 1965). In patients with a normal creatinine clearance, virtually all of the administered dose was excreted within 24 h. The excretory rate in patients with renal failure was much lower than normal and declined more slowly.

D. Debrisoquin

Debrisoquin was extensively metabolized in the rat. Approximately one-third of the injected dose appeared unchanged in the urine and feces after 24 h. The two metabolic products observed in urine retained the labeled amidine group (MEDINA et al., 1969). In two human subjects 73% of an oral dose of 50 mg of labeled debrisoquin was excreted in the urine within 24 h. This was present mainly in the form of metabolites. The total excretion of radioactivity in both subjects in eight days was 80% in the urine and 12% in the feces. No labeled pulmonary CO_2 was detectable. Chromatography of human urine showed the presence of unchanged debrisoquin and also three metabolites. In the dog, the pattern of excretion of debrisoquin was similar to that in man, a total of 90% of the dose being excreted in the urine and 10% in the feces. The dog urine contained debrisoquin plus four metabolites. Although the metabolites in both man and dog were not identified, it was shown that they were basic in nature and that all contained an intact amidine moiety (KITCHIN and TURNER, 1966).

ALLEN et al. (1975) have also shown that a high proportion of an oral dose of ^{14}C-debrisoquin sulfate is excreted in the urine by rat and man. The urinary radioactivity consisted of a mixture of unchanged drug and polar, water soluble metabolites. In both species the major metabolited was formed by 4-hydroxylation of debrisoquin. A significant proportion of the dose was excreted as acidic metabolites formed by opening the tetrahydro-isoquinoline ring and trace amounts of 5-, 6-, 7-, and 8-hydroxydebrisoquins were also excreted.

E. Guanoxan

The metabolism of ^{14}C-guanoxan in the dog as reported by CANAS-RODRIGUEZ (1966) is shown in Fig. 21. It is of interest that in addition to hydroxylation of the ring, the guanidine group of guanoxan (unlike that of other neuron blocking agents) underwent extensive transamidation. The authors indicated that this might be the major route of metabolism in the dog. In hypertensive patients, only free guanoxan and the 7-hydroxy metabolite have been found in urine samples (JACK et al., 1971).

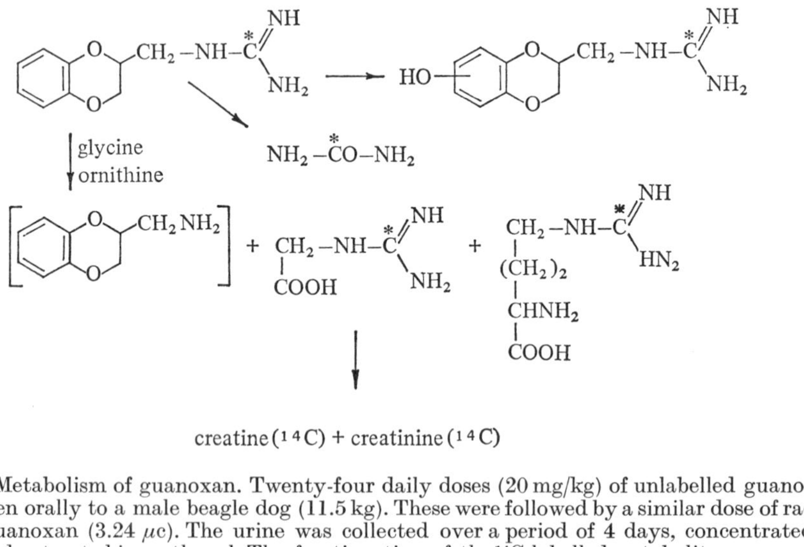

Fig. 21. Metabolism of guanoxan. Twenty-four daily doses (20 mg/kg) of unlabelled guanoxan were given orally to a male beagle dog (11.5 kg). These were followed by a similar dose of radioactive guanoxan (3.24 μc). The urine was collected over a period of 4 days, concentrated in vacuo and extracted in methanol. The fractionation of the ^{14}C-labelled metabolites was carried out by two different methods simultaneously: (a) absorption on Amberlite IRC 50 resin, buffered to pH 6.5 with disodium hydrogen phosphate, then elution of the metabolites with water, 0.5 N HCl and 1.2 N HCl in methanol successively; (b) preparative thick paper descending chromatography using n-propanol-aqueous molar ammonium carbonate-concentrated ammonia (70:30:2) as the developing solvent. From CANAS-RODRIQUEZ (1966)

VII. Actions of Adrenergic Neuron Blocking Agents in Tissues and Organs

A. General Sympathomimetic Action

Guanethidine, bretylium and related agents produce transient sympathomimetic effects in most sympathetic effector cells. Thus, the intravenous injection of guanethidine and related agents into animals produced mydriasis, piloerection, pressor responses, contraction of the nictitating membranes and spleen, positive chronotropic and inotropic responses, and increased peripheral vascular resistance. There is substantial evidence that the general sympathomimesis evoked by these agents is due to release of catecholamines directly from the adrenergic nerve endings in the effector cells (see BOURA and GREEN, 1965 and Section IV A).

B. General Potentiation of the Responses to Norepinephrine and Closely Related Pressor Amines and Inhibition of Tyramine and Other Indirectly—Acting Phenethylamines

1. Norepinephrine

In man, animals and in isolated preparations, the responses of most adrenergically innervated organs to norepinephrine and epinephrine increase in the presence of guanethidine, and other adrenergic neuron blocking agents (see BOURA and GREEN, 1965). The adrenergic neuron blockers, as a class, "fit" the amine-pump in adrenergic neurons and thus compete with pressor catecholamines for access into the neurons (see Section III B). The increased responsiveness of the effector cells in the presence of neuron blocking agents or in the presence of other inhibitors of the pump, such as cocaine and desmethylimipramine, is generally attributed to the "diversion" to the receptors of the amines which would normally be removed by the uptake mechanism (TRENDELENBURG 1963, 1966), (for a kinetic model of this phenomenon see appendix at end of this section). In addition the generalized inhibition of uptake of amines, *in vivo*, may lead to elevated plasma levels which then lead to increased responses (see for example TRENDELENBURG, 1959; HERTTING et al., 1961; FURCHGOTT et al., 1963). This theory has the great advantage of simplicity. However, it has been challenged even in the *in vitro* situation where steady state conditions can be made to apply and where its application is not complicated by many variables such as hemodynamics, metabolism and tissue binding which make interpretation of *in vivo* findings difficult. MAXWELL et al. (1966) demonstrated in rabbit aortic strips that approximately 30% reduction in binding rate of norepinephrine (from a 2×10^{-8}M solution) can be produced with guanethidine, cocaine and methylphenidate without an increase in the contractile response to the amine. In the range of 30 to 70% reduction in binding rate, the response to norepinephrine was an increasing function of the percent reduction in binding rate produced by these drugs. Guanethidine and cocaine produced additional increase in response without additional reduction in binding rate. In a series of papers, KALSNER and NICKERSON (1968a, b; 1969a–d; 1971) have argued that uptake of catecholamines by adrenergic nerve terminals represents only one among at least three other methods for inactivating catecholamines; namely, destruction by MAO, COMT and extraneuronal binding, and that shutting down the uptake pathway would lead to enchanced activity along the other paths rather than necessarily leading to elevation of physiologically potent amine levels and hence a greater response. These authors pointed out that cocaine potentiated methoxamine and histamine, neither of which is transported into adrenergic neurons by the neuronal membrane pump. KHAN and ASMAE (1968) observed that guanethidine potentiated the response of the rat fundus strip to isoproterenol to a much greater extent than it potentiated the responses to norepinephrine and epinephrine. Isoproterenol is known not to be taken up by adrenergic neurons. KHAN and ASMAE (1968) concluded that guanethidine may be acting to sensitize tissues by producing changes in the smooth muscles. GOKHALE et al. (1967) found guanethidine produced a definite, consistent and dose-related potentiation of the effects of epinephrine, norepinephrine, histamine, 5-hydroxytryptamine, aminophylline and calcium chloride in studies with the rabbit aortic strip, atrium, tracheal chain, perfused ear, ileum and with the rat hindleg. They suggested that in addition to tissue amine uptake, a direct, non-specific sensitization of the effector cells was involved in the mediation of the effect of guanethidine. GOKHALE and GULATI (1961) suggested that sensitization of the effector cells might account for the capacity of bretylium to potentiate the cardiovascular effects of epinephrine and norepinephrine.

Thus, a positive correlation between the degree of inhibition of uptake of norepinephrine or related catecholamines by nerve endings and an increase in magnitude of responses to these amines, does not necessarily prove a causal relationship.

2. Tyramine and Related Phenethylamines

Guanethidine and several other blocking agents readily suppress the actions of tyramine in effector cells while bretylium and debrisoquin are not particularly effective in this regard (Table 1 and MAXWELL et al., 1960). The general explanation for the loss of sensitivity to tyramine in the presence of some neuron blockers is based on the same rationale as used to explain the supersensitivity to norepinephrine; namely, neuron blocking agents compete with tyramine for uptake into the adrenergic neurons. Since tyramine depends largely on the release of norepinephrine from adrenergic nerve terminals for its effects, it is attenuated by agents which compete for the "amine pump".

Since bretylium and debrisoquin (see Section III B and VIII A, B) like guanethidine are also substrates for the amine pump in adrenergic neurons, the question arises as to why these two agents antagonize tyramine less effectively. Two major differences exist between guanethidine and the other two agents: 1) guanethidine is devoid of MAO inhibiting activity whereas bretylium and debrisoquin have weak activity against the isolated enzyme and significant activity in adrenergic neurons *in vivo* (Section IV C 2a) and 2) bretylium and debrisoquin show no special affinity for norepinephrine storage sites in neurons whereas guanethidine does (Section III C). This latter difference suggests that the norepinephrine which is available for release by neuron blockers is probably in the cytoplasm of the adrenergic terminals. CAMPOS et al. (1963) reported that the depletion produced by a low concentration of tyramine (ca. 10^{-5} M) was more pronounced in the supernatant fraction than in the particulate fraction (ca. $100{,}000 \times G$) of a subcellular fractionation of cat heart and suggested that the primary effect of tyramine was a mobilization of norepinephrine from the soluble fraction. In the presence of significant intraneuronal MAO inhibition, the amount of norepinephrine in the cytoplasm which is available for release is presumably enhanced. In addition, a higher level of tyramine is probably achieved in the cytoplasm since this amine is a very good substrate for MAO.

Indirect evidence supporting the hypothesis that increased norepinephrine could be expected to occur in the cytoplasm under appropriate conditions was reported by MALMFORS and ABRAMS (1970) (Section IV C2). These investigators demonstrated that bretylium, debrisoquin and nialamide, a known MAO inhibitor, all permitted the restoration of fluorescence in the iris of reserpine-pretreated rats following norepinephrine administration. Restoration of fluorescence did not occur in their absence. The restored fluorescence had a different appearance from the fluorescence observed in the untreated or in the reserpinized rats suggesting that norepinephrine was accumulating in unusual sites during inhibition of neuronal MAO. MALMFORS and ABRAMS (1970) concluded that both bretylium and debrisoquin had MAO inhibiting properties and that treatment with these agents allowed norepinephrine to accumulate outside the granule.

The available direct evidence indicates that in acute experimentation the total amount of norepinephrine in the cytoplasm (*i.e.* in the soluble fraction of a centrifugal fractionation of tissue) was not altered (CHANG et al., 1967a) or was reduced by bretylium treatment (ABBS and ROBERTSON, 1970). Presumably, therefore, some component of norepinephrine within this soluble fraction which is sensitive to tyramine-release must be increased despite the failure of the total norepinephrine in the soluble fraction to increase.

Thus, it appears that although tyramine uptake may be reduced by bretylium and debrisoquin, the overall effect of these two agents on tyramine response need not necessarily be one of inhibition. The effect would depend on the potency of the agent as a MAO inhibitor relative to its affinity for the amine pump.

KURAHASHI and SHIBATA (1971) found that pretreatment of normal, reserpinized or cold stored (and therefore functionally denervated) aortic strips with bretylium enhanced the contraction produced by tyramine and by potassium ion. These authors interpreted their results to indicate that bretylium potentiated the action of tyramine and potassium, not by a prejunctional mechanism, but by a postjunctional action, causing an increase in the sensitivity of the effector cells to the stimulus.

3. Appendix

Properties of a simple mathematical model which describes the steady-state relationship between bath concentration, binding rate and the development of local low concentrations of norepinephrine at binding sites and which also describes the influence of drugs on the system (MAXWELL et al., 1966). In isolated tissues the maximum concentration of norepinephrine that can be achieved at receptors as a result of diffusion would be a concentration equal to that in the bath. Therefore, if a drug is considered to potentiate norepinephrine by reducing its binding rate, and thus elevating norepinephrine concentration at receptors, it must follow that the concentration of norepinephrine at the receptors ($[N]_i$) is under normal circumstances lower than its concentration in the bath ($[N]_o$). Therefore, under normal circumstances $[N]_o = \text{constant} > [N]_i$. If k_d is the rate coefficient for diffusion toward and away from the receptor area and k_b is the rate coefficient for binding into stores then at steady state the rate of entry into the vicinity of the receptors = the rate of its removal from this region.

$$[N]_o k_d = [N]_i k_d + [N]_i k_b \tag{1}$$

In formulating this equation the rate coefficient for passage out of the store is considered to be negligible and is ignored. Equation 1 rearranges to:

$$\frac{[N]_o k_d}{k_b + k_d} = [N]_i \,. \tag{2}$$

Drugs such as guanethidine, bretylium or cocaine which reduce binding rate, $[N]_i k_b$, do so by reducing k_b.

It can be seen by inspection of equation 2 that when $k_b = 0$, $[N]_o = [N]_i$. It can also be seen that when $k_b \gg k_d$, $[N]_i \sim 1/k_b$ and, hence, marked changes can occur in k_b without the binding rate, $[N]_i k_b$, changing significantly. Likewise, if $k_b \ll k_d$, large reductions in k_b will result in large reductions in binding rate, $[N]_i k_b$, but will have negligible influence on $[N]_i$. Only when $k_b \cong k_d$ will the system operate so that reduction in the binding rate constant, k_b, will lead to increase in $[N]_i$ and decrease in $[N]_i k_b$.

The theoretical relationship existing between $[N]_i$ and $[N]_i k_b$ as functions of k_b, as described by Eq. (2), are plotted in Fig. 22. $[N]_o$ and k_d have been assigned values of 1 and k_b has been varied from 20 to 0.5 and the resulting relative values for $[N]_i$ calculated and plotted. The calculated value for $[N]_i$ for a given k_b was multiplied by that k_b to give a relative value for $[N]_i k_b$.

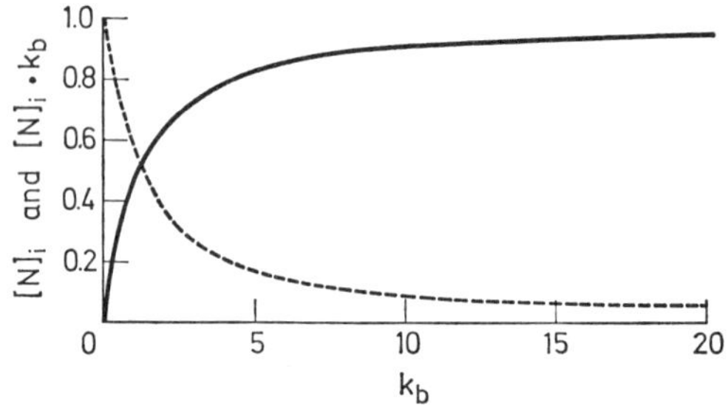

Fig. 22. Calculated theoretical values of $[N]_i$ relative to $(N)_0$ as a function of the value of k_b relative to k_d (dashed line); and values for the product of $[N]_i$ relative to $[N]_0$ times k_b relative to k_d as a function of k_b relative to k_d (solid line). Curves were determined from the equation $[N]_i = ([N]_0\, k_d) / (k_b + k_d)$ by letting $[N]_0 = 1$ and $k_d = 1$. The equation reduced to $[N]_i = 1/(k_b + 1)$. Values were assigned to k_b and $[N]_i$ was calculated. The product of these two yielded $[N]_i\, k_b$. After MAXWELL et al. (1966)

C. Vascular Smooth Muscle

Guanethidine (ABBOUD et al., 1961, 1962; MCCUBBIN et al., 1961; POLLARD and BECK, 1971) and bretylium (BLAIR et al., 1960; GREEN, 1962) have a direct vasodilator action on blood vessels which can be observed in man and animals when their indirect sympathomimetic action has waned or when reserpine has been used to deplete endogenous stores of norepinephrine. ABBOUD et al. (1961) studied the hemodynamic effects of intravenous guanethidine in dogs pretreated with reserpine. They also studied the action of intra-arterial guanethidine in the perfused foreleg of dogs. In these preparations, guanethidine produced only vasodilation. The vasodilation was due to a local action on vascular smooth muscle. This vascular relaxation did not appear to be mediated through the release of histamine or acetylcholine since standard blocking agents for these substances did not affect the vasodilator response to guanethidine. The authors concluded that the vasodilation may have resulted, at least in part, from stimulation of *beta* adrenergic receptors or other "dilator receptors" since they appeared to be blocked by dichloroisoproterenol. SOMLYO and SOMLYO (1970) suggested that the mechanism of vasodilator action of adrenergic neuron blocking agents may be related to their "local anesthetic" properties. This suggestion was made on the grounds that several reports existed that local anesthetics produced similar direct vasodilator effects, or relaxant effects in isolated blood vessel segments. For example, procaine dilated the vessels in the dog hind limb (LIPSIUS et al., 1968), and several local anesthetics relaxed the contractions of rabbit aortic strips induced by norepinephrine, histamine and acetylcholine (ASTRÖM, 1964).

Guanethidine potentiated the responses induced by catecholamines in the microcirculation of the rat mesoappendix (ZIMMERMAN and HARRIS, 1963; ALTURA and ZWEIFACH, 1966) in the rabbit aortic strip (MAXWELL et al., 1962) and in the perfused rabbit ear (MAXWELL, 1965). In the rabbit ear, 5×10^{-5} M guanethidine potentiated the response to norepinephrine while at 3×10^{-3} M it surmountably blocked the action of norepinephrine. This blocking effect at high concentrations might have been due to either a physiological antagonism or pharmacological antagonism. The blockade was readily reversible as determined by its absence after washout. The potentiating action, however, was not readily washed out (MAXWELL, 1965).

DE LA LANDE et al. (1970) demonstrated that bretylium, bethanidine and guanethidine conformed to the pattern of cocaine in greatly reducing the difference between the sensitivities of the perfused isolated rabbit ear artery to intraluminal and extraluminal norepinephrine. In the absence of drugs norepinephrine when applied intraluminally is 10 times more potent than when it is applied extraluminally. This differential is presumably caused by the adrenergic neurons at the adventitial-medial border acting as a "sponge" to take up and, thereby, prevent norepinephrine from reaching the media from the extraluminal (adventitial) side. DE LA LANDE et al. (1970) concluded that the three neuron blocking agents potentiated the effects of norepinephrine by inhibiting the uptake mechanism in adrenergic nerves.

Guanethidine in the concentration range 10^{-7} M to 5×10^{-5} M produced a dose-dependent suppression of the uptake and binding of norepinephrine by adrenergic nerves in rabbit aorta. When strips were exposed to 5×10^{-5} M guanethidine and then the guanethidine was repeatedly washed out of the bath, the capacity to potentiate norepinephrine was not diminished, but the uptake and binding were now inhibited only to the same degree as during exposure to a low, nonpotentiating dose of guanethidine (Table 16) suggesting that the potentiation of the response was not caused by the reduction in uptake (MAXWELL, 1965).

In the same communication (MAXWELL, 1965) it was demonstrated that a variety of guanidine derivatives, closely related chemically to guanethidine, produced widely differing patterns of potentiation of the responses of aortic

Table 16. *Cpm in rabbit aortic strips exposed to* 2×10^{-8} *M dl-norepinephrine-7-*H^3

Guanethidine treatment Concentration (M)	Effect on norepinephrine contraction	No.	Weight (mg)	cpm ± S.E.
A. 0	None	19	24 ± 1.1	3936 ± 224
B. 10^{-7}	None	8	26 ± 2.0	3322 ± 45
C. 5×10^{-7}	None	12	22 ± 1.2	2592 ± 264[a]
D. 5×10^{-5}	Maximum potentiation	9	23 ± 1.6	1079 ± 177[a]
E. 5×10^{-5} (then washed out)	Maximum potentiation	13	24 ± 0.8	2558 ± 197[a,b]

[a] Significantly different ($P < 0.05$) from first value in same column.
[b] Not significantly different ($P > 0.05$) from third value in same column. After MAXWELL (1965).

strips to epinephrine, epinine, norepinephrine, dopamine and tyramine. The results were difficult to rationalize solely by means of the "amine uptake inhibition hypothesis". The author suggested that guanethidine might interact with *alpha* receptors in the effector cells. The binding of guanethidine with the *alpha* receptor was not conceived of as a typical union of an agonist or antagonist with the receptor, but one which might lead to an enhancement of the affinity of the receptor for selected amines. It was speculated that such changes were brought about by altering the conformation of a receptor surface which would lead to more effective binding between selected amines and the adrenergic receptor.

MAXWELL et al. (1967) in an attempt to find evidence to support the contention of an action of guanethidine in effector cells, demonstrated that 2-(cyclohexylamino)-ethylguanidine sulfate, which is structurally similar to guanethidine and somewhat less potent as an adrenergic neuron blocking agent (RAND and WILSON, 1967c), produced a concentration-dependent contraction of the aortic strip which was not susceptible to blockade with *alpha* blocking agents or other autonomic blocking agents in reasonable doses. MAXWELL et al. (1967) suggested, that considering their structural and pharmacologic similarities, it seemed reasonable to postulate that guanethidine, like this derivative, might have a direct effect in the smooth muscle of the aortic strip but that evidence of this, as revealed by a contraction, is masked by its concommitant relaxant action on the strips.

D. Cardiac Muscle

1. Direct Inotropic and Chronotropic Actions

Guanethidine exerted a negative inotropic action (Fig. 23) in intact animals (GAFFNEY et al., 1962) and in heart-lung preparations (Fig. 24) that had been subjected to surgical procedures or to drugs which depleted myocardial stores of norepinephrine (GAFFNEY, 1961; KRAYER et al., 1962). Bretylium on the other hand evoked a small positive inotropic action in the reserpinized heart-lung preparation of the dog (GAFFNEY, 1961). In addition, GAFFNEY et al. (1962) demonstrated that in dogs with denervated hearts the increase in contractile force induced

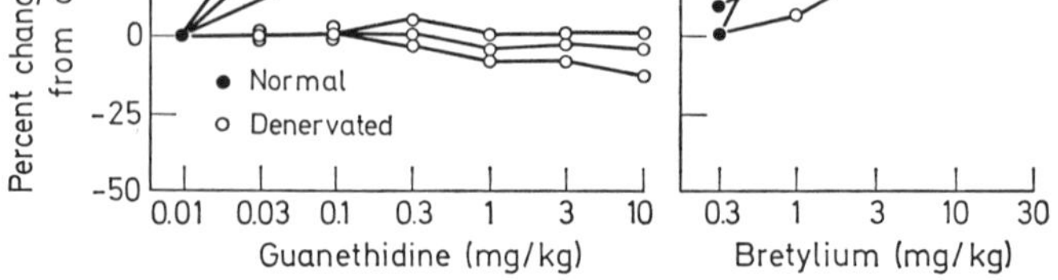

Fig. 23. Comparison of the effects of guanethidine (left) and bretylium (right) on ventricular contractile force in normal and cardiac-denervated dogs. From GAFFNEY et al. (1962) by permission of The American Heart Assiation, Inc.

by bretylium was essentially unchanged from normal, and the increase in cardiac output due to bretylium was only slightly reduced (Fig. 23). Recently, AMSTERDAM et al. (1970) reinforced the findings of GAFFNEY and his associates. In their experiments with isolated cat papillary muscles these authors observed that 10^{-4}M propranolol did not alter the contractile effects of 0.05 mg/ml ($\cong 10^{-4}$M) bretylium which included: increase in maximal isometric tension, increase in maximal rate of tension developed and an increase in maximal velocity of shortening. Bretylium did not change time to peak tension but increased the absolute refractory period.

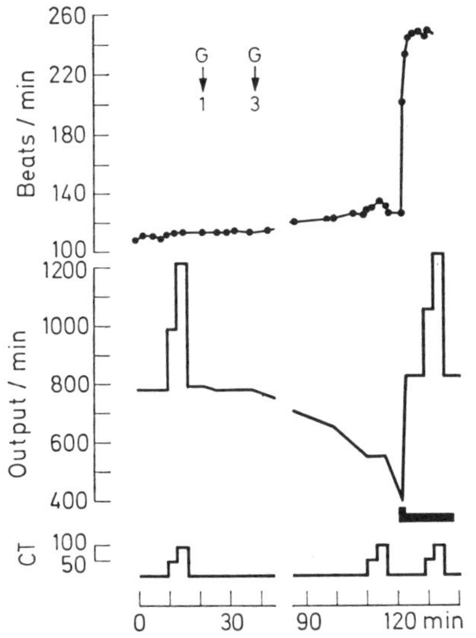

Fig. 24. Effect of guanethidine upon heart rate and systemic output in the heart-lung preparation of the reserpine pretreated dog. From top to bottom: heart rate; systemic output in ml/min; time of competence test (consisting of raising the reservoir level in two steps of 50 mm each). Dog 12 kg male, pretreated with reserpine twice 0.5 mg/kg, 48 and 24 h prior to experiment. At G, guanethidine 1 and 3 mg, respectively, was injected. The black bar at bottom indicates continuous infusion of norepinephrine first at the rate of 5 μg/min then at 3 μg/min. After KRAYER et al. (1962)

MARKIS and KOCH-WESER (1971) in contrast to GAFFNEY et al. (1961, 1962) and AMSTERDAM et al. (1970), reported that the sustained, positive, inotropic effects of bretylium in driven kitten papillary muscles and guinea pig left atrial strips were completely prevented by 10^{-6} M propranolol (Fig. 25) or by reserpine pretreatment. According to these authors the positive inotropic effect of bretylium was associated with a marked increase in rate of development of tension and a moderate decrease in the time to peak tension. MARKIS and KOCH-WESER (1971) dismissed the findings of GAFFNEY (1961) on the grounds that depletion of endogenous amines with reserpine may have been incomplete. If this were so then it would follow that the residual amine was sensitive to release by bretylium but not by guanethidine. This seems unlikely. Criticism for failure to produce complete depletion of endogenous amines could not be levelled against the work of GAFFNEY et al. (1962) since these authors presented pharmacological evidence that depletion was complete. MARKIS and KOCH-WESER (1971) also dismissed the findings of

Amsterdam et al. (1970) on the grounds that these authors used 10^{-4} M propranolol which, it was felt, would depress myocardial contractility and therefore complicate interpretation of the data.

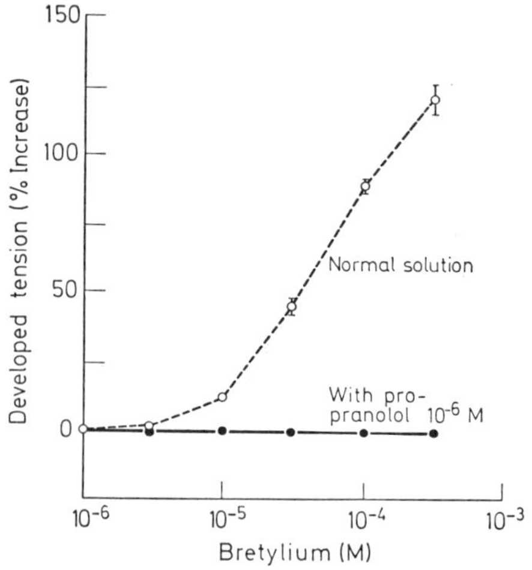

Fig. 25. Effect of propranolol on the inotropic action of bretylium. Means and standard errors of two groups of seven kitten papillary muscles. Propranolol added 45 min before exposure to bretylium. From Markis and Koch-Weser (1971)

Richmond et al. (1973) used continuous measurement of (dp/dt) IIT in order to study the effects of bretylium on the myocardium of the dog independently of its peripheral actions. Dp/dt is the maximum rate of change of left ventricular pressure and IIT is the integrated isometric tension. They found that the bretylium-induced increase in myocardial contractility was blocked by propranolol and by reserpine pretreatment (1.25 mg/kg given i.p. over 72 h) and they therefore concluded that this action of bretylium was indirect and due to catecholamine release. On the other hand, Graham and Chandler (1973) measured the rate of development of tension (dp/dt), peak active tension, and time to peak tension in cat right ventricular papillary muscle preparations and reported that the positive inotropism elicited by bretylium persisted in animals pretreated with reserpine. Graham and Chandler (1973) commented that in the experiments of Markis and Koch-Weser (1971) in which reserpine pretreatment abolished the positive inotropic action of bretylium a high dose of reserpine (1 mg/kg) had been administered. They pointed out that 0.1 mg/kg of reserpine had been shown to be adequate to remove 97% of myocardial catecholamines (Carlsson et al., 1957). They also noted that Zaimis (1961) showed that 1 mg/kg of reserpine while removing over 99% of myocardial catecholamines did so at the cost of producing histological damage and heart failure. Graham and Chandler (1973) used 0.1 mg/kg reserpine in their studies but presented no independent evidence of the completeness of catecholamine depletion in their preparations. These authors inferred that the failure of Markis and Koch-Weser (1971) to detect positive inotropism with bretylium in reserpine pre-treated animals was due to an overdose of reserpine. Graham and Chandler (1973) concluded that the positive inotropism of bretylium might be due to a direct effect on myocardium with or without release of myocardial catecholamines.

PRIOLA et al. (1973) have made some progress in resolving the conflicting results quoted above. These authors measured right ventricular and left ventriular isovolumic contractility during total heart bypass in normal dogs and dogs whose hearts had been chronically denervated. These authors found that low doses of bretylium (< 20 mg/kg, cumulative) administered *via* the arterial perfusion cannula increased contractility in normal animals but either did not change or decreased contractility in denervated animals. High doses (> 20 mg/kg, cumulative) increased contractility in both groups. Of great interest was the observation that in the denervated animals the positive inotropic responses were abolished by beta receptor blockade. These authors concluded that the positive inotropic effects of low doses of bretylium require the presence of sympathetic nerve endings whereas at high doses, bretylium produces a direct positive inotropic effect, probably by stimulating beta adrenergic receptors. It would be of great interest if this latter conclusion were given independent confirmation in the other laboratories involved in the dispute. PRIOLA et al. (1973) have attempted to rationalize the conflicting observations of GAFFNEY et al. (1962) and MARKIS and KOCH-WESER (1971) by means of their findings

It is uncertain at the present time exactly which conclusion is correct regarding the positive inotropic effects of bretylium. The conclusion of MARKIS and KOCH-WESER (1971) that the positive inotropic effect of bretylium was entirely indirect is supported by previous findings on myocardium of cats and guinea pigs (KIRPEKAR and FURCHGOTT, 1964; CERVONI et al., 1966), rats (GILLIS and NASH, 1961; BHAGAT and SHIDEMAN, 1963) and dogs (YELNOSKY and MORTIMER, 1961; GILMORE and SIEGEL, 1962).

There was general agreement in results obtained in the several preparations used by GAFFNEY (1961), GAFFNEY et al. (1962), KRAYER et al. (1962), and by MARKIS and KOCH-WESER (1971), that the positive chronotropic effects of both bretylium and guanethidine were due almost entirely to catecholamine release. Bretylium in some instances exhibited a negative chronotropic action in reserpinized preparations.

2. Antiarrhythmic Actions

Bretylium was reported to control cardiac tachyarrhythmias in animals and man (LEVEQUE, 1965; BACANER, 1966, 1968a, b; CASTANEDA and BACANER, 1969, 1970; DAY and BACANER, 1971; BERNSTEIN and KOCH-WESER, 1972). BACANER and associates demonstrated that bretylium suppressed the vulnerability of the canine ventricle to electrically-induced fibrillation. This observation was confirmed by ELLIS et al. (1968) and CERVONI et al. (1971). BUCKLEY et al. (1971) reported that bretylium reduced the vulnerability of the dog heart to fibrillation associated with hypothermia.

WIT et al. (1970) investigated the effects of bretylium on the transmembrane action potentials of canine Purkinje fibers and ventricular muscle fibers from normal and reserpine-treated dogs. Bretylium prolonged the effective refractory period solely by lengthening the action potential duration except at the highest concentration studied (4.8×10^{-5} M) where it depressed the recovery of excitability in relation to membrane potential, as indicated by a shift in the membrane response curve to the right. Bretylium, in addition, initially enhanced spontaneous depolarization of Purkinje fibers.

BIGGER and JAFFE (1971) also studied the effects of bretylium on single cell transmembrane potentials in isolated preparations of dog papillary muscle and Purkinje fibers. In concentrations of 10^{-4}M or greater, bretylium decreased the resting membrane potential, the action potential amplitude and overshoot, the maximal rate of rise of the rapid depolarization (phase zero) and the conduction velocity. Bretylium was compared with reference antiarrhythmic agents. Quinidine, procainamide, diphenylhydantoin, propranolol and lidocaine, in contrast to bretylium all exhibited two uniformly similar properties in ventricular muscle and Purkinje fiber preparations: 1) all 5 agents depressed automaticity in Purkinje fibers and 2) all 5 reference compounds caused the effective refractory period of Purkinje fibers and ventricular muscle fibers to lengthen relative to the action potential duration. This was true although some of the drugs (quinidine and procainamide) prolonged both events and some of them (propranolol, diphenylhydantoin and lidocaine) shortened both. Over a wide range of stimulation rates bretylium at 10^{-5}M and 10^{-4}M increased the duration of the action potential (Fig. 26) and of the effective refractory period of both ventricle muscle and Purkinje fibers without lengthening the effective refractory period relative to the action potential duration. Bigger and Jaffe (1971) concluded that the findings of their study suggested that the effects of bretylium on the electrophysiologic properties of the cell membrane of Purkinje and ventricular muscle fibers did not entirely explain its antiarrhythmic effects in terms of present concepts of antiarrhythmic drug action. They further suggested that the antiarrhythmic action was secondary to adrenergic neuron blockade.

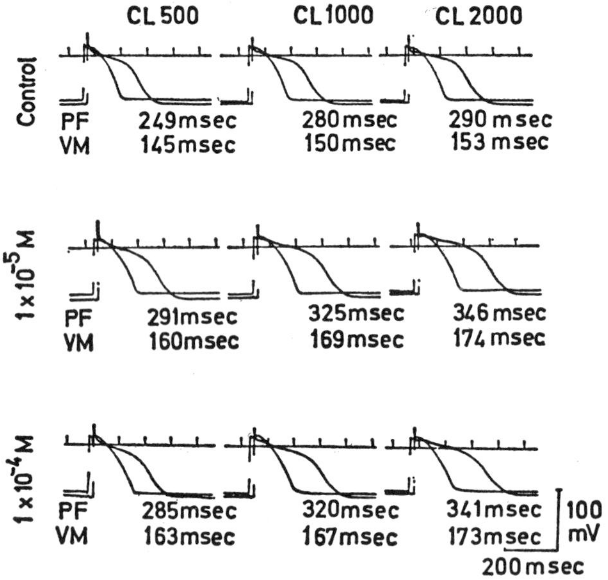

Fig. 26. Effect of bretylium tosylate on action potential duration of canine Purkinje and ventricular muscle fibers. In the top trace of each panel, time marks are repeated every 100 msec. The other 2 traces record transmembrane action potentials from ventricular muscle (shorter action potential) and a Purkinje fiber (longer action potential). The 3 vertical columns show recordings made at cycle lengths (CL) of 500 msec (left column). 1,000 msec (center column), and 2,000 msec (right column). The horizontal rows show action potentials recorded under control conditions (top row) and during exposure to bretylium tosylate in concentrations of 1×10^{-5}M (second row) and 1×10^{-4}M (third row). The action potential duration (measured to 95% repolarization(of the Purkinje fiber and ventricular muscle fiber is given under each frame. At 1×10^{-6}M, action potential duration was not significantly affected in either cell type (not shown). At 1×10^{-5}M and 1×10^{-4}M, Purkinje fiber action potential lengthened by 17% and that of the ventricular muscle cell by 12% at each drive rate. From Bigger and Jaffe (1971)

PAPP and VAUGHAN WILLIAMS (1969) studied the effects of bretylium on the single cell transmembrane potential of the driven isolated rabbit atria. They found that a concentration of approximately 5×10^{-5}M had no quinidine-like effects while approximately 5×10^{-4}M caused only a small reduction in the rate of rise of the action potential. Approximately 3×10^{-3}M and 6×10^{-3}M bretylium, after a period of changes attributed to sympathomimesis, ultimately reduced the rate of rise of the action potential, reduced the conduction velocity and maximum driving frequency, and increased the electrical threshold. These authors considered that concentrations of 5×10^{-5}M or higher were greater than would be experienced *in vivo* in the clinical situation. This is apparently the case since KUNTZMAN et al. (1970) reported plasma levels in man of approximately 4×10^{-6}M following intramuscular administration of a therapeutic dose (300 mg). PAPP and VAUGHAN WILLIAMS (1969), as did BIGGER and JAFFE (1971), speculated that it was possible that the antiarrhythmic action of bretylium was due to dampening of activity in sympathetic nerves.

ARAVINDAKSHAN and GETTES (1975) reported that in the isolated rabbit heart, bretylium ($\sim 1 \times 10^{-4}$ M) was ineffective in preventing ventricular fibrillation induced by either perfusion with low potassium solutions or by the introduction of premature stimuli. These authors concluded that the reported antifibrillatory effects of bretylium are dependent upon an intact sympathetic nervous system.

This notion was disputed by the evidence of CERVONI et al. (1971) who found that bretylium not only elevated fibrillation threshold in normal dogs, but in dogs with chronically-denervated hearts and in reserpine-treated dogs as well. BACANER (1968a) also reported that guanethidine and propranolol were ineffective in elevating ventricular fibrillation threshold.

KNIFFEN et al. (1975) reported that a structural analog of bretylium, 0-iodobenzyl trimethylammonium, had an antiarrhythmic antifibrillatory profile very similar to bretylium, yet this compound did not produce adrenergic stimulation or blockade of sympathetic neuronal activity.

WATANABE et al. (1969) described changes induced in the transmembrane potentials of isolated rabbit ventricle muscle by approximately 5×10^{-5}M bretylium which were probably due to the sympathomimetic effects of this drug.

WAXMAN and WALLACE (1972) administered bretylium to conscious dogs which had chronic implantation of recording electrodes over the SA node, bundle of His and right bundle branch. Ten to 30 min after the intravenous administration of 10 mg/kg of bretylium the effective refractory periods of atrial and ventricular muscle were prolonged by 9% and 12%, respectively. Bretylium had no effect on the excitability threshold of atrial or ventricular muscle. Surgical denervation of the heart did not abolish the electrophysiologic effects of bretylium.

Recent work by NAMM et al. in the rat (1975) has shed considerable light on the mechanism whereby bretylium exerts a specific ventricular antiarrhythmic action. Bretylium, when added to isolated rat atria and ventricle preparations at high concentrations (2×10^{-5}M to 10^{-3}M), lenthened the action potential duration (APD), and the effective refractory period, (ERP) with a resultant increase in ERP/APD, decreased the rate of rise of the action potential and suppressed the action potential amplitude. These "antiarrhythmic" actions of bretylium occurred in hearts from immunosympathectomized rats as well as in hearts from normal rats. Interestingly ventricles from innervated and immunosympathectomized rats accumulated bretylium at least 30-fold over extracellular levels. This binding of bretylium by the ventricle allows for the attainment of effective antiarrhythmic concentrations in the myocardium in the face of low plasma concentrations of the drug. In addition it accounts for the selective action on the ventricle and for the lag time characteristic of the antiarrhythmic action of bretylium. Subcellular distribution of labelled bretylium in the ventricle of immunosympathectomized rats indicated that it was bound to plasma membranes. The binding was tight but reversible. Namm et al. (1975) concluded that their results indicated that underlying the antiarrhythmic effects of bretylium is an accumulation of the drug by cardiac muscle cells and a direct effect of the drug on the electrical properties of the cardiac muscle membrane.

Guanethidine has been reported to be effective as an antiarrhythmic in several animal models (Leveque, 1964; Raines et al., 1968; Ahmad and Achari, 1967) as has bethanidine (Leveque, 1966).

3. Other Actions

Yoo and Lee (1970, 1971) reported that bretylium, guanethidine and cocaine blocked the cardiostimulant actions of phenylephrine on isolated, spontaneously-beating atria from normal rabbits but had no blocking action on phenylephrine in atria depleted of catecholamines by reserpine. The positive inotropic action of phenylephrine appeared to be direct and due to *beta* stimulant action since it was not blocked by reserpine but was blocked by 5×10^{-6}M propranolol (Yoo and Lee, (1970). If reserpine-pretreated atria were exposed to norepinephrine, the blocking effects of bretylium, guanethidine and cocaine were restored. Experiments using graded doses of reserpine showed that the greater the reduction in myocardial catecholamines the less the blockade of the inotropic actions of phenylephrine by bretylium, guanethidine and cocaine. In order to account for their results the authors proposed that bretylium, guanethidine and cocaine may combine with the catecholamine molecule and interfere with the action of phenylephrine at the cardiac *beta* adrenergic receptor. It is somewhat difficult from a chemical point of view to picture a complex that would form between 2 molecules which are not chemically reactive under physiological conditions. Alternatively, it is possible that some metabolite of norepinephrine in the adrenergic neuron having weak *beta* blocking activity was released by bretylium, guanethidine and cocaine and thereby accounted for the unusual observations of Yoo and Lee (1970, 1971). Unfortunately, there is no evidence to support this latter speculation. If the explanation of the authors is correct, it would seem that mixtures of norepinephrine with bretylium, guanethidine or cocaine added to the bath should block not only phenylephrine but standard *beta* agonists as well in reserpine-treated preparations. Additional information is needed.

E. Neuromuscular Junction

Bretylium and guanethidine produced muscle weakness in some patients (Campbell and Montuschi, 1960; Evanson and Sears, 1960; Dollery, 1961; Page, 1961; Hofmann and Spivack, 1962). Neuromuscular blockade is caused by high doses or concentrations of bretylium and guanethidine in animals and in isolated preparations. Boura and Green (1959) found that high concentrations of bretylium caused a curare-like paralysis. Thus, bretylium caused a flaccid paralysis in the chick similar to that evoked by curare and distinguishable from the paralysis produced by depolarizing drugs. On the other hand, the neuromuscular paralysis produced in the rat diaphragm preparation, in contrast to that caused by curare, was not antagonized by neostigmine. Guanethidine also produced a block of neuromuscular transmission in the rat phrenic nerve-diaphragm and cat sciatic-gastrocnemius preparations (Dixit et al., 1961). The doses required to produce these effects *in vivo* were 10 to 30 times the amount required to block the response to adrenergic nerve stimulation. These neuromuscular blocking actions were considerably shorter in duration than the neuron blockade especially after intravenous administration. Such curare-like actions are generally associated with high doses of compounds having quaternary nitrogen or basic tertiary amines, and the brief duration of this effect with neuron blocking agents *in vivo* is related to the relatively rapid fall in plasma levels of these compounds following their intravenous injection (see Section II). DIXIT et al. (1961) described a second, delayed, neuromuscular paralysis in the cat sciatic-gastrocnemius preparation for both guanethidine and bretylium which had a longer duration of action than the curariform effect. On the grounds that these agents did not block, but on the contrary, potentiated acetylcholine contracture of the frog rectus and that they exhibited only a weak, delayed, depressant effect on the response of the gastrocnemius to direct stimulation, these authors attributed the second, prolonged blockade to a prejunctional effect. GREEN and HUGHES (1966) found that the degree of neuromuscular blockade produced by bretylium increased sharply with the frequency of nerve stimulation and that choline was antagonistic in *in vitro* preparations. This was not the case with guanethidine. Guanethidine, like procaine and in contrast to bretylium, markedly reduced responses to direct stimulation of the muscle in isolated, curarized, rat diaphragm and in the gastrocnemius muscles of rabbits and cats. GREEN and HUGHES (1966) suggested that bretylium, but not guanethidine, had a presynaptic, hemicholinium-like activity. RAND and WILSON (1967a) concluded that guanethidine exerted a postjunctional neuromuscular blocking action similar to that of tubocurarine.

FERRY and NORRIS (1971) presented evidence that bretylium was a competitive inhibitor of acetylcholine at the motor end-plate in the rat phrenic nerve-diaphragm preparation in concentrations higher than 5×10^{-4}M. In addition, they demonstraed that bretylium was a competitive inhibitor of erythrocyte acetylcholinesterase, with a K_i value of 5.3×10^{-5}M. In a concentration of 5×10^{-5}M, bretylium partly reversed a curariform block of the diaphragm. Apparently bretylium exerts simultaneous facilitation and depression of neuromuscular transmission. With concentrations of approximately 5×10^{-4}M these effects offset one another.

The electrophysiologic and biochemical work of CHANG et al. (1967b) helped to unify the observations described above. Both guanethidine and bretylium initially reduced the amplitude of end-plate potentials and of spontaneous, miniature end-plate potentials without affecting the extracellularly-recorded, presynaptic nerve action potential or the muscle resting membrane potential in the rat diaphragm and frog sartorius preparations (Figs. 27 and 28). End-plate potentials in addition to being reduced were prolonged by these agents. The end-plate potentials were not further prolonged when neostigmine was added suggesting that bretylium and guanethidine prolonged the end-plate potentials by blocking cholinesterase. It is also possible that bretylium and guanethidine prolonged the end-plate potential in part because of a local anesthetic action (see Section V) as described for procaine by DEGUCHI and NARAHASHI (1971) (see Fig. 29). Delayed effects were observed by CHANG et al. (1967b) with both compounds: bretylium but not guanethidine reduced the release of acetylcholine from motor nerve endings which was evoked by nerve stimulation (Fig. 30) while guanethidine but not bretylium reduced the contractile responses to direct muscle stimulation and changed the form of the muscle action potentials (Fig. 31). CHANG et al. (1967b) felt that the delayed action of these drugs at the neuromuscular junction was more important than the acute curariform action. It is likely that the delayed effects are the clinically important entities. It appears

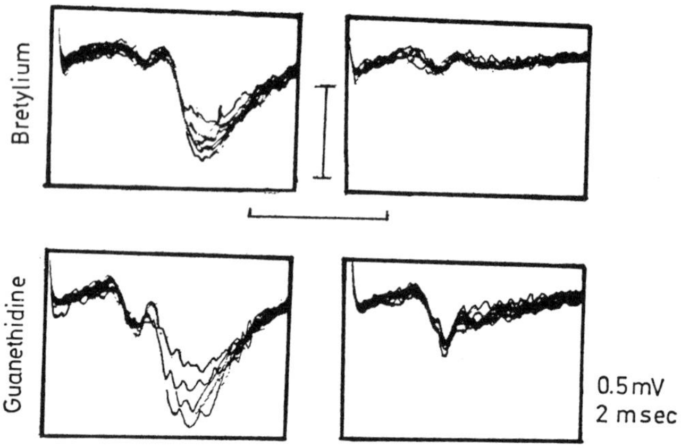

Fig. 27. Effects of bretylium and guanethidine on nerve terminal spikes and end-plate potentials. Shown in each tracing are 10 superimposed potentials extracellularly recorded in Mg-immobilized rat diaphragms upon repetitive stimulations at 100 impulses/sec. The first panel of each series shows control potentials. The second panel shows the unchanged nerve terminal spikes and complete inhibition of end-plate potentials at about 25 min after addition of 250 μg/ml, ($\cong 10^{-3}$M) each of either bretylium or guanethidine. From Chang et al. (1967b)

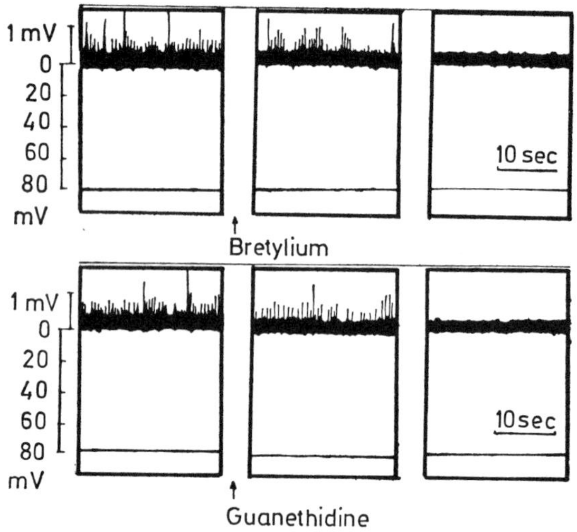

Fig. 28. Effects of bretylium and guanethidine on membrane potential and miniature end-plate potentials of the rat diaphragm. Simultaneous intracellular recordings of muscle membrane potential (lower tracing) and miniature end-plate potentials (upper tracing) from motor end-plates. At arrow, 250 μg/ml, ($\cong 10^{-3}$M) each of bretylium (upper panels) or guanethidine (lower panels) were added. The third panels were taken 4 min after addition of the drug. Note the different calibrations for miniature end-plate potentials and membrane potentials. From Chang et al. (1967b)

therefore, that bretylium and guanethidine have very different effects on the cholinergic system of skeletal muscles which may in part account for their capacity to produce muscle weakness at low and moderate dosage in man. The capacity of guanethidine to accumulate in skeletal muscle (Schanker and Morrison, 1965) may account for its effects on the responsiveness of the muscle cells (see Fig. 4 in Section II).

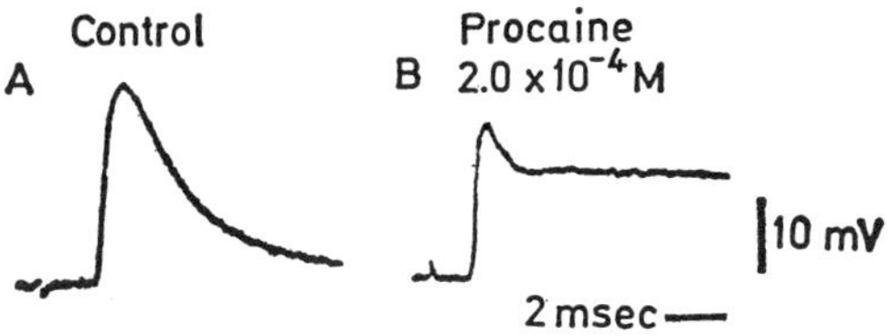

Fig. 29. Records of end-plate potentials before (control) and 32 min after application of procaine, 2.0×10^{-4}M. The two records were taken from different glycerol-treated muscle fibers. The resting potentials were —60 mV for the control muscle fiber and -76 mV for the procaine-treated muscle fiber. From DEGUCHI and NARAHASHI (1971)

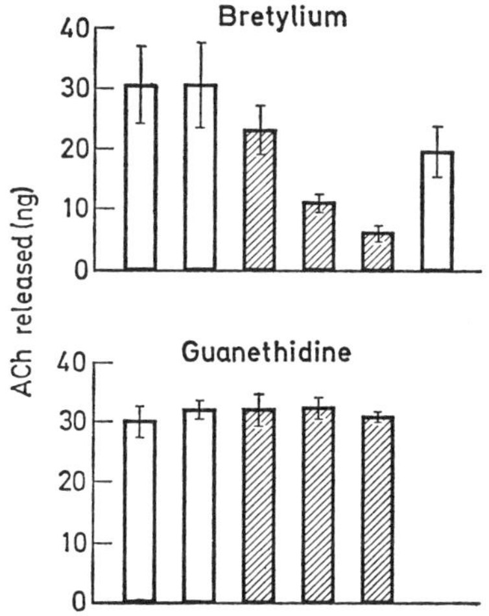

Fig. 30. Effects of bretylium and guanethidine on ACh release from the rat phrenic nerve. The amounts of ACh released upon repetitive stimulation at 50 impulses/sec for 10 min are shown with standard deviations (6 experiments). ACh release (in nanograms) before addition of drug is shown in the first two open columns. In the three hatched columns, successive ACh release after addition of 250 μg/ml, ($\simeq 10^{-3}$M) of bretylium or guanethidine is shown. The last open column shows the ACh release 20 min after washout of bretylium. From CHANG et al. (1967b)

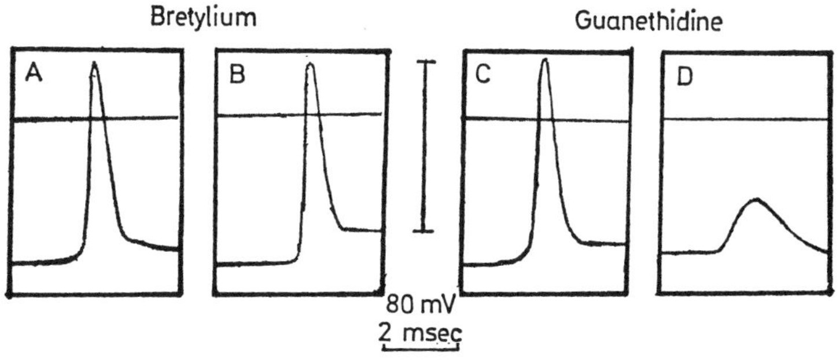

Fig. 31. Effects of bretylium and guanethidine on muscle action potentials of rat diaphragms. The first tracings (A and C) are control action potentials elicited by indirect stimulation. The second tracing for bretylium (250 μg/ml, $\simeq 10^{-3}$M) was obtained by direct stimulation after complete neuromuscular blockade (ca. 90 min), and that for guanethidine (250 μg/ml, $\simeq 10^{-3}$M) was recorded from partially paralyzed muscle for about 60 min after addition of the drug. From CHANG et al. (1967b)

The contractions of the rat isolated diaphragm which occur in response to supramaximal stimulation of the phrenic nerve at 5 shocks/min were abolished by 2 mg/ml (ca. 10^{-2}M) bethanidine but the response to direct muscle stimulation remained (BOURA and GREEN, 1963). Application of a concentration of 10 mg/ml of bethanidine directly to the phrenic nerve did not modify the muscle twitch in response to indirect stimulation applied central to the site of application. In cats anesthetized with chloralose, respiratory paralysis and abolition of the response of the gastrocnemius muscle to indirect stimulation, but not to direct stimulation, occurred concomitantly after intravenous doses of 10 to 20 mg/kg of bethanidine. Similar brief respiratory failure and paralysis of the indirectly stimulated gastrocnemius muscle has been observed in an anesthetized monkey after an intravenous dose of 10 mg/kg; however, oral doses of 50 mg/kg were well tolerated (BOURA and GREEN, 1963). GREEN and HUGHES (1966) reported that the extent of neuromuscular blockade produced by bethanidine increased with the frequency of nerve stimulation. Choline did not antagonize bethanidine effects *in vitro*.

F. Influence on Frequency-Response Curves for Several Nerve-Smooth Muscle Preparations

Differences have been reported to exist among the effects of bretylium, guanethidine and bethanidine on the responses to sympathetic nerve stimulation (BOURA and GREEN, 1959, 1962, 1963). The slopes of the curves relating frequency of sympathetic nerve stimulation to the magnitude of the resulting contraction of the nictitating membrane were depressed by bretylium, but guanethidine preferentially abolished the responses to low rates of stimulation. The effects of bethanidine of the responses of the nictitating membrane to different frequencies of sympathetic nerve stimulation were intermediate between those of bretylium and guanethidine. Similar differences between the effects of bretylium, guanethidi-

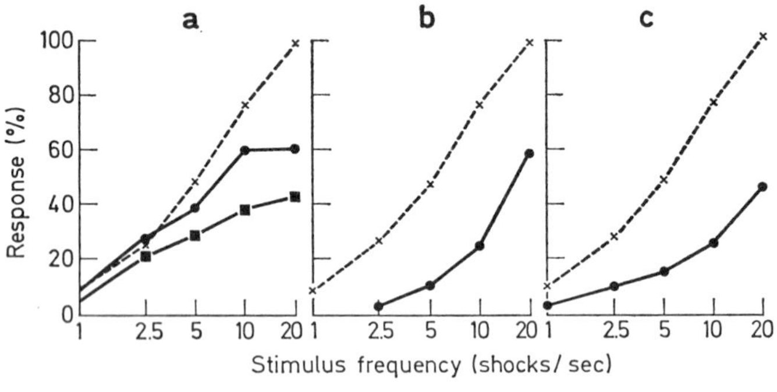

Fig. 32. The relationship of the frequency of splenic nerve stimulation (on log scale) to changes in spleen volume in anaesthetized cats. Each train of stimuli was applied for 30 sec. and adequate time was allowed for the spleen to relax fully between each train. All spleen volume changes have been expressed as a percentage of that produced by 20 shocks/sec in each animal before giving blocking agents. X——X, control responses (mean for twelve cats). (a) ●——● and ■——■, after 1.0 and approximately 2.5 mg/kg of bretylium tosylate respectively, showing depression of slope; (b) ●——●, after 0.3 mg/kg of guanethidine sulphate showing a parallel shift of the regression line; (c) ●——●, after 0.3 mg/kg of bethanidine hydrochloride which produced an effect on the regression line intermediate between those of bretylium and guanethidine. Experimental means are for groups of three cats. From GREEN and ROBSON (1964)

ne and bethanidine have been reported in studies of contraction of the spleen in anesthetized cats (Fig. 32) and in perfused rabbit ears (Green and Robson, 1964). No major distinction between bethanidine and guanethidine was found in studies of the vasoconstrictor response to sympathetic nerve stimulation in the femoral vascular bed of anesthetized cats (Green and Robson, 1964). The effects of these three agents on levels of tissue catecholamines are different (Section IV B). These differences have been related to the differing effects of these 3 compounds on frequency-response curves (Boura and Green 1962, 1963). A detailed study correlating the effects of bretylium, guanethidine and bethanidine on frequency-response curves with the uptake, storage, release and metabolism of tritiated norepinephrine would be of interest.

Differences between the effects of bretylium, guanethidine and bethanidine on curves relating frequency of adrenergic nerve stimulation to the effector responses have been used to explain differences in the incidence of postural hypotension and in the degrees of tolerance which occur during daily administration of these agents (Boura and Green, 1962; Green and Robson, 1965).

G. Actions on Excitable Membranes of Nerve Trunks

Bretylium, when applied externally to isolated adrenergic nerve trunks and to certain isolated cholinergic nerve trunks, produced partial to complete inhibition of conduction. This effect was exhibited as diminished responses of the effector organs which were innervated by these nerves and which were suspended in an organ bath (Boura and Green, 1959; Boura et al., 1960; Boyd et al., 1961). Bretylium applied in high concentrations between the point of stimulation and the effector organ blocked the response of 1) the rabbit ileum at 10 to 100 microgm/ml (41 microgm/ml = 10^{-4} M) as compared to the 1 to 3 microgm/ml required in the bath fluid and 2) the rabbit uterus at 10 to 50 microgm/ml as compared to 3 to 10 microgm/ml in the bath (Boura and Green, 1959). Boyd et al. (1961) demonstrated that 50 to 100 microgm/ml in the bath completely blocked the response of the isolated rat vas deferens to stimulation of the hypogastric nerve but that 10 mg/ml was required to be added to the nerve trunk to achieve the same effect. These authors pointed out that when bretylium was added to the bath its blocking action was slow in onset an in offset (following washout) and was concentration-dependent, whereas, the effect of procaine was essentially all or none and was rapid in its onset and in its offset following washout. The conduction block caused by topical bretylium was readily reversible by washout.

Unlike in the preparations just described, topical application of bretylium to the phrenic nerve and the preganglionic cervical sympathetics did not diminish the response of effector organs to electrical stimulation of these nerves (Boura and Green 1959; Boura et al., 1960) (see Table 17). Cholinergic and adrenergic nerve trunks took up radioactive bretylium but this was more effective in the latter group. The relationship between amount taken up by nerve trunks and nerve block was not simple as can be seen in Table 17. As pointed out by Boura et al. (1960) the differences observed after topical application of the drug were compatible with myelin acting as a diffusion barrier to the bretylium ion. Presumably fiber size was also important in relation to sensitivity to bretylium. Boura et al. (1960) speculated that bretylium may act in a manner analogous to that of the local anesthetic drugs and that its specific actions on adrenergic neurons might be related to their ability to selectively accumulate the drug, as well as to the greater sensitivity of finer and less protected fibers. The combination of a relatively weak "local anesthetic effect", selective permeability and selective uptake allowed effective doses of bretylium to be administered *in vivo* which did not produce generalized neurotoxicity. The recent work of CABRERA et al. (1966), HÄUSLER et al. (1968, 1969), MITCHELL and OATES (1970) has supported this early speculation of BOURA et al. (1960). This work has been summarized in Section V B.

Table 17. *Concentration of bretylium in nerves after topical application.* The nerve, immersed in Tyrode solution containing [^{14}C]-labelled bretylium iodide, was stimulated at 15 pulses/sec for 30 sec every 3 or 5 min. Concentration of bretylium calculated from radioactivity determination

	Response tested	Bath concentration of bretylium iodide mμmoles/ml	Immersion time in min	Inhibition of end organ response	Concentration of drug in nerve, mμmoles/g
Adrenergic nerves					
Inferior cardiac	Heart rate	500	20	Complete	600
Hypogastric	uterus	50	100	Partial	90
Hypogastric	uterus	500	75	Partial	1,270
Cholinergic nerves					
Preganglionic cervical sympathetic	Nictitating membrane	500	30	None	520
Preganglionic cervical sympathetic	Nictitating membrane	500	30	None	500
Preganglionic cervical sympathetic	Nictitating membrane	1,000	30	None	340
Preganglionic cervical sympathetic	Nictitating membrane	1,000	90	Partial	310
Greater splanchnic	Rise in B.P.	500	30	Partial	90
Greater splanchnic	Rise in B.P.	500	35	Partial	50
Phrenic	Diaphragm	500	30	None	90

From BOURA et al. (1960).

It should be pointed out that bretylium, bethanidine and guanethidine fulfill approximately the general structural criteria for local anesthetics as described by RITCHIE et al. (1970) and CHERNICK (1971); namely, a hydrophobic aromatic residue connected by an intermediate group to a hydrophilic secondary or tertiary amino group (Fig. 33). Obviously, neither guanethidine nor bretylium are structurally ideal derivatives for local anesthetic activity. The steric differences (at the charged end) between these agents and the more potent local anesthetics could alone account for the weakness of their local anesthetic activity. In the case of the neuron blockers, bretylium is a quaternary ammonium derivative and guanethidine a guanidinium derivative rather than secondary and tertiary amine derivatives. The obligatory charge on bretylium undoubtedly influences its capacity to permeate lipid membranes (other than by the specialized pumping process) and also helps to account for its lack of potency. Guanethidine, while theoretically existing to some extent in the unprotonated form, is such a strong base that it is essentially 100% charged at physiological pH. RITCHIE and GREENGARD (1966) and NARAHASHI and FRAZIER (1968) presented evidence that the charged form of local anesthetics was the active form.

The possibility exists that these charged neuronal blocking agents produced their "membrane stabilizing effects" by intimate mechanisms in excitable membranes which are quite different from those of the standard local anesthetics (s. Sec. VB).

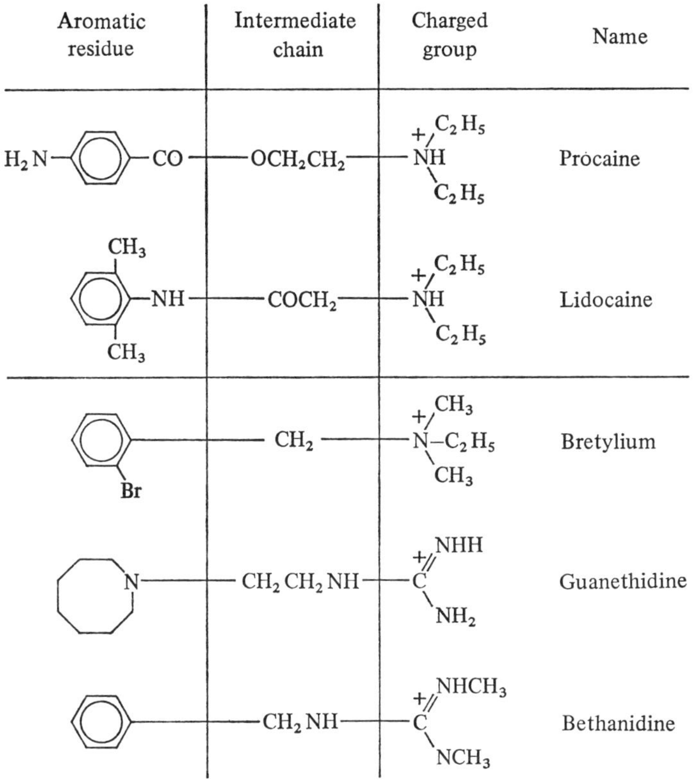

Fig. 33. Structures of the local anesthetics, procaine and lidocaine and the adrenergic neuron blocking agents, bretylium, guanethidine, and bethanidine in their protonated form

H. Effects at Synapses

Transient ganglionic blockade followed intravenous administration of bretylium (Boura and Green, 1959; Gertner and Romano, 1961), and guanethidine (Maxwell et al., 1960) (Fig. 34). In the perfused superior cervical ganglion preparation of the cat, 100 microgm of bretylium caused a small, temporary retraction of the nictitating membrane followed by a reduction of the contracting effects of preganglionic stimulation (Boura and Green, 1959). Restoration of the control

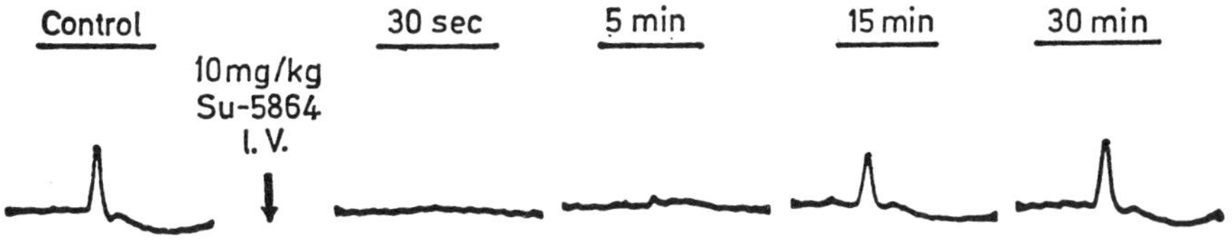

Fig. 34. The acute effect of guanethidine on the post ganglionic spike potentials which were elicited by preganglionic stimulation of the cervical sympathetic trunk in the cat anesthetized with Dial-Urethane. Note that full recovery has occurred within 30 min. Stimulation parameters: 6.5 v. 0.1 millisec; at 1 per 2 sec. From Maxwell et al. (1960)

perfusion medium led to full return of the membrane retractions. The brief nature of these ganglionic effects *in vivo* following i.v. injection was due to the high concentrations needed to evoke them and the rapid fall in plasma levels with time.

The small and temporary retraction of the nictitating membrane which occurred during perfusion of the superior cervical ganglion with bretylium suggests that bretylium might act to depolarize some cell bodies in the ganglion. It is possible that a simultaneously occurring "local anesthetic-like effect" (see Section V B and VII G) might have counteracted the tendency of bretylium to depolarize at synapses.

I. Central Nervous System

As described in Section II guanethidine and bretylium, because they are charged molecules, do not readily penetrate the blood-brain barrier. Following intravenous administration, guanethidine did not inhibit central vasomotor activity (MAXWELL, 1961; KANEKO et al., 1962). Bretylium and guanethidine when administered by oral or parenteral routes were devoid of effects on behavior attributable to central nervous actions. When injected directly into the cerebrospinal fluid in anesthetized dogs, guanethidine decreased vasomotor outflow markedly. This was reflected in a decrease in electrical activity in the splanchnic nerve and in elimination of the reflex changes in electrical activity in this nerve which normally occurred during bilateral occlusion of the common carotid arteries (KANEKO et al., 1962). Administered into the cerebral ventricles, guanethidine produced a fall in blood pressure and inhibited reflexly-mediated vasomotor responses (BHARGAVA et al., 1966).

COX and MAICKEL (1969) reported that guanethidine (200 microgm/rat) administered directly into the lateral ventricle of the rat brain, elicited pronounced behavioral effects. Hyperexcitation and enhanced responsiveness to stimuli lasted for 30 to 60 min. The rats then progressed into a prolonged depression similar to that evoked by moderate doses of reserpine. During this phase, the rats exhibited ptosis, decreased activity, and a hunched posture. Brain levels of norepinephrine and 5-hydroxytryptamine were significantly lowered and remained so for longer than 24 h (Table 18). The content of guanethidine in the brain declined over the period of 4 to 24 h at a rate indicating a half life of approximately 6.5 h. Presumably guanethidine can leave the brain although it cannot be transported into

Table 18. *Effects of intraventricular guanethidine on rat brain NE and 5HT*. Each value is the mean ± S.D. of values obtained from 4 rats given guanethidine (200 μg/rat, lateral ventricle) at time = 0. Values significantly different from time = 0 ($p < 0.05$) are indicated by #

Time (h)	Brain levels (μg/g) NE	5HT	Guanethidine
0	0.52 ± 0.04	0.69 ± 0.05	—
1	0.46 ± 0.05	0.62 ± 0.03	28.6 ± 12.8
2	0.46 ± 0.05	0.58 ± 0.05 #	—
4	0.38 ± 0.02 #	0.56 ± 0.04 #	11.6 ± 7.8
6	0.32 ± 0.03 #	0.45 ± 0.07 #	—
8	0.31 ± 0.01 #	0.49 ± 0.06 #	8.3 ± 4.0
12	0.30 ± 0.02 #	0.45 ± 0.02 #	—
18	0.30 ± 0.02 #	0.42 ± 0.02 #	3.2 ± 1.8
24	0.33 ± 0.02 #	0.52 ± 0.05 #	1.5 ± 1.1

From COX and MAICKEL (1969).

the brain to any significant degree. The data of Cox and MAICKEL (1966) indicated that central adrenergic neurons are as susceptible to guanethidine effects as are peripheral adrenergic neurons.

The uptake of several sympathomimetic amines by mouse-brain cortex slices was inhibited by guanethidine (ROSS and RENYI, 1966). Guanethidine (200 microgm) but not bretylium (100 microgm) when administered intraventricularly blocked the uptake or accumulation of intraventricularly administered tritiated norepinephrine in the brain (GLOWINSKI and AXELROD, 1965).

J. Additional Biochemical Effects

1. Effects on Mitochondrial Metabolism

Because some degree of inhibition of energy transfer had been observed with nonacidic guanidine derivatives, MALMQUIST and OATES (1968) studied the action of guanidine adrenergic neuron blocking agents on oxidative phosphorylation in isolated rat liver mitochondria. Guanethidine, bethanidine and related agents in high concentrations all inhibited mitochondrial oxygen uptake (Fig. 35). These agents also produced a parallel inhibitory effect on the disappearance of inorganic phosphate during oxidative phosphorylation. Debrisoquin, the most potent inhibitor of ADP-stimulated respiration, did not inhibit oxygen uptake when respiration was stimulated with dinitrophenol indicating that debrisoquin did not influence mitochondrial transport *per se*. MALMQUIST and OATES (1968) expressed the view that because neuron blocking drugs were concentrated within adrenergic neurons it was conceivable that their levels could become sufficient to inhibit oxidative phosphorylation. These authors felt that there may be a link between inhibition of oxidative phosphorylation and blockade of adrenergic transmission.

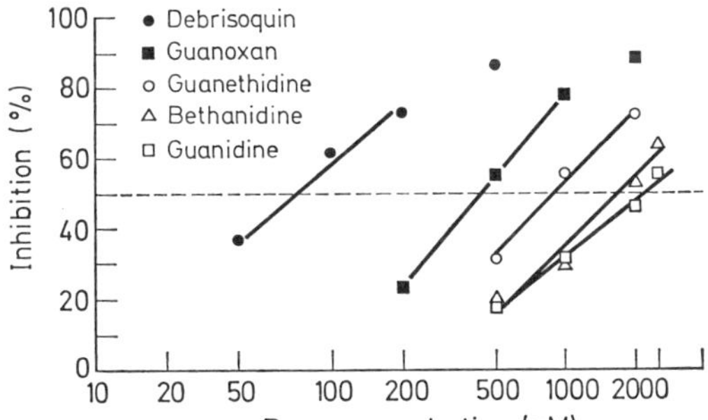

Fig. 35. Relationship between drug concentrations and extent of inhibition of mitochondrial oxygen uptake. Each point represents the average results of 2 — 6 experiments. From MALMQUIST and OATES (1968)

2. Effect on Histamine Excretion

JAQUES and LEWIS (1970) reported that when guanethidine was added to the perfusion fluid it produced an immediate release of histamine from the rat hind quarters and when injected into the peritoneum of the rat caused a dose-dependent release of histamine into the cell-free peritoneal fluid.

A single intraperitoneal injection of 10 mg/kg of guanethidine in male rats doubled the daily urinary excretion of free histamine (LE BLANC et al., 1972). Daily injection of this dose for three weeks caused a ten-fold increase. In male rats, guanethidine increased the number of mast cells in the peritoneal fluid and, in both peritoneal fluid and mesentery these cells were significantly degranulated. Guanethidine had no effect on histamine excretion in female rats. LE BLANC et al. (1972) concluded that guanethidine may block methylation of histamine by inhibiting imidazole methyl transferase since this enzyme is found in male but not in female rats.

Testosterone diminished the high histaminuria caused by guanethidine in male rats (DORÉ et al., 1974). Castration on the other hand had additive effects with guanethidine in increasing histamine excretion and decreasing methyl-histamine excretion. DORÉ et al. (1974) suggested that the action of guanethidine on imidazole N-methyltransferase might be due to a direct action on the enzyme or indirectly by an effect on testosterone secretion or activity.

Bethanidine and reserpine had no effect on histamine excretion.

K. Structural and Ultrastructural Changes in Neurons

Intraperitoneal administration of guanethidine in doses up to 5 mg/kg for 18 weeks did not affect the ultrastructure of the rat sympathetic ganglion cells (BURNSTOCK et al., 1971b; JENSEN-HOLM and JUUL, 1971). These doses were effective in producing sympatholytic effects. However, intraperitoneal administration of 5 mg/kg guanethidine for 18 weeks to rats has been reported to lead to long-lasting damage to adrenergic nerves in the male reproductive tract although adrenergic nerves in other parts of the body were not seriously affected (GANNON et al., 1971).

GERKENS (1974a) noted that treatment of rats for 19 weeks with 5 mg/kg/day i.p. guanethidine reduced the contractile responses of the vas deferens to electrical stimulation to 25% of control, potentiated the response to norepinephrine and depleted endogenous norepinephrine. Within one week after discontinuation of guanethidine treatment the responses to electrical stimulation increased to 60% of control but showed no further increase. Potentiation of the response to norepinephrine persisted for 14 weeks and endogenous levels of norepinephrine were still greatly reduced after 7 weeks. GERKENS (1974b) also reported that after 4 weeks treatment with 5 mg/kg/day guanethidine i.p. the pressor responses evoked by stimulation of the spinal sympathetic outflow were reduced by 55% and after 19 weeks treatment they were reduced by 69%. However, after cessation of treatment the responses increased to near normal within 3 weeks. JANDHYALA et al. (1975) treated dogs with 2.5 mg/kg/day for 7 to 8 months. This dose approximated the upper limit of the human therapeutic dose range. Ventricular function curves obtained in treated and placebo groups were virtually identical. Chronic guanethidine administration did not produce adverse effects on myocardial function.

JENSEN-HOLM and JUUL (1968, 1970b) described the occurrence of slowly reversible or partly-reversible, structural changes in sympathetic ganglion cells of the rat as a result of treatment for 5 to 14 days with high doses (20 mg/kg) of guanethidine. Chromatolysis of ganglion cells was observed accompanied by infiltration of a large number of small lymphocyte-like cells and macrophages. A pronounced loss of specific and non-specific cholinesterase activity and catecholamines was also seen. The dry weight and protein content of the sympathetic ganglia were increased substantially (JENSEN-HOLM and JUUL, 1970a). This dosage regimen also elicited pronounced swelling of the mitochondria of the superior cervical ganglion cells. The mitochondria also assumed round or irregular shapes (JENSEN-HOLM and JUUL, 1971). The membranes were intact but an unfolding of the crests was seen. Irregularization of the endoplasmic reticulum occurred and an increased number of dense bodies was observed. A large increase in lymphocytes was evident. The changes were reversible, with partial recovery occurring by 22 to 56 days following the cessation of treatment. The pre-and postganglionic nerve fibers, the synaptic vesicles and synapses were unaffected.

ERÄNKÖ and ERÄNKÖ (1971) reported that intraperitoneal injections of 20 mg/kg/day of guanethidine for 8 days to newborn rats, caused destruction of the superior cervical and celiac ganglia within a 3 week period.

Daily subcutaneous injections of 100 mg/kg bretylium or 15 mg/kg guanethidine to newborn mice and rats during the first few weeks of life resulted in massive destruction of immature sympathetic nerve cells (ANGELETTI and LEVI-MONTALCINI, 1972; ANGELETTI et al., 1972; CARAMIA et al., 1972).

JOHNSON and ALOE (1974) found that if nerve growth factor (2000 units/g/day) was given concurrently with 100 mg/kg/day guanethidine to newborn rats, destruction of sympathetic neurons was prevented.

Intraperitoneal administration of 25 or 30 mg/kg/day of guanethidine to rats for 6 weeks resulted in widespread sympathectomy, which persisted over long periods (BURNSTOCK et al., 1971 b). Most of the cell bodies in the superior cervical ganglia were completely degenerated. The few remaining were severely damaged. The mitochondria were the main site of neuron damage. They were swollen, the cristae were lost or severely damaged and of irregular outline.

JUUL and SAND (1973) reported that desmethylimipramine largely prevented the accumulation of guanethidine in the superior cervical ganglia and almost completely prevented the morphological effects of guanethidine on the ganglia. Reserpine only lowered the content of guanethidine in the ganglia to a small degree and likewise only slightly protected the ganglia from morphological changes. The authors concluded that the cytotoxic effect of guanethidine was due to its accumulation in ganglion nerve cells outside the norepinephrine storage granules as opposed to a mainly intragranular localization in peripheral sympathetic terminals.

JUUL and MCISAAC (1973) demonstrated that the destructive effects of repeated large doses of guanethidine on adult rat superior cervical ganglion was associated with a considerable (up to 80%) reduction of the norepinephrine of the ganglion and they reasonably assumed that the loss of norepinephrine was secondary to the chromatolysis. DOWNING and JUUL (1973) showed in isolated superior cervical ganglion from rats given repeated large doses of guanethidine that transmitted action potentials were normal in form but diminished in amplitude. Several other parameters of ganglionic transmission were measured and found to be changed in a manner consistent with a dose-dependent inactivation of a large proportion of the ganglion cells.

HILL et al. (1973) demonstrated that guanethidine in high concentrations had a direct cytotoxic effect on sympathetic neurons grown in cultures of newborn rat and embryo chick sympathetic ganglia. Guanethidine caused nerve fiber retraction.

MALMQUIST and OATES (1968) (see Section VII J) demonstrated that guanethidine as well as other adrenergic neuron blocking agents in high concentrations inhibited oxidative phosphorylation in isolated rat liver mitochondria *in vitro*. Since the destructive effect of guanethidine on adrenergic neurons is first associated with prominent changes in mitochondria, it seems highly likely that such destruction is secondary to inhibition of intraneuronal, oxidative phosphorylation by guanethidine when it is concentrated in adrenergic neurons. It is not known if neuronal destruction occurs in man. However, guanethidine has been in wide clinical use for over 10 years without reports of it producing irreversible hypotension or other effects attributed to irreversible sympathetic inhibition.

JENSEN-HOLM and JUUL (1970a) commented that in a few experiments very large doses of bethanidine (60 to 110 mg/kg daily for 10 days) reduced cholinesterase activity without affecting protein content in the superior cervical ganglion of the rat.

HAEUSLER et al. (1974) demonstrated that high doses of debrisoquin (100 to 110 mg/kg i.p.) did not seriously alter or destroy peripheral adrenergic neurons when administered to adult male rats for a period of 6 or 11 weeks.

Guanacline has been reported to produce long lasting, possibly irreversible hypotensive effects in patients following prolonged administration (BOCK and HEIMSOTH, 1969; DAWBORN et al., 1969). BURNSTOCK et al. (1971a) reported slow recovery of blood pressure following 9 to 14 weeks of intraperitoneal treatment with 5 mg/kg/day guanacline relative to recovery from a similar regimen with 5 mg/kg/day of guanethidine. Sections of sympathetic ganglion cells from rats treated with guanacline had a massive deposition of lipoprotein granules which were still present 12 weeks following cessation of treatment. Comparable changes did not occur with guanethidine treatment. BURNSTOCK et al. (1971a) suggested that the cellular effects of guanacline might account for its persistent action in man following its discontinuance. JENSEN-HOLM and JUUL (1971) confirmed the observations of BURNSTOCK et al. (1971a) and in addition reported moderate mitochondrial swelling following 20 mg/kg guanacline for 14 days.

JUUL (1973) compared the effects of 2 to 3 weeks of administration of large doses of guanethidine, guanacline, guanidine, guanoxan, debrisoquin, bethanidine, bretylium and reserpine to the adult rat on the histology, ultrastructure and cholinesterase histochemistry of the superior cervical ganglia. Of these agents only guanethidine and guanacline induced histological changes. These changes consisted of chromatolysis of the nerve cells accompanied by cellular infiltration and frank degeneration of some ganglion cells. Ultrastructural changes consisting mainly of mitochondrial swelling with partial loss of mitochondrial crests were prominent after guanethidine and guanacline and present but less prominent following bretylium, debrisoquin, bethanidine and guanoxan. Guanidine and reserpine did not produce ultrastructural changes with the doses employed. Only guanethidine and guanacline diminished cholinesterases from the cytoplasm of the nerve cells. JUUL (1973) considered that the changes observed were cytotoxic effects of the compounds, and that the differences in response were due to different potency and different extents of accumulation in the sympathetic ganglion nerve cells.

L. Effects on the Interaction Between Sympathetic and Parasympathetic Nervous Systems

PATON and VIZI (1969) demonstrated that norepinephrine and epinephrine inhibited the acetylcholine release from the parasympathetic nerve terminals of longitudinal muscle strip of guinea pig ileum during rest periods and when the frequency of field stimulation was low. This inhibitory action was blocked by *alpha* adrenergic blocking agents. VIZI and KNOLL (1971) confirmed the effect of exogenous norepinephrine in inhibiting acetylcholine release during field stimulation and demonstrated that endogenous norepinephrine released by stimulation of the periarterial sympathetic nerves to the isolated rabbit jejunum had a similar inhibitory effect. Guanethidine when added to the bath decreased the output of acetylcholine (VIZI and KNOLL, 1971) presumably due to release of norepinephrine. In tissues from animals pretreated with guanethidine (or reserpine) a rise in resting acetylcholine output and in output during stimulation at low frequencies was found (PATON and VIZI, 1969). It was concluded that acetylcholine output by the nerves in certain intestinal muscle is under the normal control of the sympathetic nerves by some form of presynaptic inhibition mediated by *alpha* adrenergic receptors. This implied that in dually-innervated organs the withdrawal of sympathetic control leads to a parasympathetic response which is not only unopposed but is enhanced.

M. Effects on Degeneration Phenomena Following Section of Post Ganglionic Sympathetic Nerves

Bretylium and *beta*-TM 10 delayed the postdenervation decline of endogenous norepinephrine in sympathetically innervated organs (see LANGER, 1966; BÁRÁNY and TREISTER, 1970; LUNDBERG, 1970, 1972; PLUCHINO et al., 1970 for references). The two agents also delayed the onset of the excitatory effects seen in denervated organs as a consequence of release of transmitter from the degenerating nerve terminals. Guanidine neuron blocking agents were only slightly effective. Phenyltrimethylammonium, a substance structurally related to bretylium but lacking its neuron blocking action, was active. The exact mechanisms by which bretylium and the other active substances delay these functional effects of nerve section are unknown.

N. Effects on Plasma Volume and Kidney Function

Guanethidine increased plasma volumes when administered to normal control subjects (WEIL and CHIDSEY, 1968) or to hypertensive patients (see SMITH, 1965, for references). In normal subjects, in contrast to hypertensive patients, the increase in plasma volume occurred in the absence of sodium retention. The increases in plasma volume in normal subjects were associated with attenuation of forearm venous sympathetic reflexes and a rise in forearm venous compliance (WEIL and CHIDSEY, 1968). These findings indicated that the changes in volume were secondary to changes in capacity of the venous system rather than to sodium retention.

Guanethidine has been reported to enhance natriuresis in saline-loaded patients (GILL et al., 1964) and in subjects deprived of dietary sodium (GILL and BARTTER, 1966).

WILLIAMS et al. (1971) studied the diuretic effects of guanethidine in the dog. Intravenous injections of guanethidine increased urine flow, osmolar clearance and saluresis. Following phenoxybenzamine, intravenous guanethidine did not elicit significant saluresis or diuresis. Direct infusion of large amounts of guanethidine into the left renal artery, after pretreatment with phenoxybenzamine, produced unilateral saluresis and diuresis although the effects were not as great as occurred from direct infusion of guanethidine in the absence of this *alpha* blocking agent. The authors concluded that guanethidine-induced saluresis appeared to result from an increased tubular rejection of sodium directly within the kidney through a sympathetic blockade of renal nerves.

O. Mast Cells and Platelets

GRIPENBERG (1972) reported that the incorporation of guanethidine into isolated rat peritoneal mast cells was dependent on temperature, the pH of the medium, and the presence of Ca ions in the medium. The incorporation also showed saturation characteristics and was inhibited by tricyclic antidepressants. The guanethidine taken up was located mainly in the amine-storing organelles. GRIPEN-

BERG (1972) concluded that the uptake of guanethidine was partly due to an active transport mechanism in the cell membrane while the incorporation into the granules was a passive process.

SOLOMON and ZIEVE (1967) demonstrated that platelets accumulated several organic bases, *i.e.*, reserpine, procaine, histamine and quinidine by physical processes and, with the possible exception of quinidine, specialized transport mechanisms did not appear to be involved. On the other hand, platelets accumulated several biogenic amines such as serotonin (HUMPHREY and THO, 1954; TRANZER et al., 1966; HUGHES and BRODIE, 1967), norepinephrine (ABRAMS and SOLOMON, 1969) and dopamine (SOLOMON, SPIRT and ABRAMS, 1970) against a concentration gradient, by a process which was saturable and was impaired by metabolic inhibitors and by lowered temperature. The findings were consistent with the existence of a transport pump for these substances in the membrane of the platelet.

Platelets also accumulated neuron blocking agents by a pump which was similar to the one that processed the amines. Guanethidine (BOULLIN and OBRIEN, 1968, 1969) and debrisoquin (BOULLIN and OBRIEN, 1968; POCELINKO and SOLOMON, 1970) were taken up against a concentration gradient and this uptake was antagonized by bretylium, tyramine and serotonin (BOULLIN and OBRIEN, 1969; POCELINKO and SOLOMON, 1970). BOULLIN and OBRIEN (1969) also demonstrated that desmethylimipramine, cocaine, amphetamine and norepinephrine inhibited the accumulation of guanethidine by the platelet. SOLOMON et al. (1968) presented kinetic data which indicated that debrisoquin inhibited the uptake of serotonin by competing for a common transport process. SOLOMON et al. (1968) suggested that the human platelet may serve as a convenient model for studying some aspects of the human adrenergic neuron.

P. Effects on Extraneuronal Uptake of Norepinephrine

IVERSEN (1963, 1965, 1967) described a second mechanism of uptake (Uptake$_2$) which occurred in isolated perfused rat hearts at high epinephrine concentrations (ca. 10^{-5} M). Unlike adrenergic neuronal uptake (designated Uptake$_1$), Uptake$_2$ became saturated only at very high external norepinephrine concentrations (ca. 4×10^{-4}M), was readily removed by washout and was blocked by normetanephrine and phenoxybenzamine. EISENFELD et al. (1967a, b) reported that *alpha*-adrenergic blocking agents, *e.g.* phenoxybenzamine, reduced the accumulation of tritiated norepinephrine and its 0-methylated and deaminated metabolites in the cocaine-treated, isolated perfused rat heart exposed to a low concentration (3×10^{-8}M) of tritiated norepinephrine. They also observed that the *alpha*-adrenergic blocking agents were potent blockers of this process even though they did not inhibit either 0-methylation or deamination in heart homogenates assayed for enzymatic activity. EISENFELD et al. (1967a, b) proposed that the adrenergic blocking agents decreased transport of norepinephrine into extraneuronal cells, thereby reducing the access of the norepinephrine to intracellular metabolizing enzymes. LIGHTMAN and IVERSEN (1969) showed that if the formation of labelled metabolites of tritiated norepinephrine was blocked by combinations of normetanephrine, metabolic inhibitors, inhibitors of neuronal uptake, MAO inhibitors, and COMT inhibitors, the accumulation of unchanged tritiated norepinephrine was increased when hearts were perfused with low concentrations of norepinephrine (ca. 2×10^{-6} M). They concluded that Uptake$_2$ operated at all norepinephrine concentration ranges in the rat heart but that in the lower concentrations ($< 10^{-5}$ M) any norepinephrine taken up by this process was rapidly metabolized. It seems likely that Uptake$_2$ and the extraneuronal uptake of EISENFELD et al. (1967a, b) are one and the same phenomenon. Extraneuronal uptake has been extensively studied (see GILLESPIE and MUIR, 1970; BURNSTOCK et al., 1971c, for references).

Guanethidine (10^{-4} M) inhibited the extraneuronal uptake of tritiated norepinephrine (3×10^{-8} M) by 70% (EISENFELD et al., 1967a, b). JACOBOWITZ et al. (1971) using histofluorescence techniques reported that guanethidine, bretylium and xylocholine (ca. 10^{-4}M) inhibited or reduced the uptake of norepinephrine into vascular smooth muscle and fibroblasts from a 2×10^{-4} M norepinephrine perfusion solution. They did not appear to have an effect on the uptake of norepinephrine into cardiac muscle or connective tissue. The physiological significance of extraneuronal uptake (and Uptake_2) and the influence of neuron blocking agents on this uptake needs further elucidation.

VIII. The Amine Pump in Peripheral Adrenergic Nerves

A. Some Problems Discussed

As described in the preceding literature review, the amine pump in the cell membrane of adrenergic neurons plays a central role in the pharmacology of adrenergic neuron blocking agents. The large number of interactions which occur among neuron blockers, catecholamines, phenethylamines and other substances such as tricyclic antidepressants and cocaine at the adrenergic neuron appear to be largely explicable in terms of competition between these agents for access to the membrane "amine pump receptor". However, several reports have appeared, especially concerning *in vivo* studies, which apparently dispute this unifying concept. Several of the more glaring exceptions require detailed discussion:

1. COSTA et al. (1966) reported that desmethylimipramine inhibited the uptake of guanethidine, metaraminol and tyramine by rat heart *in vivo* when these agents were injected in small doses, but that it did not prevent uptake of these drugs when they were given in large doses. This fact, rather than being contradictory to the possibility of competition at the pump receptor, is entirely consistent with mass law considerations for equilibrium, competitive agents. In addition, as pointed out by MITCHELL et al. (1970) desmethylimipramine inhibits the hepatic microsomal metabolism of guanethidine, and leads to elevated levels of this substance (Section VI A). This drug interaction acts to obscure the effects of desmethylimipramine in inhibiting the uptake of larger doses of guanethidine by rat heart. LEMBERGER et al. (1965) reported that tyramine was hydroxylated by rat and rabbit. Metaraminol is apparently hydroxylated by the same enzyme that hydroxylates tyramine (AXELROD, 1963). Amphetamine was also hydroxylated by the rat (AXELROD, 1954) and desmethylimipramine blocked its hydroxylation (SULSER et al., 1966; CONSOLO et al., 1967). MITCHELL et al. (1970) suggested from this array of data that guanidinium neuron blockers share a common mixed-oxygenase pathway with several sympathomimetic amines. It seems likely that desmethylimipramine action at the amine pump is overridden because of its capacity to inhibit this oxygenase and thus elevate concentrations of competing substances. Certainly this has been clearly demonstrated in the case of desmethylimipramine and guanethidine. At five hours after administration of guanethidine or bethanidine to rats, the content of these substances in the heart was much higher in the desmethylimipramine-treated group than in controls (Table 19) (MITCHELL et al., 1970), and the content of the guanidiniums in the total animal

was also elevated in the treated group (Table 15). However, as demonstrated in guinea pigs, if adequate time was allowed for the total body content of guanethidine in the desmethylimipramine-pretreated group to decline to a level equal to that of the 5 h control it was clear that the hearts from this group contained less guanethidine than those from the control group (Table 20).

Table 19. *Effect of desipramine on the concentration of guanidinium drugs in rat heart in vivo.* Control rats and rats treated with desipramine 0.5 h previously were given guanethidine (15 mg/kg i.p.) or bethanidine (15 mg/kg i.p.). Five hours after administration of the latter drugs, the animals were sacrificed and their hearts were assayed for guanidinium content. Values are means ± S.E. with number of experiments in parentheses

Treatment	Concentration of guanidinium drugs in rat heart (*μg/g*)	
	Guanethidine	Bethanidine
Control	6.29 ± 0.48 (7)	3.00 ± 0.13 (5)
Desipramine, 1 mg/kg i.p.	9.08 ± 1.07[a] (7)	
Desipramine, 30 mg/kg i.p.	13.25 ± 2.28[a] (7)	9.98 ± 0.84[b] (5)

[a] $P < 0.05$.
[b] $P < 0.001$. From MITCHELL et al. (1970).

2. OBIANWU (1969) found that administration of protriptyline, a potent inhibitor of the amine pump, to the guanethidine-treated rat only slightly restored the response to sympathetic neuron stimulation. Subsequent infusion of amphetamine substantially antagonized the guanethidine blockade. As a consequence of these findings, OBIANWU suggested that inhibition of the uptake mechanism was not an important factor in the ability of amphetamine to antagonize guanethidine-induced neuron blockade since this mechanism was already blocked by protriptyline. However, the failure of protriptyline to antagonize guanethidine probably can be explained on the grounds that it, like desmethylimipramine, inhibited metabolism of guanethidine by microsomal enzymes in the rat, and thereby elevated its concentration (MITCHELL et al., 1970). It is likewise, not surprising that on subsequent administration, amphetamine was active in reversing the blockade on the neurons since a) its action in blocking the pump would be additive with protriptyline and b) its destruction by microsomal enzymes would be inhibited by the presence of protriptyline. FEAGIN et al. (1969) demonstrated that at the same time that

Table 20. *Effect of desipramine pretreatment (30 mg/kg i.p.) on guinea-pig content of guanethidine and norepinephrine 10 h after guanethidine administration (50 mg/kg i.p.).* Values are means ± S.E. of at least eight experiments (16 animals)

Pretreatment	Heart content of guanethedine *μg/g heart*	Heart content of norepinephrine *μg/g heart*	Whole animal content of guanethidine *ug/g whole animal*
Guanethidine	10.6 ± 1.1	0.44 ± 0.10	5.3 ± 0.6
Desipramine + guanethidine	4.0 ± 0.7[a]	1.79 ± 0.23	6.0 ± 0.5
Control		2.07 ± 0.14	

[a] $P < 0.001$. From MITCHELL and OATES (1970).

protriptyline antagonized guanethidine or bethanidine hypotension in man it caused a reduction in the amount of neuronally-bound guanidinium compounds. The amount of neuronally bound guanidinium was estimated by determining the amount of guanidinium that was releasable by amphetamine at the beginning of the slow phase of excretion of the neuron blocking agents (Section II).

3. BRODIE et al. (1965) reported that pretreatment with a large dose of unlabelled guanethidine (8 mg/kg, intraperitoneally) at 30 min before the administration of a small dose of tritiated guanethidine (20 microgm/kg intravenously), markedly reduced the amount of tritiated guanethidine retained by the rat heart at 5 h. On the other hand, a large dose of unlabelled bretylium (6.2 mg/kg, intravenously), given 30 min earlier, failed to lower the retention of ^{14}C -bretylium at 5 h after administration of a small labelled dose (27 migrogm/kg intravenously). It is not known how much of the binding of the tracer dose of bretylium was neuronal and how much was extraneuronal. Also, it is likely that at 30 min the plasma level of bretylium following its intravenous injection was as low or lower than the plasma level of guanethidine following its intraperitoneal administration. MAXWELL (unpublished observations) has found that the relative potencies for guanethidine and bretylium as inhibitors of the uptake of tritiated norepinephrine in peripheral adrenergic nerves (rabbit aortic strips) *in vitro* were 6 and 1, respectively. Since these values reflect the approximate relative affinities of these two substrates for the amine pump, it is not surprising that under the conditions of the experiments of BRODIE et al. (1965) that ^{14}C -bretylium uptake might not be inhibited by intravenous bretylium under circumstances where tritiated guanethidine was inhibited by intraperitoneal guanethidine. Likewise, similar considerations of concentrations and affinities may help explain the report by BRODIE et al. (1965) that bretylium inhibited the uptake of trace amounts of tritiated guanethidine but not the uptake after pharmacological doses of guanethidine.

4. BRODIE et al. (1965) reported that pretreatment with norepinephrine, cocaine or desmethylimipramine inhibited the uptake of guanethidine into the rat heart following intravenous administration of tracer doses of guanethidine (20 microgm/kg) but not the uptake of bretylium following intravenous tracer doses of bretylium (27 microgm/kg). However, the control "uptake" of bretylium was only 1/5 that of the guanethidine and, as mentioned above, it is uncertain if this was all neuronal uptake (BOURA et al., 1960). This low uptake might not have been into neuronal stores and, therefore, it would not have been susceptible to inhibition by norepinephrine, cocaine or desmethylimipramine. The positive effect of amphetamine in reducing this small uptake of bretylium does not rule out an interaction of amphetamine with bretylium at extraneuronal sites, since amphetamine distributes readily into extraneuronal sites (THOENEN et al., 1968).

5. GLOWINSKI and AXELROD (1965) stated that guanethidine, but not cocaine or bretylium, blocked the uptake or accumulation of tritiated norepinephrine in the brain. However, their statement is based on comparisons that were made following the administration of arbitrary doses: 200 microgm/brain of guanethidine, intraventricularly: 100 microgm/brain bretylium, intraventricularly and 15 mg/kg cocaine, intraperitoneally. The failure of bretylium to block uptake can be understood if it is realized that it is probably only 1/6 as potent an inhibitor of the amine pump as guanethidine. The failure of cocaine to block uptake may also be related to factors such as its distribution and metabolism. Without knowledge of the concentration of cocaine in the brain, the report that it has no activity has little meaning.

In general, if substantial *in vitro* evidence exists for competition between 2 agents for the amine pump and if such competition can readily explain many or all of the interactions between these agents, then any *in vivo* evidence to the contrary should be taken severely to task before it is accepted. First, the relationship of doses should be adjusted to comply with the relative potencies of these agents *in vitro*. Secondly, since it is abundantly clear that drugs which interact at the amine pump also have other interactions which alter their distribution and metabolism, the only way to assess the effect of an inhibitor is to have an independent measurement of its concentration at the site being studied. Administering single, equal doses and waiting standard times before sacrifice are inadequate procedures to allow meaningful comparisons. The least that should be done is to search a wide dose range and time range *in vivo* before classifying an agent as ineffective.

6. TODA (1972) reported that the inhibition produced by bretylium of the responses of rabbit atria and aorta to transmural stimulation was prevented by cocaine and, indeed, the responses were actually potentiated. On the other hand, guanethidine blockade was prevented but the responses were not potentiated by cocaine. In addition, he reported that the neuron block produced by bretylium was not prevented in the presence of ouabain or during Na^+ deficiency or Ca^{++} excess. Ouabain and Na^+ deficiency are known to reduce the activity of the amine pump (see Section III B). The mechanism whereby excess Ca^{++} affects uptake is different (see Section III D). TODA concluded that since procedures which interfered with the amine pump did not interfere with bretylium-induced blockade, the antagonism of the neuron blocking effects of bretylium by cocaine (and desmethylimipramine) is probably associated with mechanisms other than its competition with bretylium for the amine pump. TODA's results are open to question on several counts: a) The most general criticism is that there were no independent measurements of the extent of the impairment of the amine pump produced by cocaine and the other procedures employed. b) Since cocaine is some 40 times more potent as an inhibitor of the amine pump than bretylium (see Section VIII B) it is not surprising that with the concentrations employed in TODA's study (bretylium, 2×10^{-5} M and cocaine, 3×10^{-6} M) that the influence of cocaine on the uptake of norepinephrine should determine the overall effect on the response to transmural stimulation after the neuron blocking action of bretylium has been negated. It would be revealing to know the relative effect of bretylium (2×10^{-5} M) and cocaine (3×10^{-6} M) in potentiating exogenously administered norepinephrine. c) Cocaine is only some 6–7 times more potent than guanethidine as an inhibitor of norepinephrine uptake. It appears that substantial amounts of cocaine relative to guanethidine would have to be administered in order to enhance the degree of uptake inhibition beyond that already attributable to guanethidine. Since this was apparently not the case, the failure of cocaine to enhance further the response of effector cells is understandable. In addition, guanethidine in concentrations greater than 5×10^{-5} M can inhibit contractions produced by norepinephrine and other agonists. d) The concentration of ouabain used by TODA (2×10^{-7} M) is less than 1/10th the concentration required by BERTI and SHORE (1967) to produce a 50% non-competitive inhibition of the uptake mechanism in rabbit heart. It is highly unlikely that uptake of bretylium was significantly altered by this low concentration of ouabain. Direct evidence on this point would be helpful.

TODA found that reducing Na^+ concentration to approximately 64% of normal did not influence the capacity of bretylium to produce neuronal blockade. This is not surprising since IVERSEN and KRAVITZ (1966) have demonstrated in perfused rat heart that 36% reduction in Na^+ concentration inhibited the pump by only 15%. Therefore, little inhibition of uptake of bretylium would be expected in TODA's experiments.

In addition, TODA increased Ca^{++} to 6.6 mM (3 times normal) and failed to show inhibition of bretylium block. The evidence of BOULLIN (1966) indicates that the capacity of the rat heart to concentrate guanethidine was reduced by less than 30% by 6.6 mM Ca^{++}. Furthermore, the initial rate of uptake of guanethidine was not affected at all by increasing Ca^{++} to 6.6 mM. It does not seem that the uptake and retention of bretylium should be seriously affected by this small increase in Ca^{++} which does little to guanethidine uptake and retention.

B. The "Amine Pump Receptor"

As pointed out by several authors the uptake mechanism for norepinephrine in the cell membrane of adrenergic neurons exhibits the properties of an active transport system, but the complexity of the biological systems studied does not allow direct rigorous proof of this (MITCHELL and OATES, 1970; THOENEN et al., 1968). It is usually considered to be a carrier-mediated process. The evidence for these concepts is based on stereochemical selectivity of the process, dependence on temperature and energy metabolism, uphill transport, saturation kinetics and competitive inhibition kinetics. For purposes of the present discussion we will consider the system as a carrier-mediated process.

The amine pump has been referred to as a "promiscuous pump" in that it will not only process norepinephrine but will concentrate adrenergic neuron blocking agents as well as a variety of other ring-substituted bases and is blocked by tricyclic antidepressants and cocaine (OATES et al., 1971). However, this notion of promiscuity may represent naiveté in thinking about interactions between small organic molecules and biological macromolecules. It is probably more to the point that the known substrates for the pump can all be described as having a moderately large hydrophobic group connected through a one- or two carbon chain to a positively charged basic group. The best substrates are phenethylamine derivates such as norepinephrine. Compounds having larger rings, shorter or longer chains or quaternary or guanidinium, cationic heads rather than protonated primary or secondary amines are poorer substrates (Fig. 36). Thus, in the aortic strip the approximate relative affinities for the pump as judged by ID_{50} values are norepinephrine = 25, amphetamine = 10, guanethidine = 6, and bretylium = 1 (MAXWELL, unpublished observations). All of these substrates bind to the pump receptor, but their affinities differ greatly. It is unlikely that any receptor system accepts only one specific substrate or agonist. Certainly, the *alpha* adrenergic receptor accepts agonists as widely divergent as norepinephrine, naphazoline, and tuaminoheptane (Fig. 37). Likewise, the cholinergic, muscarinic receptor receives agonists as widely divergent as acetylcholine, muscarine, and pilocarpine (Fig 38). If one considers inhibitors of the uptake mechanism one finds that the best inhibitors are generally bulkier molecules than are the substrates. Desmethylimipramine is a very potent inhibitor of the norepinephrine uptake mechanism with an affinity of approximately 1500 relative to 1 for bretylium. Cocaine is also a fair inhibitor of uptake (potency relative to bretylium = 40). Both of these substances are multi-ringed compounds (Fig. 36). Likewise, the *alpha* adrenergic blocking agents phentolamine, piperoxan and azapetine are multi-ringed compounds (Fig. 37) as are the anticholinergics atropine, procyclidine (Fig. 38) and a long list of anticholinergics (see *e. g.* CUTTING, 1969). It seems likely that these receptors have ancillary binding sites that are used by inhibitors but are not used by the substrates.

Several *in vitro* studies have been reported which concern the structure-activity relationships among substrates and inhibitors for the amine pump in the

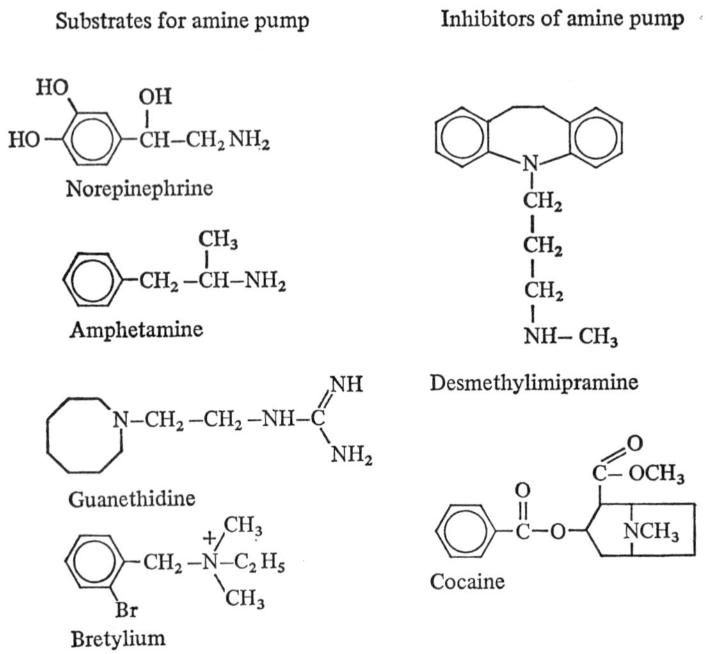

Fig. 36. Structures of several substrates and inhibitors of the "amine pump"

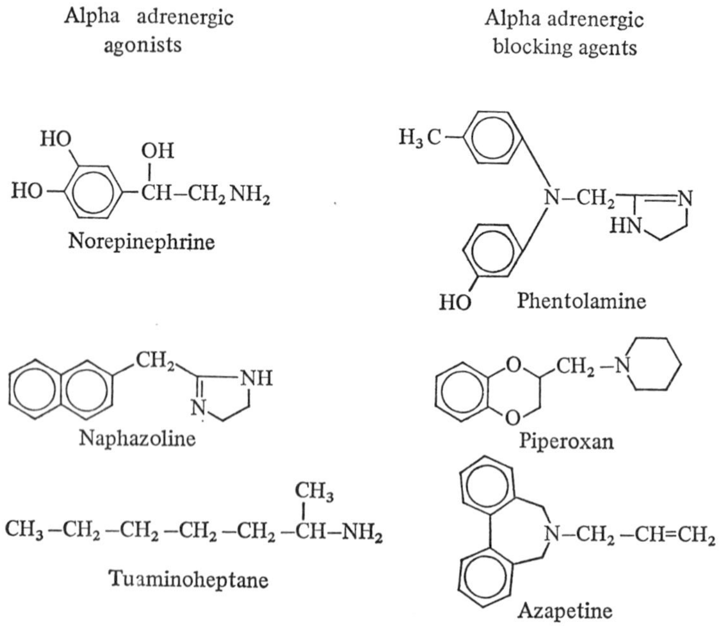

Fig. 37. Structures of several alpha adrenergic receptor agonists and alpha adrenergic blocking agents

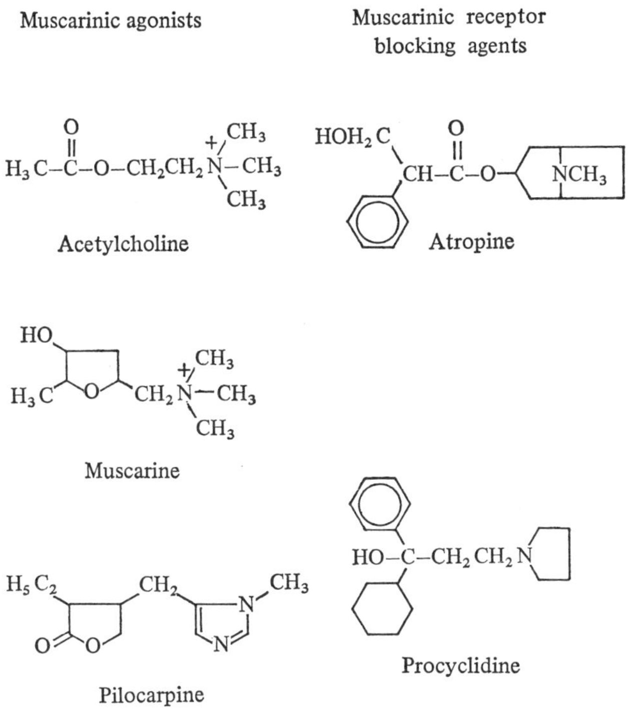

Fig. 38. Structures of several muscarinic receptor agonists and muscarinic receptor blocking agents

cell membranes of peripheral adrenergic nerves. BURGEN and IVERSEN (1965) determined the potencies of a large series of sympathomimetic amines as inhibitors (more likely competitive substrates) of the uptake of tritiated norepinephrine by the isolated, perfused rat heart. From these results they concluded that *beta* hydroxylation, N-substitution or 0-methylation decreased affinity for the neuronal uptake mechanism, but a phenolic hydroxyl group in position 3 or 4 and *alpha*-methylation increased affinity. Unfortunately in this study no attempt was made to determine if the amines had the capacity to release norepinephrine and to calculate the effect of such release on the apparent inhibitory ID_{50}'s which were generated.

CALLINGHAM (1967) studied the effects of the potent inhibitor, imipramine, and related tricyclic compounds on the uptake of norepinephrine into sympathetic nerve endings in isolated perfused rat heart. He concluded that the most potent inhibitors possessed an iminodibenzyl (imipramine) ring system. There was only 3 or 4 fold difference in potency between the most potent and the least potent tricyclic ring system. The least potent compound contained the dibenzocycloheptadiene (amitriptyline) nucleus. Increasing the length of the 3 carbon side chain by one methylene group or reducing it by one methylene group considerably weakened the activity as studied in the imipramine and desmethylimipramine series. Branching of the side chain greatly reduced potency of the compounds. Potencies varied with substitution on the terminal nitrogen such that $NHMe > NMe_2 = N^+Me_3 > NH_2$. These observations which concern potent inhibitors are important with respect to knowledge of the amine pump receptor in that they begin to suggest the chemical requirements for optimal fit.

Maxwell et al. (1969, 1970) pointed out that in a series of tricyclic antidepressants and related compounds if the rings were coplanar the compounds were relatively inactive as inhibitors of uptake into the adrenergic neurons in rabbit aorta, whereas if the phenyl rings were held at angles $> 90°$ and $< 180°$, optimal potency occurred. Furthermore, it was confirmed that N methyl substitution was associated with a 10-fold increase in potency over the NH_2 or NMe_2 derivatives. However, N-ethyl, N-isopropyl, N-butyl derivatives were only weakly active. In addition, it was found that NH_2 or NMe_2 or N^+Me_3 derivatives were approximately equipotent. The pK_a values of the potent, non-quarternary tricyclics were 8.4 or greater and therefore over 90% of the molecules were protonated and thus were present in the positively charged form at pH 7.4. It was concluded that the positively charged form was the one that fit the receptor. In support of this was the fact that the pK_a for norepinephrine, the physiologic substrate, is 9.78 and, therefore, it also is almost totally in the protonated form at physiologic pH. Several dicyclic, antihistamine compounds were found to have reasonable potency. Hence, while tricyclic structure was associated with high potency it was not an absolute requirement. Subsequent studies were carried out with the isomers

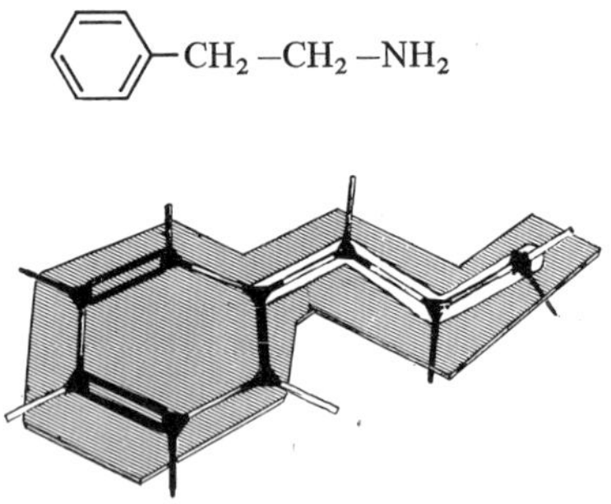

Beta–Phenethylamine

Fig. 39. Molecular model of β-phenethylamine in the planar trans-staggered conformation. Shaded overlay defines the plane of the phenethylamine. N, nitrogen. Also shown is the structural formula for β-phenethylamine. From Maxwell et al. (1970)

of methylphenidate and deoxypipradrol and with cocaine (Maxwell et al., 1970). Marked differences in potency were associated with the various stereo-isomers with one isomer containing the preponderance of activity. The 2R:2'R-(+) threo-enantiomer of methylphenidate, the R(-)-enantiomer of deoxypipradrol and the (2R:3S) enantiomer of cocaine were most active and were all superimposable on one another. Taking all these structure-activity relationships into account, the simplest explanation of the facts was that norepinephrine and other phenethylamine derivatives fit the amine pump in the planar, trans-staggered conformation (Fig. 39) and that the inhibitors took the conformations in Fig. 40. It is suggested that the phenethylamines (and the inhibitors) bind by a single phenyl ring (or part of it) to a hydrophobic surface and that the N^+ binds to a negatively charged atom within the same plane. Adjacent to the negatively charged atom is a hydrophobic area which specifically receives a methyl substitution on the chain N. Substances such as guanethidine, bretylium and bethanidine presumably can assume an approximation to this arrangement of atoms in the receptor and are capable of acceptable, though not very optimal fit. All of the more potent inhibitors bind, in addition, by a second phenyl or carbomethoxyl group to a hydrophobic surface "above" the plane of binding of the phenethylamine. Presumably one reason for the great potency of the tricyclics is that this second phenyl group is fixed in a desirable position by the bridge between it and the first phenyl group. Deoxypipradrol is

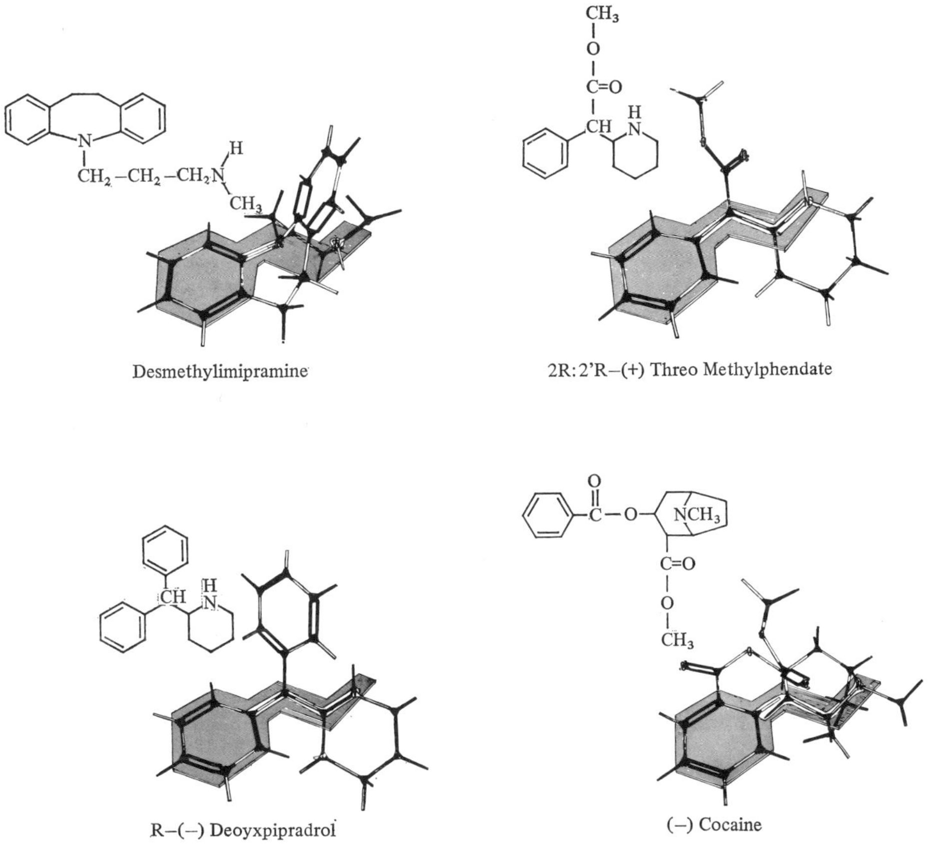

Fig. 40. Molecular models of several inhibitors of norepinephrine uptake in conformations in which one phenyl ring and the chain nitrogen take the same spatial relations as do the phenyl ring and nitrogen of β-phenethylamine in Fig. 39. Shaded overlay defines the "plane of the phenethylamine". Note that the second phenyl ring or the carbomethoxy group is above the plane of the phenethylamine in all the inhibitors. From MAXWELL et al. (1970)

weaker because the second phenyl ring is not fixed and may, therefore, be in less than an optimal conformation. Methylphenidate is still weaker because it has only a planar carbomethoxyl group instead of a second phenyl ring. Cocaine is even weaker because in addition to having the less desirable carbomethoxyl group instead of a phenyl group, the distance between its phenyl ring and the charged N^+ is not fixed by a 2 carbon linkage between these moieties as in deoxypipradrol and methylphenidate but is dependent on the assumption of a specific conformational folding for this proper spacing to occur.

IX. Authors' Perspective

From this vantage point at the end of a long literature review, the authors feel that a brief summary and a point of view are needed. The following very brief summary has been consciously "run through the wringer" of our own biases and judgements for the purpose of making a coherent picture out of sometimes contradictory information. The reader is, therefore, urged to read the rest of this monograph and to draw his own conclusions.

Much of the pharmacology of adrenergic neuron blocking agents can be comprehended on the basis that these agents in high concentrations disrupt the functioning of excitable membranes. They apparently do this by exerting a "local anesthetic-like" effect on these membranes. This action is readily reversible.

The proclivity of these agents for adrenergic neurons is due to the fact that structurally they fulfill at least the minimal requirements to fit the "amine pump" in adrenergic neuron membranes. They are, therefore, pumped into the adrenergic neuron against a concentration gradient in a manner similar to the natural substrate for the pump, norepinephrine. As a consequence of this, these agents achieve high concentrations in the adrenergic nerve terminals and disrupt the release of norepinephrine which normally occurs when action potentials come down the sympathetic neurons. There are several hypotheses as to the function which adrenergic neuron blocking agents disrupt within the nerve terminal. The authors believe that the presently-available evidence favors the view that because of their local anesthetic-like action adrenergic neuron blockers stabilize the neuronal membrane from "inside".

The usefulness of the adrenergic neuron blocking agents resides in the fact that their affinity for the amine pump, while relatively low, is sufficient to permit doses to be administered to animals and man which give rise to plasma levels that are adequate to ensure uptake and concentration in adrenergic nerve endings but which are too low to produce general depression of excitable membranes. Large doses of neuron blocking agents given by any route, or moderate doses given intravenously, produce neuromuscular blockade, ganglionic blockade and conduction blockade. These undesirable secondary effects are relatively prolonged when the doses are given by any route except the intravenous route since a prolonged absorption is thereby involved. They are relatively fleeting when given intravenously due to the rapid rise and subsequent rapid fall in plasma concentration as a result of the distribution of the drugs out of the plasma into tissues. Since the local anesthetic-like action of neuron blocking agents is readily reversible, the undesirable effects secondary to this action disappear as the plasma levels subside.

There is considerable evidence that subchronic, parenteral administration of several adrenergic neuron blocking agents, at doses greater than those needed to produce minimum neuron blockade but not great enough to produce serious secondary effects (*e.g.* neuromuscular blockade), can lead to damage or destruction of adrenergic neurons. The evidence at hand suggests quite clearly that this is due to the excessive accumulation of the blocking agents within the neuron with a consequent disruption of mitochondrial function. Apparently the neuron blocking agents vary in their predeliction for interacting with the mitochondria. It would seem a wise precaution in the therapeutic use of these agents to stick to the lowest dose which will "do the job".

The relatively transient, sympathomimetic effects of these agents are due to a transient release of norepinephrine from adrenergic nerve endings. Presumably the release is from cytoplasmic sites within the neuron rather than from the storage granules since not all of these agents interact with the storage granules.

The differing capacities of the neuron blocking agents to deplete intraneuronal norepinephrine are a result of their differing propensities to block intraneuronal MAO, and to interact with storage granules. Those agents which are known to have weak MAO-inhibiting activity *in vitro* and which do not distribute into storage granules *e.g.*, bretylium, do not deplete norepinephrine from tissues. On the other hand, guanethidine, as a prototype, interacts with storage granules and does not block MAO and is an excellent norepinephrine depleting agent.

The bulk of the experimental data presented regarding the interaction of neuron blocking agents with other drugs, *e.g.*, catecholamines, cocaine, amphetamine and tricyclic antidepressants, can be understood on the basis of competition of the various agents with the neuron blocking agents for access to the adrenergic neuron. Those data which are in apparent disagreement with this generalization, especially *in vivo* data, are explained by the fact that the neuron blocking agent and the other agent (*e.g.* desmethylimipramine) share a common degradative pathway and thus interfere with the metabolism of each other. This disturbs the relationship of the concentrations of the two agents which are presented to the amine pump and leads to conflicting results.

Acknowledgements

The authors gratefully acknowledge the many constructive criticisms which they received from their American colleagues at the Wellcome Research Laboratories, namely, Drs. R. Ferris, G. McKenzie, D. Namm, T. Tsai, C. Wang, R. Welch, and H. White; from their English colleagues at the Wellcome Research Laboratories (Beckenham, Kent, England), Drs. A. Boura and A. Green; and from Professor J. Bevan, Department of Pharmacology, U.C.L.A. Thanks are also extended to Mrs. L. Hall who patiently typed and retyped the manuscript as it progressed from rough draft to completed product.

References

Abbs, E. T.: The acute sensitization of tissues by choline 2:6-xylyl ether (TM10), bretylium and guanethidine. Life Sci. **3**, 99—103 (1962).

Abbs, E. T.: The release of catechol amines by choline 2,6-xylyl ether, bretylium and guanethidine. Brit. J. Pharmacol. **26**, 162—171 (1966).

Abbs, E. T., Dodd, M. G.: The relation between the adrenergic neuron-blocking and noradrenaline-depleting actions of some guanidine derivatives. Brit. J. Pharmacol. **51**, 237—247 (1974).

Abbs, E. T., Pycock, C. J.: The effects of bretylium on the subcellular distribution of noradrenaline and on adrenergic nerve function in rat heart. Brit. J. Pharmacol. **49**, 11—22 (1973).

Abbs, E. T., Robertson, M. I.: Selective depletion of noradrenaline: a proposed mechanism of the adrenergic neurone-blocking action of bretylium. Brit. J. Pharmacol. **38**, 776—791 (1970).

Abboud, F. M., Eckstein, J. W., Pereda, S. A.: Acute hemodynamic responses to intravenous and intra-arterial guanethidine. Amer. J. Physiol. **201**, 462—466 (1961).

Abboud, F. M., Eckstein, J. W.: Vasodilator action of guanethidine. Circulat. Res. **11**, 788—796 (1962).

Abercrombie, G. F., Davies, B. N.: The action of guanethidine with particular reference to the sympathetic nervous system. Brit. J. Pharmacol. **20**, 171—177 (1963).

Abrams, W. B., Pocelinko, R., Klausner, M., Hanauer, L., Whitman, E. N.: Clinical pharmacological studies with debrisoquin sulfate, a new antihypertensive agent. J. New Drugs **4**, 268—283 (1964).

Abrams, W. B., Pocelinko, R., Moe, R. A., Bates, H., Hanauer, L., Camacho, S.: The clinical pharmacology of postganglionic-sympathetic blocking agents. Disease Chest. **48**, 178—186 (1965).

Abrams, W. B., Solomon, H. M.: The human platelet as a pharmacologic model for the adrenergic neuron. Clin. Pharmacol. Ther. **10**, 702—709 (1969).

ABRAMSON, F. B., FURST, C. I., MCMARTIN, C., WADE, R.: The isolation, identification and synthesis of two metabolites of guanethidine formed in pig and rabbit liver homogenates. Biochem. J. **113**, 143—156 (1969).

AHMAD, M., ACHARI, G.: Anti-arrhythmic activity of guanethidine and methyldopa. J. Indian med. Ass. **49**, 363—368 (1968).

ALLEN, J. G., EAST, P. B., FRANCIS, R. J., HAIGH, J. I.: Metabolism of debrisoquine sulfate. Identification of some urinary metabolites in rat and man. Drug Metab. Dispos. **3**, 332—337 (1975).

ALTURA, B. M., ZWEIFACH, B. W.: Influence of reserpine and guanethidine on vascular reactivity and antihistamine constrictor action in the microcirculation. Angiology **17**, 493—502 (1966).

AMSTERDAM, E. A., SPANN, J. F., MASON, D. T., ZELIS, R. F.: Characterization of the positive inotropic effects of bretylium tosylate: a unique property of an antiarrhythmic agent. Amer. J. Cardiol. **25**, 81 (1970).

ANGELETTI, P. U., LEVI-MONTALCINI, R., CARAMIA, F.: Structural and ultrastructural changes in developing sympathetic ganglia induced by guanethidine. Brain Res. **43**, 515—525 (1972).

ANGELETTI, P. U., LEVI-MONTALCINI, R.: Growth inhibition of sympathetic cells by some adrenergic blocking agents. Proc. Nat. Acad. Sci. (Wash.) **69**, 86—88 (1972).

ARAVINDAKSHAN, V., GETTES, L. S.: Effects of bretylium and lidocaine on ventricular fibrillation in the isolated rabbit heart. Cardiovascular Res. **9**, 19—28 (1975).

ASTRÖM, A.: Influence of some local anesthetics upon the adrenaline contraction of isolated strips of rabbit aorta. Acta physiol. scand. **60**, 30—38 (1964).

ATHOS, W. J., MCHUGH, B. P., FINEBERG, S. E., HILTON, J. G.: The effects of guanethidine on the adrenal medulla. J. Pharmacol. exp. Ther. **137**, 229—234 (1962).

AUGSTEIN, J., GREEN, S. M.: Some new adrenergic neurone blocking agents. Nature (Lond.) (**201**), 628—629 (1964).

AXELROD, J.: Studies on sympathomimetic amines. II. The biotransformation and physiological disposition of d-amphetamine, d-p-hydroxyamphetamine and d-methamphetamine. J. Pharmacol. exp. Ther. **110**, 315—326 (1954).

AXELROD, J.: Enzymatic formation of adrenaline and other catechols from monophenols. Science **140**, 499—500 (1963).

Bacaner, M.: Bretylium tosylate for suppression of induced ventricular fibrillation. Amer. J. Cardiol. **17**, 528—534 (1966).

BACANER, M. B.: Quantitative comparison of bretylium with other antifibrillatory drugs. Amer. J. Cardiol. **21**, 504—512 (1968a).

BACANER, M. B.: Treatment of ventricular fibrillation and other acute arrhythmias with bretylium tosylate. Amer. J. Cardiol. **21**, 530—543 (1968b).

BAIN, W. A. Interference with the release of transmitter in response to nerve stimulation Boston: In: *Adrenergic Mechanisms*. Ciba Foundation Symposium. Little, Brown & Co., 1960.

BÁRÁNY, E. H., TREISTER, G.: Time relations of degeneration mydriasis and degeneration vasoconstriction in the rabbit ear after sympathetic denervation. Effect of bretylium. Acta physiol. scand. **80**, 79—92 (1970).

BATH, J., PICKERING, D., TURNER, R.: Clinical experience with bethanidine in treatment of hypertension. Brit. med. J. **1967 IV**, 519—521.

BEIN, H. J.: Some pharmacological properties of guanethidine. In: *Adrenergic Mechanisms*. Ciba Foundation Symposium. Boston: Little, Brown & Co. 1960.

BERNSTEIN, J. G., KOCH-WESER, J.: Effectiveress of bretylium tosylate against refractory ventricular arrhythmias. Circulation **45**, 1024—1034 (1972).

BERTI, F., SHORE, P. A.: A kinetic analysis of drugs that inhibit the adrenergic neuronal membrane amine pump. Biochem. Pharmacol. **16**, 2091—2094 (1967).

BEVAN, J. A., SU, C.: Distribution theory of resistance of neurogenic vasconstriction to alpha-receptor blockade in the rabbit. Circulat. Res. **28**, 179—187 (1971).

BHAGAT, B.: Modification of the effects of guanethidine on cardiac catechol-amines by various agents. Brit. J. Pharmacol. **22**, 238—245 (1964).

BHAGAT, B., SHIDEMAN, F. E.: Mechanism of the positive inotropic responses to bretylium and guanethidine. Brit. J. Pharmacol. **20**, 56—62 (1963).

BHARGAVA, K. P., JAJU, B. P., TANGRI, K. K.: Mechanism of the central hypotensive action of guanethidine. Brit. J. Pharmacol. **27**, 491—496 (1966).

BIGGER, J. T., JAFFE, C. C.: The effect of bretylium tosylate on the electrophysiologic properties of ventricular muscle and Purkinje fibers. Amer. J. Cardiol. **27**, 82—92 (1971).

BISSON, G. M., MUSCHOLL, E.: Die Beziehung zwischen der Guanethidine-Konzentration im Rattenherzen und dem Noradrenalingehalt. Naunyn-Schmiedeberg's Arch. exp. Path. Pharmak. **244**, 185—194 (1962).

BLAIR, D. A., GLOVER, W. E., KIDD, B. S. L., RODDIE, I. C.: Peripheral vascular effects of bretylium tosylate in man. Brit. J. Pharmacol. **15**, 466—475 (1960).

BOCK, K. D., HEIMSOTH, V.: Persistierende orthostatische Hypotonie nach Behandlung mit Guanacline. Dtsch. med. Wschr. **94**, 265—270 (1969).

BOGDANSKI, D. F., BRODIE, B. B.: Role of sodium and potassium ions in storage of norepinephrine by sympathetic nerve endings. Life Sci. **5**, 1563—1569 (1966).

BOULLIN, D. J.: Reduction of ^{14}C-guanethidine levels in rat heart and diaphragm by excess calcium. Brit. J. Pharmacol. **28**, 289—295 (1966).

BOULLIN, D. J.: A calcium requirement for release of ^{3}H-guanethidine by sympathetic nerve stimulation. J. Pharm. Pharmacol. **18**, 709—712 (1966).

BOULLIN, D. J.: The action of extracellular cations on the release of the sympathetic transmitter from peripheral nerves. J. Physiol. (Lond.) **189**, 85—99 (1967).

BOULLIN, D. J.: Evidence for intra-cellular guanethidine stores in the rat heart revealed after removal of calcium ions. Brit. J. Pharmacol. **32**, 145—155 (1968).

BOULLIN, D. J., COSTA, E., BRODIE, B. B.: Discharge of tritium-labeled guanethidine by sympathetic nerve stimulation as evidence that guanethidine is a false transmitter. Life Sci. **5**, 803—808 (1966).

BOULLIN, D. J., OBRIEN, R. A.: Uptake of debrisoquin and guanethidine by human blood platelets. J. Pharm. Pharmacol. **20**, 403—404 (1968).

BOULLIN, D. J., OBRIEN, R. A.: The accumulation of guanethidine by human blood platelets. Brit. J. Pharmacol. **35**, 90—102 (1969).

BOURA, A. L. A., COPP, F. C., GREEN, A. F.: New antiadrenergic compounds. Nature (Lond.) **184** B. A. 70—71 (1959a).

BOURA, A. L. A., COPP, F. C., DUNCOMBE, W. G., GREEN, A. F., MCCOUBREY, A.: The selective accumulation of bretylium in sympathetic ganglia and their postganglionic nerves. Brit. J. Pharmacol. **15**, 265—270 (1960).

BOURA, A. L. A., COPP, F. C., GREEN, A. F., HODSON, H. F., RUFFELL, G. K., SIM, M. F., WALTON, E., GRIVSKY, E. M.: Adrenergic neuron blocking agents related to choline 2,6-xylyl ether bromide (TM 10), bretylium and guanethidine. Nature (Lond.) **191**, 1312—1313 (1961).

BOURA, A. L., A. DUNCOMBE, W. G., ROBSON, R. D., MCCOUBREY, A.: The distribution and excretion by cats of a new hypotensive drug, N-benzyl-N'N''-dimethylguanidine. J. Pharm. Pharmacol. **14**, 722—726 (1962).

BOURA, A. L. A., GREEN, A. F.: The actions of bretylium: adrenergic neurone blocking and other effects. Brit. J. Pharmacol. **14**, 536—548 (1959).

BOURA, A. L. A., GREEN, A. F.: Comparison of bretylium and guanethidine: Tolerance and effects on adrenergic nerve function and responses to sympathommetic amines. Brit. J. Pharmacol. **19**, 13—41 (1962).

BOURA, A. L. A., GREEN, A. F.: Adrenergic neurone blockade and other acute effects caused by N-benzyl-N'N''-dimethylguanidine and its ortho-chloro derivate. Brit. J. Pharmacol. **20**, 36—55 (1963).

BOURA, A. L. A., GREEN, A. F.: Adrenergic neuron blocking agents. Ann. Rev. Pharmacol. **5**, 183—212 (1965).

BOURA, A. L. A., GREEN, A. F., MCCOUBREY, A., LAURENCE, D. R., MOULTON, R., ROSENHEIM, M. L.: Darenthin, hypotensive agent of new type. Lancet **1959b II**, 17—21.

BOYD, H., CHANG, V., RAND, M. J.,: The local anaesthetic activity of bretylium in relation to its action in blocking sympathetic responses. Arch. int. Pharmacodyn. **131**, 10—23 (1961).

BREST, A. N.: Hemodynamic response to antihypertensive drug therapy. J. Amer. med. Ass. **192**, 41—44 (1965).

BRODIE, B. B., KUNTZMAN, R.: Pharmacological consequences of selective deleption of catecchol amines by antihypertensive agents. Ann. N. Y. Acad. Sci. **88**, 939—943 (1960).

BRODIE, B. B., CHANG, C. C., COSTA, E.: On the mechanism of action of guanethidine and bretylium. Brit. J. Pharmacol. **25**, 171—178 (1965).

BROWN, B. G., HEY, P.: Choline phenyl ethers as inhibitors of amine oxidase. Brit. J. Pharmacol. **11**, 58—65 (1956).

BUCKLEY, J. J., BOSCH, O. K., BACANER, M. B.: Prevention of ventricular fibrillation during hypothermia with bretylium tosylate. Anesthesia and Analgesia **50**, 587—593 (1971).

BURGEN, A. S. V., IVERSEN, L. L.: The inhibition of noradrenaline uptake by sympathomimetic amines in the rat isolated heart. Brit. J. Pharmacol. **25**, 34—49 (1965).

BURN, J. H.: Release of noradrenaline from the sympathetic postganglionic fibre. Brit. med. J. **2**, 197—201 (1967).

BURN, J. H., RAND, M. J.: New interpretation of the adrenergic nerve fiber. Advanc. Pharmacol. **1**, 1—30 (1962).

BURN, J. H., WELSH, F.: The effect of calcium in removing the blocking action of bretylium and guanethidine. Brit. J. Pharmacol. **31**, 74—81 (1967).

Burnstock, G., Holman, M. E.: An electrophysiological investigation of the actions of some autonomic blocking drugs on transmission in the guinea-pig vas deferens. Brit. J. Pharmacol. **23**, 600—612 (1964).
Burnstock, G., Doyle, A. E. Gannon, B. J., Gerkens, J. F., Iwayama, T., Mashford, M. L.: Prolonged hypotension and ultrastructural changes in sympathetic neurones following guanacline treatment. Europ. J. Pharmacol. **13**, 175—187 (1971a).
Burnstock, G., Evans, B., Gannon, B. J., Heath, J. W., James, V.: A new method of destroying adrenergic nerves in adult animals using guanethidine. Brit. J. Pharmacol. **43**, 295—301 (1971b).
Burnstock, G., McLean, J. R., Wright, M.: Noradrenaline uptake by non-innervated smooth muscle. Brit. J. Pharmacol. **43**, 180—189 (1971c).
Butterfield, J. L., Richardson, J. A.: Acute effects of guanethidine on myocardial contractility and catecholamine levels. Proc. Soc. exp. Biol. (N.Y.) **106**, 259—262 (1961).
Cabrera, R., Torrance, R. W., Viveros, H.: The action of acetyl choline and other drugs upon the terminal parts of the postganglionic sympathetic fibre. Brit. J. Pharmacol. **27**, 51—63 (1966).
Calesnick, B., Sheppard, H., Bowen, N., Kamdar, J.: Direct comparison of ^{14}C-guanethidine (Ismelin) excretion following oral and subcutaneous administration. Biochem. Pharmacol. **8**, 49 (1961).
Callingham, B. A.: The effects of imipramine and related compounds on the uptake of noradrenaline into sympathetic nerve endings. In :Garattine, S., Dukes, M. (Eds.): Antidepressant drugs, pp. 35—43. Milan: Excerpta Medica Foundation, 1967.
Callingham, B. A., Cass, R.: The effects of bretylium and cocaine on noradrenaline depletion. J. Pharm. Pharmacol. **14**, 385—389 (1962).
Campbell, E. D. R., Montuschi, E.: Muscle weakness caused by bretylium tosylate. Lancet **1960 II**, 789.
Campos, H. A., Stitzel, R. E., Shideman, F. E.: Actions of tyramine and cocaine on catecholamine levels in subcellular fractions of the isolated cat heart. J. Pharmacol. exp. Therap. **141**, 290—300 (1963).
Canas-Rodriguez, A.: Preliminary studies of the metabolism of 2-guanidinomethyl-1:4-benzodioxan sulfate (Guanoxan). Experientia (Basel) **22**, 472—473 (1966).
Caramia, F., Angeletti, P. U., Levi-Montalcini, R., Caratelli, L.: Mitochondrial lesions of developing sympathetic neurons induced by bertylium tosylate. Brain Res. **40**, 237—246 (1972).
Carlsson, A.: Pharmacological depletion of catecholamine stores. Pharmacol. Rev. **18**, 541—549 (1966).
Carlsson, A., Hillarp, N.-Å., Waldeck, B.: Analysis of the Mg^{++}—ATP dependent storage mechanism in the amine granules of the adrenal medulla. Acta physiol. scand. **59**, Suppl. 215, 1—38 (1963).
Carlsson, A., Rosengren, E., Bertler, A., Nilsson, J.: Effect of reserpine on the metabolism of catecholamines. In: Garattini, S., and Ghetti, V. (Eds.): Psychotropic Drugs. Amsterdam: Elsevier Pub. Co. 1957.
Carlsson, A., Waldeck, B.: Inhibition of H^3-metaraminol uptake by antidepressive and related agents. J. Pharm. Pharmacol. **17**, 243—244 (1965a).
Carlsson, A., Waldeck, B.: Mechanism of amine transport in the cell membranes of the adrenergic nerves. Acta Pharmacol. Toxicol. **22**, 293—300 (1965b).
Carlsson, A., Waldeck, B.: The accumulation of [^{3}H] noradrenaline in the adrenergic nerve fibers of reserpine-treated mice. J. Pharm. Pharmacol. **19**, 182—190 (1967).
Cass, R., Callingham, B. A.: Some effects of drugs which influence sympathetic transmission on tissue catecholamine levels in the rat. Biochem. Pharmacol. **13**, 1619—1625 (1964).
Cass, R., Kuntzman, R., Brodie, B. B.: Norepinephrine depletion as a possible mechanism of action of guanethidine (Su-5864), a new hypotensive agent. Proc. Soc. exp. Biol. Med. **103**, 871—872 (1960).
Cass, R., Spriggs, T. L. B.: Tissue amine levels and sympathetic blockade after guanethidine and bretylium. Brit. J. Pharmacol. **17**, 442—450 (1961).
Castaneda, A., Bacaner, M.: Effect of bretylium tosylate on the prevention and treatment of postoperative arrhythmias. Amer. J. Cardiol. **25**, 461—466 (1970).
Castren, J. A., Pohjola, S.: Guanethidine and aqueous humor dynamics. Acta ophthal. (Kbh.) **40**, 348—361 (1962).
Cervoni, P., Ellis, C. H., Maxwell, R, A.: The anti-arrhythmic action of bretylium in normal, reserpine-pretreated and chronically denervated dog hearts. Arch. Int. Pharmacodyn. Therap. **190**, 91—102 (1971).
Cervoni, P., Kirpekar, S. M., Schwab, A.: The effect of drugs on uptake and release of catecholamines in the isolated left atrium of the guinea pig. J. Pharmacol. exp. Therap. **151**, 196—206 (1966).

Chamberlain, D. A., Howard, J.: Guanethidine and methyldopa: a haemodynamic study. Brit. Heart J. **26**, 528—536 (1964).

Chang, C. C., Chang, J. C.: A change in the subcellular distribution of noradrenaline in the rat isolated vas deferens effected by nerve stimulation. Brit. J. Pharmacol. **25**, 758—762 (1965).

Chang, C. C., Chang, J. C., Su, C. Y.: Studies on the interactions of guanethidine and bretylium with noradrenaline stores. Brit. J. Pharmacol. **30**, 213—223 (1967a).

Chang, C. C., Chen, T. F., Cheng, H. C.: On the mechanism of neuromuscular blocking action of bretylium and guanethidine. J. Pharmacol. exp. Therap. **158**, 89—98 (1967b).

Chang, C. C., Costa, E., Brodie, B. B.: Reserpine-induced release of drugs from sympathetic nerve endings. Life Sci. **3**, 839—844 (1964).

Chang, C. C., Costa, E., Brodie, B. B.: Interaction of guanethidine with adrenergic neurons. J. Pharmacol. exp. Therap. **147**, 303—312 (1965).

Chang, C. C., Lai, F. M., Chiueh, C. C.: Effects of calcium on smooth muscles and on the adrenergic neuron blocking action of guanethidine. Arch. int. Pharmacodyn. **190**, 34—46 (1971).

Chang, C. C., Su, C. Y.: Effect of cold stress on the subcellular distribution of noradrenaline in the rat heart. J. Pharm. Pharmacol. **19**, 73—77 (1967).

Chernick, W. S.: Local anesthetics. In: Di Palma, J. R. (Ed.): Drill's Pharmacology in Medicine, 4th ed. New York: McGraw-Hill, 1971.

Chruściel, T. L.: Sympatholytic drugs and some enzymes involved in the metabolism of catecholamines. Int. J. Neuropharmacol. **1**, 137—140 (1962).

Clarke, D. E., Leach, G. D. H.: The influence of bretylium on the interactions of infused sympathomimetic amines and tyramine in the reserpine-treated pithed rat. Brit. J. Pharmacol. **32**, 392—401 (1968).

Clarke, D. E.: Restoration of tyramine responses by bretylium, B.W. 392C60, bethanidine and monoamine oxidase inhibitors in reserpine treated rats. Brit. J. Pharmacol. **38**, 1—11 (1970).

Cohn, J. N., Liptak, T. E., Freis, E. D.: Hemodynamic effects of guanethidine in man. Circulat. Res. **12**, 298—307 (1963).

Consolo, S., Dolfini, E. Garattini, S., Valzelli, L.: Desipramine and amphetamine metabolism. J. Pharm. Pharmacol. **19**, 253—256 (1967).

Copp, F. C.: Adrenergic neurone blocking agents. Advanc. Drug Res. **1**, 161—189 (1964).

Costa, E., Boullin, D. J., Hammer, W., Vogel, W., Brodie, B. B.: Interactions of drugs with adrenergic neurons. Pharm. Rev. **18**, Part 1, 577—597 (1966).

Costa, E., Chang, C., Brodie, B. B.: Interaction of guanethidine with adrenergic neurons at a molecular level. Pharmacologist **6**, 174 (1964).

Costa, E., Kuntzman, R., Gessa, G. L., Brodie, B. B.: Structural requirements for bretylium and guanethidine-like activity in a series of guanidine derivatives. Life Sci. **1**, 75—80 (1962).

Cotton, S. G., Montuschi, E.: Side effects of guanoxan. Brit. med. J. **1966 I**, 51.

Cox, R. H., Maickel, R. P.: Effects of guanethidine on rat brain serotonin and norepinephrine Life Sci. **8**, 1319—1324 (1969).

Creveling, C. R., Daly, J. W., Witkop, B., Udenfriend, S.: Substrates and inhibitors of dopamine-β-oxidase. Biochim. Biophysica Acta (Amst.) **64**, 125—134 (1962).

Cutting, W. C.: Handbook of Pharmacology. 4th ed. New York: Appleton—Century—Crofts Division of Meredith Corp. 1969.

Dailey, J. W., Westfall, T. C.: Effect of actinomycin D on the recovery of cardiac noradrenaline after depletion with guanethidine. J. Pharm. Pharmacol. **21**, 197—198 (1969).

Dagirmanjian, R.: The effects of guanethidine on the noradrenaline content of the hypothalamus in the cat and rat. J. Pharm. Pharmacol. **15**, 518—521 (1963).

Davey, M. J., Farmer, J. B.: The mode of action of tyramine. J. Pharm. Pharmacol. **15**, 178—182 (1963).

Davey, M. J., Hayden, M. L., Scholfield, P. C.: The effects of bretylium on C fibre excitation and noradrenaline release by acetylcholine and electrical stimulation. Brit. J. Pharmacol. **34**, 377—387 (1968).

Davey, M. J., Reinert, H.: Pharmacology of the antihypertensive guanoxan. Brit. J. Pharmacol. **24**, 29—48 (1965).

Dawborn, J. K., Doyle, A. E., Ebringer, A., Howqua, J., Jerums, G., Johnston, C. I., Mashford, M. L., Parkin, J. D.: Persistent postural hypotension due to guanacline. Pharmacol. Clin. **2**, 1—5 (1969).

Day, H. W., Bacaner, M.: Use of bretylium tosylate in the management of acute myocardial infarction. Amer. J. Cardiol. **27**, 177—189 (1971).

Day, M. D., Rand, M. J.: Antagonism of guanethidine by dexamphetamine and other related sympathomimetic amines. J. Pharm. Pharmacol. **14**, 541—549 (1962).

Day, M. D., Rand, M. J.: Evidence for a competitive antagonism of guanethidine by dexamphetamine. Brit. J. Pharmacol. **20**, 17—28 (1963).

DE LA LANDE, I. S., HODGE, R. L., LAZNER, M., JELLET, L. B., WATERSON, J. G.: Pharmacological implications of the fate of noradrenaline in the artery wall. Circulat. Res. **26—27**, Supple II, 41—48 (1970).

DEGUCHI, T., NARAHASHI, T.: Effects of procaine on ionic conductances of end-plate membranes. J. Pharmacol. exp. Therap. **176**, 423—433 (1961).

DENGLER, H. J., SPIEGEL, H. E., TITUS, E. O.: Uptake of tritium-labeled norepinephrine in brain and other tissues of cat *in vitro*. Science **133**, 1072—1073 (1961).

DES PREZ, R., HELMAN, R., OATES, J. A.: Inhibition of endotoxin fever by reserpine. Proc. Soc. exp. Biol. **122**, 746—749 (1966).

DIXIT, B. N., GULATI, O. D., GOKHALE, S. D.: Action of bretylium and guanethidine at the neuromuscular junction. Brit. J. Pharmacol. **17**, 372—379 (1961).

DOLLERY, C. T.: The use of bretylium tosylate (Darenthin) in hypertension. Med. Clin. N. Amer. **45**, 429—439 (1961).

DOLLERY, C. T., EMSLIE-SMITH, D., MILNE, M. D.: Clinical and pharmacological studies with guanethidine in the treatment of hypertension. Lancet **1960 II**, 381—387.

DORÉ, F., LEBLANC, J., CÔTÉ, J.: Effects of guanethidine and imidazole on histamine metabolism. Can. J. Physiol. Pharmacol. **52**, 978—983 (1974).

DOWNING, O. A., JUUL, P.: The effect of guanethidine pretreatment on transmission in the superior cervical ganglion. Acta. Pharmacol. Toxicol. **32**, 369—381 (1973).

DOYLE, A. E., FRASER, J. R., SMITH, P. K.: Effects of bretylium tosylate on blood pressure, cardiac output and renal function in hypertension. Brit. Med. J. **1960 II**, 422—425.

DOYLE, A. E., MORLEY, A.: Studies on the absorption and excretion of [^{14}C]-bethanidine in man. Brit. J. Pharmacol. **24**, 701—704 (1965).

DUNCOMBE, W. G., MCCOUBREY, A.: The excretion and stability to metabolism of bretylium. Brit. J. Pharmacol. **15**, 260—264 (1960).

DVORNIK, D., KRAML, M., DUBUC, J., TOM, H., ZSOTER, T.: The effect of some inhibitors of the postganglionic sympathetic mechanism on monoamine oxidase. Biochem. Pharmacol. **12**, 229—240 (1963).

EISENFELD, A. J., AXELROD, J., KRAKOFF, L.: Inhibition of the extraneuronal accumulation and metabolism of norepinephrine by adrenergic blocking agents. J. Pharmacol. exp. Ther. **156**, 107—113 (1967a).

EISENFELD, A. J., LANDSBERG, L., AXELROD, J.: Effect of drugs on the accumulation and metabolism of extraneuronal norepinephrine in the rat heart. J. Pharmacol. exp. Ther. **158**, 378—385, (1967b).

ELLIS, C. H., BARNES, M., COZZI, M.: Antiarrhythmic actions of bretylium. Fed. Proc. **27**, 406 (1968).

ERÄNKÖ, L., ERÄNKÖ, O.: Effect of guanethidine on nerve cells and small intensely fluorescent cells in sympathetic ganglia of newborn and adult rats. Acta Pharmacol. Toxicol. **30**, 403—416 (1971).

EULER, V. S. VON, LISHAJKO: In: KOELLE, DOUGLAS, CARLSSON (Eds.): Proceedings of the second international pharmacological meeting, Vol. 3, 245—260. Oxford: Pergamon Press 1964.

EVANSON, J. M., SEARS, H. T. N.: Comparison of bretylium tosylate with guanethidine in the treatment of severe hypertension. Lancet **1960 II**, 387—389.

EXLEY, K. A.: The blocking action of choline 2:6-xylyl ether bromide on adrenergic nerves. Brit. J. Pharmacol. **12**, 297—305 (1957).

EXLEY, K. A.: The persistence of adrenergic nerve conduction after TM_{10} or bretylium in the cat. In "Adrenergic Mechanisms", Ciba Foundation Symposium. Boston: Little, Brown 1960.

FANN, W. E., CAVANAUGH, J. H., KAUFMANN, J. S., GRIFFITH, J. D., DAVIS, J. M., JANOWSKY, D. S., OATES, J. A.: Doxepin: Effects on transport of biogenic amines in man. Psychopharmacologia **22**, 111—125 (1971a).

FANN, W. E., JANOWSKY, D. S., DAVIS, J. M., OATES, J. A.: Chlorpromazine reversal of the antihypertensive action of guanethidine. Lancet **1971 b** II, 436—437.

FAWAZ, G.: Cardiovascular pharmacology. Ann. Rev. Pharmacol. **3**, 57—90 (1963).

FEAGIN, O. T., MITCHELL, J. R., SHAND, D. G., OATES, J. A.: Uptake and release of guanethidine and bethanidine by adrenergic neurons. J. clin. Invest. **48**, 23a (1969).

FERRY, C. B., NORRIS, B.: Actions of bretylium tosylate at the neuromuscular junction. Brit. J. Pharmacol. **41**, 607—621 (1971).

FEWINGS, J. D., HODGE, R. L., SCROOP, G. C., WHELAN, R. F.: The effects of bethanidine on the peripheral circulation in man. Brit. J. Pharmacol. **23**, 115—122 (1964).

FISCHER, J. E., WEISE, V. K., KOPIN, I. J.: Interactions of bretylium and acetylcholine at sympathetic nerve endings. J. Pharmacol. exp. Therap. **153**, 523—529 (1966).

FLEGIN, O.T., MORGAN, D.H., OATES, J.A., SHAND, D.G.: The mechanism of the reversal of the effect of guanethidine by amphetamines in cat and man. Brit. J. Pharmacol. **39**, 253P—254P (1970).

FOLLENFANT, M.J., ROBSON, R.D.: The antagonism of adrenergic neurone blockade by amphetamine and dexamphetamine in the rat and guinea-pig. Brit. J. Pharmacol. **38**, 792—801 (1970).

FURCHGOTT, R.F.: Restoration of response to tyramine in reserpinized atria pretreated with norepinephrine: Influence of MAO inhibitors and bretylium. Pharmacologist **6**, 205 (1964).

FURCHGOTT, R.F.: In Physiology and Pharmacology of Vascular Neuroeffector Systems, p. 140. Basel: Karger 1971.

FURCHGOTT, R.F., KIRPEKAR, S.M., RIEKER, M., SCHWAB, A.: Actions and interactions of norepinephrine, tyramine and cocaine on aortic strips of rabbit and left atria of guinea pig and cat. J. Pharmacol. exp. Therap. **142**, 39—58 (1963).

FURCHGOTT, R.F., SANCHEZ-GARCIA, P.: Inhibition of monamine oxidase of adrenergic nerve terminals by bretylium. Pharmacologist **8**, 176 (1966).

FURCHGOTT, R.F., SANCHEZ-GARCIA, P., WAKADE, A.R., CERVONI, P.: Interactions of bretylium and other drugs on guinea-pig atria: evidence for inhibition of neuronal monamine oxidase by bretylium. J. Pharmacol. exp. Therap. **179**, 171—185 (1971).

FURST, C.I.: Studies on the metabolism in vitro of [14C]-guanethidine including polarographic measurements of the oxygen uptake. Biochem. J. **104**, 1P (1967a).

FURST, C.I.: The biochemistry of guanethidine. Advanc. Drug Res. **4**, 133—161 (1967b).

FURST, C.I.: Studies on the distribution and excretion of a metabolite of guanethidine in the rat. Brit. J. Pharmacol. **32**, 57—64 (1968).

GAFFNEY, T.E.: Effect of guanethidine and bretylium on the dog heart-lung preparation. Circ. Res. **9**, 83—88 (1961).

GAFFNEY, T.E., BRAUNWALD, E., COOPER, T.: Analysis of the acute circulatory effects of guanethidine and bretylium. Circulat. Res. **10**, 83—88 (1962).

GAFFNEY, T.E., CHIDSEY, C.A., BRAUNWALD, E.: Study of the relationship between the neurotransmitter store and adrenergic nerve block induced by reserpine and guanethidine. Circulat. Res. **12**, 264—268 (1963).

GANNON, B.J., IWAYAMA, T., BURNSTOCK, G., GERKENS, J., MASHFORD, M.L.: Prolonged effects of chronic guanethidine treatment on the sympathetic innervation of the genitalia of male rats. Med. J. Aust. **2**, 207—208 (1971).

GARCÍA, A.G., SÁNCHEZ-GARCÍA, P.: Influence of cocaine and sodium on bretylium uptake by reserpine-treated guinea-pig left atrium. Brit. J. Pharmacol. **53**, 247—255 (1975).

GERKENS, F.: Guanethidine and guanacline on the rat vas deferens. Brit. J. Pharmacol. **52**, 191—195 (1974a).

GERKENS, J.F.: Effect of long-term treatment with guanacline or guanethidine on sympathetic function. Eur. J. Pharmacol. **26**, 143—150 (1974b).

GERKENS, J.F., MCCULLOCH, M.W., WILSON, J.: Mechanism of the antagonism between guanethidine and dexamphetamine. Brit. J. Pharmacol. **35**, 563—572 (1969).

GERTNER, S.B., ROMANO, A.: Action of guanethidine and bretylium on ganglionic transmission. Fed. Proc. **20**, 319 (1961).

GIACHETTI, A., SHORE, P.A.: Studies *in vitro* of amine uptake mechanisms in heart. Biochem. Pharmacol. **15**, 607—614 (1966).

GIACHETTI, A., SHORE, P.A.: Monoamine oxidase inhibition in the adrenergic neuron by bretylium, debrisoquin, and other adrenergic neuronal blocking agents. Biochem. Pharm. **16**, 237—238 (1967).

GIFFORD, R.W.: Bethanidine sulfate-a new antihypertensive agent. J. Amer. med. Ass. **193**, 901—905 (1965).

GILLESPIE, J.S., MUIR, T.C.: Species and tissue variation in extraneuronal and neuronal accumulation of noradrenaline. J. Physiol. (Lond.) **206**, 591—604 (1970).

GILL, J.R., BARTTER, F.C.: Importance of adrenergic nervous system for sodium conservation during sodium deprivation in normal man. J. clin. Invest. **43**, 1272 (1964).

GILL, J.R., MASON, D.T., BARTTER, F.C.: Adrenergic nervous system in sodium metabolism: effects of guanethidine and sodium retaining steroids in normal man. J. clin. Invest. **43**, 177—184 (1964).

GILLIS, C.N., NASH, C.W.: The initial pressor actions of bretvlium tosylate and guanethidine sulfate and their relation to release of catecholamines. J. Pharmacol. exp. Therap. **134**, 1—7 (1961).

GILMORE, J.P., SIEGEL, J.H.: Mechanism of the myocardial effects of bretylium. Circulat. Res. **10**, 347—353 (1962).

GLOWINSKI, J., AXELROD, J.: Effect of drugs on the uptake, release, and metabolism of H^3-norepinephrine in the rat brain. J. Pharmacol. exp. Therap. **149**, 43—49 (1965).

GOKHALE, S. D., GULATI, O. D.: Potentiation of inhibitory and excitatory effects of catechol amines by bretylium. Brit. J. Pharmacol. **16**, 327—334 (1961).
GOKHALE, S. D., GULATI, O. D., KELKAR, V. V.: Mechanism of the initial adrenergic effects of bretylium and guanethidine. Brit. J. Pharmacol. **20**, 362—377 (1963).
GOKHALE, S. D., GULATI, O. D., KELKAR, V. V.: Supersensitivity to catecholamines following guanethidine. Brit. J. Pharmacol. **30**, 445—462 (1967).
GRAHAM, J. D., CHANDLER, B. M.: The effects of lidocaine, propranolol, procaine amide and bretylium tosylate on the contractility of isolated cat papillary muscles. Can. J. Physiol. Pharmacol. **51**, 763—773 (1973).
GREEN, A. F.: Antihypertensive drugs. Advanc. Pharmacol. **1**, 161—225 (1962).
GREEN, A. F.: In: *Physiology and Pharmacology of Vascular Neuroeffector Systems*, p. 139—140. Basel: Karger 1971.
GREEN, A. F., HUGHES, R.: Effects of adrenergic neurone blocking agents on voluntary muscle stimulated at different frequencies. Brit. J. Pharmacol. **27**, 164—176 (1966).
GREEN, A. F., ROBSON, R. D.: Comparison of the effects of bretylium, guanethidine and bethanidine on smooth muscle responses to different rates of sympathetic nerve stimulation. Brit. J. Pharmacol. **22**, 349—355 (1964).
GREEN, A. F., ROBSON, R. D.: Adrenergic neurone blocking agents: tolerance and hypersensitivity to adrenaline and noradrenaline. Brit. J. Pharmacol. **25**, 497—506 (1965).
GRIPENBERG, J.: Incorporation of guanethidine into isolated rat peritoneal mast cells and mast cell granules *in vitro*. Acta physiol. scand. **88**, 516—527 (1972).
GULATI, O. D., JAYKAR, S.: Factors affecting the action of guanethidine on adrenergic neurones. Brit. J. Pharmacol. **42**, 352—363 (1971).
HARRISON, D. C., CHIDSEY, C. A., GOLDMAN, R., BRAUNWALD, E.: Relationships between the release and tissue depletion of norepinephrine from the heart by quanethidine and reserpine. Circulat. Res. **12**, 256—263 (1963).
HATTORI, K., SHIBATA, S.: The effect of cocaine on catechol-o-methyl transferase and on the response to norepinephrine of rabbit aortic strips. Japan J. Pharmacol. **21**, 559—562 (1971).
HÄUSLER, G.: In: *Physiology and Pharmacology of Vascular Neuroeffector Systems*, p. 139—140. Basel: Karger 1971.
HÄUSLER, G., HAEFELY, W., HUERLIMANN, A.: On the mechanism of the adrenergic nerve blocking action of bretylium. Naunyn-Schmiedebergs Arch. exp. Path. Pharmak. **265**, 260—277 (1969).
HÄUSLER, G., LORENZ, H. P., BARTHOLINI, G., KETTLER, R., TRANZER, J. P.: Absence of degeneration of adrenergic neurons after prolonged treatment with debrisoquin. J. Pharmacol. exp. Ther. **189**, 646—658 (1974).
HÄUSLER, G., THOENEN, H., HAEFELY, W., HÜRLIMANN, A.: Durch Acetylcholin hervorgerufene antidrome Aktivität im kardinalen Sympathicus and Noradrenalinfreisetzung unter Guanethidin. Helv. Physiol. Pharmacol. Acta **26**, CR 352—354 (1968).
HAZARD, R., BEAUVALLET, M., RENIER-CORNEC, A., LARNO, S., MOUILLÉ, P.: Effets presseurs et adrenalinosecreteurs de l'acetylcholine et du potassium chez le chien soumis á l'action de la guanethidine. C. R. Soc. Biol. **158**, 1322—1326 (1964).
HERTTING, G., AXELROD, J., PATRICK, R. W.: Actions of bretylium and guanethidine on the uptake and release of [^{3}H]-noradrenaline. Brit. J. Pharmacol. **18**, 161—166 (1962).
HERTTING, G., AXELROD, J., WHITBY, L. G.: Effect of drugs on the uptake and metabolism of H^3-norepinephrine. J. Pharmacol. exp. Therap. **134**, 146—153 (1961).
HERTTING, G., WIDHALM, S.: Über den Mechanismus der Noradrenalin-Freisetzung aus sympathischen Nervenendigungen. Naunyn-Schmiedebergs Arch. exp. Path. Pharmak. **250**, 257—258 (1965).
HEY, P., WILLEY, G. L.: Choline 2:6-xylyl ether bromide; an active quaternary local anaesthetic. Brit. J. Pharmacol. **9**, 471—475 (1954).
HIFT, H., CAMPOS, H. A.: Changes in the subcellular distribution of cardiac catecholamines in dogs dying in irreversible haemorrhagic shock. Nature (Lond.) **196**, 678—679 (1962).
HILL, C. E., MARK, G. E., ERÄNKÖ, O., ERÄNKÖ, L., BURNSTOCK, G.: Use of tissue culture to examine the actions of guanethidine and 6-hydroxydopamine. Eur. J. Pharmacol. **23**, 162—174 (1973).
HILLARP, N.-Å., MALMFORS, T.: Reserpine and cocaine blocking of the uptake and storage mechanisms in adrenergic nerves. Life Sci. **3**, 703—708 (1964).
HOFMANN, W. W., SPIVACK, A. P.: The effects of guanethidine on skeletal neuromuscular transmission. Amer. J. med. Sci. **244**, 64—69 (1962).
HORST, W. D., GATTANELL, P.: Influence of debrisoquin (Declinax) on adrenergic function and norepinephrine metabolism. Biochem. Pharmacol. **19**, 2335—2341 (1970).
HUGHES, F. B., BRODIE, B. B.: The mechanism of serotonin and catecholamine uptake by platelets. J. Pharmacol. exp. Therap. **127**, 96—102 (1959).

HUMPHREY, J. H., TOH, C. C.: Absorption of serotonin (5-hydroxytryptamine) and histamine by dog platelets. J. Physiol. (Lond.) **124**, 300—304 (1954).
HURLEY, R. E., PAGE, I. H., DUSTAN, H. P.: Bretylium tosylate as an antihypertensive drug. J. Amer. med. Assn. **172**, 2081—2083 (1960).
HUKOVIĆ, S., MUSCHOLL, E.: Die Noradrenalin-Freisetzung aus dem isolierten Herzen durch sympathische Nervenreizung. Naunyn-Schiedebergs Arch. exp. Path. Pharmak. **243**, 348 (1962).
IVERSEN, L. L.: The uptake of noradrenaline by the isolated perfused rat heart. Brit. J. Pharmacol. **21**, 523—537 (1963).
IVERSEN, L. L.: Inhibition of noradrenaline uptake by drugs. J. Pharm. Pharmacol. **17**, 62—64 (1965).
IVERSEN, L. L.: *The uptake and storage of noradrenaline in sympathetic nerves*. Cambridge: Cambridge Univ. Press, 1967.
IVERSEN, L. L.: KRAVITZ, E. A., Sodium dependence of transmitter uptake at adrenergic nerve terminals. Molec. Pharmacol. **2**, 359—362 (1966).
JAANUS, S. D., MIELE, E., RUBIN, R. P.: The action of guanethidine on the adrenal medulla of the cat. Brit. J. Pharmacol. **33**, 560—569 (1968).
JACK, D. B., STENLAKE, J. B., TEMPLETON, R.: Metabolism and excretion of guanoxan in man. J. Pharm. Pharmacol. **23**, 222S—223S (1971).
JACOBOWITZ, D., BRUS, R.: A study of extraneuronal uptake of norepinephrine in the perfused heart of the guinea-pig. Europ. J. Pharmacol. **15**, 274—284 (1971).
JANDHYALA, B. S., CAVERO, I., BUCKLEY, J. P.: Effects of chronic guanethidine administration on cardiovascular function of dogs. Res. Commun. Chem. Path. Pharmacol. **11**, 523—532 (1975).
JAQUES, R., LEWIS, G. P.: Guanethidine as a histamine liberator. Pharmacology **4**, 316—320 (1970).
JENSEN-HOLM, J., JUUL, P.: Changes of the rat superior cervical ganglion induced by guanethidine (histology and cholinesterase histochemistry). Brit. J. Pharmacol. **34**, 211P—212P (1968).
JENSEN-HOLM, J., JUUL, P.: The effects of guanethidine, pre- and post-ganglionic nerve division on the rat superior cervical ganglion: cholinesterases and protein. Acta Pharmacol. Toxicol. **28**, 270—282 (1970a).
JENSEN-HOLM, J., JUUL, P.: The effects of guanethidine, pre- and post-ganglioneic nerve division on the rat superior cervical ganglion: cholinesterases and catecholamines (histochemistry), and histology. Acta Pharmacol. Toxicol. **28**, 283—298 (1970b).
JENSEN-HOLM, J., JUUL, P.: Ultrastructural changes in the rat superior cervical ganglion following prolonged guanethidine administration. Acta Pharmacol. Toxicol. **30**, 308—320 (1971).
JOHNSON, E. M., ALOE, L.: Suppression of the *in vitro* and *in vivo* cytotoxic effects of guanethidine in sympathetic neurons by nerve growth factor. Brain Res. **81**, 519—532 (1974).
JOHNSTON, A. W., PRICHARD, B. N. C., ROSENHEIM, M. L.: Adrenergic neurone-blocking agents. Lancet **1962 II**, 996.
JOHNSTON, A. W., PRICHARD, B. N. C., ROSENHEIM, M. L.: The use of bethanidine in the treatment of hypertension. Lancet **1964 II**, 659—661.
JUUL, P.: Effects of various antihypertensive guanidine derivatives on the adult rat superior cervical ganglion: histology, ultrastructure, and cholinesterase histochemistry. Acta Pharmacol. Toxicol. **32**, 500—512 (1973).
JUUL, P., MCISAAC, R. L.: The effect of guanethidine on the noradrenaline content of the adult rat superior cervical ganglion. Acta Pharmacol. Toxicol. **32**, 382—389 (1973).
JUUL, P., SAND, O.: Determination of guanethidine in sympathetic ganglia. Acta Pharmacol. Toxicol. **32**, 487—499 (1973).
KADZIELAWA, K.: Mechanism of action of guanethidine. Brit. J. Pharmacol. **19**, 74—84 (1962).
KALSNER, S., NICKERSON, M.: A method for the study of mechanisms of drug disposition in smooth muscle. Canad. J. Physiol. Pharmacol. **46**, 719—730 (1968a).
KALSNER, S., NICKERSON, M.: Disposition of phenylephrine in vascular tissue, determined by the oil-immersion technique. J. Pharmacol. exp. Therap. **163**, 1—10 (1968b).
KALSNER, S., NICKERSON, M.: Disposition of norepinephrine and epinephrine in vascular tissue, determined by the technique of oil immersion. J. Pharmacol. exp. Therap. **165**, 152—165 (1969a).
KALSNER, S., NICKERSON, M.: Effects of reserpine on the disposition of sympathomimetic amines in vascular tissue. Brit. J. Pharmacol. **35**, 394—405 (1969b).
KALSNER, S., NICKERSON, M.: Mechanism of cocaine potentiation of responses to amines. Brit. J. Pharmacol. **35**, 428—439 (1969c).
KALSNER, S., NICKERSON, M.: Effects of a haloaklylamine on responses to and disposition of sympathomimetic amines. Brit. J. Pharmacol. **35**, 440—455 (1969d).

KALSNER, S.: The importance of the uptake mechanism of adrenergic nerves in blood vessels. In: *Physiology and pharmacology of vascular neuroeffector systems*. Basel: Karger 1971.
KANEKO, Y., MCCUBBIN, J. W., PAGE, I. H.: Central inhibition of vasomotor activity by guanethidine. J. Pharmacol. exp. Therap. **135**, 21—24 (1962).
KAUMANN, A., BASSO, N., ARAMENDIA, P.: The cardiovascular effects of N-(γ-methylamino-propyl-imino-dibenzyl)-HCl (desmethylimipramine) and guanethidine. J. Pharmacol. exp. Therap. **147**, 54—64 (1965).
KHAN, I., ASMAE, R.: Effects of reserpine and guanethidine on the responses of the isolated rat fundus strip to substituted tryptamines and catecholamines. Life Sci. **7**, 307—316 (1968)
KIRPEKAR, S. M., FURCHGOTT, R. F.: The sympathomimetic action of bretylium on isolated atria and aortic smooth muscle. J. Pharmacol. exp. Therap. **143**, 64—76 (1964).
KIRPEKAR, S. M., WAKADE, A. R., DIXON, W., PRAT, J. C.: Effect of cocaine, phenoxybenzamine and calcium on the inhibition of norepinephrine output from the cat spleen by guanethidine. J. Pharmacol. exp. Therap. **165**, 166—175 (1969).
KITCHIN, A. H., TURNER, R. W. D.: Studies on debrisoquine sulfate. Brit. med. J. **1966 II**, 728—731.
KNIFFEN, F. J., LOMAS, T. E., COUNSELL, R. E., LUCCHESI, B. R.: The antiarrhythmic and antifibrillatory actions of bretylium and its o-iodobenzyl trimethylammonium analog, UM-360. J. Pharmacol. exp. Ther. **192**, 120—128 (1975).
KOPIN, I. J., GORDON, E. K.: Metabolism of administered and drug-released norepinephrine-7-H^3 in the rat. J. Pharmacol. exp. Therap. **140**, 207—216 (1963).
KOPIN, I. J.: False adrenergic transmitters. Ann. Rev. Pharmacol. **8**, 377—394 (1968).
KRAYER, O., ALPER, M. H., PAASONEN, M. K.: Action of guanethidine and reserpine upon the isolated mammalian heart. J. Pharmacol. exp. Therap. **135**, 164—173 (1962).
KRONEBERG, G., SCHÜMANN, H. J.: Studies on the mechanism of action of guanethidine. Naunyn-Schmiedeberg. Arch. exp. Path. Pharmacol. **243**, 16—25 (1962).
KUBIKOWSKI, P., WYSOKOWSKI, J.: The influence of some hypotensive drugs and diuretics on the level of catecholamines and monoamine oxidase (MAO) activity in brain and in blood. Biochem. Pharmacol. **12**, (Suppl.), 31 (1963).
KUBO, T., MISU, Y.: Mode of action of guanethidine on adrenergic neurons and its dependence on sodium. Jap. J. Pharmacol. **24**, 307—318 (1974).
KUNTZMAN, R., COSTA, E., GESSA, G. L., BRODIE, B. B.: Reserpine and guanethidine action on peripheral stores of catecholamines. Life Sci. **1**, 65—74 (1962).
KUNTZMAN, R., JACOBSON, M. M.: Monamine oxidase inhibition by a series of compounds structurally related to bretylium and guanethidine. J. Pharmacol. exp. Ther. **141**, 166—172 (1963a).
KUNTZMAN, R., JACOBSON, M. M.: The inhibition of monoamine oxidase by benzyl and phenethylguanidines related to bretylium and guanethidine. Ann. N. Y. Acad. Sci. **107**, 945—950 (1963b).
KUNTZMAN, R., TSAI, I., CHANG, R., CONNEY, A. H.: Disposition of bretylium in man and rat. Clin. Pharmacol. Therap. **11**, 829—837 (1970).
KURAHASHI, K., SHIBATA, S.: Bretylium potentiation of the contractor responses of isolated rabbit aortic strips to potassium and tyramine. Brit. J. Pharmacol. **43**, 210—221 (1971).
LANGER, S. Z.: The degeneration contraction of the nictitating membrane in the unanesthetized cat. J. Pharmacol. exp. Therap. **151**, 66—72 (1966).
LAURENCE, D. R., ROSENHEIM, M. L.: In: *Ciba foundation symposium on adrenergic mechanisms*, pp. 201—208. Boston: Little, Brown & Co. 1960.
LAWRIE, T. D. V., LORIMER, A. R., MCALPINE, S. G., REINERT, H.: Clinical trial and pharmacological study of compound 1029 "Vatensol". Brit. med. J. **1964 I**, 402—406.
LE BLANC, J., COTÉ, J., DORÉ, F., ROUSSEAU, S.: Effects of guanethidine and related compounds on histamine excretion. Canad. J. Physiol. Pharmacol. **50**, 539—544 (1972).
LEISHMAN, A. W. D., MATTHEWS, H. L., SMITH, A. J.: Anatgonism of guanethidine by imipramine. Lancet **1963 I**, 112.
LEMBERGER, L., KUNTZMAN, R., CONNEY, A. H., BURNS, J. J.: Metabolism of tyramine to dopamine by liver microsomes. J. Pharmacol. exp. Therap. **150**, 292—297 (1965).
LEVEQUE, P. E.: Guanethidine as an anti-fibrillatory agent. Nature (Lond.) **203**, 1389 (1964).
LEVEQUE, P. E.: Anti-arrhythmic action of bretylium. Nature (Lond.) **207**, 203—204 (1965).
LEVEQUE, P. E.: Bethanidine: A new anti-fibrillatory agent. Arch. int. Pharmacodyn. **163**, 422—426 (1966).
LIGHTMAN, S. L., IVERSEN, L. L.: The role of $Uptake_2$ in the extraneuronal metabolism of catecholamines in the isolated rat heart. Brit. J. Pharmacol. **37**, 638—649 (1969).
LINDMAR, R., MUSCHOLL, E.: Die Wirkung von Pharmaka auf die Elimination von Noradrenalin aus der Perfusionsflüssigkeit und die Noradrenalinaufnahme in das isolierte Herz. Naunyn-Schmiedebergs Arch. exp. Path. Pharmak. **247**, 469—492 (1964).

LIPSIUS, M. R., SIEGMAN, M. J., KAO, C. Y.: Direct relaxant actions of procaine and tetrodotoxin on vascular smooth muscle. J. Pharmacol. exp. Ther. **164**, 60—74 (1968).
LUKAS, G.: Metabolism and Biochemical pharmacology of guanethidine and related compounds. Drug Metabo. Rev. **2** (1), 101—116 (1973).
LUNDBERG, D.: Effects of some adrenergic neuron blockers, related quaternary ammonium compounds and guanidine derivatives on degenerating adrenergic nerves in the conscious rat. Acta physiol. scand. **80**, 323—344 (1970).
LUNDBERG, D.: Bretylium and the supersensitivity to exogenous noradrenaline after sympathetic denervation studied in the conscious rat. Acta physiol. scand. **84**, 500—505 (1972).
LUNDBORG, P., STITZEL, R. E.: Studies on the dual action of guanethidine in sympathetic nerves. Acta physiol. scand. **72**, 100—107 (1968).
LURIA, M. H., FREIS, E. D.: Treatment of hypertension with debrisoquin sulfate (Declinax). Current Ther. Res. **7**, 289—296 (1965).
MAÎTRE, L., STAEHELIN, M.: Guanethidine uptake and noradrenaline depletion in noradrenaline storage particles of the rat heart. Biochem. Pharmacol. **20**, 1233—1242 (1971).
MAÎTRE, L., STAEHELIN, M., BRUNNER, H.: Antihypertensive and noradrenaline-depleting effects of guanethidine metabolites. J. Pharm. Pharmacol. **23**, 327—331 (1971).
MALMFORS, T., ABRAMS, W. B.: The effects of debrisoquin and bretylium on adrenergic nerves as revealed by fluorescence histochemistry. J. Pharmacol. exp. Ther. **174**, 99—110 (1970).
MARKIS, J. E., KOCH-WESER, J.: Characteristics and mechanism of inotropic and chronotropic actions of bretylium tosylate. J. Pharmacol. exp. Ther. **178**, 94—102 (1971).
MASON, D. T., BRAUNWALD, E.: Effects of guanethidine, reserpine and methyldopa on reflex venous and arterial constriction in man. J. clin. Invest. **43**, 1449—1463 (1964).
MALMQUIST, J., OATES, J. A.: Effects of adrenergic neuron-blocking guanidine derivatives on mitochondrial metabolism. Biochem. Pharmacol. **17**, 1845—1854 (1968).
MATSUMOTO, C., HORITA, A.: Studies of the antagonism of guanethidine by methamphetamine. Biochem. Pharmacol. **12**, 295—297 (1963).
MAXWELL, R. A.: Pharmacology of guanethidine. In: BREST, A. N., MOYER, J. H. (Ed.): *Hypertension, recent advances*. Lea & Febiger, Philadelphia, 1961.
MAXWELL, R. A.: Clinical and experimental pharmacology of sympathetic blocking agents. Conn. Med. **26**, 646—651 (1962).
MAXWELL, R. A.: Adrenergic blocking drugs, adrenergic neuron blocking drugs, and drugs altering biochemical mechanisms in adrenergic neurons. In: DI PALMA, J. R. (Ed.): *Drill's pharmacology in medicine*, 4th ed. New York: McGraw Hill 1971.
MAXWELL, R. A.: Concerning the mode of action of guanethidine and some derivatives in augmenting the vasomotor action of adrenergic amines in vascular tissues of the rabbit. J. Pharmacol. exp. Ther. **148**, 320—328 (1965).
MAXWELL, R. A., CHAPLIN, E., ECKHARDT, S. B., SOARES, J. R., HITE, G.: Conformational similarities between molecular models of phenethylamine and of potent inhibitors of the uptake of tritiated norepinephrine by adrenergic nerves in rabbit aorta. J. Pharmacol. exp. Ther. **173**, 158—165 (1970).
MAXWELL, R. A., DANIEL, A. I., SHEPPARD, H., ZIMMERMAN, J. H.: Some interactions of guanethidine, cocaine, methylphenidate and phenylalkylamines in rabbit aortic strips. J. Pharmacol. exp. Ther. **137**, 31—38 (1962).
MAXWELL, R. A., KEENAN, P. D., CHAPLIN, E., ROTH, B., ECKHARDT, S. B.: Molecular features affecting the potency of tricyclic antidepressants and structurally related compounds as inhibitors of the uptake of tritiated norepinephrine by rabbit aortic strips. J. Pharmacol. exp. Ther. **166**, 320—329 (1969).
MAXWELL, R. A., MULL, R. P., PLUMMER, A. J.: [2-(octahydro-1-azocinyl)-ethyl]-guanidine sulfate (Ciba 5864-Su), a new synthetic antihypertensive agent. Experientia (Basel) **15**, 267 (1959).
MAXWELL, R. A., PLUMMER, A. J., ROSS, S. D., PAYTAS, J. J., DENNIS, A. D.: Antihypertensive effects of the central nervous stimulant, methylphenidate. Arch. int. Pharmacodyn. **112**, 26—35 (1957).
MAXWELL, R. A., PLUMMER, A. J., ROSS, S. D., DANIEL, A. I.: Studies concerning the cardiovascular actions of the central nervous stimulant, methylphenidate. J. Pharmacol. exp. Ther. **123**, 22—27 (1958a).
MAXWELL, R. A., ROSS, S. D., PLUMMER, A. J.: Pharmacology of hexahydro-1-azepinepropionamidoxime dihydrochloride (Su-4029). J. Pharmacol. exp. Ther. **123**, 128—139 (1958b).
MAXWELL, R. A., PLUMMER, A. J., SCHNEIDER, F., POVALSKI, H., DANIEL, A. I.: Pharmacology of [2-(octahydro-1-azocinyl)-ethyl]-guanidine sulphate (SU-5864). J. Pharmacol. exp. Ther. **128**, 22—29 (1960).
MAXWELL, R. A., SCHNEIDER, F. L.: Some actions of hexahydro-1-azepinepropionamidoxime HCl (Su-4029) in certain antonomic pathways. J. Pharmacol. exp. Ther. **134**, 347—355 (1961).

MAXWELL, R. A., WASTILA, W. B., ECKHARDT, S. B.: Some factors determining the response of rabbit aortic strips to dl-norepinephrine-7-H^3 hydrochloride and the influence of cocaine, guanethidine and methylphenidate on these factors. J. Pharmacol. exp. Ther. **151**, 253—261 (1966).
MAXWELL, R. A., WASTILA, W., ECKHARDT, S. B.: A nonadrenergic musculotropic effect of 2-(cyclohexylamino)-ethylguanidine sulfate (SU-9707) in rabbit aortic strips. J. Pharmacol. exp. Ther. **158**, 248—252 (1967).
McCOUBREY, A.: Biochemical properties of bretylium. J. Pharm. Pharmacol. **14**, 727—734 (1962).
McCUBBIN, J. W., KANEKO, Y., PAGE, I. H.: The peripheral cardiovascular actions of guanethidine in dogs. J. Pharmacol. exp Ther. **131**, 346—354 (1961).
McLEAN, R. A., GEUS, R. J., PASTERNACK, J., MATTIS, P. A., ULLYOT, G. E.: Pharmacology of trimethyl[2-(2,6-dimethylphenoxy)propyl]-trimethylammonium chloride, monohydrate; compound 6890 or β TM10. J. Pharmacol. exp. Ther. **129**, 17—23 (1960).
McMARTIN, C.: The separation and detection of metabolites of guanethidine. Biochem. Pharmacol. **18**, 238—243 (1969).
McMARTIN, C., RONDEL, R. K., Vinter, J. ALLAN, B. R., HUMBERSTONE, P. M., LEISHMAN, A. W. D., SANDLER, G., THIRKETTLE, J. L.: The fate of guanethidine in two hypertensive patients. Clin. Pharmacol. Ther. **11**, 423—431 (1970).
McMARTIN, C., VINTER, J.: The preparation of high resolution microgranular carboxymethyl cellulose columns and their application to the separation of guanethidine and its metabolites in urine. J. Chromatog. **41**, 188—199 (1969).
MEDINA, M. A., GIACHETTI, A., SHORE, P. A.: On the physiological disposition and possible mechanism of the antihypertensive action of debrisoquin. Biochem. Pharmacol. **18**, 891—901 (1969).
MEYER, J. F., McALLISTER, C. K., GOLDBERG, L. I.: Insidious and prolonged antagonism of guanethidine by amitriptyline. J. Amer. med. Ass. **213**, 1487—1488 (1970).
MIELE, E.: Modificazioni della reattivita vascolare nel gatto ad opera della reserpina, guanethidinae α-methildopa. Arch. int. Pharmacodyn. **160**, 390—406 (1966).
MISU, Y., KUBO, T.: Effect of bretylium on adrenergic neurons and its relation to sodium. Jap. J. Pharmacol. **24**, 332—334 (1974).
MISU, Y., NISHIO, H., HOSOTANI, T., HAMANO, S.: A new guanidine derivative: dissociation of the adrenergic neuron blocking activity from local anesthetic activity. Jap. J. Pharmacol. **26**, 367—375 (1976).
MITCHELL, J. R., ARIAS, L., OATES, J. A.: Antagonism of the antihypertensive action of guanethidine sulfate by desipramine hydrochloride. J. Amer. med. Ass. **202**, 973—976 (1967).
MITCHELL, J. R., CAVANAUGH, J. H., DINGELL, J. V., OATES, J. A.: Guanethidine and related agents. II. Metabolism by hepatic microsomes and its inhibition by drugs. J. Pharmacol. exp. Ther. **172**, 108—114 (1970).
MITCHELL, J. R., OATES, J. A.: Guanethidine and related agents. I. Mechanism of the selective blockade of adrenergic neurons and its antagonism by drugs. J. Pharmacol. exp. Ther. **172**, 100—107 (1970).
MOE, R. A., BATES, H. M., PALKOSKI, Z. M., BANZIGER, R.: Cardiovascular effects of 3,4-dihydro-2 (1H) isoquinoline carboxamidine (Declinax). Current Ther. Res. **6**, 299—318 (1964).
MONTUSCHI, E., LOVEL, T. W. I.: Guanoxan in hypertension. Lancet **1964 II**, 1339-1340.
MONTUSCHI, E., PICKENS, P. T.: A clinical trial of two related adrenergic neurone—blocking agents: B.W. 392C60 and B.W. 467C60. Lancet **1962 II**, 897—901.
MORGAN, D. H., OATES, J. A., SHAND, D. G.: Evidence that guanethidine does not block adrenergic nerves by acting as a false transmitter. Brit. J. Pharmacol. **39**, 186P—187P (1970).
MOSER, M.: Guanethidine and bethanidine in the management of hypertension. Amer. Heart J. **77**, 423—426 (1969).
MULL, R. P., MAXWELL, R. A.: Guanethidine and related adrenergic neuronal blocking agents: In: SCHLITTER, E. (Ed.): Antihypertensive agents. New York: Academic Press 1967.
NAMM, D. H., WANG, C. M., EL-SAYAD, S., COPP, F. C., MAXWELL, R. A.: Effects of bretylium on rat cardiac muscle: Electrophysiological effects and its uptake and binding in normal and immunosympathectomized rat hearts. J. Pharmacol. exp. Ther. **193**, 194—208 (1975).
NARAHASHI, T., FRAZIER, D. T.: Site of action and active form of local anesthetics in nerve fibers. Fed. Proc. **27**, 408 (1968).
NASH, C. W., COSTA, E., BRODIE, B. B.: The actions of reserpine, guanethidine and metaraminol on cardiac catecholamine stores. Life Sci. **3**, 441—449 (1964).

NICKERSON, M.: Drugs inhibiting adrenergic nerves and structures innervated by them. In: GOODMAN, L.S., GILMAN, A. (Eds.): The Pharmacological Basis of Therapeutics, 4th ed. New York: MacMillan 1970.
OATES, J.A., MITCHELL, J.R., FEAGIN, O.T., KAUFMANN, J.S., SHAND, D.G.: Distribution of guanidinium antihypertensives—mechanism of their selective action. Ann. N. Y. Acad. Sci. **179**, 302—309 (1971).
OBIANWU, H.O.: Some studies on the mechanism by which d-amphetamine antagonizes guanethidine induced adrenergic neuron blockade. Acta physiol. scand. **75**, 102—110 (1969).
OBIANWU, H.O., STITZEL, R., LUNDBORG, P.: Subcellular distribution of [^{3}H] amphetamine and [^{3}H] guanethidine and their interaction with adrenergic neurons. J. Pharm. Pharmacol. **20**, 585—594 (1968).
OOSTERHUIS, J.A.: Guanethidine (Ismelin) in ophthalmology. 1. Observations in rabbits. Arch. Ophthalm. **67**, 592—599 (1962).
ONESTI, G., LASCHIAZZA, D., BREST, A.N., MOYER, J.H.: Cardiac and renal hemodynamic effects of debrisoquin sulfate in hypertensive patients. Clin. Pharmacol. Ther. **7**, 17—20 (1966).
OSADA, H., WESTFALL, T.C.: Influence of adrenalectomy on the recovery of norepinephrine levels following guanethidine and metaraminol. Arch. int. Pharmacodyn **180**, 162—172 (1969).
PAGE, I.H.: The prolonged use of guanethidine. Med. Clin. N. Amer. **45**, 417—420 (1961).
PAPP, J.Gy., VAUGHAN WILLIAMS, E.M.: The effect of bretylium on intracellular cardiac action potentials in relation to its anti-arrhythmic and local anaesthetic activity. Brit. J. Pharmacol. **37**, 380—390 (1969).
PATON, W.D.M., VIZI, E.S.: The inhibitory action of noradrenaline and adrenaline on acetylcholine output by guinea-pig ileum longitudinal muscle strip. Brit. J. Pharmacol. **35**, 10—28 (1969).
PFEIFER, A.K., VIZI, E.Sz., SÁTORY, E.: Studies on the action of guanethidine on the central nervous system and on the norepinephrine content of the brain. Biochem. Pharmacol. **11**, 397—398 (1962).
PHILIPPU, A., SCHÜMANN, H.J.: The effect of guanethidine and bretylium on the liberation of pyrocatecholamines. Naunyn-Schmiedebergs Arch. exptl. Path. Pharmacol. **243**, 26—35 (1962).
PLUCHINO, S., MUSKUS, A.J., PLUCHINO, R.: The mechanism of action of guanethidine on the isolated mammalian heart. J. Pharmacol. exp. Ther. **170**, 44—49 (1969).
PLUCHINO, S., VAN ORDEN, L.S., III., DRASKOCZY, P.R., LANGER, S.Z., TRENDELENBURG, U.: The effect of beta-TM10 on the pharmacological, biochemical and morphological changes induced by denervation of the nictitating membrane of the cat. J. Pharmacol. exp. Ther. **172**, 77—90 (1970).
POCELINKO, R., SOLOMON, H.M.: Accumulation of debrisoquin-^{14}C by the human platelet. Biochem. Pharmacol. **19**, 697—703 (1970).
POLLARD, A.A., BECK, L.: The distinct nature of the sustained dilator system: evidence against the pseudotransmitter hypothesis. J. Pharmacol. exp. Ther. **179**, 132—143 (1971).
POSIVIATA, M., BECKER, G., WEINER, N.: The effect of bertylium tosylate on catecholamine synthesis in the guinea pig isolated vas deferens preparation. Pharmacologist **13**, 253 (1971).
PRASAD, C.M., SHAH, D.S., GULATI, O.D.: Some factors affecting the neuron blocking action of guanethidine, xylocholine, bretylium and debrisoquin. Jap. J. Pharmacol. **23**, 805—811 (1973).
PRICHARD, B.N.C., JOHNSTON, A.W., HILL, I.D., ROSENHEIM, M.L.: Bethanidine, guanethidine, and methyldopa in treatment of hypertension: a within-patient comparison. Brit. med. J. **1968 I**, 135—144.
PRIOLA, D.V., SPURGEON, H.A., BLAUWO, II, A.S., CANNON, III, W.B., DONG, JR. E.: Mechanism of the inotropic action of bretylium tosylate on the heart. J. Pharmacol. exp. Ther. **187**, 121—132 (1973).
RAHN, K.H., DAYTON, P.G.: Studies on the metabolism of guanethidine in hypertensive patients. Biochem. Pharmacol. **18**, 1809—1816 (1969).
RAINES, A., MOROS, D., LEVITT, B.: The effect of guanethidine on ouabain-induced ventricular arrhythmia in the cat. Arch. int. Pharmacodyn **174**, 373—377 (1968).
RAND, M.J., WILSON, J.: The actions of some adrenergic neurone blocking drugs at cholinergic junctions. Europ. J. Pharmacol. **1**, 210—221 (1967a).
RAND, M.J., WILSON, J.: Receptor site of adrenergic neuron blocking drugs. Circulat. Res. **20**, **21**, Suppl. **3**, 89—99 (1967b).
RAND, M.J., WILSON, J.: The relationship between adrenergic neurone blocking activity and local anaesthetic activity in a series of guanidine derivatives. Europ. J. Pharmacol. **1**, 200—209 (1967c).

RICHARDSON, D. W., WYSO, E. M., MAGEE, J. H., CAVELL, G. C.: Circulatory effects of guanethidine. Circulation 22, 184—190 (1960).
RICHMOND, D. R., ANGUS, J. A., GOODMAN, A. H., COBBIN, L. B.: Actions of bretylium tosylate on the cardiovascular system of the dog. Cardiovascular Res. 7, 47—54 (1973).
RITCHIE, J. M., GREENGARD, P.: On the mode of action of local anesthetics. Ann. Rev. Pharmacol. 6, 405—430 (1966).
RITCHIE, J. M., COHEN, P. J., DRIPPS, R. D.: Cocaine, procaine and other synthetic local anesthetics. In: GOODMAN, L. S., GILMAN, A. (Eds.): *The pharmacological basis of therapeutics*, 4th ed. New York: MacMillan 1970.
ROBERTSON, M. I., ABBS, E. T.: Catecholamine depletion and adrenergic neurone blockade: studies with debrisoquine. J. Neurochem. 18, 1999—2001 (1971).
ROSS, S. B., GOSZTONYI, T.: On the mechanism of the accumulation of ^{3}H-bretylium in peripheral sympathetic nerves. Naunyn-Schmiedebergs Arch. Pharmacol. 288, 283—293 (1975).
ROSS, S. B., RENYI, A. L.: Uptake of some tritiated sympathomimetic amines by mouse brain cortex slices *in vitro*. Acta Pharmacol. Toxicol. 24, 297—309 (1966).
SANAN, S., VOGT, M.: Effect of drugs on the noradrenaline content of brain and peripheral tissues and its significance. Brit. J. Pharmacol. 18, 109—127 (1962).
SANNERSTEDT, R., CONWAY, J.: Hemodynamic and vascular responses to antihypertensive treatment with adrenergic blocking agents: A review Amer. Heart J. 79, 122—127 (1970).
SCHANKER, L. S., MORRISON, A. S.: Physiological disposition of guanethidine in the rat and its uptake by heart slices. Int. J. Neuropharmacol. 4, 27—39 (1965).
SCHLITTLER, E., DRUEY, J., MARXER, A.: Antihypertensive agents. Fortschr. Arzneimittelforsch. 4, 295—351 (1962).
SCHÜMANN, H. J., PHILIPPU, A.: Release of catechol amines from isolated medullary granules by sympathomimetic amines. Nature (Lond.) 193, 890—891 (1962).
SCHÜMANN, H. J., SCHNELL, K., PHILIPPU, A.: Subcelluläre Verteilung von Noradrenalin und Adrenalin im Meerschweinchenherzen. Naunyn-Schmiedeberg's Arch. exp. Path. Pharmakol. 249, 251—266 (1964).
Scriabine, A., BOOHER, K. D., PEREIRA, J. N., MCSHANE, W. K., CONSTANTINE, J. W., KOCH, R. C., MIKNIUS, S.: Pharmacological studies with guanisoquin. J. Pharmacol. exp. Ther. 147, 277—287 (1965).
SHAND, D. G., MORGAN, D. H., OATES, J. A.: The release of guanethidine and bethanidine by splenic nerve stimulation: a quantitative evaluation showing dissociation from adrenergic blockade. J. Pharmacol. exp. Ther. 184, 73—80 (1973).
SHAPIRO, A. P., KRIFCHER, E.: Pressor responses to noxious stimuli in hypertensive patients. Effects of guanethidine sulfate and alpha methyldopa. Circulation 30, 671—678 (1964).
SHEPPARD, H., ZIMMERMANN, J.: Effect of guanethidine (Su-5864) on tissue catecholamines. Pharmacologist 1, 69 (1959).
SHEPS, S. G., SCHRIGER, A., OSMUNDSON, P. J., KAVANAUGH, G. J., FAIRBAIN, J. F., BURBANK, M. K.: Experience with guanoxan in the treatment of hypertension. Mayo Clin. Proc. 41, 577—584 (1966).
SHORE, P. A., GIACHETTI, A.: Dual actions of guanethidine on amine uptake mechanisms in adrenergic neurons. Biochem. Pharmacol. 15, 899—903 (1966).
SKINNER, C., COULL, D. C., JOHNSTON, A. W.: Antagonism of the hypotensive action of bethanidine and debrisoquine by tricyclic antidepressants. Lancet 1969 II, 564—566.
SMITH, A. J.: Fluid retention by guanethidine. Circulation 31, 490—496 (1965).
SMIRK, H.: The hypotensive action of B.W. 467C60. Lancet 1963 I, 743—746.
SOLOMON, H. M., ASHLEY, C., SPIRT, N., ABRAMS, W. B.: The influence of debrisoquin on the accumulation and metabolism of biogenic amines by the human platelet, *in vivo* and *in vitro*. Clin. Pharmacol. Ther. 10, 229—238 (1969).
SOLOMON, H. M., SPIRT, N. M., ABRAMS, W. B.: The accumulation and metabolism of dopamine by the human platelet. Clin. Pharmacol. Ther. 11, 838—845 (1970).
SOLOMON, H. M., ZIEVE, P. D.: The accumulation of organic bases by the human platelet. J. Pharmacol. exp. Ther. 155, 112—116 (1967).
SOMLYO, A. P., SOMLYO, A. V.: Vascular smooth muscle. II. Pharmacology of normal and hypertensive vessels. Pharm. Rev. 22, 249—353 (1970).
SPRIGGS, T. L. B.: Peripheral noradrenaline and adrenergic transmission in the rat. Brit. J. Pharmacol. 26, 271—281 (1966).
STITZEL, R. E., CAMPOS, H. A., SHIDEMAN, F. E.: Effects of sympathetic nerve stimulation on subcellular levels of catecholamine in the heart. Int. J. Neuropharmacol. 4, 327—336 (1965).
STONE, C. A., PORTER, C. C., STAVORSKI, J. M., LUDDEN, C. T., TORTARO, J. A.: Antagonism of certain effects of catecholamine-depleting agents by antidepressant and related drugs. J. Pharmacol. exp. Ther. 144, 196—204 (1964).
SULSER, F., OWENS, M. L., DINGELL, J. V.: On the mechanism of amphetamine potentiation by desipramine (DMI). Life Sci. 5, 2005—2010 (1966).

TAYLOR, S. H., SUTHERLAND, G. R., HUTCHISON, D. C., KIDD, B. S., ROBERTSON, P. C., KENNELLY, B. M., DONALD, K. W.: The effects of intravenous guanethidine on the systemic and pulmonary circulations in man. Amer. Heart J. **63**, 239—264 (1962).

THOENEN, H., HÜRLIMANN, A., HAEFELY, W.: Interaction of phenoxybenzamine with guanethidine and bretylium at the sympathetic nerve endings of the isolated perfused spleen of the cat. J. Pharmacol. exp. Ther. **151**, 189—195 (1966).

THOENEN, H., HÜRLIMANN, A., HAEFELY, W.: Mechanism of amphetamine accumulation in the isolated perfused heart of the rat. J. Pharm. Pharmacol. **20**, 1—11 (1968).

TODA, N.: Interactions of bretylium and drugs that inhibit the neuronal membrane transport of norepinephrine in isolated rabbit atria and aortae. J. Pharmacol. exp. Ther. **181**, 318—327 (1972).

TOMLINSON, D. R., MAYOR, D.: The effects of guanethidine, bretylium and debrisoquine on the accumulation of noradrenaline in constricted postganglionic sympathetic nerves *in vitro*. Eur. J. Pharmacol. **21**, 161—170 (1973).

TRANZER, J. P., DA PRADA, M., PLETSCHER, A.: Ultrastructural localization of 5-hydroxytryptamine in blood platelets. Nature (Lond.) **212**, 1574—1575 (1966).

TRENDELENBURG, U.: The supersensitivity caused by cocaine. J. Pharmacol. exp. Ther. **125**, 55—65 (1959).

TRENDELENBURG, U.: Supersensitivity and subsensitivity to sympathomimetic amines. Pharmacol. Rev. **15**, 225—276 (1963).

TRENDELENBURG, U.: Mechanisms of supersensitivity and subsensitivity to sympathomimetic amines. Pharm. Rev. **18**, 629—640 (1966).

UDENFRIEND, S.: Tyrosine hydroxylase. Pharm. Rev. **18**, 43—51 (1966).

VEJLSGAARD, V., CHRISTENSEN, M., CLAUSEN, E.: Double-blind trial of four hypotensive drugs (methyldopa and three sympatholytic agents). Brit. med. J. **1967 II**, 598—600.

VILLARREAL, H., EXAIRE, J. E., RUBIO, V., DAVILA, H.: Effect of guanethidine and bretylium tosylate on systemic and renal hemodynamics in essential hypertension. Amer. J. Cardiol. **14**, 633—640 (1964).

VIZI, E. S., KNOLL, J.: The effects of sympathetic nerve stimulation and guanethidine on parasympathetic neuroeffector transmission; the inhibition of acetylcholine release. J. Pharm. Pharmacol. **23**, 918—925 (1971).

WALTER, I. E., KHANDELWAL, J., FALKNER, F., NIES, A. S.: The relationship of plasma guanethidine to adrenergic blockade. Clin. Pharmacol. Ther. **18**, 571—580 (1975).

WATANABE, Y., JOSIPOVIC, V., DREIFUS, L. S.: Electrophysiological mechanisms of bretylium tosylate. Fed. Proc. **28**, 270 (1969).

WATSON, P. J.: Interaction between acetylcholine and guanethidine on sensory C fibres. Europ. J. Pharmacol. **1**, 407—413 (1967).

WAXMAN, M. B., WALLACE, A. G.: Electrophysiologic effects of bretylium tosylate on the heart. J. Pharmacol. exp. Ther. **183**, 264—274 (1972).

WEIL, J. V., CHIDSEY, C. A.: Plasma volume expansion resulting from interference with adrenergic function in normal man. Circulation **37**, 54—61 (1968).

WEIL-MALHERBE, H., POSNER, H. S.: The effect of drugs on the release of epinephrine from adrenomedullary particles *in vitro*. J. Pharmacol. exp. Ther. **140**, 93—102 (1963).

WHITBY, L. G., AXELROD, J., WEIL-MALHERBE, H.: The fate of H^3-norepinephrine in animals. J. Pharmacol. exp. Ther. **132**, 193—201 (1961).

WILLIAMS, R. L., MAINES, J. E., III, PEARSON, J. E.: Direct and systemic effects of guanethidine on renal function. J. Pharmacol. exp. Ther. **177**, 69—77 (1971).

WILSON, J.: The uptake of adrenergic neurone blocking drugs. Brit. J. Pharmacol. **40**, 159P—160P (1970).

WILSON, W. R., VAN HECKE, D. C., KIRKENDALL, W. M.: Hemodynamic studies in man before and after three chemical agents which block sympathetic neural activity. J. Lab. clin. Med. **56**, 959 (1960).

WILSON, R., LONG, C.: Action of bretylium antagonized by amphetamine. Lancet **1960 II**, 262.

WIT, A. L., STEINER, C., DAMATO, A. N.: Electrophysiologic effects of bretylium tosylate on single fibers of the canine specialized conducting system and ventricle. J. Pharmacol. exp. Ther. **173**, 344—356 (1970).

YELNOSKY, J., MORTIMER, L. C.: A brief study of the sympathomimetic cardiovascular effects of bretylium. Arch. int. Pharmacodyn Ther. **130**, 200—206 (1961).

YOO, C. S., LEE, W. C.: Blockade of the cardiac action of phenylephrine by bretylium or cocaine. J. Pharmacol. exp. Ther. **172**, 274—281 (1970).

YOO, C. S., LEE, W. C.: Studies on the adrenergic blocking action of guanethidine: Arch. int. Pharmacodyn. **190**, 190—198 (1971).

ZAIMIS, E.: Reserpine induced circulatory failure. Nature (Lond.) **192**, 521—523 (1961).

ZIMMERMANN, A. M., HARRIS, L. S.: Microcirculation: effects of guanethidine and reserpine. J. Pharmacol. exp. Ther. **142**, 76—82 (1963).

Chapter 6

False Transmitters as Antihypertensive Agents

C. C. PORTER, M. L. TORCHIANA, and C. A. STONE

With 2 Figures

Early in the 1960's, it became apparent that the known ability of α-methyl aromatic amino acids to inhibit aromatic amino acid decarboxylation (SOURKES, 1954; WESTERMAN, BALZER, and KNELL, 1958; DENGLER and REICHEL, 1958; SMITH, 1960) was not solely responsible for the depression of biogenic amine concentrations in tissues following the administration of α-methyldopa or α-methyl-m-tyrosine to animals. Norepinephrine concentrations in the tissues of animals which received the amino acids returned to normal considerably more slowly than serotonin and dopamine concentrations (HESS et al., 1961; PORTER et al., 1961; STONE et al., 1961), and considerably more potent decarboxylation inhibitors had little effect upon tissue catecholamine concentrations (UDENFRIEND and ZALTZMAN-NIRENBERG, 1962).

CARLSSON and LINDQVIST (1962) identified α-methyldopamine and α-methylnorepinephrine (from methyldopa) and metaraminol (from α-methyl-m-tyrosine) in the tissues of rabbits and mice after the administration of the respective amino acids. It was suggested that the α-methylamines, especially the β-hydroxylated ones, displaced normal amines from the tissues.

DAY and RAND (1963, 1964), working with several animal species, obtained partial, organ-selective blockade of responses to nerve stimulation, and restoration of pressor responses to tyramine in reserpine-treated animals, following the administration of α-methyldopa.

From this and other evidence, it became clear that some compounds can be stored in nerve terminals and released by nervous impulses and by sympathomimetic agents, similarly to normal transmitters, and that these compounds may have less effect than normal transmitters upon receptor cells; they are designated as false, or substitute, transmitters.

The general subject of false transmitters has been reviewed extensively (CARLSSON, 1969; CROUT, 1966; KOPIN, 1968a, b; STONE, 1971; MUSCHOLL, 1972), and certain aspects of false transmitter storage and release are dealt with in other chapters of this volume (MAXWELL and WASTILA; OATES et al.; RAND and JUREVICS; all contributions see this volume). However, it is desirable to consider here a number of topics which, although discussed more extensively elsewhere, are critical to an understanding of the role of false transmitters as antihypertensive agents.

Listed in Table 1 are N- and α-methyl-, β-, 3-, and 4-hydroxy-phenethylamine derivatives which will be the main concern of the ensuing discussion. Given in the table also are some properties of these amines which govern their effectiveness

Table 1. *Phenethylamine derivatives*

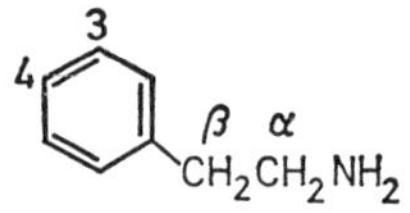

Compound number	Substituents other than H α	β	3	4	N	Type[a]	Direct potency[b] Spinal cat	Rat	Microsomal retention[c]
1						I			5
2					CH_3				
3	CH_3					I	≪		
4	CH_3				CH_3	I			
5		OH				M			13
6		OH			CH_3				
7	CH_3	OH				M	0.13		
8	CH_3	OH			CH_3	M	0.037		
9			OH			M	0.1	0.002[d]	8
10			OH		CH_3				
11	CH_3		OH			M[d]		0.02[d]	
12	CH_3		OH		CH_3				
13				OH		I	≪		5
14				OH	CH_3				
15	CH_3			OH		I			13[e]
16	CH_3			OH	CH_3	I			
17		OH	OH			D	1.5		60
18		OH	OH		CH_3	D	4.8		
19	CH_3	OH	OH			M	1.0	2.3	
20	CH_3	OH	OH		CH_3	M	0.045		
21		OH		OH		M	0.029		53
22		OH		OH	CH_3	D	0.15		
23	CH_3	OH		OH		M	0.1		56[e]
24	CH_3	OH		OH	CH_3	M	0.012		
25			OH	OH		D		0.75	77
26			OH	OH	CH_3	D			
27	CH_3		OH	OH		D[d]		1.07	
28	CH_3		OH	OH	CH_3				
29		OH	OH	OH		D	100	100	100
30		OH	OH	OH	CH_3	D	14.3		19[f]
31	CH_3	OH	OH	OH		D		57.7	
32	CH_3	OH	OH	OH	CH_3	D			

[a] I, indirect; D, direct; M, mixed. From Trendelenburg, 1963, unless noted otherwise.
[b] Potency in animals treated with reserpine. Norepinephrine taken as 100. Spinal cat data from TRENDELENBURG et al., 1962. Rat data from TORCHIANA et al., 1966.
[c] Compared with norepinephrine, 100; microsomes from rat vas deferens. from POTTER, 1967.
[d] TORCHIANA, unpublished.
[e] Rat heart granules. MUSACCHIO et al., 1965a.
[f] Rabbit heart granules. GILLIS, 1964.

1 Phenethylamine
2 N-Methylphenethylamine
3 Amphetamine; α-methylphenethylamine
4 N-Methylamphetamine; methamphetamine; desoxyephedrine; methedrine
5 Phenylethanolamine
6 N-Methylphenylethanolamine
7 Phenylpropanolamine; Norephedrine; Propadrine
8 Ephedrine
9 m-Tyramine
10 N-Methyl-m-tyramine
11 α-Methyl-m-tyramine
12 α-N,Dimethyl-m-tyramine

13 Tyramine
14 N-Methyltyramine
15 α-Methyltyramine; p-Hydroxyamphetamine; Paredrine
16 Paredrinol; Pholedrine
17 m-Octopamine; m-Norsynephrine; Norphenylephrine
18 Phenylephrine; Neosynephrine; m-Synephrine
19 α-Methyl-m-Octopamine; 3-Hydroxynorephedrine; Metaraminol; Aramine; Metadrine; m-Hydroxyphenylpropanolamine
20 m-Hydroxyephedrine
21 Octopamine; Norsynephrine
22 Synephrine; Sympatol
23 α-Methyloctopamine; 4-Hydroxynorephedrine; p-Hydroxyphenylpropanolamine
24 p-Hydroxyephedrine; Methylsympatol
25 Dopamine; 3,4-Dihydroxyphenethylamine
26 Epinine; N-Methyldopamine
27 α-Methyldopamine; α-Methyl-3,4-dihydroxyphenethylamine
28 α-N,Dimethyldopamine
29 Norepinephrine; Noradrenaline
30 Epinephrine; Adrenaline
31 Cobefrin; α-Methylnorepinephrine; α-Methylnoradrenaline; Nordefrin; Corbasil; 3,4-Dihydroxynorephedrine
32 Dihydroxyephedrine

Key to Table 1. Alphabetical

Adrenaline 30
Amphetamine 3
Aramine 19
Cobefrin 31
Corbasil 31
Desoxyephedrine 4
Dihydroxyephedrine 32
3,4-Dihydroxynorephedrine 31
3,4-Dihydroxyphenethylamine 25
α-N-Dimethyldopamine 28
α-N-Dimethyl-m-tyramine 12
Dopamine 25
Ephedrine 8
Epinephrine 30
Epinine 26
p-Hydroxyamphetamine 15
m-Hydroxyephedrine 20
p-Hydroxyephedrine 24
3-Hydroxynorephedrine 19
4-Hydroxynorephedrine 23
m-Hydroxyphenylpropanolamine 19
p-Hydroxyphenylpropanolamine 23
Metadrine 19
Metaraminol 19
Methadrine 4
Methamphetamine 4
N-Methylamphetamine 4
α-Methyl-3,4-dihydroxyphenethylamine 27
α-Methyldopamine 27
N-Methyldopamine 26
α-Methylnoradrenaline 31
α-Methylnorepinephrine 31
α-Methyl-m-octopamine 19
α-Methyloctopamine 23
α-Methylphenethylamine 3
N-Methylphenethylamine 2
N-Methylphenylethanolamine 6
Methylsympatol 24
α-Methyl-m-tyramine 11
N-Methyl-m-tyramine 10
α-Methyltyramine 15
N-Methyltyramine 14
Neosynephrine 18
Noradrenaline 29
Nordefrin 31
Norephedrine 7
Norepinephrine 29
Norphenylephrine 17
m-Norsynephrine 17
Norsynephrine 21
Octopamine 21
m-Octopamine 17
Paredrine 15
Paredrinol 16
Phenylephrine 18
Phenylethanolamine 5
Phenethylamine 1
Phenylpropanolamine 7
Pholedrine 16
Propadrine 7
Sympatol 22
m-Synephrine 18
Synephrine 22
m-Tyramine 9
Tyramine 13

as false transmitters, and which will be dealt with in some detail further on: the effective false transmitter will be the amine with principally direct action, but of low potency, and with considerable affinity for granules.

The metabolism and pharmacological effects of phenethylamine derivatives depend to a major extent upon their stereochemical configurations, a subject which has been treated adequately by others (e.g. MUSCHOLL, 1972). In the following discussion, unless otherwise noted, only amines configurationally identical to normally occurring norepinephrine, and amino acids conformationally identical to natural amino acids, will be considered.

I. Catecholamine Metabolism

The normal, preponderant pathways of catecholamine metabolism are shown in Fig. 1. Since the enzymes which catalyze the formation and destruction of norepinephrine are not specific for their normal substrates, false transmitters may

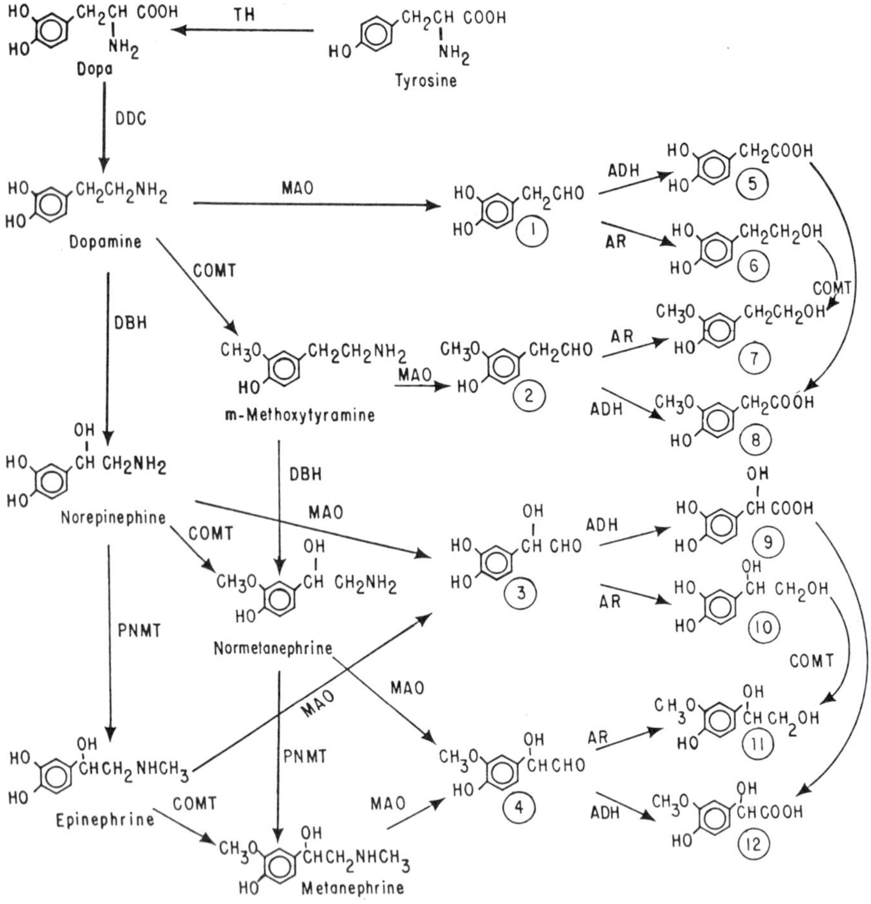

Fig. 1. Principal pathways of catecholamine metabolism. ADH, aldehydedehydrogenase; AR, aldehydereductase; COMT, catechol-O-methyltransferase; DBH, dopamine-β-hydroxylase; DDC, dopa decarboxylase; MAO, monoamine oxidase; PNMT, phenylethanolamine-N-methyltransferase; TH, tyrosine hydroxylase. 1. 3,4-Dihydroxyphenylacetaldehyde; 2. 3-Methoxy-4-hydroxyphenylacetaldehyde; 3. 3,4-Dihydroxyphenylglycolaldehyde; 4. 3-Methoxy-4-hydroxyphenylglycolaldehyde; 5. 3,4-Dihydroxyphenylacetic acid; 6. 3,4-Dihydroxyphenylethanol; 7. 3-Methoxy-4-hydroxyphenylethanol; 8. 3-Methoxy-4-hydroxyphenylacetic acid; Homovanillic acid (HVA); 9. 3,4-Dihydroxymandelic acid; 10. 3,4-Dihydroxyphenylglycol; 11. 3-Methoxy-4-hydroxyphenylglycol; 12. 3-Methoxy-4-hydroxymandelic acid; Vanillylmandelic acid (VMA)

result from the metabolism of a variety of substances, many of which also alter the operation of these enzymes on the natural substrates. For discussions of the factors which regulate catecholamine metabolism, see GOLDSTEIN et al. (1973), MOLENOFF (1974) and KOPIN (1974).

It should be emphasized that evidence for the conversion of a given substance to a known false transmitter does not mean necessarily that the reaction will lead to significant changes in neuron function. Accumulation of the false transmitter will depend not only upon its rate of formation, but also upon where it is formed, its rate of destruction, its affinity for amine storage sites and upon the rate of metabolism of normal tissue catecholamines. Duration of treatment with the precursor substance, as well as the frequency with which it is administered, also are important factors: if the metabolically-produced false transmitter becomes available more rapidly than it leaves storage sites, its concentration can be expected to reach functional levels.

A. Ring Hydroxylation

1. m-Hydroxylation: Tyrosine Hydroxylase

The conversion of tyrosine to 3,4-dihydroxyphenylalanine (dopa) is catalyzed by the enzyme tyrosine hydroxylase (NAGATSU et al., 1964a) which, although adhering to particulate matter during some purification procedures, has been shown to be a cytoplasmic enzyme (LADURON and BELPAIRE, 1968a, b; PETRACK et al., 1970; POILLON, 1971; STJÄRNE and LISHAJKO, 1967). It requires a tetrahydropteridine cofactor and is activated by ferrous ions (BRENNEMAN and KAUFMAN, 1964; ELLENBOGEN et al., 1965; NAGATSU et al., 1964a, b; POILLON, 1971).

The hydroxylation of substrates other than tyrosine has been demonstrated. Methyldopa metabolites (α-methyldopamine and α-methylnorepinephrine) were found in the brains and hearts of guinea pigs that had received α-methyltyrosine (MAÎTRE, 1965). This finding has been confirmed in experiments with radioactively labelled α-methyltyrosine (SPECTOR, 1966; UDENFRIEND et al., 1966); and *in vitro* purified tyrosine hydroxylase was shown to catalyze the conversion of α-methyltyrosine to α-methyldopa (UDENFRIEND et al., 1965). These reactions may be of biological significance, at least in some tissues (VAN ORDEN et al., 1970).

The conversion of α-methylphenylalanine to metaraminol has been shown to occur in animals (TORCHIANA et al., 1970), presumably via α-methyl-m-tyrosine and α-methyl-m-tyramine. Although the initial reaction, namely, the m-hydroxylation of α-methylphenylalanine, may be due to the action of tryptophan hydroxylase rather than to tyrosine hydroxylase (PORTER, unpublished observation), the end result is production of the false transmitter. In this connection, it is of interest to note that tyrosine hydroxylase, as well as phenylalanine hydroxylase (see below), catalyzes the p-hydroxylation of phenylalanine (IKEDA et al., 1967); thus, dopa results from the action of this enzyme upon phenylalanine.

Inhibitors of tyrosine hydroxylase are known (Table 2), for example α-methyltyrosine (NAGATSU et al., 1964b; SPECTOR et al., 1965) and α-methylphenylalanine (UDENFRIEND et al., 1965). However, of more importance to the present discussion is the fact that norepinephrine inhibits the enzyme (IKEDA et al., 1966; SPECTOR et al., 1967; UDENFRIEND et al., 1965); consequently, factors which tend to alter the concentration of norepinephrine in the nerve endings may lead to effects upon biosynthetic enzymes which oppose these alterations.

Table 2. *Inhibitors of tyrosine hydroxylase*[a]

Compound	Concentration required for 50% inhibition[b] (M)
L-Tryptophan	$>1 \times 10^{-3}$
L-Phenylalanine	2×10^{-4}
D-Phenylalanine	$>1 \times 10^{-3}$
3-Iodo-L-tyrosine	5×10^{-7}
3-Chloro-L-tyrosine	1×10^{-5}
3-Fluoro-DL-tyrosine	1×10^{-3}
3,5-Diiodo-L-tyrosine	2×10^{-5}
3,5-Dibromo-L-tyrosine	5×10^{-4}
α-Methyl-L-tyrosine	2.5×10^{-5}
α-Methyl-D-tyrosine	$>1 \times 10^{-3}$
α-Methyl-m-DL-tyrosine	$>1 \times 10^{-3}$
α-Methyl-DL-phenylalanine	8×10^{-5}
3-Iodo-α-methyl-DL-tyrosine	3×10^{-7}
3-Bromo-α-methyl-DL-tyrosine	1.5×10^{-6}
3-Chloro-α-methyl-DL-tyrosine	5×10^{-6}
3-Fluoro-α-methyl-DL-tyrosine	2×10^{-4}
3-Chloro-4-methoxy-α-methyl-DL-phenylalanine	5×10^{-4}
Catechol	5×10^{-3}
L-Norepinephrine	1×10^{-3}
3,5-Dihydroxyphenylacetamide	1×10^{-3}
3,4-Dihydroxyphenylpropylacetamide (H-22/54)	2×10^{-5}
3,4-Dihydroxy-L-phenylalanine	2×10^{-3}
3,4-Dihydroxy-D-phenylalanine	$>4 \times 10^{-3}$
α-Methyl-3,4-dihydroxy-L-phenylalanine (Aldomet)	1.5×10^{-3}
α-Methyl-3,4-dihydroxy-D-phenylalanine	$>8 \times 10^{-3}$

[a] Data from UDENFRIEND et al., 1965.
[b] Substrate, L-tyrosine, 5×10^{-5} M.

2. p-Hydroxylation

The presence of tyrosine in nutrients assures an adequate supply of the amino acid to the organism under ordinary circumstances. However, the enzyme which mediates the formation of tyrosine from phenylalanine, phenylalanine hydroxylase, catalyzes also the hydroxylation of phenylalanine derivatives. For example, p-chlorophenylalanine (GUROFF et al., 1967) and p-methylphenylalanine (DALY and GUROFF, 1968) are p-hydroxylated, with a shift of the original p-substituents to the position meta to the alanine side chain.

α-Methylnorepinephrine has been identified in the tissues of animals which received α-methyl-m-tyrosine or metaraminol (MAÎTRE and STAEHELIN, 1965); and p-hydroxylation of amines, presumably by liver microsomal enzymes, has been demonstrated for compounds such as m-tyramine, m-octopamine and N-methyloctopamine (AXELROD, 1963) and for amphetamine (ALLEVA, 1963; AXELROD, 1954; DRING et al., 1970; GOLDSTEIN and ANAGNOSTE, 1965). It appears, in fact, that m-hydroxylation, followed by p-hydroxylation, may be an alternative route from phenylalanine to dopa in mammalian species (SOURKES et al., 1961; D'IORIO et al., 1974).

B. Decarboxylation: Dopa Decarboxylase

The enzyme dopa decarboxylase, or aromatic amino acid decarboxylase, catalyzes the decarboxylation of a number of amino acids (LOVENBERG et al., 1962). It occurs not only in tissues such as liver and kidneys, but also in the cytoplasm of adrenergic neurons (HOLTZ and WESTERMAN, 1956; SHUMAN, 1956), and it requires pyridoxal phosphate as a coenzyme.

Decarboxylation is not a rate-limiting step in the biosynthesis of norepinephrine (LEVITT et al., 1965); consequently, large doses of potent decarboxylation inhibitors given to animals have minimal effects upon norepinephrine biosynthesis (UDENFRIEND and ZALTZMAN-NIRENBERG, 1962; UDENFRIEND et al., 1966). However, as discussed more fully below, under conditions of enzyme loading, as after the administration of dopa, the effect of decarboxylase inhibition can be demonstrated readily (SEE CLARK, 1963; PORTER, 1971).

Of particular pertinence to the formation of false transmitters *in vivo* are the following considerations: Compounds such as phenylalanine and tyrosine are poor substrates for the decarboxylase, while m-tyrosine and dopa are good substrates (LOVENBERG et al., 1962) (Table 3). Therefore, administered phenylalanine and

Table 3. *Substrates for dopa decarboxylase*[a]

Substrate	Relative specific activity
Dopa	6400
o-Tyrosine	4750
m-Tyrosine	2000
5-Hydroxytryptophan	1000
Tryptophan	220
Phenylalanine	104
p-Tyrosine	34
α-Methyldopa	32
α-Methyl-HTP	13
Histidine	10
α-Methyltryptophan	5
α-Methyl-m-tyrosine	4
Kynurenine	1—2
5-Methyltryptophan	<0.1
6-Methyltryptophan	<0.1
5-Methoxytryptophan	<0.1

[a] Purified guinea pig kidney enzyme. Data from LOVENBERG et al., 1962.

tyrosine escape extensive destruction in non-neuronal tissues, but after conversion to m-tyrosine or dopa in neurons, decarboxylation readily occurs to yield m-tyramine or dopamine, respectively. It should be noted, also, that although α-methyl amino acids such as methyldopa are not good substrates for dopa decarboxylase, the amines which result from their decarboxylation are resistant to destruction by monoamine oxidase (see below); consequently, these amines and their β-hydroxylated derivatives reach concentrations in the tissues of animals given the precursor amino acids sufficient to permit their functioning as false transmitters.

C. Aliphatic Side-Chain Hydroxylation: Dopamine-β-Hydroxylase

The enzyme catalyzes the conversion of dopamine to norepinephrine (FRIEDMAN and KAUFMAN, 1965; KAUFMAN and FRIEDMAN, 1965). It contains copper, and therefore it is inhibited by certain sulfhydryl compounds and chelating agents such as disulfiran, picolinic acid and α, α′-dipyridyl (GOLDSTEIN and CONTRERA, 1962; GOLDSTEIN et al., 1964; NAGATSU et al., 1967). Substrates for the hydroxylase include a variety of phenethylamine derivatives (VAN DER SCHOOT and CREVELING, 1965), for example phenethylamine itself, tyramine (CARLSSON and WALDECK, 1963), α-methyltyramine, α-methyldopamine, α-methyl-m-tyramine and p-hydroxyamphetamine (LEWANDER, 1971a, b) (see Table 4). As would be expected, substrates of the enzyme can compete with one another, thus functioning as competitive inhibitors. For example, α-methyl-m-tyramine, at a concentration equal to that of substrate (5×10^{-3} M), was found to inhibit β-hydroxylation of tyramine 20% (CREVELING et al., 1962).

Table 4. *Substrates for dopamine-β-hydroxylase*[a]

Substrate	Relative activity[b]
Phenethylamine	63
Tyramine	100
m-Tyramine	77
α-Methyltyramine	65
α-Methyl-m-tyramine	50
Dopamine	93
α-Methyldopamine	58

[a] Adapted from VAN DER SCHOOT and CREVELING, 1965.
[b] Based upon tyramine as 100.

The presence of false transmitters in neurons can inhibit the normal synthesis of norepinephrine, and dopamine β-hydroxylase may be the enzyme affected. As long as twenty-four hours after the administration of metaraminol or methyldopa (converted to α-methylnorepinephrine) to rats, the rate of norepinephrine synthesis in the myocardium may be subnormal (KOPIN et al., 1969).

Of the enzymes involved in catecholamine anabolism, dopamine-β-hydroxylase is the only one whose association with amine storage granules seems reasonably certain, not only in the adrenals (KIRSHNER, 1959), but also in noradrenergic neurons (LADURON and BELPAIRE, 1968c; POTTER and AXELROD, 1963a; STJÄRNE, 1966; STJÄRNE and LISHAJKO, 1967). Dopaminergic neurons apparently are devoid of the enzyme, and so in these cells catecholamine synthesis stops at the dopamine stage (see CARLSSON et al., 1966).

D. N-Methylation: Phenethanolamine-N-Methyl Transferase

The conversion of norepinephrine to epinephrine occurs almost exclusively in the adrenal medulla (AXELROD, 1962; MCGEER and MCGEER, 1964). However, epinephrine can be taken into sympathetic nerves from the circulation, and released by nerve stimulation (ROSELL et al., 1964), thereby acting as a false transmitter with a different balance of α- and β- receptor stimulating properties from the normal transmitter. Furthermore, other phenethanolamines (but not phenethylamines) are substrates for the enzyme (AXELROD, 1966). Although this reaction probably is of insignificant magnitude in the present context, the possibility of N-methylation contributing to false transmitter function cannot be ignored.

The enzyme catalyzes the transfer of a methyl group from S-adenosylmethionine to the phenethanolamine amino group (KIRSHNER and GOODALL, 1957); apparently it is a sulfhydryl enzyme (AXELROD, 1966). Some substrates for the enzyme are listed in Table 5.

Table 5. *Substrate for N-methyl transferase*[a]

Substrate	Relative activity (%)
l-Normetanephrine	100
dl-Phenylethanolamine	72
dl-m-Hydroxyphenylethanolamine	60
l-Norepinephrine	21
d-Norepinephrine	15
dl-Octopamine	18
dl-Neosynephrine	20
l-Norephedrine	14
l-Epinephrine	4
dl-Metanephrine	4
3-Methoxytyramine	0
Phenylethylamine	0
dopamine	0
Tyramine	0
dl-Amphetamine	0

[a] Enzyme was partially purified from monkey adrenal glands From Axelrod, 1966.

E. Amine Oxidation: Monoamine Oxidase

The catabolism of norepinephrine and closely related compounds proceeds mostly via 0-methylation (see below) and amine oxidation. Monoamine oxidase – or oxidases (Gorkin, 1966) – brings about the conversion of norepinephrine, for example, to 3,4-dihydroxyphenylglyoxal which, upon further oxidation, yields the corresponding acid, 3,4-dihydroxymandelic acid. Upon reduction, the aldehyde yields the ethylene glycol derivative, particularly in the brain (Rutledge and Jonason, 1967). It appears that dopamine has little tendency toward the latter pathway.

Monoamine oxidase is part of, or associated closely with, mitochondrial membranes, both in neuronal (Seiden and Westley, 1962) and in other tissues (Gorkin, 1966), and it attacks cytoplasmic rather than granule-bound amines (Iverson et al., 1965). It appears to be a sulfhydryl enzyme (Laguado and Sourkes, 1956), and may require a flavine cofactor (Belleau and Moran, 1963). Metal ions also influence the activity of the enzyme, but their role has not been defined precisely (Gorkin, 1966).

Monoamine oxidase catalyzes the oxidative deamination of secondary amines such as epinephrine (Blaschko et al., 1937), but not of α-methylated phenethylamines such as α-methyldopamine. However, the latter type of amine is susceptible to oxidative deamination by other enzymes, probably extraneuronal, to yield ketone derivatives (Porter and Titus, 1963). Since this process appears not to occur in neuronal tissue, the α-methyl compounds persist in this tissue more tenaciously than their non-methylated relatives.

F. m-O-Methylation: Catechol-O-Methyltransferase

Catechol-O-methyltransferase requires a divalent metal ion such as Mg^{++}, Zn^{++}, or others (Axelrod and Tomchick, 1958), and it is incapable of methylating monophenolic compounds. Its action involves the transfer of a methyl group from S-adenosylmethionine to the phenolic oxygen of the catechol ring (Axelrod, 1957). Although p-O-methylation of catechol derivatives can occur (Senoh et al., 1959), catecholamines are methylated predominantly on the m-phenolic oxygen

(Table 6). Apparently, O-methyltransferase is an extraneuronal enzyme (AXELROD, 1966; HUGHES et al., 1969; KALSMER and NICKERSON, 1969) which is responsible largely for metabolism of circulating catecholamines[1].

False transmitter catecholamines, for example α-methyldopamine (AXELROD et al., 1965), as well as non-amine catechol derivatives (ARCHER et al., 1960; DALY et al., 1962; BOOTH et al., 1959) are substrates for catechol-O-methyltransferase; and some of the latter compounds, such as pyrogallol, have been used as enzyme inhibitors (AXELROD and LAROCHE, 1956; BACQ et al., 1959; CROUT et al., 1960). Other O-methyltransferase inhibitors have been proposed, such as tropolone derivatives (BELLEAU and BURBA, 1961; MAVRIDES et al., 1963), desmethylpapaverine (BURBA and MURNAGHAN, 1964) and some O-methylated trihydroxybenzene derivatives (NIKODEJEVIC et al., 1970) (Table 7).

Table 6. *Substrates for catechol-O-methyl transferase*[a]

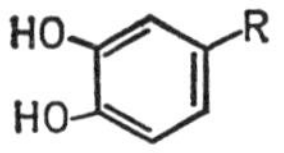

Substrate	*Meta:para* ratio	K_m	V_{max}[b]
Acidic			
R = —COOH	5.5	0.25	1.21
—CH_2COOH	7.0	0.31	1.16
—CH(OH)COOH	3.6	0.94	1.16
Neutral			
R = —$COOCH_2CH_3$	0.9	0.15	1.87
—CH_2CH_2OH	2.2	0.26	3.17
—$CH(OH)CH_2OH$	1.8	0.40	0.63
—$CH_2CH_2NH(COCH_3)$	1.7	0.52	4.94
—$CH(OH)CH_2NH(COCH_3)$	2.3	0.26	4.43
Basic			
R = —$CH_2CH_2NH_2$	6.9	0.16	0.9
—$CH(OH)CH_2NH_2$	7.03	0.26	0.66
—$CH(OH)CH_2NHCH_3$	7.2	0.38	0.49
Amphoteric			
R = —$CH_2CH_2NH_2(COOH)$	19.8		

[a] From CREVELING et al., 1970.
[b] Maximal velocity expressed as mμmoles of product formed per unit of COMT per minute (1 unit catalyzes the O-methylation of 1 mμmole of 3,4-dihydroxybenzoic acid per minute).

The administration of compounds which inhibit catecholamine catabolism has minimal effect upon normal neuronal function simply because catabolism is not the major fate of catecholamines liberated into the synaptic cleft (KOPIN and GORDON, 1962). Reuptake by presynaptic neurons seems to be the predominant mechanism in this respect (ANDÉN et al., 1964; BROWN and GILLESPIE, 1957; HERTTING et al., 1961; CROUT, 1961; STINSON, 1961).

[1] The fall of enzyme activity after denervation of some tissues (JARROTT, 1971) has been interpreted to indicate its location *in* neurons of these tissues. However, it seems probable that neuron degeneration would be accompanied by changes in the composition of synaptic cleft substances which, strictly speaking, should be considered as existing *outside* the neurons.

Table 7. *Inhibitors of catechol-O-methyl transferase*[a]

Compound	Inhibition (%)[b]
3,5-Dihydroxy-4-methoxybenzoic acid	97
3,5-Dihydroxy-4-methoxyphenethylamine	76
3-Hydroxy-4,5-dimethoxybenzoic acid	90
3-Hydroxy-4,5-dimethoxyphenethylamine	91
3,5-Dimethoxy-4-hydroxybenzoic acid	38
3,5-Dimethoxy-4-hydroxyphenethylamine	54
3-Hydroxy-4-methoxybenzoic acid	10
3-Hydroxy-4-methoxyphenethylamine	8

[a] From NIKODEJEVIC et al., 1970.
[b] Inhibitor concentration 2×10^{-4} M; substrate, 3,4-dihydroxybenzoic acid, 2×10^{-3} M.

II. Catecholamine Storage and Release[2]

False transmitters differ from normal transmitters in several important respects, including resistance to catabolism and altered affinity for storage sites (CARLSSON et al., 1965a; CARLSSON and WALDECK, 1968b; CORRODI et al., 1970). Nevertheless, the mechanisms involved are essentially similar for the two types of compounds. With proper reservations, a discussion of normal transmitter storage and release will describe adequately the storage and release of false transmitters also (ALMGREN and LUNDBORG, 1970; ALMGREN et al., 1969; MUSCHOLL and WEBER, 1965; ROSS and RENYI, 1966).

Although the metabolism, storage and release of catecholamines by adrenal medullary chromaffin cells and by adrenergic nerves have many features in common, important differences exist (HELLE et al., 1971). Insofar as possible, only information gathered from observations of nervous tissue will be utilized in this discussion.

Evidence is good that norepinephrine and also false transmitters (LEITZ and STEFANO, 1970; LUNDBORG and STITZEL, 1967a, b; LUNDBORG and WALDECK, 1966) exist in multiple – perhaps three – "pools" within postganglionic, presynaptic nerve terminals of the adrenergic system (Fig. 2). Two of these are intragranular pools, the third is an extragranular, cytoplasmic pool (MALMFORS, 1965; VAN ORDEN et al., 1967; see also CARLSSON, 1969). In addition, amines may be taken up to some degree by extraneuronal tissue (FISCHER et al., 1965b; ALMGREN and JONASON, 1971); however, the contribution to neuron function of amines so held is not known.

Quantitatively, catecholamine bound in storage granules is most significant. These particles have been isolated from several tissues beside the adrenal medulla (DE ROBERTIS et al., 1965; MICHAELSON et al., 1964; POTTER and AXELROD, 1962, 1963b; SNYDER et al., 1964; VON EULER and HILLARP, 1956; VON EULER and LISHAJKO, 1965a).

Illustrative data on the uptake of some amines by isolated granules are given in Table 1. This uptake is by two mechanisms: one, sensitive to reserpine, is activated by Mg^{++}-ATPase (not Na^{+}, K^{+}-ATPase); the other, usually less important quantitatively, is resistant to reserpine (CARLSSON, 1969; MALMFORS, 1965). The relative operation of these systems is determined, at least in part, by

[2] For excellent discussions of catecholamine storage and release, see "New Aspects of Catecholamine Storage and Release", SCHÜMANN and KRONBERG, eds. Springer, 1970; Shore, 1972.

the nature of the amine involved: the reserpine-sensitive system operates more efficiently with metaraminol than with α-methylnorepinephrine or norepinephrine, for example (LUNDBORG and STITZEL, 1967a).

Although active uptake of amines is blocked by reserpine (ANDÉN and HENNING, 1966; BHAGAT et al., 1967; DAHLSTRÖM et al., 1965), passive transport apparently is not. Therefore, administered amines can enter the granular pool and temporarily restore adrenergic function in reserpine-treated animals (DAHLSTRÖM et al., 1967). However, reserpine prevents granule amine binding more persistently

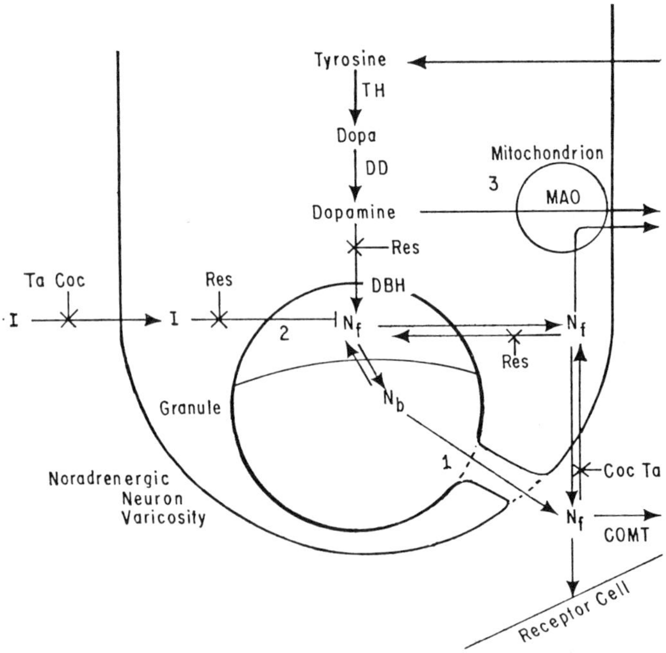

Fig. 2. Representation of the noradrenergic synapse. 1. Discharge of vesicle contents into the synaptic cleft following stimulation of the presynaptic neuron. 2. Displacement of loosely bound norepinephrine by an indirectly acting sympathomimetic agent such as tyramine. 3. Oxidative deamination of amines by mitochondrial monoamineoxidase. Coc, Cocaine; COMT, Catechol-O-methyltransferase; DBH, Dopamine-β-hydroxylase; DD, Dopadecarboxylase; I, Sympathomimetic amine; MAO, Monoamineoxidase; N_b, "Bound" norepinephrine; N_f, "Free" norepinephrine; P, 3,4-Dihydroxyphenylacetic acid; P′, 3,4-Dihydroxymandelic acid; P″, Normetanephrine; Res. Reserpine; T_a, Tricyclic antidepressants.
Note: Starting with methyldopa instead of dopa, a similar series of events can be depicted with the exception that the oxidative deamination step (3) is inoperative

than it prevents active uptake (GLOWINSKI et al., 1966), and permanent restoration of nerve function after reserpine administration may depend upon transport of fresh granules to the nerve endings (HÄGGENDAL and DAHLSTRÖM, 1970, 1971).

Storage granules are formed in neuron cell bodies and are transported to the nerve endings, possibly via microtubules (DAHLSTRÖM, 1970a, b; ERÄNKÖ and HÄRKÖNEN, 1965; FREDHOLM and SEDVALL, 1966; PELLEGRINO DE IRALDI and DE ROBERTIS, 1970; SCHMITT, 1968). Known substituents of the granules include catecholamine, adenosine triphosphate, proteins — dopamine-β-hydroxylase and "chromogranins" — and metal ions (GEFFEN et al., 1970; HELLE, 1970; HORTNAGL et al., 1969; POTTER, 1966; SMITH et al., 1969).

In vitro amines such as serotonin, norepinephrine and dopamine form complexes with ATP (WEINER and JARDETZKY, 1964) which in the presence of calcium or magnesium ions yield macromolecular aggregates, which are dispersed by increased metal ion concentrations, reserpine, tyramine and amphetamine (BERNEIS et al., 1970, 1971). The similarities between the operation of this model and the amine storage granules is striking; but undoubtedly the model is of insufficient complexity to duplicate the granules. A somewhat more complex mechanism of amine storage, including also protein, i. e., chromogranin, has been proposed (SMYTHES et al., 1971).

Release of norepinephrine into the synaptic cleft following nerve activation appears at present to follow this sequence of events (FOLKOW and HÄGGENDAL, 1970; HÄGGENDAL, 1970; STJÄRNE, 1970); membrane depolarization results in calcium mobilization (BOULLIN, 1966; DOUGLAS and KANNO, 1967; KIRPEKAR and MISU, 1967; RUBIN, 1970), possibly mediated by acetylcholine (BURN, 1971a, b)[3].

Storage granules (CHANG and CHANG, 1965) nearest to the presynaptic membrane adhere to the latter and a pore is formed through which a *part* of the granule contents, including not only norepinephrine and other amines, but also dopamine-β-hydroxylase (GEWIRTZ and KOPIN, 1970; POTTER and AXELROD, 1963b; WEINSHILBOUM et al., 1971) and chromogranins (DE POTTER et al., 1970), is discharged into the cleft. It has been suggested that Ca^{++}-dependent neurofibril contraction provides the impetus by which granules travel, via neurotubules, to the presynaptic membrane (THOA et al., 1972b). Although present in the granules, ATP apparently is not discharged as a result of nerve stimulation (STJÄRNE et al., 1970).

After discharging its contents, the granule detaches from the membrane; either its store of amine is replenished by reabsorption from the cleft and by synthesis, or it is destroyed and replaced by a new one (DE POTTER and CHUBB, 1971). At any rate, newly absorbed or synthesized amines are released in preference to older, more tightly bound ones as a consequence of nerve stimulation (CARLSSON and WALDECK, 1966b; CROUT et al., 1964; LUNDBORG, 1967). Presumably, the labile fraction of granule amine, in association with metal ions, ATP and soluble proteins, requires time to reach a state of complex formation which resists discharge.

Ordinarily, storage granules are not saturated with catecholamine, and not all of the catecholamine normally present is required for neuron function (LEE, 1967; SEDVALL and THORSON, 1965). Thus, the granules are capable of taking up moderate quantities of extraneous amines, either normal or false transmitters (MAÎTRE and STAEHELIN, 1967), without displacement of norepinephrine, and considerable amounts of norepinephrine can be displaced with little or no impairment of synaptic transmission. Displacement may be approximately one mole of false transmitter per mole of norepinephrine (PORTER et al., 1967; SCHÜMANN and GROBECKER, 1965; SHORE et al., 1964); however, synthesis inhibition, inhibition of catabolism and other factors often obscure the one for one relationship. It should be noted too that normal catecholamines can displace false transmitters from storage, if the concentration of the former is increased as, for example, by the administration of a monoamine oxidase inhibitor (CARLSSON et al., 1968a).

Finally, the relatively small quantity of norepinephrine which exists in an "unbound" state (TITUS and DENGLER, 1966; VAN ORDEN et al., 1967) in the neuron cytoplasm, is the "pool" of amine which is released readily by indirect-acting sympathomimetic agents such as tyramine (CHANG and CHANG, 1965; IVERSEN and WHITBY, 1963; LEE et al., 1967; POTTER and AXELROD, 1963c). Total norepine-

[3] The involvement of acetylcholine in adrenergic transmission has been disputed, but not irrevocably refuted (see e.g. ESTERHUIZEN et al., 1968).

phrine in the neuron exists in equilibrium among the two granule pools and the cytoplasm (MICHAELSON et al., 1964; VON EULER and LISHAJKO, 1965b), and biosynthesis of the amine regulates the overall content (VON EULER and LISHAJKO, 1967).

Displacement of cytoplasmic catecholamine by tyramine, phenethylamine and amphetamine can lead to granule depletion also (GUTMAN and WEIL-MALHERBE, 1966; JONSSON et al., 1966; MOORE and LAVIRIERE, 1963; NEFF et al., 1965), when the depleting agents are administered rather frequently. In the guinea pig, a species which does not hydroxylate amphetamine (DRING et al., 1970), administration of the amine leads to a decrease in the concentration of norepinephrine in the brain. The effect is not a persistent one, its half-life being 2.5 to 3 h (LEWANDER, 1971c). Possibly, granule depletion results from upset of the cytoplasm-granule catecholamine equilibrium.

However, in other species, metabolism of such depleting agents to compounds which have greater affinity for the granules may be involved (FISCHER et al., 1965a), that is, they may become false transmitters as illustrated by the following case. Amphetamine is metabolized to an unknown but probably a rather minor extent in both the cat and in man to yield *p*-hydroxyamphetamine (Paradrine) (CAVANAUGH et al., 1970). The latter compound undergoes *β*-hydroxylation to yield *p*-hydroxynorephedrine in man (SJOERDSMA and VON STUDNITZ, 1963), and this compound, like amphetamine (CAVANAUGH et al., 1970) has been shown to produce signs of impaired peripheral sympathetic function (GILL et al., 1967) upon chronic administration. Apparently, with continued administration of amphetamine or *p*-hydroxyamphetamine, the small amount of *p*-hydroxynorephedrine which is produced accumulates to a sufficient extent in the nerve endings to alter sympathetic function (BRODIE et al., 1970; GOLDSTEIN and ANAGNOSTE, 1965; GROPETTI and COSTA, 1969; LEWANDER, 1971b). It should be noted that the acute administration of amphetamine to man produces an increased sensitivity of the cardiovascular system, not only to tyramine but also to norepinephrine (CAVANAUGH et al., 1970). The reason for this is not known at present; however, amphetamine may decrease the uptake of norepinephrine at the nerve endings, thus making more of the transmitter available at the receptors, whether it is released by presynaptic nerves or injected.

Phenethylamine derivatives are bound in storage granules of adrenergic neurons — and are released by nerve stimulation — more readily if they are hydroxylated at the *β*-position (KOPIN, 1966; MUSACCHIO et al., 1966). However, since *β*-hydroxylation is relatively nonspecific, non-*β*-hydroxylated phenethylamines made available to the granules may be converted to the form which is bound rather easily, as *α*-methyldopamine is converted to *α*-methylnorepinephrine and *α*-methyl-m-tyramine is converted to metaraminol (CARLSSON and LINDQVIST, 1962). Compounds not bearing the *α*-methyl group, such as *m*-tyramine, also undergo *β*-hydroxylation. For example, octopamine has been found in nervous tissue of animals given monamine oxidase inhibitors (KAKIMOTO and ARMSTRONG, 1962; SNYDER et al., 1964) or tyramine (PISANO et al., 1960). It is released from the nerve ending by electrical stimulation (KOPIN et al., 1964), and in fact, it may be regarded as a normally occurring noradrenergic co-transmitter (MOLINOFF and AXELROD, 1969, 1972).

Under loading conditions, non-*β*-hydroxylated amines can enter the noradrenergic granule pool which is released by nerve stimulation, as has been shown with dopamine (ROBERTS and STREET, 1970; THOENEN et al., 1965, 1966, 1967a; WHITNACK et al., 1971; WHITSETT et al., 1970) and with *α*-methyldopamine (THOENEN, 1967b).

Ring hydroxyl groups also influence the binding of phenethylamines in storage granules (MUSACCHIO, 1965a, b). Thus, octopamine has more affinity than phenethanolamine for binding, and norepinephrine is better bound than octopamine. An α-methyl group also seems to promote binding (PHILIPPU and SCHÜMANN, 1967).

It should be emphasized here that little is known concerning structural requirements for binding in nonadrenergic systems. Presumably, important differences exist between systems (CARLSSON et al., 1965a); it has been shown that α-methyl-m-tyramine and metaraminol are bound, preferentially, in dopaminergic and noradrenergic areas, respectively, in the central nervous system (DORRIS and SHORE, 1971). It appears probable, however, that in any of the systems, relatively tightly bound compounds can be replaced in the presence of high concentrations of less firmly bound substances (CARLSSON and WALDECK, 1966a), substances related not only to the transmitter of a particular system but also to the transmitters of other systems. For example, catecholamines are taken up by serotoninergic nerves (BARRETT and BALCH, 1971), and norepinephrine is displaced from noradrenergic nerves by serotonin (FILLION and LLUCH, 1970; JESTER and HORST, 1972).

III. Uptake of Amines Through the Cell Membrane[4]

Presynaptic neuronal (synaptosomal) membranes actively transport normal and false transmitter amines into the cells (ANDÉN et al., 1964; CARLSSON et al., 1963; CARLSSON and WALDECK, 1965a, b; FUXE and HILLARP, 1964; HAMBERGER et al., 1964; MALMFORS, 1965) by a mechanism closely associated with Na^+, K^+-activated ATPase. The process is stimulated by extracellular Na^+ (BOGDANSKI and BRODIE, 1966; GILLIS and PATTON, 1967; HORST et al., 1968; IVERSEN and KRAVITZ, 1966) and inhibited by extracellular K^+ (BOGDANSKI and BRODIE, 1969; BOGDANSKI et al., 1968; COLBURN et al., 1968). Presumably, the mechanism involves a carrier which has a higher affinity for amines in the presence of Na^+ (outside membrane) than in the presence of K^+ (inside the cell) (TISSARI et al., 1969; BOGDANSKI et al., 1970).

The mechanism is blocked by a variety of compounds, notably tricyclic compounds such as imipramine, desipramine, amitriptyline and protriptyline (HORN et al., 1971; MATSUMOTO and HORITA, 1962; STONE et al., 1964). Consequently, these compounds, as well as inhibitors of catecholamine synthesis, accelerate nerve stimulation-evoked depletion of amines from the nerve ending (MALMFORS, 1964). However, it is of importance that such compounds, as has been shown for desipramine and protriptyline, block uptake into the noradrenergic, but not the dopaminergic nerves of the brain; amphetamine apparently blocks uptake by both types of nerves (CARLSSON et al., 1966; SNYDER et al., 1970).

The membrane pump is effective in transporting amines other than the normal ones, for example tyramine (GESSA and VACCA, 1965), α-methyl-m-tyramine and metaraminol (GESSA et al., 1966). If the cell is exposed to a mixture of amines, i. e. norepinephrine and a false transmitter, the amines may compete for entry, which may influence pharmacological responses in the presence of false transmitters. For example, metaraminol is more potent than α-methylnorepinephrine in preventing uptake of norepinephrine by neuronal tissue (IVERSEN, 1964). Therefore, the effectiveness of the two false transmitters might be influenced to different degrees because of less rapid uptake of impulse-released norepinephrine in the presence of one than in the presence of the other.

[4] For a review of amine uptake see IVERSEN (1971).

The more lipid soluble amines, i. e. those with fewer hydroxyl groups, pass through the membrane in both directions more rapidly than the more polar amines, *unaided* by the membrane pump. For example, it appears that metaraminol escapes from cells rather easily, and its persistence in cells depends to a considerable degree upon its return by the membrane pump. Consequently, blockade of the pump permits depletion of this amine (CARLSSON and WALDECK, 1968a; ALMGREN, 1971). Norepinephrine and α-methylnorepinephrine, being more polar, do not leak out of the cells rapidly, and their depletion is not accomplished by membrane pump blockade alone.

The gross movement of amines into and out of nervous tissue is governed by both granule and cell membrane mechanisms. The participation of the cell membrane is evident in the following case. Although metaraminol has less affinity than α-methylnorepinephrine for storage granules (LUNDBORG and STITZEL, 1967a), the two amines have comparable potency in releasing norepinephrine from the tissue (SHORE, 1966; TORCHIANA et al., 1968).

A clear demonstration of the interplay between uptake and release mechanisms of the granules and cell membranes has been presented (CARLSSON et al., 1967a). α-Methylnorepinephrine present in the brain after treatment of animals (rats) with methyldopa was decreased by the administration of tetrabenazine (an inhibitor of granule uptake) and desipramine (an inhibitor of membrane uptake), but not by either of these alone. Apparently, the false transmitter, freed from the granules by tetrabenazine and not susceptible to attack by monoamine oxidase, leaked out of the cells. Its reentry was prevented by desipramine, and therefore its concentration in the cells decreased. Similarly, the combination of drugs produced a decrease of α-methyldopamine in dopaminergic nerves. It is important to note, however, that behavioral activation observed in the methyldopa-treated animals upon the administration of tetrabenazine and desipramine was attenuated if an inhibitor of catecholamine synthesis was also given. Quite probably, release of freshly formed natural transmitter, rather than false transmitters, was responsible for the behavioral activation.

IV. False Transmitters and Sympathetic Transmission

False transmitters which are closely related structurally to the catecholamines generally are sympathomimetic agents also (Table 8). They may exert the latter type of activity by liberating the normal transmitter into the synaptic cleft (indirect action), by stimulation of the post synaptic receptors (direct action), or by a combination of both mechanisms (PATIL et al., 1965, 1967; TRENDELENBURG, 1963). It is important to note that the classification of amines in this way is not absolute. Not only the nature of the amine, but also the species and organ employed in experimentation are determinants in class assignment (STONE et al., 1966; TRENDELENBURG, 1963).

Tachyphylaxis to the initial pressor effects of indirectly acting amines develops when the normal amine pool which these agents, or their metabolites, displace is exhausted (POCH and KOPIN, 1966). If the entering agent is susceptible to attack by monoamine oxidase, and if it is not incorporated into storage granules, it is cleared from the neurons rapidly, as for example phenethylamine and tyramine. Compounds with proper structures, which resist attack by monoamine oxidase, are incorporated into the granule pools; however, if norepinephrine synthesis proceeds, the entering amine must compete with the normal one for binding sites. The fraction of newly formed norepinephrine which escapes binding either is destroyed by monoamine oxidase or leaks out of the cell, but not in a concentration great enough to cause postsynaptic stimulation.

During false neurotransmission, the storage granule amine contents released into the synaptic cleft upon stimulation of the presynaptic neuron consist of norepinephrine and the foreign amine. The ratio between the amounts of the latter two released is approximately the same as the ratio of concentrations in the neuron (CROUT and SHORE, 1964; GAFFNEY et al., 1963; HAEFLEY et al., 1967; LINDMAR et al., 1967; MUSCHOLL and MAÎTRE, 1963), and it is governed by the several factors specified above. Since the amount of norepinephrine released per granule is less than normal, granules must be liberated at a faster rate than normal in order to achieve a synaptic catecholamine concentration sufficient to stimulate the receptor cell. Thus, while a false transmitter may block low frequency-elicited nerve transmission (DAY and RAND, 1967; FARMER, 1965; KILBINGER et al., 1970; LINDMAR et al., 1967; STONE and STAVORSKI, 1963; TORCHIANA et al., 1970), high frequency stimulation may evoke normal, or nearly normal responses. However,

Table 8. *Pressor potency of sympathomimetic agents in reserpine pretreated animals*

Compound	Potency of norepinephrine = 1		
	Dog[b]	Cat[c]	Rat[b]
α-Methylnorepinephrine	0.370		0.50
Dopamine	0.005		0.004
α-Methyldopamine	0.009		0.007
Metaraminol	0.020		0.020
Octopamine		0.0002[a]	
α-Methyloctopamine		0.0010[a]	
m-Octopamine		0.0143	
α-Methyl-m-octopamine		0.0010[a]	

[a] Indirect acting sympathomimetic.
[b] Data adapted from TORCHIANA et al., 1966.
[c] Data from TRENDELENBURG et al., 1962.

metaraminol, administered as such or derived metabolically from α-methyl-m-tyrosine, was shown to block the hypertensive response to nerve stimulation in rats at frequencies ranging from 2.5 to 20 cps (SCHMITT and PETILLOT, 1970). Responses of the cat nictitating membrane to nerve stimulation after metaraminol administration were shown to be attenuated at higher frequencies (16 cps) only if the tissue was depleted of norepinephrine by 90 to 95% (STONE, 1971; TORCHIANA et al., 1970).

There are several mechanisms which operate to influence the response of receptors to the mixture of normal and false transmitters released into the synaptic cleft by nerve stimulation. First, although potency estimates vary depending upon the species, the tissue and the methods used (DAY and RAND, 1964; HAEFELY et al., 1966; SCHMITT and PETILLOT, 1970), as mentioned above, some compounds which fulfill other criteria for false transmitters exhibit direct receptor-stimulant properties, also. Second, the sensitivity of receptor cells to amines may be altered in certain situations; e. g., supersensitivity to injected norepinephrine was observed in cats which had received methyldopa or α-methyl-*m*-tyrosine (HAEFELY et al., 1966). It is of interest that in these animals responses of the nictitating membrane to nerve stimulation were either not affected (methyldopa) or reduced (α-methyl-

m-tyrosine). Apparently, supersensitivity may obscure a reduction in adrenergic response if a false transmitter with relatively strong direct sympathomimetic activity is involved.

On the other hand, a reduced response may occur in the presence of a false transmitter. This is illustrated by the finding that although the (S) isomer of α-methyldopamine, which is converted to α-methylnorepinephrine, does not alter the response to cardioaccelerator nerve stimulation, the (R) "unnatural" isomer of α-methyldopamine, which is not β-hydroxylated to the noradrenergic amine, reduces the response. Since the output of norepinephrine was the same in control and animals treated with (R) α-methyldopamine, the reduced response to nerve stimulation was attributed to a postjunctional inhibitory action of the false transmitter (KILBINGER et al., 1971).

V. False Transmitters and Blood Pressure

The effects of administered phenethylamines and their derivatives upon blood pressure can be due to influences in the periphery, in the central nervous system, or in both. False transmitters such as α-methylnorepinephrine and metaraminol administered as such do not enter the central nervous system to a great extent; and, therefore, their effects upon blood pressure are primarily peripheral in origin. Amino acids and less polar amines, such as amphetamine, do enter the central nervous system; thus, they operate both centrally and peripherally. The peripheral component can be attenuated, in the case of an amino acid, such as dopa, by administration of a substance which inhibits decarboxylation, such as carbidopa (*L*-α-methyl-α-hydrazino-3,4-dihydroxy-phenylpropionic acid) (MINSKER et al., 1971).

False transmitters in peripheral adrenergic neurons, after possible acute pressor effects, produce lowering of blood pressure mainly of the postural type. This is due to attenuation of reflex pressor impulses, occuring in afferents to the heart and blood vessels. Octopamine, for example, has been shown to be considerably less potent than norepinephrine as an arteriolar pressor agent (ALTURA, 1975). It has been suggested that the antihypertensive effect of monoamine oxidase inhibitors depends upon an accumulation of this false transmitter, formed by decarboxylation of tyrosine, followed by β-hydroxylation of the resulting tyramine, in peripheral noradrenergic neurons (KOPIN et al., 1965). The closely related compound p-hydroxynorephedrine, a metabolite of amphetamine and or p-hydroxy amphetamine, lowers blood pressure in hypertensive patients by a peripheral false transmitter mechanism (RANGNO et al., 1973).

Centrally, false transmitters may interfere with reflex arcs also. However, it is possible that inhibitory mechanisms may be *activated* centrally, particularly in the presence of amines such as α-methylnorepinephrine which have pronounced direct sympathomimetic properties.

To illustrate these mechanisms, the effects of administered methyldopa, dopa, m-tyrosine and α-methyl-m-tyrosine will be discussed.

A. Methyldopa

Methyldopa is a relatively poor substrate for dopa decarboxylase (LOVENBERG et al., 1962). Its rate of decarboxylation in peripheral tissues of the rat is rapid enough so that a small pressor response is observed after parenteral administration of a relatively large dose (100 mg/kg) of methyldopa (STONE, unpublished observation). However, in man pressor responses apparently have not been observed (BREST et al., 1961). Obviously, α-methyl-dopamine and α-methylnorepinephrine are formed metabolically in most species since they are detected in both central and peripheral tissues of animals (CARLSSON and LINDQVIST, 1962) and in the urine of animals (PORTER and TITUS, 1963) and man (BUHS et al., 1964; MUSCHOLL and RAHN, 1966) after methyldopa administration. However, sufficient amounts of the amino acid escape peripheral decarboxylation so that it enters the brain where decarboxylation also occurs.

α-Methyldopamine is converted to α-methylnorepinephrine in central as well as peripheral neurons, and it is the β-hydroxylated compound which serves as a false transmitter in the noradrenergic system. An increased realease of α-methylnorepinephrine and norepinephrine from peripheral neurons in humans who received methyldopa has been shown to occur as a result of heightened nervous activity accompanying exercise (LINDMAR et al., 1968).

Since α-methylnorepinephrine has considerable direct adrenergic activity (Table 8), its release, along with norepinephrine, by neuron activation results in only slightly attenuated receptor stimulation, at least in peripheral tissues under some conditions. In addition to its adrenergic activity, α-methylnorepinephrine inhibits the uptake of norepinephrine by presynaptic neurons (BURGEN and IVERSEN, 1965), which also may prevent the agent from clearly blocking synaptic transmission. The uptake of dopa by neurons reportedly is inhibited by methyldopa as well as by α-methyl-m-tyrosine (THOA et al., 1972a). The influence of this inhibition upon pharmacological effects of these α-methyl-amino acids is not known.

The antihypertensive effect of methyldopa in man, first reported by OATES et al. (1960), apparently is not adversely influenced by the concomitant administration of peripherally active inhibitors of dopa decarboxylase (SJOERDSMA et al., 1963; HENNING, 1968, 1969; WATANABE et al., 1971; NIJKAMP et al., 1975). Its effect, at least in animals, *is* attenuated by centrally acting decarboxylase inhibitors (DAVIS et al., 1963; HENNING, 1968, 1969; COHEN et al., 1974; DAY et al., 1973), so it can be concluded that methyldopa must be decarboxylated centrally, and that peripheral adrenergic blockade plays a minor role in its mode of action. Other evidence leading to the same conclusion can be cited (see also SCRIABINE et al., 1976):

1) Methyldopa infusion into the left vertebral artery lowers blood pressure in the cat without notably influencing catecholamine concentrations in peripheral tissues (HENNING and VAN ZWIETEN, 1968).

2) Bradycardia and decreased hind limb vascular resistance have been observed in vagotomized cats to which methyldopa was administered in such a way that the drug reached the brain but not peripheral tissue (INGENITO et al., 1970).

3) Depression of the meduallary vasomotor center in dogs by the local application of methyldopa has been observed (JAJU et al., 1966).

4) Increase of blood pressure evoked by eserin-induced stimulation of central sympathetic centers in rats is blocked by the systemic administration of methyldopa, but not by α-methyldopamine or α-methylnorepinephrine (BRUNNER er al., 1967; HEDWALL and MAÎTRE, 1971).

5) Administration of α-methyldopamine to hypertensive patients did not result in lowering of blood pressure (BUHS et al., 1964).

6) The antihypertensive effect of methyldopa lasts for a shorter time than maximum concentrations of α-methylnorepinephrine persist in peripheral tissues such as the heart (TORCHIANA et al., 1965).

Unlike the depressor responses to dopa and m-tyrosine (see below), this response to methyldopa is observed even if the brain is depleted of norepinephrine by the administration of α-methyl-m-tyrosine, and synthesis is blocked by the tyrosine hydroxylase inhibitor α-methyltyrosine methyl ester (HENNING and RUBENSON, 1971). However, blockade of dopamine-β-hydroxylase does prevent the hypotensive effect of methyldopa, as has been demonstrated in the rat (HENNING and RUBENSON, 1971; COHEN et al., 1974; DAY et al., 1973) and in the cat (TORCHIANA et al., 1972, 1973). Therefore, it seems clear that the presence of α-methylnorepinephrine in the brain causes the reduction of blood pressure following methyldopa administration. Evidence substantiating this concept has appeared. The depressor response to methyldopa is not attenuated by centrally-acting dopaminergic blocking agents, i.e., spiroperidol (HENNING and RUBENSON, 1970). However, it has been shown that the hypotensive effect of intracerebral administration of α-methylnorepinephrine is reduced by α-adrenergic blocking agents (HEISE and KRONEBERG, 1972, 1973; FINCH and HAEUSLER, 1973; VAN SPANNING and VAN ZWIETEN, 1975). Furthermore, the noncatecholamine central α-noradrenergic stimulant clonidine (SCHMITT et al., 1971) is an antihypertensive agent (ANDÉN et al., 1970; BOLME and FUXE, 1971). The antihypertensive activity of clonidine can also be decreased by α-adrenergic blocking agents (VAN ZWIETEN et al., 1975).

The above considerations may be taken to show that in the central nervous system α-methylnorepinephrine serves as a noradrenergic false transmitter with considerable stimulatory effect upon receptor neurons; that, because of its resistance to deamination, and possibly concurrent receptor supersensitivity, α-methylnorepinephrine liberated into the synapse results in increased rather than decreased stimulation of inhibitory vasomotor neurons. However, the possibility is not excluded that α-methylnorepinephrine present in the neuronal and surrounding tissue after methyldopa administration causes stimulation of receptor cells and perhaps sensitizes the latter to impulse-released norepinephrine with the net result of vasomotor inhibitory stimulation.

On the other hand, the antihypertensive effect of methyldopa may involve other mechanisms also, at least in animals. In rats, methyldopa may inhibit the response of arterioles to catecholamines, thus depressing blood pressure (ALTURA, 1974); and, in dogs, methyldopa administration leads to impaired peripheral neuronal function, at least in some organs (LOKHANDWALA et al., 1975). Involvement of α-methyldopamine in the antihypertensive action of methyldopa cannot yet be ignored entirely. WALDMEIER et al. (1975) found that the time sequence of antihypertensive activity following methyldopa administration to renal hypertensive rats paralleled the concentration of α-methyldopamine, rather than the concentration of α-methylnorepinephrine, in the brain. The data were interpreted to show that either α-methyldopamine, or *newly formed* α-methylnorepinephrine, was the active antihypertensive agent.

The acute pressor response resulting from the administration of phenethylamine derivatives is well known, and precludes the use of these compounds *per se* in the treatment of hypertension. The utility of methyldopa depends in part upon the relatively slow metabolism of the amino acid, as described above, so that the tissues are not exposed to overtly pressor concentrations of amines.

As would be anticipated, certain physiological effects, other than therapeutically useful reduction of blood pressure, appear after methyldopa administration. These effects may be due to the ability of α-methylnorepinephrine (and in some cases of α-methyldopamine) to function as a false transmitter. Since α-methylnorepinephrine has considerable potency as a direct adrenergic stimulant, the blockade of adrenergic function, at least in the peripheral tissues, is relatively minor in extent. The substitution of agents with less direct activity than α-methylnorepinephrine for norepinephrine in the nerve endings will have consequences similar in pattern to those of α-methylnorepinephrine but of different magnitude.

Galactorrhea has been observed in patients given methyldopa (Pettinger et al., 1963; Horwitz et al., 1966; Vaidya et al., 1970), and presumably is due to interference with adrenergic, or dopaminergic, hypothalamopituitary control. The development of Parkinson-like symptoms in man also has been reported (Groden, 1963; Strang, 1966; Vaidya et al., 1970); quite possibly, substitution of α-methyldopamine for dopamine in the corpus striatum is the causative factor.

Lowered plasma renin concentrations have been observed after the administration of methyldopa to human subjects (Mohammed et al., 1969; Strauss et al., 1970) and to dogs (Mohammed and Privitera, 1971). This effect is a consequence of decreased renal sympathetic nerve function due to the presence of a false transmitter (Privitera and Mohammed, 1972). However, whether the effect is a peripheral nervous system phenomenon of of central origin has not been established.

Mild orthostatic hypotension and bradycardia which have been reported to accompany methyldopa therapy in some instances (Sannerstedt et al., 1963; Dollery et al., 1962; Bayliss and Harvey-Smith, 1962) might be attributed to partial peripheral sympathetic blockade, although possible central involvement cannot be ruled out. The drowsiness often seen during the first few days of therapy (Dollery et al., 1962; Cannon et al., 1962) most likely is a central nervous system effect which cannot be satisfactorily explained at present.

Animal studies have shown that the mobilization of free fatty acids caused by tyramine administration or by stress is blocked by the prior administration of α-methyl-m-tyrosine, but not by the administration of methyldopa (Stock and Westerman, 1964; 1965). It was observed also that the β-hydroxylated amines derived from these two amino acids exhibited widely different lipolytic potencies on epididymal fat pads *in vitro*, α-methylnorepinephrine being about as potent as norepinephrine, and metaraminol being about 1/1000 th as potent. Thus, in adipose tissue metaraminol clearly functioned as a false transmitter while α-methylnorepinephrine functioned as a relatively potent substitute transmitter.

B. Dopa and m-Tyrosine

The administration of dopa to human subjects may produce hypotension (Calne et al., 1969; Cotzias et al., 1969; Godwin-Austen et al., 1969; Yahr et al., 1969), an effect which is not attenuated by peripheral decarboxylase inhibition (Watanabe et al., 1970).

In animals, dopa administration is followed by both central and peripheral adrenergic effects. As in man, prior administration of a dopa decarboxylase inhibitor which does not reach the central nervous system abolished the peripheral hypertensive response to dopa, and a hypotensive response was obtained (Henning and Rubenson, 1970; Robson, 1972; Antonaccio et al., 1974). However inhibition of decarboxylation centrally led to abolition of the hypotensive response to dopa Henning and Rubenson, 1970; Minsker, 1971; Antonaccio et al., 1974). Also, interference with another enzyme involved in the biosynthesis of norepinephrine, dopamine-β-hydroxylase, blocks dopa's ability to lower blood pressure (Henning, 1969; Torchiana et al., 1972; Rubenson, 1971). Clearly, norepinephrine must be present in the brain for dopa to exert its hypotensive effects. It follows that stimulation of noradrenergic neurons is the underlying mechanism, although the exact sequence of events following dopa administration is obscure; e.g., it is not known whether dopamine operates merely as an indirect noradrenergic agent or is converted to norepinephrine in large enough quantities to cause significant activation of noradrenergic neurons (RUBENSON, 1971). However, it has been claimed that, in the absence of monoamine oxidase inhibition, dopa stimulates central noradrenergic neurons by the indirect sympathomimetic action of the dopamine which results from its decarboxylation (ANDÉN et al., 1972). Postural hypotension following dopa administration may be due to the action of dopamine as a peripheral noradrenergic false transmitter (DHASMANA and SPILKER, 1973).

m-Tyrosine, like dopa, produces a transient pressor response when administered alone, but a prolonged depressor response when given with a peripheral decarboxylase inhibitor (RUBENSON, 1971). The depressor response was abolished by inhibition of dopamine-β-hydroxylase; and both m-tyramine and m-octopamine have been found in the brains of animals given m-tyrosine and an inhibitor of peripheral decarboxylase. Like dopa, m-tyrosine shows no depressor activity if central catecholamines are depleted and their synthesis blocked (RUBENSON, 1971).

m-Octopamine is a relatively weak sympathomimetic agent (cat nictitating membrane) with a predominantly direct type of activity (TRENDELENBURG et al., 1962; TRENDELENBURG, 1963). On the other hand, m-tyramine has significant indirect sympathomimetic activity. Thus, if the central hypotensive action of m-tyrosine depends upon the presence of norepinephrine in central neurons (RUBENSON, 1971), m-tyramine rather than m-octopamine may be the effective agent.

C. α-Methyl-m-Tyrosine

The amino acid exerts an antihypertensive effect in man (HOLTMEIER, et al., 1966; HORWITZ and SJOERDSMA, 1964). Its administration to rats leads to decreased concentrations of norepinephrine in both the brain and peripheral noradrenergic neurons (HESS et al., 1961; SOURKES et al., 1961; PORTER et al., 1961). This decrease is due largely to replacement of the catecholamine by metaraminol (CARLSSON and LINDQVIST, 1962; SHORE et al., 1964; PORTER et al., 1967). Although α-methyl-m-tyrosine is more potent than methyldopa in depleting the tissues of norepinephrine (PORTER et al., 1961) it is considerably less effective than methyldopa as an antihypertensive agent in the rat (BRUNNER et al., 1967) or in man (HORWITZ and SJOERDSMA, 1964). Metaraminol also has been reported to lower the blood pressure of hypertensive patients (CROUT et al., 1965) and of renal hypertensive rats (BRUNNER et al., 1967), in spite of the fact the amine administered systemically does not readily enter the central nervous system. It appears that metaraminol, produced in the brain by the metabolism of administered α-methyl-m-tyrosine, will have less ability than α-methylnorepinephrine to activate noradrenergic receptors, and that its mild antihypertensive activity, as well as that of metaraminol, is due to the effectiveness of metaraminol as a peripheral false transmitter.

Presumably, metaraminol serves as a false transmitter in the central nervous system also. In addition to having some direct adrenergic stimulant activity (Table 8), metaraminol blocks reuptake of norepinephrine by the presynaptic neuron (HESS, 1962; IVERSEN, 1964; ROSS and RENYI, 1964), and may have some postsynaptic sensitizing effects (HAEFELY et al., 1966). The interplay of these factors leads to no apparent centrally mediated effects on blood pressure.

References

ALLEVA, J. J.: Metabolism of tranylcypromine-C^{14} and dl-amphetamine-C^{14} in the rat. J. med. pharm. Chem. **6**, 621—624 (1963).

ALMGREN, O.: The effect of protriptyline on the disappearance and nerve impulse induced release of labelled metaraminol in the rat. Acta physiol. scand. **82**, 539—544 (1971).

ALMGREN, O., JONASON, J.: Relative importance of neuronal and extraneuronal mechanisms for the uptake and retention of noradrenaline in different tissues of the rat. Arch. exp. Path. Pharm. **270**, 289—309 (1971).

ALMGREN, O., LUNDBORG, P. G., STITZEL, R. E.: Release of ^{3}H-metaraminol from subcellular fractions of rat salivary glands by nerve stimulation. Europ. J. Pharm. **6**, 109—114 (1969).

ALMGREN, O., LUNDBORG, G.: Release of ^{3}H-metaraminol by adrenergic nerve stimulation in reserpine-treated rats. Europ. J. Pharm. **9**, 344—346 (1970).

ALTURA, B. M.: Peripheral vascular actions of α-methyldopa and its mode of action on arterioles. Proc. Soc. exp. Biol. (N. Y.) **145**, 129—134 (1974).

ALTURA, B. M.: Pharmacological effects of alpha-methyldopa, alpha-methylnorepinephrine, and octopamine on rat arteriolar, arterial and terminal vascular smooth muscle. Circulation Res. (Suppl. I) **36**, **37**, I—233—I—240 (1975).

ANDÉN, N. E., CORRODI, H., ETTLES, M., GUSTAFSSON, E., PERSSON, H.: Selective uptake of some catecholamines by the isolated heart and its inhibition by cocaine and phenoxybenzamine. Acta Pharm. (Kbh.) **21**, 247—259 (1964).

ANDÉN, N. E., CORRODI, H., FUXE, K., HÖKFELT, B., HÖKFELT, T., RYDIN, C., SVENSSON, T.: Evidence for a central noradrenaline receptor stimulation by clonidine. Life Sci. **9**, 513—524 (1970).

ANDÉN, N. E., ENGEL, J., RUBENSON, A.: Mode of action of L-dopa on central noradrenaline mechanisms. Arch. Pharm. **273**, 1—10 (1972).

ANDÉN, N. E., HENNING, M.: Adrenergic nerve function, noradrenaline level and noradrenaline uptake in cat nictitating membrane after reserpine treatment. Acta physiol. scand. **67**, 498—504 (1966).

ANTONACCIO, M. J., ROBSON, R. D., BURRELL, R.: The effects of L-dopa and L-α-methyldopa on reflexes and sympathetic nerve function. Europ. J. Pharmacol. **25**, 9—18 (1974).

ARCHER, S., ARNOLD, A., KULLNIG, R. K., WYLIE, D. W.: The enzymatic methylation of pyrogallol. Arch. Biochem. Biophys. **87**, 153—154 (1960).

AXELROD, J.: Studies of sympathomimetic amines. II. The biotransformation and physiological disposition of D-amphetamine, D-p-hydroxyamphetamine and D-methamphetamine. J. Pharmacol. exp. Ther. **110**, 315—326 (1954).

AXELROD, J.: O-Methylation of epinephrine and other catechols *in vitro* and *in vivo*. Science **126**, 400 (1957).

AXELROD, J.: Purification and properties of phenylethanolamine-N-methyltransferase. J. biol. Chem. **237**, 1657—1660 (1962).

AXELROD, J.: Enzymatic formation of adrenaline and other catechols from monophenols. Science **140**, 499—500 (1963).

AXELROD, J.: Methylation reactions in the formation and metabolism of catecholamines and other biogenic amines. Pharmacol. Rev. **18**, 95—113 (1966).

AXELROD, J., INSCOE, J. K., DALY, J.: Enzymatic formation of O-methylated dihydroxy derivatives from phenolic amines and indoles. J. Pharmacol. exp. Ther. **149**, 16—23 (1965).

AXELROD, J., LAROCHE, M. J.: Inhibition of O-methylation of epinephrine and norepinephrine *in vitro* and *in vivo*. Science **130**, 800 (1959).

AXELROD, J., TOMCHIK, R.: Enzymatic O-methylation of epinephrine and other catechols. J. biol. Chem. **233**, 702—705 (1958).

BACQ, Z. M., GROSSELIN, L., DRESSE, A., RENSON, J.: Inhibition of O-methyl-transferase by catechol and sensitization to norepinephrine. Science **130**, 453—454 (1959).

BARRETT, R. E., BALCH, T. ST.: Uptake of catecholamines into serotonergic nerve cells as demonstrated by fluorescence histochemistry. Experientia (Basel) **27**, 663—664 (1971).

BAYLISS, R. I. S., HARVEY-SMITH, E. A.: Methyldopa in the treatment of hypertension. Lancet **1962 I**, 763—768.

BELLEAU, B., BURBA, J. V.: Tropolones: A unique class of noncompetitive inhibitors of S-adenosylmethionine-catechol-O-methyltransferase. Acta Biochim. Biophys. **154**, 195—196 (1961).

BELLEAU, B., MORAN, J.: Deuterium isotope effects in relation to the chemical mechanism of monoamine oxidase. Ann. N. Y. Acad. Sci. **107**, 822—839 (1963).

BERNEIS, K. H., DA PRADA, M., PLETSCHER, A.: A possible mechanism for uptake of biogenic amines by storage organelles: incorporation into nucleotide metal aggregates. Experientia (Basel) **27**, 917—918 (1971).

BERNEIS, K. H., PLETSCHER, A., DA PRADA, M.: Phase separation in solutions of noradrenaline and adenosine triphosphate: influence of bivalent cations and drugs. Brit. J. Pharmacol. **39**, 382—389 (1970).

BHAGAT, B., BOVELL, G., ROBINSON, I. M.: Influence of cocaine on the uptake of H^3-norepinephrine and on the responses of isolated guinea-pig atria to sympathomimetic amines. J. Pharmacol. exp. Ther. **155**, 472—478 (1967).

BLASCHKO, H., RICHTER, D., SCHLOSSMAN, H.: Oxidation of adrenaline and other amines. Biochem. J. **31**, 2187—2196 (1937).

BOGDANSKI, D. F., BLASZKOWSKI, T. P., TISSARI, A. H.: Mechanisms of biogenic amine transport and storage. IV. Relationship between K^+ and the Na^+ requirement for transport and storage of 5-hydroxytryptamine and norepinephrine in synaptosomes. Acta biochim. biophys. Acad. Sci. hung. **211**, 521—532 (1970).

BOGDANSKI, D. F., BRODIE, B. B.: Role of sodium and potassium ions in storage of norepinephrine by sympathetic nerve endings. Life Sci. **5**, 1563—1569 (1966).

BOGDANSKI, D. F., BRODIE, B. B.: The effects of inorganic ions on the storage and uptake of H^3-norepinephrine by rat heart slices. J. Pharmacol. exp. Ther. **165**, 181—189 (1969).

BOGDANSKI, D. F., TISSARI, A., BRODIE, B. B.: Role of sodium, potassium, ouabain and reserpine in uptake, storage and metabolism of biogenic amines in synaptosomes. Life Sci. **7**, 419—428 (1968).

BOLME, P., FUXE, K.: Pharmacological studies on the hypotensive effects of clonidine. Europ. J. Pharmacol. **13**, 168—174 (1971).

BOOTH, A. N., MASRI, M. S., ROBBINS, D. J., EMERSON, O. H., JONES, F. T., DEEDS, F.: The metabolic fate of gallic acid and related compounds. J. biol. Chem. **234**, 3014—3016 (1959).

BOULLIN, D. J.: A calcium requirement for release of ^3H guanethidine by sympathetic nerve stimulation. J. Pharm. Pharmacol. **18**, 709—712 (1966).

BRENNEMAN, A. R., KAUFMAN, S.: The tole of tetrahydropteridines in the enzymatic conversion of tyrosine to 3,4-dihydroxyphenylalanine. Biochem. biophys. Res. Commun. **17**, 177—183 (1964).

BREST, A. N., SELLER, R., ONESTI, G., SEKINE, G., MOYER, J. H.: Preliminary observations on the antihypertensive effectiveness of α-methyldopa, a decarboxylase inhibitor. In: Hypertension, Recent Advances. Philadelphia: Lea and Febiger 1961.

BRODIE, B. B., CHO, A. K., GESSA, G. L.: Possible role of p-hydroxynorephedrine in the depletion of norepinephrine induced by d-amphetamine and in tolerance to this drug. In: International Symposium on Amphetamine and Related Compounds. New York: Raven Press 1970.

BROWN, G. L., GILLESPIE, J. S.: The output of sympathetic transmitter from the spleen of the cat. J. Physiol. (Lond.) **138**, 81—102 (1957).

BRUNNER, H., HEDWALL, P. R., MAÎTRE, L., MEIER, M.: Antihypertensive effects of alpha-methylated catecholamine analogues in the rat. Brit. J. Pharmacol. **30**, 108—122 (1967).

BUHS, R. P., BECK, J. L., SPETH, O. C., SMITH, J. L., TRENNER, N. R., CANNON, P. J., LARAGH, J. H.: The metabolism of methyldopa in hypertensive human subjects. J. Pharmacol. exp. Ther. **143**, 205—214 (1964)

BURBA, J. V., MURNAGHAN, M. F.: Catechol-O-methyltransferase inhibition and potentiation of epinephrine responses by desmethylpapaverine. Biochem. Pharmacol. **14**, 823—829 (1964).

BURN, J. H.: Acetylcholine and "auto-inhibition". J. Pharm. Pharmacol. **23**, 470—471 (1971a).

BURN, J. H.: Release of noradrenaline from sympathetic endings. Nature (Lond.) **231**, 237—240 (1971b).

BURGEN, A. S. V., IVERSEN, L. L.: The inhibition of noradrenaline uptake by sympathomimetic amines in the rat isolated heart. Brit. J. Pharmacol. **25**, 34—49 (1965).

CALNE, O. B., STERN, G. M., LAURENCE, D. R., SHARKEY, J., ARMITAGE, P.: L-Dopa in postencephalitic Parkinsonism. Lancet **1969 I**, 744—746.

CANNON, P. J., WHITLOCK, R. T., MORRIS, R. C., ANGERS, M., LARAGH, J. H.: Effect of alpha-methyldopa in severe and malignant hypertension. J. Amer. med. ass. **179**, 673—681 (1962).

CARLSSON, A.: Pseudotransmitters. J. Neuro-visceral Relations Suppl. **9**, 249—260 (1969).

CARLSSON, A., DAHLSTRÖM, A., FUXE, K., HILLARP, N.-Å.: Failure of reserpine to deplete noradrenaline neurons of α-methylnoradrenaline formed from α-methyldopa. Acta Pharmacol. (Kbh). **22**, 270—276 (1965a).

CARLSSON, A., FUXE, K., HAMBERGER, B., LINDQVIST, M.: Biochemical and histochemical studies on the effects of imipramine-like drugs and (+) amphetamine on central and peripheral catecholamine neurons. Acta physiol. scand. **67**, 481—497 (1966).

CARLSSON, A., FUXE, K., HÖKFELT, T.: Effect of desmethylimipramine, protriptyline and (+) amphetamine on fluorescence of central adrenergic neurons of rats pretreated with α-methyldopa and tetrabenazine or reserpine. Europ. J. Pharmacol. **2**, 196—201 (1967a).

Carlsson, A., Hillarp, N.Å., Waldeck, B.: Analysis of the Mg^{++}-ATP-dependent storage mechanism in the amine granules of the adrenal medulla. Acta physiol. scand. **59**, (Suppl. 215), 1—38 (1963).
Carlsson, A., Lindqvist, M.: *In vivo* decarboxylation of α-methyldopa and α-methyl-m-tyrosine. Acta physiol. scand. **54**, 87—94 (1962).
Carlsson, A., Lindqvist, M., Waldeck, B.: Mechanism of release of α-methylated noradrenaline analogues by monoamine oxidase inhibitors. Europ. J. Pharmacol. **3**, 34—39 (1968).
Carlsson, A., Waldeck, B.: β-Hydroxylation of tyramine *in vivo*. Acta pharmacol. (Kbh.) **20**, 371—374 (1963).
Carlsson, A., Waldeck, B.: Mechanism of amine transport in the cell membranes of adrenergic nerves. Acta pharmacol. (Kbh.) **22**, 293—300 (1965a).
Carlsson, A., Waldeck, B.: Inhibition of ^3H metaraminol uptake by antidepressive and related agents. J. Pharm. Pharmacol. **17**, 243—244 (1965b).
Carlsson, A., Waldeck, B.: Structure-activity relationships for release of ^{14}C octopamine from adrenergic nerves by phenylethylamines. Acta pharmacol. (Kbh.) **24**, 255—262 (1966a).
Carlsson, A., Waldeck, B.: Release of ^3H-metaraminol by different mechanisms. Acta physiol. scand. **67**, 471—480 (1966b).
Carlsson, A., Waldeck, B.: Different mechanism of drug-induced release of noradrenaline and its congenors α-methylnoradrenaline and metaraminol. Europ. J. Pharmacol. **4**, 165—168 (1968a).
Carlsson, A., Waldeck, B.: Release of α-methylated noradrenaline analogues by Nialamide. Acta pharmacol. (Kbh.) **26**, (6), 501—506 (1968b).
Cavanaugh, J.H., Griffith, J.D., Oates, J.A.: Effect of amphetamine on the pressor response to tyramine: formation of p-hydroxynorephedrine from amphetamine in man. Clin. Pharmacol. Ther. **11**, 656—664 (1970).
Chang, C.C., Chang, J.C.: A change in the subcellular distribution of noradrenaline in the rat isolated vas deferens effected by nerve stimulation. Brit. J. Pharmacol. **25**, 758—762 (1965).
Clark, W.G.: Inhibition of amino acid decarboxylases. In: Metabolic Inhibitions, Vol. I. London: Academic Press 1963.
Cohen, Y., Wepierre, J., Jacquot, C., Rapin, J.: Relation Entre l'activite antihypertensive de l'α-methyldopa et l'apparition de ses metabolites dans le coeur et le cerveau des rats hypertendus. Arch. int. Pharmacodyn. **207**, 348—360 (1974).
Colburn, R.W., Goodwin, F.K., Murphy, D.L., Bunney, W.E., Davis, J.M.: Quantitative studies of norepinephrine uptake by synaptosomes. Biochem. Pharmacol. **17**, 957—964 (1968).
Corrodi, H., Fuxe, K., Hamberger, B., Ljungdahl, A.: Studies on central and peripheral noradrenaline neurons using a new dopamine-β-hydroxylase inhibitor. Europ. J. Pharmacol. **12**, 145—155 (1970).
Cotzias, G.C., Papavasiliou, P.S., Gellene, R.: Modification of Parkinsonism— chronic treatment with L-dopa. New Engl. J. Med. **280**, 337—345 (1969).
Creveling, C.R., Dalgard, N., Shimizu, H., Daly, S.W.: Catechol-o-methyltransferase: III m- and p-o-methylation of catecholamines and their metabolites. Molec. pharmacol. **6**, 691—696 (1970).
Creveling, C.R., Daly, S.W., Witkop, B., Udenfriend, S.: Substructures and inhibitors of dopamine-β-oxidase. Acta biochim. biophys. Acad Sci. hung. **64**, 125—134 (1962).
Crout, R.: Effect of inhibiting both catechol-O-methyltransferase and monoamine oxidase on cardiovascular responses to norepinephrine. Proc. Soc. exp. Biol. **108**, 482—486 (1961).
Crout, J.R.: Substitute adrenergic transmitters: a newly appreciated mechanism of action of antihypertensive drugs. Circulation Res. **18—19** (Suppl. 1), 120—130 (1966).
Crout, J.R., Alpers, H.S., Tatum, E.L., Shore, P.A.: Release of metaraminol (Aramine) from the heart by sympathetic nerve stimulation. Science **145**, 828—829 (1964).
Crout, J.R., Creveling, C.R., Udenfriend, S.: Norepinephrine metabolism in rat brain and heart. J. Pharmacol. exp. Ther. **132**, 269—277 (1960).
Crout, J.R., Johnston, R.R., Webb, W.R., Shore, P.A.: The antihypertensive action of metaraminol (Aramine) in man. Clin. Res. **13**, 204 (1965).
Crout, J.R., Shore, P.A.: Release of metaraminol (Aramine) from the heart by sympathetic nerve stimulation. Clin. Res. **12**, 180 (1964).
Dahlström, A.: The effects of drugs on axonal transport of amine storage granules. In: Bayer Symposium II. New aspects of storage and release mechanisms of catecholamines. Berlin-Heidelberg-New York: Springer 1970a.
Dahlström, A.: Effect of mitosis inhibitors on the transport of amine storage granules in monoaminergic neurons in the rat. Acta physiol. scand. Suppl **357**, 6 (1970b).

DAHLSTRÖM, A., FUXE, K., HAMBERGER, B., HÖKFELT, T.: Uptake and storage of catecholamines in rabbit brain after chronic reserpine treatment. J. Pharm. Pharmacol. **19**, 345—349 (1967).

DAHLSTRÖM, A., FUXE, K., HILLARP, N.-Å.: Site of action of reserpine. Acta pharmacol. (Kbh.) **22**, 277—292 (1965).

DALY, J.W., AXELROD, J., WITKOP, B.: Methylation and demethylation in relation to the *in vitro* metabolism of mescaline. Ann. N. Y. Acad. Sci. **96**, 37—43 (1962).

DALY, J., GUROFF, G.: Production of m-methyltyrosine and p-hydroxymethylphenylalanine from p-methylphenylalanine by phenylalanine hydroxylase. Arch. Biochem. Biophys. **125**, 136 (1968).

DAVIS, R.A., DRAIN, D.J., HORLINGTON, M., AZARE, R.L., URBANSRA, A.: The effect of L-α-methyldopa and N-2-hydroxybenzyl-N-methylhydrazine (NSD 1039) on the blood pressure of renal hypertensive rats. Life Sci. **3**, 193—197 (1963).

DAY, M.D., RAND, M.J.: A hypothesis for the mode of action of α-methyldopa in relieving hypertension. J. Pharm. Pharmacol. **15**, 221—224 (1963).

DAY, M.D., RAND, M.J.: Some observations on the pharmacology of α-methyldopa. Brit. J. Pharmacol. **22**, 72—86 (1964).

DAY, M.D., RAND, M.J.: Mode of action of methyldopa. J. Pharm. Pharmacol. **19**, 395—396 (1967).

DAY, M.D., ROACH, A.G., WHITING, R.L.: The mechanism of the antihypertensive action of α-methyldopa in hypertensive rats. Europ. J. Pharmacol. **21**, 271—280 (1973).

DENGLER, H., REICHEL, G.: Hemmung der Dopa Decarboxylase durch α-Methyldopa *in vivo*. Arch. exp. Path. Pharmak. **234**, 275—278 (1958).

DHASMANA, K.M., SPILKER, B.A.: On the mechanism of L-dopa induced postural hypotension in the cat. Brit. J. Pharmacol. **47**, 437—451 (1973).

D'IORIO, A., BENOITON, N.L., TONG, J.H., SHARMA, S.: A new biosynthetic pathway to catecholamines via m-tyrosine. Advanc. Neurol. **5**, 265—270 (1974).

DOLLERTY, C.T., HARINGTON, M.: Methyldopa in hypertension, clinical and pharmacological studies. Lancet **1962** I, 759—763.

DORRIS, R.L., SHORE, P.A.: Localization and persistence of metaraminol and α-methyl-*m*-tyramine in rat and rabbit brain. J. Pharmacol. exp. Ther. **179**, 10—12 (1971).

DOUGLAS, W.W., KANNO, T.: The effect of amethocaine on acetylcholine-induced depolarization and catecholamine secretion in the adrenal chromaffin cell. Brit. J. Pharmacol. **30**, 612—619 (1967).

DRING, L.G., SMITH, R.L., WILLIAMS, R.T.: The metabolic fate of amphetamine in man and other species. Biochem. J. **116**, 425—435 (1970).

ELLENBOGEN, L., TAYLOR, R.J., BRUNDAGE, G.B.: On the role of pteridines as co-factors for tyrosine hydroxylase. Biochim. biophys. Res. Commun. **19**, 708—715 (1965).

ERÄNKÖ, O., HÄRKÖNEN, M.: Effect of axon division on the distribution of noradrenaline and acetylcholinesterase in sympathetic neurons of the rat. Acta physiol. scand. **63**, 411—412 (1965).

ESTERHUIZEN, A.C., GRAHAM, J.D.P., LEVER, J.D., SPRIGGS, T.L.B.: Catecholamine and acetylcholinesterase distribution in relation to noradrenaline release. An enzyme histochemical and autoradiographic study on the innervation of the cat nictitating muscle. Brit. J. Pharmacol. **32**, 46—56 (1968).

VON EULER, U.S., HILLARP, N.-Å.: Evidence for the presence of noradrenaline in submicroscopic structures of adrenergic axons. Nature (Lond.) **117**, 44—45 (1965).

VON EULER, U.S., LISHAKJO, F.: Effect of cocaine and tyramine on noradrenaline release and uptake in isolated nerve vesicles. Experientia (Basel) **21**, 342—343 (1965a).

VON EULER, U.S., LISHAJKO, F.: Free and bound noradrenaline in the rabbit heart. Nature (Lond.) **205**, 179—180 (1965b).

VON EULER, U.S., LISHAJKO, F.: Reuptake and net uptake of noradrenaline in adrenergic nerve granules with a note on the affinity for l and *d*-isomers. Acta physiol. scand. **71**, 151—162 (1967).

FARMER, J.B.: Impairment of sympathetic nerve responses by dopa, dopamine and their α-methyl analogues. J. Pharm. Pharmacol. **17**, 640—646 (1965).

FILLION, G., LLUCH, S.: Release of noradrenaline from the dog heart *in situ* following administration of 5-hydroxy-tryptamine (5-HT). Acta pharmacol. (Kbh.) **28** (Suppl. 1), 45 (1970).

FINCH, L., HAEUSLER, G.: Further evidence for a central hypotensive action of α-methyldopa in both the rat and cat. Brit. J. Pharmacol. **47**, 217—228 (1973).

FISCHER, J.E., HORST, W.B., KOPIN, I.J.: β-Hydroxylated sympathomimetic amines as false neurotransmitters. Brit. J. Pharmacol. **24**, 477—484 (1965a).

FISHER, J.E., KOPIN, I.J., AXELROD, J.: Evidence for extraneuronal binding of norepinephrine. J. Pharmacol. exp. Ther. **147**, 181—185 (1965b).

FOLKOW, B., HÄGGENDAHL, J.: Some aspects of the quantal release of thea drenergic transmitter. In: Bayer Symposium II, 1969. New aspects of storage and release mechanisms of catecholamines. New York-Berlin-Heidelberg: Springer 1970.
FREDHOLM, B., SEDVALL, G.: Influence of sympathetic nerve stimulation on noradrenaline stores in the rat salivary gland. Life Sci. **5**, 2023—2032 (1966).
FRIEDMAN, S., KAUFMAN, S.: 3,4-Dihydroxyphenylethylamine β-hydroxylase. J. biol. Chem. **240**, 4763—4773 (1965).
FUXE, K., HILLARP, N.-Å.: Uptake of L-dopa and noradrenaline by central catecholamine neurons. Life Sci. **3**, 1403—1406 (1964).
FUXE, K., SEDVALL, G.: The distribution of adrenergic nerve fibers to the blood vessels in skeletal muscle. Acta physiol. scand. **64**, 75—86 (1965).
GAFFNEY, T. E., CHIDSEY, C. A., BRAUNWALD, E.: Study of the relationship between the neurotransmitter store and adrenergic nerve block induced by reserpine and guanethidine. Circulation Res. **12**, 264—268 (1963).
GEFFEN, L. B., LIVETT, B. G., RUSH, R. A.: Immunohistochemical localization of chromogranins in sheep sympathetic neurons and their release by nerve impulses. In: Bayer Symposium II, 1969. New aspects of storage and release mechanisms of catecholamines. Berlin-Heidelberg-New York: Springer 1970.
GESSA, G. L., VARGIU, L., CRABAI, F.: Interaction of desmethylimipramine (DMI) with the adrenergic and NE releasing action of tyramine, α-methyl-*m*-tyramine and metaraminol. Life Sci. **5**, 501—507 (1966).
GESSA, G. L., VACCA, L.: Antagonismo da parte della demetilimipramina dell' effetto adrenergico della tiramina. Bol. Soc. ital. Biol. Sper. **41**, 808—813 (1965).
GEWIRTZ, G. P., KOPIN, I. J.: Release of dopamine-β-hydroxylase with norepinephrine during cat splenic nerve stimulation. Nature (Lond.) **227**, 406—407 (1970).
GILL, J. R., MASON, D. T., BARTTER, F. C.: Effects of hydroxyamphetamine (Paredrine) on the function of the sympathetic nervous system in normotensive subjects. J. Pharmacol. exp. Ther. **155**, 288—295 (1967).
GILLIS, C. N.: Characteristics of norepinephrine retention by a subcellular fraction of rabbit heart. J. Pharmacol. exp. Ther. **146**, 54—60 (1964).
GILLIS, C. N., PATTON, D. M.: Cation dependence of sympathetic transmitter retention by slices of rat ventricle. Brit. J. Pharmacol. **29**, 309—318 (1967).
GLOWINSKI, J., IVERSEN, L. L., AXELROD, J.: Storage and synthesis of norepinephrine in the reserpine-treated rat brain. J. Pharmacol. exp. Ther. **151**, 385—399 (1966).
GODWIN-AUSTEN, R. B., TOMLINSON, E. B., FREARS, C. C.: Effects of L-dopa in Parkinson's disease. Lancet **1969 II**, 165—168.
GOLDSTEIN, M., ANAGNOSTE, B.: The conversion *in vivo* of D-amphetamine to (+) *p*-hydroxynorephedrine. Acta biochem. biophys. Acad. Sci. hung. **107**, 166—168 (1965).
GOLDSTEIN, M., ANAGNOSTE, B., FREEDMAN, L. S., ROFFMAN, M., EBSTEIN, R. P., PARK, D. H., FUXE, K., HÖKFELT, T.: Characterisation, localisation and regulation of catecholamine synthesising enzymes, pp. 69—78. In: USDIN, E., SNYDER, S. H. (Eds.): Frontiers in Catecholamine Research, Strasbourg, 1973. New York: Pergamon Press 1973.
GOLDSTEIN, M., CONTRERA, J. F.: The activation and inhibition of phenylamine-β-hydroxylase. Experientia (Basel) **18**, 334 (1962).
GOLDSTEIN, M., LAUBER, E., MC KEREGHAN, M. R.: The inhibition of dopamine-β-hydroxylase by tropolone and other chelating agents. Biochem. Pharmacol. **13**, 1103—1105 (1964).
GORKIN, V. Z.: Monoamine oxidases. Pharmacol. Rev. **18**, 115—120 (1966).
GRODEN, B. M.: Parkinsonism occurring with methyldopa treatment. Brit. med. J. **1963 I**, 1001.
GROPETTI, A., COSTA, E.: Tissue concentrations of *p*-hydroxynorephedrine in rats injected with *d*-amphetamine: effect of pretreatment with desipramine Life Sci. **8**, 653—665 (1969).
GUROFF, G., DALY, J. W., JERINA, D. M., RENSON, J., WITKOP, B., UDENFRIEND, S.: Hydroxylation-induced migration: The NIH shift. Science **157**, 1524—1530 (1967).
GUTMAN, Y., WEIL-MALHERBE, H.: Kinetics of catecholamine release by tyramine in rat heart, spleen and uterus. Life Sci. **5**, 1293—1298 (1966).
HAEFELY, W., HÜRLIMANN, A., THOENEN, H.: The effect of stimulation of sympathetic nerves in the cat pretreated with reserpine, α-methyldopa and α-methyl-*m*-tyrosine. Brit. J. Pharmacol. **26**, 172—185 (1966).
HAEFELY, W., HÜRLIMANN, A., THOENEN, H.: Adrenergic transmitter changes and response to sympathetic nerve stimulation after differing pretreatment with α-methyldopa. Brit. J. Pharmacol. **31**, 105—119 (1967).
HÄGGENDAL, J.: Some further aspects on the realese of the adrenergic transmitter In: Bayer Symposium II. New aspects of storage and release mechanisms of catecholamines. Berlin-Heidelberg-New York: Springer 1970.
HÄGGENDAL, J., DAHLSTRÖM, A.: Uptake and retention of ^{3}H-noradrenaline in adrenergic nerve terminals after and axotomy. Europ. J. Pharmacol. **10**, 411—415 (1970).

HÄGGENDAL, J., DAHLSTRÖM, A.: The recovery of noradrenaline in adrenergic nerve terminals of the rat after reserpine treatment. J. Pharm. Pharmacol. **23**, 81—89 (1971).
HAMBERGER, B., MALMFORS, T., NORBERG, K. A., SACHS, C.: Uptake and accumulation of catecholamines in peripheral adrenergic neurons of reserpinized animals studied with a histochemical method. Biochem. Pharmacol. **13**, 841—844 (1964).
HEDWALL, P. R., MAÎTRE, L.: Studies on the localization of the sympathetic blockade produced by alpha-methyldopa. Arch. exp. Path. Pharmak. **270** (Suppl. 1), R 58 (1971).
HEISE, A., KRONEBERG, G.: α-Sympathetic receptor stimulation in the brain and hypotensive activity of α-methyldopa. Europ. J. Pharmacol. **17**, 315—317 (1972).
HEISE, A., KRONEBERG, G.: Central neurons α-adrenergic receptors and the mode of action of α-methyldopa. Naunyn Schmiedebergs Arch. Pharmacol. **279**, 285—300 (1973).
HELLE, K. B.: Immunological properties of chromogranin. In: Bayer Symposium II, 1969. New aspects of storage and release mechanisms of catecholamines. Berlin-Heidelberg-New York: Springer 1970.
HELLE, K. B., LAGERCRANTZ, H., STJÄRNE, L.: Biochemistry of catecholamine storage: some similarities between whole sympathetic nerve trunk vesicles and membranes of adrenomedullary vesicles. Acta physiol. scand. 81, 565—585 (1971).
HENNING, M.: Effect of different dopa decarboxylase inhibitors on the hypotensive response to α-methyldopa in rats. Brit. J. Pharmacol. **34**, 233*p* (1968).
HENNING, M.: Interaction of dopa decarboxylase inhibitors with the effect of α-methyldopa on blood pressure and tissue monoamines in rats. Acta pharmacol. (Kbh.) **27**, 135—148 (1969).
HENNING, M., RUBENSON, A.: Central hypotensive effect of L-3,4-dihydroxyphenylalanine in the rat. J. Pharm. Pharmacol. **22**, 553—560 (1970).
HENNING, M., RUBENSON, A.: Evidence that the hypotensive action of methyldopa is mediated by central actions of methylnoradrenaline. J. Pharm. Pharmacol. **23**, 407—411 (1971).
HENNING, M., VAN ZWIETEN, P. A.: Central hypotensive effect of α-methyldopa. J. Pharm. Pharmacol. **20**, 409—417 (1968).
HERTTING, G., AXELROD, J., KOPIN, I. J. WHITBY, L. G.: Lack of uptake of catecholamines after chronic denervation of sympathetic nerves. Nature (Lond.) **189**, 66 (1961).
HESS, S. M.: The releasing action of α-methyl-3-hydroxyphenylalanine (α-methyl-meta-tyrosine). Arch. int. Pharmacodyn. **138**, 584—590 (1962).
HESS, S. M., CONNAMACHER, R. H., OZAKI, M., UDENFRIEND, S.: The effects of α-methyldopa and α-methyl-*m*-tyrosine on the metabolism of norepinephrine and serotonin *in vivo*. J. Pharmacol. exp. Ther. **134**, 129—138 (1961).
HOLTMEIER, H. J., VON KLEIN-WISENBERG, A., MARONGIU, F.: Vergleichende Untersuchungen über die blutdrucksenkende Wirkung von alpha-Methyl-Dopa und alpha-Methyl-*m*-Tyrosine. Dtsch. med. Wschr. **91**, 198—205 (1966).
HOLTZ, P., WESTERMAN, E.: Über die Dopadecarboxylase und Histidindecarboxylase des Nervengewebes. Arch exp. Path. Pharmak. **227**, 538—546 (1956).
HORN, A. S., COYLE, J. T., SYNDER, S. H.: Catecholamine uptake by synaptosomes from rat brain. Structure-activity relationships of drugs with differential effects on dopamine and norepinephrine neurones. Molec. Pharmacol. **7**, 66—80 (1971).
HORST, W. D., KOPIN, I. J., RAMEY, E. R.: Influence of sodium and calcium on norepinephrine uptake by isolated perfused rat hearts. Amer. J. Physiol. **215**, 817—822 (1968).
HÖRTNAGL, H., HÖRTNAGL, H., WINKLER, H.: Bovine splenic nerve: characterization of noradrenaline-containing vesicles and other cell organelles by density gradient centrifugation. J. Physiol. (Lond.) **205**, 103—114 (1969).
HORWITZ, D., PETTINGER, W. A., ORVIS, H., THOMAS, R. E., SJOERDSMA, A.: Effects of methyldopa in fifty hypertensive patients. Clin. Pharmacol. Ther. 8, 224—234 (1966).
HORWITZ, D., SJOERDSMA, A.: Effects of alpha-methyl-meta-tyrosine intravenously in man. Life Sci. **3**, 41—48 (1964).
HUGHES, J., GILLIS, C. N., BLOOM, F. E.: The uptake and disposition of *dl*-norepinephrine in perfused rat lung. J. Pharmacol. exp. Ther. **169**, 237—248 (1969).
IKEDA, M., FAHIEN, L. A., UDENFRIEND, S.: A kinetic study of bovine adrenal tyrosine hydroxylase. J. biol. Chem. **241**, 4452—4456 (1966).
IKEDA, M., LEVITT, M., UDENFRIEND, S.: Phenylalanine as substrate and inhibitor of tyrosine hydroxylase. Arch. Biochem. **120**, 420—427 (1967).
INGENITO, A. J., BARRET, J. P., PROCITA, L.: A centrally mediated peripheral hypotensive effect of α-methyldopa. J. Pharmacol. exp. Ther. **175**, 593—599 (1970).
IVERSEN, L. L.: Inhibition of noradrenaline uptake by sympathomimatic amines. J. Pharm. Pharmacol. **16**, 435—436 (1964).
IVERSEN, L. L.: Role of transmitter uptake mechanisms in synaptic neurotransmission. Brit. J. Pharmacol. **41**, 571—591 (1971).
IVERSEN, L. L., GLOWINSKI, J., AXELROD, J.: The uptake and storage of H^3-norepinephrine in the reserpine pretreated rat heart. J. Pharmacol. exp. Ther. **150**, 173—183 (1965).

IVERSEN, L. L., KRAVITZ, E. A.: Sodium dependence of transmitter uptake of adrenergic nerve terminals. Molec. Pharmacol. **2**, 360—362 (1966).
IVERSEN, L. L., WHITBY, L. G.: The subcellular distribution of catecholamines in normal and tyramine depleted mouse hearts. Biochem. Pharmacol. **12**, 582—584 (1963).
JAJU, B. P., TANGRI, K. K., BHARGAVA, K. P.: Central vasomotor effects of α-methyldopa. Canad. J. phys. Pharmacol. **44**, 687—690 (1966).
JARROTT, B.: Occurrence and properties of catechol-O-methyl transferase in adrenergic neurons. J. Neurochem. **18**, 17—27 (1971).
JESTER, J., HORST, W. D.: Influence of serotonin on adrenergic mechanisms. Biochem. Pharmacol. **21**, 333—338 (1972).
JONSSON, J., GROBECKER, H., HOLTZ, P.: Effect of β-phenethylamine on content and subcellular distribution of norepinephrine in rat heart and brain. Life Sci. **5**, 2235—2246 (1966).
KAKIMOTO, Y., ARMSTRONG, M. D.: On the identification of octopamine in mammals. J. Biochem. **237**, 422—427 (1962).
KALSMER, S., NICKERSON, M.: Disposition of norepinephrine and epinephrine in vascular tissue, determined by the technique of oil immersion. J. Pharmacol. exp. Ther. **165**, 152—165 (1969).
KAUFMAN, S., FRIEDMAN, S.: Dopamine-β-hydroxylase. Pharmacol. Rev. **17**, 71—100 (1965).
KILBINGER, H., LINDMAR, R., LÖFFELHOLZ, K., MUSCHOLL, E.: Freisetzung von falschen Überträgerstoffen nach Infusion von (+)- und (—)-α-Methyldopamin. Naunyn-Schmiedebergs Arch. Pharmak. **266**, 370—371 (1970).
KILBINGER, H., LINDMAR, R., LÖFFELHOLZ, K., MUSCHOLL, E., PATIL, P. N.: Storage and release of false transmitters after infusion of (+) and (—) α-methyldopamine. Arch. exp. Pharmak. **271**, 234—248 (1971).
KIRPEKAR, S. M., MISU, Y.: Release of noradrenaline by splenic nerve stimulation and its dependence on calcium. J. Physiol (Lond.) **188**, 219—234 (1967).
KIRSHNER, N.: Biosynthesis of adrenaline and noradrenaline. Pharmacol. Rev. **11**, 350—357 (1959).
KIRSHNER, N., MC GOODALL, C.: The formation of adrenaline from noradrelanine. Acta biochim. biophys. Acad. Sci. hung. **24**, 658—659 (1957).
KOPIN, I. J.: Biochemical aspects of release of norepinephrine and other amines from sympathetic nerve endings. Pharmacol. Rev. **18**, 513—523 (1966).
KOPIN, I. J.: Biosynthesis and metabolism of catecholamines. Anesthesiology **29** (4), 654—660 (1968a).
KOPIN, I. J.: Flase adrenergic transmitters. Ann. Rev. Pharmacol. **8**, 377—394 (1968b).
KOPIN, I. J.: Regulation of catecholamine-synthesizing enzymes. J. Psychiat. Res. **11**, 335—338 (1974).
KOPIN, I. J., FISCHER, J. E., MUSACCHIO, J. M., HORST, W. D., WEISE, V. K.: False neurochemical transmitters and the mechanism of sympathetic blockade by monoamine oxidase inhibitors. J. Pharmacol. exp. Ther. **147**, 186—193 (1965).
KOPIN, I. J., GORDON, E. K.: Metabolism of norepinephrine-H^3 released by tyramine and reserpine. J. Pharm. exp. Ther. **138**, 351—359 (1962).
KOPIN, I. J., FISCHER, J. E., MUSACCHIO, J., HORST, W. D.: Evidence for a false transmitter mechanism for the hypotensive effect of monoamine oxidase inhibitors. Proc. nat. Acad. Sci. (Wash.) **52**, 716—721 (1964).
KOPIN, I. J., WEISE, V. K., SEDVALL, G. C.: Effect of false transmitters on norepinephrine synthesis. J. Pharmacol. exp. Ther. **170**, 246—252 (1969).
LADURON, P., BELPAIRE, F.: Evidence for an extragranular localization of tyrosine hydroxylase. Nature (Lond.) **217**, 1155—1156 (1968a).
LADURON, P., BELPAIRE, F.: Tissue fractionation and catecholamines. II. Intracellular distribution patterns of tyrosine hydroxylase, dopa decarboxylase, dopamine-β-hydroxylase, phenylethanolamine N-methyltransferase and monoamine oxidase in adrenal medulla. Biochem. Pharmacol. **17**, 1127—1140 (1968b).
LADURON, P., BELPAIRE, F.: Transport of noradrenaline and dopamine-β-hydroxylase in sympathetic nerves. Life Sci. **7**, 1—7 (1968c).
LAGUADO, J. R., SOURKES, T. L.: Inhibition of amine oxidase by metal ions and by sulphydryl compounds. Canad. J. Biochem. **34**, 1185—1194 (1956).
LEE, F. L.: The relation between norepinephrine content and response to sympathetic nerve stimulation of various organs of cats pretreated with reserpine. J. Pharmacol. exp. Ther. **156**, 137—141 (1967).
LEE, F. L., WEINER, N., TRENDELENBURG, U. :The uptake of tyramine and formation of octopamine in normal and tachyphylactic rat atria. J. Pharmacol. exp. Ther. **155**, 211—222 (1967).
LEITZ, F. H., STEFANO, F. J. E.: Desipramine-induced release of norepinephrine from heart. Biochem. Pharmacol. **19**, 1797—1801 (1970).

LEVITT, M., SPECTOR, S., SJOERDSMA, A., UDENFRIEND, S.: Elucidation of the rate-limiting step in norepinephrine biosynthesis in the perfused guinea-pig heart. J. Pharmacol. exp. Ther. **148**, 1—8 (1965).

LEWANDER, T.: Displacement of brain and heart noradrenaline by *p*-hydroxy-norephedrine after administration of *p*-hydroxyamphetamine. Acta pharmacol. (Kbh.) **29**, 20—32 (1971a).

LEWANDER, T.: On the presence of *p*-hydroxynorephedrine in the rat brain and heart in relation of changes in catecholamine levels after administration of amphetamine. Acta pharmacol. (Kbh.) **29**, 33—48 (1971b).

LEWANDER, T.: Effects of acute and chronic amphetamine intoxication on brain catecholamines in the guinea pig. Acta pharmacol. (Kbh.) **29**, 209—225 (1971c).

LINDMAR, R., MUSCHOLL, E., RANN, K. H.: Effects of rest and physical activity on the urinary excretion of noradrenaline and α-methylnoradrelanine in human subjects treated with α-methyldopa. Europ. J. Pharmacol. **2**, 317—319 (1968).

LINDMAR, R., MUSCHOLL, E., SPRENGER, E.: Funktionelle Bedeutung der Freisetzung von Dihydroxyephedrin und Dihydroxypseudoephedrin als „falschen" sympathischen Überträgerstoffen am Herzen. Arch. exp. Path. Pharmakologie **256**, 1—25 (1967).

LOKHANDWALA, M. F., BUCKLEY, J. P., JANDHYALA, B. S.: Effect of methyldopa treatment on peripheral sympathetic nerve function in the dog. Europ. J. Pharmacol. **32**, 170—178 (1975).

LOVENBERG, W., WEISSBACH, H., UDENFRIEND, S.: Aromatic 1-amino acid decarboxylase. J. biol. Chem. **237**, 89—93 (1962).

LUNDBORG, P.: Studies on the uptake and subcellular distribution of catecholamines and their α-methylated analogues. Acta physiol. scand. **72** (Suppl. 302), 3—34 (1967).

LUNDBORG, P., STITZEL, R. E.: Uptake of biogenic amines by two different mechanisms present in adrenergic granules. Brit. J. Pharmacol. **29**, 342—349 (1967a).

LUNDBORG, P., STITZEL, R. E.: Effect of reserpine and protriptyline on the subcellular distribution of ^{3}H-metaraminol in the mouse heart. Brit. J. Pharmacol. **30**, 379—384 (1967b).

LUNDBORG, P., WALDECK, B.: Two different mechanisms for incorporation of ^{3}H-metaraminol into the amine-storing granules. J. Pharm. Pharmacol. **18**, 762—763 (1966).

MAÎTRE, L.: Presence of α-methyldopa metabolites in heart and brain of guinea pigs treated with α-methyl-tyrosine. Life Sci. **4**, 2249—2256 (1965).

MAÎTRE, L., STAEHELIN, M.: Presence of α-methylnoradrenalinc (Corbasil) in the heart of guinea pigs treated with metaraminol ("Aramine"). Nature (Lond.) **206**, 723—724 (1965).

MAÎTRE, L., STAEHELIN, M.: On the norepinephrine replacement by α-methylnorepinephrine in the rat heart after treatment with α-methyldopa. Experientia (Basel) **23**, 810 (1967).

MALMFORS, T.: Release and depletion of the transmitter in adrenergic terminals produced by nerve impulses after the inhibition of noradrenaline synthesis or reabsorption. Life Sci. **3**, 1397—1402 (1964).

MALMFORS, T.: Studies on adrenergic nerves. Acta physiol. scand. **64** (Suppl. 248), 1—93 (1965).

MATSUMOTO, C., HORITA, A.: Antagonism of Bretylium by sympathomimetic amines. Nature (Lond.) **195**, 1212—1213 (1962).

MAVRIDES, C., MISSALA, K., D'ORIO, H.: The effect of 4-methyltropolone on the metabolism of adrenaline. Canad. J. Biochem. **41**, 1581—1587 (1963).

MCGEER, P. L., MCGEER, E. G.: Formation of adrenaline by brain tissue. Biochem. biophys. Res. Commun. **17**, 502—507 (1964).

MICHAELSON, I. A., RICHARDSON, K. C., SNYDER, S. N., TITUS, E. O.: The separation of catecholamine storage vesicles from rat heart. Life Sci. **3**, 971—978 (1964).

MINSKER, D. H., SCRIABINE, A., STOKES, A. L., STONE, C. A., TORCHIANA, M. L.: Effects of L-dopa alone and in combination with dopa decarboxylase inhibitors on the arterial pressure and heart rate of dogs. Experientia (Basel) **27**, 529—531 (1971).

MOHAMMED, S., FASOLA, A. F., PRIVITERA, P. J., LIPICKY, R. J., MARTZ, B. L., GAFFNEY, T. E.: Effect of methyldopa on plasma renin activity in man. Circulation Res. **25**, 543—548 (1969).

MOHAMMED, S., PRIVITERA, P. H.: The effect of methyldopa on plasma renin activity in dogs. Clin. Res. **19**, 329 (1971).

MOLINOFF, P., AXELROD, J.: Octopamine: normal occurrence in sympathetic nerves of rats. Science **164**, 428—429 (1969).

MOLINOFF, P. B., AXELROD, J.: Distribution and turnover of octopamine in tissues. J. Neurochem. **19**, 157—163 (1972).

MOLINOFF, P. B.: The regulation of the noradrenergic neuron. J. Psychiat. Res. **11**, 339—345 (1974).

MOORE, K. E., LAVIRIERE, E. W.: Effects of D-amphetamine and restraint on the content of norepinephrine and dopamine in rat brain. Biochem. Pharmacol. **12**, 1283—1288 (1963).

MUSACCHIO, J. M., FISCHER, J. F., KOPIN, I. J.: Subcellular distribution and release by sympathetic nerve stimulation of dopamine and α-methyldopamine. J. Pharmacol. exp. Ther. **152**, 51—55 (1966).

MUSACCHIO, J. M., KOPIN, I. J., WEISE, V. K.: Subcellular distribution of some sympathomimetic amines and their β-hydroxylated derivatives in the rat heart. J. Pharmacol. exp. Ther. **148**, 22—28 (1965a).
MUSACCHIO, J. M., WEISE, V. K., KOPIN, I. J.: Mechanism of norepinephrine binding. Nature (Lond.) **205**, 606—607 (1965b).
MUSCHOLL, E.: In: Handbook of Experimental Pharmacology. Berlin-Heidelberg-New York: Springer 1972.
MUSCHOLL, E., MAÎTRE, L.: Release by sympathetic stimulation of α-methylnoradrenaline stored in the heart after administration of α-methyldopa. Experientia (Basel) **19**, 658—659 (1963).
MUSCHOLL, E., RAHN, K. H.: Nachweis von α-Methylnoradrenaline im Harn von Hypertoniren während einer Behandlung mit α-Methyldopa. Klin. Wschr. **44**, 1412—1413 (1966).
MUSCHOLL, E., WEBER, E.: Die Hemmung der Aufnahme von α-Methylnoradrenalin in das Herz durch sympathomimetische Amine. Arch. exp. Path. Pharmakol. **252**, 134—143 (1965).
NAGATSU, T., KUZUYA, H., HIDAKA, H.: Inhibition of dopamine β-hydroxylase by sulfhydryl compounds and the nature of the natural inhibitors. Acta biochem. biophys. Acad. Sci. hung. **139**, 319—327 (1967).
NAGATSU, T., LEVITT, M., UDENFRIEND, S.: Tyrosine hydroxylase, the initial step in norepinephrine biosynthesis. J. biol. Chem. **239**, 2910—2917 (1964a).
NAGATSU, T., LEVITT, M., UDENFRIEND, S.: Conversion of L-tyrosine to 3,4-dihydroxyphenylalanine by cell-free preparations of brain and sympathetically innervated tissues. Biochem. biophys. Res. Commun. **14**, 543—549 (1964b).
NEFF, N. H., TOZA, T. N., HAMMER, W., BRODIE, B. B.: Kinetics of release of norepinephrine by tyramine. Life Sci. **4**, 1869—1875 (1965).
NIJKAMP, F. P., EZER, J., DEJONG, W.: Central inhibitory effect α-methyldopa on blood pressure, heart rate and body temperature of renal hypertensive rats. Europ. J. Pharmacol. **31**, 243—249 (1975).
NIKODEJEVIC, B., SENOH, S., DALY, S. W., CREVELING, C. R.: Catechol-O-methyltransferase. II. A new class of inhibitors of catechol-O-methyltransferase; 3,5-dihydroxy-4-ethoxybenzoic acid and related compounds. J. Pharmacol. exp. Ther. **174**, 83—93 (1970).
OATES, J. A., GILLESPIE, L., UDENFRIEND, S., SJOERDSMA, A.: Decarboxylase inhibition and blood pressure reduction by α-methyl-3,4-dihydroxy-DL-phenylalanine. Science **131**, 1890—1891 (1960).
ORDEN, L. S. VAN, BENSCH, K. G., GIARMAN, N. J.: Histochemical and functional relationships of catecholamines in adrenergic nerve endings. II. Extravesicular norepinephrine. J. Pharmacol. exp. Ther. **155**, 428—439 (1967).
ORDEN, L. S. VAN, SCHAEFER, J. M., BURKE, J. P., LODOEN, F. V.: Differentiation of norepinephrine storage compartments in peripheral adrenergic nerves. J. Pharmacol. exp. Ther. **174**, 357—368 (1970).
PATIL, P. N., LA PIDUS, J. B., CAMPBELL, D., TYE, A.: Steric aspects of adrenergic drugs. II. Effects of DL-isomers and desoxy derivatives on the reserpine-pretreated vas deferens. J. Pharmacol. exp. Ther. **155**, 12—23 (1967).
PATIL, P. N., TYE, A., LA PIDUS, J. B.: The effects of reserpine pretreatment of the D and L isomers of some sympathomimetic amines. J. Pharmacol. exp. Ther. **149**, 199—205 (1965).
PELLEGRINO DE IRALDI, A., DE ROBERTIS, E.: Studies on the origin of the granulated and non-granulated vesicles. In: Bayer Symposium II. New Aspects of Storage and Release Mechanisms of Catecholamines. Berlin-Heidelberg-New York: Springer 1970.
PETRACK, B., FETZER, V., SHEPPY, F., MANNING, T.: Tyrosine hydroxylase in guinea pig brain. Fed. Proc. **29**, 277 (1970).
PETTINGER, W. A., HORWITZ, D., SJOERDSMA, A.: Lactation due to methyldopa. Brit. med. J. **1963 I**, 1460.
PHILIPPU, A., SCHÜMANN, H. J.: Bildung und Speicherung von α-Methylnoradrenalin. Arch. exp. Path. Pharmakol. **256**, 183—195 (1967).
PISANO, J. J., CREVELING, C. R., UDENFRIEND, S.: Enzymic conversion of p-tyramine to p-hydroxyphenylethanolamine (norsynephrine). Biochem. biophys. Acta **43**, 566—568 (1960).
POCH, G. R., KOPIN, I. J.: The role of octopamine in tachyphylaxis to tyramine. Biochem. Pharmacol. **15**, 210—212 (1966).
POILLON, W. N.: Kinetic properties of brain tyrosine hydroxylase and its partial purification by affinity chromatography. Biochem. biophys. Res. Commun. **44**, 64—70 (1971).
PORTER, C. C.: Aromatic amino acid decarboxylase inhibitors. Fed. Proc. **30**, 871—876 (1971).
PORTER, C. C., TITUS, D.: Distribution and metabolism of methyldopa in the rat. J. Pharmacol. exp. Ther. **139**, 77—87 (1963).
PORTER, C. C., TORCHIANA, M. L., TOTARO, J. A., STONE, C. A.: Displacement of norepinephrine from the rat heart by ^{14}C-metaraminol. Biochem. Pharmacol. **16**, 2117—2124 (1967).

PORTER, C. C., TOTARO, J. A., LEIBY, C. M.: Some biochemical effects of α-methyl-3,4-dihydroxyphenylalanine and related compounds in mice. J. Pharmacol. exp. Ther. **134**, 139—145 (1961).
POTTER, L. T.: Storage of norepinephrine in sympathetic nerves. Pharmacol. Rev. **18**, 439—451 (1966).
POTTER, L. T.: Role of intraneuronal vesicles in the synthesis, storage and release of noradrenaline. Circulation Res. **21**, Supp. III, 13—24 (1967).
POTTER, L. T., AXELROD, J.: Intracellular localization of catecholamines in tissues of the rat. Nature (Lond.) **194**, 581—582 (1962).
POTTER, L. T., AXELROD, J.: Properties of norepinephrine storage particles of the rat heart. J. Pharm. exp. Ther. **142**, 299—305 (1963a).
POTTER, L. T., AXELROD, J.: Subcellular localization of catecholamines in tissues of the rat. J. Pharmacol. exp. Ther. **142**, 291—298 (1963b).
POTTER, L. T., AXELROD, J.: Studies on the storage of norepinephrine and the effect of drugs. J. Pharmacol. exp. Ther. **140**, 199—205 (1963c).
POTTER, W. P. DE, CHUBB, I. W.: The turnover rate of noradrenergic vesicles. Biochem. J. **125**, 373—376 (1971).
POTTER, W. P. DE, SCHAEPDRYVER, A. F. DE. SMITH. A. D.: Release of chromagranin A and dopamine β-hydroxylase from adrenergic nerves during nerve stimulation. Acta physiol. scand. Suppl. **357**, 7 (1970).
PRIVITERA, P. J., MOHAMMED, D.: Studies on the mechanism of renin suppression by alpha-methyldopa. In: Control of Renin Secretion New York: Plenum Press 1972.
RANGNO, R. E., KAUFMANN, J. S., CAVANAUGH, J. H., ISLAND, D., WATSON, J. T., OATES, J.: Effects of a false neurotransmitter, p-hydroxynorephedrine, on the function of adrenergic neurons in hypertensive patients. J. clin. Invest. **52**, 952—960 (1973).
ROBERTIS, E. DE, PELLERGRINO DE IRALDI, A., DE LORES ARNAIZ, G. R., ZIEHER, L. M.: Synaptic vesicles from the rat hypothalmus, isolation and norepinephrine content. Life Sci. **4**, 193—201 (1965).
ROBERTS, D. J., STREET, D. M.: Influence of pargyline on the effects of dopamine infusions on sympathetically innvervated tissues. Neuropharmacology **9**, 457—465 (1970).
ROBSON, R. D.: Utilization of enzyme inhibitors in the production and control of hypotension with L-dopa in dogs. Fed. Proc. **30**, 676 (1972).
ROSELL, S., KOPIN, I. J., AXELROD, J.: Release of tritiated epinephrine following sympathetic nerve stimulation. Nature (Lond.) **210**, 301 (1964).
ROSS, S. B., RENYI, A. L.: Blocking action of sympathomimetic amines on the uptake of tritiated noradrenaline by mouse cerebral cortex tissues *in vitro*. Acta pharmacol. (Kbh.) **21**, 226—239 (1964).
ROSS, S. B., RENYI, A. L.: Active uptake of tritiated metaraminol by mouse brain slices *in vitro*. Life Sci. **5**, 639—647 (1966).
RUBENSON, A.: Further studies on the mechanism of the central hypotensive effect of L-dopa, DL-*m*-tyrosine and L-α-methyldopa. J. Pharm. Pharmacol. **23**, 228—230 (1971).
RUBENSON, A.: Analysis of the action of *m*-tyrosine on blood pressure in the conscious rat: evidence for a central hypotensive action. J. Pharm. Pharmacol. **23**, 412—419 (1971).
RUBIN, R. P.: The role of calcium in the release of neurotransmitter substances and hormones. Pharmacol. Rev. **22**, 389—428 (1970).
RUTLEDGE, C. O., JONASON, J.: Metabolic pathways of dopamine and norepinephrine in rabbit brain *in vitro*. J. Pharmacol. exp. Ther. **157**, 493—502 (1967).
SANNERSTEDT, R., BOJS, G., VARNAUSKAS, E., WERKO, L.: Alpha-methyldopa in arterial hypertension. Acta med. scand. **174**, 53—67 (1963).
SCHMITT, H., SCHMITT, H., FENARD, S.: Evidence for an α-sympathomimetic component in the effect of catapresan on vasomotor centers. Europ. J. Pharmacol. **14**, 98—100 (1971).
SCHÜMANN, H. J.: Nachweis von Oxytyramin (Dopamin) in Sympathischen Nerven und Ganglien. Arch. exp. Path. Pharmakologie **227**, 566—573 (1956).
SCHÜMANN, H. J., GROBECKER, H.: Nachweis und Lokalization von α-Methylnoradrenalin im Meerschweinchenorgan nach Vorbehandlung mit α-Methyl-dopa. Arch. exp. Path. Pharmakologie **247**, 297 (1965).
SCHMITT, F. O.: Fibrous proteins — Neuronal organelles. Proc. nat. Acad. Sci. (Wash.) **60**, 1092—1101 (1968).
SCHMITT, H., PETILLOT, N.: Influence du replacement de la noradrenaline par des faux mediateurs et de L'inhibition de la synthesis sur L'excitabilite sympathique. J. Pharmacol. (Paris) **1**, 183—194 (1970).
SCHOOT, J. B. VAN DER, CREVELING, C. R.: Substrates and Inhibitors of dopamine-β-hydroxylase. In: Advances in Drug Research, Vol. 2. New York: Academic Press 1965.
SCRIABINE, A., CLINESCHMIDT, B. V., SWEET, C. S.: Central noradrenergic control of blood pressure. Ann. Rev. Pharmacol. Toxicol. **16**, 113—123 (1976).

SEDVALL, G., THORSON, J.: Adrenergic transmission at vasoconstrictor nerve terminals partially depleted by norepinephrine. Acta physiol. scand. **64**, 251—258 (1965).

SEIDEN, L. S., WESTLEY, J.: Partial purification of monoamine oxidase from rat brain. Acta biochim. biophys. Acad. Sci. hung. **58**, 363—364 (1962).

SENOH, S., DALY, J., AXELROD, J., WITKOP, B.: Enzymatic p-O-methylation by catechol-O-methyl transferase. J. Amer. chem. Soc. **81**, 6240—6245 (1959).

SHORE, P. A.: The mechanism of norepinephrine depletion by reserpine, metaraminol and related agents. The role of monoamine oxidase. Pharmacol. Rev. **18**, 561—568 (1966).

SHORE, P. A.: Transport and storage of biogenic amines. Ann. Rev. Pharmacol. **12**, 209—226 (1972).

SHORE, P. A., BUSFIELD, D., ALPERS, H. S.: Binding and release of metaraminol: Mechanism of norepinephrine depletion by α-methyl-m-tyrosine and related agents. J. Pharmacol. exp. Ther. **146**, 194—199 (1964).

SJOERDSMA, A., VENDSALU, A., ENGELMAN, K.: Studies on the metabolism and mechanisms of action of methyldopa. Circulation **28**, 492—502 (1963).

SJOERDSMA, A., STUDNITZ, W. VON: Dopamine-β-oxidase activity in man, using hydroxyamphetamine as substrate. Brit. J. Pharmacol. **20**, 278—284 (1963).

SMITH, A. P., POTTER, W. P. DE, SCHAEPDRYVER, A. F. DE: Subcellular fractionation of bovine splenic nerves. Arch. int. Pharmacodyn. **179**, 495—496 (1969).

SMITH, S. E.: The pharmacological actions of 3,4-dihydroxyphenyl-α-methylalanine (α-methyldopa), an inhibitor of 5-hydroxytryptophan decarboxylase. Brit. J. Pharmacol. **15**, 319—327 (1960).

SMYTHIES, J. R., ANTUN, F., YANK, G., YORKE, C.: Molecular mechanisms of storage of transmitters in synaptic terminals. Nature (Lond.) **231**, 185—188 (1971).

SNYDER, S. H., MICHAELSON, I. A., MUSACCHIO, J.: Purification of norepinephrine storage granules from rat heart. Life Sci. 965—970 (1964).

SNYDER, S. H., TAYLOR, K. M., COYLE, J. T., MEYERHOFF, J. L.: The role of brain dopamine in behavioral regulation and the actions of psychotropic drugs. Amer. J. Psychiat. **127**, 117—125 (1970).

SOURKES, T. L.: Inhibition of dihydroxyphenylalanine decarboxylase by derivatives of phenylalanine. Arch. Biochem. Biophys. **51**, 444—456 (1954).

SOURKES, T. L., MURPHY, G. F., CHAVEZ, B., ZIELINSKA, M.: The action of some α-methyl and other amino acids on cerebral catecholamines. J. Neurochem. 8, 109—115 (1961).

SOURKES, T. L., MURPHY, G. F., RABINOVITCH, S.: Conversion of DL-*m*-tyrosine to dopamine in the rat. Nature (Lond.) **189**, 577—578 (1961).

VAN SPANNING, H. W., VAN ZWIETEN, P. A.: The interaction between alpha-methyldopa and tricyclic antidepressants. Int. J. Clin. Pharmacol. **11**, 65—67 (1975).

SPECTOR, S.: Inhibitors of endogenous catecholamine biosynthesis. Pharmacol. Rev. **18**, 599—609 (1966).

SPECTOR, S., GORDON, R., SJOERDSMA, A., UDENFRIEND, S.: End-product inhibition of tyrosine hydroxylase on a possible mechanism for regulation of norepinephrine synthesis. Molec. Pharmacol. **3**, 549—555 (1967).

SPECTOR, S., SJOERDSMA, A., UDENFRIEND, S.: Blockade of endogenous norepinephrine synthesis by α-methyltryosine, an inhibitor of tyrosine hydroxylase. J. Pharmacol. exp. Ther. **147**, 86—95 (1965).

STJÄRNE, L.: Studies on noradrenaline biosynthesis in nerve tissues. Acta physiol. scand. **67**, 441—454 (1966).

STJÄRNE, L.: Quantal or graded secretion of adrenal medullary hormone and sympathetic neurotransmitter. In: Bayer Symposium II. New Aspects of Storage and release mechanisms of catecholamines. Berlin-Heidelberg-New York: Springer 1970.

STJÄRNE, L., HEDQVIST, P., LAGERCRANTZ, H.: Catecholamines and adenine neucleotide material in effluent from stimulated adrenal medulla and spleen. Biochem. Pharmacol. **9**, 1147—1158 (1970).

STJÄRNE, L., LISHAJKO, F.: Localization of different steps in noradrenaline synthesis to different fractions of a bovine splenic nerve homogenate. Biochem. Pharmacol. **16**, 1719—1729 (1967).

STINSON, R. H.: Electrical stimulation of the sympathetic nerves of the isolated rabbit ear and the fate of the neurohormone released. Canad. J. Biochem. Phys. **39**, 309—316 (1961).

STOCK, K., WESTERMAN, E.: Effect of α-methyldopa and and α-methyl-m-tyrosine on the mobilization of free fatty acids. Experientia (Basel) **20**, 495—496 (1964).

STOCK, K., WESTERMAN, E.: The significance of noradrenaline content in fatty tissue for the mobilization of unesterified fatty acids. Arch. exp. Path. Pharmak. **251**, 465—487 (1965).

STONE, C. A.: False adrenergic neurotransmission In: Proc. Symp. Physiol. Pharmacol. Vasc. Neuroeffector Systems. Basel: Karger 1971.

STONE, C. A., PORTER, C. C., STAVORSKI, J. M., LUDDEN, C. T., TOTARO, J. A.: Antagonism of certain effects of catecholamine-depleting agents by antidepressant and related drugs. J. Pharmacol. exp. Ther. **144**, 196—204 (1964).

STONE, C. A., PORTER, C. C., WATSON, L. S., ROSS, C. A.: Pharmacology of decarboxylase inhibitors. In: Hypertension-Recent Advances. Philadelphia: Lea and Febiger 1961.

STONE, C. A., STAVORSKI, J.: Comparative effects of methyldopa and reserpine on mice and phenethylamine-induced cardioacceleration in the dog. Biochem. Pharmacol. **12**, 201 (1963).

STONE, C. A., STAVORSKI, J. M., LUDDEN, C. T., WENGER, H. C., TORCHIANA, M. L.: Some direct and indirect sympathomimetic actions of metaraminol. Arch. int. Pharmacodyn. **161**, 49—60 (1966).

STRANG, R. R.: Parkinsonism occurring during methyldopa therapy. Canad. med. ass. J. **95**, 928—929 (1966).

STRAUSS, R. G., MOHAMMED, S., LOGGIE, J. M. H., SCHUBERT, W. K., FASOLA, A. F., GAFFNEY, T. E.: The effect of plasma renin activity in a child with Bartter's syndrome. J. Pediat. **77**, 1071—1074 (1970).

THOA, N. B., JOHNSON, D. G., KOPIN, I. J.: Inhibition of norepinephrine biosynthesis by α-methylamino acids in the guinea pig vas deferens. J. Pharmacol. exp. Ther. **180**, 71—77 (1972a).

THOA, N. B., WOOTEN, G. F., AXELROD, J., KOPIN, I. J.: Inhibition of dopamine-β-hydroxylase (DBH) and norepinephrine (NE) release from sympathetic nerves by colchicine, vinblastine and cytochalasin-B, and its enchancement by dibutyryl cyclic-AMP. Fed. Proc. **31**, 566A (1972b).

THOENEN, H., HAEFELY, W., GEY, K. F., HÜRLIMANN, A.: Diminished effects of sympathetic nerve stimulation in cats treated with disulfiram. Liberation of dopamine as sympathetic transmitter. Life Sci. **4**, 2033—2038 (1965).

THOENEN, H., HAEFELY, W., GEY, K. F., HÜRLIMANN, A.: Ersatz von Noradrenalin durch Dopamin als postganglionärer sympathetischer Transmitter bei Hemmung der Dopamin β-Hydroxylase durch Disulfiram. Helv. physiol. pharmacol. Acta **24**, C118—C119 (1966).

THOENEN, H., HAEFELY, W., GEY, K. F., HÜRLIMANN, A.: Quantitative aspects of the replacement of norepinephrine by dopamine as a sympathetic transmitter after inhibition of dopamine-β-hydroxylase by disulfiram. J. Pharmacol. exp. Ther. **156**, 246—251 (1967a).

THOENEN, H., HAEFELY, W., GEY, K. F., HÜRLIMANN, A.: Liberation of α-methyldopamine as a "false" sympathetic transmitter after pretreatment of cats with α-methyldopa and disulfiram. Arch. exp. Path. Pharmacol. **258**, 181—196 (1967b).

TISSARI, A. H., SCHONHOFER, P. S., BOGDANSKI, D. F., BRODIE, B. B.: Mechanism of biogenic amine transport. II. Relationship between sodium and the mechanism of ouabain blockade of the accumulation of serotonin and norepinephrine by synaptosomes. Molec. Pharmacol. **5**, 593—604 (1969).

TITUS, E., DENGLER, H. J.: The mechanism of uptake of norepinephrine. Pharmacol. Rev. **18**, 525—535 (1966).

TORCHIANA, M. L., LOTTI, V. J., BATTELLE, S., CLARK, C. M., STORMO, G., STONE, C. A.: Central hypotensive action of methyldopa and L-dihydroxyphenylalanine. Proc. Inter. Pharmacol. Congress (1972).

TORCHIANA, M. L., LOTTI, V. J., CLARK, C. M., STONE, C. A.: Comparison of centrally mediated hypotensive action of methyldopa and dopa in cats. Arch. int. Pharmacodyn. **205**, 103—113 (1973).

TORCHIANA, M. L., PORTER, C. C., STONE, C. A.: Relation between molecular configuration and certain biological actions of α-methyldopamine and α-methyl-m-tyramine and their β-hydroxylated products, α-methylnorepinephrine and metaraminol. Arch. int. Pharmacodyn. **174**, 118—134 (1968).

TORCHIANA, M. L., PORTER, C. C., STONE, C. A., HANSON, H. M.: Some biochemical and pharmacological actions of α-methylphenylalanine. Biochem. Pharmacol. **19**, 1601—1614 (1970).

TORCHIANA, M. L., PORTER, C. C., WATSON, L. S., STONE, C. A.: Relationship of cardiovascular amd antihypertensive effects of methyldopa with α-methyl-norepinephrine concentrations in the hearts of rats. Pharmacologist **7**, 145 (1965).

TORCHIANA, M. L., WENGER, H. C., STAVORSKI, J., LUDDEN, C. T., STONE, C. A.: Effect of methyldopa and related agents on pressor responses to tyramine in reserpine-pretreated rats and dogs. J. Pharmacol. exp. Ther. **151**, 242—252 (1966).

TRENDELENBURG, U.: Supersensitivity and subsensitivity to sympathomimetic amines. Pharmacol. Rev. **15**, 225—276 (1963).

TRENDELENBURG, U., MUSKUS, A., FLEMING, W. W., GOMEZ ALONSO LA SIERRA, B.: Modification by reserpine of the action of sympathomimetic amines in spinal cats; a classification of sympathomimetic amines. J. Pharmacol. exp. Ther. **138**, 170—180 (1962).

UDENFRIEND, S., ZALTZMAN-NIRENBERG, P.: On the mechanism of the norepinephrine release produced by α-methyl-metatyrosine. J. Pharmacol. **138**, 194—199 (1962).

UDENFRIEND, S., ZALTZMAN-NIRENBERG, P., GORDON, R., SPECTOR, S.: Evaluation of the biochemical effects produced *in vivo* by inhibitors of the three enzymes involved in norepinephrine biosynthesis. Molec. Pharmacol. **2**, 95—105 (1966).

UDENFRIEND, S., ZALTZMAN-NIRENBERG, P., NAGATSU, T.: Inhibitors of purified beef adrenal tyrosine hydroxylase. Biochem. Pharmacol. **14**, 837—845 (1965).

VAIDYA, R. A., VAIDYA, A. B., WOERT, M. H. VAN, KASE, N. G.: Galactorrhea and Parkinson-like syndrome: an adverse effect of α-methyldopa. Metabolism **19**, 1068—1070 (1970).

WALDMEIER, P., HEDWALL, P. R., MAÎTRE, L.: On the role of α-methyldopamine in the antihypertensive effect of α-methyldopa. Naunyn-Schmiedebergs Arch. Pharmacol. **289**, 303—314 (1975).

WATANABE, A. M., CHASE, T. N., CARDON, P. V.: Effect of L-dopa alone and in combination with an extracerebral decarboxylase inhibitor on blood pressure and some cardiovascular reflexes. Clin. Pharmacol. Ther. **11**, 740—746 (1970).

WATANABE, A. M., PARKS, L. C., KOPIN, I. J.: Modification of the cardiovascular effects of L-dopa by decarboxylase inhibitors. J. clin. Invest. **50**, 1322—1328 (1971).

WEINER, N., JARDETSKY, O.: A study of catecholamine nucleotide complexes by nuclear magnetic resonance spectroscopy. Arch. exp. Path. Pharmakol. **248**, 308—318 (1964).

WEINSHILBOUM, R. M., THOA, B. N., JOHNSON, D. G., KOPIN, I. J., AXELROD, J.: Proportional release of norepinephrine and dopamine-β-hydroxylase from sympathetic nerves. Science **24**, 1349—1351 (1971).

WESTERMAN, E., BALZER, H., KNELL, J.: Hemmung der Serotoninbildung durch α-Methyldopa. Arch. exp. Path. Pharmakol. **234**, 194—205 (1958).

WHITNACK, E., LEFF, A., MOHAMMED, S., GAFFNEY, T. E.: The effect of L-dopa on chronotropic responses to cardioaccelerator nerve stimulation in dogs. J. Pharmacol. exp. Ther. **177**, 409—414 (1971).

WHITSETT, T. L., HALUSHKA, P. V., GOLDBERG, L. I.: Attenuation of postganglionic sympathetic nerve activity by L-dopa. Circulation Res. **27**, 561—570 (1970).

YAHR, M. D., DUVOISIN, R. C., SCHEAR, M. J., BARRETT, E. E., HOEHN, M. M.: Treatment of Parkinsonism with levodopa. Arch. Neurol. (Paris) **21**, 343—354 (1969).

ZWIETEN, P. A. VAN, PAUER, M., VANSPANNING, H. W., DELANGEN, C.: Interaction between centrally acting hypotensive drugs and tricyclic antidepressants. Arch. int. Pharmacodyn. **214**, 12—30 (1975).

Chapter 7

The Pharmacology of Clonidine and Related Products

H. Schmitt

With 29 Figures

I. Introduction

Clonidine, 2-(2,6-dichlorophenylamino)-2-imidazoline, referred to as St 155, Catapresan, Catapres or Catapressan, was the first antihypertensive agent known to act on the central nervous system. Its therapeutic value as an agent for controlling high blood pressure has been well established in recent years and its clinical use is growing.

The importance of clonidine and related compounds as tools for investigating central noradrenergic mechanisms emerged progressively over the same period and rests on the hypothesis that its central and peripheral effects are linked and are due to activation of related α adrenoceptors. New concepts of the central noradrenergic mechanisms were developed as a result of this work.

Clonidine was synthesized in 1962 by Stähle as a derivative of the imidazoline series, the vasoconstrictor properties of which were well known, in the hope that it would be a nasal decongestant. The hypotensive and sedative effects of clonidine were discovered by chance in the course of early clinical trials. These effects led to a reinvestigation of the pharmacological properties of the drug, and in 1966 Hoefke and Kobinger published the first extensive report on the pharmacological properties of this interesting compound. The first clinical reports had appeared meanwhile.

Although the principal pharmacological properties of clonidine are well enough known today, many questions concerning the mechanism of action of this drug remain unanswered. I believe we are as yet in a preliminary and rudimentary stage of the pharmacological knowledge of this compound.

At the present time it appears that many central and peripheral effects of clonidine could reasonably be explained on the basis of the activation of receptors related to the classical α adrenoceptors. In addition, two main features are now apparent: (a) many other compounds structurally close to clonidine, like the classical α-sympathomimetic drugs of the imidazoline series, naphazoline and tetryzoline, have only weak central activity; (b) α adrenoceptor-blocking drugs have been shown to be selective in their ability to antagonize the peripheral and central effects of clonidine. It is not yet known whether these differences are due to differences in the structure of the receptors or to the way the drugs are distributed in the central nervous system.

Clonidine may therefore help to reveal and elucidate many aspects of the pharmacology of catecholamines on central mechanisms.

II. Chemistry

Clonidine is an imidazoline derivative substituted by a 2, 6-dichlorophenylamine group. The chloride is a white powder very soluble in water.

In its chemical structure clonidine is very close to the α-sympathomimetic agent naphazoline and the α adrenoceptor-blocking drug tolazoline.

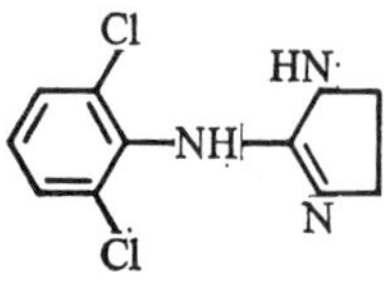
Clonidine

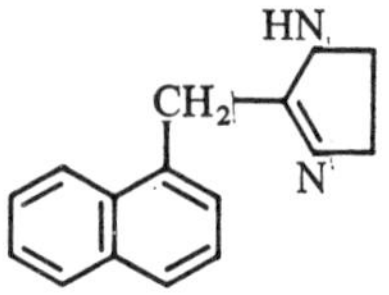
Naphazoline

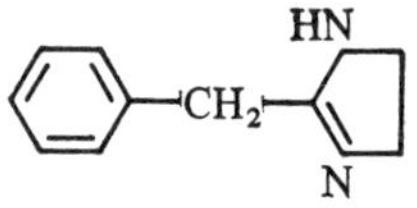
Tolazoline

III. Principal Pharmacological Properties

Clonidine appears to act on both peripheral and central structures. Peripherally clonidine is a typical α-sympathomimetic agent. Centrally clonidine is known to inhibit the sympathetic tone, to activate vagal tone, to cause sedation, to reduce secretions and to induce analgesia, hypothermia, reduction of food and water intake, and aggressivity. Table 1 summarizes the principal pharmacological properties of clonidine and gives the threshold dosage.

Table 1. *Principal pharmacological properties of clonidine*

	Threshold dosage
I. *Peripheral effects*	
Hypertension	1 μg/kg
Vasoconstriction	1 μg/kg
Contraction of the nictitating membrane	10 μg/kg
Hyperglycemia	10 μg/kg
II. *Central effects*	
Hypotension	3 to 5 μg/kg
Inhibition of the sympathetic tone	1 μg/kg
Activation of the vagal tone	2-5 μg/kg
Bradycardia	1 μg/kg
Sedation	3 to 5 μg/kg
Antinociception	500 μg/kg
Hypothermia	50 μg/kg
Inhibition of water intake	50 μg/kg
Inhibition of food intake	100 to 200 μg/kg
Aggressivity	0.5 to 3 mg/kg

Clonidine is most frequently given for its cardiovascular properties. Administered intravenously, clonidine induces biphasic changes in blood pressure: initial hypertension is followed by a long-lasting fall in blood pressure (Fig. 1). As the dosage is increased, the intensity and duration of the hypertensive effect become greater and hypotension is delayed. In addition, bradycardia and reduction in cardiac output are constant features in animals and man.

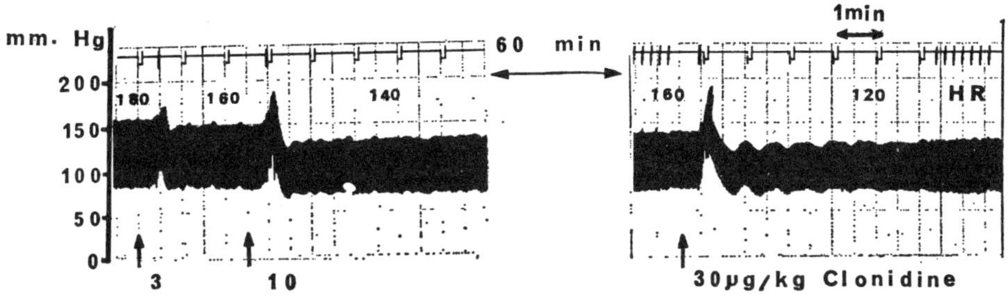

Fig. 1. Effects of clonidine on blood pressure and heart rate in monkey *(Macacca mulatta)*. Injections of 3, 10 and 30 µg/kg of clonidine induced a brief period of hypertension followed by a decrease in blood pressure, more marked in the systolic pressure, and bradycardia

IV. Effects on the Sympathetic System

A. α-Sympathomimetic Effect

The initial increase in blood pressure was early recognized as being due to the *activation of α adrenoceptors*. This effect was easier to investigate after suppression of the sympathetic tone by spinalization (KOBINGER and WALLAND, 1967b; NAYLER et al., 1968; CONSTANTINE and McSHANE, 1968), pithing (BOISSIER et al., 1968; AUTRET et al., 1971), administration of ganglion-blocking agents (BOISSIER et al., 1968; NAYLER et al., 1966, 1968), reserpine (KOBINGER and WALLAND, 1967b; BOISSIER et al., 1968; NAYLER et al., 1968), guanethidine (ROBSON and KAPLAN, 1969; ROBSON et al. 1969a, b) or bretylium (NAYLER et al., 1968). In these conditions the hypotensive effect was strikingly reduced or abolished and the hypertensive phase was potentiated (Fig. 2).

The increase in blood pressure appears to be due to *vasoconstriction*. The fact that clonidine reduces cardiac output rules out any stimulating effect on the heart as the cause of the hypertensive effect. A vasoconstrictor effect has been demonstrated on many preparations: perfused artery of the rabbit ear (HOEFKE and KOBINGER, 1966; BENTLEY and LI, 1968; BOISSIER et al., 1968), isolated aorta of rabbits (BOISSIER et al., 1968; CONSTANTINE and McSHANE, 1968), perfused hind limb of cats (KOBINGER and WALLAND, 1967b; LI and BENTLEY, 1969) and of dogs (KOBINGER and WALLAND, 1967b). In contrast, NAYLER et al. (1966) did not find any change in the perfusion pressure of isolated gracilis muscle preparation of dogs after clonidine.

Besides the vasoconstrictor and hypertensive effects, a number *of effects of clonidine could be ascribed to an activation of α adrenoceptors:* contraction of the nictitating membrane, exophthalmos, piloerection, hyperglycemia, contraction of vas deferens in guinea pig or rat (HOEFKE and KOBINGER, 1966; BENTLEY and LI, 1968; BOISSIER et al., 1968). Contraction of the spleen was reported in cats at a rather high dosage (HOEFKE and KOBINGER, 1966). Clonidine induced a contraction of rabbit pulmonary artery but the maximal effect was much weaker than those of noradrenaline (STARKE et al., 1974).

As pretreatment with reserpine or guanethidine does not change the α-sympathomimetic effects of clonidine, *an indirectly mediated effect could be excluded* (KOBINGER and WALLAND, 1967b; NAYLER et al., 1968). In pithed rats reserpinization did not change the dose-pressor response curve of clonidine, which is in agreement with these results (AUTRET et al., 1971). Clonidine, like the related drug

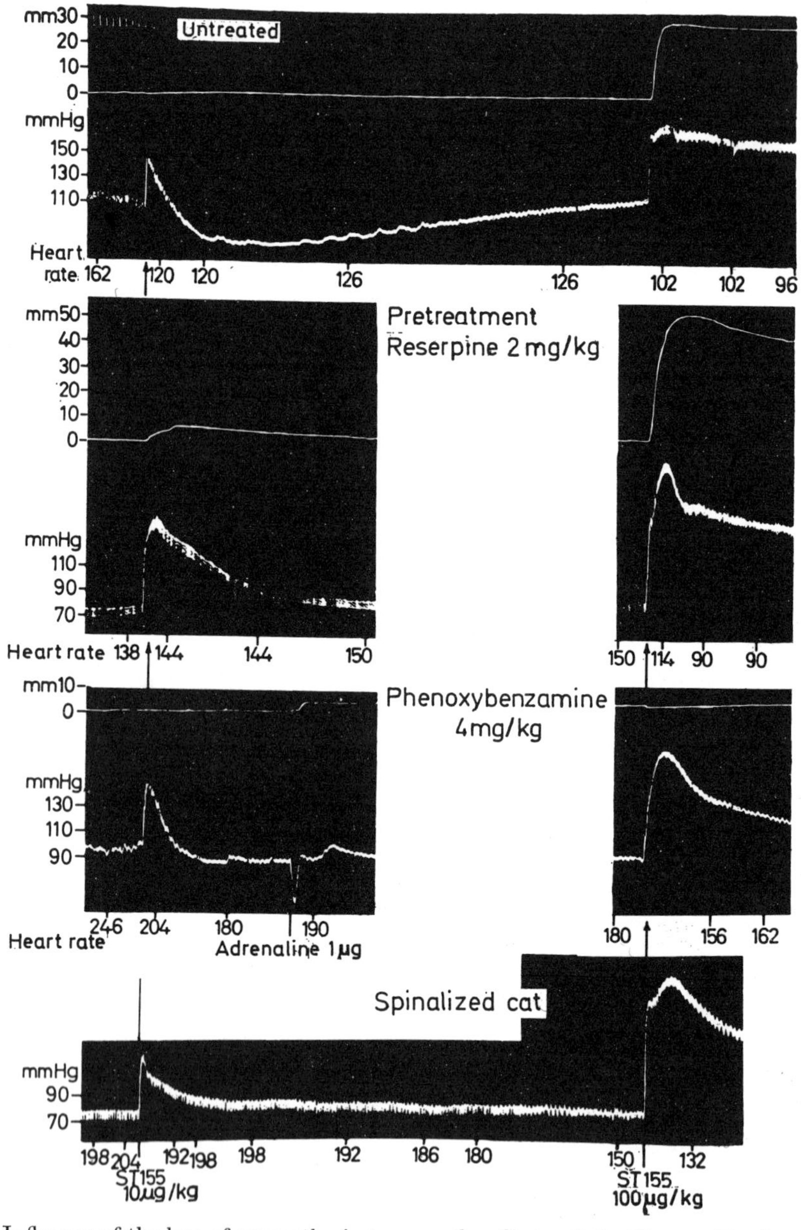

Fig. 2. Influence of the loss of sympathetic tone on the effects of clonidine on blood pressure and nictitating membrane of the cat. Phenoxybenzamine abolished the hypotensive effect of clonidine and the contraction of the nictitating membrane. After pretreatment with reserpine, clonidine induced a more marked hypertensive effect and contraction of the nictitating membrane without a fall in blood pressure. In spinal cat, only hypertension was seen. The bradycardia was suppressed only in spinal cat at the lower dosage (10 µg/kg). [KOBINGER, W., WALLAND, A.: Arzneimittel-Forsch. **17**, 293 (1967)]

BAY a 6781, did not release noradrenaline from rabbit heart even in high dosage (WERNER et al., 1972).

Pharmacological experiments revealed that clonidine acts as a *α-sympathomimetic agent* on α adrenoceptors. The hypertensive effect of clonidine was reduced by α adrenoceptor-blocking agents (KOBINGER and WALLAND, 1967b; KÜNDIG et al., 1967; NAYLER et al., 1968; BOISSIER et al., 1968; CONSTANTINE and MCSHANE, 1968; SCHMITT and SCHMITT, 1970; SCHMITT et al., 1971d; SCHMITT et al., 1973a), which also reduced or abolished the hypotensive phase.

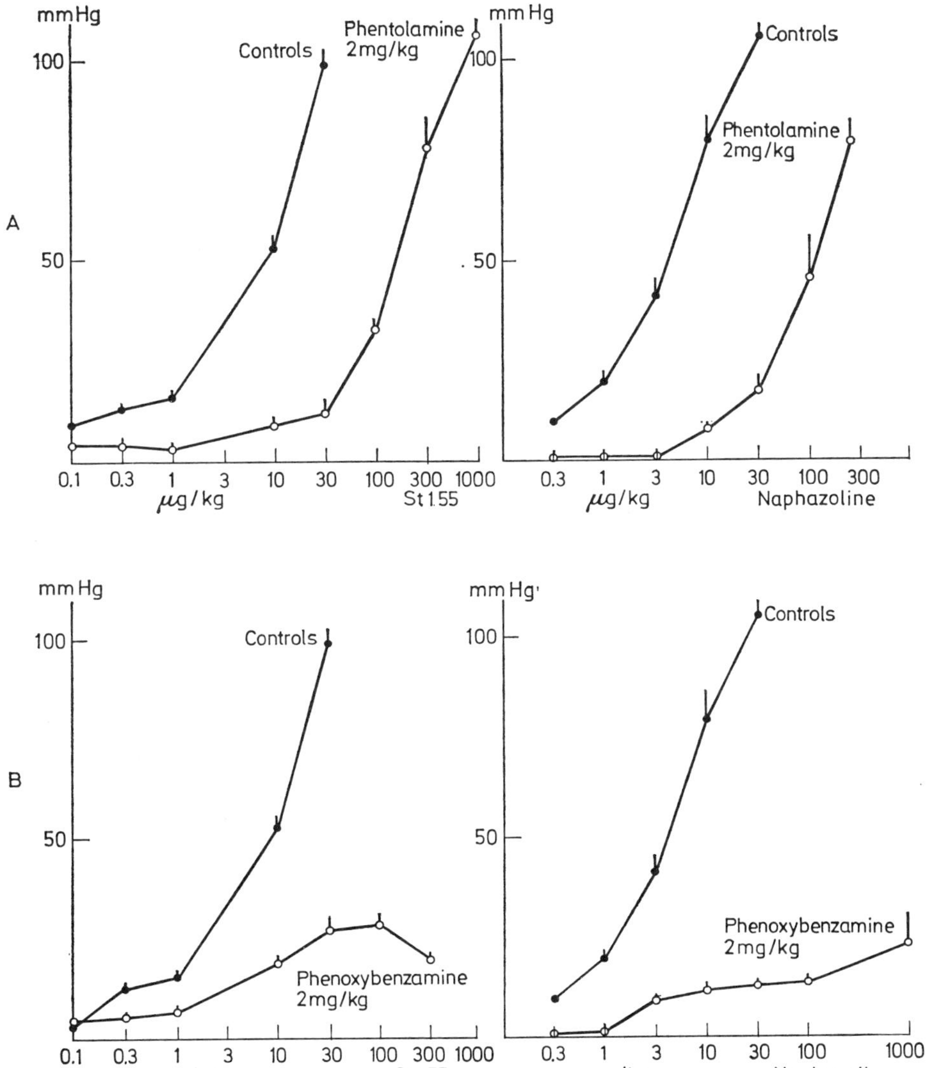

Fig. 3. Antagonism of the hypertensive effect of clonidine and naphazoline in pithed rats. Dose-response curves for clonidine and naphazoline in pithed rats: A: Phentolamine shifts the dose-response curve to the right, and B: phenoxybenzamine reduces the maximum effect. These findings indicate respectively a competitive and a nonequilibrium antagonism. [AUTRET, A.M., SCHMITT, N., FÉNARD, S., PÉTILLOT, N.: Europ. J. Pharmacol. **13**, 211 (1971)]

However, some conflicting results have been reported with phenoxybenzamine, probably because different dosages and animal species were used. Phenoxybenzamine has been reported to be poorly effective for reducing hypertension brought about by clonidine in cats (NAYLER et al., 1966; KOBINGER and WALLAND, 1967b; BOLME and FUXE, 1971), but NAYLER et al. (1968) in dogs and rabbits, and SCHMITT and SCHMITT (1970) in cats reported an antagonistic effect. In pithed rats, phentolamine caused a shift of the dose pressor-response curve of clonidine to the right; phenoxybenzamine in addition decreased the maximum effect. These effects suggest competitive and nonequilibrium antagonism, respectively. Both these α adrenoceptor-blocking agents act similarly on hypertensive effects induced by noradrenaline and α-sympathomimetic drugs of the imidazoline series, *i.e.* naphazoline, tetryzoline, tramazoline (AUTRET et al., 1971) (Fig. 3).

Clonidine produces a dose-dependent contraction of the aorta of rabbits antagonized by phentolamine and phenoxybenzamine (BOISSIER et al., 1968; CONSTANTINE and MCSHANE, 1968). However, the dose-response curve of clonidine is shifted to the right relative to adrenaline and the maximum effect is smaller, revealing weaker affinity and intrinsic activity (CONSTANTINE and MCSHANE, 1968). Clonidine was shown to protect the α adrenoceptors of rabbit isolated

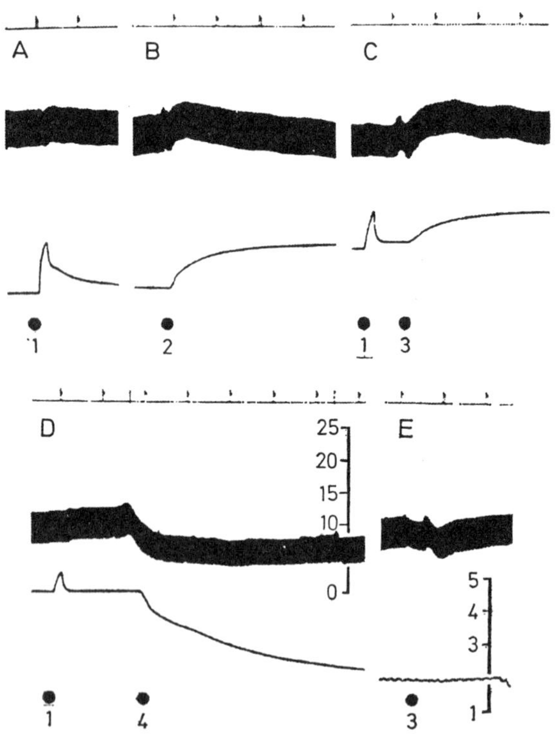

Fig. 4. Effect of clonidine on blood pressure and nictitating membrane. 1: Contraction of the nictitating membrane elicited by preganglionic stimulation of the cervical sympathetic chain. 2: Injection of clonidine (100 µg/kg). 3: Injection of clonidine (500 µg/kg). 4: Injection of phentolamine (5 mg/kg). Clonidine induced hypertension and contraction of the nictitating membrane, but did not reduce the effects of preganglionic stimulation of the cervical sympathetic chain. Phentolamine antagonized the effect of clonidine. [BOISSIER, J. R., GIUDICELLI, J.F., FICHELLE, J., SCHMITT, H., SCHMITT, HÉLÈNE: Europ. J. Pharmacol. 2, 336 (1968)]

aorta from nonequilibrium blockade induced by phenoxybenzamine (CONSTANTINE and MCSHANE, 1968). α adrenoceptor-blocking agents similarly decreased the contraction of the nictitating membrane of the cat brought about by clonidine (KOBINGER and WALLAND, 1967b; BOISSIER et al., 1968) (Fig. 4).

Although these experiments indicate that clonidine acts as an α-sympathomimetic agent, some pharmacological interactions reveal *special features*. Cocaïne, imipramine and guanethidine failed to potentiate the pressor effect of clonidine in pithed rats (AUTRET et al., 1971) and in dogs (BOISSIER et al., 1968) (Fig. 5). On the contrary, cocaïne and imipramine slightly decreased the effects of clonidine. According to current views on the mechanism of the potentiating effect of these drugs on noradrenaline, it could be suggested that clonidine is not taken up in the postganglionic sympathetic nerve terminals during the axonal uptake process.

The effects of clonidine on β *adrenoceptors* appear to be very weak or absent. In the isolated auricle of guinea pigs clonidine in high concentration increased the contractile force, but did not change the rate (HOEFKE and KOBINGER, 1966). On a heart-lung preparation of the dog (HOEFKE and KOBINGER, 1966), or the isolated heart of the cat (CONSTANTINE and MCSHANE, 1968), or of the rabbit (WERNER et al., 1972) clonidine reduced the contractile force only at high concentrations; this effect has been ascribed to the local anesthetic effect of the drug.

In conclusion, all these pharmacological investigations demonstrate that clonidine is an α-sympathomimetic agent which is probably not taken up by the sympathetic nerve terminals.

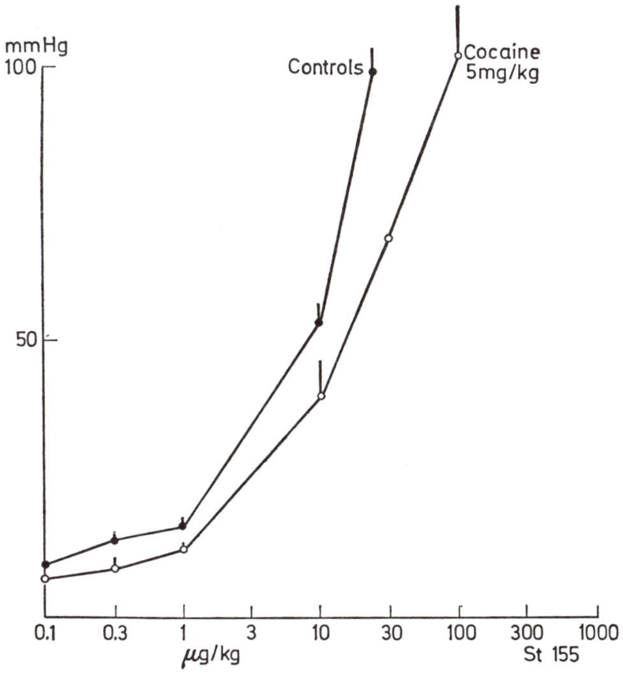

Fig. 5. Influence of cocaine on the hypertensive response to clonidine in pithed rats. The figure shows the dose-response curve of clonidine in groups of rats untreated and treated with cocaine. Cocaine shifts the dose-response curve to the right. [AUTRET, A.M., SCHMITT, H., FÉNARD, S., PÉTILLOT, N.: Europ. J. Pharmacol. 13, 212 (1971)]

B. Effects on Catecholamines

At low dosage, *clonidine did not markedly change the pharmacological effects of catecholamines.*

An increased hypertensive and bradycardic effect was reported in dogs, cats and rats after low doses of clonidine (HOEFKE and KOBINGER, 1966; SCHMITT et al., 1967; BENTLEY and LI, 1968; BOISSIER et al., 1968; RAND and WILSON, 1968; LI and BENTLEY, 1969). This potentiation may be explained—at least in part—by loss of the reflex inhibition of the sympathetic tone after clonidine; thus the vascular smooth muscle is unopposed in its response to the pressor agents. However, since noradrenaline is also potentiated after clonidine in pithed rats (BENTLEY and LI, 1968; BOISSIER et al., 1968), some peripheral component must also be involved. In man, no striking effect of clonidine on the effects of catecholamines was observed (BOCK et al., 1970; ONESTI et al., 1971).

At high dosage, clonidine reduced the effects of noradrenaline and sometimes reversed the hypertensive effects of adrenaline (KÜNDIG et al., 1967; BOISSIER et al., 1968). Clonidine reduced the contraction of guinea-pig isolated seminal vesicle induced by adrenaline (KÜNDIG et al., 1967), the contraction of rat vas deferens induced by noradrenaline (BENTLEY and LI, 1968), and the vasoconstriction induced by noradrenaline in the perfused rabbit ear (BENTLEY and LI, 1968). Clonidine caused moderate blockade of noradrenaline-induced relaxation of the human ileum but acted as a potent competitive inhibitor of noradrenaline on the saphenous vein of man (COUPAR and TURNER, 1970; COUPAR and KIRBY, 1972). COUPAR and KIRBY (1972) suggested that clonidine may cause venodilatation by blocking endogenously released noradrenaline, an effect which may contribute to the hypotensive effect of the drug. In the reviewer's opinion other evidence shows that this effect could be only of minor importance.

Clonidine appears to be a *partial agonist* on α adrenoceptors; in fact the maximum effect was less than those of noradrenaline on rabbit pulmonary artery (STARKE et al., 1974). In addition high doses of clonidine reduced the pressor response to noradrenaline and reversed the pressor response to adrenaline (BOISSIER et al., 1968); on the α adrenoceptor of the rabbit intestine similar results have been found. The intrinsic activity of clonidine determined by the maximum relaxation of pendular movements was about half the intrinsic activity of noradrenaline. The pD_2 values were respectively 5.2 for clonidine and 6.8 for noradrenaline (STRUYKER-BOUDIER et al., 1974; STRUYKER-BOUDIER, 1975). Similarly clonidine reduced the contraction of isolated pulmonary artery induced by noradrenaline (STARKE et al., 1974).

Clonidine increased the contractile force of the isolated papillary muscle of the rabbit heart. Its intrinsic activity was low (0.32 that of phenylephrine) but its affinity was higher than those of naphazoline, methoxamine, oxymetazoline and phenylephrine. The pD_2 value was 6.43 compared to 6.13 for phenylpherine. As this effect was inhibited by phentolamine, it is due to the activation of α adrenoceptors. In addition clonidine antagonized the positive inotropic effect of phenylephrine, mediated via the α adrenoceptors in the presence of 3×10^{-8} M pindolol, in a competitive manner. These results provide evidence that clonidine acts as a partial agonist on α adrenoceptors in this preparation (SCHÜMANN and ENDOH, 1976).

Clonidine antagonized the activation of adenylate cyclase induced by α-sympathomimetic agents in cortical slices revealing in this preparation α adrenoceptor blocking properties (SKOLNICK and DALY, 1975, 1976).

At low doses clonidine did not change the effects of isoproterenol, but an antagonism could be detected at high doses (BOISSIER et al., 1968; SCRIABINE et al., 1968). However, in rats KÜNDIG et al. (1967) reported potentiation of the depressor response to isoproterenol and orciprenaline after clonidine. Clonidine in high doses increased the hypertensive effect of tyramine (BOISSIER et al., 1968) but did not change the pressor response to amphetamine or guanethidine (BENTLEY and LI, 1968).

C. Influence on Noradrenaline Levels and Metabolism at Peripheral Sites

Clonidine did not change the level of noradrenaline in the heart (HOEFKE and KOBINGER, 1966). Therefore a depletion of noradrenaline stores could not account for the blood pressure-lowering effect of the drug. Clonidine inhibits the uptake of noradrenaline into the postganglionic sympathetic nerves (STARKE et al., 1972).

SALT (1973) showed that the extraneuronal uptake II process of catecholamines was very sensitive to clonidine.

Clonidine did not change the rate of synthesis of ^{3}H noradrenaline from ^{3}H tyrosine in the heart of rats (PERSSON and WALDECK, 1970). Clonidine reduced noradrenaline turnover rate in submaxillary glands of rats maintained at 22° or exposed to cold, but did not change or reduced noradrenaline turnover rate in the heart, spleen, kidneys and adrenal glands of rats maintained at 22° C. A much greater reduction was observed in rats exposed to cold (BRALET and ROCHETTE, 1973a, b). This effect has been ascribed to loss of sympathetic tone due to peripheral and central actions of the drug; that clonidine inhibits noradrenaline release, might be the cause of this effect.

Clonidine in patients reduced excretion of urinary catecholamines (HÖKFELT et al., 1968, 1969, 1970a, b; 1975) and vanillylmandelic acid (STURM and SCHEJA, 1968). This effect is believed to be due to decreased sympathetic tone.

D. Effects on Postganglionic Sympathetic Fibers

Clonidine has been reported to lower response to stimulation of the pre- and postganglionic sympathetic nerves, but only at low stimulation frequencies and rather high dosage.

Thus clonidine did not change the maximal contraction of the nictitating membrane induced by stimulation of pre- or postganglionic fibers of the cervical sympathetic chain in rabbits (HOEFKE and KOBINGER, 1966) and cats (BOISSIER et al., 1968; CONSTANTINE and MCSHANE, 1968). Similarly, clonidine did not reduce the contractions of the vas deferens of guinea pigs induced by stimulation of the hypogastric nerve (KOBINGER, 1967), or had only a weak inhibiting effect (BENTLEY and LI, 1968). In contrast, clonidine reduced the tachycardia caused in cats by stimulation of the cardiac nerve at low frequencies (KOBINGER, 1967, 1968a; SCRIABINE et al., 1968, 1970; SCRIABINE and STAVORSKI, 1976) (Fig. 6), the hypertensive effect induced in pithed rats by stimulation of the entire sympathetic system (BENTLEY and LI, 1968; BOISSIER et al., 1968), the vasoconstriction induced by stimulation of the periarterial nerves of the rabbit ear (BENTLEY and LI, 1968; BOISSIER et al., 1968), or by stimulation of the lumbar sympathetic chain in the hindquarter of cats by Melander's technique (KOBINGER and HOEFKE, 1968), the tachycardia evoked in pithed rats by stimulation of the thoracic sympathetic chain (ARMSTRONG and BOURRA, 1973; DREW, 1976). However, no effect was seen when high stimulation frequencies were used.

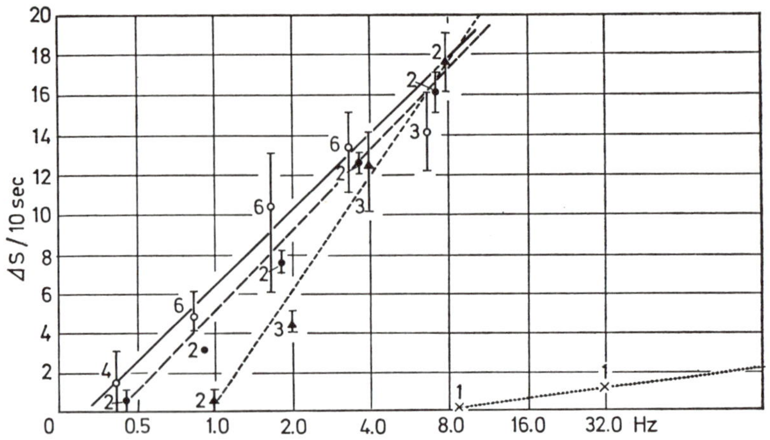

Fig. 6. Influence of clonidine on tachycardia induced in cats by stimulation of the right cardiac nerve. ●: Controls, ○ clonidine 30 µg/kg, ▲ clonidine 100 µg/kg, X guanethidine, 3.2 mg/kg. Clonidine even at high dosage reduced only the effects of the stimulation of the right cardiac nerve at low stimulation frequencies in contrast to guanethidine. [KOBINGER, W.: Arch. Pharm. exp. Path. **258**, 51 (1967)]

Thus clonidine seems to impair weakly ganglionic transmission and/or the release of noradrenaline from the postganglionic sympathetic fibers. This effect has been confirmed on the isolated iris of the rat (FARNEBO and HAMBURGER, 1971). Clonidine reduced the increased outflow of noradrenaline from the isolated perfused heart of the rabbit induced by stimulation of the postganglionic sympathetic nerves and reduced the functional responses of the myocardium (STARKE and SCHÜMANN, 1971; STARKE et al., 1971; WERNER et al., 1970, 1972) (Fig. 7). A similar effect was observed with the related compound BAY a 6781, and with this compound a decreased noradrenaline release was reported from the beef adrenal after carbachol or phenylethylamine. BAY a 6781 similarly reduced the output of noradrenaline brought about by splanchnic nerve stimulation in cats. However the drug did not change the hypertensive response, affording evidence that the decreased release of noradrenaline is not the cause of the hypotensive effect (SCHÜMANN and WERNER, 1971). STARKE et al. (1972) compared the blockade induced by clonidine, guanethidine and local anesthetics on the postganglionic sympathetic nerves of the rabbit heart. Clonidine and guanethidine, in contrast to local anesthetics, inhibit noradrenaline release much more efficiently than they depress impulse conduction. No indication was found of an accumulation of clonidine in adrenergic neurons as it was found with guanethidine. Clonidine reversibly reduces the increased noradrenaline overflow induced by sympathetic nerve stimulation or by tyramine. Amphetamine counteracts the block of adrenergic transmission induced by both clonidine and guanethidine. The authors conclude that clonidine inhibits adrenergic transmission by a specific interaction with noradrenaline release.

In recent years the concept that a *presynaptic α adrenoceptor could inhibit noradrenaline release* emerged and is now generally accepted (KIRPEKAR and PUIG, 1971; LANGER, 1973, 1974; STARKE et al., 1975). Clonidine was shown to activate presynaptic α adrenoceptors. The drug reduces noradrenaline release induced by transmural stimulation of the rabbit pulmonary artery, an effect more marked at low than at high frequency stimulation. Phentolamine increases noradrenaline release and in addition antagonizes the effect of clonidine (STARKE et al.,

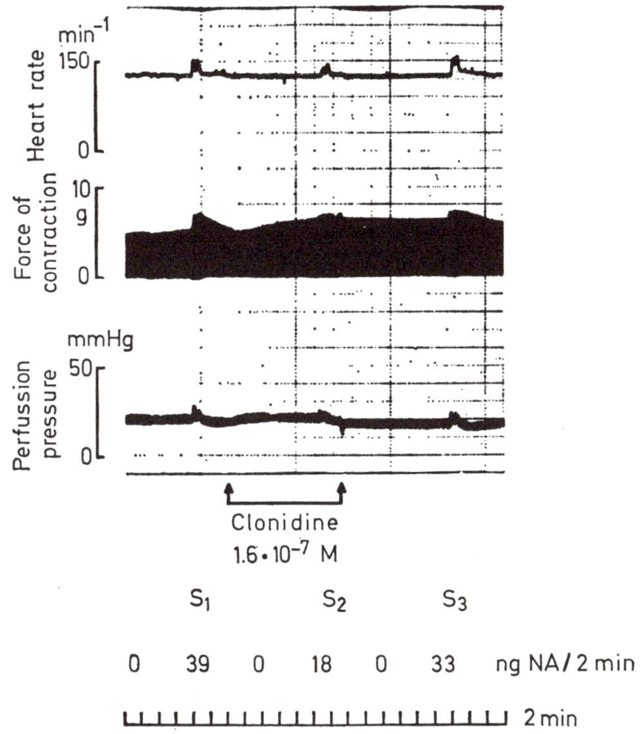

Fig. 7. Influence of clonidine on the response of an isolated rabbit heart to sympathetic nerve stimulation. $S_1 = S_2 = S_3$ = 1 min stimulation period. NA = noradrenaline. The figure shows a decreased response of the heart to sympathetic stimulation and decreased noradrenaline release. [WERNER, V., STARKE, K., SCHÜMANN, H.J.: Arch. int. Pharmacod. Thérap. **195**, 285—290 (1972)]

1974). In contrast to noradrenaline release evoked by nerve stimulation and potassium, the release evoked by tyramine or dimethyl-phenylpiperazinium is not affected (STARKE and MONTEL, 1974). As nerve impulses and potassium induce noradrenaline release only in the presence of calcium, it seems likely that α adrenoceptor agonists selectively inhibit calcium dependent processes. (STJÄRNE, 1973; STARKE and MONTEL, 1974). Although activation by low doses of α adrenoceptor agonists and blockade by α adrenoceptor blocking agents demonstrate that presynaptic α adrenoceptors resemble conventional postsynaptic ones differences in the relative pre and postsynaptic potencies of agonists have been found (STARKE et al., 1974). Thus in the rabbit pulmonary artery the apparent affinity of clonidine for presynaptic α adrenoceptors is at least ten times higher than its apparent affinity for postsynaptic α adrenoceptors (STARKE et al., 1974). Clonidine reduces in pithed rats the tachycardia evoked by stimulation of the thoracic lumbar chain (ARMSTRONG and BOURRA, 1973). In this preparation clonidine has been found to have similar potencies on pre- and postsynaptic α adrenoceptors; in contrast oxymetazoline, naphazoline, methoxamine and phenylephrine are more effective on postsynaptic receptors leading to the pressor effect and xylazine is more effective on presynaptic receptors (DREW, 1976). In dogs clonidine reduces the tachycardia induced by cardiac nerve stimulation. This effect is antagonized by high frequency stimulation of the nerve and by several α adrenoceptor blocking agents

(Scriabine and Stavorski, 1976; Antonaccio et al., 1974; Robson and Antonaccio, 1974). These experiments indicate that pre- and postsynaptic receptors might be dissimilar and that clonidine-like drugs could preferentially act on a presynaptic α-receptor. It is not yet known whether this effect might be important in the antihypertensive effect of clonidine. Using perfused hind limbs of the cats, Hauesler (1976) found that clonidine inhibits the vasoconstrictor response to stimulation of the lumbar sympathetic chain only at high dosage; the author proposed that this effect is not the major cause of the decrease in blood pressure brought about by clonidine.

The inhibitory stimulation of the sympathetic nerves has been shown to be antagonized not only by phentolamine and phenoxybenzamine but to a lesser degree by cocaine (Starke and Altmann, 1973). According to Antonaccio (1972), and Antonaccio and Robson (1973), the inhibition of the tachycardia induced by stimulation of cardiac nerves shown in intact dogs was not seen in dogs with both vagus nerves cut. Therefore the activation of the vagal tone appears to be involved in this effect. But in Kobinger's (1967) experiment in cats such an effect was not found and Scriabine und Stavorski (1973) were also unable to repeat Antonaccio and Robson's results in dogs.

E. Centrally Mediated Decrease in Sympathetic Tone as the Cause of Hypotension

Centrally mediated inhibition of sympathetic tone was suggested early as the cause of the secondary hypotension and the bradycardic effect induced in bivagotomized animals by clonidine. *The evidence was of two kinds.*

a) All procedures that abolished the sympathetic tone decreased or suppressed the hypotension brought about by clonidine. This was seen after spinalization (Kobinger and Walland, 1967b; Nayler et al., 1968) and pithing (Boissier et al., 1968; Autret et al., 1971; Armstrong and Bourra, 1973). The hypotensive effect was reduced or abolished in reserpinized animals (Kobinger and Walland, 1967b; Boissier et al., 1968; Nayler et al., 1968; Laubie and Schmitt, 1974), after administration of ganglion-blocking agents (Nayler et al., 1966, 1968), bretylium (Nayler et al., 1968), guanethidine (Rand and Wilson, 1968; Robson et al., 1969a, b; Laubie and Schmitt, 1974), or α adrenoceptor blocking agents (Kobinger and Walland, 1967b; Boissier et al., 1968; Nayler et al., 1968; Nayler and Stone, 1970; Iwata, 1969).

b) As noted previously, clonidine did not strikingly reduce the effects induced by stimulation of the sympathetic fibers (Kobinger, 1967; Boissier et al., 1968).

More direct evidence is available to support a central site of action for clonidine. Kobinger (1967), and Kobinger and Walland (1967a, c) were the first to show a *decrease in blood pressure, heart rate and cardiac output* in cats and dogs without any initial hypertension after *injection of clonidine into the cisterna magna* at doses too small to be effective by intravenous injection. These facts were confirmed repeatedly in dogs and cats (Schmitt et al., 1968; Schmitt and Schmitt, 1969 a, b; Schmitt and Fénard, 1971; Schmitt et al., 1971d; Onesti et al., 1971; Schmitt et al., 1973, 1975; Kobinger and Walland, 1971a, b, 1972a, b, c, 1973; Bogaievsky et al., 1974; Reid et al., 1973, 1975; Ganong, 1975a, b) and in rabbits (Reid and Dollery, 1972; Bogaievsky et al., 1974), (Fig. 8). In addition, intracisternal administration of clonidine at low dosage caused dilatation of the spleen, indicating a central decrease in the sympathetic tone (Kobinger and Walland, 1967c; Kobinger and Hoefke, 1968).

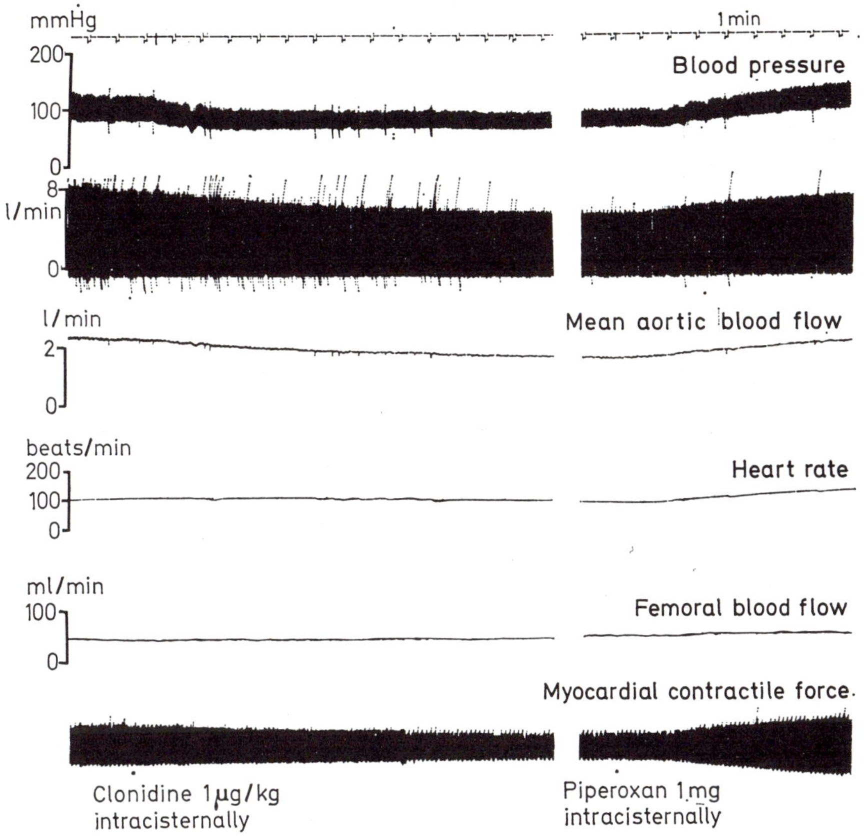

Fig. 8. Effect of intracisternal administration of clonidine in the dog. Clonidine (1 µg/kg) injected into the cisterna magna reduced blood pressure, aortic blood flow, heart rate and myocardial contractile force. Subsequent administration of piperoxan (1 mg/kg) into the cisterna magna reversed the effect. [SCHMITT, H., SCHMITT, HÉLÈNE, FÉNARD, S.: Arzneimittel-Forsch. **23**, 42 (1973b)]

Administration of the drug *into the cerebral ventricle* was another means used to localize the action to the central nervous system. SHERMAN et al. (1968) demonstrated a decrease in blood pressure in dogs without any initial hypertension after intracerebroventricular administration of clonidine at low dosage. These results were confirmed in cats and dogs (SCHMITT and SCHMITT, 1969; SCHMITT and FÉNARD, 1971; BOUSQUET and GUERTZENSTEIN, 1973) and in rabbits (TODA et al., 1969) (Fig. 9).

SATTLER and VAN ZWIETEN (1967), used a more physiological route of administration. *Infusion of clonidine at low dosage into the vertebral artery* of cats induced a dose-dependent decrease in blood pressure. CONSTANTINE and MCSHANE (1968), KATIC et al., (1972), SCHMITT et al., (1973a), LAUBIE (1975a, b) and LAUBIE and SCHMITT (1976) reported similar results in dogs, and the last authors analyzed the hemodynamic effects (Fig. 10). SHERMAN et al. (1968) used the more sophisticated method of *cross-circulation experiments* in dogs. Injection of clonidine into the cephalic circulation of a dog, the head of which was perfused by a congener and

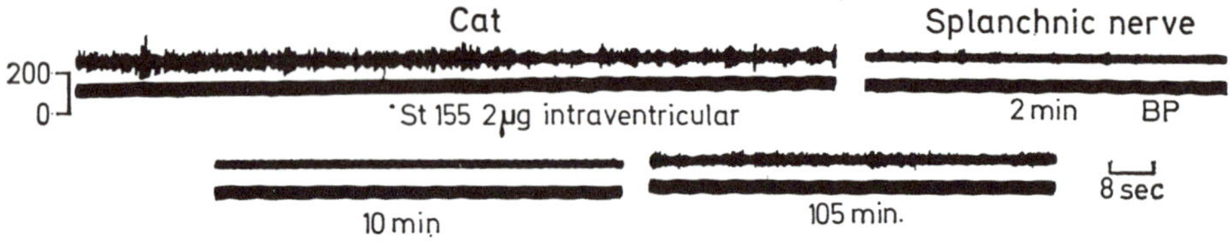

Fig. 9. Effect of intracerebroventricular injection of clonidine on blood pressure, heart rate and splanchnic discharges. The upper trace shows splanchnic discharges and the lower trace blood pressure. Injection of 2 µg/kg of clonidine into the lateral ventricle induced a progressive decrease in blood pressure and splanchnic discharges. Partial revovery occurred after 105 min. (SCHMITT, H.: In: Catapres in Hypertension, 1970, p. 31)

linked to the trunk only by the spinal cord, induced a decrease in blood pressure and heart rate in the trunk.

These results clearly show that clonidine at low dosage can inhibit the sympathetic centers, but the finding that clonidine reduces blood pressure when injected into the cisterna magna or the vertebral artery at doses which are ineffective by intravenous administration does not necessarily indicate a central mechanism of action. This hypotensive effect would not be the primary effect of clonidine when administered intravenously. It has to be shown that clonidine, after intravenous administration, is able to reduce the sympathetic traffic. To settle this point, CONSTANTINE and MCSHANE (1968) and LI and BENTLEY (1969, 1970) showed that

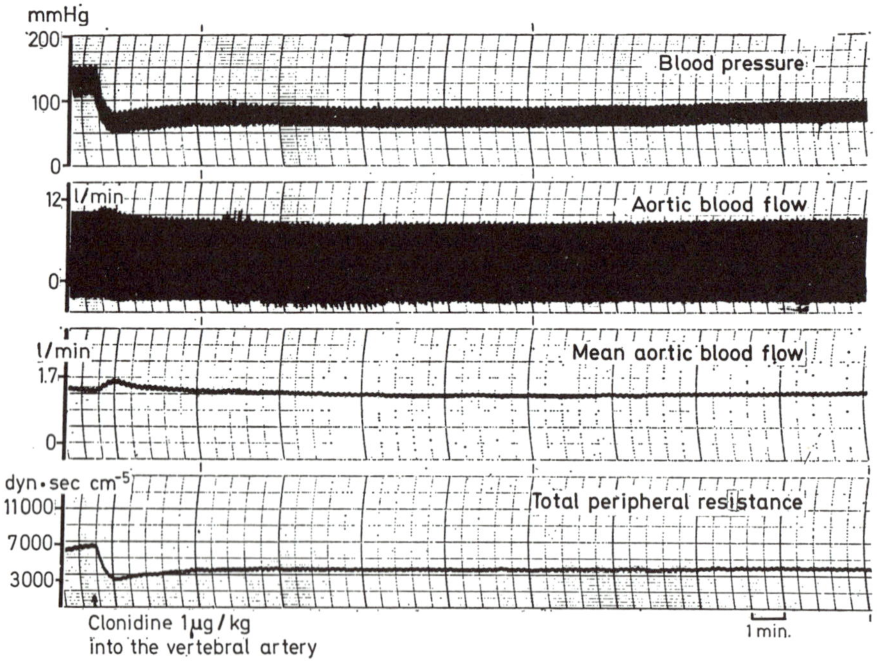

Fig. 10. Effect of clonidine injected into the vertebral artery in dogs. Clonidine (1 µg/kg) injected into the vertebral artery induced a fall in blood pressure without initial hypertension. Mean aortic blood flow increased transiently and total peripheral resistance was decreased in this dog. [SCHMITT, H., SCHMITT, HÉLÈNE, FÉNARD, S.: Arzneimittel-Forsch. **23**, 42 (1973)]

intravenous administration of clonidine decreased the perfusion pressure in the autoperfused hindquarter of a dog or a cat isolated from the trunk. Intravertebral administration elicited a similar effect, and denervation of the limb abolished the decrease in perfusion pressure (CONSTANTINE and MCSHANE, 1968). These experiments suggest that the hypotensive effect of clonidine is nervously mediated, most probably via a central mechanism. This is best demonstrated in the saline-perfused preparation, since the circulation of the hindquarters was completely isolated from the systemic circulation (LI and BENTLEY, 1969).

Recordings of the traffic in the sympathetic nerves afford a direct demonstration of the effect of the drug on the central sympathetic tone. The influence of clonidine on the electrical activity of sympathetic nerves has repeatedly been reported. Clonidine reduced or abolished the discharges in the preganglionic fibers of the splanchnic nerve or of the cervical sympathetic chain, or in the postganglionic fibers of the cardiac nerve in dogs, cats, rabbits and rats (SCHMITT et al., 1967, 1968; SCHMITT and SCHMITT, 1969, 1970; SCHMITT, 1969, 1970, 1975; SCHMITT et al., 1971, 1973; WOODHOUSE et al., 1972; HAEUSLER and FINCH, 1972; HAEUSLER, 1973a, b, c; LOEW and WAITE, 1974; WAITE, 1975; LAUBIE, 1975a, b; MCCALL and GEBBER, 1976) (Fig. 11). The central sympatho-inhibitory effect appeared

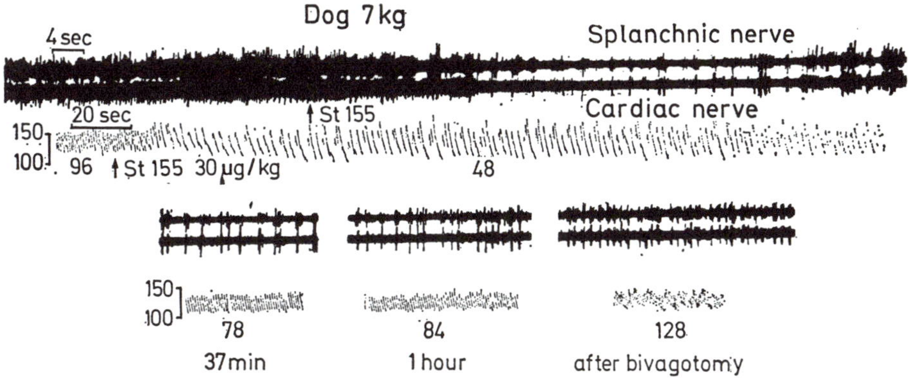

Fig. 11. Effect of clonidine on sympathetic discharges, blood pressure, and heart rate in the dog. The record shows the discharges in the preganglionic splanchnic nerve (top line), in the postganglionic cardiac nerve (second line) and on a different time scale, blood pressure (third line); the numbers give heart rate. Intravenous administration of clonidine (30 µg/kg) induced a rise in blood pressure, followed by a decrease, bradycardia, and a striking inhibition of sympathetic discharges. The last record shows that bivagotomy increased heart rate, but did not change the reduced blood pressure or sympathetic discharges. [SCHMITT, H., SCHMITT, HÉLÈNE, BOISSIER, J.R., GIUDICELLI, J.F., FICHELLE, J.: Europ. J. Pharmacol. 2, 342 (1968)]

at low doses (1 to 3 µg/kg) and was sometimes preceded by a small and transient increase in sympathetic discharges. The effect appeared to be dose-dependent (SCHMITT and SCHMITT, 1970; SCHMITT et al., 1971c, d, 1973a; LOEW and WAITE, 1974; WAITE, 1975). The inhibitory effect of clonidine on sympathetic discharges of renal nerves has been reported by HUKUHARA et al. (1968), TAUBERGER et al. (1970), AARS (1972), HAEUSLER and FINCH (1972), HAEUSLER (1973a, b, c), LAUBIE and SCHMITT (1976) and in lumbar sympathetic chain by LAUBIE and SCHMITT (1976).

Using single fibers of the splanchnic nerve, KLUPP et al. (1970) calculated the ED_{50} and reported a value of 10 µg/kg. LOEW and WAITE (1975) using multifiber preparations found an ED_{50} of 3—4 μg/kg after intravenous injection, and 1—2 μg/kg after intracerebroventricular administration.

It was desirable to confirm these results in conscious animals. A method was developed allowing splanchnic discharges to be recorded in conscious dogs (SCHMITT et al., 1974c). Small stainless steel electrodes were introduced into the splanchnic nerve and held in position with dental cement. The electrodes were soldered to Teflon-insulated stainless steel wires. The wires were passed under the skin as far as the neck and linked to a connector. Catheters were introduced into the carotid artery and the jugular vein in order to record blood pressure and to perform intravenous administration. In this manner it was possible to record blood pressure and splanchnic discharges over several weeks. Clonidine (10 μg/kg i.v.) induced the same effects as in anesthetized dogs (Fig. 12). In dogs treated twice a

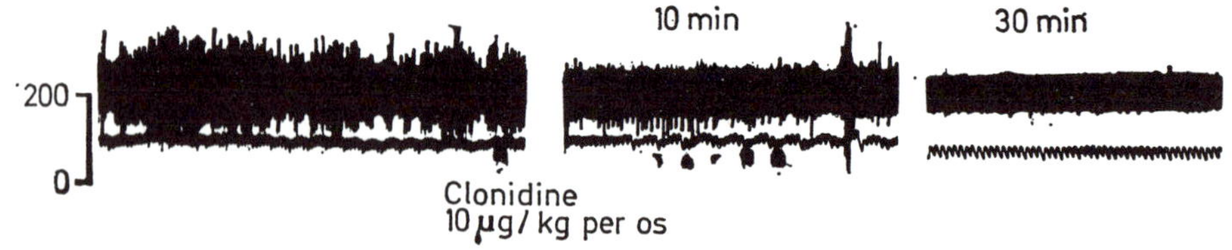

Fig. 12. Effect of clonidine (10 μg/kg) on blood pressure, heart rate, and splanchnic discharges in the conscious dog. Clonidine (10 μg/kg orally) decreased blood pressure, heart rate, and splanchnic discharges in the conscious dog, 10 and 30 min after administration. [SCHMITT, H., SCHMITT, HÉLÈNE, FÉNARD s. Neuropharmacology **13**, 248 (1974)]

day for one week with 10 μg/kg of clonidine i.v. or orally, no change was noted in the activity of the drug. Hypertension was followed by hypotension, bradycardia and a reduction in splanchnic discharges after each injection.

The recovery in blood pressure, heart rate, and splanchnic discharges appeared concomitantly, which suggests that a decrease in the sympathetic tone was the cause of the hypotensive and bradycardic effects (SCHMITT et al., 1967, 1968; SCHMITT, 1970).

A reflexly mediated decrease in the sympathetic tone could be ruled out. In fact, the sympatho-inhibitory effect of clonidine was seen in dogs after elimination of the main pathways of cardiovascular reflexes, *i.e.* denervation of the carotid sinus, cutting of both vagus nerves, and extirpation of both nodose ganglia (Fig. 13). In these preparations the blood pressure-lowering effect of clonidine was even more

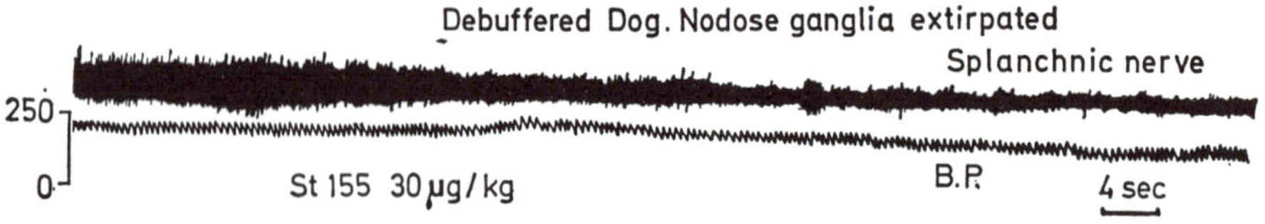

Fig. 13. Effect of clonidine on splanchnic discharges and blood pressure in a debuffered dog with both nodose ganglia extirpated. In this dog, both carotid sinus nerves and vagus nerves were cut, and both nodose ganglia were extirpated. Clonidine (30 μg/kg) induced a rise in blood pressure, followed by a decrease, the heart was slowed but less than in intact dogs, and there was inhibition of splanchnic discharges. As the main cardiovascular pathways are ruled out, a central sympatho-inhibitory effect is suggested. (SCHMITT, H.: In: Catapres in Hypertension, p. 28)

marked than in normotensive dogs but the early cardiac slowing effect was less evident (SCHMITT et al., 1967, 1968; HAEUSLER, 1973a). Injection of clonidine in small doses into the right atria did not alter blood pressure, heart rate, and sympathetic discharges (SCHMITT et al., 1967, 1968) and did not evoke firing in the afferent fibers of the vagus nerve (ZAIMIS, 1970), which eliminated a Bezold-Jarisch effect.

The reduction of sympathetic discharges was also seen after administration of clonidine in small doses into the cisterna magna or into the lateral ventricle of the brain (SCHMITT et al., 1968; SCHMITT and SCHMITT, 1969a; SCHMITT, 1970; SCHMITT et al., 1971d, 1973a; WOODHOUSE et al., 1972; WAITE, 1975) thus affording further support for the involvement of the sympathetic centers in this effect. Clonidine reduced the rate of discharges of neurons thought to be involved in cardiovascular control in the medulla oblongata (HUKUHARA et al., 1968). Similarly clonidine decreased the rate of discharges of preganglionic sympathetic neurons located in the spinal cord (DE GROAT et al., 1975).

F. Sites of Action in the Central Nervous System

Many sites of action appear to be involved in the depressor, bradycardic and sympatho-inhibitory effects of clonidine.

The *rhombencephalon* seems to be the main site of action of clonidine. In fact, transection of the brain stem above the medulla oblongata (HUKUHARA et al., 1968; SCHMITT and SCHMITT, 1969a; SINHA et al., 1973) did not reduce the effects of clonidine on blood pressure, heart rate and sympathetic discharges (Fig. 14).

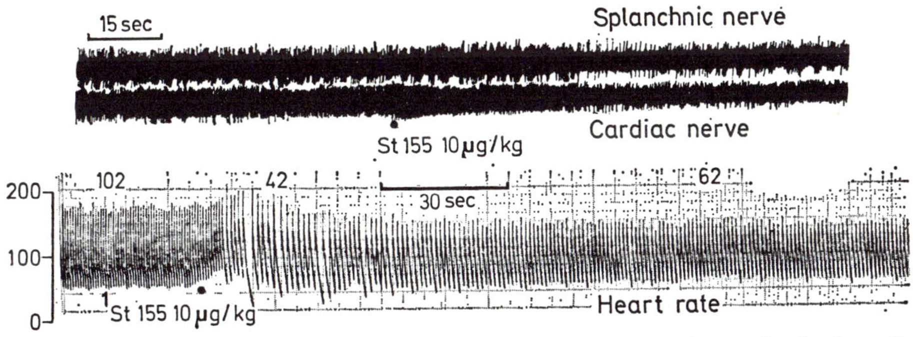

Fig. 14. Effects of clonidine on blood pressure and sympathetic discharges in the dog after transection of the brain stem between the pons and the medulla oblongata. Upper tracing: action potentials in the splanchnic nerve. Middle tracing: action potentials in the cardiac nerve. Lower tracing: blood pressure on a different time scale. At. injection of clonidine 10 μg/kg induced the usual changes: reduction of sympathetic discharges, bradycardia, brief hypertension followed, by a fall in blood pressure. [SCHMITT, H., SCHMITT, HÉLÈNE: Europ. J. Pharmacol. **6**, 10 (1969)]

Clonidine reduced, at small doses, the late component of the potential evoked in the splanchnic nerve by central sciatic stimulation. This late component is thought to be due to a spino-bulbo-spinal reflex (SINHA et al., 1973). Clonidine reduced the 3 Hz component of the sympathetic medullary cardiovascular structures (MCCALL and GEBBER, 1976). In addition clonidine induced a strong decrease in blood pressure and heart rate when injected in small doses into the vertebral artery which is known to supply the rhombencephalon, but was ineffective when administered into the internal carotid artery supplying more rostral regions (CONSTANTINE and MCSHANE, 1968; KATIĆ et al., 1972).

The *spinal cord* appears to be another site of action although less sensitive. The small electrical activity recorded in the splanchnic nerve of spinal cats was reduced by high doses of clonidine (Sinha et al., 1973; de Groat et al., 1975). Clonidine reduced the early component of the potential evoked in the splanchnic nerve by central sciatic stimulation (Sinha et al., 1973). This potential is thought to be due to a spino-spinal reflex (Coote and Downmann, 1966; Sato and Schmidt, 1971). In addition clonidine reduced the potential evoked in the splanchnic nerve by spinal cord stimulation in intact and spinalized cats (Sinha et al., 1973). In chloralose-anesthetized cats stimulation of pelvic nerve afferents to the urinary bladder evoked firing in the lumbar sympathetic outflow (hypogastric nerve). This spinal reflex was depressed by clonidine. The effect of clonidine was demonstrated in acute and spinal preparations (de Groat et al., 1975). Clonidine reduced the 10 Hz component of the sympathetic discharges which reflected the activity of spinal structures (McCall and Gebber, 1976). Clonidine reduced in spinal cats the sympathetic reflexes and the potential evoked in a sympathetic nerve by spinal cord stimulation (Neumayr et al., 1972; Franz et al., 1975). The depressing effects of clonidine on spinal reflexes were antagonized by piperoxan (Sinha et al., 1973) and tolazoline (Neumayr et al., 1972; Franz et al., 1975) suggesting an activation of α adrenoceptors by clonidine. Clonidine reduced the pressor response to spinal cord compression (Dhawan et al., 1975a, b).

However *more rostral structures* also might be accessory sites of action for clonidine. Injection of clonidine into the anterior hypothalamus—in high doses—reduced blood pressure and heart rate in rats (Struyker-Boudier and van Rossum, 1972). Midcollicular decerebration abolished the reduction of pressor responses to bulbar stimulation evoked by clonidine. This observation seems to indicate that clonidine is able to act on rostral structures involved in the excitability of the medulla oblongata (Klevans et al., 1973). Shaw et al. (1971b) examined the central actions of clonidine on unanesthetized rabbits and the findings suggest that the drug acts at diencephalic levels. There was a more pronounced fall in blood pressure in pontine preparations than in sham operated rabbits but the reverse was true for the heart rate. Other studies (Shaw et al., 1971a) showed that after section of the carotid sinus nerves and aortic nerves, clonidine produced a more marked fall in blood pressure in unanesthetized rabbits, but the bradycardia was less marked. The authors concluded that clonidine acts mainly at bulbar levels but that baroreceptor input opposes the hypotensive effect by suprabulbar mechanisms. Clonidine completely blocked the bulbar sympathetic cardioacceleration and sympathetic constrictor mechanism during mild hypoxia but during severe hypoxia, this effect was less pronounced. During severe hypoxia clonidine produced a complete blockade of the bulbar mechanism concerned with the reflex secretion of adrenaline, as estimated from the responses of the muscle bed and the arterial pH. In addition the drug blocks the diencephalically mediated inhibitory effect on cutaneous constrictor tone to the ear skin, but has little effect on the diencephalically mediated sympathetic neural constrictor mechanism normally excited during severe hypoxia. These results suggest therefore diencephalic levels of action. Clonidine was also reported—in high doses—to induce a pressor response when the drug was injected into the lateral ventricle of the brain of cats and prevented to reach the floor of the fourth ventricle by cannulation of the acqueduct of Sylvius (Bousquet and Guertzenstein, 1973), but in these experiments a leakage of the drug into the systemic circulation, leading to a stimulation of peripheral α adrenoceptors and to hypertension, was not ruled out. The pressor effect of clonidine was increased in rats by prehypothalamic section (Henning et al., 1976; Trolin, 1976). Superfusion of the posterior hypothalamus with a push-pull cannula was reported to increase the pressor response to stimulation of this structure (PHILIPPU et al., 1973a, b).

The *medullary structures* responsible for the effects of clonidine are as yet unknown in exception for those mediating the vagal bradycardia (cf. p. 338), but several areas have been suggested to be the sites of action of the drug. The *nucleus tractus solitarii* was thought to be the site of action for noradrenaline containing neurons have been found in this nucleus (DAHLSTRÖM and FUXE, 1964) and, in addition, the first synapsis of baroreceptor fibers has been localized in this structured (CRILL and REIS, 1968; SELLER and ILLERT, 1969). It was therefore tempting to suggest that a noradrenergic link was interposed in this pathway and that clonidine might mimic the effects of baroreceptor stimulation (SCHMITT et al., 1971d; HAEUSLER, 1973a, b; 1974a). Bilateral destruction of these nuclei induced in urethanized rats a rise in blood pressure and reduced the hypotensive effects of clonidine (LIPSKI et al., 1976a). Microinjection of noradrenaline in these nuclei has been reported to lower blood pressure and heart rate but clonidine was ineffective (DE JONG, personal communication). Clonidine infused in this nucleus reduced the pressor response to hypothalamic stimulation, but did not change resting blood pressure (PHILIPPU et al., 1973a, b). Infusion of clonidine in this nucleus has been reported to reduce blood pressure and heart rate (SINHA et al., 1975). However there are findings showing that the nucleus tractus solitarii is not the alone or the main site of the hypotensive action for clonidine in cats and dogs. Destruction of both nuclei tractus solitarii in cats did not change blood pressure (LAUBIE, 1975a, b; LAUBIE et al., 1976; LAUBIE and SCHMITT, 1977; ANTONACCIO and HALLEY, 1977) and increased heart rate (LAUBIE, 1975; LAUBIE et al., 1976; LAUBIE and SCHMITT, 1977). In these lesioned cats, clonidine induced a hypotension and a bradycardia no significantly different from those induced in intact animals (LAUBIE, 1975a, b; LAUBIE et al., 1976; ANTONACCIO and HALLEY, 1976). In dogs bilateral destruction of the nucleus tractus solitarii and of the vagal motor nucleus induced a fulminating hypertension and bradycardia, but the effects of clonidine on blood pressure and heart rate persisted (LAUBIE and SCHMITT, 1977). Therefore the nucleus tractus solitarii seems to be ruled out in the hypotensive and at least in part the bradycardic effect of clonidine. However there is now good evidence that clonidine induced a vagally mediated bradycardia in dogs by sensitizing at this level baroreceptor impulses (LAUBIE et al., 1976; LAUBIE and SCHMITT, 1977), although in cats other regions seem also to be involved (ANTONACCIO and HALLEY, 1976) (cf. p. 338).

The *nucleus ambiguus* does not seem to be involved in the hypotensive and bradycardic effects in dogs (LAUBIE et al., 1976) and cats (ANTONACCIO and HALLEY, 1976). Although the destruction of both motor vagus nuclei did not change the effects of clonidine (LAUBIE and SCHMITT, 1977), infusion of the drug in these nuclei decreased heart rate and blood pressure (SINHA et al., 1975). Infusion of clonidine into the reticular formation induced similar changes (SINHA et al., 1975). Destruction of the depressor area in dogs has been reported to decrease the action of clonidine (SCHMITT et al., 1973d).

BOUSQUET and GUERTZENSTEIN (1973) claimed that the site of action of clonidine is located on a small area of the *ventral surface of the medulla oblongata*, called Schläfke zone and situated 2 mm caudally to the trapezoid bodies, 4 mm laterally to the midline, on 1.2 mm length. Clonidine applied in small doses on this area induced a marked fall in blood pressure, a result confirmed by DHAWAN et al. (1975). In addition, BOUSQUET et al. (1975a, b) reported that bilateral destruction of this area, abolished the secondary depressor effect of clonidine. However other studies (LAUBIE, 1975a, b; LAUBIE and SCHMITT, 1976) performed also on pentobarbitalized cats could not confirm these results. However, more extensive destruction involving the ventral reticular formation situated between the olivary complex and the lateral reticular nucleus on 5 mm length, 4 mm lateral to the midline, from the trapezoid bodies approximately to the obex, were needed to abolish in cats the secondary depressor effect of intravenous administration of clonidine (LAUBIE, 1975a, b; LAUBIE and SCHMITT, 1977). However as the pressor effect of the drug was more transient than in spinalized animals this suggests a persisting depression of the sympathetic tone. In dogs, bilateral lesions in similar regions (4 mm lateral to the midline, from the caudal border of the trapezoid bodies to the obex) suppressed the reduction in discharges of the splanchnic, renal nerves and the lumbar sympathetic chain, but did not alter the bradycardia and blood pressure changes induced by clonidine injected intravenously. Therefore in this animal species the sites of action for reducing sympathetic discharges on one hand, and blood pressure or heart rate on the other hand seem to be different. Increased vagaltone, effect on postganglionic sympathetic fibers or activation of an active vasodilator pathway have been proposed to account for this unexpected result (LAUBIE, 1975a, b; LAUBIE and SCHMITT, 1977).

The central sympathetic inhibitory effect of clonidine is characterized by other features. Clonidine barely decreased the respiratory grouping of the sympathetic discharges and frequently changed a continuous discharge to a respiratory grouped one. The inspiratory centers were therefore still able to excite the sympathetic neurons. In cats and dogs with a low sympathetic tone respiratory grouping was predominant, and clonidine failed to decrease sympathetic discharges and blood pressure (SCHMITT et al., 1968; SCHMITT, 1970).

The reduction of the discharges induced by clonidine as well as related compounds was not similar in the various sympathetic nerves (Fig. 15). The effect of

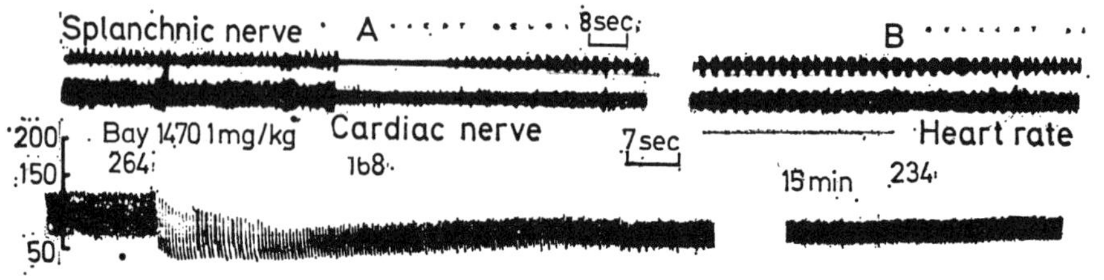

Fig. 15. Differentiated effect of xylazine on sympathetic discharges. The figure shows splanchnic discharges (top line), discharges of the cardiac nerve (second line), blood pressure (third line; on a different time scale). The animal received two previous injections of xylazine which transiently reduced the discharges in the cardiac nerve and changed the continuous discharges in the splanchnic nerve into a discharge with respiratory grouping. In A at. the injection of 1 mg/kg of xylazine (Bayer 1470) abolished the sympathetic discharges for 25 sec; they reappeared with respiratory grouping but were reduced in the cardiac nerve at 15 min. Intense bradycardia precluded the usual initial increase in blood pressure. [SCHMITT, H., FOURNADJIEV, G., SCHMITT, HÉLÈNE: Europ. J. Pharmacol. 10, 234 (1970)]

the drug was less marked on the cervical sympathetic trunk of cats and rabbits than on the splanchnic or cardiac nerves. In addition, the sympathetic activity was usually more reduced in the cardiac nerve than in the splanchnic nerve (SCHMITT et al., 1968; SCHMITT, 1970). These observations demonstrate the pharmacological heterogeneity of the central sympathetic drive and could account for some apparently paradoxical effects of clonidine. Thus the drug did not relax the nictitating membrane but always induced a contraction, an effect probably due to the predominance of the α-sympathomimetic effect over the slight reduction in the sympathetic tone of the cervical sympathetic chain. It could be rewarding to look for a differentiated effect of the sympathetic drive on arteries and veins; this could account for the low incidence of orthostatic hypotension reported in clinical trials.

Although it appears to be well established that the decrease in the sympathetic tone by clonidine is centrally mediated, other sites of action could contribute to the effect and have even been claimed as the principal causes of the hypotensive effect. LARBI and ZAIMIS (1970) and ZAIMIS (1970) reported a decreased vascular reactivity after chronic treatment with clonidine and suggested that this phenomenon could be the cause of the antihypertensive effect. However, other experiments (HODGE and ROBINSON, 1971; SAFAR et al., 1973) failed to confirm this effect in man. TANZ (1969) reported no parallel changes between cardiac output and total peripheral resistance and observed a fall in blood pressure after clonidine in spinal dogs, suggesting a peripheral site of action. SHAW et al. (1971, a) reported a fall in total peripheral resistance in rabbits after blockade of the sympathetic and parasympathetic systems, suggesting a peripheral site of action. COUPAR and KIRBY (1972) suggested that the α-adrenoceptor blocking effect of clonidine could contribute to the hypotensive effect. The inhibition of noradrenaline release could also be another contributory factor (p. 307—310).

G. Effects of Clonidine on Centrally Mediated Increases in Sympathetic Tone

Clonidine has been shown to *reduce the pressor response to stimulation of bulbar* (SCHMITT et al., 1968; DHAWAN et al., 1973; KLEVANS et al., 1973; SINHA et al., 1973) and *hypothalamic* (SCHMITT et al., 1968; SINHA et al., 1973; DHAWAN et al., 1973; HAEUSLER, 1973a, b, 1974b) *areas in cats and rats*. Increase in splanchnic nerve activity induced by these stimulations was also reduced (SCHMITT et al., 1968; HAEUSLER, 1973a, b, 1974b). The increases in blood pressure and splanchnic nerve activity induced by stimulation of the fastigial nucleus was also inhibited by clonidine (HAEUSLER, 1973a, b). KLEVANS et al., (1973) reported that decerebration reduced the inhibitory effect of clonidine on the pressor response to bulbar stimulation revealing a supramedullary site of action. However, perfusion of the nucleus tractus solitarii with clonidine at rather high concentrations by means of a pushpull cannula reduced the pressor response to stimulation of the posterior hypothalamus (PHILIPPU et al., 1973a, b), an observation which has been accounted for by a stimulation of inhibitory pathways. DHAWAN et al., (1975) found that centrally administered clonidine inhibited the threshold and maximum pressor responses evoked by both hypothalamic and medullary stimulations as well as the pressor responses following compression of the spinal cord in acute spinal animals. KLUPP et al., (1970) reported an ED_{50} of 10 μg/kg for clonidine in reducing the frequency of spontaneous discharges in single fibers of the splanchnic nerve, but 30 μg/kg were required to reduce the effect of hypothalamic stimulation by 50 p. 100 (Fig. 16). LOEW and WAITE (1974) drew the frequency or intensity curves for hypothalamic or medullary stimulations and found a decrease with clonidine at low frequencies or intensities of stimulation. KOSS and DAVISON (1976) found that clonidine reduced the electrodermal response (skin potential) evoked by stimulation of the hypothalamus only when low frequencies of stimulation were used. As this sympathocholinergic response evoked by peripheral stimulation was not changed by clonidine, a central site of action is suggested. In addition KOSS (1976) found that clonidine reduced the electrodermal response induced by hypothalamic, medullary and spinal stimulation at low frequency. Therefore the effect of clonidine is similar at each central area investigated.

Clonidine did not reduce the hypertensive effect of physostigmine in rats (SCHMITT et al., 1968) an effect assumed to be due to stimulation of sympathetic centers. However, BENTLEY and LI (1968) reported opposite results.

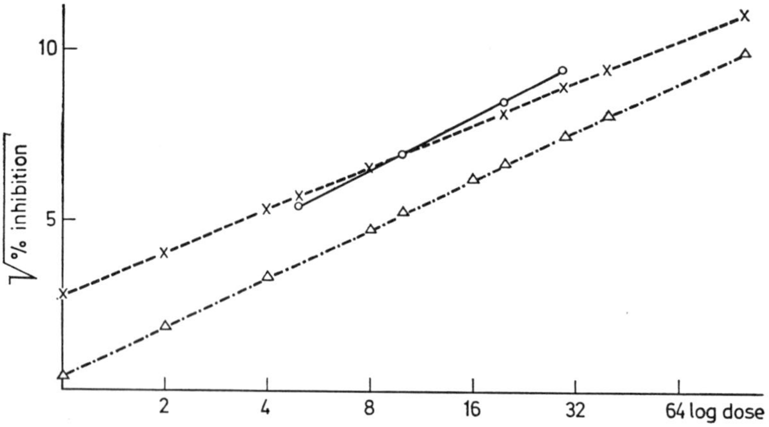

Fig. 16. Regression line of dose-dependent decrease of sympathetic activity. Abcissa: log dose; ordinate: $\sqrt{\%}$ inhibition. x—x—x decrease of spontaneous activity; o—o—o decrease of evoked impulses after stimulation of a somatic nerve; △ ... △ ... △ decrease of activity during hypothalamic stimulation. [KLUPP, H., KNAPPEN, F., OTSUKA, Y., STRELLER, I., TEICHMANN, H.: Europ. J. Pharmacol. **10**, 228 (1970)]

H. Effects of Clonidine on Centrally Mediated Depressor Responses

No results have been published on the effect of clonidine on depressor responses to central stimulation. Unpublished observations have shown that the drug given intravenously or by microinjection into the depressor bulbar area did not prevent the maximal fall in blood pressure and bradycardia induced by stimulation of the bulbar depressor area, and the absolute reduction in depressor response was thought to be due to the lower level of sympathetic tone induced by the drug.

J. Effects of Clonidine on Cardiovascular Reflexes

The effects of clonidine on a variety of cardiovascular reflexes have been investigated and an understanding of these effects could provide an interpretation for the low incidence of orthostatic hypotension found in humans.

Hypertension induced by carotid occlusion has repeatedly been reported to be decreased even during the hypertensive phase after intravenous administration; a similar reduction was found after intracisternal injections (HOEFKE and KOBINGER, 1966; KOBINGER and WALLAND, 1967b, c; BENTLEY and LI, 1968; BOISSIER et al., 1968; SCHMITT et al., 1967, 1968; SATTLER and VAN ZWIETEN, 1967; RAND and WILSON, 1968; GUT and SCHMITT, 1970; LI and BENTLEY, 1970) (Fig. 17). However, the interpretation of this effect is difficult for several reasons. Hypotension reduces the pressure on the walls of the carotid sinus and consequently decreases baroreceptor firing. If fewer baroreceptor fibers may cease to fire during carotid occlusion, the effect appears to be lessened. On the other hand, vasoconstriction of the sinus walls induced by the drug could cause the baroreceptor fibers to fire even during low intrasinusal blood pressure and so abolish the effect. Taking the percentage of increase in blood pressure as an index of the reflex, TANZ (1969) did not find any reduction in hypertension due to carotid occlusion by clonidine. A similar observation was made recently with low doses of clonidine (10 μg/kg), but an inhibition at higher dosage was seen in cats even when blood pressure remained at the same level (SCHMITT, 1975). However, clonidine seems to sensitize to the bradycardic effects of sinusal stimulation. Cardiac slowing induced by an

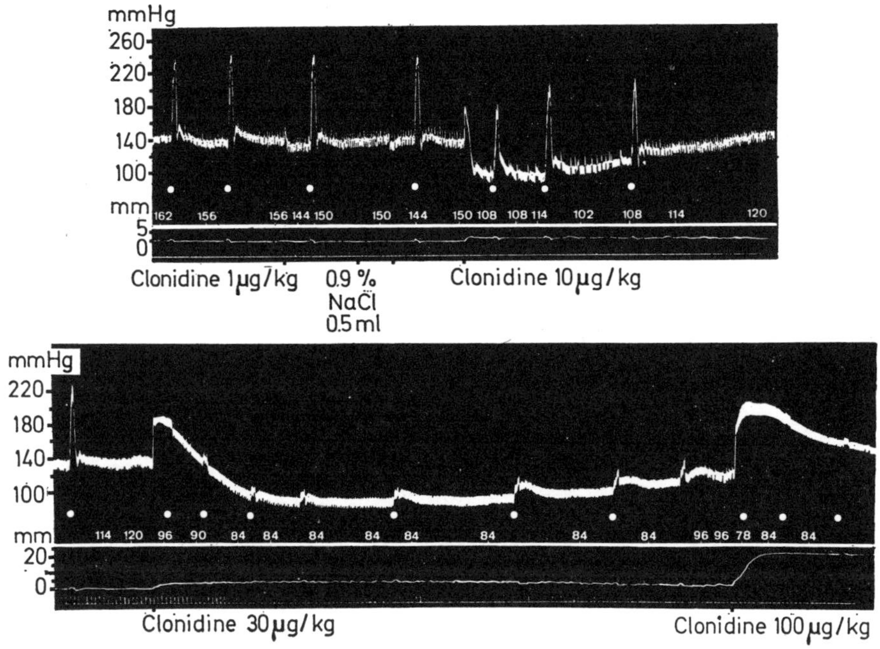

Fig. 17. Effect of clonidine on carotid sinus reflex in dogs. Clonidine reduced the carotid sinus reflex. [HOEFKE, W., KOBINGER, W.: Arzneimittel-Forsch. **16**, 1039 (1966)]

increase in blood pressure was potentiated by clonidine (ROBSON et al., 1969a, b; NAYLER and STONE, 1970; KOBINGER and WALLAND, 1971a, b, 1972a, b, c). HUKUHARA et al., (1968) found that clonidine prolonged the initial inhibition of the sympathetic discharges during carotid occlusion and reduced the secondary increase, suggesting that it has an effect of its own on this reflex.

Tests of the effects of clonidine on *chemoreceptor reflexes* have given conflicting results. No effect was reported by SCHMITT et al. (1968) and SCHMITT (1970) on the increased sympathetic discharges induced by stimulation of chemoreceptors by nicotine, 5-hydroxytryptamine, piribedil, or angiotensin, or on asphyxia in dogs. In contrast, SATTLER and VAN ZWIETEN (1967) noted a less marked effect of clonidine on the carotid sinus reflex in cats ventilated with oxygen than in cats ventilated with air, and suggested that chemoreceptor reflexes might be more susceptible to the drug than baroreceptor reflexes. On the other hand, clonidine inhibited the pressor effect induced by injection of cyanide into the carotid artery. SCHMITT (1970) mentioned that the increased sympathetic discharges induced in animals by vasodilators such as papaverine, phentolamine, tolazolinc or diazoxide were not changed by clonidine (Fig. 18). It is surprising that stimulations that increase the sympathetic tone by removing the inhibitory influences of the baroreceptors on sympathetic centers could still be effective when these centers were inactivated. Perhaps the fall in carotid blood pressure induced some hypoxia stimulating the chemoreceptors and therefore the sympathetic centers. Yet respiratory stimulation due to intrasinusal hypotension was not impaired by clonidine and the inspiratory center was able to stimulate the sympathetic centers.

The *hypertensive effect induced by stimulation* of *the central end of the vagus nerve* in dogs was reduced by high doses of clonidine (HOEFKE and KOBINGER, 1966; BOISSIER et al., 1968). In cats, HUKUHARA et al. (1968) reported increased initial inhibition and reduced secondary stimulation of the sympathetic discharges induced by central vagal stimulation after clonidine in cats.

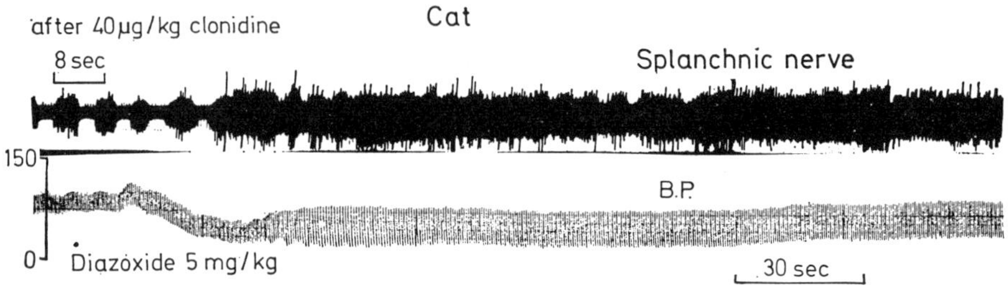

Fig. 18. Failure of clonidine to inhibit increased sympathetic discharges induced by diazoxide. In a cat treated with 40 µg/kg of clonidine, diazoxide induced a decrease in blood pressure and reflexly mediated increase in sympathetic discharges

Less work has been done on the excitation of afferent fibers *in somatic nerves.* No effect was found on hypertension induced in rabbit by central sciatic stimulation (GUT and SCHMITT, 1970). However, in cats, KLUPP et al. (1971) found that the same dose of clonidine reduced the electrical response in the splanchnic nerve to stimulation of the saphenous nerve also the spontaneous activity (Fig. 16). The authors accounted for this result by postulating a medullary site of action for both effects. Clonidine in cats and dogs reduced the hypertension induced by central sciatic nerve stimulation but at rather high doses (30 µg/kg); the effect was more marked when the frequency of stimulation was low (SINHA et al., 1973).

The effect of clonidine on the *compensatory reflexes* during tilting or Valsalva's maneuver is of special interest. Many authors found no impairment of these reflexes after clonidine in man and animals (ANTONACCIO, 1971; BOCK et al., 1966, 1968, 1970; KNOBLOCH and MORR, 1966; KOCHSIEK and FRITSCHE, 1966; MICHEL, 1968; BARNETT and CANTOR, 1968; GRABNER et al., 1968; BREST, 1970; MUIR et al., 1969; MUIR 1970; KROETZ et al., 1970; SAFAR et al., 1973). However, in rats MALING et al., (1968) with rather high doses of clonidine found abolition of the compensatory reflexes to tilting. According to CONSTANTINE and MCSHANE (1968) clonidine abolished these reflexes in the monkey but not in the dog. KOBINGER and ODA (1969) and KOBINGER (1969, 1970) studied the influence of several antihypertensive drugs on the diving reflex in ducks. This reflex is characterized by pronounced bradycardia and reduced cardiac output without any fall in mean blood pressure, indicating an increase in the vasoconstrictor tone. In contrast to guanethidine and bretylium, which caused the mean blood pressure to fall, clonidine and α methyldopa were devoid of any significant action on this reflex.

On the other hand, clonidine did not markedly change the increase in blood pressure and cardiac output during *exercise* in man (MUIR, 1970; ONESTI et al., 1971; SAFAR et al., 1973).

The effects of clonidine on *vasodepressor reflexes* have been studied less. A sensitization of the cardiac slowing to increased intrasinusal pressure has already been mentioned (p. 321). Low doses of clonidine which have virtually no influence on pre- and postganglionic sympathetic nerve activity and blood pressure potentiated the effect of sinus nerve stimulation on these parameters. After high doses of clonidine, when sympathetic nerve activity was markedly depressed and blood pressure considerably lowered, sinus nerve stimulation yielded no further decrease in these parameters (HAEUSLER, 1973a, b, 1974b). The maximum fall in blood pressure induced by stimulation of central end of the aortic nerve or sciatic nerve in rabbits and cats was not changed by clonidine, and the reduction in the absolute hypotension was explained by the prior diminution in the sympathetic tone brought about by the drug (GUT and SCHMITT, 1970). However, LI and BENTLEY (1969), using the autoperfused hind limb of cats, reported a decrease in vasodilator response to injection in the trunk of noradrenaline, adrenaline, dopamine and veratrine, but an increased vasoconstrictor response to histamine. The authors proposed impairment of cardiovascular centers, since the reduction was apparent at the initial perfusion pressure. However, this kind of reasoning does not appear correct since the hind limb was not isolated and clonidine was able to reach the vascular bed, exert its vasoconstrictor effect, and maintain the perfusion pressure. The spontaneous sympathetic tone was diminished and any stimulus reducing this tone could cause only a reduced response. However, clonidine did not change the maximum fall in blood pressure induced by centripetal stimulation of sciatic, splanchnic or vagal nerves, or by veratrine in dogs, cats and rabbits. The reduced absolute change must therefore also be due to the decrease in sympathetic tone produced by clonidine (unpubl. observations).

In summary, the effects of clonidine on cardiovascular reflexes, other than those of the carotid sinus, appear weaker than its effects on spontaneous sympathetic tone. This could in part furnish a reasonable explanation for the low incidence of orthostatic hypotensions in man.

K. Evidence for Activation of a Central α-Sympathomimetic Mechanism as the Cause of the Sympatho-Inhibitory Effect of Clonidine

It is tempting to link the central sympatho-inhibitory effect of clonidine with its peripheral α-sympathomimetic properties. It was suggested very early that the *inhibitory effect of clonidine on spontaneous sympathetic activity was also mediated by activation of medullary α adrenoceptors* (SCHMITT et al., 1968).

However, it has been difficult to find definite evidence for this view. The antagonism exerted by α adrenoceptor blocking agents seems to depend on the route of administration and on animal species. These agents could be classified in several groups as far as antagonism with clonidine is concerned.

i) *Two classic α adrenoceptor blocking agents, piperoxan and yohimbine,* were found to be strong antagonists of the sympatho-inhibitory effect of clonidine. The demonstration was based on evidence of several kinds. Not only they were found to prevent the sympatho-inhibitory effect of clonidine, but they reversed it when it is fully developed (SCHMITT et al., 1971d, 1973a; HAEUSLER and FINCH, 1972; HAEUSLER, 1973a, b).

a) Piperoxan (1 to 2 mg/kg) and yohimbine (0.5 to 1 mg/kg) slightly reduce spontaneous sympathetic activity and the dose of clonidine needed to reduce splanchnic discharges and blood pressure is higher (Fig. 19).

b) Intravenous injection of piperoxan and yohimbine once the sympatho-inhibitory effect of clonidine has been fully established leads to a rapid recovery in splanchnic discharges, heart rate, and blood pressure. Subsequently the dosage of clonidine required to reduce splanchnic discharges has to be increased. The process of recovery by piperoxan or yohimbine and depression of the sympathetic activity by clonidine could be repeated by increasing the dose (Fig. 20).

c) Intracisternal administration of clonidine at low doses (1 to 2 μg/kg) decreases blood pressure, heart rate, and sympathetic discharges. The administration of piperoxan or yohimbine at low doses, after the effects of clonidine have been fully established, leads to a rapid recovery in splanchnic discharges, heart rate, and blood pressure and the dose of clonidine has to be increased to elicit the same effects as before (Fig. 21). In dogs the decrease in blood pressure, heart rate, aortic blood flow and myocardial contractions induced by clonidine administered at low doses into the cisterna magna is antagonized by subsequent administration of piperoxan or yohimbine by the same route (cf. Fig. 8).

Pretreatment with intraventricular administration of piperoxan antagonized the hypotensive effect of intraventricular clonidine in conscious renal hypertensive cats (FINCH et al., 1974, 1975b) or in conscious hypertensive rats (FINCH, 1975a).

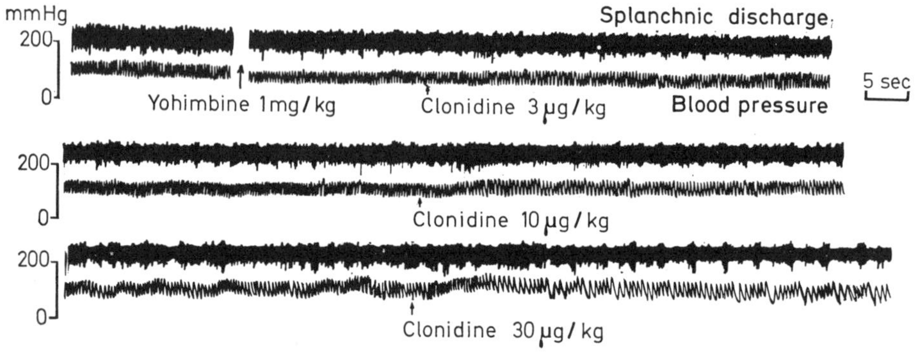

Fig. 19. Antagonism of the central sympatho-inhibitory effect of clonidine by yohimbine. Yohimbine (1 mg/kg) abolished the effect of clonidine (3 to 10 μg/kg) on splanchnic discharges. A higher dose (30 μg/kg) was necessary to induce a decrease in splanchnic discharges. [SCHMITT, H., SCHMITT, HÉLÈNE, FÉNARD, S.: Arzneimittel-Forsch. **23**, 41 (1973)]

d) Administration of clonidine into the vertebral artery of dogs induces a dose-dependent decrease in blood pressure and a dose-response curve could be drawn for the hypotensive effect. Low doses of piperoxan or yohimbine injected by the same route shift the dose-response curve of clonidine to the right which strongly suggests a competitive antagonism (Fig. 22).

ii) Besides piperoxan and yohimbine, *several other α adrenoceptor blocking agents* were investigated for their ability to antagonize the central sympatho-inhibitory effect of clonidine after intravenous administration. However, many of these agents themselves induce a strong inhibition of the sympathetic activity so precluding any increase in the dose to give a clear demonstration of antagonism to clonidine. Only a reduction in the effects of clonidine at low doses could be seen. Such an effect was found with tolazoline and phentolamine (SCHMITT and SCHMITT, 1970), with the benzodioxane derivatives, 883F, dibozane and ethomoxane and with azapetine, thymoxamine, chlorpromazine and amitriptyline (SCHMITT et al., 1973a). Phenoxybenzamine (SCHMITT and SCHMITT, 1970) and ergot alkaloids (SCHMITT and FÉNARD, 1970c) reduce sympathetic discharges only at high doses and do not antagonize the sympatho-inhibitory effect of clonidine. However, in man tolazoline was found to antagonize the effects of clonidine (BOCK et al., 1970).

Taking the decrease in blood pressure as an index of the central sympatho-inhibitory effect of clonidine, BOLME and FUXE (1971) found an antagonistic effect for phenoxybenzamine and haloperidol. Unfortunately, the decrease in blood pressure is not a reliable index of central antagonism between α adrenoceptor-blocking agents and clonidine, since blockade of peripheral α adrenoceptors precludes any further lowering of blood pressure by a centrally mediated reduction of the

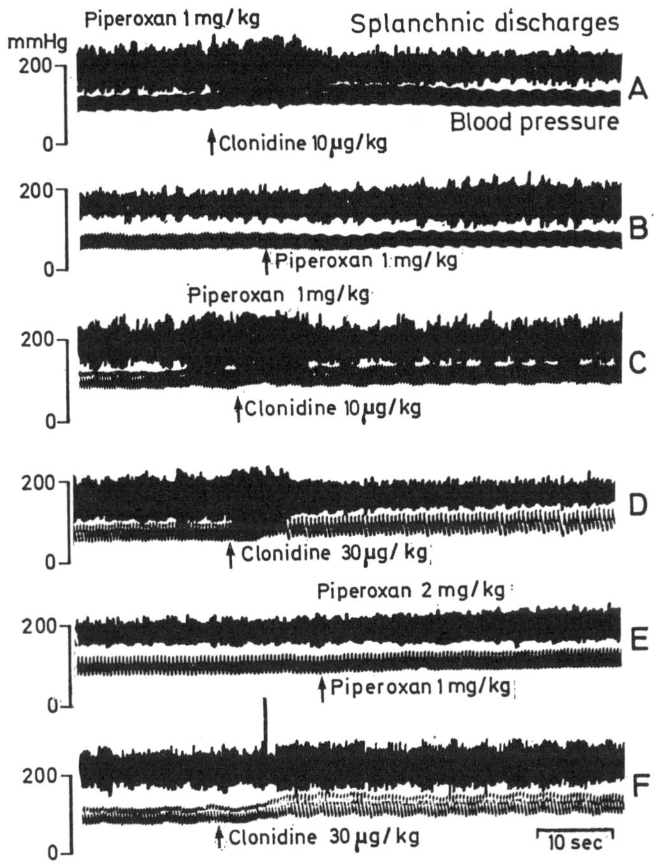

Fig. 20. Antagonism by piperoxan of the sympatho-inhibitory effect of clonidine in the cat. The cat was treated with 1 mg/kg of piperoxan. 3 µg/kg of clonidine was ineffective. At A, 10 µg/kg of clonidine induced the usual changes: hypertension followed by hypotension, bradycardia and decrease in splanchnic discharges. In B, piperoxan (1 mg/kg) induced a recovery in blood pressure, heart rate and sympathetic discharges. In C, 10 µg/kg of clonidine was ineffective, but 30 µg/kg (in D) reduced splanchnic discharges. Subsequent administration of piperoxan (1 mg/kg three times) produced a recovery (E) and after another dose of piperoxan (1 mg/kg), clonidine (30 µg/kg) no longer reduced splanchnic discharges but increased them (F). [SCHMITT, H., SCHMITT, HÉLÈNE, FÉNARD, S.: Arzneimittel-Forsch. **23**, 40—45 (1973)]

sympathetic tone. Perfusion of the third and the fourth ventricles of cats with phentolamine or phenoxybenzamine has been reported to decrease the hypotensive effect of xylazine, a congener of clonidine administered by the same route (HEISE et al., 1971). Phentolamine has been reported to prevent and to reverse the hypotensive effect of another congener of clonidine, BAY a 6781, when both drugs were administered into the lateral ventricle of the brain (JACOBS et al., 1972).

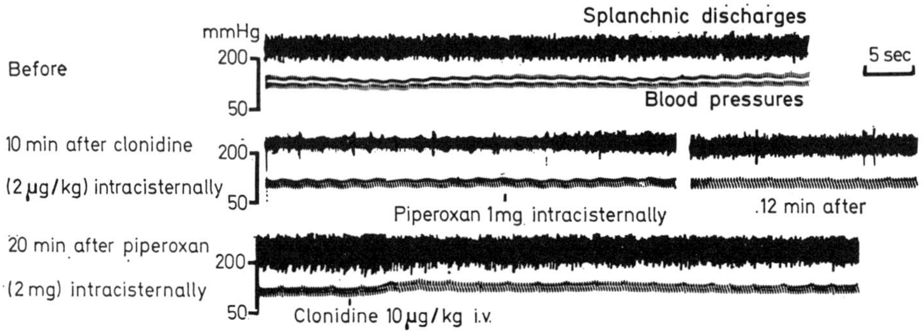

Fig. 21. Antagonism by intracisternal administration of the effects of clonidine. The figure shows: control, after injection of 1 µg/kg of clonidine into the cisterna magna, splanchnic discharges were reduced, blood pressure down; piperoxan (1 mg) injected into the cisterna magna induced a recovery. Clonidine (10 µg/kg) injected intravenously no longer reduced splanchnic discharges and blood pressure. [SCHMITT, H., SCHMITT, HÉLÈNE, FÉNARD, S.: Arzneimittel-Forsch. **23**, 41 (1973)]

Injection of α adrenoceptor blocking agents and clonidine into the cerebral cavities showed that antagonism could occur. Thus injection of phentolamine (FINCH, 1974; FINCH et al., 1975a, b; DAY and ROACH, 1974) into the lateral ventricle of normotensive, renal hypertensive cats or hypertensive rats abolished the effects of intraventricular clonidine. Injection of phentolamine, tolazoline, phenoxybenzamine, 883 F, dibozane, ethomoxane or azapetine into cisterna magna of rats induced a decrease in blood pressure and after recovery the effects of clonidine administered by the same route were reduced. Thymoxamine reduced blood pressure, but did not block the effect of clonidine. In rabbits, the intracisternal admini-

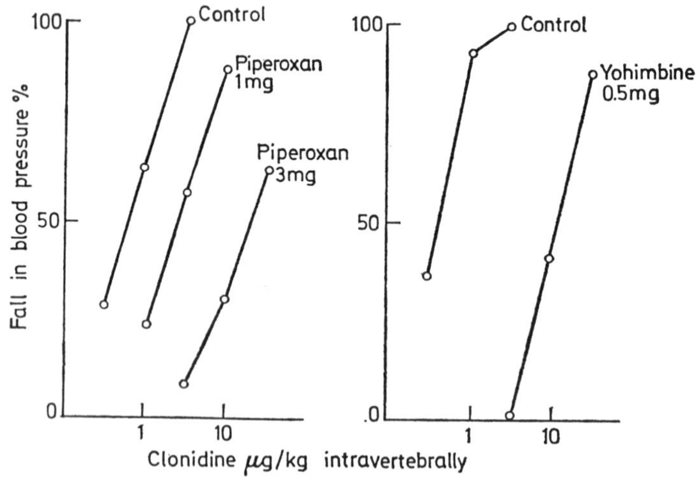

Fig. 22. Competitive antagonism of yohimbine and piperoxan on the decrease in blood pressure induced by intravertebral administration of clonidine in the dog. The figure shows the decrease in blood pressure induced by cumulative doses of clonidine into the vertebral artery of the dog. Piperoxan (left) and yohimbine (right) shift the dose-response curve to the right; this indicates a competitive antagonism. [SCHMITT, H., SCHMITT, HÉLÈNE, FÉNARD, S.: Arzneimittel-Forsch. **23**, 42 (1973)]

stration of clonidine reduced blood pressure, and phentolamine, tolazoline and phenoxybenzamine administered via the same route abolished the hypotensive effect of clonidine. In dogs, phentolamine and tolazoline injected into the cisterna magna did not change blood pressure but abolished the hypotensive effect of clonidine. Phenoxybenzamine and thymoxamine did not change the effects of clonidine. Dibenamine and dibozane were shown to antagonize the hypotensive effect of clonidine. Azapetine reduced blood pressure which precluded any further information on the effect of clonidine (BOGAÏEVSKY et al., 1974; unpublished results). These results suggest that clonidine activates central α adrenoceptors different from the peripheral ones, and varying according to the animal species.

Pimozide and spiroperidol, at doses which blocked central dopamine but not noradrenaline receptor sites, did not block the hypotensive effects of clonidine thus ruling out any involvement of central dopaminergic receptors (BOLME and FUXE, 1971). However pimozide was reported to prevent the hypotensive effect of clonidine to appear when both drugs were applied on the ventral surface of the medulla oblongata (BLOCH et al., 1974).

β adrenoceptors do not seem to be involved in the central sympatho-inhibitory effects of clonidine since the β adrenoceptor blocking agents, propranolol, pindolol and Kö 1366, do not alter the effects of clonidine on splanchnic discharges (SCHMITT et al., 1971b), and the blood pressure lowering effects of the drug (NAYLER et al., 1968; RAND and WILSON, 1968). WOODHOUSE et al., (1972) reported however, that centrally administered propranolol (0.1 to 0.5 µg/kg) reduced spontaneous efferent nerve activity and prevented both the neural and hypotensive effects of clonidine. It is strange that such a low dose of propranolol could be effective. A transient, but definite inhibitory effect of this drug on sympathetic nerve activity could be detected at doses of 1 to 2 mg/kg i.v. (SCHMITT et al., 1971b). But DAY and ROACH (1974) reported that responses to intracerebroventricular administration of clonidine in conscious cats were unaffected by prior intracerebroventricular administration of the β adrenoceptor blocking agents, (—) propranolol and (−) alprenolol, each given in a much higher dose than in the experiments of WOODHOUSE et al. (1972).

It has been proposed that clonidine did not act directly on central α adrenoceptors but indirectly by releasing noradrenaline or inhibiting its release. In fact, clonidine has been shown to reduce the overflow of ^3H noradrenaline caused by stimulation of cortical slices *in vitro*. This effect was more marked at low than at high frequency stimulation. Clonidine antagonized the increase in ^3H noradrenaline overflow induced by phentolamine or phenoxybenzamine. Therefore α adrenoceptors appear to be involved in this effect. On the other hand, clonidine reduced the ^3H 5-hydroxytryptamine overflow induced by electrical stimulation of cortical slices (STARKE and MONTEL, 1973a, b). REID and DOLLERY (1972) and DOLLERY and REID (1973) found that in rabbits pretreated by intracerebroventricular administration of 6-hydroxydopamine the level of noradrenaline in the brain was reduced to 22% of normal; intracisternal administration of clonidine did not reduce blood pressure and intravenous administration induced 50% less hypotension than in untreated animals. The authors concluded that a peripheral mechanism was partly responsible for the blood pressure lowering effect of the drug and that central adrenergic neurons were involved in the effects of clonidine. However in dogs, pretreatment with intracisternal administration of 6-hydroxydopamine or of reserpine did not reduce the inhibitory effect of clonidine on splanchnic discharges (SCHMITT et al., 1972c). Desipramine has been reported to reduce the central hypotensive effect of clonidine in rabbits (BRIANT and REID, 1972). Similarly administration of several antidepressant agents (imipramine, desmethylimipramine, nortriptyline) into the vertebral artery of cats antagonized the hypotensive effect of clonidine injected by the same route (Van Spanning and Van Zwieten, 1973; Van Zwieten, 1975b). Intracisternal administration of imipramine, desipramine, clomipramine and amitriptyline antagonized the hypotension induced by clonidine administered by the same route in rats. However desmethylimipramine was ineffective and amitriptyline was effective in rabbits (unpubl. observations). Dibenzepine, another antidepressant agent, did not reduce, but potentiated in DOCA hypertensive rats, the hypotensive effect of clonidine and of the related drug B.S. 100–141 (Scholtysik and Salzman, 1973). The interactions between antidepressant agents and clonidine deserve therefore further work. In fact the centrally mediated reduction in sympathetic nerve activity and the centrally mediated bradycardia induced by clonidine do not appear to be mediated by alterations of noradrenaline release. Pretreatment of cats with reserpine and α-methyl-p-tyrosine in order to deplete noradrenaline and to block the synthesis of the neurotransmitter did not markedly change the reduction in sympathetic nerve activity induced by clonidine (Haeusler, 1974a, c; Kobinger and Pichler, 1976). In rats similarly pretreated, clonidine potentiated the bradycardia induced by a rise in blood pressure as the drug did in normal rats (Kobinger and Pichler, 1974, 1975b).

Evidence has also been found for a facilitation of vagal bradycardia by an action of clonidine on α adrenoceptors: in dogs treated with a β adrenoceptor-blocking agent or with guanethidine vagal cardiodepressor reflex induced by angiotensin or noradrenaline administration i.v. was shown to be potentiated by small doses of clonidine injected into the cisterna magna and this effect was antagonized by phentolamine (Kobinger and Walland, 1971a, b, 1972a, c), chlorpromazine and haloperidol (Kobinger and Walland, 1972c), but not by phenoxybenzamine (Kobinger and Walland, 1972c). However neither of these drugs reversed the hypotensive and bradycardic effects of clonidine (Kobinger and Walland, 1972c). The same potentiation of the vagal cardio-depressor reflex elicited in conscious dogs by inflating a cuff placed around the descending aorta has been reported (Walland and Kobinger, 1973; Walland et al., 1974). Phentolamine decreased by itself the bradycardia induced by angiotensin in dogs treated with a β adrenoceptor blocking agent, but was ineffective in dogs pretreated with reserpine and a β adrenoceptor-blocking agent. It was concluded that a noradrenergic component could modulate the baroreceptor pathway leading to a vagal bradycardia (Kobinger and Walland, 1973).

L. Discrepancies Between the Decrease in Blood Pressure and the Reduction in Sympathetic Nerve Activity

The centrally mediated fall in blood pressure induced by clonidine has been ascribed to a reduced sympathetic tone which was reflected by the decrease in spontaneous nerve activity. This inhibition was shown to be dose-dependent after intravenous injection of clonidine (Klupp et al., 1970; Loew and Waite, 1974; Waite, 1975) or after injection of clonidine in to the third ventricle of the brain in cats (Waite, 1975). However some results did not fit well with this assumption.

Injection of clonidine into the vertebral artery of dogs usually induced a rapid and marked fall in blood pressure but the reduction in sympathetic nerve activity was less than expected. In fact a primary fall in blood pressure appeared and was not associated with a reduction in splanchnic and cardiac discharges. This phase was followed by an incomplete recovery, and finally a prolonged hypotension occured. Even during the last phase and in spite of a marked hypotension, sympathetic nerve activity was not abolished and sometimes not changed (SCHMITT, 1975; LAUBIE et al., 1976). After large destruction in the ventral surface of the medulla oblongata in dogs, intravenous injections of clonidine induced the usual secondary decrease in blood pressure, but did not change the discharges recorded in the splanchnic nerve, in the cardiac nerve or in the lumbar sympathetic chain (LAUBIE, 1975; LAUBIE et al., 1976a).

In some cats the discharges recorded in the splanchnic nerve were respiratory grouped. The inspiratory bursts were separated by periods of electrical silence. In these cats injection of clonidine into the cisterna magna induced a decrease in blood pressure without reducing splanchnic nerve activity (LAUBIE et al., 1976a).

In rabbits and rats, the discharges of the splanchnic nerve were usually respiratory grouped. The respiratory bursts were separated by periods of electrical silence or by periods of small electrical activity. However blood pressure does not have this periodicity. In both animal species clonidine induced the usual biphasic changes in blood pressure: an initial and brief increase in blood pressure followed by a prolonged hypotension. However the splanchnic electrical activity was not changed by the lower doses and decreased by 30 μg/kg of clonidine. Intracisternal administration of clonidine reduced blood pressure without changing splanchnic discharges (LAUBIE et al., 1976a; BOGAÏEVSKY, unpublished observations).

LOMBARDI et al. (1976) mentioned that in cats, intravenous infusion of low doses of clonidine reduced blood pressure but did not change the discharges in the white rami communicantes of the thoracic sympathetic chain. As these doses of clonidine reduced the effects of the stimulation of the sympathetic nerves, a peripheral action has been proposed for clonidine. Although this explanation was probably correct in the conditions of the authors, it does not account for the discrepancies found after central injection by other authors.

Clonidine might have reduced nerve activity in sympathetic nerves supplying other vascular beds, which activity was not recorded in the experiments. Clonidine (SCHMITT, 1970, 1975) and the related drug xylazine (SCHMITT et al., 1970) differentially reduced the activity in various sympathetic nerves. Another possibility is that clonidine might centrally stimulate an active vasodilator mechanism. Active vasodilatation was ruled out in the past for the control of blood pressure. However BECK (1961) reported experiments suggesting the involvement of vasodilator fibers present in the sympathetic nerves in dilatation.

M. Interferences Between Clonidine, Neuroleptic and Antidepressant Agents

Today it is difficult to predict from animal experiments the interferences of neuroleptics and antidepressant agents with clonidine. In fact, in animals, the interferences seem to depend on the route of administration of the drug and possibly on the access of the drug to the site(s) of action of clonidine.

VAN ZWIETEN (1975b) examined the influence of several neuroleptic agents on the hypotensive effects of clonidine when both drugs were injected into the vertebral artery of cats. He showed that neuroleptic agents decreased the hypotensive effect of clonidine. In contrast chlorpromazine administered intravenously reduced sympathetic nerve activity but did not alter to a great extent the inhibition of this activity elicited by clonidine (SCHMITT et al., 1973a) and similar results have been found with pimozide and haloperidol (LAUBIE, unpublished results). However intracisternal administration of chlorpromazine did not change blood pressure but antagonized the hypotensive effect of clonidine administered by the same route. Pimozide injected at small doses into the cisterna magna reduced and even reversed the hypotensive effect of intracisternal administration of clonidine, a result which is in agreement with those reported by BLOCH et al. (1974). But other neuroleptic agents-perphenazine, haloperidol, spiroperidol, thioridazine and clozapine-did not change the hypotensive effect of clonidine (TSOUCARIS KUPFER, BOGAÏEVSKY, BOGAÏEVSKY, HUCHET and SCHMITT, unpublished results). Similarly FINCH (1974) reported that intracerebroventricular administration of haloperidol did not change the hypotensive effect of intracerebroventricular injection of clonidine.

Desipramine has been reported to antagonize the antihypertensive effect of clonidine in man (BRIANT et al., 1973). Intracisternal administration of desipramine has been reported to abolish the secondary decrease in blood pressure induced by intravenous injection of clonidine (BRIANT and REID, 1972; DOLLERY and REID, 1973). SPANNING and VAN ZWIETEN (1974) and VAN ZWIETEN (1975b) reported that many antidepressant agents injected into the vertebral artery of cats reduced the hypotensive effect of clonidine injected by the same route. This antagonism has been taken as an evidence that the effects of clonidine were indirectly mediated by noradrenergic mechanisms (BRIANT and REID, 1972; DOLLERY and REID, 1973) or ascribed to the blockade of central α adrenoceptors by antidepressant agents (VAN ZWIETEN, 1975b). However HOEFKE and WARNKE-SACHS (1974) could not detect an antagonism in rabbits when desipramine and clonidine were injected intravenously. Intravenous administration of imipramine or amitryptiline reduced sympathetic nerve activity in cats and dogs, but did not significantly change the reduction of this activity induced by clonidine administered intravenously (SCHMITT et al., 1973a; LAUBIE, unpublished results).

Therefore the extrapolation of these conflicting results to man seems to be impossible.

V. Effects on the Parasympathetic System

A. Increase in Vagal Tone

The fact that cardiac slowing is induced by clonidine after inhibition of the sympathetic tone and its reduction by atropine or by cutting both vagus nerves suggest that it effects a centrally or reflexly mediated *increase in vagal tone*. Evidence for this is given below (p. 339). In addition WOODHOUSE et al. (1972), STRELLER (personal communication) found increased discharges in the cardiac efferent fibers of the vagus nerve after clonidine.

Another apparent *effect of clonidine on vagal activity is to antagonize the inhibition of vagal activity brought about by some procedures*. KATIĆ et al. (1972) demonstrated the antagonistic effect of clonidine injected into the vertebral artery on the tachycardia and hypertension induced by carotid occlusion and intravertebral infusion of angiotensin in morphine-chloralosed dogs with low heart rate. The effects of angiotensin and carotid occlusion were apparent after spinal transection but much reduced by cutting both vagus nerves, therefore inhibition of vagal activity was suggested. Phentolamine injected by the same route antagonized the effect of clonidine, an observation consistent with the results of KOBINGER and WALLAND (1971a, b; 1972a, b, c). However, tolazoline and phenoxybenzamine – as well as methamphetamine, imipramine and propranolol – were ineffective. More surprisingly, bethanidine, bretylium and guanethidine administered intravenously antagonized this central effect of clonidine, although these drugs are not thought to cross the blood-brain barrier. However, the tracings published by the authors showed an increase in blood pressure after these three postganglionic blocking agents, possibly due to their indirect sympathomimetic effect. As the value of carotid occlusion is strongly dependent on the basal blood pressure, no definite conclusion can be drawn from this test.

B. Effects on the Action of Acetylcholine and Vagal Stimulation

No parasympatholytic effect was detected, for clonidine did not change the effect induced by stimulation of the peripheral vagus nerve (SCRIABINE et al., 1968). A slight inhibition of the cardiovascular effects of acetylcholine by clonidine was found only in rats (BENTLEY and LI, 1968). Clonidine has been found to cause weak inhibition of acetylcholine-induced contractions of ileum and colon (HOEFKE and KOBINGER, 1966; BENTLEY and LI, 1968; COUPAR and KIRBY, 1972; WERNER et al., 1972). In contrast, the related compound xylazine has been reported to reduce the effect of peripheral vagal stimulation (KRONEBERG et al., 1967).

C. Effects on Parasympathetic Postganglionic Fibers

SCRIABINE and STAVORSKI (1970), DECK et al. (1971), and WERNER et al. (1972) reported that clonidine *reduced* the contraction of transmurally stimulated guinea-pig ileum, also *the release of acetylcholine* into the bath caused by this stimulation. The effect was antagonized by phentolamine and phenoxybenzamine and was therefore considered to be an α-sympathomimetic effect. The related compounds, BAY 1470 (OBERDORF and KRONEBERG, 1968, 1969, 1970) and BAY a 6781 (WERNER et al., 1972), as well as naphazoline (OBERDORF and KRONEBERG, 1970), showed similar properties. PATON and VIZI (1969) described a similar kind of presynaptic inhibition with noradrenaline but the effect did not seem sufficient to block the action of peripheral vagal stimulation (SCRIABINE et al., 1968).

It is tempting to speculate that the neurotransmitter could inhibit the release of the neurotransmitter of the opposite system, thereby enhancing its own effect. In fact acetylcholine has been shown to reduce the release of noradrenaline by a muscarinic effect (LINDMAR et al., 1968; LÖFFELHOLZ and MUSCHOLL, 1969).

D. Interactions with Cholinolytic and Cholinergic Agents

Certain pharmacological experiments *revealed some interactions with cholinergic mechanisms*. Administration of atropine during the hypotension induced by clonidine produced a prompt increase in heart rate and blood pressure (MAXWELL, 1969; ZAIMIS, 1970). However this effect was found only when the cardiac slowing induced by clonidine was very marked and the increase in heart rate elevated aortic blood flow and blood pressure; the total peripheral resistance did not change (SCHMITT and FÉNARD, 1970a). Administration of ganglion-blocking agents—such as hexamethonium or mecamylamine—or bilateral vagotomy during this hypotensive phase induced an increase in blood pressure and heart rate; the mechanism of this effect was quite different, for increased total peripheral resistance occured with only a slight effect on aortic blood flow (SCHMITT and FÉNARD, 1970a, b) (Fig. 24).

Other experiments indicate central interactions between atropine and clonidine. In half of the experiments atropine administered when the full effect of clonidine has been established led to prompt recovery not only in blood pressure and heart rate but also in splanchnic discharges (Fig. 23). Administration of atropine pro-

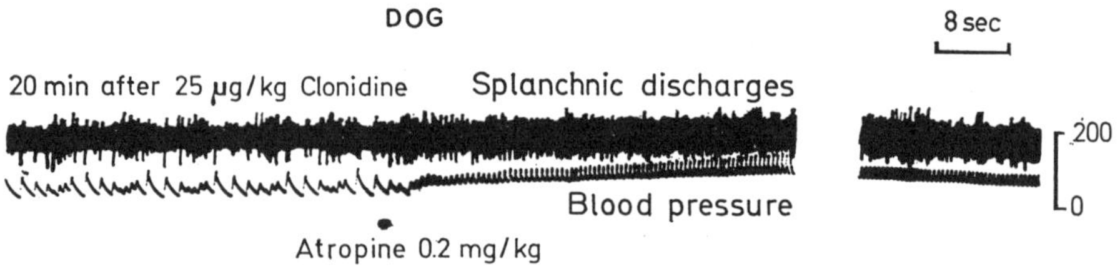

Fig. 23. Effect of atropine on blood pressure and splanchnic discharges after clonidine in the dog. Atropine (0.2 mg/kg) increased heart rate, blood pressure, and sympathetic discharges in a dog previously treated by clonidine (25 µg/kg). After administration of 25 µg/kg of clonidine, blood pressure, and heart rate were decreased; splanchnic discharges were reduced. The administration of 0.2 mg/kg of atropine increased heart rate, blood pressure, and splanchnic discharges. This type of action occured in about half of the experiments. [Schmitt, H. Fénard, S.: J. Pharmacol. (Paris) **1**, 365 (1970)]

tracted the hypotensive effect of clonidine and the inhibitory action on splanchnic discharges (Schmitt and Fénard, 1970a, b) and prolonged the hypertension (Kobinger and Walland, 1967b).

Scriabine and Stavorski (1970) reported that physostigmine reduced the hypotensive effect of clonidine in debuffered dogs. This result was interpreted as a consequence of the elevation of acetylcholine levels in the brain by inhibition of cholinesterases, and clonidine was thought to decrease acetylcholine release as it does at peripheral sites. The reduction in the sympathetic tone could be due to the reduced acetylcholine release. However, taking splanchnic discharges as an index of the central sympathetic tone, Schmitt et al. (1972a, b) were able to demonstrate an antagonistic effect of physostigmine on clonidine only when small doses of clonidine

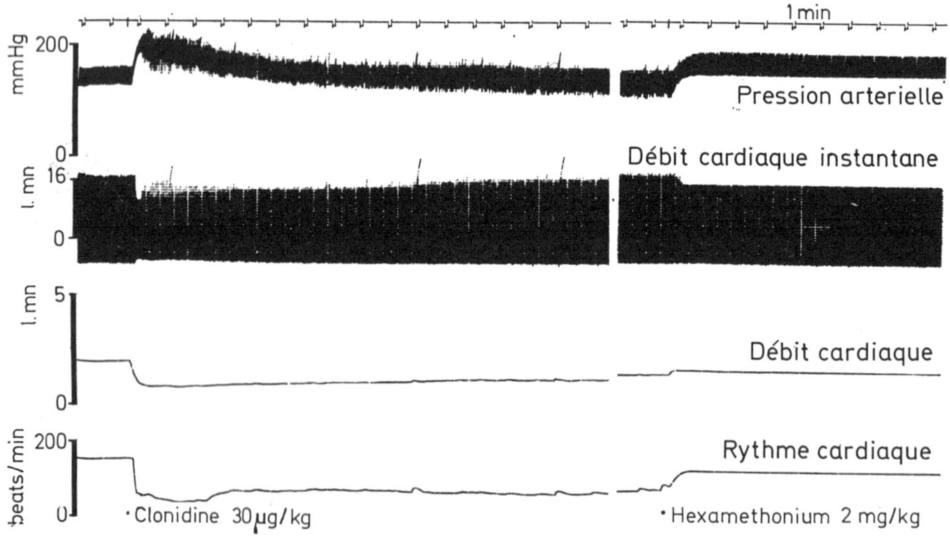

Fig. 24. Effect of clonidine on hemodynamics in the dog. Clonidine (30 µg/kg) induced an initial increase in blood pressure followed by a decrease. Heart rate and aortic blood flow were strongly reduced. Instaneous blood flow was decreased. Hexamethonium (2 mg/kg) reversed the effect of clonidine. [Schmitt, H., Fénard, S.: J. Pharmacol. (Paris) **1**, 304 (1970)]

were used. The ganglion-blocking drug mecamylamine did not change the effects of clonidine on sympathetic discharges.

More recently, LAUBIE (1975a, b) found a clear *antagonism between clonidine and cholinomimetic agents after central administration*: i) Vertebral artery administration of clonidine induced a dose-dependent decrease in heart rate and blood pressure. When the effect of clonidine was fully established, intracisternal administration of oxotremorine, of physostigmine, or of acetylcholine and physostigmine in small doses induced a prompt recovery in blood pressure, heart rate and sympathetic discharges. Subsequent administration of atropine in low doses into the vertebral artery induced bradycardia, hypotension and reduced sympathetic discharges, likely allowing the effects of clonidine to reappear.

ii) Previous administration of oxotremorine, physostigmine or acetylcholine and physostigmine into the cistana magna did not change blood pressure and heart rate in pentobarbitalized dogs. However these drugs shifted the hypotensive or bradycardic dose-responses curves to clonidine to the right. Atropine allowed the effect of clonidine to reappear.

However the antagonism exerted by cholinomimetic drugs did not appear to be specific. In fact a similar antagonism has been found with morphine-like drugs, such as dextromoramide and fentanyl, which have been shown to reduce blood pressure and heart rate by a central action (LAUBIE et al., 1974).

VI. Effects on Angiotensin and Plasma Renin Activity

The effects of angiotensin were reported to be changed in two ways by clonidine in rats: in pithed rats, clonidine increased the pressor response to low doses of angiotensin (BENTLEY and LI, 1968; BOISSIER et al., 1968), an effect seen with many sympathomimetic agents; in intact rats, clonidine reduced the hypertensive effect of low doses of angiotensin and this effect was assumed to be due to the absence of stimulation of the sympathetic centers by angiotensin (BOISSIER et al., 1968). In dogs, clonidine only slightly reduced the response to angiotensin (NAYLER et al., 1966; SCHMITT et al., 1968). In man, clonidine did not alter the pressor response to angiotensin (ONESTI et al., 1971). Clonidine has been reported to inhibit the tachycardia and hypertension which were assumed to be due to a centrally mediated decrease in the parasympathetic tone induced by intravertebral infusion of low doses of angiotensin in morphine-chloralosed dogs (KATIĆ et al., 1972).

Several investigators have reported that *clonidine suppresses renin secretion in dogs* (ONESTI et al., 1971; REID et al., 1973, 1974, 1975; GANONG et al., 1975). Intravenous administration of clonidine (ONESTI et al., 1971; REID et al., 1973, 1974, 1975) resulted in a consistent decrease in renal vein plasma renin activity. However there was no correlation with renal perfusion pressure in the experiments of ONESTI et al. (1971). The suppression of renin secretion appeared before any change in blood pressure and continued during the depressor effect of the drug. Decrease in renal perfusion pressure is a known stimulus for renin release. But in these experiments the clonidine induced fall in perfusion pressure was associated with a significant decrease in renin release. The most likely explanation of the renin suppression by clonidine is that it is due to sympathetic inhibition. However according to REID et al. (1975), intravenous clonidine reduced in dogs renin secretion only when renal perfusion pressure was prevented to change. That the sympathetic system is involved in the suppression of renin release by clonidine was substantiated by the failure of clonidine to change renin secretion after denervation of the kidney. This result would be expected if the suppression of renin secretion was mediated by way of renal nerves. However renin secretion was markedly reduced by renal denervation and non-neural mechanisms could also be involved. Vasopressin is known to reduce renin release; however clonidine induced in these dogs diuresis probably due to reduced vasopressin secretion. Clonidine reduced renin release in hypophysectomized dogs (REID et al., 1975). Although plasma potassium concentration was slightly elevated after clonidine, it was unlikely that this small change could be responsible for renin suppression (REID et al., 1975). In addition clonidine did not change the rate of renin release *in vitro* (NOLLY et al., 1974) suggesting that clonidine did not affect renin secretion directly.

The possibility of interference with a *central mechanism of renin regulation* was suggested by the ability of clonidine to decrease renin release after injection into the cerebral cavities. ONESTI et al. (1971) showed a decrease in blood pressure and in renin secretion after intracisternal injection of clonidine in low doses (1 μg/kg) in spite of the reduction in renal perfusion pressure. However REID et al. (1975) could demonstrate a reduction in renin secretion after injection of a low dose of clonidine into the third ventricle of dogs only when the renal perfusion pressure was maintained. The reason why in this investigation, but not in ONESTI et al's investigation, sympathetic inhibition did not override the effect of renal perfusion pressure is not known.

Several investigators reported *in man a decrease in plasma renin activity* (HÖKFELT et al., 1968, 1970a, b; 1975; BAER et al., 1971; ONESTI et al., 1971; BROD et al., 1972; SAFAR et al., 1973) accompanied by a reduced urinary aldosterone (HÖKFELT et al., 1968, 1970b; BAER et al., 1971) or no change in plasma aldosterone (SAFAR et al., 1973). The decrease in plasma renin activity was reported to occur after the reduction in catecholamine excretion, suggesting that the inhibition of sympathetic activity was responsible for the renin suppression (HÖKFELT et al., 1970b). Sympathetic inhibition was also in man capable of overcoming the stimuli for an increase in renin release exerted by a decrease in renal perfusion pressure, alteration in renal circulation and effects on the receptors of the juxtaglomerelar apparatus. That clonidine reduces the spontaneous stimulus for renin secretion without impairing the effect of some normal stimuli, is indicated by the elevated plasma renin induced by sodium restriction in clonidine treated patients (HÖKFELT et al., 1970a, 1975) or by upright position (HÖKFELT et al., 1975). However in contrast to untreated subjects who responded to hypoglycaemia by insulin with a marked increase in catecholamines and renin, clonidine treated patients did not show this response. The increased production of catecholamines during hypoglycemia is mediated via a mechanism located in the central nervous system and clonidine exerts an inhibitory effect on this mechanism (HÖKFELT et al., 1975).

However the results are not so clear in rats. Plasma renin activity has been shown to be increased (ROSENTHAL et al., 1970) or decreased (PETTINGER et al., 1976) in conscious rats, increased in urethanized rats (ALEXANDRE et al., 1973a; CHEVILLARD et al., 1976), but reduced in pentobarbitalized rats (KIRCHERTZ and PETERS, 1973). In pithed rats clonidine (3 to 30 μg/kg) as well as the classical α sympathomimetic agent naphazoline (15 to 45 μg/kg) increased plasma renin activity and phentolamine abolished this effect. Thus in this preparation-at least-activation of α adrenoceptors seems to induce renin release. The administration of clonidine into the cisterna magna induced a progressive decline in blood pressure but did not change plasma renin activity. Hypotension reduced renal perfusion pressure and this decrease is a known stimulus for renin release. In this study the clonidine induced fall in perfusion pressure was not associated with a rise in plasma renin activity. The most likely explanation for this discrepancy is that it is due to a central block of the stimulus. In intact rats activation of peripheral α adrenoceptors could overcome this inhibition (CHEVILLARD et al., 1976).

PETTINGER et al. (1976) investigated the effects of clonidine on plasma renin activity on spontaneous hypertensive rats and found that the drug reduced dose-dependently renin release. This reduction in plasma renin release was ascribed to an α sympathomimetic mechanism for it was abolished by α adrenoceptor blocking agents such as phentolamine, phenoxybenzamine and clozapine. However a peripheral mechanism appears to be involved as drugs known to inhibit the sympathetic tone such as guanethidine or chlorisondamine did not abolish the inhibitory effect of clonidine on renin release.

The observation that clonidine can lower plasma renin activity raises the possibility that this effect may also contribute to the antihypertensive efficacy of the drug; however, the possible therapeutic implications of the effect of clonidine on renin remain speculative.

VII. Effects on 5-Hydroxytryptamine and Histamine

Clonidine did not alter the cardiovascular effects of 5-hydroxytryptamine (SCHMITT et al., 1968). However COUPAR and KIRBY (1972) reported weak inhibition of the vasoconstrictor effect of 5-hydroxytryptamine on human saphenous veins. Clonidine has been shown to increase the vasoconstrictor effect of tryptamine and 5-hydroxytryptamine on the isolated ear artery of the rabbit (FOZARD, 1973).

Clonidine did not change the hypotensive effect of histamine in cats but increased the reflex tachycardia induced by the drug (LI and BENTLEY, 1969). Clonidine has been reported to be a nonequilibrium antagonist of histamine on strips of gastrointestinal tract (COUPAR and KIRBY, 1972).

Clonidine has been reported to *activate histamine H_2 receptors.* In the presence of theophylline, clonidine stimulated the production of cyclic AMP by minced gastric tissue of guinea pigs in a dose-dependent manner. On the other hand, clonidine increased the secretion of gastric acid. These effects were competitively antagonized by the histamine H_2 receptor blocking agent burimamide but not by the histamine H_1 receptor blocking agent diphenhydramine (KARPPANEN and WESTERMANN, 1973). Clonidine has been found to increase the rate and the myocardial force of guinea pigs and this effect was antagonized by the histamine H_2 receptor blocking agent, burimamide (CSONGRADY and KOBINGER, 1974).

Clonidine induced a concentration-dependent accumulation of cyclic AMP in the hippocampus of guinea-pigs. This effect was not antagonized by the α adrenoceptor blocking agent phentolamine, by the β adrenoceptor blocking agent timolol or the H_1 histamine antagonist mepyramine. However the H_2 histamine antagonist metiamide antagonized the effects of clonidine (AUDIGIER et al., 1976).

Intracerebroventricular injection of metiamide into the lateral ventricle of the brain in rats has been reported to reduce the secondary fall in blood pressure induced in urethanized rats by intravenous and intracerebroventricular administration of clonidine (KARPPANEN et al., 1976, 1977[1]) and it has been suggested that H_2 receptors are involved in the hypotensive effect of clonidine. Injection of metiamide into the cisterna magna of urethanized rabbits antagonized the hypotensive

[1] KARPPANEN, H., PAAKKARI, I., PAAKARI, P. Further evidence for central H_2-receptor involvement in the hypotensive effect of clonidine in the rat. Europ. Pharmacol. **42**, 299—302 (1977).

effect of intracisternal clonidine (HOEFKE, personal communication). In conscious renal hypertensive cats, intracerebroventricular injection of metiamide did not change the hypotensive effect of intracerebroventricular administration of clonidine (FINCH and HICKS, 1976). Similarly injection of metiamide in high doses into the cisterna magna of dogs did not change the maximum hypotensive effect of intracisternal injection of clonidine; on the other hand 4-methylhistamine, a stimulant of H_2 receptors injected into the cisterna magna of dogs did not induce hypotension (DELBARRE, HUCHET and SCHMITT, unpublished results).

Therefore the antagonistic effect of metiamide against the hypotensive effect of clonidine does not seem to be a general property and could not be explained at the present time.

VIII. Clonidine and Cyclic Adenosine 3',5'-Monophosphate Formation

α adrenoceptor as well as β adrenoceptor stimulating agents have been shown to activate cerebral adenylate cyclase and therefore to increase the levels of cyclic AMP in cerebral slices (CHASIN et al., 1971; PALMER et al., 1973; SATTIN et al., 1975; SKOLNIK and DALY, 1975). Were α adrenoceptors in the brain activated by clonidine, it would be expected that the drug induces also an increase in cyclic AMP in cortical slices. However clonidine has no significant effect on basal levels of cyclic AMP in incubated slices of rat cerebral cortex, but this drug and oxymetazoline antagonize noradrenaline elicited accumulation of cyclic AMP to a degree which corresponds to the α adrenergic component of the noradrenaline response. Clonidine completely antagonizes the formation of cyclic AMP elicited by the α adrenoceptor stimulating agent, methoxamine. Clonidine does not antagonize the accumulation of cyclic AMP elicited by maximum concentrations of the β adrenergic agonist, isoproterenol, and markedly potentiated the stimulatory effects of submaximum concentrations of this agonist. These results indicate that clonidine and oxymetazoline function as potent antagonists with respect to noradrenaline and methoxamine stimulated formation of cyclic AMP in brain tissue, presumably at an α adrenergic locus. In addition, clonidine and oxymetazoline appear to interact synergically with the β adrenergic component of cyclic AMP generating system (SKOLNICK and DALY, 1975). Pretreatment with 6-hydroxydopamine does not change the inhibitory effects of clonidine on noradrenaline-stimulated accumulation of cyclic AMP and the stimulatory effects of this agent on isoproterenol-elicited accumulation of cyclic AMP. These results are consistent with the hypothesis that both effects are exerted at postsynaptic α adrenoceptors (SKOLNICK and DALY, 1976a).

Clonidine has been shown to increase the levels of cyclic AMP in cerebral slices of guinea pig, presumably by an activation of H_2 histamine receptors (AUDIGIER et al., 1976).

Thus in these biochemical findings, it was not possible to obtain evidence that clonidine acts as an α adrenoceptor agonist, but unexpectandly the drug appears to act as an antagonist on some systems. Clonidine has been reported to decrease cyclic guanosine 3',5'-monophosphate content in the medial forebrain and cerebellum of mice *in vivo* (BARTMUS et al., 1976).

IX. Baroreceptor Mechanisms

Baroreceptor mechanisms appear to be involved in the hemodynamic effects of clonidine, but there are not perfectly understood.

Sensitization of baroreceptor pathways appears to be responsible for the *bradycardia transmitted by way of the vagus nerves*. Clonidine increased the reflexly mediated cardiac slowing induced by catecholamines and angiotensin (ROBSON and KAPLAN, 1968, 1969; ROBSON et al., 1969a, b) or by an increase in blood pressure in dog heart lung bypass preparation (NAYLER and STONE, 1970). This effect disappeared after stellate gangliectomy and bilateral vagotomy, but was still present, although reduced after administration of propranolol; atropine reduced or even abolished the potentiation of cardiac slowing induced by clonidine. Thus both sympathetic and parasympathetic systems appear to be involved in this effect (NAYLER and STONE, 1970). This effect may be – in part – the cause of the bradycardia seen during the hypertensive phase when the sympathetic tone has been eliminated (ROBSON and KAPLAN, 1968, 1969; ROBSON et al., 1969a, b).

The potentiating effect of clonidine may be due to *a direct effect on baroreceptors*, sensitizing those to their natural stimuli. Clonidine increased the rate of the discharges of the baroreceptor fibers in the aortic nerve of the rabbit (which did not contain chemoreceptor fibers) (AARS, 1972; KORNER et al., 1974, 1976; SLEIGHT et al., 1975). This effect was ascribed by AARS (1972) to a dilatation of the aorta. In dogs, intravenous administration of clonidine changed the pulse-synchronous pattern of discharges of the sino-carotid nerve into a continuous pattern during the hypertensive phase; during the hypotensive phase, the pulse synchronous discharges reappeared, but amplified and for a given level of blood pressure the discharges were greater. Therefore the gain at the level of baroreceptors appears to have been elevated by clonidine (LAUBIE et al., 1976b; LAUBIE and SCHMITT, 1977).

The *vagally mediated bradycardia* appears to be due *to a sensitization to baroreceptor impulses* – at least in dogs, cats and men. Intravenous administration of clonidine reduced heart rate and induced a hypertension in dogs with the spinal cord transected at C_2; this bradycardia did not occur in dogs with the spinal cord transected and in addition with both carotid sinus nerves and both aortic nerves cut (LAUBIE et al., 1976b; LAUBIE and SCHMITT, 1977). Clonidine was shown to increase vagal discharges in cats and this effect disappeared after deafferentiation (STRELLER, 1976, personal communication). Similarly in paraplegic men clonidine administered orally did not change blood pressure but reduced heart rate and this effect disappeared after local anaesthesia of both carotid sinuses (REID, personal communication).

In addition to an effect on baroreceptors, clonidine appears to *potentiate the vagally mediated bradycardia by an action on the central nervous system*. Administration of low doses of clonidine into the cisterna magna of dogs treated with a β-adrenoceptor blocking agent, or with guanethidine reduced heart rate and potentiated the bradycardia elicited by the rise in blood pressure induced by angiotensin (KOBINGER and WALLAND, 1971a, b, 1972a, b, c). In conscious dogs, intracisternal injection of low doses of clonidine was shown to potentiate the bradycardia elicited by a rise in aortic blood pressure induced by inflating a cuff placed on the descending thoracic aorta (WALLAND et al., 1974). Similarly, injection of clonidine into the vertebral artery of dogs treated with a β adrenoceptor blocking agent or with guanethidine, induced cardiac slowing (LAUBIE et al., 1976b; LAUBIE and SCHMITT, 1977). The potentiation of the bradycardia induced by the hypertensive effect of angiotensin was shown to be antagonized by injection of low doses of phentolamine or chlorpromazine into the cisterna magna; however phenoxybenzamine injected intravenously was a poor antagonist, but haloperidol antagonized this effect. It is interesting to note that neither of these drugs induced a recovery in the basal heart rate (KOBINGER and WALLAND, 1971c, 1972a). The α adrenoceptors involved in this potentiation of the cardiodepressor reflex have been localized by transection experiments into the medulla oblongata (KOBINGER and PILCHER, 1974).

In dogs treated with a β adrenoceptor blocking agent or guanethidine or in dogs with the spinal cord transected at C_2, and after deafferentiation performed according to the method described by EDIS and SHEPHERD (1971), clonidine decreased no longer heart rate, demonstrating that the central part of the vagally mediated bradycardia depends also on baroreceptor impulses (LAUBIE et al., 1976b; LAUBIE and SCHMITT, 1977).

Clonidine has been reported to have differentiated effects on sino-carotid and aortic baroreceptors (ANTONACCIO et al., 1975). In unilaterally sinusectomized dogs, with the other carotid sinus perfused, an increase in perfusion pressure of the sinus reduced blood pressure and heart rate. However, intravenous administration of noradrenaline did not change the pressure into the sinus, but reflexly reduced heart rate. Clonidine abolished the heart slowing induced by rising the pressure into the carotid sinus, but did not change the bradycardia induced by intravenous administration of noradrenaline. In bilaterally sinusectomized dogs clonidine increased the bradycardic response to intravenous injection of noradrenaline, and this effect was abolished by aortic stripping. Clonidine seems therefore to reduce the reflex response to an hypertension into the carotid sinus, but to potentiate the response to an increase in pressure into the aortic arch. In addition, clonidine was claimed to reduce the depressor and bradycardic response to the stimulation of the carotid sinus nerve (ANTONACCIO et al., 1975).

However in other studies (LAUBIE et al., 1976b; LAUBIE and SCHMITT, 1977) clonidine injected into the vertebral artery was found to potentiate the bradycardia elicited by stimulation of the carotid sinus nerve in dogs treated with a β adrenoceptor blocking agent. This effect was seen—especially—at high frequencies of stimulation. As clonidine did not change the bradycardia induced by stimulation of the nucleus tractus solitarii or of the nucleus ambiguus, the *site of action of the drug was suggested to be at the level of the nucleus tractus solitarii.* In dogs, bilateral destruction of the nucleus tractus solitarii induced a fulminating rise in blood pressure and heart rate. In these dogs, β adrenoceptor blockade reduced blood pressure and heart rate, did not change the hypotensive effect of clonidine injected into the vertebral artery, but prevented the bradycardic effect of the drug (LAUBIE and SCHMITT, 1977). The nucleus tractus solitarii has been shown to be the site of the first synapsis of the fibers coming from baroreceptor areas (MIURA and REIS, 1969). Therefore clonidine, and consequently a noradrenergic mechanism appear either to reduce the release of the unknown neurotransmitter from the first afferent fibers, or to facilitate its effects on the postsynaptic membrane of the second order neurons.

However in cats pretreated with propranolol, the destruction of both nuclei tractus solitarii reduced the bradycardia induced by noradrenaline and its potentiation by clonidine, but did not change the bradycardic and hypotensive effects of clonidine. Bilateral destruction of the nucleus ambiguus did not alter the hypotensive or bradycardic effects of clonidine or the normal reflex bradycardia to noradrenaline but completely prevented the enhancement of reflex bradycardia to noradrenaline caused by clonidine. These results therefore suggest that in cats the hypotensive and vagal components of the bradycardia caused by clonidine are not reliant upon activation of nucleus tractus solitarii or of nucleus ambiguus cell bodies. Furthermore normal reflex bradycardia requires an intact nucleus tractus solitarii but not nucleus ambiguus whereas reflex enhancement by clonidine requires both an intact nucleus tractus solitarii and nucleus ambiguus (ANTONACCIO and HALLEY, 1976). Therefore, some differences in the site of action seem to exist between dogs and cats. However, in cats clonidine seems to act on the nucleus tractus solitarii; in fact, the drug increases the potential evoked in this structure by stimulation of the carotid sinus nerve (LIPSKI and SOLNICKA, 1976b).

Moreover, BENTLEY and LI (1968) reported a quicker and shorter hypotensive effect of clonidine in deafferentiated cats, a result consistent with increased baroreceptor discharges due to clonidine. A greater decrease in blood pressure and a smaller bradycardic effect were seen in dogs (SCHMITT et al., 1968), in cats (HUKUHARA et al., 1968; MAGUS and LONG, 1968) and in rabbits (SHAW et al., 1971a) with carotid sinus and aortic nerves cut. This effect was ascribed to a greater sympathetic discharge and higher blood pressure than in normal animals. However, the potentiation of the hypotensive effect occured in animals with only carotid sinus nerves cut and with normal blood pressure (MAGUS and LONG, 1968; LAUBIE and SCHMITT, 1974). It therefore appears that sinusal mechanisms counteract the effect of clonidine on blood pressure, which is the opposite of its effect on heart rate.

The fall in cardiac output induced by clonidine was reduced in deafferentiated rabbits (SHAW et al., 1971a) and in dogs with both carotid sinus nerves cut (LAUBIE and SCHMITT, 1974). As the decrease in heart rate was also less marked, this reduced cardiac slowing could be the cause of the less reduced cardiac output.

As the hemodynamic effect was similar in deafferentiated and pontine rabbits, SHAW et al (1971b) suggested that baroreceptor mechanisms counteract the blood pressure decrease at suprabulbar level.

X. Hemodynamic Effects

As mentioned previously, rapid intravenous injection of clonidine induced biphasic changes in blood pressure: initial and transient hypertension was followed by a long-lasting fall in blood pressure; heart rate was slowed and values as low as 40 beats per minute were recorded in anesthetized dogs and in man. It is to be noted that the initial hypertensive effect has been encountered in man after rapid intravenous injection (BOCK et al., 1968, 1970; VORBURGER et al., 1967a, b, 1968; KROETZ et al., 1970; FINNERTY, 1970; MCRAVEN et al., 1971; ONESTI et al., 1971). An analysis of the hemodynamic effects of clonidine has been carried out; this is the subject of this chapter.

A. Bradycardia

The cardiac slowing induced by clonidine in animals and man is a well-known effect but the mechanism of this action has not been entirely elucidated.

Clonidine *has no direct bradycardic effect on the heart.* In fact the drug has no significant effect on the beat frequency of isolated atria (NAYLER et al., 1969), isolated spontaneously beating Langendorff perfused heart (CONSTANTINE and MCSHANE, 1968; KAPLAN et al., 1969; NAYLER et al., 1969; SCRIABINE et al., 1970; STARKE et al., 1972), heart-lung preparations of dogs (HOEFKE and KOBINGER, 1966), or recently transplanted cardiac homografts (NAYLER et al., 1969). Similarly, clonidine has been reported to leave heart rate unchanged in spinal cats (KOBINGER and WALLAND, 1967b; RAND and WILSON, 1968) although bradycardia occurs in spinal dogs (NAYLER et al., 1968). The effect of clonidine on the heart rate of intact animals cannot therefore be accounted for simply in terms of a direct negative chronotropic effect.

The cardiac slowing induced by clonidine appears to be caused *by decreased sympathetic tone and increased vagal activity.* This conclusion is supported by the following facts: the bradycardic effects of clonidine on heart rate in dogs and rabbits is greatly reduced or abolished by stellate gangliectomy and bilateral vagosympathectomy (MAGUS and LONG, 1968; NAYLER et al., 1969), by the simultaneous blockade of parasympathetic and sympathetic systems by ganglion-blocking agents (NAYLER et al., 1966; SCRIABINE et al., 1968), or by simultaneous administration of atropine and β adrenoceptor-blocking agents (SHAW et al., 1971a; LAUBIE and SCHMITT, 1974). Similarly in reserpinized dogs, cutting of both vagus nerves prevented the cardiac slowing effect of clonidine (LAUBIE and SCHMITT, 1974). In bivagotomized cats cutting of cardiac nerves prevented heart slowing (KOBINGER, 1967). In intact dogs, in which clonidine-induced bradycardia has been established, cutting the vago-sympathetic and excising the stellate ganglia resulted in the heart rate returning almost to control levels (NAYLER et al., 1969).

There are some discrepancies regarding the respective roles of the increased vagal activity and the reduced sympathetic activity in the mechanism of the bradycardic effect of clonidine.

The effect of clonidine on heart rate in intact animals is decreased but not abolished by bilateral vagotomy or by prior administration of either atropine or propantheline (HOEFKE and KOBINGER, 1966; KOBINGER and WALLAND, 1967a, b; SCHMITT et al., 1967, 1968; NAYLER et al., 1968; NAYLER and STONE, 1970; SCRIABINE et al., 1968; SCHMITT and FÉNARD, 1970a,b; LAUBIE and SCHMITT, 1974). Its effect on heart rate cannot, therefore, be explained only in terms of increased vagal control. The effect of clonidine in producing prolonged bradycardia was prevented by pretreatment with propranolol or pronethalol (NAYLER et al., 1966; SCRIABINE et al., 1968; NAYLER and STONE, 1970; RAND and WILSON, 1968; ROBSON and KAPLAN, 1969), reserpine (KOBINGER and WALLAND, 1967b), or guanethidine (SCRIABINE et al., 1968; KAPLAN et al., 1969; ROBSON and KAPLAN, 1969). These drugs have in common the action of impairing the sympathetic innervation of the heart by blockade of the β adrenoceptors, by depletion of noradrenaline stores, or by prevention of noradrenaline release, respectively. Since the prolonged bradycardic effect of clonidine depends on the integrity of the cardiac sympathetic innervation, it follows that the effect is due to a reduction of sympathetic effects on the heart. However, after these drugs, clonidine produced a transient bradycardia, which accompanied the pressor response and was abolished by bivagotomy; it may be ascribed to increased vagal activity and is quite distinct from the more pronounced and long-lasting bradycardia produced by clonidine when the sympathetic innervation of the heart is not impaired by drugs. According to SCRIABINE et al. (1970), this increased vagal activity appeared at rather high dose levels.

However, some facts could not be accounted for by the hypothesis that vagal tone was increased only during the initial phase of clonidine action and decreased sympathetic tone was the sole cause of the delayed effect. Bretylium did not abolish the delayed cardiac slowing induced by clonidine in dogs (NAYLER et al., 1968). A similar observation was reported in dogs treated with a β adrenoceptor blocking agent (LAUBIE and SCHMITT, 1974). In dogs pretreated with reserpine clonidine, even at low dosage, induced a marked and prolonged bradycardia that was abolished by cutting both vagus nerves (LAUBIE and SCHMITT, 1974). In bivagotomized dogs both phases of cardiac slowing were significantly less marked than in control dogs (LAUBIE and SCHMITT, 1974). Thus the increased vagal tone appears, at least in dogs and for some doses (15 µg/kg or more), to be present in both phases of action of clonidine and to account for the bradycardia seen after exclusion of the sympathetic tone.

Some results suggest that clonidine can reduce heart rate by a *peripheral action*. Clonidine has been reported to slow heart rate when injected into the sinus node artery at doses that are ineffective by systemic administraton, *i.e.* as low as

0.1 µg (SCRIABINE et al., 1970), but KAPLAN et al. (1969) could not find this effect. Clonidine slowed the heart rate in bilaterally vagotomized dogs with the spinal cord sectioned at C2 at a time when the sympathetic tone was high and blood pressure was falling (SCRIABINE et al., 1970). Clonidine reduced cardiac acceleration caused by low-frequency stimulation of cardiac postganglionic sympathetic fibers or of stellate ganglion (KOBINGER, 1967; SCRIABINE et al., 1968, 1970). Sympathetic fibers have been assumed to discharge at these low frequencies (ÜVNAS, 1960) although more recent experiments on single cardiac sympathetic fibers indicate a somewhat higher frequency of discharges (GREEN and HEFFRON, 1968). In addition, clonidine antagonized the increase in heart rate caused by the muscarinic ganglionic stimulant Nc NA 343 (SCRIABINE et al., 1968, 1970; ANTONACCIO, 1972; ANTONACCIO and ROBSON, 1973) and theophylline (SCRIABINE et al., 1968). Therefore an involvement of peripheral sympathetic blocking action in the mechanism of clonidine induced cardiac slowing is suggested. Recent experiments seem to show that clonidine may reduce heart rate by stimulating presynaptic α adrenoceptors. Clonidine reduced the tachycardia induced by stimulation of the thoracic sympathetic chain in pithed rats and this effect was antagonized by α adrenoceptor blockade (DREW, 1976) (p. 309).

Many experiments suggest that clonidine influences *central structures* to reduce heart rate. Clonidine induced bradycardia after administration into the cisterna magna at low dosage (KOBINGER, 1967; KOBINGER and WALLAND, 1967c; SCHMITT et al., 1968; SCHMITT and SCHMITT, 1969a; SCHMITT et al., 1971c, d, 1973a; ONESTI et al., 1971), into the lateral ventricle of the brain (SHERMAN et al., 1968; SCHMITT and SCHMITT, 1969a; SCHMITT and FÉNARD, 1970a, b, c, 1971), into the vertebral artery (SATTLER and VAN ZWIETEN, 1971; CONSTANTINE and MCSHANE, 1968; SCHMITT et al., 1973a), or into the cephalic circulation in cross circulation experiments (SHERMAN et al., 1968). As with blood pressure, these experiments do not necessarily prove that central structures are the primary sites of action of clonidine, yet the reduction in discharges of the cardiac nerve (SCHMITT et al., 1967, 1968; SCHMITT and SCHMITT, 1969a; WOODHOUSE et al., 1972) provides strong support for the view that it acts on centers regulating heart rate and is at least a contributory factor in the bradycardic effect of clonidine.

A sensitization of the bradycardic effect of sino-carotid reflexes has been suggested by ROBSON and KAPLAN (1969a, b; ROBSON et al. 1969) and NAYLER and STONE (1970) to play a role, at least in high doses. Clonidine increased the reflexly mediated cardiac slowing induced by catecholamines and angiotensin (ROBSON and KAPLAN, 1969a, b; ROBSON et al., 1969; KOBINGER and WALLAND, 1972a, b, c, 1973) or by increasing blood pressure in heart-lung bypass preparations of the dog (NAYLER and STONE, 1970). This effect disappeared after stellate gangliectomy and bilateral vagotomy, but could be seen in a reduced form after administration of propranolol; atropine reduced or abolished the cardiac slowing sensitization induced by clonidine. Thus both sympathetic and parasympathetic systems appear to be involved in this effect (NAYLER and STONE, 1970), which could be the cause of the cardiac slowing seen during the hypertensive phase when the sympathetic tone has been eliminated (ROBSON and KAPLAN, 1969a, b). However, it is not apparent how clonidine could further reduce the sympathetic tone when this tone has been already abolished by the drug. The potentiating effect of clonidine could be due to a central action for intracisternal administration of the drug, increased cardiac slowing being induced by angiotensin and noradrenaline; this effect is abolished by intracisternal administration of phentolamine, suggesting a central noradrenergic mechanism responsible for this effect (KOBINGER and WALLAND, 1971b, 1972b, c,, 1973).

In dogs with both vagus nerves intact but with both carotid sinuses denervated, the cardiac slowing induced by clonidine was significantly less than in intact dogs, which indicates sensitization of the impulses coming from the carotid sinus to their natural stimuli. As the bradycardia was of the same magnitude as in bivagotomized dogs, it was concluded that sensitization of the carotid sinus walls could account for the increased vagal tone (LAUBIE and SCHMITT, 1974). Similar observations were made in cats by MAGUS and LONG (1968) and in rabbits by SHAW et al. (1971b).

However, the sensitization of sino-carotid reflexes cannot by itself explain the bradycardia seen after sino-carotid denervation (SCRIABINE et al., 1968, 1970; ROBSON et al., 1969a, b) or combined with bivagotomy (SCRIABINE et al., 1968, 1970; SCHMITT et al., 1967, 1968). Other mechanisms of action must therefore be involved.

Recently it has been demonstrated that the vagal part of the bradycardia induced by clonidine results in dogs from a peripheral and central sensitization to baroreceptor impulses. The central part is exerted at the level of nucleus tractus solitarii (LAUBIE et al., 1976b; LAUBIE and SCHMITT, 1977) (p. 338).

It could be concluded from these experiments that reduction in sympathetic discharges and increased vagal activity both normally contribute to the bradycardia produced by clonidine. Peripheral, central and reflex sites of action could all be effective in initiating the effect.

B. Cardiac Output

A *reduction in cardiac output* after clonidine has been reported in dogs (HOEFKE and KOBINGER, 1966; KOBINGER and WALLAND, 1967b; NAYLER et al., 1966, 1968; LAUBIE and SCHMITT, 1969; MAXWELL, 1969; SCHMITT and FÉNARD, 1970a, b AUTRET et al., 1971; LAUBIE and SCHMITT, 1974); monkeys (CONSTANTINE and MCSHANE, 1968; BOLME et al., 1975), rabbits (NAYLER et al., 1968; SHAW et al., 1971a, b) and rats (BRALET et al., 1974). The decrease in cardiac output was more marked during the hypertensive phase than in hypotension (KOBINGER and WALLAND, 1967b; AUTRET et al., 1971). However, occasionally in dogs blood pressure fell without any change in cardiac output (LAUBIE and SCHMITT, 1974).

In hypertensive patients a decrease in cardiac output was usually reported (GRABNER et al., 1966; MICHEL et al., 1966; SCHNEIDER and GATTENLÖHNER, 1966; BARNETT and CANTOR, 1968; GRABNER and MICHALEK, 1968; SCHNEIDER, 1968; STENBERG et al., 1968; VORBURGER et al., 1967a, b, 1968; ZIMMERMANN et al., 1968; KROETZ et al., 1970; BREST, 1970; MUIR, 1970; REUBI et al., 1970; KOCH, 1971; MCRAVEN et al., 1971; ONESTI et al., 1971). However, in some clinical trials no significant change in cardiac output was found (KOCHSIECK and FRITSCHE, 1966) or even an increase (DAVIDOV et al., 1967; FINNERTY, 1970). In long term treatment, cardiac output was reported to recover its initial value (REUBI et al., 1970; SAFAR et al., 1973).

The causes of the reduction in cardiac output appear to be multiple and as yet imperfectly understood. Loss of sympathetic tone, increased vagal activity, α-sympathomimetic effects, and hemodynamic changes could all play a role. *The reduction of central sympathetic tone* appears to be one of the main factors. a) Clonidine decreased cardiac output when administered at low doses into the cisterna magna or the vertebral artery of dogs in order to limit the effect to central structures; however, the initial effect was smaller than after intravenous administration (KOBINGER and WALLAND, 1967c; SCHMITT and FÉNARD, 1971; SCHMITT et al., 1971d, 1973a; ONESTI et al., 1971). Clonidine reduced cardiac output when injected into the cerebral ventricles of monkeys (BOLME et al., 1975). b) The fall in cardiac output was reduced through not abolished, at least in the delayed phase, by some processes which excluded the sympathetic system, *i.e.* ganglion blockade (NAYLER et al., 1968) or β adrenoceptor blockade (KOBINGER and WALLAND, 1967 b), or pretreatment with reserpine (LAUBIE and SCHMITT, 1974).

Some experiments suggest that *increased vagal tone* could account, at least partly, for the decrease in cardiac output seen after exclusion of the sympathetic system. (a) In fact, parasympathetic blockade with atropine has been reported to reduce the decrease in cardiac output induced by clonidine, at least initially (KOBINGER and WALLAND, 1967 b). In bilaterally vagotomized dogs the decrease in cardiac output was significantly smaller than in intact animals (LAUBIE and SCHMITT, 1974). (b) Pretreatment of dogs with reserpine caused clonidine to induce marked bradycardia, fall in cardiac output, and greater increases in blood pressure and total peripheral resistance than in intact dogs (KOBINGER and WALLAND, 1967 b). LAUBIE and SCHMITT (1974) reported similar experiments, but the decrease in heart rate and cardiac output found in their investigations were so great that they prevented blood pressure from rising. In contrast, in reserpinized and bilaterally vagotomized dogs, clonidine did not change heart rate and cardiac output in spite of potentiation of the hypertensive effect (LAUBIE and SCHMITT, 1974). These experiments clearly indicate that the increased vagal tone may be the cause of the fall in cardiac output induced by clonidine, at least in certain circumstances, especially when increased vagal activity slows the heart to such low frequencies that cardiac output is strongly dependent on heart rate.

Nevertheless it is doubtful whether this bradycardia plays any role in the reduction of cardiac output in normal animals, for pacing of the heart did not significantly increase cardiac output in animals treated with clonidine (LAUBIE and SCHMITT, 1974).

The carotid sinus may be involved in the reduction of cardiac output. In fact in dogs with carotid sinus denervation, clonidine induced a greater hypotensive effect, but smaller decreases in heart rate and cardiac output than in normal dogs (LAUBIE and SCHMITT, 1974). According to SHAW et al. (1971 b), in normal animals a supramedullary baroreceptor mechanism counteracts the decrease in blood pressure and cardiac output.

The *loss in sympathetic tone and increased vagal tone* – in some circumstances – seems to be the predominant factors in reducing cardiac output. After a simultaneous β adrenoceptor blockade with the β adrenoceptor-blocking agent S. 2395 and parasympathetic blockade with atropine, or reserpinization and bilateral vagotomy clonidine did not significantly change cardiac output in dogs (LAUBIE and SCHMITT, 1974). In bypass preparations of dogs, NAYLER et al. (1968) and FEHN et al. (1972) reported a decreased venous return after clonidine and ascribed this effect to loss of the sympathetic tone towards the great veins increasing the volume of the capacitance vessels.

As α-sympathomimetic agents have been shown to *reduce venous return* (LEWIS and WEIL, 1969), the activation of α adrenoceptors by clonidine could be involved in reducing cardiac output. This effect could account for the early fall in cardiac output, occuring before any change in blood pressure, an effect also seen with other α-sympathomimetic agents (AUTRET et al., 1971). Thus loss of sympathetic tone acting on β receptors of the veins, which have been shown to increase venous return (LEWIS and WEIL, 1969) and activation of α adrenoceptors could both contribute to the cardiac output-reducing effect of clonidine. These effects could explain the lack of effects of clonidine after phentolamine (KOBINGER and WALLAND, 1967b), although a central antagonistic effect of phentolamine could not be excluded. The delayed reduction of cardiac output seen after injection of clonidine into the vertebral artery of dogs could also be accounted for by the absence of activation of peripheral α adrenoceptors (SCHMITT et al., 1973a).

It was possible to eliminate a direct depressive effect on the heart as the cause of the reduced cardiac output because in heart-lung preparations of the dog clonidine did not change cardiac output, even in high concentrations (HOEFKE and KOBINGER, 1966).

In summary, clonidine appears to decrease cardiac output predominantly by a reduction in the sympathetic tone; in some circumstances the strong bradycardia may contribute to the effect. The increased aortic blood pressure could also initially reduce the cardiac output, and there could be a reduction in venous return by activation of α adrenoceptors or loss of stimulation of β adrenoceptors.

C. Stroke Volume

In spite of the reduced cardiac output, *stroke volume* appears to remain *unchanged* or is even *slightly increased* in animals because the bradycardia compensates for the decrease in cardiac output (KOBINGER and WALLAND, 1967b; AUTRET et al., 1971; LAUBIE and SCHMITT, 1974). It was only during the hypertensive phase that a reduction was seen, probably due to the impairment of systolic ejection (AUTRET et al., 1971).

In man, conflicting results have been reported: no change (GRABNER et al., 1966; GRABNER and MICHALEK, 1968; STENBERG et al., 1968), a decrease (SCHNEIDER and GATTENLÖHNER, 1966; MICHEL et al., 1966; MICHEL, 1968; ZIMMERMANN et al., 1968; VORBURGER et al., 1968; KOCH, 1971; MCRAVEN et al., 1971; ONESTI et al., 1971), and even an increase (SCHNEIDER and GATTENLÖHNER, 1966; SCHNEIDER, 1968).

D. Ventricular Volumes

In dogs neither the end-systolic ventricular volume or the end-diastolic ventricular volume were changed by clonidine (LAUBIE and SCHMITT, 1974). Perhaps the increased diastolic filling time compensates for the reduced venous return. However, as the left ventricular end-diastolic pressure was found to be increased (LAUBIE and SCHMITT, 1974), it is difficult to account for this discrepancy.

E. Atrial and Left Ventricular End-Diastolic Pressures

In dogs *left atrial pressure has been found to be elevated by clonidine* (NAYLER et al., 1968). Similarly, *left ventricular end-diastolic pressure was increased* in dogs after clonidine and this effect was more marked during the hypertensive phase (LAUBIE and SCHMITT, 1974).

During the pressor phase the increased aortic pressure probably opposes the ejection of the blood, so increasing left ventricular end-diastolic pressure. This conclusion is supported by the fact that this pressure is elevated in all circumstances. The increased left ventricular end-diastolic pressure found in the hypotensive phase is more difficult to account for. The reduced sympathetic tone alone could not account for this elevation, for it was seen in reserpinized dogs (LAUBIE and SCHMITT, 1974). Conversely the increased vagal tone could be involved, but is not the sole factor, for the elevation of left ventricular end-diastolic pressure was also seen in bilaterally vagotomized dogs but, surprisingly, it was not found in dogs with both carotid sinus nerves cut. In the latter case the fall in blood pressure was more marked than after bivagotomy and it could be that hypotension facilitates ejection. It is clear that the cardiac slowing is involved in this effect because a decrease in left ventricular end-diastolic pressure is induced by pacing of the heart after full establishment of the clonidine effect. On the other hand, after procedures abolishing the bradycardia induced by clonidine: reserpinization combined with cutting both vagus nerves, simultaneous sympathetic and parasympathetic blockade with the β adrenoceptor blocking agent S 2395, and atropine, there was no delayed rise in left ventricular end-diastolic pressure (LAUBIE and SCHMITT, 1974).

In conclusion, cardiac slowing seems to be the main cause of this increase and a fall in blood pressure could antagonize the effect. It is possible that the reduced venous return found by NAYLER et al. (1966, 1968) could also oppose the effect of bradycardia.

In man right atrial pressure tends to fall (KROETZ et al., 1970; MUIR, 1970; MCRAVEN et al., 1971) or remains unchanged (STENBERG et al., 1968; GRABNER and MICHALEK, 1968). No change in right and left ventricular end-diastolic pressure at rest, but a slight decrease during exercise has been found by KOCH (1971) in man, which suggests that the myocardial contractions are not impaired by the drug at the doses used.

F. Blood Volume

In man, no change in blood volume was found (BOCK et al., 1970), but the cardio-pulmonary blood volume was reduced (MUIR, 1970). It is likely that circulatory blood volume is decreased and that some trapping of the blood occurs, accounting for the latter effect and the reduced venous return.

G. Heart Work

Clonidine did not significantly change left and right heart work in the hypertensive phase, but a decrease was seen during the secondary fall in blood pressure owing to the hypotensive effect and the reduced cardiac output. Stroke work was also decreased (LAUBIE and SCHMITT, 1969; MAXWELL, 1969; AUTRET et al., 1971; LAUBIE and SCHMITT, 1974).

H. Myocardial Performance

The decrease in cardiac output brought about by clonidine is not due to a direct negative inotropic effect of the drug. In fact, clonidine is without effect on isolated heart (CONSTANTINE and MCSHANE, 1968; NAYLER et al., 1969; SCRIABINE et al., 1970), on isolated atria of rats, rabbits and men (NAYLER et al., 1969), on papillary muscles of dogs and men (NAYLER et al., 1969), and on heart-lung preparations of dogs (HOEFKE and KOBINGER, 1966).

Therefore any change in myocardial performance in intact animals would be due to such indirect effects as loss of sympathetic tone, increased vagal activity, and hemodynamic effects.

Surprisingly few studies have been devoted to the effects of clonidine on the performance of the heart. *Clonidine reduced the contractile force* of the left ventricle measured isometrically with a strain gauge after intravenous (BOISSIER et al., 1968) as well as intracisternal administration (SCHMITT et al., 1971d, 1973a) (see Fig. 8). Although this decrease could be partly accounted for by the bradycardia, this seems unlikely in view of the fact that pacing of the heart did not change the reduced maximal rate of rise in left ventricular pressure induced by clonidine (LAUBIE and SCHMITT, 1974). The decrease in myocardial contractions appears therefore to be due to central mechanisms, probably loss of the sympathetic tone.

Other indices of myocardial performance used by some workers *were also found to be reduced in intact animals by clonidine.* This was shown for the maximal rate of rise in left ventricular pressure, the velocity of the blood in the ascending aorta, the pressure/time index, and the indice max *dp/dt/IP* (LAUBIE and SCHMITT, 1969; AUTRET et al., 1971; LAUBIE and SCHMITT, 1974). However, the period of systolic ejection was not significantly changed (LAUBIE and SCHMITT, 1974). Clonidine increased left ventricular end-diastolic pressure in dogs, the effect being more pronounced during the hypertensive phase. An increase in left ventricular end-diastolic pressure at a time when stroke work was reduced must indicate a decrease in myocardial performance (LAUBIE and SCHMITT, 1969, 1974). Similarly, NAYLER et al. (1968) found an increase in left atrial pressure with decreased stroke work; however, when left atrial pressure was kept low no depression of myocardial performance could be detected by these authors.

Changes in blood pressure did not seem to account for the decreased myocardial performance. Hypertension would be expected to increase max *dp/dt*, which did not occur. During the hypotensive phase, the curve relating *dp/dt* to the developed ventricular pressure was strongly depressed and shifted to the right; thus hypotension was not the cause of the decreased myocardial performance. The heart slowing induced by clonidine did not appear to be a major factor in reducing myocardial performance. In fact, pacing of the heart did not change the reduced maximal rate of rise in left ventricular pressure induced by clonidine (LAUBIE and SCHMITT, 1974).

A reduction in the size of the heart did not seem to play a role, as left ventricular end-diastolic and end-systolic volumes were unchanged in dogs after clonidine (LAUBIE and SCHMITT, 1974).

Changes in autonomic tone thus appear to be the main cause of reduced myocardial performance after clonidine, in particular loss of the sympathetic tone. Elimination of the sympathetic tone in dogs by pretreatment with reserpine abolished or reduced the decrease in the maximal rate of rise in left ventricular pressure after clonidine, whereas cutting of both vagus nerves or both carotid sinus nerves did not alter this decrease. These experiments indicate further that heart slowing or activation of the vagal tone are not factors in reducing myocardial performance (LAUBIE and SCHMITT, 1974). After simultaneous β adrenoceptor blockade and parasympathetic blockade, clonidine did not significantly decrease the maximum rate of rise in left ventricular pressure (LAUBIE and SCHMITT, 1974).

In man the pre-ejection period of the systole was lengthened as was the mean rate of the left ventricular ejection index; the decrease in these indices may be caused either by a negative inotropic effect on the left ventricle or by a decrease in end-diastolic fiber length (KROETZ et al., 1970; MCRAVEN et al., 1971). Animal experiments suggest the first explanation is more likely. The pressure time index was reduced, reflecting decreased myocardial oxygen consumption (KROETZ et al., 1970; MCRAVEN et al., 1971).

In conclusion, the centrally mediated decrease in sympathetic tone appears to be the main factor in reducing myocardial performance after clonidine and inducing hypokinetic circulation also found in man (HAAN, 1966, 1968).

J. Total Peripheral Resistance

Clonidine administered intravenously *altered total peripheral resistance in two ways*. In dogs, an increase seen during the hypertensive phase was probably due to peripheral vasoconstriction (KOBINGER and WALLAND, 1967a, b, c; LAUBIE and

SCHMITT, 1969; AUTRET et al., 1971; LAUBIE and SCHMITT, 1974) but during the hypotensive phase total peripheral resistance was usually unchanged in dogs (KOBINGER and WALLAND, 1967b, c ; LAUBIE and SCHMITT, 1969; AUTRET et al., 1971; LAUBIE and SCHMITT, 1974) and rats (BRALET et al., 1974). In man, total peripheral resistance was usually reported to remain unchanged after clonidine (GRABNER et al., 1966; ZIMMERMANN et al., 1966; VORBURGER et al., 1968; KROETZ et al., 1970; BREST, 1970; REUBI et al., 1970; KOCH, 1971; MCRAVEN et al., 1971; ONESTI et al., 1971).

Changes in total peripheral resistance are well known to result from two factors: active changes in the diameter of the vessels induced by alterations in the sympathetic tone, and passive stretching of the walls of these vessels by the volume of ejected blood. Clonidine could act on the vessels in opposite ways, because the centrally mediated decrease in sympathetic tone is opposed by direct vasoconstriction and reduced cardiac output. The latter factor appears to dominate over the reduced sympathetic tone. Thus, intracisternal or intravertebral administration of clonidine at low dosage produced a decrease in blood pressure and cardiac output but did not change the total peripheral resistance, eliminating the vasoconstrictor effect as a possible cause of the absence of decrease (KOBINGER and WALLAND, 1967b, c; SCHMITT and FÉNARD, 1971; SCHMITT et al., 1973a; ONESTI et al., 1971).

It is of interest to note that in certain circumstances a fall in peripheral resistance occurs, affording evidence for a fall in the sympathetic tone of vascular bed when clonidine was administered intravenously or into the vertebral artery (CONSTANTINE and MCSHANE, 1968; BENTLEY and LI, 1969). Injection of clonidine into the vertebral artery of dogs induced a primary phase of hypotension and maintained aortic blood flow with a fall in total peripheral resistance.In some dogs the decrease in total peripheral resistance appeared to be the main cause of the hypotensive effect (SCHMITT et al., 1973a) (see Fig. 10). Even in intact animals and with clonidine by the intravenous route, a fall in total peripheral resistance was found in monkeys (CONSTANTINE and MCSHANE, 1968), in rabbits (SHAW et al., 1971a), and occasionally in dogs (LAUBIE and SCHMITT, 1974). In dogs treated with the β adrenoreceptor-blocking agent toliprolol, which prevents the cardiac effects of clonidine on the heart brought about by the reduced sympathetic tone, total peripheral resistance was found to be decreased at a delayed phase (KOBINGER and WALLAND, 1967b). However, after β adrenergic blockade with S 2395 and parasympathetic blockade with atropine, clonidine induced a fall in blood pressure and cardiac output without significantly changing total peripheral resistance (LAUBIE and SCHMITT, 1974). In dogs with both carotid sinuses denervated but with intact vagus nerves, clonidine induced a greater hypotensive effect but a similar fall in cardiac output and heart rate as in intact dogs. The total peripheral resistance was therefore slightly but no significantly decreased (LAUBIE and SCHMITT, 1974).

In some clinical trials too, total peripheral resistance was found to be lowered by clonidine (DAVIDOV et al., 1967; GRABNER and MICHALEK, 1968; KOCHSIECK and FRITSCHE, 1966; SCHNEIDER and GATTENLÖHNER, 1966). BREST (1970), ONESTI et al. (1971) reported no change in the supine position, but a decrease in the erect position. In chronic treatment total peripheral resistance has been found to be reduced (REUBI et al., 1970; SAFAR et al., 1973), but MICHEL et al. (1966) mentioned increased total peripheral resistance after clonidine.

In conclusion, the unchanged total peripheral resistance seen in the hypotensive phase seems to be the result of a decreased stretch on the walls of the vessels opposing the reduced sympathetic tone.

K. Pulmonary Circulation

Pulmonary pressure has been reported to be unchanged in dogs (LAUBIE and SCHMITT, 1969; DUHAULT and SCHMITT, unpubl. observations) *or slightly but significantly decreased* (MAXWELL, 1969) *during the hypotensive phase.* However, in all these experiments pulmonary vascular resistance rose due to the fall in cardiac output. Left ventricular end-diastolic pressure (LAUBIE and SCHMITT, 1969, 1974; AUTRET et al., 1971) and left atrial pressure (NAYLER et al., 1968) were elevated, hence a reduction in pressure gradient occured and no definite conclusion could be drawn on the state of the pulmonary vessels.

During the hypertensive phase pulmonary pressure rose markedly with a reduction in the pulse pressure and probably vasoconstriction of the pulmonary vessels. A similar feature was seen with many other α-sympathomimetic agents (AUTRET et al., 1971; DUHAULT and SCHMITT, unpubl. observations).

In hypertensive patients either no significant changes in pulmonary pressure have been reported (KOCHSIEK and FRITSCHE, 1966) or a decrease in pulmonary and wedge pressures (MICHEL et al., 1966; GRABNER and MICHALEK, 1968; STENBERG et al., 1968; ZIMMERMANN et al., 1968; KROETZ et al., 1970; MUIR, 1970; KOCH, 1971; MCRAVEN et al., 1971) with variable changes in pulmonary vascular resistance.

L. Coronary Circulation

The effect of clonidine on coronary circulation has so far been poorly investigated. HOEFKE and KOBINGER (1966) reported in dogs changes in coronary blood flow parallel to the blood pressure changes: *coronary blood flow increased during the hypertensive phase and was reduced during hypotension.* LAUBIE and SCHMITT (1969) and MAXWELL (1969) measured coronary blood flow in dogs during the hypotensive phase and found a decrease in this flow without any change in coronary vascular resistance. The myocardial fraction of cardiac output was decreased in rats by clonidine but the nutritional blood flow was not changed (BRALET et al., 1974). In dogs with surprisingly high coronary blood flow and on extracorporeal circulation NAYLER et al. (1966) found that coronary flow was increased after clonidine. Coronary blood flow per beat increased in all these experiments due to the strong bradycardia.

The oxygen content of the coronary sinus blood either did not change (LAUBIE and SCHMITT, 1969) or was slightly increased (MAXWELL, 1969). Consequently oxygen extraction was either unchanged or decreased. Both groups of authors found a striking reduction in myocardial oxygen consumption and in carbon dioxide production without any significant change in the cardiac respiratory quotient. No change in lactate or pyruvate consumption by the heart was found in dogs; this eliminated the possibility of an anaerobic metabolism (LAUBIE and SCHMITT, 1969). The index of efficiency was found by MAXWELL (1969) to be reduced. It has been suggested that the decreased oxygen consumption was the result of hemodynamic changes: decrease in heart work, bradycardia, reduction in myocardial contractions (LAUBIE and SCHMITT, 1969).

A direct action of clonidine on coronary vessels was seen by HOEFKE and KOBINGER (1966); on injecting low doses of clonidine into the coronary artery, they found that coronary blood flow was decreased. In contrast, NAYLER et al. (1960) found increased coronary flow and decreased coronary resistance after injection of clonidine into the coronary artery. The effect was not suppressed by phentolamine. The increased coronary flow by intravenous injection was ascribed to direct and to indirect effects. These surprising results are difficult to account for.

M. Cerebral Circulation

Using a thermoelectric method to estimate changes in cerebral blood flow in cats, ZAÏMIS (1970) and ZAÏMIS and HANINGTON (1969) reported *a decrease in this flow*. In dogs cerebral blood flow was measured by the N_2O method and a similar decrease was found without any significant alteration in cerebral vascular resistance (LAUBIE and SCHMITT, 1969). In rhesus monkeys cerebral blood flow has been measured by an electromagnetic probe placed on the carotid artery after tying the external carotid artery and this flow was found to be decreased after clonidine (unpubl. observations).

In unanesthetized rabbits clonidine did not change cerebral blood flow in normocapnia but reduced the increase induced by hypercapnia (COSNIER et al., 1973). In rats, using labeled microspheres, BRALET et al. (1974) found decreased cerebral blood flow and increased cerebral resistance. In monkeys by the use of a similar technique, clonidine has been shown to reduce cerebral blood flow after intravenous or intracerebroventricular injections (BOLME et al., 1975).

Similarly, cerebral blood flow has been found to be decreased in man by clonidine (DIESENHAMMER and KLAUSBERGER, 1966; SKINHØJ, 1968; JAMES et al., 1970). This effect associated with a "stabilization of cerebral vasomotricity" (ZAÏMIS, 1970) led various authors to propose clonidine as a treatment of migraine (WILKINSON, 1969; SJAASTAD and STENSRUD, 1971).

No significant change in cerebral oxygen consumption or carbon dioxide production was found after clonidine, but during the first thirty minutes a trend towards increased oxygen consumption was observed (LAUBIE and SCHMITT, 1969).

N. Renal Blood Flow

The effect of an antihypertensive agent *on renal blood flow* is of considerable interest for clinical use.

In renal hypertensive dogs, LAUBIE and SCHMITT (1969) reported a decrease in renal blood flow, limited to the renal plasma blood flow without any change in renal vascular resistance or glomerular filtration rate. NAYLER et al. (1966) detected variable changes in bypass preparations and BARAC (1971) found in dogs a decreased renal blood flow due to vasoconstriction. BRALET et al. (1974) did not find changes in renal fraction of cardiac output or in the renal nutritional blood flow in rats. In monkeys renal blood flow was found to be maintained or increased after intravenous or intracerebroventricular administration of clonidine (BOLME et al., 1975).

However, in man no significant changes in renal blood flow or even a slight increase are usually mentioned. The absence of effects was seen in both acute and chronic treatment, and in supine or erect posture. Renal vascular resistance was therefore decreased (BAUM, 1966; BOCK et al., 1966, 1968, 1970; LUDWIG, 1968; GRABNER et al., 1966; BREST, 1970; ONESTI et al., 1971). REUBI et al. (1970) found a decreased renal blood flow in man in acute experiments. The same observation was made by FRANK and LOEWENICH-LAGOIS (1966), BUCHT et al. (1970), GRABNER and MICHALEK (1968), VORBURGER et al. (1967a, b, 1968), WILLIS and WILLIAMSON (1969).

O. Splanchnic Blood Flow

LAUBIE and SCHMITT (1969) measured *the mesenteric blood flow* in renal hypertensive dogs and found a decrease after clonidine but without any alteration in mesenteric vascular resistance, in oxygen consumption or carbon dioxide production, or in the respiratory quotient. BRALET et al. (1974) did not find a decrease in splanchnic blood flow in rats. Hepatic blood flow has been found to be increased in monkeys after intravenous or intracerebroventricular administration of clonidine (BOLME et al., 1975).

However, in man, GRABNER et al. (1966) and GRABNER and MICHALEK (1968) did not detect any change in hepatic blood flow in spite of a decrease in cardiac output, and NAYLER et al. (1966) in bypass preparations of dogs found no change in splanchnic blood flow.

P. Gastric Blood Flow

OTTENJANN (1968) measured *gastric blood flow* in man with a thermosonde and found it to be decreased after clonidine.

Q. Bone-Marrow Blood Flow

Blood flow in bone marrow was decreased by clonidine (GRABNER and MICHALEK, 1968).

R. Peripheral Circulation

A *reduced femoral blood* flow was repeatedly reported after clonidine in animals (HOEFKE and KOBINGER, 1966; KOBINGER and WALLAND, 1967 b; CONSTANTINE and MCSHANE, 1968; KOBINGER and HOEFKE, 1968; LI and BENTLEY, 1969; LAUBIE and SCHMITT, 1969) and man (BOCK et al., 1966, 1968, 1970). The effect was also seen after intra-arterial injection of clonidine at low dosage (KOBINGER and WALLAND, 1967 b); and could consequently be due to a direct vasoconstrictor effect. The femoral vascular resistance rose after intravenous administration of clonidine but no change was found in oxygen consumption, carbon dioxide production, or respiratory quotient (LAUBIE and SCHMITT, 1969). Clonidine has been shown to reduce muscular and skin blood flow in monkeys by use of labelled microspheres (BOLME et al., 1975).

In man vasoconstriction occurs in cutaneous (BOCK et al., 1966, 1968, 1970; GRABNER and MICHALEK, 1968; HILD and DIETZ, 1968), but not in muscular vessels (BOCK et al., 1966, 1968, 1970; ONESTI et al., 1971) and could be the cause of the pallor seen after intravenous administration of the drug. Intra-arterial administration of clonidine in man decreased blood flow in the forearm, but intravenous administration has been found to cause an increase, probably through a central effect (EHRINGER, 1966).

In hypertensive patients, Raynaud's syndrome was reported during the first days of treatment; this could reflect vasoconstriction in muscle vascular beds (WINCHESTER and KENNEDY, 1971).

On measuring the segmental resistance values in the hind limb of dogs CONSTANTINE and MCSHANE (1968) found that the initial increase and secondary decrease in total peripheral resistance seen when the perfusion rate was kept constant were due predominantly to changes in the resistance of the small vessels and arterial segments; venous resistance remained essentially constant. The results of these experiments show that peripheral vasodilatation occured during the depressor phase of drug response and that the dilatation was confined mainly to "resistance" rather than to "capacitance vessels".

However, in dogs with extracorporeal circulation, NAYLER et al. (1966, 1968) found venodilatation responsible for the decrease in venous return. OWEN (pers. comm.), using Mellander's technique in cats, found increased resistance in capacitance vessels after intra-arterial administration of clonidine; the effect was very similar to that of the ergot alkaloids known to be α-sympathomimetic agents.

In man, venous capacity was found to be increased after intra-arterial and intravenous administration of clonidine (EHRINGER, 1966) but peripheral venous pressure did not change (ONESTI et al., 1971).

S. Changes in Vascular Reactivity

In 1970 LARBI and ZAÏMIS presented evidence that chronic treatment with clonidine changed vascular reactivity to vasodilator and vasoconstrictor agents. In cats treated with clonidine (10 to 20 μg/kg for 1 to 4 weeks) the vasoconstriction of the femoral bed induced by adrenaline or noradrenaline and the vasodilatation induced by isoproterenol were reduced. It was suggested that the loss of the vasoconstrictor effect of catecholamines could account for the antihypertensive action, and that the centrally mediated inhibition of the sympathetic tone could only be effective in acute experiments. However, experiments performed chronically in man (HODGE and ROBINSON, 1970) could not confirm this effect. Moreover, chronic treatment of dogs with fine electrodes inserted into the splanchnic nerve and a catheter in the aorta failed to reveal changes in the effect of the drug on blood pressure and splanchnic discharges (SCHMITT et al., 1974).

SHAW et al. (1971a) found decreased peripheral resistance in rabbits after injection of a bolus of clonidine followed by a perfusion. Muscular resistance was decreased but cutaneous resistance was increased. The effect persisted after sectioning of carotid sinus and aortic nerves and postganglionic blockade and was ascribed to a peripheral effect.

T. ECG.

The effect of clonidine on the ECG did not appear to be predominant. Soon after the intravenous administration cardiac irregularities appear, such as pulsus alternans and bi- or trigeminism, and in dogs there was increased respiratory arrhythmia (BOISSIER et al., 1968). The latter effect could be due to increased vagal tone in rabbits. PQ and PT intervals were slightly increased, but QS intervals remained unchanged after clonidine (HOEFKE and KOBINGER, 1966). In man, no effect on the ECG has been mentioned (BOCK et al., 1966; HAAN, 1966; GRABNER et al., 1966).

Clonidine has been reported to exert a central antiarrhythmic effect against ouabain in cats an effect which has been related to the decreased sympathetic tone brought about by the drug (GILLIS et al., 1971, 1972). In doses from 0.4 to 1 mg/kg clonidine inhibited the ventricular arrhythmias produced in mice by halothane and adrenaline (DANNENBERG, pers. comm.).

XI. Effects on Respiration

The effects of clonidine on the respiratory tract have been only poorly investigated. However, bronchoconstriction would be expected owing to the three main actions of clonidine: activation of the parasympathetic system, activation of α adrenergic receptors, which some authors have shown to cause bronchoconstriction (CASTRO DE LA MATA et al., 1962), and loss of the sympathetic tone predominant on β adrenoceptors, as the use of β adrenoceptor-blocking drugs has shown.

In experiments performed on dogs, clonidine in dosage from 10 to 25 μg/kg *did not significantly change respiratory rate, respiratory volume* (LAUBIE and SCHMITT,

1969; MAXWELL, 1969), pulmonary resistance, and compliance (DUHAULT and SCHMITT, unpubl. observations). These experiments seem to rule out the possibility of bronchoconstriction by clonidine. However, at 50 μg/kg, clonidine did increase pulmonary resistance during the hypertensive phase, an effect possibly due to activation of α adrenoceptors (DUHAULT and SCHMITT, unpubl. observations). In clinical trials, no respiratory trouble has been reported. In rats a depression in respiration has been reported and it was suggested to be due to the stimulation of central α adrenoceptors (BOLME and FUXE, 1973). In adult fowls clonidine was shown to cause tachypnea (MARLEY and NISTICO, 1975).

LAUBIE and SCHMITT (1969) did not find any change in total oxygen consumption or carbon dioxide production in renal hypertensive dogs anesthetized with pentobarbital, but MAXWELL (1969) reported a decrease in both values in chloralosed dogs. The respiratory quotient was unchanged.

Conflicting results have been reported in man. Some authors found no change in respiration (KOCHSIEK and FRITSCHE, 1966; STAUCH, 1968a, b; KOCH, 1971). In other investigations, a slight decrease in ventilation per minute and in tidal volume occured without any change in respiratory frequency. Oxygen consumption was reduced, but carbon dioxide production was not significantly decreased; respiratory quotient remained unchanged (KIRCHHOFF, 1968; STENBERG et al., 1968; KROETZ et al., 1970; MCRAVEN et al., 1971).

The decreased oxygen uptake was accompanied by an increased arteriovenous oxygen difference. Thus, oxygen extraction was more efficient, so compensating for the fall in cardiac output. As arterial lactate and pyruvate levels did not change, there was no evidence of anaerobic metabolism (KOCH, 1971).

XII. Effects on Gastro-Intestinal Tract

Few studies have been devoted to the effects of clonidine on the gastro-inte s tinal tract. Contraction of the isolated ileum of guinea pig has been shown by HOEFKE and KOBINGER (1966), and a decrease in the response to acetylcholine was seen without any change for histamine or barium chloride effect. A conflicting result was published by BOISSIER et al. (1970), who found decreased effects of 5-hydroxytryptamine and histamine without any effect on acetylcholine.

In man, clonidine was reported to induce constipation. Clonidine reduced the antral motility as measured with a microballoon, even when stimulated by metochlorpropamide (OTTENJANN, 1968).

XIII. Effects on Secretions

Clonidine has been shown to *reduce salivary, gastric, pancreatic and sudoral secretions*, but the mechanism of this effect is as yet poorly understood. In addition, in some experimental conditions, clonidine was shown to increase gastric secretion.

A *reduction in salivary secretion* is a common side-effect of the therapeutic use of clonidine, and dryness of the mouth is sometimes severe enough to warrant interruption of the antihypertensive treatment. Clonidine did not change the effect on salivary secretion of pilocarpine and of stimulation of chorda tympani (RAND et al., 1969). As clonidine reduced salivary responses to a conditioned stimulus in dogs, a central site of action was suggested (RAND et al., 1969).

In man, clonidine has been found to reduce secretion of the parotid glands which has been previously increased by citric acid. The potassium level in the secretion was elevated and the secretion was more viscous. It is possible that this effect could be correlated with the parotid pain experienced by hypertensive patients after clonidine. Other antihypertensive drugs, *e.g.* reserpine or guanethidine, did not show this effect (BOCK et al., 1970). A concentration of clonidine in the salivary glands (CHO et al., 1969) might be involved in this effect.

In conscious pylorus-ligated rats, clonidine *reduced the volume and acidity of the gastric content* (HOEFKE and KOBINGER, 1966; WALZ and VAN ZWIETEN, 1970; BRODIE et al., 1970; HOEFKE, 1975). Swallowing of the alkalin saliva is a known stimulus for gastric secretion in rats. However the decrease in salivary secretion induced by clonidine is not the alone cause of the reduced gastric secretion. In fact gastric secretion was further reduced in rats and dogs in which a gastric fistula drained immediately the swallowed saliva (JENNEWEIN, 1977). BRODIE et al. (1970) found that an intracerebroventricular administration of clonidine was less effective than an intravenous injection for reducing gastric secretion in pylorus-ligated rats and they ruled out a central site of action as the cause of the effect. Nevertheless PASCAULT and ROGER (1976) reported a greater effectiveness of clonidine after intracerebroventricular than after subcutaneous administration, but the difference was not impressive. Therefore a central site of action was not entirely ruled out. In conscious stomach lumen perfused rats clonidine reduced gastric acid secretion induced by insulin and vagal stimulation. JENNEWEIN (1977) proposed that clonidine acts at peripheral sites of action by inhibiting the release of acetylcholine. Likewise in conscious dogs with a denervated pouch, clonidine did not reduce the secretion induced by carbachol, but in dogs with a gastric fistula clonidine abolished the secretory effects of insulin (JENNEWEIN, 1977). In gastric fistula rats, PASCAULT and ROGER (1976) reported that clonidine did not change the increase in gastric secretion induced by metacholine, but abolished the effects of histamine, pentagastrin and 2-desoxyglucose. In man, clonidine reduced antral acidity, but did not diminish the increase induced by histamine according to OTTENJANN (1968) and GELINOV and BELOVEJDOC (1970). A similar reducing effect has been found in unconscious patients with pathologically increased gastric secretion (NEUHAUS and HUMPERT, 1968).

KAESS and MIKULICZ-RADECKI (1971) investigated the effect of clonidine on gastric secretion in man. The acidity was not affected, but basic gastric secretion and also betazol, pentagastrin-, and insulin-induced gastric secretion were decreased after the intravenous administration of 4 μg/kg of clonidine. The effect was very similar to that of parasympatholytic agents. It is noteworthy that in other tests clonidine was found to be devoid of parasympatholytic properties and to decrease gastric secretion induced by central vagal stimulation (hypoglycemia induced by insulin). Although the cardiovascular effects of the drug preclude its general use in the treatment of ulcers, this effect could be advantageous in hypertensive and ulcerous patients, in contrast to the increased gastric secretion brought about by reserpine or guanethidine.

Large intravenous doses of clonidine have been shown to cause an *increase of acid secretion* in the perfused stomach of anesthetized rats and guinea-pigs. These effects were similar to those observed with the other sympathomimetic agents, such as naphazoline; they were inhibited by phentolamine and tolazoline and were ascribed to the stimulation of α adrenoceptors (WALZ and VAN ZWIETEN, 1970). However KARPPANEN and WESTERMANN (1973) found that the increased gastric acid secretion induced by clonidine in perfused stomach of guinea pigs was inhibited by burimamide, a H_2 histamine receptor blocking agent. JENNEWEIN (1977) reported an antagonistic effect of cimetidine, another H_2 histamine receptor blocking agent in perfused stomach of anesthetized rats against clonidine. In addition clonidine increased the level of cyclic AMP in minced gastric tissue after treatment with clonidine and the effect was also antagonized by burimamide. Both effects seem therefore to be due to an activation of H_2 histamine receptors (KARPPANEN and WESTERMANN, 1973). Administration of clonidine in conscious dogs with Heidenhain pouch caused a dose-related increase in gastric acid secretion and in the maximum secretory rate to pentagastrin. A concomitant increase in gastric blood flow was found. The effects have been ascribed to the loss of the sympathetic tone (CURWAIN and ENDERSBY, 1974).

Clonidine reduced gastric ulcerations produced by reserpine, histamine, ligature of the pylorus or restraint (HOEFKE and KOBINGER, 1966; BOISSIER et al., 1970; BRODIE et al., 1970), but did not reduce hemorrhage produced by cold plus restraint. The protective effect of clonidine, mepyramine, atropine, hexamethonium, phenoxybenzamine, phentolamine and phenobarbital were compared on different kinds of experimental ulcers in rats and BOISSIER et al. (1970) found a similar protective effect with clonidine and phenobarbital. They concluded that the site of action was central.

However BRODIE et al. (1971) found that intracerebroventricular administration of clonidine was less effective than intravenous one in inhibiting cold plus restraint hemorrhage.

KAESS and MIKULICZ-RADECKI (1971) found a *decrease* in basic and secretin-induced *pancreatic secretion.* Although the bicarbonate concentration was not altered, bicarbonate secretion was reduced.

Reduction of sudoral secretion was reported in man and this could be troublesome in hot climates. Return to the initial rectal temperature after exercise was delayed (WENDT and CASPERS, 1968).

XIV. Effects on the Kidney

Clonidine (0.3 to 1 μg/kg) has been shown to increase diuresis and elimination of sodium, potassium and chloride in rats (HOEFKE and KOBINGER, 1966; LE DOUAREC et al., 1972a, b). Clonidine reduces water intake (LE DOUAREC et al., 1972a, b), resulting in a negative water balance. These effects are found also with other α-sympathomimetic agents (LEHR et al., 1967) and could be a particular response of the rat to this type of drugs.

However, in dogs, clonidine has only a slight effect on diuresis (HOEFKE and KOBINGER, 1966; LAUBIE and SCHMITT, 1969). Clonidine has repeatedly been reported *to increase diuresis in dogs* (KOBINGER, 1968; CHRYSTANS and LAVENDER, 1975; REID et al., 1975; OLSEN, 1976). Cosm was not changed (KOBINGER, 1968), but free water clearance was increased (KOBINGER, 1968; OLSEN, 1976). The glomerular filtration rate was unchanged (KOBINGER, 1968; LAUBIE and SCHMITT, 1969; ONESTI, 1971; CHRYSTANS and LAVENDER, 1975) or slightly decreased (HOEFKE and KOBINGER, 1966; ONESTI et al., 1971) and renal plasma flow was reduced (LAUBIE and SCHMITT, 1969; ONESTI et al., 1971; CHRYSTANS and LAVENDER, 1975). The excretion of sodium was found to be decreased (ONESTI et al., 1971; CHRYSTANS and LAVENDER, 1975), increased (OLSEN, 1975), unchanged (REID et al., 1975) or increased then decreased (LAUBIE and SCHMITT, 1969). The excretion of potassium was unchanged (LAUBIE and SCHMITT, 1969, CHRYSTANS and LAVENDER, 1975) or increased (REID et al., 1975). The excretion of chloride has been found unchanged (LAUBIE and SCHMITT, 1969; OLSEN, 1976) or reduced (CHRYSTANS and LAVENDER, 1975). BARAC (1971) using high doses of clonidine in dogs observed an oliguria followed by increased diuresis.

Intracisternal administration of clonidine reduced renal plasma flow and sodium excretion without changing the glomerular filtration rate suggesting that the effects were probably a consequence of the centrally induced loss in the sympathetic tone (ONESTI et al., 1971).

KOBINGER (1968) suggested that clonidine could inhibit ADH release. In dogs deprived of water, clonidine induced diuresis and the osmolarity of the urine fell below that of the plasma; a positive free water clearance was seen without any change in osmolar clearance. In dogs in water diuresis clonidine transiently reduced the volume of urine and free water clearance and increased urine osmolarity; the effect of vasopressin was not changed by clonidine. These results led to the suggestion of inhibition of ADH release by clonidine. In fact clonidine has been reported to reduce ADH secretion (HUMPHREY and REID, 1975) although the drug did not seem to change urinary ADH excretion (OLSEN, 1976). It is however doubtful that the alone inhibition of ADH secretion could account for increased diuresis and free water clearance induced by clonidine. In fact infusion of clonidine at low doses into the renal artery of dogs increased diuresis and free water clearance, reduced renal blood flow without changing the glomerular filtration rate and the excretion of sodium, potassium and chloride (CHRYSTANS and LAVENDER, 1975). CHRYSTANS and LAVENDER (1975) ascribed these results to an increase in oncontic pressure in peritubular capillaries or to a redistribution of blood from the outsalt wasting nephrons towards deeper salt retaining corticomedullary nephrons. The increased sodium reabsorption by the ascending limb of Henle loop could account for the increase in free water clearance. However, it was not possible to explain the increased diuresis on these bases and reduction of the secretion of ADH was suggested. OLSEN (1976) reported that after the administration of ADH clonidine increased no longer urinary flow, and sodium excretion and did not increase osmolar clearance. According to this author, after the administration of indomethacine in order to inhibit the prostaglandine synthetase system clonidine reduced diuresis, sodium, potassium and chloride excretion but did not change osmolar clearance. As clonidine increased prostaglandine excretion, OLSEN (1976) ascribed to the release of theses substances the increase in urinary flow and in free water clearance.

In dogs with hypotonic diuresis clonidine reduced water, sodium, potassium and chloride excretion, osmolar clearance, free water clearance, glomerular filtration rate and plasma renal flow. These changes could be due to a vasoconstriction of the renal vessels induced by the drug, to a redistribution of the renal blood flow or to an action on the reabsorption of the electrolytes or water. This latter suggestion was supported by the fact that clonidine enhanced water reabsorption in a greater extent and for a longer duration that electrolytes absorption. The reduced sodium, potassium and chloride excretion was followed by an increase (unpublished results).

Thus the effects of clonidine on kidney of dogs appear to be complex and poorly understood.

In man, clonidine has been reported to leave the glomerular filtration rate unchanged (BOCK et al., 1966; BAUM, 1966; ONESTI et al., 1971) or to decrease it (FRANK and LOEWENICH-LAGOIS, 1966; GRABNER et al., 1966; GRABNER and MICHALEK, 1968; VORBURGER et al., 1968). Renal plasma blood flow has been found to be unchanged (BOCK et al., 1966, 1968), decreased (FRANK and LOEWENICH-LAGOIS, 1966; GRABNER et al., 1966; GRABNER and MICHALEK, 1968; VORBURGER et al., 1968), or increased (BAUM, 1966).

Urinary volume was decreased and excretion of sodium and chloride was reduced, but the excretion of potassium remained unchanged (DAVIDOV et al., 1967; GRABNER et al., 1966; GRABNER and MICHALEK, 1968; VORBURGER et al., 1968; BREST, 1970; REUBI et al., 1970). However, BOCK et al. (1966) and BAUM (1966) did not detect any change. KOCHSIEK and FRITSCHE (1966) made a similar observation in spite of a small elevation in blood sodium and chloride and a slight decrease in bicarbonate. Sodium retention may be responsible for the weight gain. Sodium retention was ascribed to enhanced tubular reabsorption of sodium and water, for the rejected fraction of filtered sodium was found to be decreased (REUBI et al., 1970). C_{H_2O} has been found to be decreased but the change was too small to be ascribed to an effect in the ascending limb of the loop of Henle (VORBURGER et al., 1968).

XV. Effects on the Eyes

Clonidine in high doses *induced mydriasis, exopthalmos and contraction of the nictitating membrane* in animals (HOEFKE and KOBINGER, 1966; BOISSIER et al., 1968), effects which were ascribed to the α-sympathomimetic properties of the drug. The mydriatic effect has been shown to be dose-dependent in rats and to decrease somewhat with subsequent injections of high doses. This tolerance was ascribed to the α adrenoceptor-blocking effects of the drug (WALLAND and KOBINGER, 1971). Clonidine in high doses caused retinal damage in rats but not in dogs and monkeys. This effect was ascribed to light. In fact, light does induce retinal damage in rats, and it is to be expected that mydriasis would increase this effect. In rats with one eye sutured, retinal damage was found in the unsutured eye but not in the closed eye (WEISE et al., 1971).

In man, a low dosage of clonidine (75 to 150 μg) did not change the diameter of the pupilla the myotic action of pilocarpine and did not alter the accommodation. Blood pressure in the ophthalmic artery was lowered and the decrease was related to systemic hypotension. *Clonidine reduced intraocular pressure* in normal subjects and in glaucomatous patients (HASSLINGER, 1969; HEILMANN, 1969, 1970, 1971; JUENEMANN and SCHMIDT, 1970; EDELHAUSER, 1971; JUENEMANN and PAUST, 1971; MAKABE, 1966, 1968). The effect was assumed to result from either decreased production of intraocular fluid (MAKABE, 1966, 1968) or an increased drainage of intraocular fluid (HASSLINGER, 1969). In rabbits, clonidine decreased intraocular pressure as did other α-sympathomimetic agents (HOEFKE, pers. comm.).

XVI. Sedative Effects

The *sedative effect of clonidine* was mentioned in the first pharmacological report on the drug (HOEFKE and KOBINGER, 1966) and confirmed repeatedly in clinical trials. This effect may be troublesome, at least at the beginning of treatment. However, tolerance rapidly appeared.

Clonidine *reduced spontaneous activity* without inducing sleep in mice and rats (HOEFKE and KOBINGER, 1966; BOISSIER et al., 1970; LAVERTY and TAYLOR, 1969; MALING et al., 1968, 1969; MAJ et al., 1972); the drug antagonized the stimulating effect of amphetamine (MALING et al., 1969) and prolonged the duration of sleep induced by chloral hydrate and barbiturates (HOEFKE and KOBINGER, 1966; MALING et al., 1969; BOISSIER et al., 1970; LAVERTY and TAYLOR, 1969). Clonidine together with subhypnotic doses of chloral hydrate will induce sleep (DELBARRE and SCHMITT, 1969, 1971, 1973).

In cats and dogs clonidine decreased spontaneous activity, induced exophthalmos and piloerection, muscular relaxation, ataxia and catatonia at the high dose of 1 mg/kg (HOEFKE and KOBINGER, 1966; TRAN QUANG LOC et al., 1974). Clonidine delayed the sedation and catatonia induced by reserpine but did not antagonize the sedative effects of the alkaloid once they were fully developed

(HOEFKE and KOBINGER, 1966). However a stimulating effect was sometimes recognized. In reserpinized rats clonidine injected into the nucleus accumbens potentiated the increase in locomotor activity induced by injection of apomorphine into the same nucleus (ANDÉN et al., 1976).

Clonidine disrupted, even in small dosage, conditioned avoidance reflexes in black and Long Evan rats (LAVERTY and TAYLOR, 1969; DELBARRE and SCHMITT, 1974) but appears to be less effective in Wistar rats.

Clonidine increased the latency for intracranial self-stimulation in rats in which the electrode was inserted into the hypothalamic median forebrain bundle; in addition clonidine prolonged the increased latency induced by α-methyl p-tyrosine. Clonidine did not alter the latency for the cessation of intracranial self-stimulation. The increased latency for intracranial self stimulation has been ascribed to the activation of central α adrenoceptors (HUNT et al., 1976).

The *effects of clonidine on EEG* have been surprisingly little investigated. GOGOLAK and STUMPF (1966) reported high slow waves in rabbits after clonidine; the threshold for the arousal reaction induced by electrical stimulation of the mesencephalic reticular formation was elevated. The action appears to be very similar to that of naphazoline. The same high slow-wave pattern was seen in rats after clonidine had been given intravenously or intracerebroventricularly (HOLMAN et al., 1971; FLORIO et al., 1975), in rabbits and cats (TRAN QUANG LOC et al., 1973, 1974; FLORIO et al., 1975). In cats, clonidine induced a sleep-like pattern in the neocortex, but an arousal reaction in the paleocortex (F. KUHN, pers. comm.). This interesting dissociation has been previously reported for the related agent, xylazine (HOFFMEISTER, 1968). Clonidine increased the duration of after-discharges induced by stimulation of the amygdala and the duration of after-discharges produced by stimulation of the hippocampus, in contrast to xylazine which shortened the duration of after-discharges after stimulation of the amygdala (F. KUHN, pers. comm.). The significance of these changes is not known. In cats, the high slow-wave pattern and behavioral sedation induced by clonidine disappear with repeated administration, affording evidence of tolerance (TRAN QUANG LOC et al., 1974).

In rats clonidine suppressed REM sleep, prolonged the sleeping time (KLEINLOGEL et al., 1975). In man 300 μg of clonidine given at the evening reduced or abolished REM sleep and prolonged the stages III and IV of sleep (AUTRET et al., 1977). Clonidine reduced ponto-geniculo-occipital spikes in cats after a depletion of noradrenaline with injection of the benzoquinolizine Ro4-1284 or of 5-hydroxytryptamine with p-chlorophenylalanine (HAEFELY et al., 1972; RUCH-MONACHON et al., 1975).

In view of the peripheral α-sympathomimetic properties of clonidine, it was of interest to determine *whether activation of receptors having some properties in common with the classical α adrenoceptors could induce sleep*. Such an investigation could provide some indications concerning the possible classification of these receptors and perhaps the role of noradrenaline in the central nervous system.

In order to investigate this possibility, it was necessary to use tests easy to quantify. For this reason chickens were used at first. In 1970 ZAÏMIS reported that clonidine caused sleep in chickens. These animals therefore allow a comparison of some α-sympathomimetic agents. Clonidine and the related compound LD 2855 were the most active drugs. Naphazoline, tramazoline and xylazine were much less potent. Tetryzoline was only slightly potent. It was not possible to compare the effect of oxymetazoline, for the dose-response curve for this agent was not parallel to the dose-response curve of other α-sympathomimetic drugs, possibly due to its greater toxicity. It appears therefore that the order of potency for the α-sympathomimetic drugs is different from the order established for vascular receptors (AUTRET et al., 1971). It could therefore be concluded that there is some difference in the receptors involved in the two types of action (DELBARRE and SCHMITT, 1969, 1971). FÜGNER and HOEFKE (1971) compared the sedative action of noradrenaline, α-methylnoradrenaline and clonidine in chickens. They found clonidine to be the most potent agent. Sensitivity to clonidine increased with age, whereas sensitivity to noradrenaline did not change and that of adrenaline decreased. 5-Hydroxytryptamine was weakly effective and isoproterenol was only very slightly active.

In the second part of these experiments, chickens were treated with adrenoceptor and cholinoceptor blocking agents and ten minutes later with clonidine, naphazoline or tetryzoline. The results were very clear. The classical α adrenoceptor-blocking drugs—yohimbine, tolazoline, phentolamine, piperoxan and dibenamine—reduced in a dose-related manner the duration of sleep induced by the three α-sympathomimetic agents. Yohimbine and piperoxan are the most effective agents. Some other α adrenoceptor agents found to be ineffective or only weakly effective were phenoxybenzamine, 883 F, dibozane, ethomoxane, azapetine and thymoxamine (DELBARRE and SCHMITT, 1969, 1971, 1973). HOLMAN et al. (1971) also reported an antagonistic effect of phentolamine on sleep induced by clonidine. FÜGNER (1971) showed that phentolamine and tolazoline, but not phenoxybenzamine, were competitive antagonists of clonidine. In chickens, chlorpromazine and imipramine did not induce sedation but they antagonized the sedative effects of clonidine, naphazoline and tetryzoline. Haloperidol, a neuroleptic agent assumed to block preferentially the dopaminergic receptors, reduced only the effects of tetryzoline. In contrast to the antagonistic effects of α adrenoceptor-blocking agents, β adrenoceptor-blocking drugs—propranolol, pindolol, Kö 1366, S 2395, alprenolol, sotalol and practolol—as well as atropine and mecamylamine had no antagonistic effects. These results strongly suggest that, at least in chickens, the sedative effects of clonidine are due to the activation of central receptors having some properties in common with peripheral receptors. The ineffectiveness of some classical α adrenoceptor-blocking agents provides further evidence that there is some difference in the structure of the central and peripheral receptors (DELBARRE and SCHMITT, 1971, 1973). MARLEY and NISTICO (1974, 1975) found that injection of clonidine as well as of noradrenaline into the III ventricle or the hypothalamus of adult fowls induced behavioral and electrocorticographic sleep. Injected during the awaking effects of dexamphetamine clonidine reversed the action of the amine. The effects of intrahypothalamically injected clonidine have been reported to be blocked by phentolamine and phenoxybenzamine infused into the hypothalamus, but propranolol, methysergide, atropine and p-chlorophenylalanine were ineffective.

It would be of interest to have some indication that a similar mechanism operates in mammals. For this purpose, the duration of the sleeping time induced in mice by a combination of the α-sympathomimetic agent and a subhypnotic dosage of chloral hydrate was used as a test. The order of activity of the sympathomimetic agents was the same as in chickens. The α adrenoceptor-blocking compounds—tolazoline, phentolamine, piperoxan, dibenamine, 883 F, yohimbine—antagonize the effect. Piperoxan and yohimbine are the most potent agents. In contrast, phenoxybenzamine, dibozane, ethomoxane, azapetine and thymoxamine were ineffective. The β adrenoceptor blocking drugs, propranolol and sotalol did not change the potentiating effect of clonidine on sleep induced by chloral hydrate; pindolol and practolol increased the duration of sleep induced by clonidine and chloral hydrate. In contrast Kö 1366, S 2395, alprenolol and dichloroisoproterenol shortened this time. It is not yet possible to account for these discrepancies. In contrast to chickens, atropine and mecamylamine reduced the potentiating effects of α-sympathomimetic agents in chloral hydrate-induced sleep. It has been proposed that the cholinergic pathways responsible for the sedative effect are present in mammals but not in chickens. Possibly reticulo-cortical pathways could account for this discrepancy (Delbarre and Schmitt, 1971, 1973) (Fig. 25).

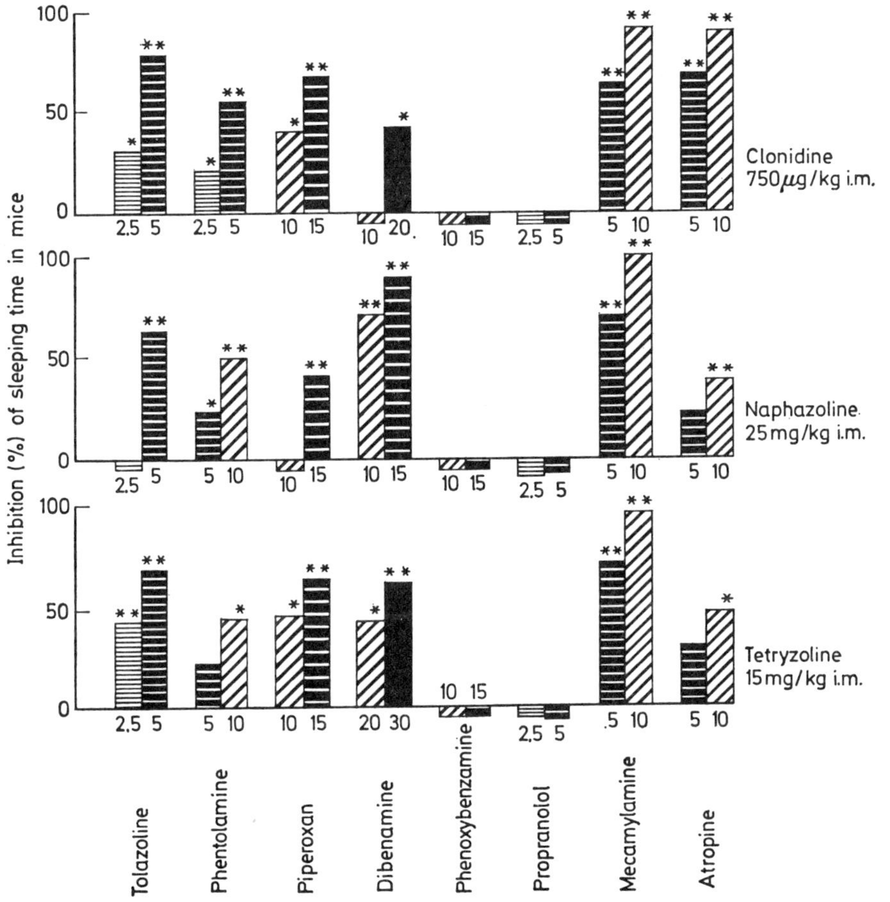

Fig. 25. Antagonistic effects of the sedative action of clonidine, naphazoline, and tetryzoline in mice. Antagonism is expressed as a percentage of the potentiating effect of clonidine, naphazoline and tetryzoline on a subhypnotic dose of chloral (250 mg kg^{-1}). Tolazoline, phentolamine, piperoxan, dibenamine, administered i.m. show a definite antagonism. Phenoxybenzamine and propranolol were ineffective. Atropine and mecamylamine antagonized also the effect (*$p > 0.05$ **$p > 0.01$). [Delbarre, B., Schmitt, H.: Europ. J. Pharmacol. **13**, 359 (1971)]

Piperoxan and yohimbine antagonized the disruption of conditioned reflexes in a shuttle-box induced in Long Evans rats by clonidine (Delbarre and Schmitt, 1974). The disruption of conditioned reflexes in a shuttle-box induced by clonidine was antagonized by atropine, as were the effects of α adrenoceptor-blocking agents (Delbarre and Schmitt, 1974). This observation raises the question of whether clonidine and α adrenoceptor-blocking drugs have some common effects on the central nervous system. Similarly, the decrease in locomotor activity induced by low doses of clonidine has been shown to be antagonized by atropine and scopolamine, but not by atropine methylbromide or scopolamine butylbromide in mice and rats. Clonidine selectively increased acetylcholine levels in the striatum without affecting acetylcholine content in the cortex, thalamus, pons or medulla oblongata (MAJ et al., 1972).

Clonidine and apomorphine depressed response rates in rats trained to bar-press on a schedule for water reinforcement. Frontal cortical lesions did not alter the effect of clonidine but potentiated the effect of apomorphine. These results suggest that the frontal cortex modulates the activity of dopaminergic but not of noradrenergic neuronal pathways (GLICK and COX, 1976).

In another investigation it was shown that piperoxan, yohimbine and to a lesser degree tolazoline, could reverse or prevent the high slow wave pattern and behavioral sedation induced by clonidine in rabbits and cats (Fig. 26). Dibenamine

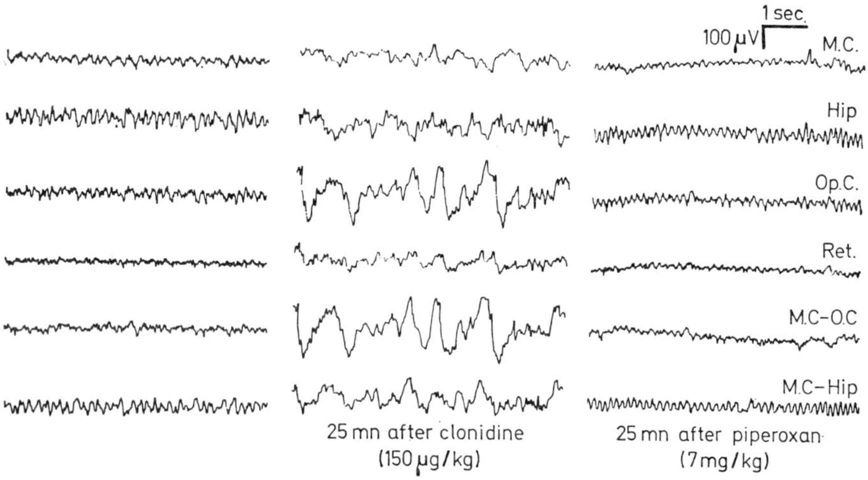

Fig. 26. Effect of clonidine on EEG of rabbits and its antagonism by piperoxan. Clonidine (150 µg/kg) induced in rabbits a pattern of high slow waves; 7 mg/kg of piperoxane reversed this effect. M.C. = motor cortex; Hip = hippocampus; Op.C. = optic cortex; Ret = reticular formation; M.C.—O.C. = motor cortex—optic cortex; Mc-Hip = motor cortex—Hippocampus

and phenoxybenzamine reversed the high slow waves activity in a record of arousal, but did not antagonize the behavioral sedation, particularly the muscular relaxation. Phentolamine and azapetine did not alter the behavioral and EC_0G effect of clonidine (TRAN QUAN LOC et al., 1973, 1974). FLORIO et al. (1975) reported that tolazoline, phentolamine and yohimbine, but not phenoxybenzamine prevented the behavioral and EEG sedation induced by clonidine in rats and rabbits and that yohimbine antagonized the effects of clonidine in cats.

An α-sympathomimetic effect for clonidine was also disclosed by the reduction in ponto-geniculo-occipital waves induced in cats by central noradrenaline or 5-hydroxytryptamine depletion (HAEFELY et al., 1972; RUCH-MONACHON et al., 1975).

These experiments clearly demonstrate that the peripheral and sedative effects of clonidine are related and due to the activation of receptors with some common properties. However, the difference in order of potency of α-sympathomimetic agents and the ineffectiveness of some α adrenoceptor-blocking agents on central actions suggest that the two groups of receptors are not alike.

HOLMAN et al. (1971) investigated the possible intervention of tryptaminergic mechanisms in sleep induced by clonidine. According to JOUVET and RENAULT (1966) and MOURET et al. (1968), slow-wave sleep was due to the activity of raphe median nuclei, which are assumed to release 5-hydroxytryptamine. In chickens, pretreatment with p-chlorophenylalanine, a drug known to inhibit tryptophan-hydroxylase and to reduce the level of 5-hydroxytryptamine in the brain of mammals, did not change the sleep-inducing effect of clonidine. As this drug did not reduce the level of 5-hydroxytryptamine in the brain of chickens, complementary experiments were performed in rats, an animal species in which this pretreatment reduces the level of 5-hydroxytryptamine in the brain. The effect of intravenous or intraventricular injection of clonidine was not altered. The blockade of tryptaminergic receptors by methysergide did not change the sleep-inducing effect of clonidine. While lysergamide (LSD 25) reduced this effect, the result could be accounted for by the own stimulating effect of the drug. It was concluded that the sleep-like pattern induced by clonidine did not involve tryptaminergic mechanisms and that factors other than 5-hydroxytryptamine must play a role in initiating slow-wave sleep. However clonidine was shown to be able to reduce the frequency of discharges in neurons of the raphe median nuclei, an effect indirectly mediated for it was not seen after pretreatment with 6-hydroxy-dopamine (SVENSSON et al., 1975).

To account for the discrepancies between the results obtained with clonidine and the generally accepted concept of a stimulating effect of endogeneous noradrenaline and of a maintaining effect of the amine on REM sleep, it has been postulated that clonidine either reduces noradrenaline release by activating presynaptic α adrenoceptors (ANDÉN et al., 1976) or activates postsynaptic adrenaline receptors located on the noradrenergic neurons of the locus coeruleus inhibiting their discharges (BOLME et al., 1974). However some observations seem to indicate a postsynaptic site of action. In reserpinized rats in which electrocorticogramm was not different from that of untreated rats clonidine induced a EC_0G synchronisation. In rats treated with α-methyl-p-tyrosine in order to inhibit catecholamine synthesis clonidine induced a more marked behavioral depression than in untreated rats but surprisingly did not induce EC_0G synchronisation (FLORIO et al., 1975). Were these observations confirmed a reappraisal of the role of noradrenaline in wakefulness and in REM sleep is needed.

XVII. Antinociceptive Action

In animals *clonidine reduced responses to pain* at a dosage higher than the doses that act on blood pressure. This action was shown in several tests, *i.e.* hot plate in mice, electrical stimulation of the rat's tail. Clonidine is some 3 to 10 times more potent than morphine (HOEFKE, pers. comm.; SCHMITT et al., 1974a). The related compound xylazine was found to be as potent as morphine (KRONEBERG et al., 1967; HOFFMEISTER, 1968; PAALZOW, 1974; SCHMITT et al., 1974a). Other α-sympathomimetic agents like naphazoline, tetryzoline or oxymetazoline had no antinociceptive action when given by the parenteral route of administration, but were effective in both tests after intracerebroventricular administration (SCHMITT et al., 1974a; Fig. 27). The mechanism seems to be different from those of morphine, as naloxone failed to antagonize the antinociceptive effect of clonidine (PAALZOW and PAALZOW, 1976).

The antinociceptive action of clonidine was antagonized by yohimbine but phenoxybenzamine was ineffective and chlorpromazine increased the effect (PAALZOW and PAALZOW, 1976). The effect of xylazine was easily antagonized by two

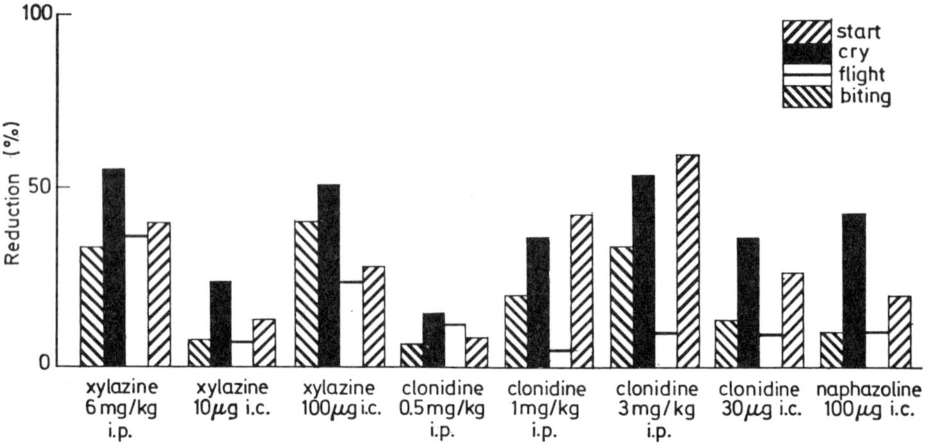

Fig. 27. Antinociceptive action of sympathomimetic agents. The figure shows the reduction of startle, cry, flight and biting of the electrodes induced by xylazine (6 mg/kg I.P.; 100 μg intracerebroventricularly), clonidine (1—3 mg/kg I.P.; 30 μg intracerebroventricularly) and naphazoline (100 μg intracerebroventricularly). [LE DOUAREC, J.C., SCHMITT, H.: Neuropharmacology **13**, 291 (1974)]

α adrenoceptor-blocking agents, piperoxan and yohimbine, at doses from 1 to 7 mg/kg. Three other benzodioxane derivatives—ethomoxane, dibozane and 883 F—showed partial antagonism but at higher dosage. Tolazoline and dibenamine were found to antagonize the antinociceptive effects of xylazine but at high dosage. In contrast, four classical α adrenoceptor-blocking agents—phentolamine, phenoxybenzamine, azapetine and thymoxamine—were ineffective or slightly effective (only inhibiting biting of the electrodes). The β adrenoreceptor-blocking agent propranolol was ineffective even in high dosage. Pindolol, a β adrenoceptor-blocking agent ten times more potent than propranolol, antagonized only the effects of xylazine on the starttle reaction, but Kö 1366 was an effective antagonist (SCHMITT et al., 1974b).

Endogeneous stores of noradrenaline did not seem to be involved in the antinociceptive effect of clonidine. Inhibition of tyrosine hydroxylase by α-methyl-*p*-tyrosine reduced the effect of clonidine on the threshold for vocalisation after-discharges but increased the threshold for vocalisation. Inhibition of dopamine-β-hydroxylase by FLA 63 or depletion of monoamine stores by reserpine did not change the effects of clonidine (PAALZOW and PAALZOW, 1976).

However 5-hydroxytryptamine mechanisms appear to oppose the effects of clonidine. 5-hydroxytryptophane reduced the threshold for vocalisation after-discharges and inhibition of tryptophane hydroxylase by p-chlorophenylalanine increased the effects of clonidine. However lysergamide was ineffective (PAALZOW and PAALZOW, 1976).

Atropine and mecamylamine were ineffective against the antinociceptive effect of xylazine (SCHMITT et al., 1974b) but atropine was reported to increase the effects of clonidine (PAALZOW and PAALZOW, 1976).

PAALZOW and PAALZOW (1976) discused several possibilities to account for these results: reduced noradrenaline release by an action on an α presynaptic adrenoceptor, stimulation of an adrenaline receptor according to the concept of BOLME et al. (1974). SCHMITT et al. (1974b) suggested an activation of central α adrenoceptors of a special kind.

Clonidine has an influence on the naloxone-induced withdrawal signs in morphine-dependent rats. Clonidine inhibited precipited shakes and potentiated escape attempts induced by naloxone. Clonidine injected intracerebroventricularly reduced body temperature in morphine dependent rats and placebo pellet implanted rats. Naloxone reduced body temperature only in morphine dependent rats. It has been suggested that clonidine modulates morphine withdrawal signs by potentiating the behavior associated with heat dissipation and inhibiting the behavior associated with heat gain. These effects may occur via stimulation of central noradrenergic mechanisms (TSENG et coll., 1975).

In mice, investigations were performed by the hot-plate method to distinguish any influence of adrenoceptor- and cholinoceptor-blocking agents administered intraperitoneally on the effects of xylazine injected either intraperitoneally (10 mg/kg) or intracerebroventricularly (10 μg). Some α adrenoceptor-blocking agents antagonized the effects of xylazine at doses below 10 mg/kg. Such an effect was detected for piperoxan, dibozane, ethomoxane, yohimbine, tolazoline, phentolamine, 883 F, dibenamine and chlorpromazine. Propranolol was shown to be devoid of any effect but surprisingly enough three potent β adrenoceptor-blocking agents – pindolol, Kö 1366 and S 2395 – antagonized the antinociceptive effect of xylazine. Atropine and atropine methylnitrate were both shown to be antagonistic agents but mecamylamine was ineffective. It is noteworthy that three α adrenoceptor-blocking agents – phenoxybenzamine, azapetine and thymoxamine – were ineffective. Imipramine was slightly effective but clomipramine was much more potent. When both groups of drugs were administered intracerebroventricularly the similarities with the experiments performed in rats were more striking. Tolazoline, piperoxan, yohimbine, ethomoxane and chlorpromazine were found to be good antagonistic agents. With other classical α adrenoceptor-blocking agents – phentolamine, dibenamine, phenoxybenzamine, 883F, dibozane, azapetine and thymoxamine – no definite antagonism could be detected. Kö 1366 was an effective antagonistic agent, but pindolol was ineffective. Atropine and atropine methylnitrate decreased the antinociceptive effect of xylazine, suggesting the involvement of muscarinic mechanisms (SCHMITT et al., 1974b).

These experiments suggest that the *receptors involved in the antinociceptive effect of xylazine, and probably of clonidine have some properties in common with the classical α adrenoceptors, but are quite dissimilar*. A peripheral mechanism seems to be involved in the action where the hot-plate test is used, but not in the test of electrical stimulation of the rat's tail (SCHMITT et al., 1974b).

XVIII. Water Intake

Clonidine reduced water intake in rats and induced diuresis at the same time, leading therefore to a negative water balance (Le Douarec et al., 1971a, b). Other α-sympathomimetic drugs elicited similar effects (Lehr et al., 1967; Le Douarec et al., 1971a, b).

The decrease in water intake by clonidine was prevented or even reversed by the α adrenoceptor-blocking agents: tolazoline, phentolamine, piperoxan and dibenamine. In contrast, phenoxybenzamine was ineffective. β Adrenoceptor-blocking drugs were also ineffective, as were atropine and mecamylamine. It appears therefore that this effect of clonidine is also due to the activation of receptors that have some properties in common with α adrenoceptors (Fig. 28).

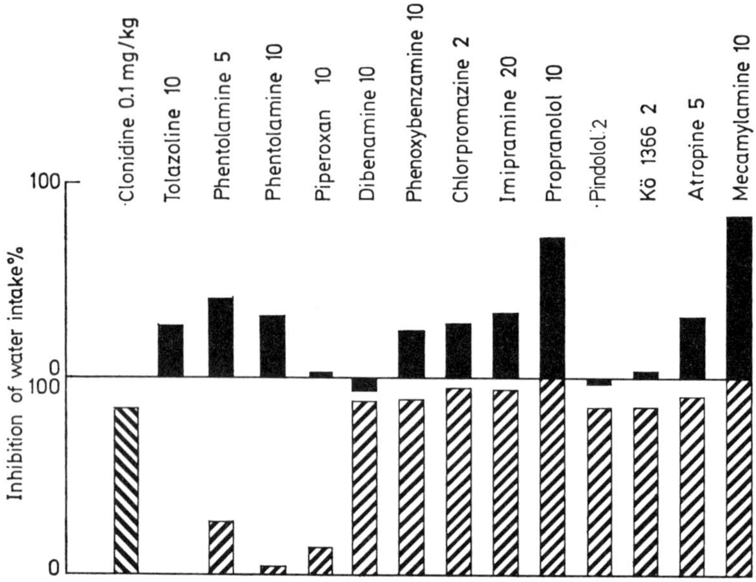

Fig. 28. Influence of adrenergic and cholinergic blocking agents on water intake in deprived rats. The figure shows the percentage inhibition of water intake. Block columns: effect of adrenergic and cholinergic blocking agents; striped columns effect of clonidine (0.1 mg/kg) and influence thereon of adrenergic and cholinergic blocking agents. Tolazoline, phentolamine and piperoxan decreased the effect of clonidine. [Le Douarec, J.C., Schmitt, H., Lucet, B.: J. Pharmacol. (Paris) **2**, 435—444 (1971)]

XIX. Food Intake

Parenteral or oral administration of *clonidine decreased food intake* in rats. Some other α-sympathomimetic agents, *e.g.* naphazoline and L.D. 2855, induced a similar effect, but tetryzoline was ineffective. Clonidine is the most potent agent so far known for decreasing food intake in rats. However, the doses required were much higher than doses reducing blood pressure (Le Douarec et al., 1972).

This effect of clonidine was shown to be decreased by some α adrenoceptor-blocking agents: piperoxan, 883F, yohimbine and to a lesser extent phentolamine and tolazoline. But many α adrenoceptor-blocking drugs failed even in high doses to antagonize the appetite suppressant effect of clonidine; dibozane, ethomoxane, azapetine, thymoxamine and chlorpromazine did not show any activity. Imipramine was also ineffective, as well as the β adrenoceptor-blocking agents, propranolol, pindolol and Kö 1366, and the anticholinergic drugs atropine and mecamylamine. It appears that the type of receptors involved in the effect had some properties in common with the classical α adrenoceptors yet were dissimilar (LE DOUAREC et al., 1972) (Fig. 29).

The reduction in food intake is not the sole effect of clonidine. In dogs small doses increased food intake, but a trend to a decrease was shown at higher dosage. *Injection of clonidine into the anterior hypothalamus of rat increased food intake* and induced grooming, stereotypy and hypothermia (LE DOUAREC et al., 1972).

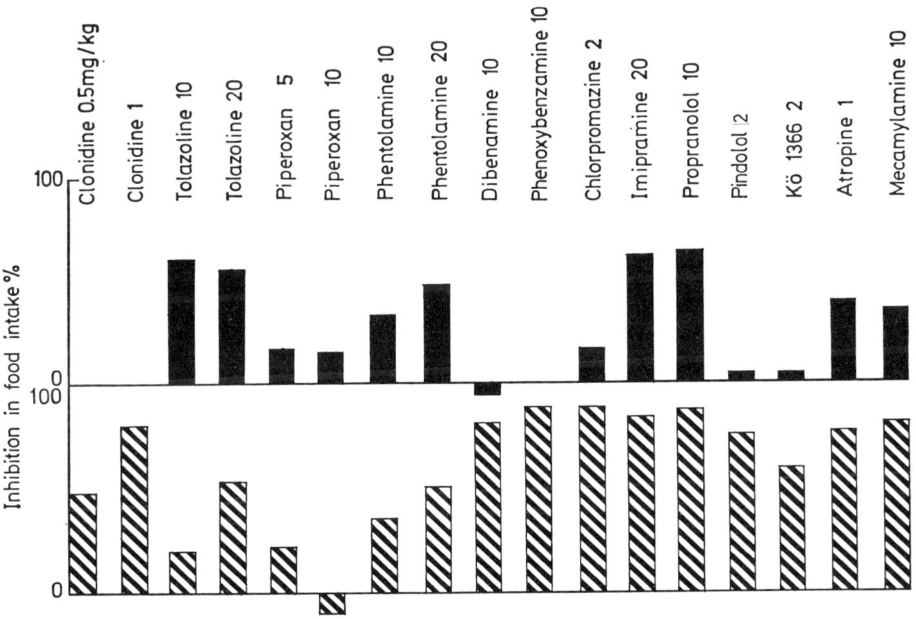

Fig. 29. Influence of adrenergic and cholinergic blocking agents on food intake in rats. The figure shows percentage reduction in food intake. Black columns: effect of adrenergic and cholinergic blocking agents; striped columns: effect of clonidine (0.5 mg/kg and 1 i.p.) and influence thereon of adrenergic and cholinergic blocking agents. Tolazoline, phentolamine and piperoxan decreased the effects of clonidine. Yohimbine has the same effect. 883 F, thymoxamine, azapetine, dibozane, ethomoxane were found ineffective. For antagonistic studies, clonidine at the dosage of 1 mg/kg was used. [LE DOUAREC, J. C., SCHMITT, H., LUCET, B.: J. Pharmacol. (Paris) **3**, 187—198 (1972)]

The other α-sympathomimetic agents naphazoline and tetryzoline have the same effect. BROEKKAMP and VAN ROSSUM (1972) reported similar results with noradrenaline, clonidine and oxymetazoline inducing an increased food intake in rats after administration into the anterior hypothalamus. Phentolamine blocked the effect of clonidine, suggesting an α-sympathomimetic effect. A similar effect of clonidine was reported after intracerebroventricular administration. In half of the animals the large increase in food intake masked the hypnotic effect of the drug (HOLMANN et al., 1971). Similar effects have been obtained in cats by local application of clonidine. Intracerebroventricular injections of clonidine (1 to 10 μg) increased the food intake of satiated cats. In contrast to this, the food intake was reduced after systemic administration (F. KUHN, pers. comm.). BROEKKAMP et al. (1975) suggest the existence of two noradrenergic pathways to control food intake: one leading to an increase and the other to a decrease.

XX. Hypothermic Effect

In doses far higher than clinical ones but well below the toxic dose, *clonidine induced dose-related hypothermia in rats*. The degree and duration of the hypothermia increased with increasing dose (LAVERTY and TAYLOR, 1969).

This response was compared in rats with the effect of other α-sympathomimetic agents, for LOMAX and FORSTER (1969) had reported a fall in body temperature with naphazoline and tetryzoline. In fact, clonidine and L.D. 2855 were the most potent agents. Naphazoline, tramazoline and xylazine were less effective, and tetryzoline was the least active compound. The dose-response curve of oxymetazoline was significantly different from the parallelism that might have been due to toxicological effects (SCHMITT et al., 1971e; TSOUCARIS-KUPFER and SCHMITT, 1972a, b).

It is of interest that intraventricular administration of clonidine in sheep and goats could induce either hypothermia or hyperthermia according to the ambient temperature (MASKREY et al., 1970). At temperatures above the neutral point, hypothermia occured, but at a temperature of 18° C hyperthermia could be observed. The authors discussed the involvement of noradrenergic mechanisms in this response and possible cutaneous vasodilation induced by the inhibition of the sympathetic centers. In rabbits clonidine induced a rise in body temperature as did intracerebroventricular injection of noradrenaline.

In rats the site of action of the hypothermic effect was sought. Intracerebroventricular administration of clonidine did not alter the body temperature, but injection of a small dose of clonidine into the cisterna magna induced a rapid fall in body temperature. Similarly injection of clonidine into the anterior hypothalamus at a dose lower than that required to induce hypothermia by parenteral administration caused a rapid fall in body temperature. However, since with the same dose the hypothermia was lower than after intracisternal injection, other sites of action could be involved (TSOUCARIS-KUPFER and SCHMITT, 1972a, b).

The antagonism between clonidine and adrenoceptor- and cholinoceptor-blocking agents was investigated. Prior administration of tolazoline, phentolamine, dibenamine, phenoxybenzamine and piperoxan reduced the hypothermic effect of clonidine. Chlorpromazine exerted the same effect, probably due to its α adrenoceptor-blocking properties. Imipramine was not effective. The β adrenoceptor-blocking agents propranolol, pindolol and Kö 1366 slightly but significantly decreased this effect, as did atropine, but mecamylamine was ineffective. The same pattern of antagonism was found by intrahypothalamic administration of the drugs but the antagonism was more apparent, in particular for the β adrenoceptor-blocking agents and for atropine. Adrenergic mechanisms were postulated in this effect and also muscarinic ones. It was suggested that both the adrenoceptor-blocking compounds and atropine more easily block the part of the activity due to central actions than that due to peripheral ones (TSOUCARIS-KUPPER and SCHMITT, 1972a, b). Noradrenergic but no dopaminergic mechanisms have been shown to be involved in the hypothermia induced by clonidine and the reserve was seen for piribedil, a dopaminergic agonist (REID et al., 1975).

XXI. Glycemia

In rats *clonidine induces a rise in blood sugar*. This hyperglycemia is caused by two different actions: increased hepatic glycogenolysis (REHBINDER and DECKERS, 1968) and reduced insulin secretion (SENFT et al., 1968). The utilization of glucose is therefore reduced (REHBINDER and DECKERS, 1968). Both phenomena resulted from the activation of peripheral α adrenoceptors (REHBINDER and DECKERS, 1968; SENFT et al., 1968). Clonidine also reduced the increased insulin secretion brought about by glucose; as this effect is antagonized by phentolamine, it must be an α-sympathomimetic one (SENFT et al., 1968).

Adrenalectomy, ganglion-blocking agents and resepine do not alter the hyperglycemic effect of clonidine, thus ruling out adrenal and ganglionic sites of action or noradrenaline release as the cause of this effect (IWATA, 1969). BOCK and VAN ZWIETEN (1971a, b) reported that intravertebral administration of clonidine in rather high dosage induced hypotension, bradycardia and hyperglycemia. This action was localized at central sites, for the same doses administered intravenously did not produce hyperglycemia. This hyperglycemia was reduced by phentolamine, haloperidol and atropine. Previous bilateral adrenalectomy diminished the hyperglycemic effect. BOCK and VAN ZWIETEN (1971b) made the very interesting observation of an increase in the plasma level of somatotropin after clonidine, which could account for the dual central action of the drug, involving hyperglycaemia followed by moderate hypoglycemia. These results suggest that clonidine could be an important tool for investigating the central regulation of glycemia.

In man, clonidine at clinical doses did not change glycemia, insulin levels in blood, and tolerance to glucose or to hypoglycemic sulfonamides (KRAMER et al., 1968; KRAUSE, 1968; WAHL, 1968).

XXII. Spinal Reflexes

In spite of the claim that in cats activation of α adrenoceptors increases the monosynaptic spinal reflexes (BAKER and ANDERSON, 1970), little work has been done on the effects of clonidine on the spinal reflexes. In decerebrate cats, *clonidine reduces the mass polysynaptic reflexes at doses far below those required to reduce monosynaptic reflexes* as measured electrophysiologically (F. KUHN, pers. comm.). The related compound xylazine has also been reported to decrease the flexor reflex at doses far below those required to reduce the patellar reflex in cats anesthetized with chloralose-urethane. The drug was more potent than chlordiazepoxide (KRONEBERG et al., 1967).

The effects of clonidine on spinal reflexes have recently been extensively studied in spinal cats by WAROT (1976). Clonidine infused intravenously in rather high doses (250 μg/kg during 30 minutes) or locally applied on the spinal cord (2 to 5 per 1000) does not change monosynaptic reflexes induced in ventral roots by stimulation of flexor or extensor nerves. In contrast clonidine strongly reduces polysynaptic reflexes induced in ventral roots by stimulation of flexor or extensor nerves. In addition clonidine depresses the variations of activity produced at the level of flexor and extensor motoneurons by means of various influences. Thus clonidine reduces the facilitation of flexor monosynaptic reflexes induced by stimulation of the plantar nerve and the inhibition of extensor monosynaptic reflexes produced by stimulation of the same nerve. In addition the drug reduces the facilitation exerted by stimulation of Ib afferents of an extensor nerve on flexor motoneurons, but does not change the inhibition exerted by stimulation of Ia afferents on these motoneurons. Clonidine antagonizes the Ib inhibition exerted by an extensor nerve on the motoneurons of the agonistic nerve. The drug does not change the amplitude of dorsal root potentials induced by stimulation of Ia flexor and extensor muscular afferents. Clonidine produces a delayed activation of motoneurons to the prolonged stimulation of the ipsilateral sural nerve. L-dopa- and apomorphine have been shown to produce effects similar to those of clonidine.

The effects of clonidine are also seen in reserpinized cats and were therefore suggested to be due to a direct activation of postsynaptic α adrenoceptors. The classical α adrenoceptor-blocking agents, phenoxybenzamine, phentolamine, yohimbine and chlorpromazine, antagonize the effects of clonidine and apomorphine. The dopaminergic blocking agent, pimozide, antagonizes the effects of apomorphine but does not change the effects of clonidine. The 5 HT receptor blocking agent, methysergide, does not change the effects of clonidine and apomorphine. It was therefore concluded that clonidine activates classical α adrenoceptors in the spinal cord, but apomorphine might acts by activation of dopaminergic receptors.

ANDÉN et al. (1970) found that clonidine facilitated flexor reflexes induced by pinching of the paw in spinal rats. High doses of phenoxybenzamine antagonized this effect. Haloperidol has been reported to induce a similar antagonism, but the classical α adrenoceptor blocking agents, phentolamine, yohimbine, piperoxan and tolazoline, were only slightly effective. In contrast yohimbine, piperoxan, and tolazoline, but not phenoxybenzamine or haloperidol markedly antagonized the disappearance of noradrenaline in the spinal cord and brain of rats and in the brain of mice induced by α-methyl-p-tyrosine treatment. Therefore it was concluded that the postsynaptic functional effects and the biochemical effects of clonidine may be due to stimulation on different α adrenoceptors (ANDÉN et al., 1976).

XXIII. Neuro-Endocrine Effects

Although noradrenergic mechanisms have been involved in the secretion of pituitary hormones, the effects of clonidine on these mechanisms has been rarely investigated. *Clonidine has been shown to reduce corticosteroid secretion* from the adrenal glands after intravenous injection as well as after administration into the third ventricle of pentobarbitalized dogs; this reduction in ACTH secretion was abolished by phenoxybenzamine administered into the third ventricle (GANONG et al., 1975a, b). *Clonidine increased the level of somatotropin in the plasma* after intravenous administration, but even in high doses the drug was ineffective after injection into the third ventricle of pentobarbitalized dogs. However the effect of clonidine on somatotropin release is thought to be centrally mediated for administration of low dose of phenoxybenzamine into the third ventricle abolished this effect (GANONG et al., 1975a, b). In acromegalic man, clonidine has been shown to increase the level of somatotropin in the plasma and this effect was not prevented by a small dose of yohimbine (GILBERT et al., 1976). Clonidine has been reported to inhibit vasopressin secretion (KOBINGER, 1968; HUMPHREY and REID, 1975), (p. 355).

XXIV. Aggressivity

In 1968 Morpurgo reported *aggressivity* (biting attacks) in *mice after high doses of clonidine*. This effect was antagonized by neuroleptic drugs and diazepam. This observation was of considerable interest. Aggressivity after clonidine has been shown in other animal species. In chronic experiments, clonidine (0.2 mg/kg) reduced nocturnal activity in white rats but induced violent bouts of activity consisting of fighting behavior involving some and occasionally all members of the group. Black rats were irritable and difficult to handle after clonidine, but did not show this violent fighting behavior (Laverty and Taylor, 1969). Renal hypertensive dogs were irritable and attacked the experimenter in chronic treatment (Laubie and Schmitt, unpubl. observations). Kuhn (pers. comm.) found that cats became aggressive after clonidine and made the very interesting observation that this type of aggressive behavior resembles that encountered after destruction of the septal nucleus which induces theta rhythm in the hippocampus of intact animals. Clonidine has been shown to induce at very high doses automutilation in mice (Razak et al., 1975).

In contrast, clonidine seems to reduce some other types of aggressive behavior. Pain-induced aggression is reduced in black rats by clonidine, perhaps due to the antinociceptive action of the drug (Laverty and Taylor, 1969). In Carroll and Lim's method clonidine reduced all the behavioral responses to pain to about the same extent; biting of the electrodes, which could be considered as a manifestation of pain-induced aggressive behavior was also reduced (Schmitt et al., 1974b). In the cat, clonidine does not reduce the aggressivity induced by amygdaloid stimulation (F. Kuhn, pers. comm.).

Pretreatment with atropine or other parasympatholytic agents very markedly increases the aggressive behavior induced by clonidine or xylazine (unpubl. observations). Lithium chloride has been reported to increase in mice the aggressive behavior caused by clonidine (Ozawa et al., 1975).

XXV. Actions on Neurons in the Central Nervous System

Three investigations were concerned with the effects of clonidine on the firing of neurons. Anderson and Stone (1973a, b) applied clonidine and noradrenaline by microiontophoresis to single neurons of the cerebral cortex and medullary reticular formation of anesthetized rats. Most of the units responded in the same manner to both noradrenaline and clonidine. The usual response was a depression of the firing rate. Bulbocapnine antagonized some responses to clonidine and noradrenaline whilst leaving unaffected similar responses to 5-hydroxytryptamine. On 13% of the cells clonidine produced an increase of firing rate. It was concluded that clonidine could have an action on noradrenaline receptors in the brain. Svensson et al. (1975) studied the effects of clonidine on the cells of the locus coeruleus and of the raphe median. Clonidine was shown to reduce the firing rate of the neurons in both nuclei. Pretreatment with intacerebroventricular 6-hydroxydopamine did not change the effects on the neurons of the locus coeruleus, but suppressed the effects on the neurons of raphe median nucleus. These latter were thought to be due to an effect exerted by noradrenergic or adrenergic pathways. As the cells of the locus coeruleus contrained noradrenaline it was suggested that clonidine acts on adrenaline receptors (cf. p. 361) reducing noradrenaline release and inducing therefore sedation. Skolnick et al. (1976b) found that clonidine reduced by a nonspecific effect the firing rate of cerebellar Purkinje cells and did not change the depressant effect of noradrenaline. In this investigation clonidine was thought to be an α adrenoceptor-blocking agent in view of previous biochemical experiments (SKOLNICK and DAVY, 1975, 1976a). However the possibility remains that in this system clonidine could mimic the effects of noradrenaline.

XXVI. Effects of Clonidine on Excitation and Excitation-Contraction Coupling

A strong local anesthetic effect was noted for clonidine by HOEFKE and KOBINGER (1966), although the concentrations used far exceeded those used in animal and man; this finding was confirmed (WASHIZU, 1971; STARKE et al., 1972).

WASHIZU (1971) reported that clonidine broadened the action potential of the isolated sensory neurons of the crayfish stretch-receptor organ. The amplitude and the rate of rise and fall of the action potential were decreased by clonidine at concentrations of 0.5 to 2 mM, although the critical firing level was not changed. A clear increase in membrane resistance was observed at 2 mM. The effect was very similar to that of procaine. Blockade of antidromic conduction was seldom observed following administration of clonidine or procaine, in spite of the great retardation of the rising phase of action potential.

Some differences were found in the action of clonidine on atrium and ventricular papillary muscles. A low concentration of clonidine increased the contractile force of spontaneously beating atrium (HOEFKE and KOBINGER, 1966; WASHIZU, 1970), but no action was found on atrium driven by electrical pulses (WASHIZU, 1972). In contrast, clonidine increased the contractile force of ventricular papillary muscle driven by electrical pulses (WASHIZU, 1972). With high concentrations a decrease in the contractile force and the rate was seen for both tissues. In atrial cells the duration of the action potential was found to be increased; the most prominent effect was the prolongation of the falling phase; the effect of clonidine was relatively greater at zero membrane potential level than at the half-height of the action potential. These effects on the action potential appeared even when the contractile force was depressed. They could be reversed by increasing the calcium level, although the ion had a more marked mechanical effect (WASHIZU, 1970). The positive inotropic effect was explained by a lengthening of the mechanically effective period of the action potential, and the bradycardia by the retardation of repolarization. The negative inotropic effect was due to the decoupling of the action potential and contraction resulting from inhibited calcium activity. The action was explained by a delayed recovery of sodium conductance, which increased during the rising phase of the action potential (WASHIZU, 1970).

The effect of clonidine on ventricular papillary muscle cells was in low concentration to shorten the action potential and to slow the late rising phase, an action similar to that of noradrenaline; the prolongation of the action potential appeared at much higher concentrations than with the atrium. The differences on the contractile force could be explained by a decoupling effect of the drug which prevailed on the atrium over the effect of prolongation of action potential (WASHIZU, 1972).

These effects could hardly play a role *in vivo*, due to the high concentrations used.

XXVII. Influence on Monoamine Metabolism in the Brain

Clonidine does not change the level of catecholamines in the brain (HOEFKE and KOBINGER, 1966; LAVERTY and TAYLOR, 1969; ANDÉN et al., 1970; PERSSON, 1970; PERSSON and WALDECK, 1970; BRALET et al., 1973a, b, c). A slight increase in noradrenaline or dopamine levels has occassionally been reported after high doses of clonidine (LAVERTY and TAYLOR, 1969; PERSSON and WALDECK, 1970). The increased dopamine levels in the corpus striatum could account for the stereotypies seen with high doses of the drug (PERSSON and WALDECK, 1970).

However, clonidine is not without any action on catecholamine metabolism. In fact, clonidine *slowed the disappearance of noradrenaline in the brain* after inhibition of tyrosine hydroxylase with α-methyl-*p*-tyrosine (ANDÉN et al., 1970, 1976; BRALET et al., 1973a, b, c; ROCHETTE et al., 1974). Phenoxybenzamine at high dosage was devoid of any action of its own on noradrenaline metabolism but antagonized the effects of clonidine (ANDÉN et al., 1970). Piperoxan and yohimbine were more potent to antagonize this effect that phenoxybenzamine was. The reverse was true for the inhibition of the increase of flexor reflex in spinalized rats. ANDÉN et al. (1976) hypothesized that clonidine activates presynaptic α adrenoceptors in the brain. BOLME et al. (1975) suggested that clonidine acts on adrenaline receptors located on noradrenergic neurons. Both phenomena have been proposed to be responsible for the reduction of noradrenaline release (p. 361). These facts provide evidence of a reduced turnover rate after clonidine probably due to an α-sympathomimetic effect. They were taken to indicate activation of α adrenoceptors in the brain by clonidine, which in turn decreased the turnover rate of noradrenaline by a transsynaptic effect. Clonidine at high dosage increased the storage of ^{3}H-noradrenaline without changing the concentration of metabolites (LAVERTY and TAYLOR, 1969).

Since this effect was more apparent in the medulla obongata, it was suggested that this area is the main site of action of the drug which would explain the suppression of sympathetic tone. Clonidine reduces the release of noradrenaline in the brain of rats and also reduces the concentration of *m*-methoxy-*p*-hydroxyphenylglycol (BRAESTRUP, 1974).

Clonidine does not change and sometimes increases dopamine levels in the brain (ANDÉN et al., 1970; PERSSON and WALDECK, 1970).

Dopamine turnover showed only a slight reduction under the influence of clonidine, an effect antagonized by phenoxybenzamine, thus indicating that noradrenaline receptor stimulation, directly or to a certain extent indirectly, may inhibit the neural activity of the dopamine neurons (ANDÉN et al., 1970; ROCHETTE and BRALET, 1975).

Clonidine reduces the turnover rate of 5-hydroxytryptamine measured by the rate of disappearance of the amine after inhibition of tryptophan hydroxylase with dopacetamide. The reduced turnover rate of 5-hydroxytryptamine after treatment with clonidine could be counteracted by injecting phenoxybenzamine or haloperidol before clonidine. As these agents act by blocking noradrenaline but not 5-hydroxytryptamine receptors, the clonidine-induced retardation of 5-hydroxytryptamine turnover may be due to the loss of the inhibition of 5-hydroxytryptamine neurons normally exerted by noradrenaline (ANDÉN et al., 1970).

XXVIII. Metabolism

Investigations of *the metabolism of clonidine* were difficult owing to the small effective dosage.

Experiments were performed with ^{14}C-clonidine in rats, dogs, monkeys and man (CHO and CURRY, 1969; REHBINDER and DECKERS, 1966, 1968, 1969; DECKERS and REHBINDER, 1968; REHBINDER, 1970; EHRHARDT, 1972a, b). The gastrointestinal absorption of the drug was shown to be rapid and peak plasma concentrations were reached in 1 to 2 h, the elimination constant being 0.23 h^{-1}.

Clonidine is distributed all over the body; the highest concentrations were found in the organs of elimination: kidney, gut and liver. Clonidine was also found in high concentrations in the spleen and in the submaxillary glands, where a concentration 40 to 60 times that in plasma was reached (CHO et al., 1969). Surprisingly, the concentration in the brain was the lowest found, but was twice the plasma concentration (EHRHARDT, 1972b).

The high concentration found in the gut suggests an entero-hepatic cycle, and indeed, in rats clonidine has been shown to be excreted into the bile at rather high concentrations.

In the blood of rats 40 to 50% of clonidine is bound to plasma protein (CHO and CURRY, 1969).

Clonidine is metabolized and up to the present at least seventeen derivatives have been detected (REHBINDER and DECKERS, 1966, 1968, 1969; EHRHARDT, 1972b; HODGES, 1976). The percentage of the drug metabolized varies with animal species, being greater in rats and monkeys than in man and dogs. In rats, clonidine is parahydroxylated and *p*-hydroxyclonidine and its glycuroconjugate were found to be the principal metabolites. In this animal species two other metabolites appear to be oxidation products of *p*-hydroxyclonidine. *p*-Hydroxyclonidine injected intravenously has been found in the brain of the rat to only a small extent, suggesting that clonidine is metabolized at a peripheral site (EHRHARDT, 1972b). *p*-Hydroxy clonidine has not been detected in dogs and man, although several metabolites of clonidine were found. *p*-Hydroxyclonidine was reported to lack the pharmacological properties of clonidine, but EHRHARDT (1972b) has detected peripheral and central effects for the compound: *p*-hydroxyclonidine injected parenterally increased blood pressure in rats without any secondary decrease in blood pressure; injected into the cisterna magna, *p*-hydroxyclonidine induced a fall in blood pressure. These experiments suggest that *p*-hydroxyclonidine does not cross the blood-brain barrier (EHRHARDT, 1972b). Recently 2,6-(dichlorophenyl)guanidine has been shown to be a metabolite of clonidine (HODGES, 1976).

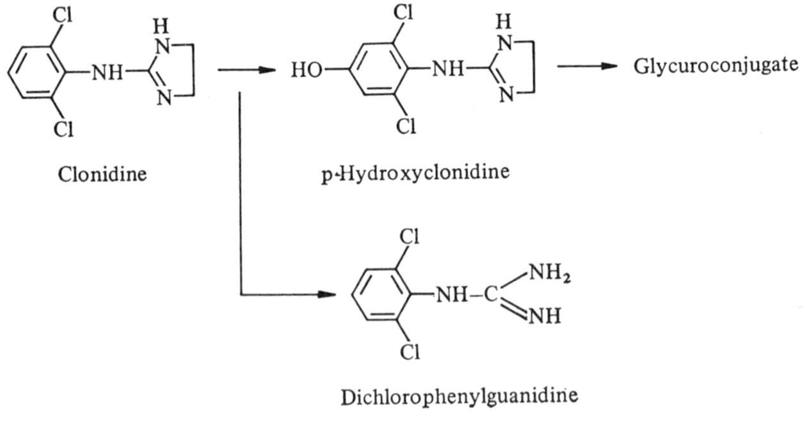

Clonidine is eliminated in urine and in part in feces; in rats 46% of the total radioactivity is eliminated in urine after 6 h and 33% in feces after 48 h. Two thirds of the clonidine in urine and one third in feces is unchanged; 10 to 20% is eliminated in the bile. In dogs and man, elimination is slower but the percentage eliminated by each route seems to be the same.

The half-life of clonidine has been reported to be 3 h in rats (CHO and CURRY, 1969), 10 h (REHBINDER, 1970) in dogs, and about 20 h in monkeys and man (DARDA, 1975; FRYDMAN et al., 1975; DOLLERY et al., 1976). In rats two curves of decay has been found in the liver and in the blood ($k_1 = 0.693$ and $k_2 = 0.077$); in the brain only a curve has been found (EHRHARDT, 1972b).

XXIX. Related Compounds

Many derivatives of clonidine have been mentioned in patents, but detailed pharmacological data are available for only a few. WERMUTH et al. (1973) and recently TIMMERMANS (personal communication) compared the pharmacological properties of a number of imidazoline derivatives, and in addition their lipophilicity. He presented interesting speculations on their structure from the view point of quantum chemistry.

LAVERTY (1970) compared the antihypertensive and behavioral effects of some imidazoline derivatives. In fact these compounds were less potent than clonidine was. *St600* [2-(2-methyl-5-fluorophenylamino)-2-imidazoline] has been mentioned to be about 10 times less potent than clonidine in animals and man but the sedative effects for an equipotent antihypertensive action have been reported to be less than those of clonidine (KHO et al., 1975a, b). However a reappraisal of the effects of the drug leads to the conclusion that the difference was due to a slight liposolubility of St600, leading to a slow accumulation into the brain. When the equilibrium between the levels in plasma and brain are reached the effects appear similar to those of clonidine (BOERHINGER, Ingelheim, personal communication).

St91 [2-(2,6-diethylphenylamino)-2-imidazoline] is an interesting compound. Intravenous injection of this drug induces only a pressor response, a bradycardia and a fall in cardiac output, but the secondary fall in blood pressure seen with clonidine is not seen (HOEFKE et al., 1975; TISNÉ-VERSAILLES, personal communication). The discharges of the sino-carotid nerve are increased after St91 even when blood pressure recovered control values (TISNÉ-VERSAILLES, personal communication). Injected into the cisterna magna of cats, St91 reduces blood pressure, but at higher doses than those of clonidine (HOEFKE et al., 1975; KOBINGER and PILCHER, 1975c; SCRIABINE et al., 1975), but conflicting results have been reported (TISNÉ-VERSAILLES, personal communication). In dogs intracisternal administration of St91 does not change blood pressure and sympathetic discharges (KOBINGER and PILCHER, 1975c; TISNÉ-VERSAILLES, personal communication). However by this route, St91 potentiates the bradycardic response to an increase in blood pressure (KOBINGER and PILCHER, 1975c) as clonidine does. It has been suggested that lack of depressor response was due to a difficulty of the compound to cross the blood brain (HOEFKE et al., 1975c). However this explanation does not seem to be the alone one, as St91 does not induce sleep in chickens, in which the blood brain barrier is lacking. This compound, on the other hand induces slow-wave sleep in mammals (TISNÉ-VERSAILLES, pers. com.).

Tiamenidine (Hoe-440,2-methyl-4-chlorothiophene-2-phenylamino)-2- imidazoline) was reported to be ten times less potent than clonidine as an antihypertensive agent, but the sedative action induced by the drug was found to be less pronounced than those produced by clonidine for a similar reduction in blood pressure (LINDNER and KAISER, 1974; SIMON et al., 1976).

Some *oxazoline* derivatives have been shown to possess properties similar to those of clonidine. LD 2855 (2,6-dimethylphenylamino) 2-Δ_2-oxazoline) was probably the first agent described with clonidine like properties (BEAUVALLET et al., 1958; GIUDICELLI et al., 1958). GIUDICELLI and SCHMITT (1970) reported a more extensive study of this compound. The pharmacological properties of LD 2855 were found to be similar to those of clonidine qualitatively and quantitatively.

The pharmacology of Bay a 6781, an oxazoline compound has not been reported in details; its effect in inhibiting noradrenaline release has been described (WERNER et al., 1970, 1972). The drug reduces blood pressure when injected in small doses into the cerebral ventricle of the brain in cats. This effect has been reported to be antagonized by the α adrenoceptor blocking compound phentolamine (JACOBS et al., 1972).

Xylazine [2-(2,6-dimethylphenylamino)-4H-5-6-dihydro 1,3 thiazine] is a drug, the pharmacological properties of which were described by KRONEBERG et al. (1966, 1967). It has been reported at first as a blocker of noradrenergic and cholinergib fibers and the hypotensive activity was ascribed to this action. However SCHMITT et al. (1970) reported a decrease in sympathetic nerve activity with this compound even in debuffered animals. The effects are very similar to those of clonidine and the main site of action has been localized into the medulla oblongata by transection experiments. HEISE and KRONEBERG (1970, 1971) reported a decrease in blood pressure when xylazine was infused into the cisterna magna and the third ventricle of the brain of cats. This effect was antagonized by previous infusion in these cavities of phentolamine or phenoxybenzamine. These experiments afford further support for the activation of a noradrenergic receptor in this effect. Xylazine increases the vagal tone and the activity of the baroreceptor reflex in dogs by a central action (ANTONACCIO et al., 1973). Xylazine has been shown to reduce the effects of the stimulation of postganglionic sympathetic fibers, probably by an action on presynaptic α adrenoceptors (ANTONACCHIO et al., 1973). The sedative and antinociceptive effects of xylazine were shown to be very pronounced in regard to the antihypertensive action (KRONEBERG et al., 1967). The compound was used in anesthesiology in man and in veterinary medicine. Xylazine appears therefore to have properties very similar to those of clonidine, although at higher doses. However some actions appear to be different. Xylazine reduced the duration of after-discharges induced by amygdaloïd stimulation, but like clonidine, increased the duration of after-discharges induces by hippocampal stimulation (KUHN, personal communication).

Guanabenz (2,6-dichlorobenzylidene aminoguanidine, Wy 8678) is an α-sympathomimetic agent of a different chemical structure. Its effects on the cardiovascular system were shown to be very similar to those of clonidine (BAUM et al., 1969, 1970; NATOFF et al., 1968; NATOFF and STANTON, 1969). The drug reduces sympathetic discharges in the cat (BAUM and SHROPHIRE, 1970; BAUM et al., 1970; BAUM and SHROPSHIRE, 1976). This effect has been shown to be reduced by phentolamine (BAUM and SHROPSHIRE, 1976). Unlike to clonidine, guanabenz does not amplify the discharges of the sino-carotid nerve in cats (BAUM and SHOPSHIRE, 1976). Gunabenz reduces the turnover rate of noradrenaline in the brain, an effect suggested to be the consequence of stimulation of α adrenoceptors (BOLME et al., 1973).

SAH 43663 is a hydroxylated derivative of guanabenz. It was found to be 10 times less effective than clonidine was. However its pharmacological properties do not appear to be different.

Lofexidine is another derivative with activity quantitatively and qualitatively similar to those of clonidine.

BS 100-41 is another drug inducing cardiovascular actions similar to those of clonidine. It reduces sympathetic nerve activity after intravenous as well after intracerebroventricular administration. The drug was found about 20 to 40 times

Related compounds

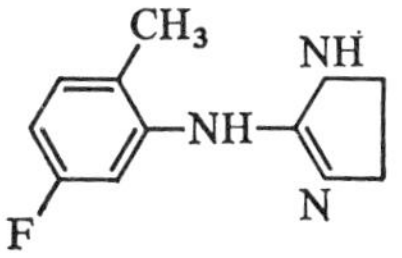

St 600

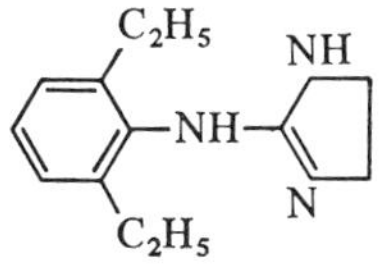

St 91

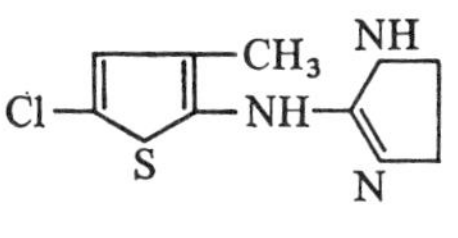

Thiamenidine (Hoe 440)

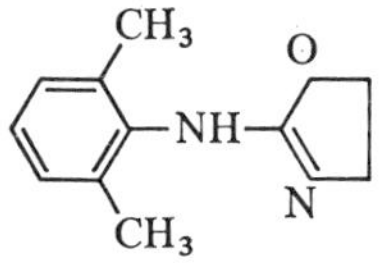

L.D. 2855

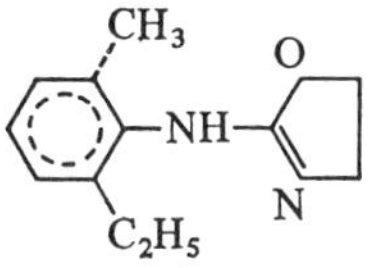

Bay a 6781

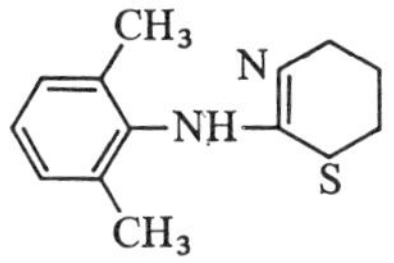

Xylazine (Bay 1470)

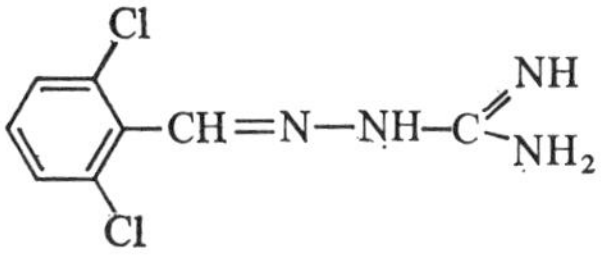

Guanabenz (Wy 8678)

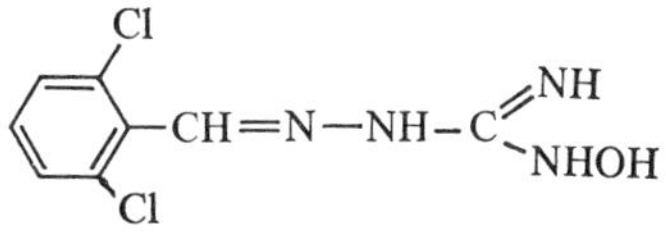

SAH 43 663

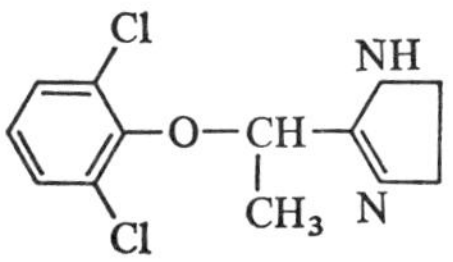

Lofexidine (Ba 160)

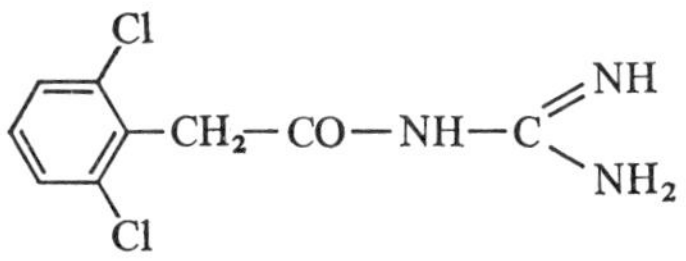

BS 100·141 (Sandoz)

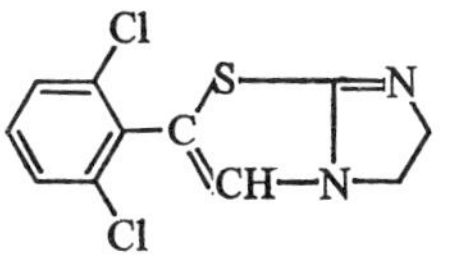

44.549/1. (Sandoz USA)

less potent than clonidine was (SCHOLTYSIK, 1974; SAAMELI et al., 1975). The drug reduces the effects of postganglionic sympathetic fibers stimulation (PACHA et al., 1975). However the mechanism of action of the drug appears to be different. In contrast to clonidine, the application of the drug on the S zone of the ventral surface of the medulla oblongata does not induce a fall in blood pressure (SCHOLTY-

SICK, 1974). BS 100-141 has been reported in cats to suppress paradoxical sleep, but in contrast to clonidine, it does not increase the duration of the total sleep (KLEINLOGEL et al., 1975).

44.594/15 (Sandoz USA) appears to be a very effective drug for reducing centrally blood pressure (VAN ZWIETEN, 1975a), but its other pharmacological properties were not described.

XXX. Conclusion

As mentioned at the beginning of this review, clonidine appears to be a valuable tool for investigating central noradrenergic mechanisms. The proposal that clonidine is a central as well as a peripheral α-sympathomimetic agent is based on several kinds of evidence: (a) there is a natural trend to link the different actions of drugs; (b) clonidine decreases the noradrenaline turnover rate in the central nervous system (ANDÉN et al., 1970) and this effect is generally accepted as due to the activation of adrenergic receptors, which by a negative feedback mechanism lead to decreased noradrenaline synthesis; (c) the central effects of clonidine were shown to be antagonized by some α adrenoceptor-blocking agents; the decreased noradrenaline turnover rate was also abolished by phenoxybenzamine at high dosage (ANDÉN et al., 1970).

However, were such a hypothesis accepted, it would imply that the central receptors were different from the peripheral ones, and that several kinds of central receptors were involved. This assumption is based (a) on the different potency of α-sympathomimetic agents in eliciting central responses and activating peripheral adrenergic receptors, and (b) on the selectivity of α adrenoceptor-blocking drugs in antagonizing the central effects of clonidine.

In the peripheral sympathetic system clonidine has been shown to activate pre- as well as postsynaptic α adrenoceptors. Some workers suggested that—at least—some central actions of clonidine might be due to an activation of central presynaptic α adrenoceptors. Clonidine reduced noradrenaline release in cortical slices likely by an effect on presynaptic α adrenoceptors; in fact, this effect was antagonized by some α adrenoceptor blocking agents (STARKE and MONTEL, 1973a, b). Desipramine was shown—in some circumstances—to antagonize the central hypotensive effect of clonidine and this antagonism was ascribed to an indirectly mediated effect of the drug (BRIANT et al., 1973; REID et al., 1973). However VAN SPANNING and VAN ZWIETEN (1973), VAN ZWIETEN (1975b) suggest that desipramine blocked central postsynaptic α adrenoceptors. Pretreatment of rabbits with intracerebroventricular administration of 6-hydroxydopamine has been reported to reduce the hypotensive effect of intracisternal injection of clonidine, suggesting an indirectly mediated effect for clonidine (DOLLERY and REID, 1973); however in this investigation, blood pressure of treated rabbits was lower than blood pressure of control rabbits precluding any definite conclusion. In fact other workers found evidence against an indirectly mediated effect for clonidine. Pretreatment of cats with reserpine and α-methyl-*p*-tyrosine in order to deplete noradrenaline and to inhibit catecholamine synthesis did not change the reducing effect of clonidine on sympathetic discharges (HAEUSLER, 1973a, b; KOBINGER and PICHLER, 1976) or the potentiation of the vagal cardiodepressor reflex induced by the drug (KOBINGER and PICHLER, 1974, 1975b).

ANDÉN et al. (1976) suggest that some central effects of clonidine might be due to an activation of central presynaptic α adrenoceptors, but that other effects might be due to an activation of central postsynaptic α adrenoceptors. In fact clonidine was less potent in stimulating hind limbs flexor reflex activity of spinal rats than in inhibiting the α-methyl-*p*-tyrosine induced disappearance of noradrenaline in the spinal cord and in the whole brain. The increase in flexor activity due to clonidine was virtually completely inhibited by phenoxybenzamine and haloperidol but was only partially inhibited by yohimbine and piperoxan in high doses and was not changed by tolazoline. The potentiation by clonidine of the apomorphine induced locomotor stimulation of reserpine treated mice was almost completely inhibited by phenoxybenzamine, not affected by yohimbine and only slightly inhibited by tolazoline. The inhibition of the α-methyl-*p*-tyrosine induced disappearance of noradrenaline in the spinal cord and in the whole brain was reduced by yohimbine, piperoxan or tolazoline, but not by phenoxybenzamine or haloperidol. Clonidine caused an inhibition of the accumulation of L-dopa after dopa-decarboxylase inhibition in noradrenaline rich regions of the rat central nervous system. This effect is antagonized by yohimbine, piperoxan and tolazoline but not by phenoxybenzamine. Thus phenoxybenzamine seems to act mainly on postsynaptic α adrenoceptors as the drug inhibited the effects of clonidine after reserpinization. ANDÉN et al. (1976) suggested that the biochemical effects of clonidine might be due to an activation of presynaptic α adrenoceptors and that yohimbine, piperoxan and tolazoline might preferentially block these receptors. Accordingly the effect of clonidine preferentially blocked by phenoxybenzamine might be due to the activation of postsynaptic α adrenoceptors, but the effects of clonidine more easely blocked by yohimbine, piperoxan and tolazoline might be ascribed to the stimulation of presynaptic α adrenoceptors. However BOLME et al. (1974) proposed another concept. Piperoxan and yohimbine blocked the hypotensive and respiratory effects of clonidine in chloralosed rats at doses which did not change clonidine induced increase in flexor activity. Furthermore piperoxan and yohimbine increased brain noradrenaline turnover. The authors suggest that clonidine acts on "adrenaline receptors" which mediate hypotensive and respiratory effects. Piperoxan and yohimbine were thought to block these adrenaline receptors.

However, clonidine does not activate cerebral adenylate cyclase as do α-sympathomimetic agents. On the contrary the drug has been shown to antagonize the accumulation of cAMP elicited by noradrenaline and methoxamine. Therefore the drug seems to act as an α adrenoceptor blocking agent on this biochemical system (SKOLNICK and DALY, 1975). On the other hand clonidine potentiated the accumulation of cAMP induced by isoproterenol and this effect was antagonized by some α adrenoceptor blocking agents, suggesting the activation of central α adrenoceptors in this effect (SKOLNICK et al., 1975; 1976a).

As pimozide – an assumed specific dopaminergic receptor blocking agent – antagonizes the hypotensive effect of clonidine applied on the ventral surface of the medulla oblongata, an activation by clonidine of dopaminergic receptors has been suggested (BLOCH et al., 1974). However recently BLUMBERG et al. (1975) questioned the specificity of pimozide for blocking dopaminergic receptors; in fact pimozide was shown to block the activation of central adenylate cyclase induced by noradrenaline but did not change the activation caused by dopamine or 5-hydroxytryptamine. Piperoxan, but not pimozide blocked the behavioral effects of clonidine and the reverse was true for those of apomorphine (TSOUCARIS-KUPFER et al., 1973).

Some interactions between *clonidine and dopaminergic mechanisms* have been detected. Clonidine enhanced the stereotyped behavior elicited by apomorphine, L-dopa and *d*-amphetamine in animals pretreated with reserpine, α-methyl-*p*-tyrosine and the specific dopamine-β-hydroxylase inhibitor FLA 63 (ANDÉN et al., 1970, 1973, 1976; MAJ et al., 1972). The combination of apomorphine and clonidine also increased locomotor activity in mice (MAJ et al., 1972). However in parkinsonian patients clonidine was found to reduce the therapeutic effect of L-dopa and piribedil (Shoulson and Chase, 1976). Early clinical trials of clonidine in psychotic patients suggest that clonidine reduced hallucinations in delusional states and anxiety (Daskalopoulos et al., 1977; unpublished results).

Clonidine might activate histamine H_2 receptors in the brain (p. 335) and in some conditions histamine H_2 antagonists were able to block the hypotensive effects of clonidine by a central action (Karppanen et al., 1976). However the implications of these experiments are not known.

The central effects of clonidine seem to be at best explained by an activation of α adrenoceptors present in the brain. Some of these receptors ressemble the classical peripheral postsynaptic α adrenoceptors, but many other are alike the peripheral presynaptic α adrenoceptors. In fact, yohimbine and piperoxan were found to antagonize strongly the central effects of clonidine as well as the effects on the presynaptic α adrenoceptors (Drew, 1976), but the potent α adrenoceptor blocking agent thymoxamine is ineffective on the central and presynaptic (Drew, 1976) receptors. It is not yet known whether all the central receptors are located presynaptically or whether some are situated postsynaptically. The activation of these central α adrenoceptors might modify the functioning of other biochemical systems, but the implications of these alterations are not as yet understood.

The activation of central α adrenoceptors seems to account for the effects of clonidine. However, other effects seem also to be involved buth their inportance is not explained.

References

Aars, H.: Effects of clonidine on aortic diameter and aortic baroreceptor activity. Europ. J. Pharmacol. **20**, 52—59 (1972).

Alexandre, J.-M., Chevillard, C., Ménard, J., Schmitt, H.: Rôle des récepteurs α-adrénergiques dans la sécrétion de rénine du rat. J. Pharmacol. (Paris) **4** 412—413 (1973).

Andén, N. E., Corrodi, H., Fuxe, K., Hökfelt, B., Hökfelt, T., Rydin, K., Svensson, T.: Evidence for a central noradrenaline receptor stimulation by clonidine. Life Sci. **9**, 513—523 (1970).

Andén, N. E., Grabowska, M., Strömbom, W.: Different alpha-adrenoceptors in the central nervous system mediating biochemical and functional effects of clonidine and receptor blocking agents. Arch. Pharmacol. **292**, 43—52 (1976).

Andén, N. E., Strömbom, U., Svensson, T. H.: Dopamine and noradrenaline receptor stimulation: reversal of reserpine induced suppression of motor activity. Psychopharmacologia (Berl.) **29**, 289—298 (1973).

Anderson, C., Stone, T. W.: The effect on clonidine on single cortical and medullary neurones Brit. J. Pharmacol. **49**, 176—177P (1973a).

Anderson, C., Stone, T. W.: On the mechanism of action of clonidine: effects on single central neurones. Brit. J. Pharmacol. **51**, 259—365 (1973b).

Antonaccio, M. J.: Reflex responses to vertical tilting in dogs: a comparison with bilateral carotid occlusion. Pharmacologist **13**, 192 (1971).

Antonaccio, M. J.: The effect of clonidine (St155) on adrenergic nerve function in intact and vagotomized animals. Fifth International Congress on Pharmacology, Abstracts of volunteer papers, **8**, 44 (1972).

Antonaccio, M. J., Haley, J.: Studies on the mechanism and brain stem site of action of the hypotensive, bradycardic and reflex-enhancing actions of clonidine in cats. Fed. Proc. **35**, 323 (no. 655) (1976).

Antonaccio, M. J., Halley, J., Kerwin, L.: Functional significance of α-stimulation and α-blockade on responses to cardiac nerve stimulation in anesthetized dogs. Life Sci. **15**, 765—777 (1974).

Antonaccio, M. J., Robson, R. D.: The effect of clonidine on adrenergic nerve function in vagotomized and non vagotomized animals. J. Pharmacol. exp. Ther. **184**, 631—640 (1973).

Antonaccio, M. J., Robson, R. D., Burrell, R.: Effects of clonidine on baroreceptor function in anesthetized dogs. Europ. J. Pharmacol. **30**, 6—14 (1975).

ANTONACCIO, M. J., ROBSON, R. D., KERWIN, L.: Evidence for increased vagal tone and enhancement of baroreceptor reflex activity after xylazine, (2-(2,6-dimethylphenylamino)-4H-5,6 dihydro-1,3 thiazine) in anesthetized dogs. Europ. J. Pharmacol. **23**, 311—315 (1973).

ARMSTRONG, J. M., BOURA, A. L. A.: Effects of clonidine and guanethidine on peripheral sympathetic nerve function in the pithed rat. Brit. J. Pharmacol. **47**, 850—852 (1973)

AUDIGIER, Y., VIRION, A., SCHWARTZ, J. CH.: Stimulation of cerebral histamine H_2-receptors by clonidine. Nature (Lond.) **262**, 307—308 (1976).

AUTRET, A., MINZ, M., BELLEVAIRE, T., CACHERA, H. P., SCHMITT, H.: The REM sleep suppressing effect of α adrenostimulation in human C.N.S. Europ. J. of Clin. Pharmacol. (in press).

AUTRET, A. M., SCHMITT, H., FÉNARD, S., PÉTILLOT, N.: Comparison of haemodynamic effects of α-sympathomimetic drugs. Europ. J. Pharmacol. **13**, 208—217 (1971).

BAER, L., BRUNNER, H. R., BARD, R., LARAGH, J. H.: Suppression of renin and aldosterone by clonidine. Ann. intern. Med. **74**, 830 (1971).

BAKER, R. G., ANDERSON, E. G.: The antagonism of the effects of L-3-4-dihydroxy-phenylalanine on spinal reflexes by adrenergic blocking agents. J. Pharmacol. exp. Ther. **173**, 224—231 (1970).

BARAC, G.: Effect immédiat de la 2-(2,6-dichlorophénylamino)-2-imidazoline (St 155) sur la diurèse et le débit sanguin rénal chez le chien. C.R. Soc. Biol. (Paris) **164**, 2406—2409 (1971).

BARNETT, A. J., CANTOR, S.: Observations on the hypotensive action of Catapres (St 155) in man. Med. J. Aust. **1**, 87—91 (1968).

BARTMUS, D., GUMULKA, S. W., DINNENDAHL, V., SCHONHOFER, P. S.: Brain cyclic nucleotides and adrenolytics: effects on amphetamine and apomorphine induced changes. Arch. Pharmacol. **294** (Suppl.) R 11 (1976).

BAUM, P.: Experimentelle Untersuchungen zur Nieren-Hämodynamik und zum Verhalten der Elektrolyte nach einmaliger Verabreichung von 2-(2,6-Dichlorophenylamino)-2-Imidazolin-hydrochlorid. Arzneimittel-Forsch. **16**, 1162—1165 (1966).

BAUM, T., ECKFELD, D. K., METZ, N., DINISH, J. L., ROWLES, G., VAN PELT, R., SHROPSHIRE, A. J., FERNANDEZ, S. P., GLUCKMAN, M. I., BRUCE, N. F.: 2,6-Dichlorobenzylidene aminoguanidine acetate (W-8678) a new hypotensive agent. Experientia (Basel) **25**, 1066—1067 (1969).

BAUM, T., SHROPSHIRE, A. T.: Inhibition of spontaneous sympathetic nerve activity by the antihypertensive agent, Wy-8678. Neuropharmacology **9**, 503—506 (1970).

BAUM, T., SHROPSHIRE, A. T.: Studies on the centrally mediated hypotensive action of guanabenz. Europ. J. Pharmacol. **37**, 31—44 (1976).

BAUM, T., SHROPSHIRE, A. T., ROWLES, G., VAN PELT, R., FERNANDEZ, S. P., ECKFELD, D. K., GLUCKMAN, M. I.: General pharmacologic actions of the antihypertensive agent 2—6 dichrobenzylidene aminoguanidine acetate (Wy 8678). J. Pharmacol. exp. Ther. **171**, 276—287 (1970).

BEAUVALLET, M., GIUDICELLI, R., CHABRIER, P., NAJER, H.: Sur l'action vasculaire de quelques amino 2-oxazolines N-substituées. J. Physiol. (Paris) **51**, 397—398 (1959).

BECK, L.: Active reflex vasodilatation in the innervated hind limb of the dog. Amer. J. Physiol. **201**, 123—128 (1961).

BENTLEY, G. A., LI, D. M. F.: Studies on the new hypotensive drug St 155. Europ. J. Pharmacol. **4**, 124—134 (1968).

BLOCH, R., BOUSQUET, P., FELDMAN, J., VELLY, J., SCHWARTZ, J.: Action hypotensive de la clonidine appliquée sur la surface ventrale du bulbe rachidien: analogie avec la dopamine. Thérapie **29**, 251—259 (1974).

BLUMBERG, J. B., TAYLOR, R. E., SULSER, F.: Blockade by pimozide of a noradrenaline sensitive adenylate cyclase in the limbic forebrain: possible role of limbic noradrenergic mechanisms in the mode of action of antipsychotics. J. Pharm. Pharmacol. **27**, 125—128 (1975).

BOCK, J. U., VAN ZWIETEN, P. A.: Central hyperglycaemic action of clonidine. Arch. Pharmakol. **270**, Suppl., R 11 (1971a).

BOCK, J. U., VAN ZWIETEN, P. A.: The central hyperglycaemic effect of clonidine. Europ. J. Pharmacol. **16**, 303—310 (1971b).

BOCK, K. D., HEIMSOTH, V., MERGUET, P., SCHÖNERMARK, J.: Klinische und klinisch-experimentelle Untersuchungen mit einer neuen blutdrucksenkenden Substanz: Dichlorophenylaminoimidazolin. Dtsch. med. Wschr. **91**, 1761—1770 (1966).

BOCK, K. D., MERGUET, P., BRANDT, T., MURATA, T.: Experimental studies with clonidine hydrochloride in normotensive and hypertensive subjects. In: CONOLLY, M. E. (Ed.): Catapres in hypertension, pp. 101—112. London: Butterworths 1970.

BOCK, K. D., MERGUET, P., MURATA, T., HEIMSOTH, V.: Klinisch-experimentelle Untersuchungen über die Wirkungen von Dichlorophenylaminoimidazolin. In: HEILMEYER, HOLTMEIER, PFEIFFER (Eds.): Hochdrucktherapie, pp. 28—38. Stuttgart: Thieme 1968.

Bogaievsky, D., Bogaievsky, Y., Tsoucaris-Kupfer, D., Schmitt, H.: Blockade of the central hypotensive effect of clonidine by α adrenoceptor antagonists in rats, rabbits and dogs. Clin. exp. Physiol. Pharmacol. **1**, 527—534 (1974).

Boissier, J.-R., Giudicelli, J.-F., Fichelle, J., Schmitt, H., Schmitt, Hélène: Cardiovascular effects of 2-(2,6-dichlorophenylamino)-2-imidazoline hydrochloride (St 155). I. Peripheral sympathetic system. Europ. J. Pharmacol. **2**, 333—339 (1968).

Boissier, J.-R., Giudicelli, J.-F., Larno, S., Fichelle, J.: Action du St 155 sur la sécrétion gastrique et l'ulcère expérimental. J. Pharmacol. (Paris) **1**, 109—122 (1970).

Bolme, P., Corrodi, H., Fuxe, K., Hökfelt, T., Lidbrink, P., Goldstein, M.: Possible involvement of central adrenaline neurons in vasomotor and respiratory control. Studies with clonidine and its interactions with piperoxane and yohimbine. Europ. J. Pharmacol. **28**, 89—94 (1974).

Bolme, P., Corrodi, H., Fuxe, K.: Possible mechanism of the hypotensive action of 2,6-dichlorobenzylidene aminoguanidine: evidence for central noradrenaline stimulation. Europ. J. Pharmacol. **23**, 175—182 (1973).

Bolme, P., Forsyth, R. P., Ishizaki, T., Melmon, K. L.: Hemodynamic effects of systemic and central administration of clonidine in the monkey. Amer. J. Physiol. **228**, 1276—1279 (1975).

Bolme, P., Fuxe, K.: Pharmacological studies on the hypotensive effects of clonidine. Europ. J. Pharmacol. **13**, 168—174 (1971).

Bolme, P., Fuxe, K.: Pharmacological studies on a possible role of central noradrenaline neurons in respiratory control. J. Pharm. Pharmacol. **25**, 351—352 (1973).

Bousquet, P., Feldman, J., Velly, J., Belhadj-Mostefa, H., Bloch, R., Schwartz, J.: Rôle de la surface ventrale du bulbe rachidien dans la régulation de la pression artérielle et dans l'action hypotensive de la clonidine. C. R. Soc. Biol. (Paris) **169**, 1359—1365 (1975a).

Bousquet, P., Feldman, J., Velly, J., Bloch, R.: Role of the ventral surface of the brain stem in the hypotensive action of clonidine: Europ. J. Pharmacol. **34**, 151—156 (1975b).

Bousquet, F., Guertzenstein, P. G.: Localization of the central cardiovascular action of clonidine. Brit. J. Pharmacol. **49**, 573—579 (1973).

Braestrup, C.: Effects of phenoxybenzamine, aceperone and clonidine on the level of 3-methoxy-4-hydroxy phenylglycol (MOPEG) in rat brain. J. Pharm. Pharmacol. **26**, 139—141 (1974).

Bralet, J., Rochette, L.: Influence du traitement par la clonidine sur la synthèse des cathécholamines dans le coeur, les glandes sous-maxillaires et la surrénale du rat. Biochem. Pharmacol. **12**, 3173—3180 (1973a).

Bralet, J., Rochette, L.: Effect of clonidine on the turnover rate of noradrenaline in peripheral tissues of the rat. Europ. J. Pharmacol. **23**, 239—244 (1973b).

Bralet, A. M., Rochette, L., Bralet, J.: Influence de la clonidine sur les débits sanguins nutritionnels et les résistances vasculaires régionales chez le rat normotendu et hypertendu. J. Pharmacol. (Paris), **5**, 87—100 (1974).

Bralet, J., Rochette, L., Bralet, A. M.: Influence de la clonidine sur la synthèse et la libération de la noradrénaline chez le rat. J. Pharmacol. (Paris) **4**, 416—417 (1973c).

Brest, A. N.: Pharmacodynamic effects of Catapress. In: Conolly, M. E. (Ed.): Catapress in hypertension, pp. 71—77. London: Butterworths 1970.

Briant, R. H., Reid, J. L.: Desmethylimipramine and the hypotensive action of clonidine in the rabbit. Brit. J. Pharmacol. **46**, 563P.—564P. (1972).

Briant, R. H., Reid, J.-L., Dollery, C. T: Interaction betweens clonidine and desipramine in man. Brit. Med. J. **1973 I**, 522.

Brod, J., Horbach, L., Just, H, Rosenthal, J., Nicolescu, R.: Acute effects of clonidine and central and peripheral haemodynamics on plasma renin activity. Europ. J. Clin Pharmacol. **4**, 107—111 (1972).

Brodie, D. A., Lotti, V. J., Bauer, B. G.: Drug effects on gastric secretion and stress gastric hemorrhage in the rat. Amer. J. dig. Dis. **15**, 111—120 (1970).

Broekkamp, C. L. E., Struyker-Boudier, H. A. J., van Rossum, J. M.: The involvement of catecholaminergic receptors in the regulation of feeding behavior. In: Milliez, P., Safar, M. (Eds.): Recent Advances in Hypertension. Vol. **2**, pp. 99—106. Reims: Société Aliena 1975.

Broekkamp, C., Van Rossum, J. M.: Clonidine-induced intrahypothalamic stimulation of eating in rats. Psychopharmacologia **25**, 162—168 (1972).

Bucht, H., Bergquist-Poppen, M., Bergstrom, J., Bozovic, L., Castenfors, J.: The effect of Catapresan on the renal circulation and the plasma renin activity. In: Heilmeyer, Holtmeier, Pfeiffer (Eds.): Hochdrucktherapie, pp. 124—128. Stuttgart: Thieme 1968.

Castro de la Mata, R., Penna, M., Aviado, D. M.: Reversal of sympathomimetic bronchodilatation by dichloro-isoproterenol. J. Pharmacol. exp. Ther. **135**, 197—303 (1962).

CHASIN, M., RIVKIN, I., MAMRAK, F., SAMANIAGO, S. G., HESS, S. M.: α- and β-adrenergic receptors as mediators of accumulation of cyclic adenosine 3′,5′ monophosphate in specific areas of guinea pig brain. J. biol. Chem. **246**, 3037—3041 (1971).
CHEVILLARD, C., PASQUIER, R., ALEXANDRE, J. M., SCHMITT, H.: Actions périphériques et centrales d'agents alpha-sympathomimétiques (clonidine et naphazoline) sur l'activité rénine plasmatique du rat. J. Pharmacol. (Paris) **7**, 457—467 (1976).
CHO, A. K., CURRY, S. H.: The physiological disposition of 2-(2,6 dichloro-anilino)-2-imidazoline (St 155). Biochem. Pharmacol. **18**, 511—520 (1969).
CHO, A. K., CURRY, S. H., JACOBSEN, S.: Localisation of basic drugs in the submaxillary gland. Biochem. Pharmacol. **18**, 2323—2330 (1969).
CHRYSTANS, S. G., LAVENDER, A. R.: Direct renal hemodynamic effects of clonidine. Arch. int. Pharmacodyn. Therap. **218**, 202—211 (1975).
CONSTANTINE, J. W., MCSHANE, W. K.: Analysis of the cardiovascular effects of 2-(2,6-dichlorophenylamino)-2-imidazoline hydrochloride (Catapres®). Europ. J. Pharmacol. **4**, 109—123 (1968).
COOTE, J. H., DOWNMANN, C. B. B.: Central pathways of some autonomic reflex discharges. J. Physiol. (Lond.) **183**, 714 (1966).
COSNIER, D., GRIMAL, J., CHEUCLE, M., STREICHENBERGER, G.: Influence de l'hypercapnie sur les effects circulatoires cérébraux de la clonidine chez l'animal éveillé. J. Pharmacol. (Paris) **4**, 505—519 (1973).
COUPAR, I. M., KIRBY, M. J.: The effect of clonidine on human isolated smooth muscle. Europ. J. Pharmacol. **17**, 50—58 (1972).
COUPAR, I. M., TURNER, P.: Relative affinities of some α-adrenoreceptor blocking drugs in isolated human smooth muscle. Brit. J. Pharmacol. **40**, 155P—157P (1970).
CRILL, W. E., REIS, D. J.: Distribution of carotid sinus and depressor nerves in cat brain stem. Amer. J. Physiol. **214**, 269—276 (1968).
CSONGRADY, A., KOBINGER, W.: Investigations into the positive inotropic effect of clonidine in isolated hearts. Arch. Pharmacol. **281**, 123—128 (1974).
CURWAIN, B. P., ENDERSBY: Enhancement of pentagastrin induced gastric acid secretion by clonidine in the conscious dog. Brit. J. Pharmacol. **50**, 431—434 (1974).
DAHLSTRÖM, A., FUXE, K.: Evidence for the existence of monoamine-containing neurones in the central nervous system. Acta physiol. scand. **62**, Suppl. 232 (1964).
DARDA, S.: Pharmacokinetics of clonidine. In: MILLIEZ, P., SAFAR, M. (Eds.): Recent advances in hypertension. Vol. 2, pp. 375—388. Reims: Société Aliéna 1975.
DAVIDOV, M., KAKAVIATOS, N., FINNERTY, FA. JR.: The antihypertensive properties of an imidazoline compound (St 155). Amer. J. Cardiol. **19**, 125—126 (1967).
DAY, M. D., ROACH, A. G.: Central α- and β-adrenoceptors modifying arterial blood pressure and heart rate in conscious cats. Brit. J. Pharmacol. **51**, 525—533 (1974).
DASKALOPOULOS, N. TH., SCHMITT, H., COTTEREAU, M.-J., DENIKER, P.: Unpublished data (1977).
DECK, R., OBERDORF, A., KRONEBERG, G.: Die Wirkung von 2-(2,6-Dichlorophenylamino)-2-imidazolin-hydrochlorid (Clonidin) auf die Kontraktion und die Acetylcholin-Freisetzung am isolierten, koaxial elektrisch gereizten Meerschweinchenileum. Arzneimittel-Forsch. **21**, 1580—1584 (1971).
DECKERS, W., REHBINDER, D.: Resorption, Verteilung, Ausscheidung und Metabolismus von Catapresan. In: HEILMEYER, HOLTMEIER, PFEIFFER (Eds.): Hochdrucktherapie, S. 17—26. Stuttgart: Thieme 1968.
DEGROAT, W., DOUGLAS, J., LALLEY, P.: Effects of clonidine, L-dopa and L-5-HTP on spinal and supraspinal sympathetic reflexes elicited by visceral and somatic afferent stimulation. Sixth International Congress of Pharmacology, Helsinski Abstract n° 1262, p. 52 (1975).
DELBARRE, B.: Sedative effects of α-sympathomimetic agents. In: MILLIEZ, P., SAFAR, M. (Eds.): Recent advances in hypertension, Vol. 2, pp. 87—97. Reims: Société Aliéna 1975.
DELBARRE, B., SCHMITT, H.: Influences pharmacologiques exercées sur la durée du sommeil provoqué chez le poussin par la 2-(2,6-dichlorophénylamino)-2-imidazoline (St 155, Catapresan®) C. R. Soc. Biol. (Paris) **163**, 1922—1926 (1969).
DELBARRE, B., SCHMITT, H.: Sedative effects of α-sympathomimetic drugs and their antagonism by adrenergic and cholinergic blocking drugs. Europ. J. Pharmacol. **13**, 356—363 (1971).
DELBARRE, B., SCHMITT, H.: A further attempt to characterize sedative receptors activated by clonidine in chickens and mice. Europ. J. Pharmacol. **22**, 355—359 (1973).
DELBARRE, B., SCHMITT, H.: Action of clonidine and α-adrenoreceptor blocking agents on conditioned avoidance reflexes in rats: their interactions and antagonism with atropine. Psychopharmacologia **35**, 195—202 (1974).
DELBRÜCK, O.: Ergebnisse toxikologischer und teratologischer Tierversuche mit 2-(2,6-Dichlorophenylamino)-2-Imidazolin-hydrochlorid. Arzneimittel-Forsch. **16**, 1053—1055 (1966).

DHAWAN, B. N., JOHRI, M. B., SRIMAL, R. C., VISWESARAM, D.: A study in cat of the effect of clonidine on central vasomotor loci. Arch. Pharmacol. **279**, Suppl. R22 (1973).
DHAWAN, B. N., JOHRI, M. B., SING, G. B., SRIMAL, R. C., VISWERAMAN, D.: Effect of clonidine on the excitability of vasomotor loci in the cat. Brit. J. Pharmacol. **54**, 17—21 (1975a).
DHAWAN, B. N., SINGH, G. B., SRIMAL, R. C.: The effect of clonidine on some centrally evoked cardiovascular responses. In: MILLIEZ, P., SAFAR, M. (Eds.): Recent Advances in Hypertension. Vol. 1, pp. 111—124. Reims: Société Aliéna 1975b.
DIESENHAMMER, E., KLAUSBERGER, E. M.: Die cerebrale Hämodynamik unter der Einwirkung von 2-(2,6-Dichlorophenylamino)-2-Imidazolin-hydrochlorid. Arzneimittel-Forsch. **16**, 1161—1162 (1966).
DOLLERY, C. T., DAVIES, D. S., DRAFFAN, G. H., DARGIE, H. J., DEAN, C. R., REID, J. L., CLARE, R. A., MURRAY, S.: Clinical pharmacology and pharmacokinetics of clonidine. Clin. Pharmacol. Therap. **19**, 11—17 (1976).
DOLLERY, C. T., REID, J. L.: Central noradrenergic neurones and the cardiovascular actions of clonidine in the rabbit. Brit. J. Pharmacol. **47**, 206—216 (1973).
DREW, G. M.: Effects of α-adrenoceptor agonists and antagonists on pre- and post-synaptically located α-adrenoceptors. Europ. J. Pharmacol. **36**, 313—320 (1976).
DUCHÊNE-MARULLAZ, P., DELORT, P., COSNIER, D.: De l'action bradycardisante de la clonidine (St155). J. Pharmacol. (Paris) **1**, 425 (1970).
EDIS, A. J., SHEPHERD, J. T.: Selective denervation of aortic arch baroreceptors and chemoreceptors in dogs. J. appl. Physiol. **30**, 294—296 (1971).
EDELHAUSER, E. M.: Erfahrungen mit der lokalen Applikation von Clonidin beim Glaukom. Klin. Mbl. Augenheilk. **158**, 514—517 (1971).
EHRHARDT, J. D.: Synthèse de la clonidine marquée et étude de son métabolisme chez le rat. J. Pharmacol. (Paris) **3**, 256—267 (1972a).
EHRHARDT, J. D.: Métabolisme du Catapressan: Action hypotensive du 4-hydroxy-catapressan. Thérapie **27**, 947—954 (1972b).
EHRINGER, H.: Die Wirkung von 2-(2,6-Dichlorophenylamino)-2-Imidazolin-hydrochlorid auf die Extremitätendurchblutung, den Blutdruck und die Venenkapazität bei Normotonikern, Arzneimittel-Forsch. **16**, 1165—1169 (1966).
FARNEBO, L. D., HAMBURGER, B.: Drugs-induced changes in the release of ^{3}H-noradrenaline from field stimulated rat iris. Brit. J. Pharmacol. **43**, 97—106 (1971).
FEHN, P. A., LINDSAY, L. A., KIRSTEN, W.: Evidence for a decreased venous return caused by clonidine. Fifth International Congress on Pharmacology. Abstracts of Volunteer papers p. 67 (398) (1972).
FINCH, L.: The cardiovascular effects of intraventricular clonidine and BAY 1470 in conscious hypertensive cats. Brit. J. Pharmacol. **52**, 333—338 (1974).
FINCH, L., BUCKINGHAM, R. E., MOORE, R. A., BUCHER, T. J.: Evidence for a central α-sympathomimetic action of clonidine in the rat. J. Pharm. Pharmacol. **27**, 181—185 (1975a).
FINCH, L., HERSOM, A., HICKS, P.: The central regulation of blood pressure by sympathomimetics. In: MILLIEZ, P., SAFAR, M. (Eds.): Recent Advances in Hypertension, Vol. 1, pp. 73—83. Reims: Société Aliéna 1975b.
FINCH, L., HICKS, P. E.: No evidence for central histamine-receptor involvement with the hypotensive effects of clonidine in cats. Europ. J. Pharmacol. **40**, 365—368 (1976).
FINNERTY, F. A.: Evaluation of the anti-hypertensive effects of Catapres in man. In: CONOLLY, M. E. (Ed.): Catapres in hypertension, pp. 155—165. London: Butterworths 1970.
FLORIO, V., BIANCHI, L., LONGO, V. G.: A study of the central effects of sympathomimetic drugs: EEG and behavioural investigations on clonidine and naphazoline. Neuropharmacology **14**, 707—714 (1975).
FOZARD, J. R.: Clonidine and methysergide: effects on isolated artery. Arch. Pharmacol. **279** Suppl. R21 (1973).
FRANK, H., LOEWENICH-LAGOIS, K. VON: Therapeutische Prüfung und Untersuchungen zur Nierenfunktion mit einer neuen blutdrucksenkenden Substanz (St155). Dtsch. med. Wschr. **91**, 1680—1686 (1966).
FRANZ, D. N., HARE, B. D., NEUMAYR, R. J.: Reciprocal control of sympathetic preganglionic neurons by monoaminergic, bulbospinal pathways and a selective effect of clonidine. In: MILLIEZ, P., SAFAR, M. (Eds.): Recent Advances in Hypertension, Vol. 1, pp. 85—96. Reims: Editions Aliéna 1975.
FRYDMAN, A., WEISS, Y., SAFAR, M., ALEXANDRE, J. M.: Pharmacokinetics of clonidine in man (preliminary results). In: MILLIEZ, P., SAFAR, M. (Eds.): Recent Advances in Hypertension, Vol. 2, pp. 369—374. Reims: Société Aliéna 1975.
FÜGNER, A.: Antagonism of the drug-induced behavioural sleep in chicks. Arzneimittel-Forsch. **21**, 1350—1352 (1971).
FÜGNER, A., HOEFKE, W.: A sleep-like state in chicks caused by biogenic amines and other compounds: quantitative evaluation. Arzneimittel-Forsch. **21**, 1243—1247 (1971).

GANONG, W. F.: Brain amines and the control of ACTH and growth hormone secretion. In: MOTTA, M., CROSIGNANI, P. G., MARTINI, L. (Eds.): Hypothalamic Hormones, pp. 237—248. London-New York-San Francisco: Academic Press 1975a.
GANONG, W. F., REID, I. A., LOVINGER, R. D., KAPLAN, S. L.: Neuroendocrine effects of clonidine. Sixth International Congress of Pharmacology, Abstracts, p. 93 (n° 200). Helsinki, Finland (1975b).
GELINOV, CHR., BELOVEJDOC, N.: Klinische Untersuchungen über die Beeinflussung der Acidität der Magensekretion durch Catapresan. Verh. dtsch. Ges. inn. Med. **76**, 160—163 (1970).
GILBERT, J. C., RIBEYRO, F., GRAISLEY, B., TOUBOUL, J. P.: Régulation monoaminergique centrale de l'hormone de croissance (submitted).
GILLIS, R. A., DIONNE, R. A., STANDAERT, F. G.: Suppression by clonidine (St 155) of digitalis-induced arrhythmias. Pharmacologist **13**, 225 (1971).
GILLIS, R. A., DIONNE, R. A., STANDAERT, F. G.: Suppression by clonidine (St 155) of digitalis induced arrhythmias. J. Pharmacol. exp. Therap. **182**, 218—226 (1972).
GIUDICELLI, R., BEAUVALLET, M., CHABRIER, P., NAJER, H.: Sur l'action vasculaire de quelques amino-2-oxazolines N-substituées. C. R. Acad. Sci. (Paris) **247**, 891—893 (1958).
GIUDICELLI, R., SCHMITT, H.: Propriétés antihypertensives et mécanisme d'action de la (di-méthyl-2-6-phénylamino)-2 Δ_2-oxazoline-1,3. J. Pharmacol. (Paris) **1**, 339—358 (1970).
GLICK, S. D., COX, R. D.: Differential sensitivity to apomorphine and clonidine following cortical damage in cats. Europ. J. Pharmacol. **36**, 241—246 (1976).
GOGOLAK, G., STUMPF, CH.: Wirkung von 2-(2,6-Dichlorophenylamino)-2-Imidazolin-hydrochlorid auf die EEG-Weckreaktion beim Kaninchen. Arzneimittel-Forsch. **16**, 1050—1052 (1966).
GRABNER, G., MICHALEK, P.: Einige experimentelle Erfahrungen mit Catapresan. In: HEILMEYER, HOLTMEIER, PFEIFFER (Eds.): Hochdrucktherapie, S. 49—55. Stuttgart: Thieme 1968.
GRABNER, G., MICHALEK, P., POKORNY, D., VORMITTAG, E.: Klinische und experimentelle Untersuchungen mit der neuen blutdrucksenkenden Substanz 2-(2,6-Dichlorophenylamino)-2-Imidazolin-hydrochlorid. Arzneimittel-Forsch. **16**, 1174—1176 (1966).
GRAUBNER, W., WOLF, M.: Kritische Betrachtungen zum Wirkungsmechanismus des 2-(2,6-Dichlorophenylamino)-2-Imidazolin-hydrochlorids. Arzneimittel-Forsch. **16**, 1055—1058 (1966).
GREEN, J. R., HEFFRON, P. F.: Studies upon patterns of activity in single postganglionic sympathetic fibres. Arch. int. Pharmacodyn. Therap. **173**, 232—243 (1968).
GUT, J.-P., SCHMITT, H.: Action de la 2-(2,6-dichlorophénylamino)-2-imidazoline (St 155, Catapresan®) sur quelques réflexes cardiovasculaires du lapin. C. R. Soc. Biol. (Paris) **164**, 880—883 (1970).
HAAN, D.: Kontinuierliche automatische Blutdruckregistrierung nach Verabreichung einer neuen antihypertensiven Substanz. Arzneimittel-Forsch. **16**, 1180—1183 (1966).
HAAN, D.: Cardiale Kontraktionskraft und kontinuierliche Langzeitkontrolle der Kreislaufwerte unter 2-(2,6-Dichlorophenylamino)-2-Imidazolin-hydrochlorid. In: HEILMEYER, HOLTMEIER, PFEIFFER (Eds.): Hochdrucktherapie, S. 55—60. Stuttgart: Thieme 1968.
HAEFELY, W. E., JALFRE, M., MONACHON, M. A.: Drug-induced PGO wawes: a neuropharmacological method for evaluating agents which interact with central norepinephrine (NE) and serotonin (5 HT) neurons or receptors. Fifth international Congress on Pharmacology. Volunteer papers p. 93, (558) (1972).
HAEUSLER, G.: Activation of the central pathway of the baroreceptor reflex, a possible mechanism of the hypotensive action of clonidine. Arch. Pharmacol. **278**, 231—246 (1973a).
HAEUSLER, G.: Clonidine and the baroreceptor reflex. Arch. Pharmacol. **279**, Suppl. R 22, 31 (1973).
HAEUSLER, G.: Sympathetic nerve activity after noradrenaline depletion and its alteration by clonidine. Arch. Pharmacol. **282**, R 29 (1974a).
HAEUSLER, G.: Further similarities between the action of clonidine and a central activation of the depressor baroreceptor reflex. Arch. Pharmacol. **285**, 1—14 (1973b).
HAEUSLER, G.: Clonidine induced inhibition of sympathetic nerve activity: no indication for a central presynaptic or indirect sympathomimetic mode of action. Arch. Pharmacol. **286**, 97—111 (1974c).
HAEUSLER, G.: Studies on the possible contribution of a peripheral presynaptic action of clonidine and dopamine to their vascular effects under *in vivo* conditions. Arch. Pharmacol. **295**, 191—202 (1976).
HAEUSLER, G., FINCH, L.: On the nature of the central hypotensive effect of clonidine and α methyldopa. J. Pharmacol. (Paris) **3**, 544—545 (1972).
HAEUSLER, G., LEWIS, P.: The baroreceptor reflex and its relations to central adrenergic mechanisms. In: MILLIEZ, P., SAFAR, M. (Eds.): Recent Advances in Hypertension, Vol. 1, pp. 17—26. Reims: Société Aliéna 1975.

HASSLINGER, C.: Catapresan [2-(2,6-Dichlorophenylamino)-2-Imidazolin-hydrochlorid], ein neues augendrucksenkendes Medikament. Klin. Mbl. Augenheilk. **154**, 95—105 (1969).

HEILMANN, K.: Catapresan and Catapresan-Kombination in der Glaukombehandlung. Sitzungsbericht der 120. Versammlung der Verein. Rhein. Westf. Augenärzte (1969).

HEILMANN, K.: Untersuchungen über Wirkung von Catapresan auf den intraokulären Druck. 1. Mitteilung. Klin. Mbl. Augenheilk. **157**, 182—192 (1970).

HEILMANN, K.: Untersuchungen über die Wirkung von Catapresan auf den intraokularen Druck. 2. Mitteilung. Klin. Mbl. Augenheilk. **158**, 493—500 (1971).

HEISE, A., KRONEBERG, G.: Periphere und zentrale Kreislaufwirkung des α-Sympathomimeticums 2-(2,6-Xylidino)5,6-dihydro-4H-1-3-thiazinhydrochlorid (BAY 1470). Arch. Pharmakol. **266**, 350—351 (1970).

HEISE, A., KRONEBERG, G., SCHLOSSMANN, K.: α-sympathomimetische Eigenschaften als Ursache der blutdrucksteigenden und blutdrucksenkenden Wirkung von BAY 1470 (2-(2,6-Xylidino)5-6-dihydro 4H-1-3-thiazin-hydrochlorid. Arch. Pharmakol. **208**, 348—360 (1971).

HENNING, M., STOCK, G., TROLIN, G.: Circulatory effects of clonidine after prehypothalamic section of the brain stem. Acta Pharmacol. Toxicol. **38**, 376—381 (1976).

HILD, R., DIETZ, R.: Über die Wirkung von Catapresan auf die Volumenpulsamplitude der Haut, den Blutdruck und die Pulsfrequenz bei Gesunden. In: HEILMEYER, HOLTMEIER, PFEIFFER (Eds.): Hochdrucktherapie, S. 60—63. Stuttgart: Thieme 1968.

HODGE, R. L., ROBINSON, S. M.: Vascular actions of clonidine in man. Brit. J. Pharmacol. **40**, 573P—574P (1970).

HODGES, P.: Identification of 2,6-dichlorophenylguanidine as a metabolite of clonidine. J. Pharm. Pharmacol. **28**, 61—62 (1976).

HOEFKE, W.: Effects of clonidine and clonidine-like substances on gastric secretion in rats Sixth International Congress of Pharmacology. Abstracts, p. 119 (n° 278) (1975).

HOEFKE, W., KOBINGER, W.: Pharmakologische Wirkungen des 2-(2,6-Dichlorophenyiamino)-2-Imidazolin-hydrochlorids, einer neuen antihypertensiven Substanz. Arzneimittel-Forsch. **16**, 1038—1056 (1966).

HOEFKE, W., KOBINGER, W., WALLAND, A.: Relationship between activity and structure in derivatives of clonidine. Arzneimittel-Forsch. **25**, 786—793 (1975).

HOEFKE, W., WARNKE-SACHS, E.: Influence of desmethylimipramine on the hypotensive effect of clonidine. Arzneimittel-Forsch. **24**, 1046—1047 (1974).

HOFFMEISTER, F.: On the possible relations between postganglionic adrenergic and cholinergic neurone blockade demonstrable in the peripheral autonomous system and central analgesia. The analgesic activity of BAY 1470 and its relation to morphine analgesia. In Pain: SOULAIRAC, A., CAHN, J., CHARPENTIER, J. (Eds.), pp. 281—298. London-New York: Academic Press 1968.

HÖKFELT, T., DYMLING, J. F., HEDELAND, H.: The effect of Catapresan on urinary catecholamines, plasma renin and urinary aldosterone in hypertensive patients. In: HEILMEYER, HOLTMEIER, PFEIFFER (Eds.): Hochdrucktherapie, S. 105—108. Stuttgart: Thieme 1968.

HÖKFELT, B., HEDELAND, H., DYMLING, J. F.: Studies on catecholamines, renin and aldosterone following Catapresan® [2-(2,6-dichlorophenylamino)-2-imidazolin] in hypertensive patients. Europ. J. Pharmacol. **10**, 389—397 (1970a).

HÖKFELT, B., HEDELAND, H., DYMLING, J. F.: The influence of Catapresan on catecholamines, renin and aldosterone in man. In: CONOLLY, M. E. (Ed.): Catapresan in Hypertension, pp. 85—98. London: Butterworths 1970b.

HÖKFELT, B., HEDELAND, H., HANSSON, B. G.: The effects of clonidine and penbutolol, respectively on catecholamines in blood and urine, plasma renin activity and urinary aldosterone in hypertensive patients. Arch. int. Pharmacol. Therap. **213**, 307—321 (1975).

HOLMAN, R. B., SHILLITO, E. E., VOGT, M.: Sleep produced by clonidine [2-(2,6-dichlorophenylamino)-2-imidazoline hydrochloride]. Brit. J. Pharmacol. **43**, 685—695 (1971).

HUKUHARA, T. J., OTSUKA, Y., TADEKA, R., SAKAI, F.: Die zentralen Wirkungen des 2-(2,6-Dichlorophenylamino)-2-Imidazolin-hydrochlorids. Arzneimittel-Forsch. **18**, 1147—1153 (1968).

HUMPHREY, M. H., REID, I. A.: Acute effect of clonidine on renal water excretion. Clin. Res. **22**, 532A (1974).

HUNT, G. E., ATRENS, D. M., CHESCHER, G. B., BELCKER, F. T.: α-noradrenergic modulation of hypothalamic self-stimulation; studies employing clonidine, l-phenylephrine and α-methyl-p-tyrosine. Europ. J. Pharmacol. **37**, 105—111 (1976).

IWATA, Y.: Hyperglycaemic action of 2-(2,6-dichlorophenylamino)-2-imidazoline hydrochloride in relation to its hypertensive effects. Jap. J. Pharmacol. **19**, 249—259 (1969).

JACOBS, F., WERNER, U., SCHÜMANN, H. J: Zum Mechanismus der antihypertensiven Wirkung des Oxazolin-Derivates BAY a 6781. Arzneimittel-Forsch. **22**, 1124—1126 (1972).

JAMES, I.M., LARBI, E., ZAIMIS, E.: The effect of the acute intravenous administration of clonidine (St155) on cerebral blood flow in man. Brit. J. Pharmacol. **39**, 198P—199P (1970).

JENNEWEIN, H.M.: The effect of clonidine on gastric acid secretion in rats and dogs. Arch. Pharmacol. **297**, 85—90 (1977).

JOUVET, M., RENAULT, J.: Insomnie persistante après lésions des noyaux du raphé chez le chat. C. R. Soc. Biol. (Paris) **160**, 1461—1465 (1966).

JUENEMANN, G., PAUST, E.: Über Wirkungsweise und Wirkungsprinzip des Catapresan in der Glaukomtherapie. Klin. Mbl. Augenheilk. **158**, 501—513 (1971).

JUENEMANN, G., SCHMIDT, G.: Zur Catapresanwirkung am Glaucomatosenauge. Klin. Mbl. Augenheilk. **157**, 193—201 (1970).

KAESS, H., MIKULICZ-RADECKI, J. VON: Der Einfluß von 2-(2,6-Dichlorophenylamino)2-Imidazolin-hydrochlorid (Catapresan®) auf die Funktion von Magen und Pankreas. Europ. J. clin. Pharmacol. **3**, 97—101 (1971).

KAPLAN, H.R., LASALA, S.A., SIMON, A., ROBSON, R.D.: St155-induced cardiac slowing in dogs. Europ. J. Pharmacol. **6**, 193—196 (1969).

KARPPANEN, H., PAAKKARI, I., PAAKKARI, P., HUOTARI, R., ORMA, A.L.: Possible involvement of central histamine H_2-receptors in the hypotensive effect of clonidine. Nature (Lond.) **259**, 587—588 (1976).

KARPPANEN, H.O., WESTERMANN, E.: Increased production of cyclic AMP in gastric tissue by stimulation of Histamine (H_2) receptors. Arch. Pharmacol. **279**, 83—87 (1973).

KATIĆ, F., LAVERY, H., LOWE, R.D.: The central action of clonidine and its antagonism. Brit. J. Pharmacol. **44**, 779—787 (1972).

KHO, T.L., SCHALEKAMP, A.D.H., ZAAL, G.A., WESTER, A., BIRGENHÄGER, W.H.: Comparison between the effects of St 600 and Catapres. Arch. int. Pharmacod. Therap. **214**, 347—350 (1975).

KHO, T.L., SCHALEKAMP, A.D.N., ZAAL, G.A., WESTER, A., BIRGENHÄGER, W.H.: Comparison between the effects of St 600 and clonidine. Arch. int. Pharmacod. Therap. **217**, 162—169 (1975).

KIRCHERTZ, E.J., PETERS, G.: The effect of clonidine (Catapres®) and other hypotensive agents on plasma renin activity. Experientia (Basel) **29**, 764 (Abst.) (1973).

KIRCHHOFF, H.W.: Lungenfunktionsprüfungen und leitungsmedizinische Untersuchung über die Wirkung von Catapresan bei gesunden Versuchspersonen. In: HEILMEYER, HOLTMEIER, PFEIFFER (Eds.): Hochdrucktherapie. Stuttgart: Thieme 1968.

KIRPEKAR, S.M., PUIG, M.: Effect of flow stop on noradrenaline release from normal spleens and spleens treated with cocaine, phentolamine or phenoxybenzamine. Brit. J. Pharmacol. **43**, 359—369 (1971).

KLEINLOGEL, H., SCHOLTYSIK, C., SAYERS, A.C.: Effects of clonidine and BS 100-141 on the EEG sleep pattern in rat. Europ. J. Pharmacol. **33**, 159—163 (1975).

KLEVANS, L.R., KEPNER, K., KOVACS, J.C.: Role of forebrain in clonidine-induced suppression of cardiovascular responses. Europ. J. Pharmacol. **24**, 262—265 (1973).

KLUPP, H., KNAPPEN, F., OTSUKA, Y., STRELLER, I., TEICHMANN, H.: Effects of clonidine on central sympathetic tone. Europ. J. Pharmacol. **10**, 225—229 (1970).

KNOBLOCH, H., MORR, H.: Einzeldosisstudien zur Wirkung von 2-(2,6-Dichlorophenylamino) 2-Imidazolin-hydrochlorid auf Blutdruck und Puls bei Hypertonikern und zur Verträglichkeit. Arzneimittel-Forsch. **16**, 1169—1174 (1966).

KOBINGER, W.: Über den Wirkungsmechanismus einer neuen antihypertensiven Substanz mit Imidazolinstruktur. Arch. Pharm. exp. Path. **258**, 48—68 (1967).

KOBINGER, W.: Die Wirkung von 2-(2,6-Dichlorophenylamino)-2-Imidazolin-hydrochlorid (St155, Catapres®) auf die Harnausscheidung von osmotisch freiem Wasser. Arch. Pharm. exp. Path. **260**, 153—154 (1968).

KOBINGER, W.: Die Beeinflussung des Tauchreflexes durch sympathicushemmende Antihypertensiven. Arch. Pharm. exp. Path. **264**, 256—257 (1969).

KOBINGER, W.: Comparison of peripheral and central effects of Catapres® (St155, 2-(2,6-dichlorophenylamino)-2-imidazolin hydrochloride) on the sympathetic nervous system. In: CONOLLY, M.E. (Ed.): Catapres in Hypertension, pp. 43—50. London: Butterworths 1970.

KOBINGER, W.: In: KIM, K.E., MOYER, J.H. (Eds.): Pharmacological basis of the cardiovascular actions of clonidine in hypertension: Mechanism and Management. G.ONESTI, pp. 369—380. New York-London: Grune & Stratton 1971.

KOBINGER, W., HOEFKE, W.: Pharmakologische Untersuchungen über den Angriffspunkt und Wirkungsmechanismus eines neuen Hochdruckmittels. In: HEILMEYER, HOLTMEIER, PFEIFFER (Eds.): Hochdrucktherapie, S. 4—17. Stuttgart: Thieme 1968.

KOBINGER, W., ODA, M.: Effects of sympathetic blocking substances on the diving reflex of ducks. Europ. J. Pharmacol. **7**, 289—295 (1969).

KOBINGER, W., PICHLER, L.: Evidence for direct α-adrenoceptor stimulation of effector neurons in cardiovascular centers by clonidine. Europ. J. Pharmacol. **22**, 151—154 (1974).

KOBINGER, W., PICHLER, L.: Localization into the central nervous system of adrenoceptors which facilitate a cardioinhibitory reflex. Arch. Pharmacol. **286**, 371—377 (1975a).

KOBINGER, W., PICHLER, L.: The central modulatory effect of clonidine on the cardiodepressor reflex after suppression of synthesis and storage of noradrenaline. Europ. J. Pharmacol. **30**, 56—62 (1975b).

KOBINGER, W., PICHLER, L.: Investigation into some imidazoline compounds. with respect to peripheral α-adrenoceptor stimulation and depression of cardiovascular centers. Arch. Pharmacol. **291**, 175—191 (1975c).

KOBINGER, W., PICHLER, L.: Centrally induced reduction in sympathetic tone—a postsynaptic α-adrenoceptor stimulating action of imidazolines. Europ. J. Pharmacol. **40**, 311—320 (1976).

KOBINGER, W., WALLAND, A.: Untersuchungen über den Wirkungsmechanismus von 2-(2,6-Dichlorophenylamino)-2-Imidazolin-hydrochlorid (Catapresan, St 155). Arch. Pharm. exp. Path. **257**, 291—292 (1967a).

KOBINGER, W., WALLAND, A.: Circulatory studies with 2-(2,6-dichlorophenylamino)-2-imidazoline hydrochloride. Arzneimittel-Forsch. **17**, 292—300 (1967b).

KOBINGER, W., WALLAND, A.: Investigations into the mechanism of the hypotensive effect of 2-(2,6-dichlorophenylamino)-2-imidazoline HCl. Europ. J. Pharmacol. **2**, 155—162 (1967c).

KOBINGER, W., WALLAND, A.: Involvement of adrenergic receptors in central vagus activity. Europ. J. Pharmacol. **16**, 120—122 (1971a).

KOBINGER, W., WALLAND, A.: Enhancement of vagal reflex bradycardia by clonidine: peripheral or central nervous effect? Acta pharmacol. **29**, suppl. 4,25 (1971b).

KOBINGER, W., WALLAND, A.: Involvement of adrenergic neurones within the CNS in vagally mediated cardiodepressor reflexes. Arch. Pharmakol. **274**, Suppl., R 67 (1972a).

KOBINGER, W., WALLAND, A.: Evidence for a central activation of a vagal cardiodepressor reflex by clonidine . Europ. J. Pharmacol. **19**, 203—209 (1972b).

KOBINGER, W., WALLAND, A.: Facilitation of vagal bradycardia by an action of clonidine on central α-receptors. Europ. J. Pharmacol. **19**, 210—217 (1972c).

KOBINGER, W., WALLAND, A.: Modulating effect of central adrenergic neurones on a vagally mediated cardioinhibitory reflex. Europ. J. Pharmacol. **22**, 344—350 (1973).

KOCH, G.: Hemodynamic effects of 2-(2,6-dichlorophenylamino)-2-imidazoline hydrochloride (St 155) at rest and during exercise with special respect to the pulmonary circulation. Arzneimittel-Forsch. **21**, 57—61 (1971).

KOCHSIEK, J., FRITSCHE, H.: Die Wirkung eines Imidazolin-Derivates auf den arteriellen Blutdruck, die Hämodynamik und die Ventilation. Arzneimittel-Forsch. **16**, 1154—1160 (1966).

KORNER, P., OLIVER, J., SLEIGHT, P., CHALMERS, J., ROBINSON, J.: Effects of clonidine on the baroreceptor heart rate reflex and on single aortic baroreceptor fibre discharge. Europ. J. Pharmacol. **28**, 189—198 (1974).

KORNER, P., OLIVER, J., SLEIGHT, P., ROBINSON, S., CHALMERS, J.: Assessment of cardiac autonomic excitability in renal hypertensive rabbits using clonidine induced resetting of the baroreceptor heart rate reflex. Europ. J. Pharmacol. **37**, 381—384 (1976).

KOSS, M.C.: Studies on the site of action of clonidine utilizing a sympathetic cholinergic system. Europ. J. Pharmacol. **37**, 381—384 (1976).

KOSS, M.C., DAVISON, M.H.: The electrodermal response as a model for central sympathetic reactivity: the action of clonidine. Europ. J. Pharmacol. **37**, 71—78 (1976).

KRAEMER, D., KRAUSE, W., RENNER, H.: Bericht über eine Langzeitprüfung mit 2-(2,6-Dichlorophenylamino)-2-Imidazolin-hydrochlorid unter besonderer Berücksichtigung der Wirkung auf den Blutdruck und des Kohlenhydrat-Stoffwechsels. Arzneimittel-Forsch. **20**, 519—521 (1970).

KRAUSE, W.: Catapresanbehandlung mit Funktionprüfung des Inselorgans (Tolbutamid-Test) bei nicht diabetischen Hypertoniken. In: HEILMEYER, HOLTMEIER, PFEIFFER (Eds.): Hochdrucktherapie, S. 147—148. Stuttgart: Georg Thieme 1968.

KROETZ, F.W., MCRAVEN, D., KIOSCHOS, J.M., KIRKENDALL, W.M.: The acute effects of Catapres on cardiac haemodynamics of hypertensive man. In: CONOLLY, M.E. (Ed.): Catapres in hypertension, pp. 59—70. London: Butterworths 1970.

KRONEBERG, G., OBERDORF, A., HOFFMEISTER, F., WIRTH, W.: Adrenergisch-cholinergische Neuronhemmstoffe. Naturwissenschaften **53**, 502 (1966).

KRONEBERG, G., OBERDORF, A., HOFFMEISTER, F., WIRTH, W.: Zur Pharmakologie von 2-(2,6-Dimethylphenylamino) 4H 5,6 dihydro-3-thiazin (Bayer 1470), eines Hemmstoffes adrenergischer und cholinergischer Neurone. Arch. Pharm. exp. Path. **256**, 257—280 (1967).

KÜNDIG, H., MONNIER, H., LEVIN, N.W., CHARLTON, R.W.: Mechanism of action of St155 on the blood pressure in rats. Arzneimittel-Forsch. **17**, 1440—1444 (1967).

KULJAK, S., STERN, P.: Catapresan—induced tremor and its characteristics. Pharmacol. Res. **2**, 17—22 (1970).

LANGER, S.Z.: The regulation of transmitter release elicited by nerve stimulation through α presynaptic feed-back mechanism. In: USDIN, E., SNYDER, S.H. (Eds.): Frontiers in Catecholamines Research, pp. 543—549. New York-Toronto-Oxford-Sidney-Braunschweig: Pergamon Press 1973.

LANGER, S.Z.: Presynaptic regulation of catecholamine release. Biochem. Pharmacol. **23**. 1773—1800 (1974).

LARBI, E., ZAIMIS, E.: The effect of the chronic administration of clonidine (St155) on vascular smooth muscle. Brit. J. Pharmacol. **39**, 221P (1970).

LAUBIE, M.: Interactions between cholinergic and noradrenergic pathways in central control of blood pressure. In: MILLIEZ, P., SAFAR, M. (Eds.): Recent Advances in Hypertension, Vol.2, pp. 49—59. Reims: Société Aliéna 1975.

LAUBIE, M.: Pharmacological evidence for interactions of cholinergic and noradrenergic mechanisms in central cardiovascular control. Proceedings of the Sixth International Congress of Pharmacology. Volume 4, Drug Therapy, pp. 79—85. Helsinki, Finland, 1975.

LAUBIE, M., DELBARRE, B., BOGAÏEVSKY, D., BOGAÏEVSKY, Y., TSOUCARIS-KUPFER, D., SENON, D., SCHMITT, HÉLÈNE, SCHMITT, H.: Pharmacological evidence for a central α-sympathomimetic mechanism controlling blood pressure and heart rate. Circulation Res. **38**, (suppl. II) 35—41 (1976a).

LAUBIE, M., SCHMITT, H.: Effects hémodynamiques du St155, (2-(2,6-dichlorophenylamino)-2-imidazoline) hydrochloride, chez le chien hypertendu. Arch. int. Pharmacodyn. Thérap. **179**, 23—35 (1969).

LAUBIE, M., SCHMITT, H.: Influence of autonomic blockade on the reduction in myocardial performance produced by clonidine. Europ. J. Pharmacol. **25**, 56—65 (1974).

LAUBIE, M., SCHMITT, H.: Sites of action of clonidine: centrally mediated increase in vagal tone, centrally mediated hypotensive and sympatho-inhibitory effects. In: Hypertension and Brain Mechanisms, de Jongh ed., pp. 337-348, Elsevier, 1977.

LAUBIE, M., SCHMITT, H., CANELLAS, J., ROQUEBERT, J., DEMICHEL, P.: Centrally mediated bradycardia and hypotension induced by narcotic analgesics: dextromoramide and fentanyl. Europ. J. Pharmacol. **28**, 66—75 (1974).

LAUBIE, M., SCHMITT, H., DROUILLAT, M.: Action of clonidine on the baroreceptor pathways and medularry sites mediating vagal bradycardia. Europ. J. Pharmacol. **38**, 293—303 (1976b).

LAVERTY, R.: A comparison of the behavioural effects of some hypotensive imidazoline derivatives in rats. Europ. J. Pharmacol. **9**, 163—169 (1970).

LAVERTY, R., TAYLOR, K.M.: Behavioural and biochemical effects of 2-(2,6-dichlorophenylamino)-2-imidazoline hydrochloride (St155) on the central nervous system. Brit. J. Pharmacol. **35**, 253—264 (1969).

LE DOUAREC, J.-C., SCHMITT, H., LUCET, B.: Influence of clonidine and other α-sympathomimetic agents on water intake in rats. J. Pharmacol. (Paris) **2**, 240—241 (1971a).

LE DOUAREC, J.-C., SCHMITT, H., LUCET, B.: Influence de la clonidine et des substances α-sympathomimétiques sur la prise d'eau chez le rat assoiffé. J. Pharmacol. (Paris) **2**, 435—444 (1971b).

LE DOUAREC, J.-C., SCHMITT, H., LUCET, B.: Effects de la clonidine et d'autres agents sympathomimétiques sur la prise de nourriture: Antagonisme par des agents adrénolytiques. J. Pharmacol. (Paris) **3**, 187—198 (1972).

LEHR, D., MALLON, J., KROKOWSKI, M.: Copious drinking and stimultaneous inhibition of urine flow elicited by beta adrenergic stimulation and contrary effects of alpha adrenergic stimulation. J. Pharmacol. exp. Ther. **158**, 150—163 (1967).

LEWIS, C.H., WEIL, M.H.: Haemodynamic spectrum of vasopressor and dilator drugs. J. Amer. med. Ass. **20P**, 1391—1398 (1969).

LI, D.M., BENTLEY, G.A.: The effect of St155 on the active reflex vasodilatation induced by adrenaline, noradrenaline and veratrine. Europ. J. Pharmacol. 8, 39—46 (1969).

Li, D. M. P., Bentley, G. A.: The effects of various antihypertensive drugs on the reflex responses to vasoactive substances. Europ. J. Pharmacol. **12**, 24—34 (1970).

Lindmar, R., Löffelholz, K., Muscholl, E.: A muscarinic mechanism inhibiting the release of noradrenaline from the peripheral adrenergic nerve fibres by nicotinic agents. Brit. J. Pharmacol. **32**, 280—294 (1968).

Lindner, E., Kaiser, J.: Tiamenidine (Hoe 440), a new antihypertensive agent. Arch. int. Pharmacol. Therap. **211**, 305—325 (1974).

Lipski, J., Przybylski, J., Solnicka, E.: Reduced hypotensive effect of clonidine after lesions of the nucleus tractus solitarii in rats. Europ. J. Pharmacol. **38**, 19—22 (1976a).

Lipski, J., Solnicka, E.: The effect of activation of central adrenergic receptors by clonidine on the excitability of the solitary tract neurons in cats. Acta physiol. pol. **27**, 309—316 (1976b).

Loew, D. N., Waite, R.: A quantitative assessement of the effects of clonidine on preganglionic sympathetic nerve activity in the cat. Brit. J. Pharmacol. **50**, 456P—457P (1974).

Löffelholz, K., Muscholl, E.: A muscarinic inhibition of noradrenaline release evoked by postganglionic sympathetic nerve stimulation. Arch. Pharmakol. **265**, 1—5 (1969).

Lomax, P., Forster, R. S.: Temperature changes induced by imidazoline sympathomimetics in the rat. J. Pharmacol. exp. Ther. **167**, 159—165 (1969).

Lombardi, F., Malliani, A., Portillo-Nunez, P., Zaïmis, E., Zanchetti, A.: Peripheral vascular effect of clonidine independent of a reduction in sympathetic activity. Brit. J. Pharmacol. **57**, 448P—449P (1976).

Ludwig, H.: Der Einfluß der Langzeitbehandlung mit 2-(2,6-Dichlorophenylamino)-2-Imidazolin HCl auf die Nierenhämodynamik beim arteriellen Hochdruck. Arzneimittel-Forsch. **18**, 600—604 (1968).

McCall, R. B., Gebber, G. L.: Differential effect of baroreceptor reflexes and clonidine on frequency components of sympathetic discharge. Europ. J. Pharmacol. **36**, 69—78 (1976).

McRaven, D. R., Kroetz, F. W., Kioschos, J. M., Kirkendall, W. M.: The effect of clonidine on hemodynamics in hypertensive patients. Amer. Heart. J. **81**, 482—489 (1971).

Magus, R. D., Long, J. P.: Mechanism of the hypotensive action of 2-(2,6-dichlorophenylamino)-2-imidazoline hydrochloride (St 155) in the cat. J. pharm. Sci. **57**, 594—598 (1968).

Maj, J., Sowinska, H., Baran, L., Karturkiewicz, Z.: The effect of clonidine on locomotor activity in mice. Life Sci. **11**, 483—491 (1972).

Makabe, R.: Ophthalmologische Untersuchungen mit Dichlorophenylamino-Imidazolin unter besonderer Berücksichtigung des Einflusses auf den intraokularen Druck. Dtsch. med. Wschr. **91**, 1686—1688 (1966).

Makabe, R.: Einfluß von Catapresan auf den Ophthalmica und Augeninnendruck. In: Heilmeyer, Holmeier, Pfeiffer (Eds.): Hochdrucktherapie, S. 64—67. Stuttgart: Thieme 1968.

Maling, H. M., Cho, A. K., Horokova, Z., Williams, M. A.: The pharmacologic effects of St 155 (Catapres) and related imidazolines in the rat. Pharmacology **2**, 337—351 (1969).

Maling, H. M., Cho, A., Williams, M. A.: Some central effects of St 155 (Catapres) and related imidazolines in the rat. Pharmacologist **10**, 157 (1968).

Marley, E., Nistico, G.: Sleep and hypothermic effects of clonidine in fowls. Brit. J. Pharmacol. **52**, 434P—435P (1974).

Marley, E., Nistico, G.: Central effects of clonidine, 2-(2,6-dichlorophenylamino)-2-imidazoline hydrochloride, in fowls. Brit. J. Pharmacol. **55**, 459—473 (1975).

Maskrey, M., Vogt, M., Bligh, J.: Central effects of clonidine [2-(2,6-dichlophenylamino)-2-imidazoline hydrochloride, St 155] upon thermoregulation in the sheep and goat. Europ. J. Pharmacol. **12**, 297—302 (1970).

Maxwell, G. M.: The effects of 2-(2,6-dichlorphenylamino)-2-imidazoline hydrochloride (Catapres®) upon the systemic and coronary haemodynamics and metabolism of intact dogs. Arch. int. Pharmacodyn. Therap. **181**, 7—14 (1969).

Michel, D.: Erfahrungen mit Catapresan in der Hochdrucktherapie. Dtsch. med. Wschr. **93**, 1375 (1968).

Michel, D., Zimmermann, W., Nassehi, A., Seraphim, P.: Erste Beobachtungen über einen antihypertensiven Effekt von 2-(2,6-Dichlorophenylamino)-2-Imidazolin-hydrochlorid am Menschen. Dtsch. med. Wschr. **91**, 1540—1547 (1966).

Miura, M., Reis, D. J.: Termination and secondary projections of carotid sinus nerve in the cat brain stem. Amer. J. Physiol. **217**, 142—153 (1969).

Morpurgo, C.: Aggressive behaviour induced by large doses of 2-(2,6-dichlorophenylamino)-2-imidazoline hydrochloride (St 155) in mice. Europ. J. Pharmacol. **3**, 374—377 (1968).

MOURET, J., BOBILLIER, P., JOUVET, M.: Effects de la p-chlorophénylalanine sur le sommeil du rat. C. R. Soc. Biol. (Paris) **161**, 1600—1603 (1968).

MUIR, A. L.: The circulatory effects of Catapres at rest and exercise. In: CONOLLY, M. E. (Ed.): Catapres in hypertension, pp. 79—83. London: Butterworths 1970.

MUIR, A. L., BURTON, J. L., LAWRIE, D. M.: Circulatory effects at rest and exercise of clonidine, an imidazoline derivate with hypotensive properties. Lancet **1969 II**, 181—184 (1969).

NATOFF, I. L., KATZUNG, B. G., WEIR, F., KOOMA, J. K.: Cardiovascular properties of 1-(2,6-dichlorobenzylidene) aminoguanidine hydrochloride (SD 15.488). Pharmacologist **10**, 157 (1968).

NATOFF, I. L., STANTON, N. C.: Comparative study of the cardiovascular properties of 2-(2,6-dichlorophenylamino)-2-imidazoline hydrochloride (Catapres) and 2-(2,6-dichlorobenzylidene) aminoguanidine hydrochloride (SD 15.488). Fourth international Congress on Pharmacology. (Abstracts) 312 (1969).

NAYLER, W. G., MCINNES, I., STONE, J., CARSON, V., LOWE, T. E.: Catapres (St155) induced changes in coronary vascular resistance. Cardiovasc. Res. **4**, 457—465 (1970).

NAYLER, W. G., PRICE, J. M., STONE, J., LOWE, T. E.: Further observations on the cardiovascular effects of St155 (Catapres). J. Pharmacol. exp. Ther. **166**, 364—373 (1969).

NAYLER, W. G., PRICE, J. M., SWANN, J. B., MCINNES, I., RACE, D., LOWE, T. E.: Effect of the hypotensive drug St155 (Catapres) on the heart and peripheral circulation. J. Pharmacol. exp. Ther. **164**, 45—59 (1968).

NAYLER, W. G., ROSENBAUM, M., MCINNES, I., LOWE, T. E.: Effect on a new hypotensive drug, St155, on the systemic circulation. Amer. Heart J. **72**, 764—770 (1966).

NAYLER, W. G., STONE, J.: An effect of St155 (clonidine), 2-(2,6-dichlorophenylamino)-2-imidazoline hydrochloride, (Catapres®), on relationship between blood pressure and heart rate in dogs. Europ. J. Pharmacol. **10**, 161—167 (1970).

NEUHAUS, G. A., HUMPERT, U.: Die Beeinflussung der gesteigerten Magensaftsekretion unter intramuskulärer Gabe von 2-(2,6-Dichlorophenylamino-)-2-Imidazolin-hydrochlorid. In: HEILMEYER, HOLTMEIER, PFEIFFER (Eds.): Hochdrucktherapie, S. 205—210. Stuttgart: Thieme 1968.

NEUMAYR, R. J., HARE, B. D., FRANZ, D. N.: Depression of spinal vasomotor pathways by L-dopa and by clonidine. Fifth International Congress on Pharmacology; Abstracts of Volunteer Papers p. 167, (997) (1972).

NOLLY, H. L., REID, I. A., GANONG, W. F.: Effects of adrenergic agents on renin release *in vitro*. Fed. Proc. **33**, 253 (1974).

OBERDORF, A., KRONEBERG, G.: Weitere Untersuchungen zum Wirkungsmechanismus von 2-(2,6-Dimethylphenylamino) 4H-5-6-dihydro 1-3-thiazin (Bayer 1470) am isolierten Meerschweinchen nach Paton. Arch. Pharm. exp. Path. **260**, 183 (1968).

OBERDORF, A., KRONEBERG, G.: The relationship between α and β receptor function and the liberation and action of acetylcholine on the coaxially stimulated guinea pig ileum. Fourth Int. Congress of Pharmacology, Abstracts. 144—145 (1969).

OBERDORF, A., KRONEBERG, G.: Alpha- und Beta-sympathicomimetische Wirkungen am elektrisch gezreizten isolierten Meerschweinchenileum. Arch. Pharmakol. **267**, 195—207 (1970).

OLSEN, V. B.: Clonidine induced increase of renal prostaglandin activity and water diuresis in conscious dogs. Europ. J. Pharmacol. **36**, 95—102 (1976).

ONESTI, G., SCHWARTZ, A. B., KIM, K. E., PAR-MARTINEZ, V., SCHWARTZ, C.: Antihypertensive effect of clonidine. Circulat. Res. **28**, Suppl. 2, 53—69 (1971).

OTTENJANN, R.: Sekretion, Motilität und Schleimhautdurchblutung des Magens unter dem Einfluß von Dichlorophenylaminoimidazolin. In: HEILMEYER, HOLTMEIER, PFEIFFER (Eds.): Hochdrucktherapie, S. 202—205. Stuttgart: Thieme 1968.

OZAWA, H., MIYAUCHI, T., SUGAWARA, K.: Potentiating effect of lithium chloride on aggressive behaviour induced in mice by nialamide plus L-dopa and by clonidine. Europ. J. Pharmacol. **34**, 169—180 (1975).

PAALZOW, G., PAALZOW, L.: Clonidine antinociceptive activity: effects of drugs influencing central monoaminergic and cholinergic mechanisms in the rat. Arch. Pharmacol. **292**, 119—126 (1976).

PAALZOW, L.: Analgesia produced by clonidine in mice and rats. J. Pharm. Pharmacol. **26**, 361—363 (1974).

PACHA, W., SALZMANN, R., SCHOLTYSIK, G.: Inhibitory effects of clonidine and BS 100-141 on responses to sympathetic nerve stimulation in cats and rabbits. Brit. J. Pharmacol. **53**, 513—516 (1975).

Palmer, G. C., Sulser, F., Robinson, G. A.: Effects of neurohumoral and adrenergic agents on cyclic AMP levels in various areas of the rat brain *in vitro*. Neuropharmacology **12**, 327—337 (1973).

Pascaud, X. B., Roger, A. R.: Is the gastric antisecretory property of clonidine in rats of central origine? Brit. J. Pharmacol. **58**, 419—420 (1976).

Paton, W. D. M., Vizi, E. S.: The inhibitory action of noradrenaline and adrenaline on acetylcholine output by guinea pig ileum longitudinal muscle strip. Brit. J. Pharmacol. **35**, 10—28 (1969).

Persson, T.: Drug induced changes in ^{3}H catecholamine accumulation after ^{3}H tyrosine. Acta pharmacol. Toxicol. **28**, 378 (1970).

Persson, T., Waldeck, B.: Further studies on the possible interaction between dopamine and noradrenaline containing neurons in the brain. Europ. J. Pharmacol. **11**, 315—320 (1970).

Pettinger, W. A., Keeton, K. E., Campbell, W. B., Harper, D. C.: Evidence for a renal α-adrenoceptor inhibiting renin release. Circulation Res. **38**, 338—346 (1976).

Philippu, A., Roensberg, W., Przuntek, H.: Pressor response to hypothalamic stimulation as influenced by drugs affecting adrenergic receptors. Arch. Pharmacol. **277** Suppl., R 55 (1973a).

Philippu, A., Roensberg, W., Przuntek, H.: Effects of adrenergic drugs on pressor responses to hypothalamic stimulation. Arch. Pharmacol. **278**, 273—286 (1973b).

Rand, M. J., Rush, M., Wilson, J.: Some observations on the inhibition of salivation by St 155 [2-(2,6-dichlorophenylamino)-2-imidazoline hydrochloride, Catapres. Catapresan]. Europ. J. Pharmacol. **5**, 168—172 (1969).

Rand, M. J., Wilson, J.: Mechanism of the pressor and depressor actions of St 155 [2-(2,6-dichlorophenylamino-2-imidazoline hydrochloride, Catapres®]. Europ. J. Pharmacol. **3**, 27—33 (1968).

Razak, A., Fusiwara, M., Ueki, S.: Automutilation induced by clonidine in mice. Europ. J. Pharmacol. **30**, 356—359 (1975).

Rehbinder, R.: The metabolism of clonidine (Catapres, St 155). In: Conolly, M. E. (Ed.): Catapres in Hypertension, pp. 227—233. London: Butterworths 1970.

Rehbinder, D., Deckers, W.: Biochemische Untersuchungen zur Resorption, Verteilung und Ausscheidung des 2-(2,6-Dichlorophenylamino)-2-Imidazolin-hydrochlorids bei der Ratte. Arzneimittel-Forsch. **16**, 1052—1053 (1966).

Rehbinder, D., Deckers, W.: Stoffwechseleffekte des Catapresan®. Arch. Pharmakol. exp. Path. **261**, 162—175 (1968).

Rehbinder, D., Deckers, W.: Untersuchungen zur Pharmakokinetik und am Metabolismus des 2-(2,6-Dichlorophenylamino)-2-Imidazolin-hydrochlorid (St 155). Arzneimittel-Forsch. **19**, 169—176 (1969).

Reid, I. A., MacDonald, D. M., Ganong, W. F.: Suppression of renin secretion by clonidine. Fed. Proc. **32**, 765 (1973).

Reid, I. A., MacDonald, D. M., Pachnis, B., Ganong, W. F.: Studies concerning the mechanism of suppression of renin secretion by clonidine. J. Pharmacol. exp. Therap. **192**, 713—721 (1975).

Reid, I. A., Pachnis, B., Ganong, W. F.: Mechanism of suppression of renin secretion by clonidine. Fed. Proc. **33**, 543 (1974).

Reid, J. L., Briant, R. H., Dollery, C. T.: Desmethylimipramine and the hypotensive action of clonidine in the rabbit. Life Sci. **12**, 459—467 (1973).

Reid, J.-L., Dollery, C. T.: Central noradrenergic neurons and the hypotensive actions of clonidine. Fifth International Congress on Pharmacology. Abstracts of Volunteer Papers, p. 190 (1135) (1972).

Reid, J. L., Lewis, P. L., Myers, M. G.: Role of central dopaminergic mechanisms on piribedil and clonidine induced hypothermia in the rat. Neuropharmacology **14**, 215—220 (1975).

Reubi, F. C., Vorburger, C., Bütikofer, E.: A comparison of the short-term and long-term haemodynamic effects of antihypertensive drug therapy. In: Conolly, M. E. (Ed.): Catapres in Hypertension, pp. 113—125. London: Butterworths 1970.

Robson, R. D., Antonaccio, M. J.: Effects of clonidine on responses to cardiac nerve stimulation as a function of impulse frequency and stimulus duration in vagotomized dogs. Europ. J. Pharmacol. **29**, 182—186 (1974).

Robson, R. D., Kaplan, H. R.: A reflex cholinergic involvement of St 155 [2-(2,6-dichlorophenylamino)-2-imidazoline hydrochloride]. Pharmacologist **10**, 157 (1968).

Robson, R. D., Kaplan, H. R.: An involvement of St 155 [2-(2,6-dichlorophenylamino)-2-imidazoline hydrochloride, [Catapres®] in cholinergic mechanims. Europ. J. Pharmacol. **5**, 328—337 (1969).

Robson, R. D., Kaplan, H. R., Laforce, J.: An analysis of the bradycardic effect of St155 [2-(2,6-dichlorophenylamino-2-imidazoline hydrochloride]. Fed. Proc. **28**, 738 (1969a).

Robson, R. D., Kaplan, H. R., Laforce, S.: An investigation into the bradycardic effects of St155 [2-(2,6-dichlorophenylamino)-2-imidazoline HCl] in the anesthetized dog. J. Pharmacol. exp. Ther. **169**, 120—131 (1969b).

Rochette, L., Bralet, J.: Effects of clonidine on the synthesis of cerebral dopamine. Biochem. Pharmacol. **24**, 303—305 (1975).

Rochette, L., Bralet, A. M., Bralet, J.: Influence de la clonidine sur la synthèse et la libération de la noradrénaline dans différentes structures cérébrales du rat. J. Pharmacol. (Paris) **5**, 209—220 (1974).

Rosenthal, J., Hoefke, W., Wolff, H. P.: Die Wirkung von 2-(2,6-Dichlorophenylamino)-2-Imidazolin HCl auf Blutdruck und Plasmareninaktivität bei Ratten. Pflügers Arch. **312**, R85—R86 (1969).

Ruch-Monachon, M. A., Jalfre, M., Haefely, W.: Drugs and PGO waves in the lateral geniculate body of the curarised cat. III. PGO waves and brain catecholamines. Arch. int. Pharmacol. Therap. **219**, 287—307 (1976).

Saameli, K., Scholtysik, G., Waite, R.: Pharmacology of BS 100-141, a centrally acting antihypertensive drug. Clin. exp. Pharmac. Physiol., suppl. **2**, 207—212 (1975).

Safar, M. E., Weiss, Y. A., Levenson, J. A., London, G. M., Milliez, P. L.: Antihypertensive effect of clonidine and salt depletion in severe hypertension. Clinical and hemodynamic study. Europ. J. clin. Pharmacol. **5**, 203—209 (1973).

Salt, J. L.: Inhibition of uptake$_2$ in the isolated rat heart by steroïds, clonidine and methoxylated phenylethylamines. Europ. J. Pharmacol. **20**, 329—340 (1972).

Sato, A., Schmidt, R. F.: Spinal and supraspinal components of the reflex discharges into lumbar and thoracic white rami. J. Physiol. (Lond.) **212**, 839—850 (1971).

Sattin, A., Rall, T. W., Zanella, J.: Regulation of cyclic adenosine 3,5′ monophosphate levels in guinea-pig cerebral cortex by interaction of α-adrenergic and adenosine receptor activity. J. Pharmacol. exp. Therap. **192**, 22—32 (1975).

Sattler, R. W., Van Zwieten, P. A.: Acute hypotensive action of 2-(2,6-dichlorophenylamino)-2-imidazoline hydrochloride (St155) after infusion into the cat's vertebral artery. Europ. J. Pharmacol. **2**, 9—13 (1967).

Scheja, H. W., Sturm, A. Jr.: Klinische Untersuchungen zum Wirkungsmechanismus der 2-(2,6-Dichlorophenylamino)-2-Imidazolin HCl (Catapresan). Verh. dtsch. Ges. inn. Med. **74**, 559—562 (1968).

Schmitt, H.: Reduction of central sympathetic tone by two new drugs. Central action of 2-(2,6′-dichlorophenylamino)-2-imidazoline and reflex action of (pyrimidyl-2"-(1-methylene-dioxy-3′-4′-benzyl-4-piperazine). In: Bertelli, A. (Ed.): Circulatory drugs, pp. 153—154. Amsterdam: North Holland Publ. Com. 1969.

Schmitt, H.: Centrally mediated decrease in sympathetic tone induced by 2-(2,6-dichlorophenylamino)-2-imidazoline (St155, Catapres). In: Conolly, M. E. (Ed.): Catapres in Hypertension, pp. 23—41. London: Butterworths 1970.

Schmitt, H.: On some unexplained effects of clonidine. In: Milliez, P., Safar, M. (Eds.): Recent Advances in Hypertension, Vol. 2, pp. 63—72. Reims: Société Aliéna 1975.

Schmitt, H., Delbarre, B., Autret, A.-M.: Antagonism of the action of clonidine on EEG. J. Pharmacol. (Paris) **2**, 242 (1971a).

Schmitt, H., Fénard, S.: Interaction de la clonidine (St155) avec l'atropine, la mécamylamine et la bivagotomie. J. Pharmacol. (Paris) **1**, 424—425 (1970a).

Schmitt, H., Fénard, S.: Influence de l'atropine, des ganglioplégiques et de la bivagotomie sur les effects hémodynamiques de la clonidine. J. Pharmacol. (Paris) **1**, 359—368 (1970b).

Schmitt, H., Fénard, S.: Effects des alcaloïdes de l'ergot de seigle sur les centres vasomoteurs et leur inhibition par la clonidine. C. R. Soc. Biol. (Paris) **164**, 1006—1009 (1970c).

Schmitt, H., Fénard, S.: Effects des substances sympathomimétiques sur les centres vasomoteurs. Arch. int. Pharmacodyn. Thérap. **190**, 229—240 (1971).

Schmitt, H., Fénard, S., Schmitt, Hélène: Influence d'agents β-bloquants sur les effects inhibiteurs exercés par la clonidine sur les centres vasomoteurs. J. Pharmacol. (Paris) **2**, 369—372 (1971b).

Schmitt, H., Fournadjiev, G., Schmitt, Hélène: Central and peripheral effects of 2-(2,6-dichlorophenylamino)4H 5—6 dihydro 1—3 thiazine (Bayer 1470) on sympathetic system. Europ. J. Pharmacol. **10**, 230—238 (1970).

Schmitt, H., Le Douarec, J.-C., Pétillot, N.: Antinociceptive effects of some α-sympathomimetic agents. Neuropharmacology 13, 289—294 (1974a).

Schmitt, H., Le Douarec, J.-C., Pétillot, N.: Antagonism of the antinociceptive action of xylazine, an α-sympathomimetic agent by adrenoceptor and cholinoceptor blocking agents. Neuropharmacology 13, 295—303 (1974b).

Schmitt, H., Schmitt, Hélène: Localization of the hypotensive effect of 2-(2,6-dichlorophenylamino)-2-imidazoline hydrochloride (St155, Catapresan). Europ. J. Pharmacol. 6, 8—12 (1969a).

Schmitt, H., Schmitt, Hélène: α-sympathomimetic drugs with centrally mediated hypotensive effect. Fourth International Congress on Pharmacology. Abstracts 315—316 (1969b).

Schmitt, H., Schmitt, Hélène: Interactions between 2-(2,6-dichlorophenylamino)-2-imidazoline hydrochloride (St155, Catapresan®) and α-adrenergic blocking drugs. Europ. J. Pharmacol. 9, 7—13 (1970).

Schmitt, H., Schmitt, Hélène, Boissier, J.-R., Giudicelli, J.-F.: Centrally mediated decrease in sympathetic tone induced by 2(2,6-dichlorophenylamino)-2-imidazoline (St155, Catapresan®). Europ. J. Pharmacol. 2, 147—148 (1967).

Schmitt, H., Schmitt, Hélène, Boissier, J.-R., Giudicelli, J.-F., Fichelle, J.: Cardiovascular effects of 2-(2,6-dichlorophenylamino)-2-imidazoline hydrochloride (St155). II. Central sympathetic structures. Europ. J. Pharmacol. 2, 340—346 (1968).

Schmitt, H., Schmitt, Hélène, Fénard, S.: Influence of some α-adrenergic blocking drugs on the inhibitory effect of clonidine on vasomotor centres. J. Pharmacol. (Paris) 2, 192 (1971c).

Schmitt, H., Schmitt, Hélène, Fénard, S.: Evidence for an α-sympathomimetic component in the effects of Catapresan on vasomotor centres: antagonism by piperoxan. Europ. J. Pharmacol. 14, 98—100 (1971d).

Schmitt, H., Schmitt, Hélène, Fénard, S.: Action de l'ésérine, de l'oxotrémorine et de la mécamylamine sur les centres sympathiques et interférence avec les effects inhibiteurs de la clonidine. J. Pharmacol. (Paris) 3, 118—119 (1972a).

Schmitt, H., Schmitt, Hélène, Fénard, S.: Action de l'ésérine, de l'oxotrémorine et de la mécamylamine sur les centres sympathiques et interférence avec les effects inhibiteurs de la clonidine. J. Pharmacol. (Paris) 3, 423—434 (1972b).

Schmitt, H., Schmitt, Hélène, Fénard, S.: Influence of some drugs interfering with catecholamines on splanchnic discharges and blood pressure in conscious dogs. Fifth International Congress on Pharmacology. Abstracts of Volunteer papers, p. 204 (1222) 1(1972e).

Schmitt, H., Schmitt, Hélène, Fénard, S.: Action of α-adrenergic blocking drugs on the sympathetic centres and their interactions with the central sympatho-inhibitory effect of clonidine. Arzneimittel-Forsch. 23, 40—45 (1973a).

Schmitt, H., Schmitt, Hélène, Fénard, S.: Decrease in the sympatho-inhibitory action of clonidine after destruction of the sympatho-inhibitory area. Experientia (Basel) 29, 1247—1249 (1973b).

Schmitt, H., Schmitt, Hélène, Fénard, S.: A technique for recording splanchnic discharges in unanaesthetized dogs. Neuropharmacology 13, 247—250 (1974c).

Schmitt, H., Tsoucaris-Kupfer, D., Pétillot, N.: Hypothermia induced in rats by clonidine and related compounds: Inhibition by adrenergic blocking agents. J. Pharmacol. (Paris) 2, 241 (1971e).

Schneider, K. W.: Cardialhämodynamik im akuten Versuch, nach chronischer Behandlung und im Belastungstest mit St155. In: Heilmeyer, Holtmeier, Pfeiffer (Eds.): Hochdrucktherapie, S. 78—83. Stuttgart: Thieme 1968.

Schneider, K. W., Gattenlöhner, W.: Hämodynamische Untersuchungen nach St155 [2-(2,6-Dichlorophenylamino-2-Imidazolin-hydrochlorid] beim Menschen. Dtsch. med. Wschr. 91, 1533—1539 (1966).

Scholtysik, G.: Inhibition of effects of accelerator nerve stimulation in cats and rabbits by BS 100-41 and guanabenz. Naunyn-Schmiedebergs Arch. Pharmacol. 282, R86 (1974).

Scholtysik, G., Salzmann, R.: Interaction between antidepressant and centrally antihypertensive drugs. Arch. Pharmacol. 279, Suppl., R. 23 (1973).

Schümann, H. J., Endoh, M.: α-Adrenoceptors in the ventricular myocardium: clonidine, naphazoline and methoxamine as partial α-agonists exerting a competitive dualism in action to phenylephrine. Europ. J. Pharmacol. 36, 413—421 (1976).

Schümann, H. J., Werner, U.: Hemmung der Hormonfreisetzung aus dem Nebennierenmark durch BAY a 6781, eine antihypertensiv wirksame Substanz. Arch. Pharmakol. 268, 71—82 (1971).

SCRIABINE, A., STAVORSKI, J. M.: Effect of clonidine on the electrically-induced contraction of the isolated guinea-pig ileum. Fed. Proc. **29**, 149 (1970).

SCRIABINE, A., STAVORSKI, J. M.: Effect of clonidine on cardiac acceleration in vagotomized dogs. Europ. J. Pharmacol. **24**, 101—104 (1973).

SCRIABINE, A., STAVORSKI, J. M.: Effects of phentolamine, phenoxybenzamine and desipramine on clonidine blockade induced of cardiac acceleration in the dog. Europ. J. Pharmacol. **42**, 63—70 (1977).

SCRIABINE, A., STAVORSKY, J., WENGER, H. C., TORCHIANA, M. L., STONE, C. A.: Cardiac slowing effects of clonidine (St155) in dogs. J. Pharmacol. exp. Ther. **171**, 256—264 (1970).

SCRIABINE, A., STONE, C. A., STAVORSKI, J. M.: Studies on the mechanism of St155-induced cardiac slowing in dogs. Pharmacologist **10**, 156 (1968).

SCRIABINE, A., SWEET, C. S., LUDDEN, C. T., STAVORSKI, J. M.: Central vs peripheral cardiovascular effects of 2-(2,6-diethyl-phenylamino)-2-imidazoline hydrochloride (St 91). Sixth International Congress of Pharmacology Abstracts p. 636 (n° 1549) (1975).

SELLER, H., ILLERT, M.: The localization of the first synapse in the carotid sinus baroreceptor reflex pathway and its alteration by the afferent input. Pflügers Arch. **306**, 1—19 (1969).

SENFT, G., SIFT, R., LOSERT, W., SCHULTZ, G., HOFFMANN, W.: Hemmung der Insulininkretion durch Alpha-Receptoren-stimulierende Substanzen. Arch. Pharm. exp. Path. **260**, 309—323 (1968).

SHAW, J., HUNYOR, S. N., KORNER, P. I.: The peripheral circulatory effects of clonidine and their role in the production of arterial hypotension. Europ. J. Pharmacol. **14**, 101—111 (1971a).

SHAW, J., HUNYOR, S. N., KORNER, P. I.: Sites of central nervous action of clonidine on reflex autonomic function in the unanaesthetized rabbit. Europ. J. Pharmacol. **15**, 66—78 (1971b).

SHERMAN, G. P., GREGA, G. J., WOODS, R. J., BUCKLEY, J. P.: Evidence for a central hypotensive mechanism of 2-(2,6-dichlorophenylamino)-2-imidazoline (Catapresan, St155). Europ. J. Pharmacol. **2**, 326—328 (1968).

SHOULSON, I., CHASE, T. N.: Clonidine and the antiparkinsonian response to L-dopa. Neuropharmacology **15**, 25—27 (1976).

SIMON, P., CHERMAT, R., BOISSIER, J. R.: Comparaison des effects sédatifs de deux α-sympathomimétiques antihypertenseurs: la clonidine et la tiaménidine. Thérapie **30**, 855—861 (1975).

SINHA, J. N., ATKINSON, J. M., SCHMITT, H.: Effects of clonidine and L-dopa on spontaneous and evoked splanchnic nerve discharges. Europ. J. Pharmacol. **24**, 113—119 (1973).

SINHA, J. N., TANGRI, K. K., BHARGAVA, K. P., SCHMITT, H.: Central sites of sympatho-inhibitory effects of clonidine and L-dopa. In: MILLIEZ, P., SAFAR, M. (Eds.): Recent Advances in Hypertension, Vol. 1, pp. 97—109. Société Aliéna 1975.

SJAASTAD, O., STENSRUD, P.: 2-(2,6-dichlorophenylamino)-2-imidazoline hydrochloride (St155 or Catapresan) as a prophylactic remedy against migraine. Acta neurol. scand. **47**, 120—122 (1971).

SKINHØJ, E.: Die zerebrale hämodynamische Wirkung eines Imidazolin-Derivates mit blutdrucksenkender Wirkung. In: HEILMEYER, HOLTMEIER, PFEIFFER (Eds.): Hochdrucktherapie. Stuttgart: Thieme (1968).

SKOLNICK, P., DALY, J. W.: Stimulation of adenosine 3,'5' monophosphate formation by alpha and beta adrenergic agonists in rat cerebral cortical slices: effects of clonidine. Molec. Pharmacol. **11**, 545—561 (1975).

SKOLNICK, P., DALY, J. W.: Interaction of clonidine with pre and postsynaptic adrenergic receptors of rat brain: Effects on cyclic AMP generating systems. Europ. J. Pharmacol. **39** 11—21 (1976a).

SKOLNICK, P., DALY, J. W., FREEDMAN, R., HOFFER, J.: Interelationship between catecholamine-stimulated formation of adenosine 3,5′ monophosphate in cerebellar slices and inhibitory effects on cerebellar Purkinje cells: antagonism by neuroleptic compounds. J. Pharmacol. exp. Therap. **197**, 280—292 (1976b).

SLEIGHT, P., WEST, M., KORNER, P., OLIVER, J., CHALMERS, J., ROBINSON, J.: The action of clonidine on the baroreflex control of heart rate in conscious animal and man and on single aortic baroreceptor discharge in the rabbit. Arch. inter. Pharmacod. Thérap. **214**, 4—11 (1975).

STARKE, K., ALTMANN, K. P.: Inhibition of adrenergic neurotransmission by clonidine: an action on prejunctional α-receptors. Neuropharmacology **12**, 339—347 (1973).

STARKE, K., MONTEL, H.: Involvement of α-receptors in clonidine induced inhibition of transmitter release from central monoamine neurones. Neuropharmacology **12**, 1073—1080 (1973a).

Starke, K., Montel, H.: Alphareceptor-mediated modulation of transmitter release from central noradrenergic neurones. Naunyn-Schmiedeberg's Arch. Pharmacol. **279**, 53—60 (1973a).

Starke, K., Montel, H.: Influence of drugs with affinity for α-adrenoceptors on noradrenaline release by potassium, tyramine and dimethylphenylpiperazinium. Europ. J. Pharmacol. **27**, 273—280 (1974).

Starke, K., Montel, H., Endo, T., Taube, H.D.: Pharmacological consequences of the presynaptic control of noradrenaline release. In: Milliez, P., Safar, M. (Eds.): Recent Advances in Hypertension, Vol. 2, pp. 75—84. Reims: Société Aliéna 1975.

Starke, K., Montel, H., Gayk, W., Merker, R.: Comparison of the effects of clonidine on pre and postsynaptic adrenoceptors in the rabbit pulmonary artery. Naunyn-Schmiedeberg's Arch. Pharmacol. **285**, 133—150 (1974).

Starke, K., Schümann, A.J.: Zur peripheren sympathikushemmenden Wirkung des Clonidins. Experientia (Basel) **27**, 70—71 (1971).

Starke, K., Wagner, J., Schümann, H.J.: Characterization of the peripheral antiadrenergic effect of clonidine. Arch. Pharmakol. **270**, Suppl. I, R1361 (1971).

Starke, K., Wagner, J., Schümann, H.J.: Adrenergic neuron blockade by clonidine: comparison with guanethidine and local anesthetics. Arch. int. Pharmacod. Thérap. **195**, 291—308 (1972).

Stauch, M.: Einfluß von Dichlorophenylaminoimidazolin (Catapres) auf die alveolare Ventilation und die Kurzschlußdurchblutung der Lunge. Klin. Wschr. **46**, 505—507 (1968a).

Stauch, M.: Die Wirkung von 2-(2,6-Dichlorophenylamino)-2-Imidazolin HCl auf die arterielle Sauerstoffspannung und den Blutdruck in Ruhe und bei Belastung. Arzneimittel-Forsch. **18**, 597—600 (1968b).

Stenberg, J., Holmberg, S., Naets, E., Varnauskas, E.: The hemodynamic effects of Catapresan. Central circulation at rest. Circulation at rest and during exercise. In: Heilmeyer, Holtmeier, Pfeiffer (Eds.): Hochdrucktherapie, pp. 68—75. Stuttgart: Thieme 1968.

Stjärne, L.: Mechanisms of catecholamine secretion. In: Usdin, E., Snyder, S.H. (Eds.): Frontiers in Catecholamine Research, pp. 491—496. New York-Toronto-Oxford-Sydney-Braunschweig: Pergamon Press 1973.

Struyker-Boudier, H.A.J.: Catecholamines receptors in nervous tissue. The release of neuronal catecholamine and receptors in the mode of action of dopaminergic and antihypertensive drugs. Nijmegen: Stiching Studentenpren 1975.

Struyker-Boudier, H.A.J., Van Rossum, J.M.: Clonidine induced cardiovascular effects following stereotaxic application in the hypothalamus of rats. J. Pharm. Pharmacol. **24**, 410—411 (1972).

Struyker-Boudier, H., Smeets, G., Brauwer, G., van Rossum, J.: Central and peripheral alpha adrenergic activity of imidazoline derivates. Life Sci. **15**, 887—899 (1974).

Sturm, A. Jr., Scheja, H.W.: Zur Wirkung des Catapresans auf den Blutdruck und die Ausscheidung des Hauptkatecholaminmetaboliten. In: Heilmeyer, Holtmeier, Pfeiffer (Eds.): Hochdrucktherapie, S. 99—104. Stuttgart: Thieme 1968.

Svensson, Th., Bunney, B.S., Aghajanian, G.K.: Inhibition of both noradrenergic and serotoninergic neurons in brain by the adrenergic agonist clonidine. Brain Res. **92**, 291—306 (1975).

Tanz, R.D.: On the mechanism of Catapresan induced hypotension and bradycardia. Pharmacologist **11**, 270 (1969).

Tauberger, G., Kuhn, P., Brus, M.: Untersuchungen der zentralen sympathicusdämpfenden Wirkungen von Reserpin, Methyldopa und Clonidin. Arch. Pharmakol. **266**, 464—465 (1970).

Toda, N., Fukuda, N., Shimamoto, K.: The mode of hypotensive action of 2-(2,6-dichlorophenylamino)-2-imidazoline in the rabbit. Jap. J. Pharmacol. **19**, 199—210 (1969).

Tran Quang Loc, Delbarre, B., Tsoucaris-Kupfer, D., Schmitt, H.: Antagonisme des effects de la clonidine sur l'électrocorticogramme du lapin et du chat par des substances adrénolytiques α. J. Pharmacol. (Paris) **4**, 415 (1973).

Tran Quang Loc, Tsoucaris-Kupfer, D., Bogaievsky, Y., Bogaievsky, D., Delbarre, B., Schmitt, H.: Antagonisme de l'action sédative de la clonidine par quelques α adrénolytiques: étude électrocorticographique et comportementale chez le lapin et le chat. J. Pharmacol. (Paris) **5**, 51—62 (1974).

Trolin, G.: Effect of pentobarbitone and decerebration on the clonidine induced circulatory changes. Europ. J. Pharmacol. **34**, 1—7 (1976).

TSENG, L. F., LOH, K. H., WEI, E. T.: Effects of clonidine on morphine withdrawal signs in the rat. Europ. J. Pharmacol. **30**, 93—99 (1975).

TSOUCARIS-KUPFER, D., DELBARRE, B., SCHMITT, H.: Actions antagonistes du pimozide et du pipéroxane sur les récepteurs dopaminergiques et noradrénergiques du système nerveux central. J. Pharmacol. (Paris) **4**, 408—409 (1973).

TSOUCARIS-KUPFER, D., SCHMITT, H.: Action hypothermisante de substances α-sympathomimétiques: Antagonisme avec quelques adrénolytiques et cholinolytiques. C. R. Acad. Sci. (Paris) **274**, 607—610 (1972a).

TSOUCARIS-KUPFER, D., SCHMITT, H.: Hypothermic effect of α-sympathomimetic agents and their antagonism by adrenergic and cholinergic blocking agents. Neuropharmacology **11**, 625—635 (1972b).

ÜVNAS, B.: Central cardiovascular control. Handbook of Physiology, Neurophysiology Vol. 2, pp. 1131—1162, 1960.

VAN SPANNING, H. W., VAN ZWIETEN, P. A.: The interference of tricyclic antidepressants with the central hypotensive effect of clonidine. Europ. J. Pharmacol. **24**, 402—404 (1973).

VAN ZWIETEN, P. A.: Centrally induced hypotension by 2-(2,6-dichlorophenyl)-5,6-dihydroimidazo(2,1-b)thiazole fumarate (compound 44.594/15). Pharmacology **13**, 352—353 (1975a).

VAN ZWIETEN, P. A.: Interaction between centrally acting hypotensive drugs and tricyclic antidepressants. Arch. int. Pharmacod. Thérap. **214**, 12—30 (1975b).

VORBURGER, G., BUTIKOFER, E., REUBI, F.: Die akute Wirkung von St 155 auf die cardiale und renale Hämodynamik. In: HEILMEYER, HOLTMEIER, PFEIFFER (Eds.): Hochdrucktherapie, S. 86—93. Stuttgart: Thieme 1968.

VORBURGER, G., BUTIKOFER, E., WEISS, S.: Die akute Wirkung von Catapresan, einem neuen Hypotensiven, auf die cardiale und renale Hämodynamik. Thirty-fifth Annual Meeting of the Schweizerische Gesellschaft für Kardiologie, p. 69—71 (1967a).

VORBURGER, C., BUTIKOFER, E., WEISS, S., DIACON, C.: Die akute Wirkung von St 155, einem neuen Hypotensiven auf kardiale und renale Hämodynamik. Helv. med. Acta **34**, Suppl. 47, 133—134 (1967b).

WAHL, P.: Über die Wirkung von Catapresan auf den intravenösen Glucosetoleranztest. In: HEILMEYER, HOLTMEIER, PFEIFFER (Eds.): Hochdrucktherapie, S. 150—151. Stuttgart: Thieme 1968.

WAITE, R.: Inhibition of sympathetic nerve activity resulting from central alpha adrenoceptor stimulation. In: MILLIEZ, P., SAFAR, M. (Eds.): Recent Advances in Hypertension, pp. 27—36. Reims: Société Aliéna 1975.

WALLAND, A.: Blutdruck und Herzfrequenz der Ratte nach wiederholter Behandlung mit 2-(2,6-Dichlorophenylamino)-2-imidazolin. Arzneimittel-Forsch. **18**, 833—836 (1968).

WALLAND, A., KOBINGER, W.: On the problem of tolerance of 2-(2,6-dichlorophenylamino)-2-imidazoline. Arzneimittel-Forsch. **21**, 61—65 (1971).

WALLAND, A., KOBINGER, W.: Investigations upon the vagal regulation of the heart rate in conscious dogs. Arch. Pharmacol. **277**, Suppl. R 87 (1973).

WALLAND, A., KOBINGER, W., CSONGRADY, A.: Action of clonidine on baroreceptor reflexes in conscious dogs. Europ. J. Pharmacol. **26**, 184—190 (1974).

WALZ, A., VAN ZWIETEN, P. A.: The influence of 2-(2,6-dichlorophenylamino)-2-imidazoline hydrochloride (Clonidine) and some related compounds on gastric secretion in the anesthetized rat. Europ. J. Pharmacol. **10**, 369—377 (1970).

WAROT, D.: Clonidine et contrôle noradrenergique des activités spinales réflexes. Thèse de médecine, Paris 1976.

WASHIZU, Y.: St 155 on excitation-contraction in guinea pig-atrium. Arch. int. Pharmacod. Thérap. **188**, 356—363 (1970).

WASHIZU, Y.: Some effects of clonidine, procaine and tetrodotoxin on crayfish sensory neuron. Europ. J. Pharmacol. **14**, 384—388 (1971).

WASHIZU, Y.: Differential effects of clonidine on guinea-pig atrial and papillary muscles. Arch. int. Pharmacod. Thérap. **196**, 184—191 (1972).

WEISE, J., STOETZER, H., KNAPPEN, F., WALLAND, A.: The effect of clonidine on the pupil diameter and the retina in rats, assessed in relation to the intensity of light. Arzneimittel-Forsch. **21**, 821—825 (1971).

WENDT, F., CASPERS, I.: Körpertemperatur und Schweißsekretion bei körperlicher Belastung unter dem Einfluß von 2-(2,6-Dichlorophenylamino)-2-Imidazolinhydrochlorid. In: HEILMEYER, HOLTMEIER, PFEIFFER (Eds.): Hochdrucktherapie, S. 197—201. Stuttgart: Thieme 1968.

WERMUTH, C. G., SCHWARTZ, J., LECLERC, G., GARNIER, J. P., ROUOT, B.: Conformation de la clonidine et hypothèses sur son interaction avec un récepteur α adrénergique. Chim. Thérap. **1**, 115—116 (1973).

WERNER, U., STARKE, K., SCHÜMANN, H. J.: Wirkungen von Clonidin (St 155) und BAY a 6781 auf das isolierte Kaninchenherz. Arch. Pharmakol. **266**, 474—475 (1970).

WERNER, U., STARKE, K., SCHÜMANN, H. J.: Actions of clonidine and 2-(2-methyl-6-ethyl-cyclohexylamino)-2-oxazoline on postganglionic autonomic nerves. Arch. int. Pharmacodyn. **195**, 282—290 (1972).

WILKINSON, M.: Clonidine for migraine. Lancet **1969 II**, 430.

WILLIS, L. R., WILLIAMSON, H. E.: The effect of Catapres on renal blood flow. Clin. Res. **17**, 559 (1969).

WINCHESTER, J., KENNEDY, A. C.: Iatrogenic Raynaud's Phenomenon. Brit. med. J. **1971 III**, 113.

WOODHOUSE, B. L., RAM, N., GARVEY, H. L.: Influence of St 155 (Catapres) upon efferent autonomic nerve activity. Fed. Proc. **31**, 563 (Abstr.) (1972).

ZAÏMIS, E.: On the pharmacology of Catapres (St 155). In: CONOLLY, M. E. (Ed.): Catapres in hypertension, pp. 9—22. London: Butterworths 1970.

ZAÏMIS, E., HANINGTON, E.: A possible pharmacological approach to migraine. Lancet **1969 II**, (9) 298—300.

ZIMMERMANN, W., MICHEL, D., SERAPHIN, P. H.: Zur Wirkung von Catapres auf den kleinen Kreislauf. In: HEILMEYER, HOLTMEIER, PFEIFFER (Eds.): Hochdrucktherapie, S. 97—104. Stuttgart: Thieme 1968.

Chapter 8

Drugs Acting on Arteriolar Smooth Muscle (Vasodilator Drugs)

F. GROSS

The Section "III. Nitroprusside" was written by V. A. W. KREYE and F. GROSS

With 8 Figures

I. Introduction

Drugs that reduce arteriolar smooth muscle tone directly are often called vasodilators, but it must be kept in mind that reduction in sympathetic tone or stimulation of β-adrenergic receptors also results in a dilation of the resistance vessels. Nevertheless, it has become customary to reserve the term "vasodilator drug" for those agents that act directly on the vasculature without interfering with the autonomic innervation. For a long time, attempts have been made to lower blood pressure by drugs that relax arteriolar smooth muscle directly and in this way reduce total peripheral resistance. Papaverine was the first agent to be used; it was followed by various others, but—with two exceptions—results were disappointing. However, these two drugs were not considered as being of practical value for the treatment of hypertension, because they had only a short duration of action, were difficult to administer, and one of them had already an established place in therapeutics other than the treatment of high blood pressure. The two compounds are sodium nitroprusside and nitroglycerine, the former described as a vasodilator nearly 50 years ago (JOHNSON, 1929), the latter having been used to relieve anginal pain for about 100 years.

The first effective vasodilator in the treatment of hypertension was hydralazine (GROSS et al., 1950), which, although discovered in Europe, has first been clinically investigated and then generally applied as an antihypertensive in the USA (SCHROEDER, 1951). It is surprising that hydralazine and, together with it, dihydralazine have remained the only vasodilators widely used in the treatment of high blood pressure for nearly 25 years. Various efforts have been made to develop new agents that act on arteriolar muscle similarly to hydralazine but cause less unpleasant side reactions. However, until recently, nearly all attempts have failed. One exception was diazoxide (RUBIN et al., 1962; FINNERTY et al., 1963), which is a potent antihypertensive but elicits, besides sodium retention, hyperglycaemia, which prevents its administration in the long-term treatment of hypertension (DOLLERY et al., 1962; BARTORELLI et al., 1963; WILSON and OKUN, 1963).

Some years ago, various compounds of quite different chemical structures were characterized as directly acting vasodilators, such as guancydine (CUMMINGS et al., 1969), minoxidil (DUCHARME et al., 1973), or prazosin (SCRIABINE et al., 1968). All three were selected for studies in man and underwent clinical pharmacologic investigations and therapeutic trials. Prazosin has been marketed in various countries recently, but this drug can no longer be considered as a directly acting vasodilator. On the basis of experimental and clinical studies it is an α-adrenergic blocking agent rather than a typical vasodilator (BOLLI et al., 1975). On the other hand, fusaric acid and some of its derivatives, such as bupicomide, which inhibit dopamin-β-hydroxylase, seem to act as direct vasodilators (HIDAKA et al., 1969; KORBUDA et al., 1973; VELASCO et al., 1975). However, they have not been introduced as therapeutics so far.

Since drugs acting directly on arteriolar smooth muscle do not reduce but increase sympathetic reflex activity, all vasodilators in doses that lower blood pressure induce an increase in heart rate and cardiac output, stimulate renin release from the kidney and may favor sodium retention and plasma volume expansion (KOCH-WESER, 1974). Occasionally also an increase of pressure in the pulmonary circulation may occur. Hence, in long-term treatment of hypertension, vasodilators have to be given together with β-adrenergic blocking agents and saluretics. At the time when hydralazine was introduced, neither of these two types of drug was known, and it was not until 1954 that (di-)hydralazine was associated with reserpine (reserpine-hydralazine, Serpasil-Apresolin, reserpine-dihydralazine, Adelphan) in order to reduce its stimulating effect on heart rate and to enhance its antihypertensive action. Five years later, when hydrochlorothiazide became available, it was added to the reserpine-(di-)hydralazine combination, but until then only occasionally a mild sodium and fluid retention had been observed with hydralazine.

The degree of the positive chronotropic effect varies for individual drugs as well as in different species, being least pronounced with sodium nitroprusside (see p. 440). Sodium nitroprusside also reduces venous return to the heart as a consequence of venous pooling (SCHLANT et al., 1962; BHATIA and FROHLICH, 1973), whereas all the other vasodilators increase rather than decrease venous return. The rise in cardiac output counteracts to a certain degree the hypotensive effect. During anesthesia, the reflex tachycardia may be suppressed, and therefore the fall in blood pressure is in general more marked than in conscious animals or man. Hemodynamically, the tachycardic response imposes an additional work load upon the heart, for which the reduction in total peripheral resistance only partially makes up. When vasodilators are used in the treatment of hypertension, an already impaired oxygen supply to the myocardium may be further diminished by the rise of cardiac output and anginal attacks may be provoked, as has been observed with hydralazine, diazoxide or minoxidil. On the other hand, the elevated heart rate counteracts orthostatic reactions, as not infrequently experienced as a side-effect of antihypertensives which act on the efferent sympathetic system, especially ganglionic blockers or guanethidine.

Increase in reflex sympathetic activity may also be responsible for the stimulation of renin release from the kidney, which results in an elevated plasma renin or angiotensin II concentration (KÜCHEL et al., 1967; UEDA et al., 1968). Although the significance of this finding for the course of hypertension is not at all clear, it cannot be considered an adverse reaction that would diminish the hypotensive effect of vasodilators. The increase in plasma renin activity is the consequence of a regulatory process induced by sympathetic activation (KOCH-WESER, 1974). In most cases such a rise in plasma renin activity has as little influence on the effectiveness of vasodilators as the activation of the renin-angiotensin system caused by diuretics or a low sodium diet. Beta-adrenergic blockers may suppress the activation of the renin-angiotensin system provoked by vasodilators, but this effect contributes little or nothing to the antihypertensive effect of that class of drugs.

One pharmacologic feature that may be brought up in favour of various vasodilator drugs is that most of them are free from central effects, and do not induce fatigue nor diminish vigilance. So far, no drugs are known that lower blood pressure by acting directly on the vasculature and affecting central areas that are responsible for blood pressure regulation. Nevertheless, it cannot be excluded that such types of drug exist.

In general, it may be expected that vasodilators will have an increasing share in the drug treatment of hypertension, especially if some of the newly developed agents become available (KOCH-WESER, 1973, 1974). It is, however, already evident by now that in antihypertensive therapy the trend towards peripherally acting drugs favors also the wider use of hydralazines, especially since it is possible to abolish the unwanted effects on the heart by the simultaneous administration of β-adrenergic antagonists.

II. Hydralazines

The synthesis of hydralazine occurred as a consequence of making use of a heterocyclic ring (phthalazine) which was considered to be of interest from a chemical point of view (DRUEY, personal communication). The hydrazine derivative of phthalazine was prepared without having in mind a special therapeutic activity, also not as an antihistaminic, as it has been incorrectly stated in various papers, and the substance was screened by standard methods which rapidly revealed its remarkable action on blood pressure. The hypotensive effect of hydralazine, which is characterized by its gradual onset, limited degree, and long duration, was observed in the laboratory as early as 1945, but only four years later was the first paper on this new group of blood pressure-lowering substances published (GROSS et al., 1950). One of the reasons for the delay was the disappointing results during the first period of clinical trials; investigators had reported unpleasant acute side effects, such as headache, nausea, vomiting, flushing, tachycardia, and angina. These were considered so severe that some leading Swiss clinicians recommended the abandoning of the drug, which, in their opinion, could never be used as a therapeutic agent.

Pharmacologic and clinical studies were then taken up in the United States, where meanwhile the experimental results had been confirmed (CRAVER et al., 1951), and where hydralazine met with the interest of clinical specialists. Some clinicians considered the drug a most valuable antihypertensive, since, after the ganglionic blockers, it was the first synthetic compound that was effective in lowering blood pressure and could be used in antihypertensive therapy (SCHROEDER, 1951; PAGE, 1951). Subsequently, because of the favourable reports published in the United States, hydralazine attracted attention in some European countries, and one of its derivatives, dihydralazine, was further clinically investigated and eventually marketed (ESSELIER et al., 1953). However, in Europe, except in Sweden, neither hydralazine nor dihydralazine ever gained a position in the treatment of hypertension comparable to that of hydralazine in the United States and some other countries, mainly Japan. Only in combination with reserpine and later with reserpine and hydrochlorothiazide dihydralazine was and still is widely used in some European countries, whereas in the United States and various other countries, hydralazine is combined with the other two drugs.

Various related compounds, including hydrazinopyridazines, had been submitted to clinical trials, especially with respect to finding a better tolerated compound. However, those attempts failed, and neither the antihypertensive action nor the tolerability was superior to those of hydralazine or dihydralazine

(Gross et al., 1950; Druey and Tripod, 1967; personal observations). Other groups of investigators synthetized and studied hydrazinophthalazines, such as N_1-carbethoxy-N_2-hydrazinophthalazine, Binazin, (Biniecki et al., 1958a, b) which has been clinically studied in Poland and found to have an activity similar to that of hydralazine (Gamski, 1972). The substance is probably metabolized to hydralazine in the organism. Among the hydrazinopyridazines, the 3-hydrazino-6-[N, N- bis (2-hydroxyethyl) amino] pyridazine (L 6150) has recently been reported to have a similar hypotensive action as hydralazine, but a lower animal toxicity (Baldoli et al., 1971). It remains to be demonstrated whether these compounds really present advantages over (di-)hydralazine. Another pyridazine derivative JSF 2123 has been synthetized by Pifferi et al. (1975). Hence, "molecular manipulation" has not been successful with hydralazine so far, which 30 years after its synthesis, still holds its place as an antihypertensive and (until now) has not been superseded by another vasodilator in the treatment of high blood pressure. Recently hydralazine has aroused new interest, since it is possible to reduce the tachycardic response by β-adrenergic blockers. More than 1000 papers have been published on the experimental and clinical findings with hydrazinophthalazines, and only some of them may be considered in the context of this review. A former review is found in Antihypertensive Agents (E. Schlittler ed. 1967).

A. Pharmacodynamics

1. Cardiovascular Actions

Action on Blood Pressure and Blood flow. The characteristic action of hydralazine is the lowering of blood pressure, which in all species studied, including man, is very similar. The onset of action is gradual, the maximum response is reached after 10 to 20 min, the degree of blood pressure reduction is limited, and the duration of action is long. A dose-response relationship for the hypotensive effect is obtained within a relatively narrow dosage range only, which, in rabbits and cats, is between 0.1 and 1.0 mg/kg. Higher doses do not induce a more marked fall in blood pressure, but a prolongation of the effect, which lasts for several hours (Gross et al., 1950; Bein et al., 1953). The diastolic pressure may be somewhat more lowered than the systolic one. In dogs, both anesthetized and conscious, a similar long-lasting lowering of blood pressure was observed as in rabbits and cats (Craver et al., 1951; Moyer et al., 1951; Walker et al., 1951), but later it was found that the acute hypotensive effect is less pronounced than that in other species, such as rats (Bein and Brunner, 1965). In the spinal cat, in which the basal blood pressure is reduced to about 50 to 60 mm Hg, hydralazine does not induce a further hypotensive effect. From this observation it was erroneously concluded that the drug would have a central site of action. If, however, the blood pressure of the spinal cat is re-established to "normal values" by vasopressor substances, such as ephedrine or ergotamine, hydralazine lowers it in the same way as in normotensive animals (Gross et al., 1950; Bein et al., 1953).

The reduction in peripheral vascular resistance is the consequence of a general vasodilation of the precapillary resistance vessels (Åblad and Johnson, 1963; Mellander and Johansson, 1968). The degree of vasodilation differs in the various vascular beds, but it was demonstrated in the femoral, the mesenteric, the renal, and the carotid arteries (Gross et al., 1950; Bein et al., 1953). A dilation of the coronary arteries could also be shown (Bein et al., 1952; Brunner et al., 1965a). The splanchnic blood flow is definitely increased (Hoobler and Dontas, 1953; Marks et al., 1955). The effect on the capacitance vessels is much less pronounced than that on the resistance vessels (Åblad, 1963; Åblad and

MELLANDER, 1963), being in contrast to the action of nitrates or sodium nitroprusside, which have a definite dilating effect on the capacitance system (ÅBLAD and JOHANSSON, 1963; FROHLICH and BHATIA, 1973). In acute studies in man together with the fall in blood pressure an increase in pulse pressure was observed and circulation time (measured by the intravenous injection decholine) was shortened (SCHMID and KELLNER, 1953).

Right from the beginning, the increase in renal blood flow despite the fall in blood pressure has been considered a special feature of hydralazine (GROSS et al., 1950). Very soon, REUBI (1950a, b) showed it also in human beings by means of the indirect clearance method. When hydralazine in relatively large doses (5 mg) was injected directly into the renal artery of dogs, an initial vasoconstriction was obtained, which was then followed by a long-lasting vasodilation (PAGE and McCUBBIN, 1953). The hemodynamic effects of hydralazine in this and other respects are similar to those induced by pyrogens (FREIS, 1961).

Hydralazine, when injected in doses of 0.30 to 0.55 mg into a brachial artery in man, induced a decrease in vascular resistance of the hand and forearm on the injected side, but not on the contralateral one (ÅBLAD et al., 1962; ÅBLAD, 1963). The maximum effect was obtained 12 to 20 min after the administration. After cold exposure of the hand, the vasoconstrictor effect was not reduced by the intra-arterial injection of hydralazine, whereas phenoxybenzamine and guanethidine diminished the vasoconstriction by about 40 to 60% (ÅBLAD, 1963).

Action on the Heart. Simultaneously with the fall in blood pressure, an increase in heart rate and cardiac output occurs, as a consequence of enhanced peripheral sympathetic activity. The increase in heart rate is more pronounced in the conscious animal than in the anesthetized one and is of shorter duration than the fall in blood pressure (CRAVER et al., 1951; BEIN et al., 1953; ÅBLAD, 1963; MEIER et al., 1965a; BRUNNER et al., 1967). The tachycardia was markedly diminished by cutting the cardiac sympathetic nerves, indicating that the increase in heart rate is the consequence of reflex sympathetic activation (GRIMSON et al., 1952). In anesthetized dogs hydralazine did not increase heart rate (BRUNNER et al., 1965a). Since hydralazine has only a weak action on the capacitance vessels, venous return is not diminished and cardiac output increases simultaneously with the rise in heart rate (FREIS et al., 1953; SCHMID and KELLNER, 1953; ÅBLAD, 1963; ZACEST et al., 1972). Besides tachycardia, some uncharacteristic electrocardiographic changes such as a high and prolonged *P* wave were observed in conscious dogs; the long-lasting increase in heart rate was not related to the fall in blood pressure (SCHAPER and JAGENEAU, 1961). In anesthetized dogs an increase in myocardial contractility was reported, which could be inhibited by β-adrenergic blockade (BARRETT et al., 1965). To a certain degree, the increase in heart rate and cardiac output counteracts the hypotensive action of hydralazine, an effect that could be demasked either by administering β-adrenergic blockers (pronethalol) or by anesthesia (BRUNNER et al., 1965a, 1967). In conscious dogs pronethalol reduced tachycardia but also counteracted the lowering of blood pressure induced by hydralazine. Anesthesia abolished the increase in heart rate and enhanced the hypotensive effect of hydralazine, which was similarly intensified by β-adrenergic blockade (BRUNNER and HEDWALL, 1965; BRUNNER et al., 1965a, 1967). Continued use of pronethalol and hydralazine reduced oxygen consumption of the heart (BRUNNER and HEDWALL, 1965a; MEIER et al., 1965b). In conscious rats, both tachycardia and fall in blood pressure were inhibited by β-adrenergic blockers (BRUNNER et al., 1965, 1967). Of course, other β-adrenergic blockers would act similarly to pronethalol.

In the isolated perfused heart of the rabbit, hydralazine and dihydralazine, in concentrations of 10^{-6} g/ml, had no effect on the frequency, but reduced the amplitude of contraction (Bein et al., 1953; Tripod and Meier, 1954, 1958). The coronary arteries were dilated by concentrations of 10^{-7} to 10^{-6} g/ml and coronary flow increased (Barrett et al., 1952). No information is available about a direct stimulating effect of hydralazine on the isolated heart.

Effects on Sympathetic Vascular Reflexes. It was observed early that the carotid occlusion reflex, elicited in cats, was inhibited by hydralazine. Furthermore, the pressor responses produced by stimulation of the proximal end of the cut vagus nerve as well as of the central part of the cut sciatic nerve were also inhibited by hydralazine (Bein et al., 1953). The increase in blood pressure during anoxia was found to be unaffected (Grimson et al., 1950) or suppressed (Bein et al., 1953). In dogs, either an inhibition (Grimson et al., 1950) or only a slight reduction of the carotid occlusion reflex was seen (Walker et al., 1951). Other investigators could not fully confirm these observations, in particular they were unable to demonstrate a stronger inhibitory effect of hydralazine against the pressor effect elicited by nerve stimulation as compared with that induced by the injection of adrenaline or noradrenaline (Kirpekar and Lewis, 1957).

The increase in efferent sympathetic activity following the administration of hydralazine has been demonstrated by various techniques (Åblad, 1963). In the cross-circulated dog kidney with intact innervation, hydralazine, when injected into the donor animal connected with the kidney being studied produced a decrease in renovascular resistance. However, when hydralazine was given to the receptor dog, it reduced the blood pressure, and the resistance of the cross-circulated kidney was elevated as a consequence of the increased sympathetic-fiber discharge to the kidney (Page and McCubbin, 1953). The vasconstrictor response was abolished when the depressor and the sinus nerves of the recipient dog were cut. It was concluded that hydralazine, by a reflex mechanism, had stimulated the vasconstrictor fiber discharge (Åblad, 1963). In cats after close intracarotid or after i. v. injection, chemoreceptor activity was increased, whereas splanchnic activity remained unaffected (Dontas, 1957). Perfusion of the isolated head of the dog, according to the technique of Heymans, did not reveal a depression of cardiovascular reflexes after hydralazine administration (Walker et al., 1951). In other cross-circulation experiments, using the head of the dog, the results seemed to indicate an inhibition of sympathetic outflow (Tangri and Bhargava, 1960), but the interpretation of these results was not conclusive. In later studies Gupta and Bhargava (1965) claimed that the diminution of sinus nerve activity and of efferent sympathetic pathways to the heart did not prevent tachycardia after hydralazine. On the other hand, the increased activity of sympathetic cardiac fibers has been made responsible for the transient reduction in noradrenaline stores in the rat heart (Linét et al., 1969).

Åblad and associates (1962) undertook studies in normal man in order to investigate the effect of hydralazine on the vascular resistance in the forearm, excluded temporarily from the circulation. While in the arm with the nonoccluded circulation, hydralazine produced the expected decrease in vascular resistance, an increase in resistance was found in the occluded arm. The latter effect was attributed to an increased vasoconstrictor fiber discharge to the hand (Åblad et al., 1962). Several years earlier, it had already been reported that, in patients who had no sympathetic innervation of one or both legs, hydralazine increased the blood flow in the leg without sympathetic innervation, while the flow on the innervated side was decreased or unchanged (Stunkard et al., 1954).

Studies in Experimental Hypertension. The first studies on the antihypertensive action of hydralazine were started only after the drug had already been widely used as a therapeutic agent. In the eclampsia-like syndrome, elicited in the rats by high doses of DOCA, salt, and renin, a protective effect of hydralazine was demonstrated (GAUNT and RENZI, 1953). A systematic study in various types of experimental hypertension revealed that prophylactic and therapeutic use of hydralazine delayed the development of DOCA hypertension or normalized blood pressure in the already established form. Cortisone-induced hypertension could also be suppressed. However, it was not possible to obtain an antihypertensive effect in experimental renal hypertension (GROSS et al., 1955). Later on, a blood pressure-lowering effect of hydralazine could be demonstrated also in rats and in dogs with hypertension caused by renal artery stenosis, when 3 mg/kg were administered by mouth (BEIN and BRUNNER, 1965). In rats the hypotensive effect of hydralazine could be completely prevented by a β-adrenergic blocking agent (pronethalol or propranolol [BRUNNER et al., 1965b, 1967)].

Adrenal regeneration hypertension of the rat also responds well to hydralazine (GARDNER and BROOKS, 1962). In spontaneously hypertensive rats (OKAMOTO-AOKI strain), hydralazine lowers blood pressure (NAGAOKA et al., 1969), but the most effective treatment was achieved with a combination of hydralazine, reserpine, and chlorothiazide, which was added to the drinking water. The doses were 1.4 mg reserpine, 80 mg hydralazine, and 1000 mg chlorothiazide per liter of water for male rats and half the concentration for females (FREIS, 1972). It can be stated that common types of experimental hypertension respond well to hydralazine or some of its derivatives, the effectiveness of the treatment depending on the dosage, the dose intervals, and the administration of the drug.

2. Antagonistic Effects on Vascular Smooth Muscle

Hydralazine diminishes the response to various vasoconstrictor substances, both *in vitro* and *in vivo*, without having a specific adrenolytic activity (GROSS et al., 1952; BEIN et al., 1953). In aortic strip preparations from rabbits, hypertensin (at the time the experiments were carried out, angiotensin was still called hypertensin and was not available in synthetic form) was antagonized by low concentrations of hydralazine, whereas higher concentrations were necessary to obtain a similar effect against adrenaline, noradrenaline, tyramine, or isoamylamine (SCHROEDER et al., 1953; SCHROEDER, 1959). In the same preparation, concentrations of 10^{-6} g/ml hydralazine slightly inhibited contractions induced by adrenaline, but higher concentrations were less effective (PERRY and CAMEL, 1960). The tone of isolated strips of horse carotid arteries was diminished by hydralazine. In the same preparation a nonspecific partial antagonistic effect against various vasoconstrictors such as adrenaline, noradrenaline, 5-hydroxytryptamine, histamine, acetylcholine, barium chloride and potassium chloride was observed (KIRPEKAR and LEWIS, 1958a). It was supposed that hydralazine may have some affinity for adrenergic receptors, but no further data are available to support such an assumption. In the isolated bovine mesenteric artery preparation ÅBLAD (1963) demonstrated that hydralazine reduced the vasoconstrictor action of noradrenaline under aerobic conditions, whereas under anaerobic conditions the action of hydralazine was reversed and the vasoconstriction enhanced. Similar results were obtained when contractions were elicited by either histamine or barium chloride. In contrast papaverine and sodium nitrite antagonized noradrenaline also in the absence of oxygen. In the isolated perfused hind limb-preparation of the rabbit, hydralazine, in concentrations of 10^{-6} g/ml, diminished the vasoconstriction induced by sympathomimetic drugs, by histamine, which acts as a constrictor at maximum dilation, or by barium chloride (Bein et al., 1953); the most pronounced effect was obtained against barium chloride (Tripod et al., 1954). In the isolated perfused heart of the rabbit an antagonistic effect of hydralazine against barium chloride and pitressin was demonstrable (Tripod and Meier, 1954), and, in the intact cat the coronary constriction induced by pitressin was abolished (Bein et al., 1952). Intermediates of carbohydrate metabolism such as pyruvate or succinate and also of protein- and fat metabolism protected to a certain degreee against the hydralazine-induced depression of vasoconstrictor responses of horse carotid artery strips. This effect was interpreted as the consequence of a nonspecific depression of tissue metabolism produced by hydralazine, but no further results are available that could favor such a hypothesis (Kirpekar and Lewis, 1958b).

In the whole animal, the adrenolytic effect of hydralazine is not pronounced; neither the pressor effect of adrenaline or noradrenaline, nor that after stimulation of the splanchnic nerve could be completely inhibited, but was only reduced (Gross et al., 1950; Moyer et al., 1951; Kirpekar and Lewis, 1957; Bein et al., 1953). Similarly the hypertensive responses to pitressin (Bein et al., 1952) and to angiotensin were diminished (Meier et al., 1957). In man it was shown that, after intra-arterial injection of hydralazine into one brachial artery, the vasoconstrictor response, induced by an intra-arterial or i. v. infusion or noradrenaline, could not be prevented, whereas it was markedly inhibited by phenoxybenzamine (Åblad, 1963).

On the basis of the data available, the hydralazines are characteristic vasodilators, which to a certain degree reduce the response of the arterioles to various vasoconstrictor stimuli. On the basis of different responses of isolated arteries under aerobic and anaerobic conditions it had been suggested that hydralazine might react with two different types of receptors, one being responsible for the vasodilator action and being stimulated by low concentrations, and the other, which favors vasoconstriction, being affected by high concentrations of the drug (Åblad, 1963). This interesting hypothesis has not been followed up further, but in view of the fact that in the whole animal and in man no "reversal" of the hypotensive action of hydralazine has been observed by increasing the doses, it is doubtful whether the effect observed with isolated artery strips is of significance for the response to hydralazine *in vivo*.

3. Other Pharmacodynamic Actions

Action on the Kidney. Despite the fact that increase in renal blood flow has been observed in early experimental studies and also in man (Reubi, 1950), little has been done in further investigating the action of hydralazine on renal function. No change in glomerular filtration rate was found and tubular function as measured by *Tm*-glucose was not affected in dogs (Moyer et al., 1951). Together with the increase in renal plasma flow the filtration fraction is reduced (Wilkinson et al., 1952; Stein and Hecht, 1955). Clinical observations on fluid retention and mild edema formation have been reported by various authors (Moyer, 1953; Wilkinson et al., 1952; Koch-Weser, 1974), but have not stimulated further studies on the effects hydralazine may have on the kidney. It may be that proximal tubular reabsorption is enhanced as with other vasodilators such as minoxidil, but to a lesser degree. However, no quantitative data or dose-response curves are available. Like other vasodilators hydralazine stimulates renin release from the kidney which results in an increase in plasma renin activity (Ueda et al., 1968; Gottlieb et al., 1972).

Other Effects. Together with the fall in blood pressure and the corresponding sympathetic stimulation, an increase in respiratory rate is observed in conscious and anesthetized experimental animals (BEIN et al., 1953). The isolated intestine of the rabbit is paralyzed by a concentration of 10^{-5} g/ml, while the seminal vesicle or the uterus of guinea pigs is not affected by this concentration (TRIPOD and MEIER, 1958). The guinea pig ileum is contracted by dihydralazine, which also reduced the response to acetylcholine (WERLE et al., 1955). An antagonism against barium chloride in the rabbit intestine, against histamine in the guinea pig intestine, and against adrenaline in the guinea pig seminal vesicle was only demonstrable with concentrations of 10^{-3} and 10^{-4} g/ml, respectively. An inhibitory effect on the transmission within the upper cervical ganglion of the cat was claimed, the block being similar to that induced by iproniazid or β-phenylisopropyl-hydrazine (GERTNER and ROMANO, 1962). Acetylcholine was still released on preganglionic nerve stimulation. On the other hand, it was possible to demonstrate a restitution of sensitivity against ganglionic blocking drugs by the administration of hydralazine (BEIN et al., 1953).

4. Biochemical Effects

Inhibition of Enzymes. Hydralazine inhibits various enzymes, such as diaminooxydase (histaminase) (GROSS et al., 1952; SCHULER and WYSS, 1960) and monaminooxydase (SCHULER and MEIER, 1955), but this enzyme inhibition is not correlated with the effect on blood pressure. Other hydrazine derivatives, which have no hypotensive action, inhibit these enzymes even more effectively (WERLE et al., 1955; SCHULER and WYSS, 1960). Also the inhibition of dopa-decarboxylase activity and the subsequent reduction of the concentration of dopamine or noradrenaline in various tissues are not related to the action of hydralazine on blood pressure (WERLE et al., 1955; SANO et al., 1960). Histidine decarboxylase activity was also diminished by various hydrazines and guanylhydrazines which indicates that these interferences with various enzyme activities are not correlated to the hypotensive or other specific pharmacodynamic activities (WERLE et al., 1955).

A transient reduction of catecholamine concentrations in various tissues of the rat was seen after repeated administration of dihydralazine (BYGDEMAN and STJÄRNE, 1959), but these authors could reproduce their results only in part (1960). However, several years later it was reported that the noradrenaline content of the rat heart was transiently diminished after hydralazine and less marked after dihydralazine. It was presumed that this effect was not caused by an interference of hydralazine with the binding mechanism of noradrenaline in the tissues, but rather be the consequence of the increased activity of cardiac sympathetic fibers elicited by the fall in blood pressure (LINÉT et al., 1969).

Recently, an inhibitory effect of hydralazine on dopamine-β-hydroxylase, isolated from bovine adrenal glands, has been described, and this effect was related to the chelating of copper ions, which activate the enzyme (LIU et al., 1974). On the basis of the scant data available, it is not possible to decide whether this effect is related to the vasodilating action of hydralazine. Hydralazine was found to inhibit acetylation of sulfanilamide and glucosamine in pigeon liver extracts. This inhibition is the consequence of a competition for acetyl coenzyme *A* of hydralazine and other acetylated drugs (DOUGLASS et al., 1957). Oxygen uptake of preparations from brain, liver, and kidney of rats and from rabbit aorta was depressed by hydralazine in all tissues studied. Hydralazine also depleted the brain of energy-rich phosphates when given in sublethal doses but had no similar effect on heart, liver or skeletal muscle (KIRPEKAR and LEWIS, 1959a).

Chelating Activity of Hydralazine. Various metals combine with hydralazine, such as Fe^{2+}, Fe^{3+}, Cu^{2+}, Mn^{2+}, Sn^{2+}, Al^{3+}, Cr^{3+}, Co^{2+}, Ag^{2+}, Hg^{2+}, V^{3+}, and V^{5+} (PERRY, 1953; PERRY and SCHROEDER, 1954). Of these, copper is the one most strongly bound. The complexes formed with Fe^{2+} and Fe^{3+} have been studied from a chemical point of view by FALLAB (1962) and FALLAB and ERLENMEYER (1963), but from their work no conclusions can be drawn with respect to the significance that metal chelating may have for the action of hydralazine on smooth muscle. Fe^{3+} rapidly oxydizes hydralazine to phthalazine and molecular N_2. A hydralazine-iron complex was studied pharmacologically, but the results obtained were disappointing insofar as they did not give any information about the significance of the chelating process (KIRPEKAR and LEWIS, 1959b). Various trace metals, bound to hydralazine, are excreted in the urine during treatment with the drug. Of these, copper was eliminated in twice the amount as compared with the period before treatment (77 ± 25 γ/day before, and 166 ± 92 γ/day during treatment), whereas no significant changes were found for iron, cobalt, cadmium, rubidium, and various others (WESTER, 1975).

Like other hydrazines, hydralazine also binds with various carbonyl and aldehyde groups, such as pyruvic acid, acetaldehyde, and α-ketoglutaric acid, but not with glucose, lactic acid, or propionic acid (PERRY and SCHROEDER, 1953; SCHROEDER, 1959; EDITORIAL 1977). Similarly, mercaptans, such as cystine, reduced glutathione, or 2,3-dimercaptopropanol (BAL), are also bound. When incubated with serum, egg albumin, or mashed arterial tissue, hydralazine slowly combines with these proteins and loses its hypotensive activity (MEIER et al., 1954). Plasma protein binding is about 88 to 89% (WAGNER and HEDWALL, 1975). It is unknown what percentage of hydralazine administered is irreversibly bound to plasma proteins. Whether the various reactions demonstrable *in vitro* are of biological significance has not been extensively studied, in particular not with respect to their possible significance for inducing adverse reactions (see 436).

5. Mechanism of Action

Although on the basis of the first pharmacologic studies of hydralazine it was supposed that the drug acted directly on the arteriolar smooth muscle, some data were available that suggested that there was also a central site of action (GROSS et al., 1950; CRAVER et al., 1951; BEIN et al., 1953). From experiments in cats, in which only an enhanced chemoreceptor activity was observed after intracarotid injection, but no increased splanchnic activity after i. v. administration, it is obvious that hydralazine behaved like a slowly acting peripheral vasodilator (DONTAS, 1957). From the extensive studies of ÅBLAD and associates (1963) it became evident that hydralazine and related compounds exert their hypotensive effect by means of a direct action on the vascular smooth muscle and have no influence on centers regulating blood pressure. The increased sympathetic fiber discharge which occurs as a consequence of the vasodilation, has to be considered a reflex adjustment to vasodilation.

In further studies on a possible central mechanism of action, hydralazine was administered into the fourth cerebral ventricle or the carotid arteries of cats, and the hypotensive response obtained was taken as an indication that the drug acted centrally (LIM et al., 1955). However, other investigators reported contradictory results. When hydralazine was injected into the cisterna magna or the third cerebral ventricle of cats, only a slight fall in blood pressure was observed, accompanied by a reduced pressor response to i. v.-injected adrenaline (SCHMITT and GICQUEL, 1956). Furthermore, injection of hydralazine into the vertebral artery of the cat caused a similar hypotensive response to an i. v. injection (REIS and VAN ZWIETEN, 1967; VAN ZWIETEN, 1968). In the case of a central mechanism of action, the intravertebral injection should induce a more pronounced hypotensive reaction than the i. v. injection. When the isolated brain of the cat was perfused in situ, hydralazine, added to the perfusion fluid, produced a fall in blood pressure and bradycardia together with a decrease in hind limb vascular resistance (INGENITO et al., 1969). The central components of the cardiovascular reflexes, elicited by changes of pressure in the carotid sinus, and cerebral blood flow were not affected by hydralazine. On the other hand, an increase in brain noradrenaline concentration was observed. It was presumed that the vasodilation of the hind limbs was caused by a central mechanism (INGENITO et al., 1969). Direct application of hydralazine on the floor of the fourth cerebral ventricle induced tachycardia in conscious and anesthetized dogs. In view of these findings and since tachycardia could not be prevented by eliminating efferent sympathetic pathways to the heart, it was concluded that hydralazine suppressed cardioinhibitory centers located in the dorsal medulla (GUPTA and BHARGAVA, 1965).

In renal hypertensive rats, a comparative study of hydralazine, methyldopa, and guanethidine with respect to their site of action was undertaken. The recording of the nerve activity from an intact lumbar sympathetic chain showed a reduction of spontaneous sympathetic outflow both with methyldopa and with hydralazine, which was much more pronounced with the former drug than with the latter. Furthermore, an increase of the hydralazine dose from 1 to 2 mg/kg, which resulted in a greater fall in blood pressure, produced no significant reduction of spontaneous sympathetic outflow (BAUM et al., 1972). These authors concluded that, in contrast to methyldopa, the central activity of hydralazine is unimportant in comparison with its peripheral activity.

If the data available today are summarized, it is evident that hydralazine exerts its hypotensive action mainly by a direct action on the smooth arteriolar muscle, and that a central mechanism of action contributes to the reduction of peripheral resistance only to a minor, if any, degree. The sympathetic reflex mechanisms are not at all affected, and, consequently, the sympathetic discharge to the resistance vessels and to the heart is increased. When sympathetic stimulation is suppressed by either ganglionic blockers or drugs acting on the postganglionic adrenergic transmission, such as reserpine, guanethidine, or β-adrenergic blockers, the full vasodilating effect of hydralazine becomes "unmasked", and, correspondingly, the total peripheral resistance will be further reduced. Hence, it is not only the suppression of reflex tachycardia, but also the abolishment of reflex vasoconstrictor tone by sympatholytic drugs or β-adrenergic receptor blockers, which intensify the hypotensive effect of hydralazine.

Action on Vascular Smooth Muscle. So far, it is not clear how hydralazine interferes with the smooth muscle tone in the arteriolar wall. In various investigations it was shown that, after i. v. injection of labeled ^{14}C-hydralazine in rats and mice, the drug, or a metabolite, accumulates in the vessel walls both of arteries and veins. The discovery that hydralazine is concentrated in the arterial wall resulted from studies with ^{14}C labeled material in mice (PERRY et al., 1962). The concentration of hydralazine in the arteries of various organs of mice (kidney, liver, spleen, heart, lung, brain and muscles) was demonstrated by means of radioautography (MOORE-JONES and PERRY, 1966). In the arteries the concentration of radioactivity was somewhat higher than in the veins (WAGNER and HEDWALL, 1972, 1975). The half-life of radioactivity in the vessel walls was more than 30 h and exceeded that in other organs or tissues, where it was between 2 and 8 h. The concentration of radioactivity in the aorta or the carotid artery at 6 and 24 h after the i. v. injection of labeled hydralazine was about 500 to 600 times higher than the concentration in plasma. Autoradiographic studies in mice revealed that the radioactivity was associated with the elastic elements in the small blood vessels of lung, liver, spleen, and kidney (WAGNER and HEDWALL, 1975). Although it cannot be affirmed that the radioactivity found in the vessels represents the unchanged drug, *in vitro* studies with mesenteric artery preparations of the rat suggest that hydralazine itself accumulates in the arteries. When mesenteric arteries were perfused with solutions of increasing hydralazine concentrations, a level of saturation of the vasoconstrictor response to electrical stimulation was obtained with much lower concentrations, the threshold being in the range of 2 to 5 μg/kg (WAGNER and HEDWALL, 1975). No correlation could be found between the concentration of hydralazine or its metabolites in the walls of the resistance vessels and the hypotensive effect, but the presence of radioactivity in the arteries and arterioles corresponds better to the duration of the effect on the blood pressure than the plasma concentration of hydralazine (WAGNER and HEDWALL, 1975).

The strong chelating activity of hydralazine has been related to the hypotensive effect. Already SCHROEDER and associates (SCHROEDER et al., 1955; SCHROEDER, 1959) supposed that the binding of copper by hydralazine might be of significance for its hypotensive effect. In this context, the observation that hydralazine inhibits dopamine-β-hydroxylase, which is activated by copper, may be of significance (LIU et al., 1974). It has been supposed that hydralazine reduces smooth muscle tone in the arterioles by means of an interference with enzymes that either depend on the presence of metal ions or contain metals, such as tyrosinase, which is a copper-containing enzyme, but is not inhibited by hydralazine (SCHROEDER, 1959). Despite extensive studies, no conclusive results are available on the effect of hydralazine on enzymes or coenzymes containing metals, but further studies in this direction should be undertaken.

B. Pharmacokinetics

First studies on the distribution of ^{14}C labeled hydralazine were done in mice and revealed a rapid excretion of radioactivity by the kidney. A relatively high concentration of radioactivity was found in the aorta, which decreased slowly, whereas activity in the kidneys fell rapidly (PERRY et al., 1962). In man, after administration by mouth, hydralazine is well absorbed, and the maximum hypotensive effect is demonstrable within one hour (ZACEST and KOCH-WESER, 1972). The plasma concentrations after i. v. injection are higher than those after ingestion, either as a consequence of incomplete absorption or as the result of a first-pass effect through the liver. Plasma hydralazine was measured by SCHULERT (1961), and later on, an improved method was described, which is more sensitive and allows to measure plasma concentrations as low as 0.05 γ/ml (ZACEST and KOCH-WESER, 1972).

The plasma half-life in healthy volunteers ranged from 2.2 to 7.8 h, being in the same range after either i. v. or oral administration. Other investigators found the plasma half-life of the unchanged drug being 2.25 h and the binding to plasma protein was 88 to 89% (WAGNER and HEDWALL, 1975). In plasma hydrazones are formed and an equilibrium exists between hydrazine and hydrazones. By means of gaschromatography determination of unchanged hydralazine in the plasma of rats and man is possible. Procedures have also been developed for the analysis of acid hydrolysable conjugates in plasma (ZAK et al., 1977). In patients with hypertension, the plasma concentration depended upon the period between the ingestion and the taking of blood, but was not related to the daily dose (REIDENBERG et al., 1973). In patients with impaired renal function, the plasma concentration was higher than in those with a normal kidney function, which is in agreement with the fact that hydralazine is mainly eliminated by the kidney. In dogs, the plasma half-life was 3 to 4 h when measured either by a chemical method or by radioactivity; and hydralazine is less bound to plasma proteins than in man (LESSER et al., 1973).

Studies on the metabolism of hydralazine were undertaken first in rats and rabbits by means of ^{14}C labeled drug (McISAAC and KANDA, 1964). Radioactivity was rapidly excreted by the kidney and within 24 h 75% of the total amount administered appeared in the urine. In addition to the unchanged substance the O-glucuronide and the N-acetyl-1-hydrazinophthalazine were isolated as metabolites in the urine. A competitive inhibition of acetylation may occur, when other drugs which are acetylated are simultaneously administered with hydralazine (DOUGLASS et al., 1957).

Other metabolites isolated from human urine were 3-methyl-*s*-triazolo (3,4-*a*)-phthalazine and the corresponding 3-hydroxymethyl-derivative (DOUGLASS and HOGAN, 1959; EDWARDS and MARQUARDT, 1969; ZIMMER et al., 1973, 1975). Also S-triazolo (3,4-*a*)-phthalazine and 1-phthalazinone have been found (ZAK et al., 1974a, b). A diagram of the metabolism of hydralazine is given in Fig. 1. Within 2 days, 80% of the administered radioactivity was excreted in the urine and 10% in the feces. Similar results have been reported by WAGNER and HEDWALL (1975), who found within 5 days 86% of radioactivity in the urine and 11%

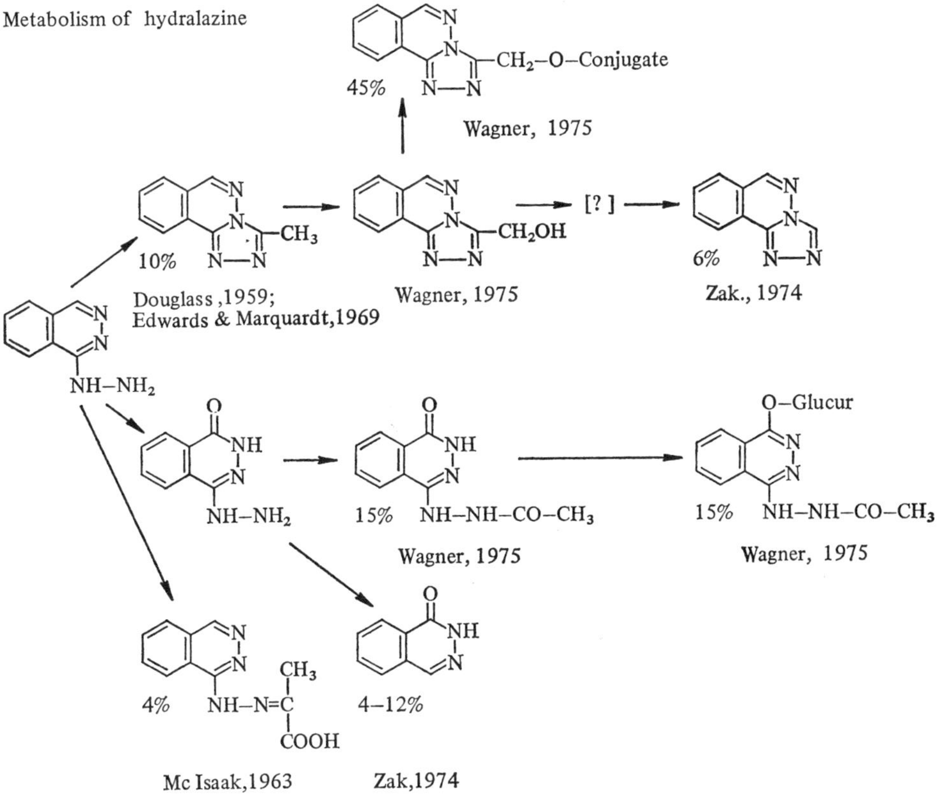

Fig. 1. Metabolism of hydralazine (WAGNER and HEDWALL, 1975)

in the feces. Only about 7% of the material found in the urine was unchanged hydralazine.

Since a major way of metabolism is N-acetylation, hydralazine inactivation was studied in fast and slow acetylators (ZACEST and KOCH-WESER, 1972). It was found that the acetylation phenotype was a major determinant of the plasma concentration of hydralazine, being, after oral administration, about 1.7 times higher in slow acetylators than in fast ones (Fig. 2). A good correlation between

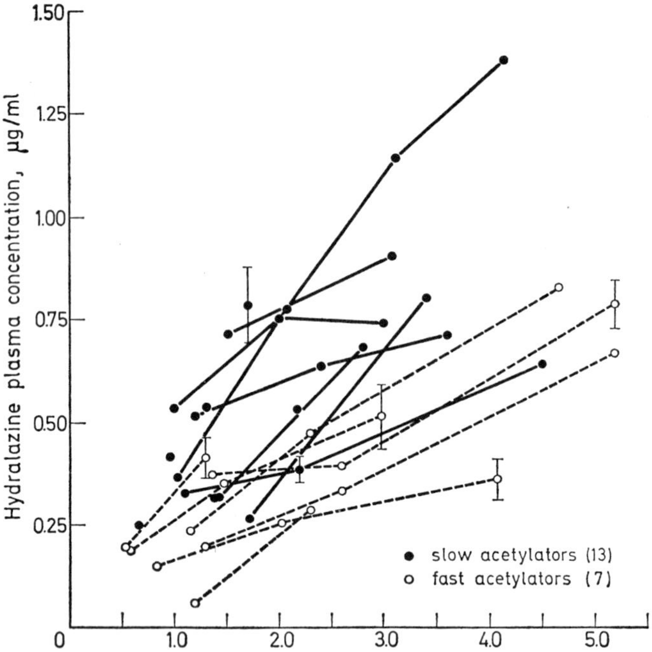

Fig. 2. Relation of daily dose of hydralazine to plasma concentration in 20 patients. Points indicate means of one to six determinations, standard deviations indicated for means of four or more determinations. Points for patients who received more than one daily dose are connected (ZACEST and KOCH-WESER, 1972)

the plasma concentration and the hypotensive effect was found, but fast acetylators needed about 60% higher doses to control their blood pressure than slow acetylators. In another study on the significance of the acetylator phenotype for the blood pressure response to hydralazine, fast acetylators needed about 40% higher doses (ZACEST and KOCH-WESER, 1972; JOUNELA et al., 1975; ZACEST and STANLEY, 1975). The metabolism by the intestinal wall and the first-pass absorption by the liver are also related to the genetic acetylator phenotype (REIDENBERG et al., 1973). These findings explain why, after i. v. injection, similar plasma concentrations were found in fast and slow acetylators (ZACEST and STANLEY, 1975). Besides, there is a renal elimination process, which is unrelated to the acetylator phenotype.

When hydralazine was given together with propranolol, slow acetylators needed an average dose of 2.4 mg/kg for a satisfactory blood pressure control whereas fast acetylators required 3.7 mg/kg (ZACEST and KOCH-WESER, 1972). Despite the fact that fast acetylators need higher doses of hydralazine than slow ones, no adverse reactions were observed during one year of treatment, when average doses of 1.4 mg/kg were given. It was stated that within such a dosage range, hypertensive patients may be treated successfully with hydralazine without knowing their acetylator phenotype, but when hydralazine is given over a prolonged period, it is preferable to determine the phenotype, so as to be warned of an increased risk (JOUNELA et al., 1975).

The difference in dosages between slow and fast acetylators cannot explain the discrepancies in the amounts of hydralazine given by various investigators. Today, a more careful increase in the doses is usual than 20 years ago, and the possibility to combine hydralazine with reserpine, β-adrenergic blockers or diuretics reduces the need for excessive doses. In general, it will hardly be necessary to go beyond 150 to 200 mg a day, a dose that is well tolerated, in most cases also when acetylation is slow.

1. Therapeutic Use

SCHROEDER was the first to use hydralazine systematically in the treatment of high blood pressure, both alone and in combination with ganglionic blockers, the only active hypotensive drugs available in 1950 (SCHROEDER, 1951, 1952a). The so-called hyphex (*hy*dralazine-*hex*amethonium) combination was effective in controlling successfully the blood pressure in two-thirds of patients with severe hypertension (SCHROEDER, 1952b, 1953, 1957, 1959; SCHROEDER et al., 1953; PERRY and SCHROEDER, 1954). For the first time it was possible to treat malignant hypertension effectively, not only by reducing the blood pressure, but also by reversing severe organ lesions, such as renal damage, congestive heart failure, or retinopathy (SCHROEDER, 1953; PERRY and SCHROEDER, 1956). Heroic doses of hydralazine (up to 900 mg daily) and of hexamethonium (up to 4.5 g) were given at that time. Several years later, a study of the survival rates of patients with severe hypertension who had been treated with the "hyphex" combination was presented, from which it was evident that long-term results of that treatment were also favourable, some of the patients having been considered cured (SCHROEDER and PERRY, 1960). Although in some studies the results were much less encouraging than those reported by SCHROEDER and his associates (JOHNSON et al., 1952; HOOBLER and DONTAS, 1953) most investigators confirmed the efficacy of hydralazine in the treatment of hypertension (TAYLOR et al., 1952; MERRILL and KENYON, 1953; MOYER, 1953; FREIS et al., 1953), and despite some reservation the use of hydralazine rapidly spread out in the United States. It was especially suggested for cases with reduced renal function (PERRY and SCHROEDER, 1956), although some authors did not confirm beneficial effects in chronic renal failure (MERRILL and KENYON, 1953).

In Europe, dihydralazine was found to be of similar effectiveness as hydralazine, although it was used in lower dosages right from the beginning (ESSELIER et al., 1953; SCHAUB et al., 1964).

After the ganglionic blockers had been replaced by more specifically acting drugs, hydralazine was mostly used in combination with other antihypertensives, such as reserpine (e.g. HUGHES et al., 1955; LEE et al., 1956; HOOBLER and BLAQUIER, 1959; SCHAUB et al., 1964) and later on hydrochlorothiazide or related diuretics. When given together with reserpine, the increase in heart rate can be suppressed completely or in part. In addition, as a consequence of the different mode of action the antihypertensive effect is enhanced by the simultaneous administration of the two drugs. In view of the toxic reactions seen with high doses given during a prolonged period the daily doses have been limited to between 100 to 200 mg. Today hydralazine is hardly ever used alone and is not considered suitable and sufficiently active for monotherapy.

Hydralazine, when injected i.v., elicited an increase in plasma renin activity (PRA) which was more pronounced in salt depleted patients (UEDA et al., 1968). A similar response of PRA was found with minoxidil, but the hypotensive effect of the two vasodilators was not diminished by the release of renin (GOTTLIEB et al., 1972) (Fig. 3). It was suggested that use should be made of the increase in PRA

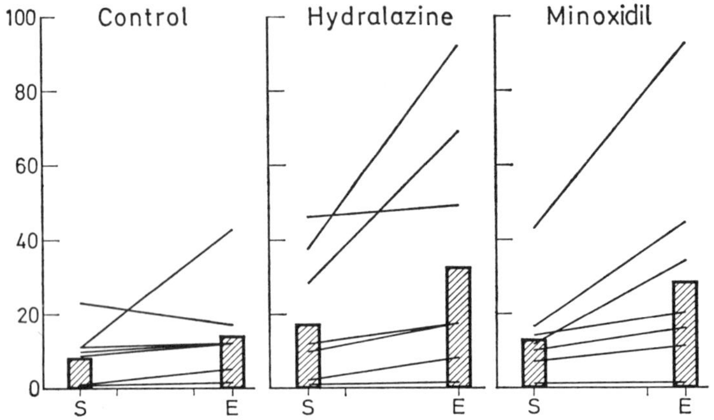

Fig. 3. Plasma renin activity (mμg/ml/h) as measured with patients in both supine (*S*) and erect (*E*) positions in all three study periods. The mean and individual values are given (GOTTLIEB et al., 1972)

induced by hydralazine in the diagnosis of various forms of hypertension (UEDA et al., 1968), but experiences made since with the renin or angiotensin assay do not support such a procedure (GROSS, 1976).

In the treatment of hypertensive emergencies, the drug being administered either i.v. or i.m., and also in toxemia of pregnancy, favourable results have been reported (ASSALI et al., 1952; SCHROEDER, 1953; REUTTER, 1965). It may still be used occasionally for this purpose, in doses of 10 to 25 mg i.v. or i.m., but more effective drugs are available now (KOCH-WESER, 1973).

A review on how intensive therapy has affected mortality and morbidity in hypertension was published by PERRY, SCHROEDER and associates in 1966. In the long-term treatment of high blood pressure, hydralazine still keeps its place in combination with other drugs, the same being the case for dihydralazine (SCHAUB et al., et al., 1964). Convincing results on the control of blood pressure have been reported in the Veterans Administration Cooperative Study, in which the effects of drug treatment (a combination of reserpine, hydralazine, and hydrochlorothiazide-SER-AP-ES) and of placebos have been compared (FREIS, 1967, 1970). During a follow-up period of 20 months, in the group treated with the antihypertensive drugs, only 1 of 73 patients had a major cardiovascular complication and one died, whereas in the group of 70 patients who received placebos, four deaths and 23 major complications occurred (FREIS, 1967). In patients with less severe hypertension (diastolic pressure 90 to 114 mm Hg) the treatment was continued for up to five years. The death rate in the placebo group was 19, against eight in the treated group, and – similarly – major complications had developed in 56 of the control patients, but in only 22 of the treated ones (FREIS, 1970). In 20 patients of the control group. the diastolic blood pressure rose to values of 125 mm Hg or more, and therefore these patients had to be excluded from the study and submitted to effective treatment. The combination of hydralazine with reserpine and hydrochlorothiazide has been found useful also in other studies on the treatment of moderate hypertension (CLARK and TROOP, 1972).

Recently, the combination of hydralazine with β-adrenergic blocking drugs and hydrochlorothiazide has been proposed (ZACEST and KOCH-WESER, 1972; ZACEST et al., 1972; GOTTLIEB et al., 1972). In this way, the reflex activation of the sympathetic discharge is prevented, especially the stimulating effect on the heart. The blood pressure was lowered to normal values in both supine and standing position, and the patients preferred propranolol to sympatholytic drugs, which caused more unpleasant side effects. Dihydralazine has also been combined with propranolol for the treatment of ambulatory hypertensive patients (KATILA and FRICK, 1970). In other studies, the combined administration of dihydralazine and alprenolol has been investigated both with respect to hemodynamic changes and the antihypertensive effect (SANNERSTEDT et al., 1971, 1972). It has been suggested that hydralazine or dihydralazine may be the first drug added, when monotherapy with either a β-adrenergic blocker or a diuretic does not suffice to control blood pressure (WERKÖ, 1975). The doses of either hydralazine or dihydralazine should not exceed the range of 100 to 150 mg daily since it is not to be expected that with higher doses a more effective lowering of blood pressure will be obtained, but only an increased risk of adverse reactions.

2. Adverse Reactions

Side effects and adverse reactions, induced by hydralazine, can be divided into acute, unpleasant symptoms, which occur immediately after the beginning of treatment, delayed responses, observed after 10 to 14 days of treatment, and reactions seen only after the drug has been administered for prolonged periods of several months or even years.

Acute Side Effects. Most of the symptoms are the consequence of the acute vasodilation and the fall in blood pressure. Headache, often occipital subsequent to intracranial vasodilation, flushing, conjunctivitis, nasal congestion, nausea, and vomiting may occur. Headache could be relieved by vasoconstrictors such as ergotamine (YONKMAN and FREIS, 1952), but this type of treatment has not found acceptance. In addition, tachycardia, palpitation, and—in patients with coronary heart disease—anginal attacks may be provoked (TAYLOR et al., 1952; MOYER, 1953; JUDSON et al., 1956), and the T wave of the electrocardiogram may be flattened or reversed (REUBI, 1950). The acute side reactions, except those of cardiac origin, even though very unpleasant in the beginning, will decrease in most cases after several days and may be less marked when the doses are increased gradually (SCHROEDER, 1959). Tachycardia with all its consequences can be controlled by the simultaneous administration of β-adrenergic blocking drugs, which have a synergistic effect on blood pressure. Quite a few patients who initially complain of the acute side-effects tolerate hydralazine well after several weeks. Postural hypotension is very rare (ROWE et al., 1955; SCHROEDER, 1959; ÅBLAD, 1963).

After a few days, edema formation in nondependent parts of the body may occur, which is a consequence of increased sodium reabsorption in the proximal tubules (MOYER, 1953; WILKINSON et al., 1952; ZACEST et al., 1972). This effect is less pronounced with hydralazine than with other vasodilators, such as diazoxide or minoxidil, even of high doses of hydralazine are given. It has to be remembered that for quite some time when hydralazine already had its established place in the treatment of high blood pressure (*e.g.*, SCHROEDER, 1959), chlorothiazide or similar drugs were not available, and that mild retention of water and salt, which occasionally was observed, was not then considered a major problem of hydralazine therapy.

Delayed Reactions. After administration for 10 to 20 days, a febrile reaction may occur, which has similarities with serum sickness (ALARCÓN-SEGOVIA et al., 1967; PERRY, 1973). This so-called early febrile reaction, which is seen after the absorption of between 2.5 and 10.0 g of hydralazine, has been observed in 15 of 441 patients followed up by PERRY (1973). Fever may be accompanied by severe arthralgia and myalgia, rash, and lymphadenopathy. The symptoms disappeared when the hydralazine treatment was stopped, and they did not reappear in 11 of 15 patients when the drug was given again. In the remaining four patients, re-exposure to the drug elicited anew a febrile reaction. In 6 of the 11 patients who had been re-exposed, the late toxicity syndrome developed after 5 to 6 months of therapy (PERRY, 1973).

Late Toxicity Syndrome. After prolonged treatment with high doses of hydralazine a lupus erythematosus-like syndrome or rheumatoid arthritis was first described in 1953 (MORROW et al., 1953; DUSTAN et al., 1954; PERRY and SCHROEDER, 1954; HENN et al., 1955; MULLER et al., 1955; HILDRETH et al., 1960; PIGEON and GENEST, 1960). The so-called hydralazine syndrome was thought to be specific for hydralazine, but later it was found that other drugs, such as procainamide or diphenylhydantoin, could provoke similar reactions in man (LEE and SIEGEL, 1968). The syndrome is characterized by arthralgia, muscle pain, fever, high erythrocyte sedimentation rate, and the presence of lupus erythematosus (LE) cells in the peripheral blood. Leukopenia (below 4000 leucocytes per mm^3), anemia (hemoglobin below 11.5 g/100 ml) and thrombocytopenia were other hematologic symptoms. Dermatosis in the form of an erythematous rash has also been observed. It was stated that the syndrome was indistinguishable—clinically, serologically, and pathologically—from systemic lupus erythematosus (SLE), except that it disappeared when the drug was discontinued (SCHROEDER, 1959; BENDERSKY and RAMIREZ, 1960; PIGEON and GENEST, 1960; ALARCÓN-SEGOVIA, 1967; ALKALAY and BULLARD, 1971; PERRY, 1973). It seems that women are more susceptible than men and that patients often belong to families in which rheumatic diseases are frequent (LEE and SIEGEL, 1968).

The most careful long-term follow-up of patients who developed a hydralazine syndrome was done by PERRY (1973), who reported that out of 371 patients treated for prolonged periods with hydralazine and ganglionic blockade 44 had developed the LE-like syndrome after receiving doses of between 100 and 1600 mg hydralazine daily. Of these 44 patients, 14 had severe toxic reactions, which appeared within 3 to 20 months of treatment. In 12 of 15 patients, antinuclear antibodies were found in the original series, but in another series of 15 patients, studied more recently, all had antinuclear antibodies. Another review has been published by ALARCÓN-SEGOVIA et al. (1967) who reported on 50 patients with hydralazine syndrome. It was stated that 74% of the manifestations were possibly indicative of an underlying lupus diathesis.

From the data collected by these two groups of investigators it is evident that the syndrome may develop in between 8 and 13% of patients who receive high doses of hydralazine, but in another review the percentage among exposed patients was only 1 to 2% (LEE and SIEGEL, 1968). In general, doses below 200 mg daily may be considered safe, but a few cases have also been observed on doses of 100 mg or less (McNicol and Hutchinson, 1956; Reynolds and Caldwell, 1957). Other investigators have stated that late toxic reactions of hydralazine are rare when doses below 400 mg daily are given (Pigeon and Genest, 1960). It is not known whether patients in whom relatively low doses elicited the syndrome were slow phenotype acetylators, who run a higher risk than fast acetylators.

According to Perry, four phases may be distinguished in the development of the hydralazine syndrome: The first phase of two to 72 months, which is an asymptomatic period of hydralazine intake prior to the earliest symptoms; the second phase of two weeks to 40 months, during which the blood pressure is well controlled, but during which arthralgia, myalgia, and effusions may occur; the third phase lasting from a few days to four years, during which, after withdrawal of hydralazine the toxic reactions disappear; and the fourth phase, during which hypertension is no longer controlled after withdrawal. This latter phase can be avoided by the administration of antihypertensive drugs other than hydralazine. Antibodies against hydralazine have been demonstrated by means of a hemagglutinine test in the serum of one patient after prolonged treatment (Friedman and Heine, 1963). In another study circulating antibodies to hydralazine were found in patients with active lupus erythematosus induced by the drug. In one case antibodies against hydralazine appeared when symptoms of lupus were present and disappeared during asymptomatic periods (Hahn et al., 1972). Antibodies to native DNA appeared only during the asymptomatic period.

An unexplained feature of the late toxic reaction is that it generally affects patients in whom the blood pressure is well controlled. It has even been claimed that there is a reciprocal relationship between the hydralazine syndrome and blood pressure control (Perry, 1973), and that in patients with toxic reactions, the diastolic blood pressure was lower and the survival rate longer than in patients without the syndrome. Furthermore, it has been observed that toxic reactions were followed by prolonged and complete remissions of blood pressure (Perry et al., 1966; Miller et al., 1975).

In the group followed up by Perry hydralazine was not discontinued in all patients who developed toxic symptoms. Of those with severe toxic reactions, five continued to take reduced doses of the drug for more than 18 months and had a well-controlled diastolic pressure. After re-exposure, the syndrome may not reappear, particularly when low doses are given. In hypertensive patients who suffered from idiopathic LE, hydralazine (mean dose 203 mg daily) was given for a mean duration of 21 months, together with prednisone and azathioprine. No new symptoms nor exacerbation of the pre-existing systemic lupus occurred (Reza et al., 1975). Hence idiopathic LE is not a contraindication against the use of hydralazine, although other antihypertensives should be preferred.

After the hydralazine syndrome had first been reported in man, various attempts were made to reproduce it in experimental animals, so as to be able to study the conditions that might favour the manifestation of the syndrome as well as its underlying mechanism. However, it was not possible to find an animal model that closely corresponded to the clinical observations made in man. A syndrome, characterized by anorexia and lassitude, was produced in dogs, in which also LE-like cells, anemia, and leukopenia were found as well as a thickening of the glomerular basement membrane (Comens, 1956a, 1960). Comens (1956b) ascribed part of the effects to a manganese depletion caused by the chelating activity of hydralazine. However, the feeding of manganese or copper could not prevent the syndrome (Schroeder, 1959). Other investigators did not consider these changes characteristic for the hydralazine syndrome or SLE (Gardner, 1957) or failed to demonstrate such effects in dogs (Alarcón-Segovia and Osmundson,

1965). In the studies of ALARCÓN-SEGOVIA, neither LE-cells nor antinuclear antibodies were detectable, and also at autopsy, no lesions were found in any of the dogs which had received between 26 and 45 g of hydralazine (ALARCÓN-SEGOVIA et al., 1967). In another series of dogs, elevated β-globulin levels and a false, positive Wassermann reaction occurred, which has also been reported in man, but no LE-cells were detected (BLAS ZINGALE et al., 1960). On the other hand, spontaneous SLE has been described in dogs without their being given hydralazine (LEWIS et al., 1965).

Also in guinea pigs, experiments were undertaken to produce the hydralazine syndrome, and LE-cells have been found in a certain percentage of animals, together with anemia, leukopenia, and changes in plasma proteins (SIGUIER et al., 1958). Similar observations have been made by BRAVERMAN and LERNER (1962), who found LE-cells in 17% of guinea pigs that received hydralazine and could also demonstrate antinuclear antibodies and thickened glomerular basement membranes. MONIER (1960) found LE-cells in rats, but this had not been the case in another study (MÖLLERBERG, 1958), and also attempts to induce the hydralazine syndrome in the pig failed (MCCOY and LEACH, 1959). Hence, in summary, the attempts to induce a hydralazine syndrome in experimental animals have not been successful, and it may be concluded that similar reactions, which may be caused in man by other drugs, cannot be excluded on the basis of animal toxicity studies, not even of prolonged duration.

The pathogenesis of the drug-induced SLE is not clear at all (ZBINDEN, 1976). Although it was an attractive idea to relate the syndrome to the chelating activity of the substance, it was not possible to demonstrate a depletion or binding of any one essential metal. It has been suggested that a predisposition to SLE exists, which has been called lupus diathesis (ALARCÓN-SEGOVIA et al., 1967), but no definition of such a diathesis was given, except the statement that it may end in manifest SLE. It is supposed that those patients who develop the hydralazine syndrome have a lupus diathesis, which is then activated by hydralazine or other drugs, such as procainamide or diphenylhydantoin. Other authors too have discussed an intrinsic factor which is activated by certain drugs (LEE and SIEGEL, 1968). However, from the data of PERRY it is obvious that hydralazine can induce the syndrome also in the absence of an alleged diathesis. Nevertheless, since antibodies to native DNA which are characteristic for SLE appear also in hydralazine-induced lupus, similarities between the spontaneous disease and the adverse drug reaction may be explained. The observation that hydralazine can be given to hypertensive patients suffering from primary LE without causing a deterioration in their state tells against the activation of an underlying disease (DUBOIS, 1966; REZA et al., 1975).

In vitro hydralazine can combine with aldehyde groups of collagen to from a hydrazine. The drug could act as a hapten which makes collagen antigenic (PAZ and SEIFTER 1972; EDITORIAL 1977), but such a mechanism has not been demonstrated *in vivo*.

Besides the characteristic hydralazine syndrome, polyneuropathy has also been reported in connection with long-term hydralazine treatment (KIRKENDALL and PAGE, 1958; RASKIN and FISHMAN, 1965). It was presumed that pyridoxine deficiency, caused by the binding of pyridoxine to hydralazine, was responsible for this reaction, which was considered comparable to the polyneuropathy induced by INH. By the formation of the pyridoxal-hydralazine complex (a hydrazone) the coenzyme could be inactivated and excreted in the urine. However, cases of polyneuropathy caused by hydralazine seem to be rare, and no similar observations have been published since.

C. Some Hydralazine Derivatives

In a group of new phthalazine derivatives synthesized by BINIECKI and coworkers (1958a, b), the N_1-carbethoxy-N_2-hydrazinophthalazine (binazine) was found to be of special interest. The compound has a four to six times lower acute toxicity than hydralazine, but the hypotensive effect is also slightly reduced as compared with that of hydralazine. The pharmacodynamic profile of binazine is very similar to that of hydralazine: lowering of blood pressure, increase in renal blood flow, and a diminished pressor response to various vasoconstrictors, such as adrenaline, noradrenaline, or vasopressin. It was claimed that the drug acted on hypothalamic vasopressor centres (GAMSKI, 1973), but such an explanation of the blood pressure-lowering effext may be based on a similar erroneous interpretation of experimental data as has been the case for hydralazine. It was presumed that binazine is rapidly hydrolyzed in the organism to hydralazine, which then is the substance responsible for the pharmacologic effects of binazine.

Similar results have been obtained with the phthalazine derivative DJ 1461 (1-[2-(1,3 dimethyl-2-butenylidene) hydrazino] phthalazine), which also has about one-fourth of the hypotensive activity of hydralazine (AKASHI et al., 1974). The drug was said to have no cardiac stimulating activity, and a dissociation between the hypotensive and the tachycardic effect was claimed. DJ 1461 reduced blood pressure in spontaneous hypertensive rats in a way similar to that of hydralazine, but the increase in heart rate in these experiments was definitely less with the new drug. As long as these results obtained in rats are not confirmed by studies in other animals species or in man, it is not possible to draw any conclusions as to the therapeutic significance of this observation.

Recently, L6150 (DL150IT), a hydrazinopyridazine, has been extensively studied pharmacologically and compared with hydrazinophthalazine (BALDOLI et al., 1971, 1972, 1974; SARDI et al., 1973). Whereas, in normotensive and spontaneously hypertensive rats, the compound was less hypotensive than hydralazine, it was about four times as active in lowering blood pressure in renal hypertensive dogs. However, no difference was observed with respect to the duration of action. At a comparable degree of blood pressure reduction, tachycardia was more pronounced by L6150 than by hydralazine. The relative increase in coronary blood flow was higher than with hydralazine, both in conscious and in anesthetized dogs, and it was claimed that for the same increase in cardiac output the increase in coronary flow would be relatively greater with L6150 than with hydralazine. Toxicity studies in various animal species revealed a lower acute toxicity for the pyridazine derivative as compared with hydralazine, and also in long-term toxicity studies the new compound was tolerated in higher doses. Hemodynamic effects in man are comparable to those of hydralazine (DE PONTI et al., 1976). Some clinical studies have been undertaken in which an antihypertensive action was demonstrated (BROD et al., 1976, WESTER et al., 1976), but the data available do not suffice to definitely compare the therapeutic usefulness with that of hydralazine. Time has been too short to decide yet whether L6150 may be less prone than hydralazine to induce symptoms of rheumatoid arthritis or LE when given to patients in corresponding doses over a prolonged period.

Other hydrazinopyridazines, e.g., the 3-hydrazino-6-(2-hydroxypropyl)methylamino-pyridazine, have been described recently (CARPI and DORIGOTTI, 1974; PIFFERI et al., 1975). Substance JSF2123 has a definite hypotensive effect in various animal species and increases blood flow in various vascular beds, including that of the kidney. The heart rate increased as a consequence of the fall in blood pressure. It was claimed that the drug would be 6 to 10 times more active than hydralazine, but would be less toxic. No clinical results have been published so far. The same is the case with a series of other hydrazinopyridazines (LECLERC et al., 1976). It has also still to be demonstrated whether the acute side-effects, such as headache, nausea, vomiting, flushing or tachycardia induced by L6150 or JSF2123 are less unpleasant than those occurring with hydralazine, but on the basis of former clinical studies with hydrazinopyridazines, such as compound 6084 (DRUEY and TRIPOD, 1967), it remains doubtful that L6150 is really superior to the well-established hydralazine. Nothing is known for the new compounds on the incidence of adverse reactions such as rheumatoid arthritis, myalgia or SLE.

For the time being hydralazine and dihydralazine have maintained their position as the only vasodilators to be widely prescribed in the treatment of hypertension, and it may be expected that this situation will not change within the next few years. Minoxidil is more effective, but if it is marketed, its use will certainly be more restricted than that of hydralazine. After 25 years of experience with hydralazine the handling of the drug, especially when given together with other antihypertensives, is well known and it will take time until a comparable amount of information for a possible replacement becomes available.

III. Nitroprusside

V. A. W. KREYE and F. GROSS

Nitroprusside, in the form of its sodium salt, is one of the most potent blood pressure-lowering drugs, but its short duration of action and the fact that it has to be administered by i.v. infusion have limited its use to the treatment of hypertensive emergencies. The substance was for the first time synthetized by PLAYFAIR in 1849 and toxicologic studies were already made by HERMANN in 1886 and by DAVIDSOHN in 1887 who also described the hypotensive effect. However, only 40 years later, the first careful pharmacologic and toxicologic analysis was published by JOHNSON (1929). Until then, nitroprusside had mainly been considered to be a toxic substance that acts by releasing cyanide ions, and JOHNSON mentioned for the first time the possibilities of its therapeutic use in diseases such as hypertension, angina, bronchial asthma, and spasms of sphincters within the gastrointestinal tract. Subsequently, nitroprusside fell into oblivion again, and it took another 25 years until PAGE and his associates reported on its cardiovascular actions, especially on high blood pressure (PAGE et al., 1955). Although the effectiveness of nitroprusside as a powerful blood pressure-lowering agent, suitable for the treatment of hypertensive emergencies, had clearly been demonstrated, the use of the drug remained restricted to a few specialists. However, new interest arose in 1970, when not only the use of nitroprusside as an antihypertensive was recommended by various investigators (WILBRANDT et al., 1970; MANI, 1971; PARADE, 1972), but also its favourable effect in patients with left ventricular failure was described, which in based on a reduction of left ventricular afterload (FRANCIOSA et al., 1972). Simultaneously, studies on the pharmacology, pharmacokinetics and toxicology were taken up, and short reviews on the drug were published by TUZEL (1974) and PALMER and LASSETER (1975).

A. Pharmacodynamics

1. Cardiovascular Effects

In the whole animal, the marked hypotensive effect is the outstanding pharmacologic feature of nitroprusside (DAVIDSOHN, 1887; JOHNSON, 1929; PAGE et al., 1955; KYNCL, 1971; ROSS and COLE, 1973a, b; ADAMS et al., 1973, 1974; ROWE and HENDERSON, 1974; KOMAREK and MANSFELD, 1976). The reduction of the mean arterial pressure by nitroprusside in conscious dogs is the result of an almost parallel decrease in systolic and diastolic blood pressures (ROSS and COLE, 1973b). The blood pressure begins to fall within a few seconds after the start of an i.v. injection and may be maintained at a reduced level by continuous infusion. After a bolus injection, the blood pressure returns to the initial level within 2 to 5 min, depending on the dose and the degree of blood pressure reduction (Fig. 4). This hypotensive effect is similar in rats, rabbits, cats and dogs.

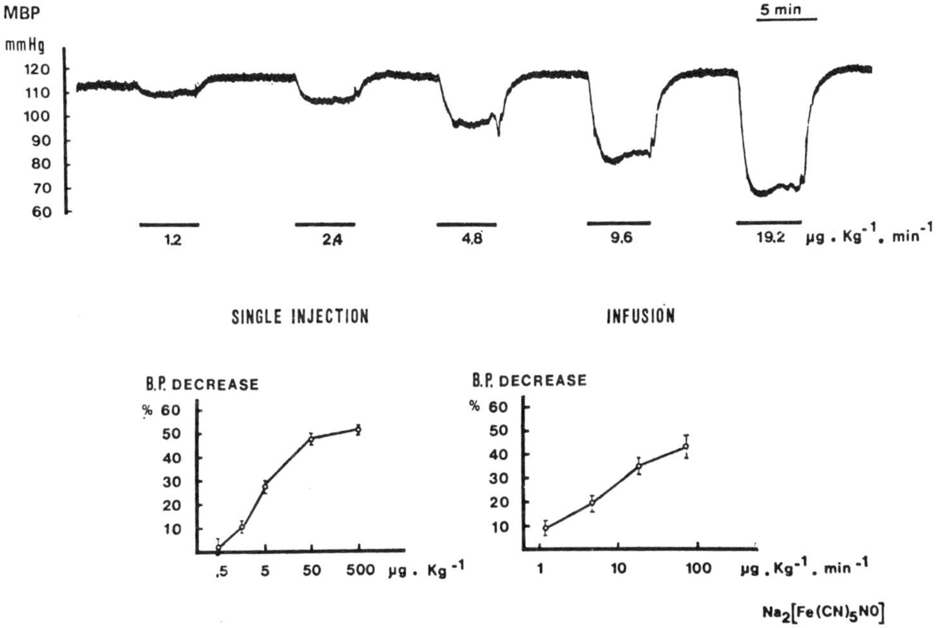

Fig. 4. Effect of increasing doses of sodium nitroprusside on mean blood pressure of a normotensive rat anesthetized with urethane. Below: Dose-response curves for bolus injections *(left)* and for infusions of 5 min each *(right)* (KYNCL, 1971)

During sustained hypotension produced by an infusion of nitroprusside, responses to vasoconstrictor substances (noradrenaline, vasopressin) were found to be moderately diminished in the dog (PAGE et al., 1955), whereas KYNCL (1971) observed no distinct reduction of the pressor response to adrenaline, noradrenaline, or angiotensin in the rat during infusion of medium doses of nitroprusside. Similarly, HILTON (1959) reported an unaltered pressor response to adrenaline during nitroprusside-induced reduction of blood pressure in dogs, but the maximum rise of blood pressure produced by adrenaline was diminished equivalent to the degree of the fall in blood pressure induced by nitroprusside. In rats the carotid occlusion reflex was suppressed, but, after cessation of the infusion, an overshooting response, which in its intensity corresponded to the degree of the preceding suppression, was obtained (Kyncl, 1971).

The fall in arterial blood pressure induced by nitroprusside is invariably associated with a striking reduction in the total peripheral resistance (Miller and Van Maanen, 1968; Bastron and Kaloyanides, 1972; Adams et al., 1973, 1974; Ross and Cole, 1973a, b; Rowe and Henderson, 1974), which in anesthetized dogs amounted to as much as 60% (Adams et al., 1974) or even 77% (Ross and Cole, 1973b) above control values. Pulmonary arterial pressure was reduced in dogs (Adams et al., 1974; Rowe and Henderson, 1974), but only the latter authors reported a consistent fall in pulmonary resistance.

Regional blood flow reflects the balance between local vascular resistance and perfusion pressure. By its hypotensive effect, nitroprusside reduces perfusion pressure indirectly; by its vasodilator action, it directly affects resistance in individual vascular beds. Since the degree of these effects depends on the experimental conditions chosen, divergent findings on changes in regional blood flow during the infusion of nitroprusside have been reported. In dogs, a significant decrease in the blood flow to the stomach, spleen, and skeletal muscle was noted, but a moderate increase was found in renal blood flow (Robie and McNay, 1974). Whereas the isolated dog kidney responded to nitroprusside by a 10% increase in blood flow, in the whole animal marked reductions in *p*-aminohippurate and inulin clearances as well as in sodium excretion pointed towards an impaired renal perfusion during nitroprusside-induced hypotension. In dogs with moderate lowering of blood pressure, mesenteric and femoral blood flows had increased, but they were decreased when blood pressure fell to lower levels (Ross and Cole, 1973b). Komarek and Mansfeld (1976) reported a reduced femoral blood flow during the infusion of nitroprusside. Whereas an increased coronary blood flow was measured by Tountas et al. (1965), Ross and Cole (1973b), Rowe and Henderson (1974), da Luz et al. (1974) and Cohn et al. (1974), no consistent changes or even slight reductions in myocardial blood flow were described by Luka et al. (1974) and Franciosa et al. (1973).

The hypotensive effect of nitroprusside is modified by drugs that act on the arteriolar smooth muscle, resulting in either an additive, a synergistic, or an antagonistic effect. In the rat, both a smooth muscle stimulant, such as barium chloride, or a relaxant, such as papaverine, diminished the hypotensive response to nitroprusside in a similar way, although, in the case of barium chloride, the blood pressure level was higher and, in the case of papaverine, lower than the basal blood pressure (Kyncl, 1971). Inversely, in the dog, the prior administration of nitroprusside antagonized the hypotensive response to histamine (Hilton and Tumlinson, 1960). Other antihypertensive substances which act on the arteriolar muscle, such as dihydralazine or diazoxide, enhanced the blood pressure-lowering effect of nitroprusside. On the other hand atropine, α-adrenergic blocking agents or antihistaminics did not inhibit the depressor action of nitroprusside (Page et al., 1955; Kyncl, 1971).

Action on the Heart

Heart rate may either increase, remain unaltered or decrease during nitroprusside-induced hypotension. In anesthetized dogs, heart rate increased (Miller and Van Maanen, 1968; Adams et al., 1973, 1974; Rowe and Henderson, 1974), but other investigators observed no consistent changes (Page et al., 1955; Ross and Cole, 1973a, b). An initial increase, followed by a decrease in heart rate has been seen during the course of nitroprusside infusions (KOMAREK and MANSFELD, 1976). In concious rats, simultaneously with the fall in blood pressure, heart rate increased but it was little or not at all affected in anesthetized animals (KYNCL, 1971). Since, during nitroprusside infusion, heart rate increased in dogs despite β-adrenergic blockade with propranolol, an inhibition of vagal tone rather than a stimulation of efferent sympathetic fibers was assumed to play the major role in the control of heart rate (ADAMS et al., 1974); ROSS and COLE, 1973b). The suppression of reflex tachycardia during anesthesia has been claimed to be responsible for a more pronounced hypotensive response to nitroprusside (KYNCL, 1971) (Fig.5). Similar to anesthesia, drugs or regimens that prevent or reduce the reflectory rise in heart rate during the fall of blood pressure, such as ganglionic blocking agents, β-adrenergic blockers (propranolol), or surgical sympathectomy intensify the hypotensive response to nitroprusside (PAGE et al., 1955; KYNCL, 1971). Equivocal results have been published when cardiac performance was studied in dogs. MILLER and VAN MAANEN (1968) described an initial increase in contractile force during nitroprusside infusion which later returned to control values. During β-adrenergic or ganglionic blockade, nitroprusside reduced the contractile force of the heart. A reduction in left ventricular stroke work and stroke volume and an unchanged cardiac output have been reported by LUKA et al. (1974), and a reduc-

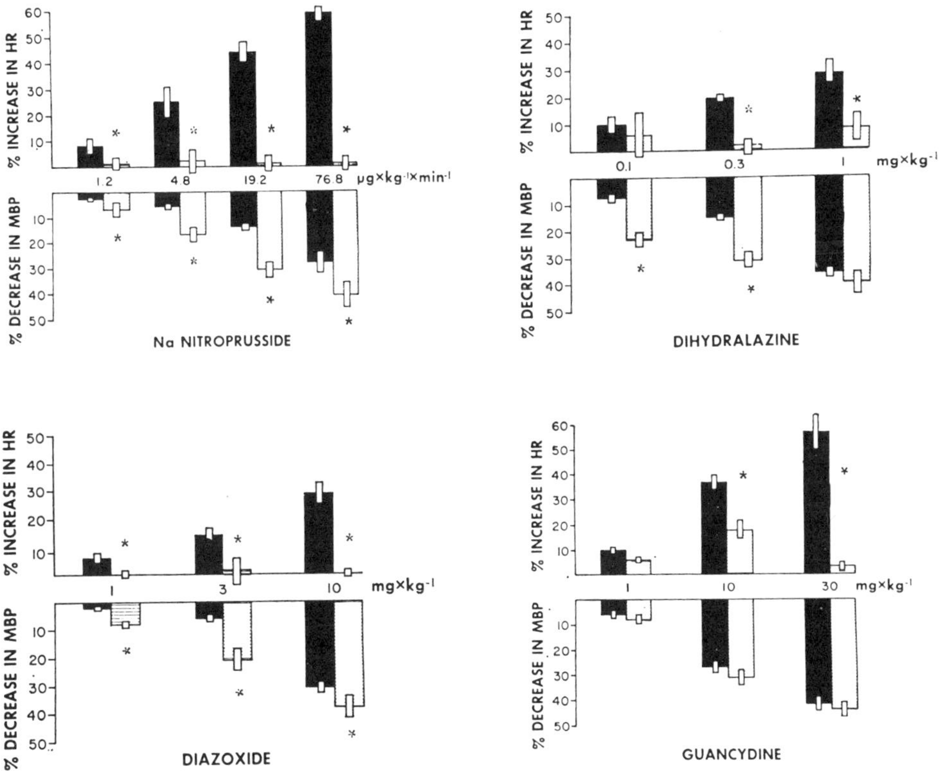

Fig. 5. Increase in heart rate *(HR)* and decrease in mean blood pressure *(MBP)* in conscious *(black bars)* and in anesthetized (urethane) rats *(white bars)*. Doses of the various drugs are indicated in the middle of each graph (KYNCL, 1971)
. $p \leqq 0.05$ by paired t-test

tion in cardiac output and stroke volume was seen when heart rate was kept constant (Komarek and Mansfeld, 1976). From measurements of dP/dt, the latter authors concluded a negative inotropic effect at least with high doses of nitroprusside. Similarly, reduced myocardial contractile force was seen during infusions of nitroprusside (Schlant et al., 1962), but since this occurred 1 to 2 min later than the fall in blood pressure, the authors presumed that it was caused by an indirect effect of the drug. Although stroke volume decreased by 28% cardiac output was unaltered ouring to an increase in heart rate by 30% (Adams et al., 1973). An increase in cardiac output was observed without adverse effects on myocardial contractility or variuos parameters of cardiac work (Ross and Cole (1973a,b) and Rowe and Henderson (1974.)

When nitroprusside was administered to dogs with experimental myocardial infarction favourable effects on various cardiac parameters have been reported (Franciosa et al., 1973; Cohn et al., 1974; Mueller et al., 1974a, b; Da Luz et al., 1974). The encouraging results of these experimental studies and similar investigations in patients (see "Therapeutic Use") are the rationale for applying sodium nitroprusside in patients suffering from cardiac failure or acute myocardial infarction with severe impairment of cardiac function. Several authors have measured in animal experiments metabolic parameters such as myocardial oxygen consumption, the ratio of oxygen supply to demand (i.e., coronary sinus flow/ myocardial O_2 consumption), and lactate handling. From the results of these studies it can be deduced that nitroprusside may enhance the oxygen utilisation of the failing heart, especially when coronary dilation induced by nitroprusside can still compensate for the fall in coronary perfusion pressure subsequent to hypotension induced by the drug. In view of the metabolic improvement seen mainly in the ischemic zones, the size of the infarct might decrease under the influence of nitroprusside (Mueller et al., 1974a,b).

2. Effects on Smooth Muscle and the Mechanism of Action

Nitroprusside has a relaxant effect on various smooth muscle preparations (Thienes, 1926; Johnson, 1929), which is much more pronounced in smooth muscle of the tonic type such as vascular and tracheal smooth muscle, than in smooth muscle of the phasic type from the splanchnic region (Kreye et al., 1975). Helical strips from rat aorta, contracted by $10^{-8}M$ noradrenaline or 40 mM KCl, started to relax with concentrations as low as $10^{-10}M$ nitroprusside. However, whereas nitroprusside completely relaxed vascular smooth muscle in which tone was induced by drugs, the tone produced by depolarising concentrations of potassium was partially resistant even to very high concentrations of nitroprusside. This divergent effect of nitroprusside on noradrenaline- and potassium-induced contractions has also been described with isolated pulmonary artery of rabbits (Häusler and Thorens, 1975b). Any inhibitory or stimulating effects of nitroprusside on α- or β-adrenoceptors, respectively, could be excluded, and the drug also relaxes rat aorta contracted by angiotensin II, Phe^2-Lys^8-vasopressin, or barium chloride. The action of nitroprusside on the isolated rat aorta is rapid, since realaxation starts 15 to 30 s after its addition to the organ-bath, and a new plateau of reduced tone is obtained after 3 to 5 min (Kreye et al., 1975). Strips of canine saphenous vein are similarly relaxed by nitroprusside as arterial preparations, and the drug does not alter the efflux or noradrenaline from these preparations when they are stimulated electrically (Verhaege and Shepherd, 1975). Thus, the drug does not inhibit the release of transmitter from nerve endings.

Smooth muscle preparations from the splanchnic region which have varying degrees of phasic contractility are less sensitive than aortic strips and develop tachyphylaxis (portal vein, duodenum of the rat), or are unresponsive to sodium nitroprusside (vas deferens, uterus of the rat). GOLENHOFEN (1976) who discriminates between "*P*- and *T*-mechanisms" (phasic and tonic) of smooth muscle activation concluded, on the basis of results obtained with the gastric fundus of the rat, that nitroprusside predominantly suppresses the "*T*-mechanism". It clearly differs from drugs such as verapamil which selectively act on the "*P*-mechanism" (GOLENHOFEN, 1976; BOEV et al., 1976). Nitroprusside inhibits the excitation-contraction coupling in vascular smooth muscle and this effect is more pronounced on the pharmacomechanical coupling than on the electromechanical coupling induced by potassium (KREYE and LÜTH, 1976). A concentration-dependent hyperpolarisation of vascular smooth muscle may be of significance for the vasodilator activity of nitroprusside (HÄUSLER and THORENS, 1976). This hyperpolarisation may be the result of an inhibitory effect on chloride permeability (KREYE, 1977b). The finding of an "antagonism" between calcium and nitroprusside in contraction studies with isolated preparations of vascular smooth muscle suggested that nitroprusside might interfere directly with the handling of calcium ions by the cell (KREYE et al., 1975; HÄUSLER and THORENS, 1976). Conflicting results have been reported on the question whether nitroprusside, like verapamil, inhibits calcium influx into the cells of vascular smooth muscle. KREYE et al. (1975) found that nitroprusside inhibited the ^{45}Ca influx induced by potassium depolarisation, but HÄUSLER and THORENS (1975) saw no effect of the drug on calcium uptake by K^+-depolarized preparations, whereas the initial ^{45}Ca uptake in response to noradrenaline was reduced. In the presence of nitroprusside an augmented calcium uptake by K^+-depolarized rabbit aortic strips was reported (VAN BREEMEN, 1975).

It is now generally agreed that the inhibition of calcium influx into vascular smooth muscle is not necessary for the action of nitroprusside. Nitroprusside depressed the noradrenaline-induced contraction of the rabbit aorta and canine saphenous vein in a calcium-free medium to which either lanthanum chloride or verapamil had been added in order to abolish calcium influx (KREYE et al., 1975; VERHAEGE and SHEPHERD, 1975). When nitroprusside was present in the rinsing fluid, the K^+-depolarized rat aorta relaxed twice as rapidly as without the drug. This effect was independent of the extracellular calcium concentration (KREYE and LÜTH, 1976). These findings indicate that nitroprusside may interfere with the intracellular activation of calcium either by inhibiting the release of calcium from storage sites (e.g., sarcoplasmatic reticulum, or mitochondria), by facilitating the extrusion of intracellular calcium, or by an enhanced sequestration of intracellular calcium (e.g., activation of uptake by sarcoplasmatic reticulum, or mitochondria). However, in a microsomal fraction from rabbit aorta which should have contained sarcoplasmatic reticulum membranes, it was not possible to demonstrate an increase in the Mg-ATP-dependent calcium binding in the presence of sodium nitroprusside (BARON and KREYE, 1973). No measurable decrease in the cellular concentration of ATP was found in homogenates of rat aortic strips incubated with nitroprusside in concentrations which induced maximal relaxation (KREYE et al., 1975).

Various smooth muscle relaxants, such as papaverine or isoproterenol, increase the cellular content of cAMP, and this "second messenger" may play a causal role in the relaxation induced by these drugs. However, incubation with nitroprusside in concentrations of 10^{-7} and $10^{-5} M$ had no effect on the concentration of cAMP in rat aortic tissue (KREYE et al., 1975). The Mg-ATP-induced tone of "glycerinated" preparations of rabbit aorta (which is an experimental model of the contractile proteins) was not affected by nitroprusside, which indicates that the drug has no direct action on the contractile proteins (KREYE et al., 1975).

In the isolated, electrically driven cat papillary muscle, no direct positive or negative inotropic effects were seen with nitroprusside up to a concentration of $10^{-4} M$, but with $10^{-3} M$ a slight (10%) reduction in contractile force was obtained (CHATTERJEE et al., 1973). Similarly, nitroprusside in concentrations up to $10^{-3} M$ had no effect on frequency or amplitude of isolated guinea pig auricles (KREYE et al., 1975).

3. Other Effects

Both *in vivo* and *in vitro* nitroprusside inhibited the aggregation of rabbit platelets in a dose-dependent manner, the underlying mechanism being still unknown (GLUSA et al., 1974). This effect was no longer demonstrable 20 min after cessation of the nitroprusside infusion. In mice, nitroprusside produced hypothermia which could not be prevented by atropine (BURKE and MANN, 1970).

4. Structure-Activity Relationships

Despite various efforts to identify the part of the nitroprusside molecule that is responsible for the relaxant effect on arteriolar smooth muscle, the available data give only limited information. To both the nitroso group (JOHNSON, 1929) and the iron-nitroso group (PAGE et al., 1955) the specific activity had been attributed, but NO as well as Fe^{++} can be substituted in the molecule without complete loss of the vasodilator activity (KREYE, 1974). To various derivatives in which the nitroso group was replaced by a nitro-, an aquo-, an amino- or a cyano-group and the iron by either molybdenum, manganese, or ruthenium, aortic strips of the rat responded as shown in Table 1. Blood pressure-lowering activities had been described previously for aquo- and aminopentacyanoferrate (JUNG and PETSCH, 1967) and for nitropentacyano-ferrate (CAUJOLLE et al., 1968; JUNG and PETSCH, 1967), the latter and the corresponding nitroso-sulfo-compound having activities only slightly inferior to that of nitroprusside. However, both compounds may have no activity of their own since in aqueous solution and at neutral pH they change into nitroprusside (KREYE, 1974).

Since nitroprusside is rapidly metabolized in the body, the question arises whether intermediates or final breakdown products rather than the parent compound are responsible for its vasodilator action. Therefore, the relaxant effect of known or assumed metabolites of nitroprusside, i.e., CN^-, SCN^-, aquopentacyanoferrate, NO_2^-, Fe^{++}, and Fe^{+++}, and of a donator of NO-radicals, i.e., di-tert.-butylnitroxyl, were studied on rat aortic strips contracted by noradrenaline. None of these substances had a relaxant effect comparable to that of nitroprusside (Table 1; KREYE, 1974). Thus, the vasodilator action of nitroprusside seems to be a feature of the whole molecule and its characteristic conformation. The fact that its activity is maintained, at least to a certain degree, when the ligands or the central iron atom are substituted may be explained by the assumption that such changes induce only slight differences in the conformation of the substance.

B. Pharmacokinetics

After cessation of a nitroprusside infusion in therapeutic doses, blood pressure returns to preinfusion levels within 2 to 5 min indicating the rapid metabolization of the substance. As early as 1886, HERRMANN reported an odor of cyanide on dissection of experimental animals which had been poisoned by the oral administration of nitroprusside. This finding was confirmed by several authors either in experimental animals or in a few patients who had committed suicide with nitro-

Table 1. Comparative activity of sodium nitroprusside in aortic strips of the rat. Relaxation of the noradrenaline-induced contraction. (+) equivocal effect, + slight, ++ definite, +++ complete relaxant effect

Compounds	Molarity of compounds								Remarks
	10^{-10}	10^{-9}	10^{-8}	10^{-7}	10^{-6}	10^{-5}	10^{-4}	10^{-3}	
$Na_2[Fe(CN)_5NO] \cdot 2\ H_2O$	(+)	+	++	+++					Sodium nitroprusside (NP)
$Na_4[Fe(CN)_5NO_2] \cdot 10\ H_2O$		+	++	+++					Converts to NP at pH 7.4
$Na_4[Fe(CN)_5NOS]$			+	++	+++				Rapid conversion to NP?
$Na_2NH_3[Fe(CN)_5NH_3] \cdot x\ H_2O$				(+)	+	+++			
$Na_3[Fe(CN)_5H_2O^8 \cdot H_2O$				(+)	+	+++			
$K_4[Fe_{II}(CN_6] \cdot 3\ H_2O$							+	+++	
$K_3[Fe_{III}(CN)_6]$						+	+++		
$K_4[Mo(CN)_5NO] \cdot 2\ H_2O$			(+)	+	++	+++			Rapid breakdown
$K_3[Mn(CN)_5NO]$						+	++		
$K_2[Ru(CN)_5NO]$			+	++	+++				

prusside. Furthermore, the toxic effects of parenterally administered nitroprusside are suppressed by antidotes to cyanide (SMITH and KRUSZYNA, 1974; KREYE et al., 1976). Breakdown of nitroprusside by the release of cyanide groups is supposed to be the primary metabolic step, but this process is not well understood. Since nitroprusside is stable at plasma pH, simple hydrolysis cannot be responsible for its *in vivo* inactivation (SMITH and KRUSZYNA, 1974). Several investigators have shown that nitroprusside is decomposed on contact with homogenates from various tissues (HILL, 1942; CASINELLI, 1956; SMITH and KRUSZYNA, 1974); this reaction is of a nonenzymatic nature since it persists after heating of the homogenates to 90° C. When nitroprusside was incubated with various amino acids only those containing SH-groups such as methionine and cysteine cleaved cyanide from the drug (PAGE et al., 1955). Consequently it was supposed that the reaction of iron in nitroprusside with SH-groups of tissue proteins was the underlying mechanism of the breakdown of the molecule. HILL (1942), CASINELLI (1956) and SMITH and KRUSZYNA (1974), who measured release of cyanide, as well as RESKE (1976) who, by a bioassay method, measured the amount of non-inactivated nitroprusside, all described a breakdown of nitroprusside when incubated with whole blood. Since erythrocyte ghosts were inactive and hemolyzed blood more active than whole blood, SMITH and KRUSZYNA (1974) concluded that nitroprusside reacted with hemoglobin in a way that an electron be transferred from the former to the latter. As a consequence methemoglobin may be formed as well as an unstable form of nitroprusside which then dissociates all its cyanide. However, the inactivation of nitroprusside by blood from different species is a slow process (after 60 min of incubation: mouse 33%, rat 35 to 47%, human 7.5% (SMITH and KRUSZYNA, 1974); rat 68% (RESKE, 1976), and cannot account for the rapid *in vivo* inactivation. When nitroprusside was infused into various vascular beds of the rat, it was found, that in the cerebral and portal circulation as well as in the hind limb 30 to 35% of nitroprusside were extacted during one single passage (RESKE, 1976). By comparison of blood pressure responses to nitroprusside of acutely nephrectomized and of sham-operated rats, an extraction rate in the renal vascular bed of up to 66% was calculated. After i.v. injection of ^{14}C-nitroprusside in rats, HÖBEL et al. (1974) recovered 11.3% of the total radioactivity in the urine within 24 h. At 0 to 6 h, 4.5%; at 6 to 12 h, 3.5%; at 12 to 18 h, 2.0%; and at 18 to 24 h, 1.5%. By means of thin layer chromatography, the radioactivity recovered during the first period of urine collection (0 to 6 h) was located in spots with Rf-values of nitroprusside (19.2%), CN^- (24.6%), and SCN^- (56.2%) (RAITHELHUBER and HÖBEL, 1976), whereas only negligible amounts of ^{14}C were found in the feces (HÖBEL et al., 1974; HÖBEL and RAITHELHUBER, 1976).

It is generally accepted that cyanide, once released from nitroprusside, is rapidly converted to thiocyanate by rhodanese (LANG, 1933), a reaction which is limited by the amount of mobile sulfur present in the organism. The reverse reaction, from thiocyanate to cyanide, catalyzed by thiocyanate oxidase (GOLDSTEIN and RIEDERS, 1953), plays no role in the metabolism of nitroprusside. Thiocyanate, with its long half-life of about 8 days, is slowly eliminated from the body.

C. Therapeutic Use

1. Hypertensive Emergencies

The usefulness of nitroprusside in hypertensive emergencies had already been recommended by PAGE et al. (1955), but at that time no commercial preparations were available and therefore the use remained limited. This situation has changed recently and various brands of nitroprusside are marketed now. Nitroprusside is administered by i.v. infusion, the dosage depending on the response of the individual patient. Doses between 70 and 400 μg/min may be given initially, and after the fall of the blood pressure, the reduced level may be maintained by the infusion of smaller doses. The duration of the infusion depends on the individual circumstances and may last from 1 h up to several weeks. In a study on 57 patients total doses of between a few milligrams and nearly 10 grams (during a period of 45 days) were given (WILBRANDT et al., 1970). The rate of infusion depends on the response of blood pressure and a "titration" of the dose is necessary in each patient. Infusion rates usually range from 15 to 500 μg/min (PAGE et al., 1955; GIFFORD, 1961; KANEKO et al., 1967; KATZ and WOLF, 1971; WILBRANDT et al., 1970; AHEARN and GRIM, 1974), the highest reported rate being 800 μg/min (TUZEL, 1974). It is generally agreed that this high infusion rate should not be exceeded in order to prevent acute symptoms of toxicity. In view of the high potency of nitroprusside, expert supervision preferably in an intensive care unit and frequent blood pressure controls are requested (AMA Statement, 1974). In most of the reported cases sodium nitroprusside was administered to patients with hypertensive crises in the course of severe essential or renovascular hypertension who had developed signs of encephalopathy. Other conditions such as phentolamine-resistant pheochromocytoma (KATZ and WOLF, 1971; NOUROK et al., 1963), hyperaldosteronism (KATZ and WOLF, 1971), ergotamine-induced hypertension with severe peripheral ischemia (CARLINER et al., 1974), and hypertensive crises caused by an exaggerated blood pressure response to mephentermine or metaraminol (MORACA et al., 1962) have also been successfully treated by the drug.

The advantages of nitroprusside in the treatment of hypertensive emergencies are the instantaneous onset of action, its consistent effectiveness even in patients in whom other antihypertensives have failed, the possibility to maintain any desired level of blood pressure for lengthy periods simply by adjusting the rate of infusion, and if necessary, the rapid reversibility within a few minutes.

The effects of nitroprusside infusions in hypertensive patients are comparable to those found in experimental animals. In 23 severely hypertensive patients, unfusions of nitroprusside at various doses and lengths of periods induced a mean decrease of systolic blood pressure by 36.7%, and of the diastolic pressure by 38.2% (WILBRANDT et al., 1970). A similar parallelism of systolic and diastolic blood pressure changes was shown by GIFFORD (1961), whereas a more prominent effect on the systolic blood pressure was described by KATZ and WOLF (1971) and FRANCIOSA (1972). Hypertensive patients have been found to be more sensitive than normotensive patients (PAGE et al., 1955), but other investigators did not confirm that observation (SCHLANT et al., 1962). A considerable drop in total peripheral resistance has been calculated (SCHLANT et al., 1962; GUIHA et al., 1972; BHATIA and FROHLICH, 1973).

2. Controlled Hypotension

MORACA et al. (1962) were the first who administered nitroprusside during general anesthesia in patients undergoing cardiovascular (coarction of aorta) and brain surgery. The rationale for administering vasodilators in surgery is the prevention of frank bleeding or oozing of blood which might obscure the field of operation. Nitroprusside has now widely replaced the ganglionic blockers formerly used for this purpose. Advantages are the rapid onset of action and the prompt return of blood pressure when the infusion is stopped, furthermore it has no adverse effects on the heart. Conscious patients, premedicated with pethidine and promethazine, showed no changes in heart rate, stroke volume and cardiac output, although nitroprusside considerably reduced their arterial blood pressures and systemic vascular resistance. After induction of anesthesia, they responded to nitroprusside with an increase in cardiac output at constant stroke volumes (Styles et al., 1973). Identical findings were reported by Wildsmith et al. (1973) who applied nitroprusside for "controlled hypotension" during surgery at the ear. Patients who had undergone open-heart surgery and postoperatively required vasodilators responded to nitroprusside with an increase in stroke and cardiac indexes (Stinson et al., 1975).

Nitroprusside has been successfully applied during surgery of cerebral aneurisms and other cerebrovascular malformations (Siegel et al., 1971; Griffiths et al., 1974), in microsurgery of the ear and transsphenoidal hypophysectomy (Taylor et al., 1970), and in orthopedic as well as urologic surgery (prostatectomy, partial cystectomy and nephrectomy; Schiffmann and Fuchs, 1966). Another application has been its use during renal arteriography of unanesthetized hypertensive patients: By lowering their blood pressure, a better filling and visualization of the renal arteries was obtained than during the hypertensive state, and smaller doses of contrast media could be applied (Moraca et al., 1962; Schiffmann and Fuchs, 1966).

3. Left Ventricular Failure

Recently, nitroprusside has been tried in the treatment of congestive heart failure refractory to digitalis and diuretic therapy. In normotensive patients with cardiac failure, nitroprusside, while reducing heart rate, total peripheral resistance and pulmonary capillary wedge pressure, considerably increased cardiac output, stroke work, and urinary sodium excretion (Guiha et al., 1972). In patients with acute myocardial infarction, the substance reduced left ventricular filling pressure (LVFP) by 50%, and cardiac output rose consistently in patients at the beginning of cardiac failure or shock. A reduction in afterload rather than in preload was assumed to underly the decrease in LVFP, although a reduction in cardiac filling because of venous pooling also probably played a role in the hemodynamic response to the drug (Franciosa et al., 1972, 1973). Nitroprusside reduced stroke work index in patients with myocardial infarction whose LVFP was below 15 mm Hg, but it increased both stroke work and cardiac index and decreased LVFP in patients who had an initial LVFP above 15 mm Hg (Chatterjee et al., 1973).

Several other reports have been published according to which in cases of myocardial infarction with severe impairment of cardiac function "agressive therapy" with nitroprusside is favoured either alone (Forrester et al., 1973; Bleifeld and Hanrath, 1975; Mukherjee et al., 1976) or in combination with external counterpulsation (Parmley et al., 1974). However, although a dramatic improvement of cardiac performance is regularly seen when nitroprusside is given in moderate doses (30 to 200 μg/min) to these patients, proof is lacking so far that this regimen reduces mortality of severe cardiac infarction.

a) Tolerance and Tachyphylaxis

Several authors who had used nitroprusside exclusively to treat hypertensive emergencies have claimed that primary tolerance to the drug does not exist, and that tachyphylaxis does not develop during the course of long-term infusions. However, since nitroprusside is used more frequently to induce "controlled hypotension" during anesthesia, the number of reports on nitroprusside tolerance and tachyphylaxis has increased. Moraca et al. (19 62) were the first to describe tolerance to the drug in 5 out of 20 normotensive patients. LOWSON (1972) and EPPENS (1973) reported that tachyphylaxis occurred almost regularly in young patients, but reraly in the elderly. A severe case of tachyphylaxis has been described by AMARANATH and KELLERMEYER (1976). DAVIES et al. (1975b), applied nitroprusside to children who underwent surgery, and subdivided "abnormal responses to nitroprusside" into three types: constant high dose response, resistance, and tachyphylaxis. Whereas the mechanism of primary tolerance to nitroprusside is unknown, it has been suggested by these authors that a disorder in the detoxification of cyanide may underly the development of tachyphylaxis. This assumption was supported by the observation that tachyphylaxis to nitroprusside could be abolished by the administration of thiosulfate, an antidote to cyanide. Recently this hypothesis was substantiated by the finding that sodium cyanide abolishes the relaxant effect of nitroprusside on isolated vascular smooth muscle (KREYE 1977a).

Both tolerance and tachyphylaxis are of a high potential risk, since, when ignored or overlooked, toxic doses of nitroprusside may be administered.

b) Adverse Reactions

If nitroprusside is too rapidly infused, blood pressure may fall too quickly resulting in a circulatory collapse (reviewed by TUZEL, 1974). However, such an overshooting response can be reversed within a few minutes after discontinuation of the infusion. Nevertheless, sodium nitroprusside is a drug which is not easy to handle and may be dangerous. Reports on three fatalities related to nitroprusside administration were published recently (JACK, 1974; MERRIFIELD and BLUNDELL, 1974; DAVIES et al., 1975a). All three patients were young males without cardiovascular diseases who received nitroprusside for hypotensive anesthesia and developed tachyphylaxis and metabolic acidosis. The fatal doses ranged from 400 to 750 mg, and were infused during relatively short periods (80 to 300 min). Based on evidence from toxicologic experiments in animals (SMITH and KRUSZYNA, 1974; McDOWALL et al., 1974; KREYE et al., 1976; POSNER et al., 1976) it is probable that these patients died from subacute poisonin*)* with cyanide, which is cleaved from nitroprusside. Since its has been shown that antidotes to cyanide such as thiosulfate or hydroxocobalamine effectively protect against the acute toxicity of nitroprusside (SMITH and KRUSZYNA, 1974; KREYE et al., 1976; POSNER et al., 1976) these substances should always be at hand when nitroprusside is to be administered. Sodium thiosulfate in a dose at least fourfold that of the administered nitroprusside should be injected intravenously when a patients shows signs of acute toxicity (KREYE et al., 1976).

Thiocyanate, the final breakdown product of the *in vivo* inactivation of nitroprusside, is slowly excreted by the kidney at a half-life of about 8 days. Thus, when nitroprusside is given for prolonged periods, the plasma thiocyanate may rise steadilly and reach toxic levels. Symptoms such as fatigue, nausea, anorexia, headaches, skin rashes, disorientation, psychotic behaviour, and muscle spasms may appear at plasma levels of 5 to 10 mg/100 ml and death may occur at 20 mg/100 ml (PALMER and LASSETER, 1975). Therefore, during chronic treatment with nitroprusside, the plasma thiocyanate level should be regularly controlled, especially when renal function is impaired (PAGE et al., 1955). Treatment should be interrupted when the thiocyanate level attains between 8 and 12 mg/100 ml (GIFFORD, 1961; AMA Statement, 1974). Toxic plasma levels of thiocyanate may be rapidly reduced by peritoneal dialysis (PALMER and LASSETER, 1975).

Rare side effects of nitroprusside therapy reported are hypothyroidism probably caused by thiocyanate (NOUROK et al., 1964), and methaemoglobinemia (BOWER and PETERSON, 1975). Finally, it has to be mentioned that nitroprusside may interfere with the metabolism of vitamin B_{12}, and may cause symptoms of B_{12} deficiency in patients with low plasma levels of B_{12}, impaired liver function and Leber's optic nerve atrophy; administration of vitamin B_{12} in its hydroxo-form has been recommended in these cases (VESEY et al., 1974).

c) Dosage and Preparations

Until recently nitroprusside solutions for infusion had to be prepared by hospital pharmacies. Appropriate procedures have been described by SHEPS (1971) and VORBURGER (1967). Today, brands of sodium nitroprusside are available, such as:

Nipride; 1 ampoule contains 44 mg of dehydrated nitroprusside, equivalent to 50 mg sodium nitroprusside

Nipruss; 1 ampoule contains 52.75 mg of dehydrated nitroprusside, equivalent to 60 mg sodium nitroprusside.

The lyophilized substance is to be dissolved in the solvent which is delivered together with the drug. Appropriate amounts of the solution should be added to 5% glucose to prepare the concentration desired for the infusion. Since nitroprusside is unstable in light (ANDERSON and RAE, 1972), the infusion bottle or syringe must be wrapped with a sheet of aluminium foil or black paper. Infusions either by constant drip or by a pump at a rate of about 3 µg/kg/min (range: 0.5 to 8 µg/kg/min), equivalent to 200 µg/min (range: 20 to 400 µg/min), will normally suffice to reduce blood pressure to the desired level. It must be warned against exceeding an infusion rate of 800 to 900 µg/min, even in cases of partial or complete tolerance to nitroprusside or of tachyphylaxis developing during its administration.

IV. Diazoxide

When the antihypertensive activity of benzothiadiazine diuretics was first observed, it soon became evident that it could not exclusively be explained by the diuretic and natriuretic actions and their consequences for plasma and extracellular fluid volume, but that an effect on arteriolar smooth muscle also contributed to the lowering of elevated blood pressure. Numerous derivatives of benzothiadiazine were synthetized in an attempt to dissociate the diuretic and antihypertensive activities (WOHL, 1970a, b; TOPLISS and YUDIS, 1972). Diazoxide, chemically related to chlorothiazide, in which the sulfamoyl group in position 7 is replaced by chlorine, was found to be the most promising compound (RUBIN et al., 1961, 1962, 1963). Although the strong blood pressure-lowering activity of diazoxide was rapidly observed, both in experimental animals and in man, it took more than 10 years until the drug was released for the treatment of hypertensive crises. The reason for the delay was the strong hyperglycemic effect of diazoxide, which was already observed during the extended period of clinical trials (DOLLERY et al., 1962; LOCKWOOD et al., 1963; TABACHNIK et al., 1964). The inhibitory effect on the release of insulin (WALES et al., 1967; FRERICHS et al., 1968; TABACHNIK and GULBENKIAN, 1968) had the consequence that diazoxide was tried in the treatment of hyperinsulinism due to insulin-secreting tumors (FAJANS et al., 1966).

In contrast to the saluretic effect of benzothiadiazine diuretics, diazoxide induces sodium and water retention, which leads to an increase in plasma volume and extracellular fluid volume (FINNERTY et al., 1963; BARTORELLI et al., 1963; BAER et al., 1969). The edema-producing activity of the drug is more marked than that of other antihypertensives, including those which, like diazoxide, act directly on vascular smooth muscle, such as hydralazine and dihydralazine. However, some other vasodilators such as minoxidil also cause sodium and fluid retention which makes it necessary to give diuretics simultaneously (GILMORE et al., 1970; LIMAS and FREIS, 1973, see also 4). Although, for several years, the effect on carbohydrate tolerance and other metabolic effects seemed to prevent the use of diazoxide as an antihypertensive, its blood pressure-lowering effect turned out to be so promising that it was marketed in several countries during the past years in its injectable form, mainly for the treatment of hypertensive crises.

A. Pharmacodynamics

1. Cardiovascular Actions

In various animal species, such as dogs, cats, and rats, diazoxide lowers normal and elevated blood pressure. In normotensive unanesthetized dogs (CONWAY et al., 1961) as well as in anesthetized cats and dogs, 1 to 10 mg/kg diazoxide, given i.v., elicit a rapid fall in blood pressure, which returns to basic levels within a period of half an hour to several hours, the duration as well as the degree of the effect being dose-dependent (RUBIN et al., 1961, 1962). In rats with metacorticoid hypertension the blood pressure-lowering effect was more pronounced than in normotensive rats (STANTON and WHITE, 1973). Simultaneously with the decrease in blood pressure, heart rate and cardiac output increase, both in unanesthetized and anesthetized dogs (CONWAY et al., 1961; ROWE et al., 1963; RUBIN et al., 1963). Some authors also observed an increase in stroke volume (CONWAY et al., 1961; ZITOWITZ and RUBIN, 1962; RUBIN et al., 1963). The transient rise in heart rate is of a reflex nature, but elevated cardiac output and stroke volume may be related to the peripheral vascular changes, which are the consequence of a uniform peripheral arteriolar dilation (ZITOWITZ and RUBIN, 1962; RUBIN et al., 1962, 1963). After repeated administration of 5 mg/kg or single injections of 10 to 20 mg/kg, a decrease in heart rate has been observed (RUBIN et al., 1962). This "paradoxical" effect might be explained by an inhibitory action that diazoxide, when given in high doses, may have on the activity of sympathetic structures in the brainstem (SCHMITT et al., 1968). When diazoxide was compared with sodium nitrite, both drugs were found to lower systemic arterial blood pressure and to elevate heart rate, but stroke volume and cardiac output did not increase after sodium nitrite, which induced a mild reduction in myocardial contractile force, whereas diazoxide had no such effect (RUBIN et al., 1963). On the other hand, a reduced capacity of the left ventricle for external work was obtained with diazoxide in the heart-lung bypass preparation of the dog (NAYLER et al., 1968).

The increase in stroke volume and cardiac output may—at least in part—be the consequence of a stimulation of catecholamine release, which may act on β-adrenergic receptors. Such an interpretation is supported by the finding that propranolol inhibited tachycardia and elevated cardiac output in dogs (RAMASWAMY and RICHARDSON, 1968). However, in rabbits only a transient reduction of heart rate was obtained when propanolol was given together with diazoxide (SPONER et al., 1976) (see Fig. 6). The blood pressure-lowering effect was not diminished by propranolol or, in other studies, by propranolol or sotalol (NAYLER et al., 1968; RAMASWAMY and RICHARDSON, 1968; SPONER et al., 1976). On the other hand, various authors demonstrated that diazoxide stimulates the release of catecholamines from the adrenals (TABACHNIK et al., 1965; STAQUET et al., 1965) and from extra-adrenal tissues (LOUBATIERES et al., 1968).

2. Effects on Various Vascular Beds

The vasodilating effect of diazoxide was demonstrable in all vascular beds that have been studied. When injected directly into the main arteries or i.v., it increases the flow in skeletal muscle, in the kidneys, in the coronary circulation, or the pulmonary circulation. The resistance in the forelimb vessels of the dog is reduced after intra-arterial injection (Rubin et al., 1962) and intra-arterial infusion into the gracilis muscle of dogs results in a fall of vascular resistance by about 36% (Powell et al., 1971). In intact dogs, a transient increase in coronary flow, with concomitant elevation in oxygen content of coronary sinus blood, and decreased or unchanged myocardial oxygen consumption have been observed (Rowe et al., 1963; Schmitt et al., 1968; Scott and Cowley, 1969). Direct injection into the coronary circulation of conscious dogs reduced resistance in the coronary vascular bed, but had no influence on heart rate or cardiac output. However, when administered intravenously, diazoxide induced a more pronounced increase in coronary flow, probably as a consequence of its effect on heart rate (Scott and Cowley, 1969). It is, however, difficult to compare the effects of doses given by different routes. In the heart-lung bypass preparation of the dog, Nayler et al. (1968) also found an increased coronary flow as part of a change in percentage distribution of total blood flow to various vascular beds, but no change in myocardial oxygen consumption was obtained. Besides the coronary circulation, the regional circulation of the upper and lower vena cava received more blood, whereas, in the azygous vein, renal and splanchnic regions, the percentage of total blood flow was reduced, After i. v. injection, a decrease in pulmonary resistance and in pulmonary artery pressure was found in dogs (Rowe et al., 1963).

Whether the action on coronary circulation, which is demonstrable experimentally, is of possible therapeutic value has not been shown so far. Like other drugs that increase coronary flow in unanesthetized or anesthetized dogs with intact coronary arteries, also diazoxide will cause no therapeutically useful dilation of the coronary arteries in patients with coronary atherosclerosis.

3. Effects on Nonarteriolar Smooth Muscle

Smooth muscles other than that in the arterial wall are also relaxed by diazoxide. Myometrial strips from pregnant and nonpregnant women lose their spontaneous activity when exposed to diazoxide, and oxytocin-induced uterine contractions are inhibited by diazoxide (Landesman and Wilson, 1968; Landesman et al., 1968). During labor, the drug suppressed uterine contractions both in intensity and frequency in a dose-dependent manner (Landesman et al., 1969). The inhibitory effect of isoprenaline on the isolated rabbit ileum was enhanced (Wilkenfeld and Levy, 1969), and ureteral peristalsis was inhibited in dogs, the intensity of the effect depending on the dose (Boyarsky and Labay, 1968). It is not known whether a comparable effect on the ureter occurs also in man, but clinical data do not indicate any practical significance of such an action.

4. Effects on the Kidney

In the first papers, a depression of urinary volume and electrolyte excretion was described which was dose-dependent (10 to 50 mg/kg) and demonstrable both in dogs and rats (Rubin et al., 1962; Taylor and Rubin, 1964). In conscious dogs, the antinatriuretic effect occurred with some delay, even after i.v. injection (Milton and Taylor, 1962), whereas in anesthetized dogs it was observed immediately after administration of the drug (Taylor, 1963). The decrease in sodium excretion seems to be the consequence of an effect on tubular sodium reabsorption and is not directly related to the blood pressure-lowering effect. Glomerular filtration rate remained unchanged, and renal plasma flow was reduced in rats (TAYLOR and RUBIN, 1964) and dogs (RUBIN et al., 1962). Free water clearance was diminished during water diuresis in dogs (TAYLOR and RUBIN, 1964). Infusion of diazoxide into the renal artery produced diuresis and natriuresis, together with an increased glomerular filtration rate, probably as a consequence of the vasodilation of the renal vascular bed (GREENE, 1967).

In patients with vasopressin-deficient diabetes insipidus, diazoxide induced a reduction in urinary volume, free water clearance, and sodium excretion. In these patients, an increased proximal tubular reabsoprtion of sodium and water was supposed, which may have been the consequence of peripheral vasodilation (POHL et al., 1972a).

In hypertensive patients, diazoxide, in a dose of 4 mg/kg i.v., caused, besides the fall in blood pressure, a reduction in para-aminohippurate- and inulin clearances as well as in uric acid clearance, but no correlation was observed between the antinatriuretic effect and the changes in renal hemodynamics or blood pressure (JOHNSON, 1971).

5. Mechanism of Antihypertensive Action

Right from the beginning, diazoxide was characterized as a drug that acts on the arteriolar smooth muscle (RUBIN et al., 1962, 1963). The vasodilation is independent of a direct stimulation of β-adrenergic receptors (NAYLER et al., 1968; RAMASWAMY and RICHARDSON, 1968; POWELL et al., 1971). The contrasting observation made with strips from pregnant and nonpregnant human uterus, in which the relaxant effect of diazoxide was reversed by both α- and β-adrenergic blocking drugs (LANDESMAN and WILSON, 1968) cannot be related to the arteriolar muscle.

In isolated preparations of rat aorta, diazoxide showed a competitive-type inhibition of vasoconstriction induced by barium chloride (WOHL et al., 1967). It was suggested that, in vascular smooth muscle, the drug competes with barium ions for a specific receptor site, which is normally activated by calcium ions. This receptor is located more closely to the site of the excitation-contraction coupling than the α-adrenergic receptors. In the latter, diazoxide induces a non-competitive blockade of noradrenaline (WOHL et al., 1968). In aortic strips from rabbits, diazoxide produced a more pronounced shift of the dose-response curve for phenylephrine than for barium chloride. The antagonism against phenylephrine by a combination of phentolamine and diazoxide was comparable to what should be expected if diazoxide acted on the phenylephrine induced contraction, both at the α-receptor level and beyond it. From these data it was concluded that diazoxide, besides acting directly on arteriolar muscle, would also act on α-receptors (TAYLOR and GREEN, 1970), but no similar observations have been reported by other investigators. Also in patients, who were treated with diazoxide, no adrenolytic activity has been demonstrated. Furthermore, in aortic strips from normotensive rats, the diazoxidebarium interaction was less pronounced than in aortic strips from rats with DOCA hypertension. Similar studies with noradrenaline did reveal such a difference between aortic strips from normo- and hypertensive rats. It was supposed that the increased potency of diazoxide in arterial tissue from hypertensive rats and the corresponding antihypertensive effect may be due to a difference in calcium transport in arteriolar smooth muscle cells of normotensive and hypertensive rats (WOHL et al., 1968). On the other hand diazoxide had a similar relaxing activity on KCl-induced contraction of aortic strips from spontaneously hypertensive rats and their corresponding controls (Okamoto-Aoki Strain). In this respect the drug was related to verapamil (LEVY, 1975). It was concluded that diazoxide and verapamil affected transmembrane fluxes in the tonic phase of KCl-induced contraction equally in aortic tissue from spontaneous hypertensive and normotensive control rats. Comparable results were obtained in young rats with spontaneous hypertension (JANIS and TRIGGLE, 1973).

In other studies it was shown that diazoxide inhibited phosphodiesterase in a way similar to that of theophylline, and an interference with the metabolism of cyclic 3′5′-adenosine monophosphate (cAMP) was made responsible for the relaxing effect on smooth muscle (MOORE, 1968). It was also demonstrated that diazoxide, like theophylline, potentiated the inhibiting response of the isolated rabbit ileum to isoprenaline (WILKENFELD and LEVY, 1969). However, the constriction of mesenteric artery strips by noradrenaline was diminished by diazoxide, but not by isoprenaline, which also increased the concentration of cyclic AMP in aortic tissue (MCNEILL et al., 1969). On the basis of these observations it is improbable that diazoxide exerts its vasodilator effect by interfering with the breakdown of cyclic AMP, but probably by either depleting an intracellular calcium pool or by inhibiting the release of calcium from such a pool.

6. Metabolic Effects

Besides affecting vascular resistance and blood pressure, diazoxide acts on carbohydrate and fat metabolism. Hyperglycemia was first observed in man (DOLLERY et al., 1962), and was subsequently also demonstrated in dogs and rats (LANGDON and WOLFF, 1962; WOLFF, 1964). The increase in blood sugar is already seen in acute experiments and is caused by both pancreatic and extrapancreatic effects. Large single doses of diazoxide, administered i.v. in dogs (50 mg/kg) or i.p. in rabbits, rats, and mice (80 to 100 mg/kg), produce an increase in blood glucose levels within one to several hours and a return to control levels within 24 h (TABACHNIK et al., 1964). A rise in plasma glucose level in dogs was already seen with the infusion of 15 mg/kg (SAUBAR et al., 1967). It was suggested by some authors that the hyperglycemic response was related to the lowering of blood pressure, and this hypothesis was supported by the finding that sodium nitroprusside induced an increase in blood sugar levels when given in doses that elicited a comparable fall in blood pressure (STAQUET et al., 1965). However, no other reports on a hyperglycemic response to sodium nitroprusside have been published so far, nor has the drug a hyperglycemic effect in man that is comparable to that of diazoxide.

A direct effect on the release of insulin has been reported by various groups. In incubated pancreatic tissue from rats, rabbits or minipigs, the glucose-induced release of insulin was inhibited by concentrations between 5 and 50 pg/ml of diazoxide, the pancreatic tissue of minipigs being more sensitive than that of rats or rabbits (FRERICHS et al., 1966, 1968; TABACHNIK and GULBENKIAN, 1968). In rats, a hyperglycemic response was demonstrable after single oral doses of 200 to 500 mg/kg or i.v. administration of 50 to 200 mg/kg (FRERICHS et al., 1967). Reduced secretion of insulin has also been shown in dogs, in which it was possible to stimulate insulin secretion by tolbutamide and to overcome in this way the diazoxide-induced hyperglycaemia (WALES et al., 1967).

It is difficult to relate the inhibition of insulin release to the interference of diazoxide with phosphodiesterase activity, since the resulting increase in cyclic

3′5′ AMP within the β-cells of pancreatic islets should stimulate insulin secretion. Hence it is doubtful if the effect of diazoxide on insulin release has anything to do with the effect of the drug on phosphodiesterase activity.

7. Catecholamine Release

Diazoxide stimulates the release of catecholamines from the adrenal medulla and extra-adrenal tissue. An increase in plasma catecholamine concentration has been found in dogs after 35 mg/kg i.v. (STAQUET et al., 1965), and also in rats the plasma catecholamine levels rose after very high doses (400 mg/kg) similarly as those of blood glucose (ZARDAY et al., 1966; LOUBATIÈRES et al., 1968). It was tempting to relate the stimulated release of catecholamines to the diazoxide-induced hyperglycemia, and the fact that ganglionic blockers (chlorisondamine) or sympathetic inhibitors (bretylium) attenuated the hyperglycemic response favored the opinion that catecholamines were at least in part responsible for the increase in blood glucose. That the release of catecholamines is not only of a reflex nature in response to the fall in blood pressure was shown by direct stimulation of the adrenal medulla after intra-adrenal injection of diazoxide in the dog (LOUBATIÈRES et al., 1968). On the other hand the hyperglycemic response to diazoxide was similar in intact rats and in rats with adrenal demedullation (JANES et al., 1964). When given together with guanethidine diazoxide provoked a marked hyperglycemia in intact rats but not in rats with adrenal demedullation.

It may be concluded that the release of catecholamines contributes to the hyperglycemic action of diazoxide, but that the mechanism mainly responsible is an inhibition of insulin secretion. The possible role of released catecholamines is also evident from observations made with various β-adrenergic blocking drugs. Sotalol as well as propranolol reduce the hyperglycemic effect of diazoxide without completely preventing it (TABACHNIK and GULBENKIAN, 1968; WALFISH et al., 1970; SPONER et al., 1976) (Fig. 6). The α-adrenergic blocking agents phenoxybenzamine and phentolamine diminish the inhibition of insulin release (TABACHNIK and GULBENKIAN, 1968; BLACKARD and APRILL, 1967), a finding that suggests that the diazoxide-induced reduction of insulin release is mediated by an α-adrenergic mechanism within the β-cells of the pancreatic islets, whereas the extrapancreatic effect on carbohydrate metabolism is the consequence of β-adrenergic stimulation. However, the significance of the sympathetic nervous system for the hyperglycemic response has not yet been fully elucidated.

The fact that insulin and tolbutamide prevent or reverse the hyperglycemic effect of diazoxide demonstrates that the responsiveness to insulin is maintained and that diazoxide has no antagonistic action against insulin (WELLER and BORONDY, 1965). In rats and mice, acute and chronic hyperglycemic effects of diazoxide could be antagonized by insulin and tolbutamide (WOLFF, 1964; WALES et al., 1967; TABACHNIK and GULBENKIAN, 1968). In addition, it was demonstrated that diazoxide reversed the tolbutamide-induced hypoglycemia (LOUBATIÈRES et al., 1968). The antagonistic action of sulfonylurea derivatives has also been shown in isolated rat pancreatic tissue, where diazoxide (7.5 μg/100 ml) did not inhibit the stimulating effect of much higher concentrations of glibenclamide (5 μg/ml) or glycodiazin (200 μg/ml) (MALAISSE and MALAISSE-LAGAE, 1970). So far, it is not clear whether diazoxide and tolbutamide act on the same receptor in the β-cells of the pancreatic islets when inhibiting or stimulating the release of insulin. It is obvious that, despite the fact of a maintained response to insulin or tolbutamide, the hyperglycemia provoked by diazoxide limits its therapeutic use in hypertension.

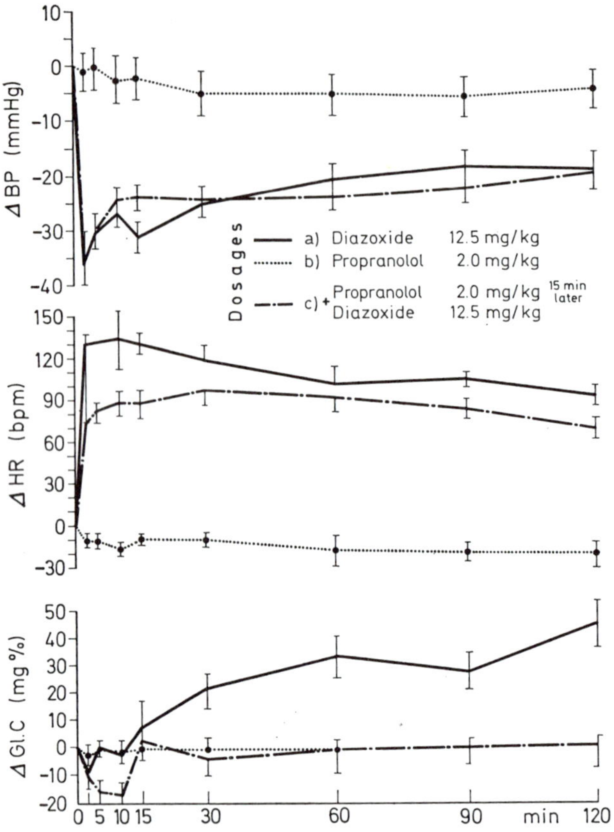

Fig. 6. Inhibitory effect of propranolol on the hyperglycemic response to diazoxide in rabbits. Fall in blood pressure is not affected and increase in heart rate only slightly reduced. Ordinates: above: Fall in blood pressure (mm Hg), medium: Increase in heart rate (beats per min), below: Increase in blood glucose concentration mg-%). Abscissae: Time after injection of diazoxide. In c: Propranolol was injected 15 min before diazoxide (Sponer et al., 1976)

8. Lipolytic Effect

An increase in plasma-free fatty acids has been found in rats (Tabachnik et al., 1965) and similar observations have been reported in dogs (Tabachnik et al., 1965; Spitzer and Scott, 1970). An increased myocardial uptake of released free fatty acids has been observed (Spitzer and Scott, 1970) but it is not clear whether this effect is related to the action of diazoxide on the heart. No effect on lipolysis has been demonstrated *in vitro* (Tabachnik and Gulbenkian, 1968), and the effect may be mediated indirectly by the increased release of catecholamines. Such an interpretation is in agreement with the partial inhibition of lipolysis by propanolol (Blackard and Aprill, 1967). In contrast to the hyperglycemic action, the increase in plasma-free fatty acids is only of minor significance for the use of diazoxide as a therapeutic agent in man.

9. Stimulation of Renin Release

Like other vasodilating drugs, diazoxide stimulates the release of renin from the kidneys. This effect was first demonstrated in hypertensive patients, in whom plasma renin activity after diazoxide injection rose three- to fourfold

(KÜCHEL et al., 1967; SUZUKI, 1970). Patients with a suppressed renin activity did not respond with an increase in plasma renin activity. In patients with essential hypertension and suppressed renin response, the effect of diazoxide on plasma renin activity is diminished similarly to that of other procedures that usually stimulate renin release, such as upright posture or salt restriction. The effect of diazoxide on renin release is independent of changes in plasma and extracellular fluid volume (BAER et al., 1969) and can also be demonstrated in isolated kidneys perfused at constant pressure with a cell-free perfusion medium. Under these experimental conditions diazoxide induced a dose-dependent increase in renal perfusate flow and glomerular filtration rate; urinary sodium excretion was increased in contrast to the sodium retaining-effect of the drug in intact animals and man. (Fig. 7). Renin release was stimulated up to 460% of control values at 5 min after the start of the diazoxide infusion, which suggests that the rise of plasma renin concentration observed *in vivo* is caused by a direct intrarenal effect of the drug (HOFBAUER et al., 1976). No data are available to

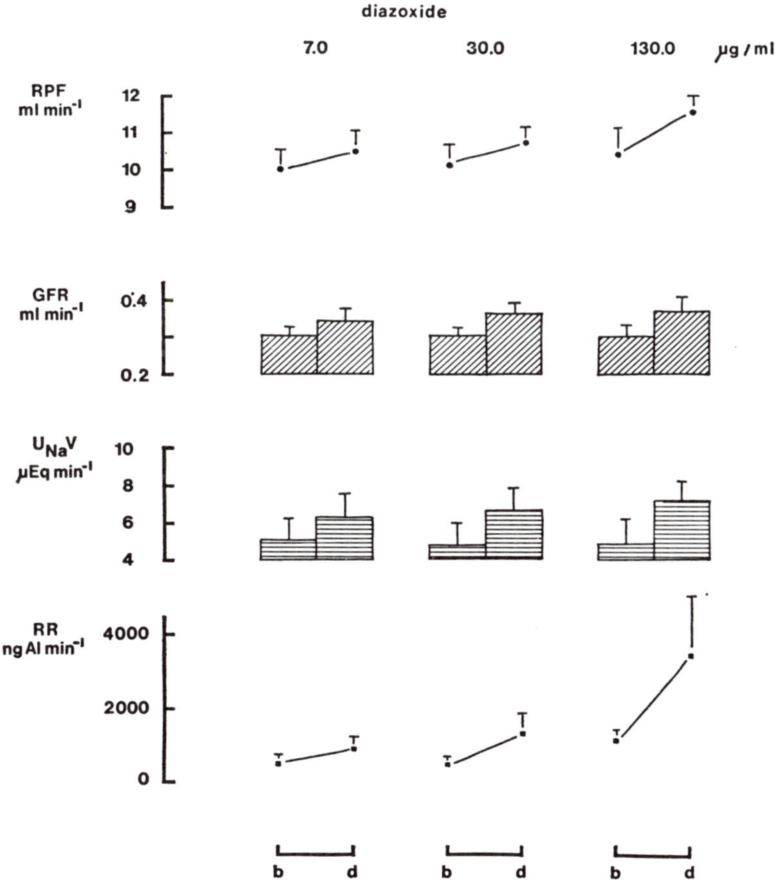

Fig. 7. Isolated rat kidney. Effect of increasing doses of diazoxide *(upper line)* on renal perfusion flow *(RPF)*, glomerular filtration rate *(GFR)*, urinary sodium excretion ($U_{Na}V$) and renin release(*RR*) in ng angiotensin II per min. *b*: before, *d*: during perfusion with diazoxide (HOFBAUER, 1976)

show whether the sodium and fluid retention, which is induced by diazoxide, affects the stimulation of renin release as should be expected, according to the findings that expansion of intravascular volume reduces plasma renin activity.

B. Pharmacokinetic Studies

Several pharmacokinetic studies with diazoxide have revealed that the drug has a long plasma half-life of about 30 h, and that it is strongly bound to serum albumin (Symchowicz et al., 1967; Sellers and Koch-Weser, 1969; Pruitt et al., 1973; Koch-Weser, 1976). In another study, however, a shorter plasma half-life of 10 to 19 h was measured (Crout et al., 1970). Plasma half-life exceeds the blood pressure-lowering effect, and when the drug is administered at intervals of 4 to 10 h, it accumulates in the body, where plasma concentrations up to 100 μg/ml may be reached after the administration of 300 mg every 8 h. As usual plasma concentration protein binding is approximately 90%, and the concentration in plasma is about twice as high as that in the red blood cells (Sellers and Koch-Weser, 1969). After rapid i.v. injection, an initial distribution phase of about 10 min can be separated from the postdistribution phase during which plasma concentration falls slowly, corresponding to the long plasma half-life. The initial decline of plasma concentration is caused by diffusion into the extracellular fluid volume and probably also into the cells of the arterioles (Sellers and Koch-Weser, 1973). During the postdistribution phase, no correlation between plasma concentration and the degree of hypotension is observed, since the latter depends on the concentration of diazoxide in the resistance vessels (Sellers and Koch-Weser, 1973; Koch-Weser, 1974). The concentration that reaches the arteriolar smooth muscle cells within the first distribution phase is larger when the drug is injected rapidly than when it is given in the form of a slow infusion, because of lower initial binding to plasma albumin. However, in rabbits no difference in blood pressure-lowering activity was observed when diazoxide was rapidly or slowly injected (Sponer et al., 1976). Effective blood concentration is about 10 μg/ml (Calesnik et al., 1965). It has been suggested that the more pronounced hypotensive response after rapid injection be caused by an irreversible binding of diazoxide to the receptor during a short period of high concentration (Crout et al., 1970). However, the escape of complete albumin binding is the more likely explanation of an initially higher diffusion rate of free, active diazoxide which reaches the arteriolar receptors (Sellers and Koch-Weser, 1973; Koch-Weser, 1976). The observation of a more marked fall in blood pressure after rapid injection (Finnerty et al., 1967; Hamby et al., 1968; Miller et al., 1969; Mroczek et al., 1971) is in contrast to that of a crossover study in seven patients in whom a similar reduction in blood pressure was obtained when diazoxide was given within 10 s and within 10 min (Crout et al., 1970). The majority of clinical investigators agree that rapid i.v. injection results in a better therapeutic response in the treatment of hypertensive emergencies, especially in patients with uremia. It has been observed that in non-uremic patients the blood pressure-lowering effect of diazoxide does not depend on the speed of injection (Lee et al., 1975a), whereas it does in uremic patients (Mathew and Kincaid-Smith, 1971). In any case, diazoxide should be administered with care also in patients with hypertensive crises.

Diazoxide was well absorbed when given by mouth, and plasma levels of between 5 and 10 μg/ml were obtained (Calesnik et al., 1965). Very high levels of 80 to 100 μg/ml have been described in patients with renal failure (Neary et al., 1973). It was little metabolized to the hydroxymethyl- and carboxy derivatives, but most of the unchanged drug was eliminated by the kidney (SELLERS and KOCH-WESER, 1969; SYMCHOWICZ et al., 1967; PRUITT et al., 1971, 1973; KOCH-WESER, 1976). After administration of 600 mg, other investigators found only 12% of the unchanged drug in the urine within 24 h, and in addition a metabolite (CROUT et al., 1970), which was not identified. The excretion occurred by glomerular filtration and was slow, according to the strong binding to plasma albumin. No tubular secretion was observed, but tubular reabsorption was shown in children, in whom the renal clearance was 2.4 ml/min or less (PRUITT et al., 1971, 1973). In renal failure, the plasma half-life was prolonged in relation to the decrease in glomerular filtration rate (SELLERS and KOCH-WESER, 1969).

As a strongly albumin-bound drug, diazoxide may interact with other drugs. Coumarin derivatives may be displaced from their binding sites on serum albumin, and, consequently, their doses have to be reduced (SELLERS and KOCH-WESER, 1970; KOCH-WESER, 1976). Like benzothiadiazine diuretics diazoxide may induce hyperuricemia, since it suppresses tubular secretion of uric acid. However, this interaction is mild and seems to be without clinical significance when the drug is given for a few days only (LOCKWOOD et al., 1963; JOHNSON, 1971; KOCH-WESER, 1976).

C. Therapeutic Use

Diazoxide is a potent blood pressure-lowering compound, and it would have found a prominent place in the treatment of high blood pressure if it were devoid of its hyperglycemic action, which is a severe obstacle to the chronic administration of the drug. Until recently, the drug was available for investigational purposes only, and its use was limited to small groups of specialists in various countries. The consequence of such a long period of clinical trial is that the large number of publications available does not correspond to the practical significance of the drug. Since the drug has been marketed now in several countries, and despite the fact that, at least for the time being, its use is limited to the treatment of hypertensive emergencies, its place in the treatment of high blood pressure may be better defined in a few years.

The blood pressure-lowering effect is demonstrable both in normotensive subjects and in hypertensive patients. The average dose used is 300 mg or 5 mg/kg, administered i.v. After i.v. injection, the blood pressure falls rapidly; the maximum effect is seen within 3 to 5 min and then it is maintained for some time. The blood pressure may return within several hours (5 to 12) to the original level, but the duration of action may vary, depending upon the severity and the type of hypertension. After smaller doses of 2 to 4 mg/kg diazoxide, a duration of action of between 3 and 4 h was observed (KAKAVIATOS and FINNERTY, 1962; KAKAVIATOS et al., 1962; FINNERTY et al., 1963). Compared with hydralazine, the onset of the hypotensive response is prompter, and blood pressure-lowering is more pronounced (OKUN et al., 1963). Total peripheral resistance is diminished, and relaxation of the arterioles affects all vascular beds (WILSON and OKUN, 1963). In the skin, the vasodilator effect is less pronounced than that of hydralazine, and therefore flushing is only a minor problem. The dilatory effect is not extended to the veins (THIRWELL and ZSOTER, 1972). Simultaneously with the decrease in blood pressure, heart rate and cardiac output increase (KAKAVIATOS and FINNERTY, 1962; FINNERTY et al., 1963; ROWE et al., 1963; OKUN et al., 1963; GUEDON et al., 1972; BHATIA and FROHLICH, 1973; KOCH-WESER, 1974, 1976). The main indication for diazoxide is the treatment of hypertensive emergencies, when a prompt and rapid fall of blood pressure has to be achieved

(FINNERTY et al., 1963, 1967; FINNERTY, 1974; WILSON and KIRKENDALL, 1964; MILLER et al., 1969; MATHEW and KINCAID-SMITH, 1971; MROCZEK et al., 1971; BHATIA and FROHLICH, 1973). This has been especially the case when hypertension was associated with cerebrovascular hemorrhage or encephalopathy (GIFFORD, 1971). Also in children diazoxide has been successfully used in severe hypertensive episodes (MCLAINE and DRUMMOND, 1971). In hypertension during pregnancy effective lowering of blood pressure was obtained (FINNERTY, 1970; PENNINGTON and PICKER, 1972) although labor may be temporarily affected as a consequence of the relaxing effect diazoxide has on the uterus (FINNERTY, 1970; LANDESMAN et al., 1968).

It has been claimed that by repeated injection a prolonged reduction of blood pressure could be achieved (FINNERTY et al., 1967, 1968; DAVIDOV et al., 1974), but other investigators were unable to modify the course of severe hypertension by diazoxide (BEAMER and MCDONALD, 1970). A beneficial effect was reported in hypertensive patients with renal failure (MROCZEK et al., 1969; POHL and THURSTON, 1971) even when the drug was given by mouth for a prolonged period (POHL et al., 1972b; SWALES et al., 1972; THURSTON et al., 1973). In view of the strong albumin binding of diazoxide care has to be taken that the drug is not accumulated in patients with impaired renal function (NEARY et al., 1973).

When compared with sodium nitroprusside, the fall in blood pressure and the increase in heart rate is similar for 300 diazoxide and an infusion of 60 μg/ml of sodium nitroprusside, but cardiac output and left ventricular ejection rate increase with diazoxide only, whereas they are slightly reduced during sodium nitroprusside infusion (BHATIA and FROHLICH, 1973). This difference in hemodynamics was ascribed to the venous pooling occurring with nitroprusside whereas diazoxide has no effect on the capacitance vessels (THIRWELL and ZSOTER, 1972). In the treatment of hypertensive patients with recent myocardial infarction diazoxide may be dangerous, since immediately after injection of the drug electrocardiographic changes have been observed which indicated an increase in myocardial injury (O'BRIEN et al., 1975).

As with other drugs, such as hydralazine, which act directly on arteriolar smooth muscle and stimulate heart rate, anginal attacks may be provoked and also myocardial infarction has been observed (KUMAR et al., 1976) in patients with coronary heart disease. The increase in cardiac output cannot be ascribed exclusively to the increase in heart rate, since the cardiac index still rose after heart rate had already returned to normal (JUST and STEIN, 1969). Since cardiovascular reflexes are maintained and the initial increase in cardiac output at the time the fall in blood pressure is most marked, orthostatic hypotension is not or only rarely seen with diazoxide (FINNERTY et al., 1963; LOCKWOOD et al., 1963; KOCH-WESER, 1974). The hypotensive effect that corresponds to the true reduction in total peripheral resistance can be obtained when the increase in heart rate is reduced by β-adrenergic blocking drugs, such as propanolol, which not only enhances the blood pressure-lowering effect, but also improves cardiac tolerance in patients with coronary or myocardial disease (BAER et al., 1969; KOCH-WESER, 1976). Whereas, in the treatment of hypertensive emergencies, the simultaneous administration of a β-adrenergic blocker is not necessary, this would be the case if diazoxide were given repeatedly over a period of several days or weeks (KINCAID-SMITH et al., 1973). In one study, when diazoxide was administered during β-adrenergic blockade, neither the hypotensive effect nor the increase in heart rate induced by diazoxide were affected (LEE et al., 1975b; MROCZEK et al., 1976).

D. Adverse Reactions

1. Carbohydrate Metabolism

Hyperglycemia has been observed shortly after the beginning of clinical studies (DOLLERY et al., 1962; THOMSON et al., 1962; LOCKWOOD et al., 1963; OKUN et al., 1963). This was a severe setback for the wide use of the drug, which, for several years, was hardly given at all. However, the blood pressure-lowering effect looked interesting enough to take up clinical work again, and it turned out that disturbance of carbohydrate metabolism is no problem when diazoxide treatment is limited to a few days. Furthermore, it was observed that hyperglycemia induced by diazoxide responds well to tolbutamide and other sulfaurea derivatives as well as to insulin (FINNERTY, 1970). In patients with latent or manifest diabetes, antidiabetic treatment may have to be started or the doses of oral antidiabetic drugs or of insulin may have to be increased (UPDIKE and HARRINGTON, 1969; CHARLES and DANFORTH, 1971). Similarly, in patients with chronic renal failure, hyperglycemia may appear within a short term of treatment, and antidiabetic therapy may be necessary (POHL and THURSTON, 1971; CHARLES and DANFORTH, 1971). Without antidiabetic treatment severe hyperglycemia together with hyperosmolar, non-ketoacidotic coma has been described (UPDIKE and HARRINGTON, 1969; CHARLES and DANFORTH, 1971; BALSAM et al., 1971). The mechanism underlying the hyperglycemic response in man corresponds to that observed in experimental animals. After the administration of glucose, either by mouth or by injection, the insulin response was decreased when diazoxide was given (STEINKE and SOELDNER, 1968). In healthy subjects who were pretreated with chlorpropamide, diazoxide (600 mg) and the benzothiadiazine diuretic trichlormethiazide (6 to 10 mg daily) produced hyperglycemia and a decrease in plasma insulin concentration (FAJANS et al., 1966). It may be concluded that, in man as in experimental animals, diazoxide suppresses insulin release from the pancreas.

This hyperglycemic effect was used therapeutically in patients with insulin-secreting tumours, in whom diazoxide caused a fall in the elevated plasma levels of insulin (GRABER et al., 1966; WEGIENKA et al., 1968). The reduction in insulin release could be maintained for several weeks, when diazoxide, together with trichlormethiazide, was given daily by mouth (FAJANS et al., 1966). Also in leucine-sensitive hyperglycemia diazoxide has been tried (GREEN and BERGER, 1968). Various investigators have given diazoxide by mouth during prolonged periods in the treatment of hypertension without reporting hyperglycemia or other disturbances of carbohydrate metabolism (POHL et al., 1972b; KINCAID-SMITH et al., 1973; THURSTON et al., 1973). So far, it is not known what other factors besides the well-known inhibition of insulin release and the extrapancreatic stimulation of catecholamine secretion may be responsible for the manifestation of the diabetic syndrome provoked by diazoxide. Possibly—as in experimental animals—the simultaneous administration of β-adrenergic blocking drugs may reduce the incidence and degree of hyperglycemic response, but further studies are necessary before such a conclusion may be drawn and recommendations are made.

The excretion of cortisol was found to be diminished in healthy subjects who received diazoxide in daily oral doses of 200 to 400 mg for 1 or 2 weeks. Aldosterone excretion remained unchanged, and no variations in serum electrolytes were observed (EHRLICH, 1970). No corresponding studies on the cortisol secretion rate have been undertaken, and clinical experience does not give any evidence for adrenocortical activity to be significantly affected by diazoxide treatment.

2. Retention of Sodium

Even during early clinical trials, it was evident that diazoxide, unlike the benzothiadiazine saluretics, produced retention of salt and water, with subsequent weight gain and edema formation (HUTCHEON and BARTHALMUS, 1962; THOMSON et al., 1962; BARTORELLI et al., 1963; LOCKWOOD et al., 1963). Later on, this observation was confirmed by all investigators. Glomerular filtration rate (inulin or creatinine clearance) and renal plasma flow (para-aminohippurate) may decrease immediately after administration of diazoxide in hypertensive subjects (JOHNSON, 1968, 1971; LEONETTI et al., 1970). However, 1 to 2 h after the injection of diazoxide (300 mg), both glomerular filtration rate and renal plasma flow are increased, although blood pressure is still reduced (HAMBY et al., 1968). Urine volume and sodium excretion fall after administration of diazoxide (BARTORELLI et al., 1963; HAMBY et al., 1968; KAKAVIATOS et al., 1967, 1968; THOMSON et al., 1966; LEONETTI et al., 1970). The mechanism underlying sodium retention is an enhanced tubular reabsorption (JOHNSON, 1968; HAMBY et al., 1968). Excretion of other electrolytes, such as potassium, chloride and bicarbonate, is also reduced. Urinary pH may decrease subsequent to a diminished excretion of bicarbonate (BARTORELLI et al., 1963; THOMSON et al., 1966). There is no escape from the sodium-retaining effect of diazoxide, and therefore the administration of diuretics may become necessary, especially if renal function is impaired (MROCZEK et al., 1969; FINNERTY, 1971). Development or unmasking of cardiac failure has been observed with diazoxide when no diuretic therapy was given on time (BEAMER et al., 1970).

FINNERTY et al. (1970) reported that the hypotensive response to diazoxide as well as to hydralazine and reserpine may be diminished when plasma and extracellular fluid volumes are increased. Patients who have developed tolerance to diazoxide may become responsive again when furosemide or other diuretics are given (FINNERTY, 1971). In view of the sodium and fluid retention regularly observed during diazoxide therapy, it is indicated to give a diuretic right from the beginning, in order to avoid the increase in plasma and extracellular fluid volumes and the development of tolerance (KOCH-WESER, 1974, 1976).

With other antihypertensive drugs, such as reserpine or hydralazine, retention of fluid and salt has also been described, but this effect is more pronounced with diazoxide, probably as a consequence of its direct effect on the renal tubules. The release of antidiuretic hormone by diazoxide has been suggested (JOHNSON, 1968), but there is no experimental or clinical evidence for such an action. The effect of diazoxide in patients with diabetes insipidus may be explained by the increase in sodium and water reabsorption in the proximal tubules (POHL et al., 1972a).

The tubular effect of diazoxide is also demonstrable with respect to uric acid, the secretion of which is suppressed (LOCKWOOD et al., 1963; JOHNSON, 1968). However, hyperuricemia is not a clinical problem during diazoxide treatment of short duration. In hypertensive patients treated for several days or even weeks with diazoxide given by mouth, extrapyramidal symptoms have been observed in a relatively high percentage of patients (15%), when daily doses of 200 to 400 mg were given (NEARY et al., 1973). This was especially the case in patients with impaired renal function in whom very high plasma levels of diazoxide were reached. The symptoms could be controlled by either reducing the dose or by giving anti-Parkinson drugs of the anticholinergic type (procyclidine) or diazepam. Other investigators have warned against giving diazoxide by mouth to hypertensive patients with renal failure (DE BROE et al., 1972).

3. Other Side Effects

Hirsutism has been seen in some female patients and prepubertal children during prolonged oral therapy (Koch-Weser, 1976). After cessation of treatment, hypertrichosis disappeared (Koblenzer and Baker, 1968; Muller, 1969). This observation is of interest, since hirsutism also occurs during the administration of minoxidil, but is not seen with hydralazine or dihydralazine. Hence, it is improbable that hypertrichosis is related to the vasodilating effect on the skin.

During long-term treatment, hematological side effects were also described, mainly granulocytopenia and thrombopenia (Wales and Wolff, 1967).

The fact that the administration of diazoxide has so far been limited in most cases to a few days may have prevented the occurrence of side reactions, which may become visible only during prolonged treatment.

When administered parenterally, the drug has to be injected strictly i.v., because paravenous injection or leaking of the alkaline solution from the vein results in a severe burning sensation due to the high pH of the solution. Diazoxide is soluble only in alkaline solutions (pH: 11), the concentration being 1.5% (300 mg in 20 ml).

E. Combination With Other Drugs

The combined use of diazoxide with β-adrenergic blockers to prevent tachycardia and with diuretics to inhibit salt and water retention has already been mentioned. No fixed dose ratios can be recommended in view of the fact that diazoxide is reserved—at least for the time being—to the treatment of hypertensive emergencies or special cases, such as hypertension in patients with renal failure or acute hypertension in pregnancy (Finnerty, 1970; Pohl and Thurston, 1971; Pohl et al., 1972b). Severe hypotension was observed when diazoxide was given prior or subsequent to hydralazine or sympathetic inhibitors such as reserpine or methyldopa (Henrich et al., 1977).

Despite the various inconveniences of diazoxide, it is to be expected that the drug may be increasingly used in the treatment of hypertension. However, whether the oral form, which is not generally available so far, will receive broad distribution remains doubtful. A wider usage of the drug may, to a certain degree. depend on the results obtained with other antihypertensive drugs that act directly, on the arteriolar muscle and are now in clinical trials or have just been marketeld Although it is highly improbable that diazoxide will become a first-choice antihypertensive drug, it may stay in the first row of second-choice drugs and may keep a place in the treatment of hypertensive emergencies. From all the data available it is evident that the blood pressure-lowering effect of diazoxide differs from that of the benzothiadiazide diuretics both quantitatively and qualitatively. Hence it can be stated that the original goal to separate the diuretic from the hypotensive effect of the benzothiadiazines has not been achieved, since the action of diazoxide on blood pressure has nothing in common with that of the benzothiadiazine diuretics.

V. Minoxidil

The most interesting of the recently developed vasodilators is the piperidinopyrimidine derivative minoxidil (6-imino-1,2-dihydro-1-hydroxy-2-imino-4-piperidino-pyrimidine, U10858), which originated from the triazine derivative U7720 (2,4-diamino-6-(diallylamino-3-triazine) or diallylmelamine, DAM). The latter compound had a marked hypotensive activity in unanesthetized dogs (Freyburger et al., 1965). Subsequently, it was shown that, in various species,

DAM was transformed to several metabolites, of which a ring N-oxide of the parent molecule seemed to be responsible for the reduction in blood pressure (ZINS, 1965; ZINS et al., 1968). Starting from this metabolite, numerous compounds were synthesized, of which minoxidil was most intensely studied and later on clinically investigated.

Most of the pharmacodynamic and toxicologic studies have been done in the Upjohn Company (DUCHARME et al., 1973), whereas clinical pharmacology has been pioneered by Chidsey and associates (GILMORE et al., 1970; GOTTLIEB et al., 1972a, b; CHIDSEY, 1973). Recently, the compound has undergone extensive clinical investigation, and the overall results look encouraging with respect to therapeutic activity, whereas toxicity poses several problems (MARTIN et al., 1975).

A. Pharmacodynamics

1. Cardiovascular Actions

In unanesthetized rats, dogs, and rhesus monkeys, the compound has a dose-dependent, protracted blood pressure-lowering effect in normotensive as well as in hypertensive animals. When given by mouth, the maximum hypotensive effect was seen between 4 and 6 h after administration, and only after 24 to 48 h, depending upon the dose, blood pressure returned to its original level (Fig. 8). When given by mouth once daily in doses of 0.5 to 2.0 mg/kg over a period of 3 weeks to renal hypertensive dogs, blood pressure could be maintained on reduced levels, the degree of lowering depending on the dose. After cessation of treatment, blood pressure returned to the previous values within 1 week (DUCHARME et al., 1973). In rats, after i.p. injection of a large dose (10 mg/kg), maximum hypotension occurred within 30 min and blood pressure had not returned to the initial level within 12 h (PLUSS et al., 1972); when orally administered, blood pressure was definitely decreased 4 h after drug intake and the effect persisted for more than 24 h (DUCHARME et al., 1973).

Simultaneously with the occurrence of hypotension, heart rate and cardiac output rise. The effect on the heart is not only of reflex origin, since, in dogs, it was demonstrable even with doses (0.125 mg/kg orally) that did not lower blood pressure. With the high dose of 2.0 mg/kg, a more than two- to threefold increase in both heart rate and cardiac output occurred, and after 48 h the two parameters were still markedly elevated (DUCHARME et al., 1973). In conscious dogs an enhanced myocardial blood flow was observed which was independent of changes in cardiac work (HUMPHREY et al., 1974).

The carotid occlusion reflex in unanesthetized dogs was diminished during a treatment period of 1 week, when 3 mg/kg were administered daily by mouth. In addition, in these animals, minoxidil had a synergistic effect on the hypotension induced by hexamethonium, which did not lower blood pressure by itself in a dose of 5 mg/kg i.v., but produced a marked hypotension during the administration of minoxidil (DUCHARME et al., 1973).

In the blood-perfused hind limbs of dogs, minoxidil reduced perfusion independently of whether sympathetic innervation was intact or functionally eliminated by crushing the lumbar sympathetic trunk on one side at the height of the third lumbar vertebra (DUCHARME et al., 1973). The vasodilator action of various drugs administered intra-arterially, such as acetylcholine, glyceryltrinitrate or histamine, was not affected, but the reponse to isoproterenol was slightly reduced. Vasoconstriction induced by sympathetic nerve stimulation was diminished after i.v. administration of minoxidil, whereas no effect was

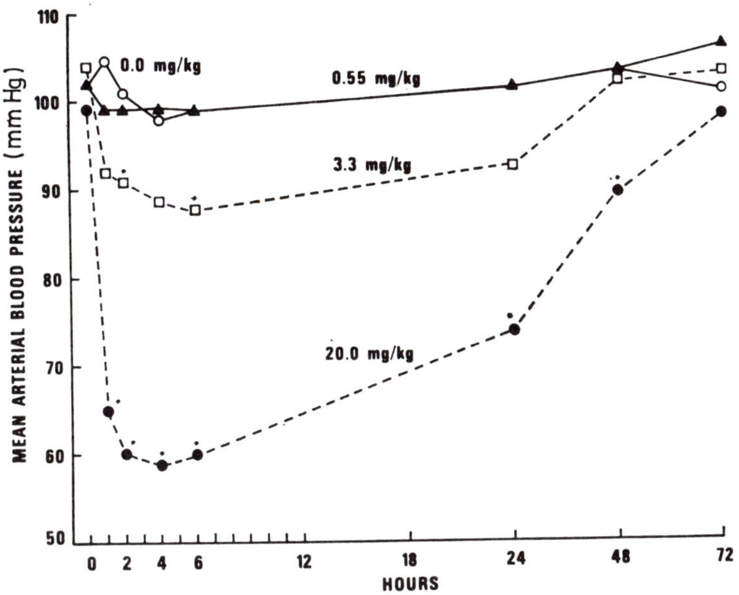

Fig. 8. Dose-response effect of minoxidil on mean arterial blood pressure of unansthetized, notmotensive rhesus monkeys. Each point represents the average effect of four monkeys. Asterisks indicate the values which are significantly different ($P < 0.05$) from the 0.0 mg/kg dose group at the corresponding time. Standard deviations ranged from ± 3.85 to ± 11.16 mm Hg (DuCharme et al., 1973)

demonstrable on noradrenaline-induced vasoconstriction (DuCharme et al., 1973). The vasodilating effect of minoxidil was not affected by atropine, propranolol, or the antihistaminic tripelennamine, which indicates that its action is not mediated by cholinergic, β- adrenergic or histaminergic mechanisms.

2. Other Actions

Little has been reported so far on other pharmacodynamic effects of minoxidil. In dogs, an increase in sodium reabsorption was found in the proximal tubules (Humphrey et al., 1971); total renal blood flow was decreased, and this effect could not be reversed by propranolol (Humphrey et al., 1974). In rats, oral doses of 1.5 mg/kg or more induced an increase in plasma glucose concentration, and with the high dose of 100 mg/kg a reduced glucose tolerance was seen in fasted rats (DuCharme et al., 1973).

Acute toxicity was studied in rats and mice; the LD50 in rats was 759 mg/kg after i.p. and 1321 mg/kg after oral administration; in mice, the i.p. LD50 was 1317 mg/kg. Subacute toxicity studies of one month's duration were done in dogs, rhesus monkeys, and minipigs; with a daily oral dose of 20 mg/kg, no gross or microscopic changes were observed in the two latter species. However, in dogs, a degenerative lesion was found in the right atrium, which histologically revealed acute and chronic hemorrhages, degeneration of muscle cells and proliferation of blood vessels and connective tissue. In other species, even under more prolonged treatment and with higher doses, no similar changes have been found (Carlson and Feenstra 1977). In dogs, a one-year treatment with daily oral doses of 3, 10 and 30 mg/kg resulted in similar lesions of the right atrium, but no other toxic symptoms were detectable. In rats, neither 10 mg/kg nor 30 mg/kg were toxic when given daily mouth for one year, but, when 100 mg/kg were given, increases in liver, kidney, adrenal and heart weight were observed, and changes in the hemogram had occurred (DuCharme, 1973).

3. Mechanism of Action

The mode of action of minoxidil has not yet been elucidated, but from the data available it can be concluded that the drug exerts its vasodilating action mainly by a direct effect on the arteriolar smooth muscle. It was suggested that minoxidil, besides its musculotropic action, may also slightly suppress the sympathetic vasoconstrictor tone, but like other vasodilators it produces a reflex increase of sympathetic tone consequently to the reduction of vascular resistance and also increases renin release from the kidney (Gottlieb et al., 1972b; Pettinger and Mitchell, 1973; Velasco et al., 1974). The synergistic effect of minoxidil and hexamethonium on blood pressure was taken as an indication that minoxidil alone stimulates vasoconstrictor tone by a reflex mechanism (DuCharme et al., 1973).

On the subcellular level, minoxidil—like other vasodilators—may interfere with the release of calcium and in this way prevent calcium from reaching its receptor site. Studies with vascular smooth muscle preparations of the rat tail artery, depolarized with potassium, revealed that the response to calcium and to noradrenaline was antagonized by minoxidil (Bonaccorsi et al., 1973). However, data available are insufficient to support the hypothesis that minoxidil acts by preventing calcium penetration through the plasma membrane.

B. Pharmacokinetics

In normotensive rats, studies with labeled minoxidil (^{14}C-labeled in the pyrimidine ring) revealed a rapid clearance of the drug after i.p. injection. Twelve hours after administration, plasma concentration had fallen to less than 1% of the maximum measured 30 min after the injection, but mean blood pressure was still reduced by 16%. Most (92%) of the total radioactivity found in plasma at 12 h corresponded to minoxidil, which at 2 h accounted only for 16% of the total radioactivity. Hence, an increasingly large proportion of metabolized minoxidil was in the plasma during the first hours after administration (Pluss et al., 1972). In the kidney, where the highest extractable radioactivity was found, the percentage of minoxidil activity also increased from 27.1% after 30 min to 56.4% after 12 h. The drug was accumulated to a certain degree in the arterial tissue, where, after 12 h, four times the plasma concentration of minoxidil was demonstrable. Hence, minoxidil seems to be retained in the arterial tissue, a fact that might explain why the effect on blood pressure outlasts the plasma clearance of the drug (Pluss et al., 1972). Other vasodilating drugs, such as hydralazine (Perry et al., 1962) also concentrate in the arterial wall, but to a much more marked degree, as has been demonstrated by extraction and autoradiographic studies (Wagner and Hedwall, 1972, 1975; Wagner, 1973). It is, however, not known whether the proportion of unchanged to metabolized hydralazine in plasma is similarly shifted in favor of the unmetabolized compound as is the case with minoxidil.

In man, the pharmacokinetics of minoxidil have also been studied with ^{14}C-labeled material. After oral administration of an average dose of 6 mg, an initial distribution phase was observed, followed by an exponential decline of the plasma concentration curve, the calculated half-life being 4.2 h (Gottlieb et al., 1972b). Within 24 h, 80% of the administered radioactivity were recovered from the urine, of which only a small fraction (9.8 ± 7%) was unmetabolized drug. Of the metabolites, the major part was a glucuronide conjugate of minoxidil, whereas two other metabolites could not be identified. The excretion of the unidentified metabolites increased relatively to the excretion of the glucuronide conjugate and the unmetabolized drug. The renal clearance contributed only 10% to the rapid total body clearance of the drug. This may be of practical importance, since, for the disposition of the drug, glomerular filtration rate is not of major significance as compared with the metabolism of the drug. In patients with renal failure, accumulation of the drug may be limited. In patients who received minoxidil for a week, the disappearance rate of labeled material from plasma was slightly accelerated (GOTTLIEB et al., 1972b) but there was no indication for an enzyme induction.

As in rats, the duration of the antihypertensive effect in man was longer than would have been expected on the basis of plasma half-life and the rapid clearance and metabolization. The protracted lowering of blood pressure might be due to the presence of unmetabolized minoxidil in the arterial and arteriolar smooth muscle, where even a relatively low concentration may suffice for a sustained relaxing effect.

C. Therapeutic Use

Various reports on the use of minoxidil in the treatment of hypertension have been published, from which the powerful antihypertensive activity in man is evident (GILMORE et al., 1970; GOTTLIEB et al., 1972a; LIMAS et al., 1972; LIMAS and FREIS, 1973; PETTINGER and MITCHELL, 1973; LIEBAU et al., 1974; WERNER et al., 1974; HARTNETT et al., 1975; MROCZEK et al., 1975; ZACEST et al., 1976). However, it has been stressed that minoxidil has to be combined with β-adrenergic blockers to suppress the tachycardic effect, and preferably with a diuretic to prevent fluid retention. Minoxidil has been compared with hydralazine with respect to its antihypertensive activity in the same patients and has been found superior in therapeutic efficacy (GOTTLIEB, 1972a). Whereas daily doses of hydralazine were in the order of 200 to 800 mg, minoxidil was given in doses of 2.5 to 30 mg per day and produced a better response of blood pressure which could be lowered by 35 mm Hg and more (GILMORE et al., 1970; GOTTLIEB et al., 1972a). Propranolol and hydrochlorothiazide were added to either vasodilator. Various authors have reported that high blood pressure resistant to other antihypertensive drugs responded when minoxidil was given (LIMAS et al., 1972; LIMAS and FREIS, 1973); DORMOIS et al., 1975; KINCAID-SMITH, 1976; ZAGEST et al., 1976).

In order to achieve rapid control of blood pressure, "aggressive" treatment with minoxidil was performed by giving, after an initial dose of 5 mg, the same dose at 6-h intervals until a fall in blood pressure was observed. By this mode of treatment blood pressure was reduced to normal levels within 24 to 42 h (O'MALLEY and MCNAY, 1975). In another study the same authors tried to individualize the dosage scheme using pharmacodynamic parameters, mainly blood pressure, to establish the loading dose, maintenance dose and dose frequency (SHEN et al., 1975; O'MALLEY and MCNAY, 1975; GIBALDI, 1975). It was found that loading dose requirements increased with mean arterial baseline pressure, whereas maintenance doses were largely independent upon the height of blood pressure.

Remarkable results have been obtained in patients suffering from severe or malignant hypertension with renal failure (LIMAS and FREIS, 1973; PETTINGER and MITCHELL, 1973; WILBURN et al., 1975; MEHTA et al., 1975; MUTTERPERI et al., 1976; BRYAN et al., 1977). In combination with propranolol and hydrochlorothiazide or similar diuretics, minoxidil turned out to be more effective than other antihypertensive drugs that had been given before and had not achieved blood pressure control. In various patients, administration of minoxidil in daily doses of 20 to 40 mg prevented nephrectomy, which had to be envisaged in view of the unresponsive severe hypertension (O'Malley et al., 1975b; Pettinger and Mitchell, 1973). The fact that it was possible to administer the drug in the usual doses despite severely impaired renal function demonstrates that kidney function is of minor importance for the disposition of the drug. On the other hand, it has also been reported that in patients with renal failure it may not be possible to control overload heart failure and that it was necessary to interrupt treatment with minoxidil despite satisfactory reduction of blood pressure (Redmond et al., 1974).

The increase in plasma renin activity which has been described by various investigators (Gottlieb et al., 1972a; Pettinger and Mitchell, 1973; Velasco et al., 1974; Redmond et al., 1974; O'Malley et al., 1975a) does not influence the blood pressure-lowering effect. The stimulation of renin release from the kidney is similar to that caused by other vasodilators, but according to the pronounced hypotensive effect of minoxidil it seems to be more pronounced than with hydralazine. One group did not see an effect on plasma renin activity (Bryan et al., 1977). Such an assumption is confirmed by studies in which, besides a sympathetic stimulation of renin release, which is sensitive to propranolol, a second mechanism is involved that is not blocked by propranolol and probably the consequence of a decrease in renal perfusion pressure (O'Malley et al., 1973, 1975a).

D. Adverse Reactions

Tolerability of minoxidil was considered to be satisfactory, but fluid retention, tachycardia and headaches may occur. Propranolol or another β-adrenergic blocker should be added, together with a diuretic, preferably furosemide in doses of 160 to 500 mg. When the dose of propranolol was correctly titrated, heart rate could be maintained at the usual level. Congestive heart failure has been observed during minoxidil treatment probably as a consequence of fluid retention, and heart size may increase despite the control of blood pressure (Martin et al., 1975; Sannerstedt et al., 1975). Pulmonary hypertension has also been observed during minoxidil treatment (Wilburn et al., 1975). An unpleasant side reaction observed by several investigators is hypertrichosis especially in the face but also on arms and legs (Gottlieb et al., 1972a; Pettinger and Mitchell, 1973; Mehta et al., 1975; Mutterperl et al., 1976; Bryan et al., 1977). The mechanism underlying this effect is unknown; similar hair growth has been observed with diazoxide (Muller, 1969; Koblenzer and Baker, 1968; Zacest et al., 1976), but not with hydralazine.

Considering all the data available it is highly probable that minoxidil represents a progress in the group of antihypertensive vasodilators, provided that it will be used in the proper way, i.e., in combination with β-adrenergic blockers and diuretics. It is more powerful than hydralazine and has no effect on insulin release or carbohydrate metabolism like diazoxide. If applied carefully minoxidil will be a welcome addition to the group of antihypertensive drugs, but as a consequence of its potency its use will be restricted to the treatment of severe hypertension which is refractory to drugs with a less pronounced action on blood pressure.

VI. Guancydine

The compound has a simple chemical structure, including a guanidino group, to which a cyano group is bound. Obviously guancydine (1-cyano-3-tert.-amyl-guanidine) and other cyanoguanidines were synthesized with the aim of developing antihypertensive agents with a mode of action similar to that of guanethidine. However, it turned out that drugs of that type that are chemically more closely related to guanethidine had no blood pressure-lowering activity (GADEKAR et al., 1968), which was mainly limited to aliphatic derivatives. The first pharmacologic reports on guancydine stressed an antagonistic activity to angiotensin, and it was claimed that the drug was not a directly acting vasodilator (CUMMINGS et al., 1968, 1969). However, it soon became evident that the hypothesis of a semiselective antagonism to angiotensin was untenable, and that guancydine acted directly on the smooth arteriolar muscle, exerting a nonspecific, noncompetitive, insurmountable antagonism to various drugs producing contractions of different types of smooth muscle (WORCEL et al., 1971).

The results of preliminary clinical studies looked promising, but the more extended and more prolonged use revealed an increasing incidence of side reactions, mainly mental instability and hyperexcitability. Today, the situation for marketing the drug is not promising, but, nevertheless, guancydine is of theoretical and practical interest as another type of drug affecting smooth muscle.

A. Pharmacodynamics

1. Cardiovascular Action

After i.v. injection in anesthetized dogs, a fall in blood pressure and an increased flow in the mesenteric and renal vascular beds was observed; simultaneously, renal vascular resistance was diminished (CUMMINGS et al., 1968). In normotensive dogs, doses of 8 to 15 mg/kg, given by mouth, did not affect blood pressure, but 30 mg/kg caused hypotension, tachycardia, and an increase in cardiac output. The lower doses were effective in reducing blood pressure in hypertensive dogs, without increasing heart rate. In normotensive rats, oral administration of guancydine caused a dose-related lowering of blood pressure. Vasopressor responses to angiotensin, renin, and phenylethylamine were markedly reduced, whereas responses to adrenaline and noradrenaline were less diminished and those to vasopressin or barium chloride not affected at all (CUMMINGS et al., 1968). In rats, propanolol blocked the hypotensive response partially (CUMMINGS et al., 1968). In contrast, in human beings, when reflex tachycardia was prevented by propanolol or other β-adrenergic blockers, the fall in blood pressure was more pronounced than with guancydine alone (STENBERG et al., 1971).

In metacorticoid hypertension, repeated doses of guancydine reduced mean blood pressure and the degree of cardiac hypertrophy. Chronic treatment with 80 mg/kg daily diminished the concentration of noradrenaline in the rat heart, whereas 20 mg/kg were ineffective. In the brain neither noradrenaline nor serotonin concentration was diminished (ELLENBOGEN et al., 1972). In spontaneously hypertensive rats, no effect on catecholamine synthesis or storage was observed, despite a lowering of blood pressure, and similar results were obtained in metacorticoid hypertension (ELLENBOGEN et al., 1972, 1974). Hence it was concluded that guancydine does not lower blood pressure by interfering with adrenergic transmitters.

A more detailed study on the angiotensin antagonism revealed that the pressor response to angiotensin in rats could be inhibited by guancydine that was administered 2 h previously. In this way, guancydine also diminished the response to renin, to noradrenaline, and to a lesser degree to adrenaline (WELTER and GRACE, 1967; CUMMINGS et al., 1969). In nephrectomized rats, the response to angiotensin was no longer blocked, although the drug still induced a fall in blood pressure. However, when the nephrectomized rats were cross-circulated with intact rats, the reduction in angiotensin response produced by guancydine was re-established (CUMMINGS and GRACE, 1969). After repeated administration the angiotensin antagonism was diminished, whereas that to phenylethylamine remained unchanged, and so was the hypotensive effect (CUMMINGS et al., 1969). Vasoconstriction induced by angiotensin in the renal vascular bed of dogs could be inhibited by pretreatment with guancydine (WELTER and GRACE, 1967; CUMMINGS et al., 1969).

On the basis of these data it was presumed that guancydine is a semiselective antagonist to angiotensin. However, studies of various smooth muscle organs, such as the uterus and the colon of rats or of rabbit aortic strips, revealed that not only the actions of angiotensin, but also those of noradrenaline, 5-hydroxytryptamine, or acetylcholine were blocked by guancydine (WORCEL et al., 1971). A nonspecific reduction of vasoconstrictor response has also been reported for other drugs acting directly on the arteriolar muscle, such as hydralazine (DRUEY and TRIPOD, 1967). It was suggested that such a nonspecific antagonism against various drugs which stimulate smooth muscle may be caused by an interference with the excitation-contraction coupling or the contraction process of the smooth muscle, but no extensive studies have been undertaken with guancydine to prove such a hypothesis.

In man, no effect of guancydine on the pressor response to angiotensin was demonstrable (HAMMER et al., 1971; VILLARREAL et al., 1971). It may be that higher doses than those tolerated in man are necessary to obtain a reduced responsiveness of the resistance vessels to vasoconstrictor agents.

2. Other Effects

Fluid and salt retention was observed with guancydine in animals. The effect is mainly the consequence of an increased sodium reabsorption in the proximal tubules, which is independent of adrenocortical hormones and may be caused by a decrease in glomerular filtration rate and perhaps an intrarenal shunting of blood (GUSSIN et al., 1969, 1970, 1971). An effect on the release of antidiuretic hormone could be ruled out. The fluid retention was compared with that induced by either reserpine or hydralazine, which both differ in their mechanisms of action from that of guancydine. Possibly, the increased tubular sodium reabsorption is similar to that caused by diazoxide or minoxidil, although less pronounced. In the frog's bladder epithelium, guancydine inhibited the effect of oxytocin on net water influx (WORCEL et al., 1971).

B. Pharmacokinetics

Little is known about pharmacokinetics in man. After oral administration, the drug is well absorbed. The plasma half-life is in the order of 4 h (HAMMER et al., 1971), and the drug is administered at intervals of 6 to 8 h. Preliminary studies did not reveal a good correlation between the dose and the blood level, nor between blood level and the hypotensive response (HAMMER et al., 1971). Nothing is known as to how the drug is metabolized.

C. Therapeutic Use

In patients with various types of hypertension, guancydine can diminish systolic and diastolic blood pressure by 10 to 30 mm Hg in both supine and standing position (WERNING et al., 1970; HAMMER et al., 1971; CLARK and

GOLDBERG, 1972; STENBERG et al., 1971; VILLARREAL et al., 1971; RUSSO and MENDLOWITZ, 1972). After oral administration, the blood pressure begins to fall gradually within 30 min and the maximum effect is seen after 1 to $1^1/_2$ h (HAMMER et al., 1971). The hypotensive effect seems to be somewhat more pronounced than that of hydralazine (HAMMER et al., 1971), but definitely less than that obtained with diazoxide or minoxidil. Heart rate and cardiac output rise as with other drugs that do not interfere with sympathetic cardiovascular reflexes, such as hydralazine. The enhanced cardiac output counteracts in part the hypotensive effect (HAMMER et al., 1971), and for this reason combinations with other drugs that prevent tachycardia and increase in cardiac output have been suggested. HAMMER et al. (1971) found small doses of reserpine satisfactory; CLARK and GOLDBERG (1972) gave guanethidine or β-adrenergic blocking drugs. As for other drugs of this mechanism of action, combination with β-adrenergic blocking drugs will result in the most satisfactory lowering of blood pressure. Fluid and salt retention produced weight gain and edema formation (HAMMER et al., 1971; WERNING et al., 1970; STENBERG et al., 1971; RUSSO and MENDLOWITZ, 1972; VILLARREAL et al., 1971), and therefore the simultaneous administration of a diuretic is recommended. Quinethazone was given by CLARK and GOLDBERG (1972), whereas HAMMER et al. (1971) used chlorothiazide or hydrochlorothiazide. The simultaneous use of a diuretic not only prevents the retention of salt and water, but also has an additive hypotensive effect. Glomerular filtration rate and renal plasma flow remained unchanged or varied only slightly, but urinary sodium excretion was diminished (VILLARREAL et al., 1971). The retention of salt and water was more pronounced after guancydine than usually seen after hydralazine, which, during its much wider and longer use has only rarely produced a definite retention of sodium and water and oedema formation. Plasma renin activity was found to be elevated (WERNING et al., 1970).

In a well-controlled study, the duration of guancydine treatment was 4 weeks, and doses between 500 and 1500 mg per day were given by mouth. A good summary of the clinical findings has been prepared by KOCH-WESER (1974).

D. Adverse Reactions

Guancydine causes various unpleasant side reactions, mainly of central nature, such as headache, hyperexcitability, restlessness (FREIS and HAMMER, 1969; CLARK and GOLDBERG, 1972; HAMMER et al., 1971; STENBERG et al., 1971; VILLARREAL et al., 1971), feelings of anxiety, mental confusion, asthenia, and paraesthesia (CLARK and GOLDBERG, 1972). One patient showed a state of depression after a 2-week treatment, and another felt intoxicated (STENBERG et al., 1971). These side effects may be due to the diffusion of guancydine through the blood-brain barrier, but no studies have been undertaken to determine whether the drug enters the brain, and if so, where it may act there. Gynecomastia has been observed in three male patients and galactorrhoea in one female patient who had previously shown a similar response to spironolactone (CLARK and GOLDBERG, 1972). All these side reactions were reversible after discontinuation of the drug. However, the central nervous effects are so unpleasant that they prevent the extensive use of the drug in the treatment of high blood pressure.

As a consequence of tachycardia and increased cardiac output in patients with already existing myocardial lesions, electrocardiographic changes, indicating myocardial ischemia, may occur, with or without anginal pain (CLARK and GOLDBERG, 1972). This has also been reported with other vasodilators. Concomitant administration of β-adrenergic blocking drugs may prevent this type of adverse reaction. As it was pointed out by WERKÖ (1971) a major disadvantage of guancydine like that of similarly acting drugs is the induction of a hyperkinetic circulation. In addition the retention of sodium and water may result in edema formation and therefore the simultaneous administration of β-adrenergic blockers and of diuretics are necessary in order to obtain a satisfactory therapeutic response.

In conclusion it may be stated that the adverse reactions of guancydine, mainly those of the central nervous system, are so severe that clinical studies with the drug have been abandoned. Since little is known on the biotransformation of the drug it is not possible to indicate if the drug itself or one of its metabolites are responsible for the central side effects. On the other hand, the substance is sufficiently active to justify its use as an antihypertensive agent. It could be worthwhile to study the metabolism of the drug with respect to pharmacokinetics both in animals and man in order to find out what the reason for the side effects might be. Possibly a better tolerated drug could be found in that series of compounds.

VII. Prazosin

In 1968, a group of aminoquinazolines was described that had antihypertensive activities (SCRIABINE et al., 1968). The most active of these derivatives was CP12299-1, which was first called furazosin and later on, when it was studied clinically, prazosin. It has been claimed that prazosin represents "the culmination of a systematic synthesis and pharmacological development effort, which had as its goal the development of an agent that would lower blood pressure by direct vasodilation" (HESS, 1974), but one wonders how much of such a bold statement is really valid for the explanation of the antihypertensive action of prazosin. The hypothesis has little substantial support, and—as in other cases—the fact that prazosin was found is good luck rather than the result of systematic planning.

The blood pressure-lowering effect of prazosin is only partly caused by a direct effect on the arteriolar smooth muscle, resulting in a reduction of total peripheral resistance. In addition, there are some pharmacologic data that indicate an interference with peripheral sympathetic function mainly the α-adrenergic receptors (CONSTANTINE, 1974). However, the latter activity is not well defined, and the data reported in favour of it are not convincing.

Prazosin was marketed as an antihypertensive in various countries during the second half of 1974, although the pharmacologic results that had been published were only those from the manufacturer's laboratories (SCRIABINE et al., 1968; CONSTANTINE et al., 1973; CONSTANTINE, 1974). Pharmacokinetic data were scarce, and only very few clinical publications had appeared in well known and widely distributed journals. Some clinical papers were given at a symposium in Geneva in March 1974 and later were published in a monograph (1974), which is not easily accessible to the average doctor. It is remarkable that, today, a new antihypertensive for chronic treatment was accepted for marketing by the drug regulatory authorities on the basis of little published information, and one also wonders why so few data have been produced during the 6 years that have passed since the first experimental and clinical publications (RICHARDSON et al., 1968).

A. Pharmacodynamics

1. Cardiovascular Actions

In anesthetized normotensive dogs, prazosin, in doses of 0.1 and 0.4 mg/kg, caused a rapid fall in blood pressure, which was subsequently maintained at the low level for more than 1 h. The maximum hypotensive effect was dose-dependent in the limited range studied, being 20 mm Hg with the low and 45 mm Hg with the high dose. Heart rate increased transiently when blood pressure fell, but returned to the basal value within several minutes, although blood pressure had not returned to the pre-injection level. Cardiac output and stroke volume increased after the higher dose only, and total peripheral resistance was reduced. Arterial blood flow in various vascular beds, such as the femoral, mesenteric, as well as renal arteries, was elevated, whereas no significant change was seen in the flow of the internal carotid artery (CONSTANTINE et al., 1973; CONSTANTINE, 1974).

After single doses given by mouth to rats and dogs in which hypertension had been elicited by renal artery stenosis, a dose-dependent fall in blood pressure occurred. The duration of the maximum pressure reduction was approximately 6 h, but even after 24 h blood pressure had not returned to the values measured prior to the administration of the drug. By daily oral doses (0.625 mg/kg) a reduced blood pressure could be maintained, without significant changes in heart rate (CONSTANTINE et al., 1973; CONSTANTINE, 1974). When compared with hydralazine (1 mg/kg i.v.) prazosin (0.1 mg/kg i.v.) produced a greater fall of blood pressure in renal hypertensive dogs (MASSINGHAM and HAYDEN, 1975).

In the perfused forelimb of the dog, a reduction of vascular resistance was calculated after intra-arterial infusion, which, occurred mainly at the level of the small vessels (93%) and, to a much lesser degree (7%), in the paw arteries; venous resistance was not affected. Similar results were obtained in innervated dog hind leg (CAVERO 1976). This pattern is comparable to that observed with diazoxide, whereas compounds such as sodium nitrite or phentolamine induced a higher decrease in vacular resistance of the large arteries, which contributed 24% and 29% respectively to the reduction in total peripheral resistance. No direct vasodilator effect was observed in denervated legs of rats (WOODS et al., 1975).

In aortic strips of rabbits, prazosin showed a competitive antagonism to noradrenaline; the dose-response curve for noradrenaline was shifted to the right by increasing concentrations of prazosin. On the other hand, a noncompetitive type of antagonism was found against barium chloride-induced contractions (CONSTANTINE et al., 1973; CONSTANTINE, 1974).

In anesthetized rats and dogs, prazosin induced a "reversal" of the blood pressure response to adrenaline, whereas no influence was observed on the effect of noradrenaline or of angiotensin. Strangely enough, the authors of the pharmacologic study did not explain the divergent effects of prazosin on the pressor activity of adrenaline and noradrenaline and do not give dose-response curves for an antagonism of prazosin to α-adrenergic stimulants *in vivo*. In dogs anesthetized with chloralose, 0.05 mg/kg of prazosine reduced the carotid occlusion reflex (CONSTANTINE, 1974; CAVERO 1976).

2. Other Actions

The contractions of the cat's nictitating membrane, elicited by either pre- or postganglionic electrical stimulation, were similarly diminished, indicating that prazosin does not influence intraganglionic transmission.

Little has been published on the effects of prazosin on smooth muscle other than vascular, e.g., the tracheobronchial system, intestine, or uterus. It has only been mentioned that prazosin does not possess bronchodilator activities (HESS,

1974). In rats an increase in plasma renin concentration was obtained 30 and 120 min after administration, but the rise was less pronounced in renal hypertensive rats than in normotensive controls (FERNANDEZ et al., 1975). In renal hypertensive dogs prazosin did not change plasma renin concentration, whereas in the same animals hydralazine produced an increase in PRC (MASSINGHAM and HAYDEN, 1975).

Cyclic AMP phosphodiesterase was inhibited by prazosin in a concentration-dependent manner. The phosphodiesterase preparations were isolated from rat heart (low affinity, high Km: $10^4 M$) and rat aorta (low Km: $10^{-6} M$). The latter enzyme was more strongly inhibited by prazosin than by theophyllin or hydralazine, which had only about $^1/_{100}$ the activity of prazosin (HESS, 1974). This inhibitory effect of prazosin on phosphodiesterase activity was related to the vasodilator action of the drug, but further data are necessary in order to support such a presumption.

3. Mechanism of Action

On the basis of the available data it was suggested that prazosin acts mainly by its direct relaxing effect on vascular smooth muscle. In addition, prazosin interferes with peripheral sympathetic function, but it is not yet clear in which way it acts on α-adrenergic receptors. The vasodilating effect of prazosin is diminished by pretreatment with hexamethonium, which does not influence the effect of diazoxide, guancydine or papaverine, whereas it inhibits that of phentolamine. From this observation it was concluded that prazosin, at least in part, would produce vasodilation by acting on the postganglionic adrenergic fibers. It was also demonstrated that prazosin had some protective effect on the phenoxybenzamine blockade of α-adrenergic receptors, but was less active in this respect than phentolamine (CONSTANTINE et al., 1973; CONSTANTINE, 1974).

The claim was made that prazosin, unlike phentolamine, does not occupy α-adrenergic receptors (CONSTANTINE, 1974), although it behaves like a competitive α-adrenergic blocker in the isolated aortic strip contracted by noradrenaline. Subsequently, it was suggested that prazosin might exert its action at "a site distal to the α-adrenergic receptor", with the result of functional impairment of the receptor. However, no further explanation has been given for this hypothesis based on exclusion rather than on evidence. Recently, prazosin has been defined as a selective antagonist of post-synaptic α-adrenoceptors (CAMBRIDGE et al., 1977). Correctly it was supposed that prazosin acts on the smooth vascular muscle at some other site than diazoxide, which forms weak molecular bonds at three anionic sites on the receptor and may compete there with calcium ions (WOHL, 1970).

The available results and their interpretation make it difficult to state whether prazosin acts on blood pressure and total peripheral resistance mainly on the basis of a direct effect on the arteriolar muscle or whether the "impairment of peripheral sympathetic function" contributes mainly to these activities. The results available clearly demonstrate that prazosin is not a typical vasodilator but is more closely related to α-adrenolytics (CAVERO 1976). The fact that reflex tachycardia is much less pronounced than with diazoxide or hydralazine, or completely lacking, indicates some effect on the sympathetic innervation, but more work is necessary to reveal the type of antisympathetic activity and its significance for the overall action of prazosin.

B. Pharmacokinetics

Little is known about the pharmacokinetics of prazosin, in particular its fate in the organism. Plasma half-life in man seems to be similar to that in dogs, i.e., 1 to 2 h. Studies in dogs on the tissue distribution of 2-C^{14} labeled prazosin revealed that, 30 min after i.v. injection, the concentrations in various arteries, including the coronaries, exceeded plasma concentration by three to six times, but the radioactive compounds were not identified. Various metabolites of prazosin have been isolated from bile and urine of rats and dogs, including 6-O-demethylated, hydroxylated, and also hydrolysed derivatives, which, as the unchanged prazosin, are excreted in part as glucuronides. Gastrointestinal absorption was said to be complete (HESS, 1974), but no data have been published as yet. After oral administration of labeled prazosin, about 6% to 10% of radioactive material is excreted in the urine within 24 h, the remaining amount in the feces after biliary excretion (HESS, 1974). Major metabolites are the 6-O-demethyl and 7-O-demethyl derivatives of prazosin (ALTHUIS and HESS 1977).

C. Therapeutic Use

There is no doubt that prazosin lowers blood pressure in patients with mild and moderate hypertension, and that it is active when given by mouth in daily doses of 3 to 20 mg, occasionally up to 40 mg (PITTS, 1974). In the beginning the usual dosage scheme was three tablets a day, but in controlled studies it was shown that results with a twice-daily regimen were similar to those obtained with t.i.d. or q.i.d. schedules (OKUN, 1974). Most investigators who have published on their experience with the drug, although often limited, agree that it is an active antihypertensive (COHEN, 1970; KINCAID-SMITH et al., 1973; HAYES et al., 1974; MROCZEK et al., 1974; OKUN, 1974; ONESTI et al., 1974; STOKES and WEBER, 1974; VENABLES and DUFF, 1974; PAUL et al., 1976). However, some authors found only a weak activity with well-tolerated doses and observed unpleasant side-effects when the dose was increased (AMERY et al., 1974; THULIN et al., 1974), especially severe orthostatic reactions.

The activity was compared with that of α-methyldopa in some studies, and the effect on blood pressure was similar (MROCZEK et al., 1974; ONESTI et al., 1974; STOKES and WEBER, 1974; VENABLES and DUFF, 1974; ADRIAENSEN and VRYENS, 1975; BLOOM et al., 1975), but α-methyldopa was often given in relatively low doses (750 mg per day), and therefore it is difficult to estimate the antihypertensive potential of the two drugs. In a double blind crossover trial of prazosin and hydralazine, good control of blood pressure was achieved with the two drugs when combined with diuretics and β-adrenergic blockers. The antihypertensive effect of 25 mg hydralazine was somewhat stronger than that of 1 mg prazosin (KINCAID-SMITH and HUA, 1974). During long-term treatment no tolerance to the drug developed (BOLLI and SIMPSON, 1974; PITTS, 1974).

All investigators found little or no increase in heart rate or cardiac output, and in hemodynamic studies a fall in total peripheral resistance was calculated (LUND-JOHANSEN, 1974; MASONI et al., 1974). When a single i.v. injection of 2 mg was compared with repeated oral administration of up to 20 mg daily for 10 days, the blood pressure response was much less pronounced when the drug was given by mouth and cardiac index remained unchanged (SAFAR et al., 1974). Reduction of blood pressure was more marked during standing or exercise than in the recumbent position (SAFAR et al., 1974; LUND-JOHANSEN, 1974). Plasma renin activity did not change (SAFAR et al., 1974), which is in contrast to the increase induced by vasodilators such as diazoxide (KÜCHEL et al., 1967), by minoxidil (PETTINGER and KEETON, 1973), or hydralazine.

The antihypertensive action is enhanced by the simultaneous administration of either diuretics (SAFAR et al., 1974; AMERY et al., 1974; ONESTI et al., 1974; KINCAID-SMITH, et al., 1973; PAUL et al., 1976; SCHIRGER and SHEPS 1977) or of β-adrenergic blockers (AMERY et al., 1974; STOKES and WEBER, 1974; HUA et al., 1976; Schirger and Sheps 1977). In the latter case the effect on heart rate is negligible. In contrast to diazoxide and minoxidil, prazosin produces little or no sodium retention (Safar et al., 1974; Hua et al., 1976), and a tendency to weight gain together with a decrease in hematocrit has only occasionally been reported (Thulin et al., 1974).

In patients with chronic renal failure and hypertension, prazosin was found to be active, provided that the dose is carefully controlled. In patients with impaired renal function prazosin did not deteriorate it (Hua et al., 1976). Daily doses of 1 mg may be sufficient, and 6 mg should not be exceeded (Curtis, 1974; Hayes et al., 1974). In these patients the addition of 3 mg daily to the antihypertensive regimen may produce a significant fall of blood pressure (Curtis and Bateman, 1975).

D. Adverse Reactions

The main side reactions seem to be dizziness and severe orthostatic response, which can be severe enough to make withdrawal of the drug necessary (Amery et al., 1974; Thulin et al., 1974; Kellaway, 1976). In a summarizing report on 934 patients, postural dizziness has been observed in 13.7%, palpitations in 5.3%, and edema in 4.1% (Pitts, 1974). Headache and nausea, frequently seen with hydralazine, have been reported in 7.8% and 4.9% of the patients respectively (Fernandes et al., 1975). Tachycardia was rare (0.2%), and nothing was said about the provocation of anginal attacks. At the time of introduction, the drug was considered to be well tolerated but soon afterwards quite a few reports have been published on severe orthostatic reactions (Gabriel et al., 1975b; Bendall et al., 1975). It was said that orthostatism is less pronounced when treatment is started with 2 mg daily, but other investigators found already this dose too high (Gabriel et al., 1975a,b; Rosendorf, 1976; Graham et al., 1976). With 0.5 mg daily, mild dizziness has been seen as side-effect in 4.6% of patients, whereas with 2 mg per day, 16% of the patients had severe reactions to the first dose (Rosendorf, 1976; Stokes et al., 1977). The data available are not yet sufficient to make a definite statement with respect to the tolerability of the drug and how to avoid initial overshooting responses, which seem to subside with protracted treatment (Graham et al., 1976). However, it is evident that at the time of introduction too high doses had been recommended for the beginning of treatment. Particular care has to be taken in sodium-depleted patients (Stokes et al., 1977). In a double blind crossover study with α-methyldopa (750 mg daily) in elderly patients prazosin in a dose of three times 1 mg daily for 4 to 6 weeks was considered to be safe and effective and no orthostatic reaction had been observed (Adriaensen and Vryens, 1975; Paul et al., 1976). The variation in experiences and opinions on the tolerability of prazosin is remarkable. Whereas some investigators consider prazosin to be dangerous (Gabriel, 1975a, b; Thulin et al., 1974) others stress the lack of side effects (Hayes et al., 1974; Adriaensen and Vryens, 1975; Bolli et al., 1975; Hua et al., 1976). The discrepancy is difficult to explain but probably not only caused by the administration of too high does at the beginning of treatment. Even if this were the case then prazosin would have a narrow margin of safety which would be in contrast with most of the other antihypertensives. Acute febrile polyarthritis has been reported as a further possible complication of prazosin treatment (Cairns and Jordans, 1976).

In summarizing one can say that prazosin is an interesting antihypertensive agent, which merits further studies, especially in combination with diuretics and ß-adrenergic blocking drugs. For the time being it is not possible to determine where the drug has to be classified among the other antihypertensive agents, both with respect to efficacy and safety. Additional studies on its pharmacology, its mechanism of action, on pharmacokinetics, its therapeutic usefulness, and the incidence of side effects after prolonged treatment are advisable.

References

Section I Introduction

BARTORELLI, C., GARGANO, N., LEONETTI, G., ZANCHETTI, A.: Hypotensive and renal effects of diazoxide, a sodium retaining benzothiadiazine compound. Circulation **27**, 895—903 (1963).

BHATIA, S. K., FROHLICH, E. D.: Hemodynamic comparison of agents useful in hypertensive emergencies. Amer. Heart J. **85**, 367—373 (1973).

BOLLI, P., WOOD, A. J. PHELAN, E. L., LEE, D. R., SIMPSON, F. O.: Prazosin: preliminary clinical and pharmacological observations. Clin. Sci. molec. Med. **48**, Suppl. II, 177s—179s (1975).

CUMMINGS, J. R., WELTER, A. N., GRACE, JR., J. L., GRAY, W. D.: Angiotensin blocking actions of guancydine. J. Pharmacol. exp. Ther. **170**, 334—346 (1969).

DOLLERY, C. T., PENTECORT, B. L., SAMAAN, N. A.: Drug-induced diabetes. Lancet **1962 II**, 735—737.

DUCHARME, D. W., FREYBURGER, W. A., GRAHAM, B. E., CARLSON, R. G.: Pharmacologic properties of minoxidil: a new hypotensive agent. J. Pharmacol. exp. Ther. **184**, 662—670 (1973).

FINNERTY, F. A., JR., KAKAVIATOS, N., TUCKMAN, J., MAGILL, J.: Clinical evaluation of diazoxide; a new treatment for acute hypertension. Circulation **28**, 203—208 (1963).

GROSS, F., DRUEY, J., MEIER, R.: Eine neue Gruppe blutdrucksenkender Substanzen von besonderem Wirkungscharakter. Experientia (Basel) **6**, 11—12 (1950).

HIDAKA, H., NAGATSU, T., TAKEYA, K., TAKEUCHI, T., SUDA, H., KOJIRI, K., MATSUSAKI, M., UMEZAWA, H.: Fusaric acid, a hypotensive agent produced by fungi. J. Antibiot. **22**, 228—230 (1969).

JOHNSON, C. C.: The actions and toxicity of sodium nitroprusside. Arch. int. Pharmacodyn. **35**, 480—496 (1929).

KOCH-WESER, J.: Vasodilation for vasospastic hypertension. New Engl. J. Med. **289**, 213—214 (1973).

KOCH-WESER, J.: Vasodilator drugs in the treatment of hypertension. Arch. intern. Med. **133**, 1017—1027 (1974).

KORDUBA, C. A., VEALS, J., WOHL, A., SYMCHOWITZ, S., TABACHNIK, J. J. A.: SCH 10595, an effective dopamine-β-hydroxylase inhibitor and a hypotensive agent. J. Pharmacol. exp. Ther. **184**, 671—677 (1973).

KÜCHEL, O., FISHMAN, L. M., LIDDLE, G. W., MICHELAKIS, A.: Effect of diazoxide on plasma renin activity in hypertensive patients. Ann. intern. Med. **67**, 791—799 (1967).

RUBIN, A. A., ROTH, F. E., TAYLOR, R. M., ROSENKILDE, H.: Pharmacology of diazoxide, an antihypertensive, non-diuretic benzothiadiazine. J. Pharmacol. exp. Ther. **136**, 344—352 (1962).

SCHLANT, R. C., TSAGARIS, T. S., ROBERTSON, R. J., JR.: Studies on the acute cardiovascular effects of intravenous sodium nitroprusside. Amer. J. Cardiol. **9**, 51—59 (1962).

SCHROEDER, H. A.: Effects on hypertension of sulfhydryl and hydrazine compounds. J. clin. Invest. **30**, 672—673 (1951).

SCRIABINE, A., CONSTANTINE, J. W., HESS, H. J., MCSHANE, W. K.: Pharmacological studies with some new antihypertensive aminoquinazolines. Experientia (Basel) **24**, 1150—1151 (1968).

UEDA, H., YAGI, S., KANEKO, Y.: Hydralazine and plasma renin activity. Arch. intern. Med. **122**, 387—391 (1968).

VELASCO, M., GILBERT, C. A., RUTLEDGE, C. O., MCNAY, J. L.: Antihypertensive effect of a dopamine-beta-hydroxylase inhibitor, bupicomide: A comparison with hydralazine. Clin. Pharmacol. exp. Ther. **18**, 145—153 (1975).

WILSON, W. R., OKUN, R.: Acute hemodynamic effects of diazoxide in man. Circulation **28**, 89—93 (1963).

Section II Hydralazines

ÅBLAD, B.: A study of the mechanism of the hemodynamic effects of hydralazine in man. Acta pharmacol. toxicol. (Kbh.) **20**, Suppl. 1, 1—53 (1963).

ÅBLAD, B., JOHNSSON, G.: Comparative effects of intraarterially administered hydralazine and sodium nitrite on blood flow and volume of forearm. Acta pharmacol. toxicol. (Kbh.) **20**, 1—15 (1963).

ÅBLAD, B., MELLANDER, J.: Comparative effects of hydralazine, sodium nitrite and acetylcholine on resistance and capacitance blood vessels and capillary filtration in skeletal muscle in the cat. Acta physiol. scand. **58**, 319—329 (1963).

ÅBLAD, B., JOHNSSON, G., HENNING, M.: The effects of hydralazine administered into the brachial artery on adrenergic vasoconstrictor stimuli in the hand. Acta pharmacol. toxicol. (Kbh.) **19**, 165—180 (1962)

Akashi, A., Chiba, T., Kasahara, A.: Antihypertensive activity of 1[2-(1,3-dimethyl-2-butenylidene)-hydrazino] phthalazine (DJ-1461), a new phthalazine derivative. Europ. J. Pharmacol. **29**, 161—164 (1974).
Alarcón-Segovia, D., Osmundson, P. J.: Peripheral vascular syndromes associated with systemic lupus erythematosus. Ann. intern. Med. **62**, 907 (1965).
Alarcón-Segovia, D., Worthington, J. W., Ward, L. E., Wakim, K. G.: Lupus diathesis and the hydralazine syndrome. New Engl. J. Med. 272, 462—466 (1965).
Alarcón-Segovia, D., Wakim, K. G., Worthington, J. W., Ward, L. E.: Clinical and experimental studies on the hydralazine syndrome and its relationship to systemic lupus erythematosis. Medicine **46**, 1—33 (1967).
Alkalay, J., Bullard, J. C.: Systemic lupus erythematosus following prolonged treatment with hydralazine. Ann. Allergy **29**, 35—36 (1971).
Assali, N. S., Kaplan, J., Oighenstein, S., Inymoto, R.: Hemodynamic effects of 1-hydrazinophthalazine (Apresoline) in human pregnancy: results of intravenous administration. J. clin. Invest. **32**, 922—930 (1952).
Baldoli, E., Sardi, A., Bianchi, G.: Hypotensive action of 3-hydrazino-6-N,N-bis-(2-hydroxyethyl) amino pyridazine dihydrochloride (L 6150) in normotensive and hypertensive animals. Naunyn Schmiedebergs Arch. Pharmak. **269**, 391—392 (1971).
Baldoli, E., Sardi, A., Dezulian, V., Capellini, M., Bianchi, G.: On the pharmacology of 3-hydrazino-6-[N,N-bis(2-hydroxyethyl)amino]-pyridazine-dihydrochloride (L 6150), Arzneimittel-Forsch. **23**, 1591—1595 (1973).
Barrett, W., Reitze, W., Plummer, A. J., Yonkman, F. F.: Coronary dilating action of L-hydrazinophthalazine (BA 5968) (Apresoline) in the canine heart-lung preparation. Fed. Proc. **2**, 320—321 (1952).
Barrett, W. E., Povalski, H., Rutledge, R.: A hypothesis concerning the mechanism of action of hydralazine HU. Fed. Proc. **24**, 712 (1965).
Baum, T., Shropshire, A. T., Vasner, L. L.: Contribution of the central nervous system to the action of several antihypertensive agents (Methyldopa, Hydralazine, and Guanethidine). J. Pharmacol. exp. Ther. **182**, 135—144 (1972).
Beelar, V. P.: Rheumathoid arthritis-like syndrome during apresoline therapy. Med. Ann. D. C. **22**, 651—652 and p. 696 (1953).
Bein, H. J., Brunner, H.: Mode of action of antihypertensive drugs. In: Gross, F. (Ed.): Antihypertensive Therapy, pp. 15—28. Heidelberg-Berlin-New York: Springer 1965.
Bein, H. J., Tripod, J., Meier, R.: Zur Kreislaufwirkung des 1-hydrazinophthalazins. Experientia (Basel) 8, 74—75 (1952).
Bein, H. J., Gross, F., Tripod, J., Meier, R.: Experimentelle Untersuchungen über die Kreislaufwirkung der blutdrucksenkenden Hydrazinophthalazinderivate Apresolin und Nepresol. Schweiz. med. Wschr. **83**, 336—340 (1953).
Bendersky, G., Ramirez, C.: Hydralazine poisoning. Review of the literature and autopsy study of persons with massive intestinal bleeding. J. Amer. med. Ass. **173**, 1789—1794 (1960).
Bhatia, S. K., Frohlich, E. D.: Hemodynamic comparison of agents useful in hypertensive emergencies. Amer. Heart J. **85**, 367—373 (1973).
Biniecki, S., Rylski, L.: Synthèse de la 1-hydrazino 6-chlorphthalazine et de la 1-hydrazino-7-chlorphthalazine. Ann. pharm. franç. **16**, 21—26 (1958).
Biniecki, S., Moll, M., Rylski, L.: Synthèse de la 1-hydrazino 5-chlorphthalazine et de la 1-hydrazino 8-chlorphthalazine. Ann. pharm. franç. **16**, 421—428 (1958).
Blas Zingale, S., Canepa, L., Roldan, H. J.: Intento de production experimental en perros del lupus hidralazinico. Medicina (B. Aires) **20**, 135 (1960).
Braverman, I. M., Lerner, A. B.: Hydralazine disease in the guinea pig as an experimental model for lupus erythematosus. J. invest. Derm. **39**, 317—327 (1962).
Brod, J., Bahlmann, J., Cachovan, M., Dahlgrün, H., P. Pretschner, Futterová, M.: Clinical and haemodynamic study of a new vasodilator drug L 6150 (3-[bis-(2-hydroxaethyl) amino]-6-hydrazinopyridazine dihydrochloride). Clin. Sci. molec. Med. **51**, Suppl. 3, 601 s—603 s, 1976.
Brunner, H., Hedwall, P. R., Meier, M.: Inhibition of acute effects of hydralazine by an adrenergic beta-receptor blocking agent. Experientia (Basel) **21**, 136—137 (1965a).
Brunner, H., Hedwall, P. R., Meier, M.: Influence of an adrenergic beta-receptor blocking agent on the effect of various hypotensive agents in the hypertensive rat. Experientia (Basel) **21**, 231—232 (1965b).
Brunner, H., Hedwall, P. R., Meier, M.: Influence of adrenergic beta-receptor blockade on the acute cardiovascular effects of hydralazine. Brit. J. Pharmacol. **30**, 123—133 (1967).
Bygdeman, M., Stjärne, L.: Effects of 1,4 dihydralazinophthalazine in organ content and adrenal medullary secretion of catecholamines. Nature (Lond.) **184**, 1646—1647 (1959).
Bygdeman, M., Stjärne, L.: Effects of 1,4-dihydrazinophthalazine on the catecholamines. Nature (Lond.) **186**, 82—83 (1960).

CARPI, C., DORIGOTTI, L.: Antihypertensive activity of a new 3-hydrazinopyridazine derivative: ISF 2123. Brit. J. Pharmacol. **52**, 459 (1974).
CLARK, G. M., TROOP, R. C.: One-tablet combination drug therapy in the treatment of hypertension. J. chron. Dis. **25**, 57—64 (1972).
COMENS, P.: Experimental hydralazine disease and its similarity to disseminated lupus erythematosus. J. Lab. clin. Med. **47**, 444—454 (1956a).
COMENS, P.: Manganese depletion as an etiologic factor in hydralazine disease. Amer. J. Med. **20**, 944—945 (1956b).
COMENS, P.: Chronic intoxication from hydralazine resembling disseminated lupus erythematosus and its apparent reversal by manganese. In: Metal-binding in Medicine, pp. 312—320. Philadelphia: Lippinerk 1960.
CONDEMI, J. J., MOORE-JONES, D., VAUGHAN, J. H., PERRY, H. M., JR.: Antinuclear antibodies following hydralazine toxicity. New Engl. J. Med. **276**, 486—491 (1967).
CRAVER, B. N., BARRETT, W., CAMERON, A., YONKMAN, F. F.: The activities of 1-hydrazinophthalazine (Ba 5968) a hypotensive agent. J. Amer. pharm. Ass. sci. Ed. **40**, 559—564 (1951).
DE MARCO, P., SHOHOV, P., KRESKY, B., ZAINO, E. C.: Disseminated lupus erythematosus in a 28 month old infant with onset during hydralazine therapy. Clin. Pediat. **3**, 308—310 (1964).
DE PONTI, C., BARDI, U., MARCHETTI, M.: A Comparative Study of the hemodynamic effects of single intravenous doses of 3-hydrazino-6-[N,N-bis-(2-hydroxyethyl)-amino]-pyridazine-dihydrochloride and hydrazine. Arzneimittelforsch. **26**, 2089—92, 1976.
DONTAS, A. S.: Effects of reserpine and hydralazine on carotid and splanchnic nerve activity and blood pressure. J. Pharmacol. exp. Ther. **121**, 1—7 (1957).
DOUGLASS, C. D., HOGAN, R.: A metabolite of 1-hydrazinophthalazine (hydralazine). Proc. Soc. exp. Biol. (N. Y.) **100**, 446—448 (1959).
DOUGLASS, C. D., DILLAHA, C. J., DILLAHA, J., KOMITZ, S. L.: Inhibition of biologic acetylation by 1-hydrazinophthalazine. J. Lab. clin. Med. **49**, 561—565 (1957).
DRUEY, J., TRIPOD, J.: Hydralazines. In: SCHLITTLER, E. (Ed.): Antihypertensive Agents, pp. 223—262. New York-London: Academic Press 1967.
DUBOIS, E. L.: Lupus erythematosus, p. 148. New York: McGraw Hill 1966.
DUSTAN, H. P., TAYLOR, R. D., LORCORAN, A. C., PAGE, I. H.: Rheumatic and febrile syndrome during prolonged hydralazine treatment. J. Amer. med. Ass. **154**, 23—29 (1954).
Editorial: Hydrallazine, Lancet 1977/I, 342—343.
EDWARDS, S., MARQUARDT, F. H.: The metabolism of 1-hydrazinophthalazine: the correct structure of the pseudo "N-acetyl-1-hydrazinophthalazine". Hoppe Seylers Z. physiol. Chem. **350**, 85—86 (1969).
ESSELIER, A. F., LUSCHER, W., MORANDI, L.: Hydrazinophthalazine bei Hypertension. Schweiz. med. Wschr. **83**, 28—37 (1953).
FALLAB, S.: Reaktivität von Koordinationsverbindungen. VIII. Zur Bildung von Eisen (II)-Chelaten des Phthalazyl-(1)-hydralazyl-Radikals. Helv. chim. Acta **45**, 1057—1063 (1962).
FALLAB, S., ERLENMEYER, H.: Zum Wirkungsmechanismus des chemischen Strahlenschutzes. Experientia (Basel) **19**, 374—376 (1963).
FANNER, R. G., GIFFORD, R. W., JR., HINES, E. A., JR.: Effect of medical treatment of severe hypertension. Arch. intern. Med. **112**, 118—128 (1963).
FREIS, E. D.: Hydralazine: Pharmacology and clinical application. In: BREST, A. N., MOYER, J. H. (Eds.): Hypertension: Recent Advances. The 2nd Hahnemann Symposium on Hypertensive Disease, pp. 291—295. Philadelphia: Lea & Febiger 1961.
FREIS, E. D.: Veterans administration cooperative study group on antihypertensive agents. Effect of treatment on morbidity in hypertension: results in patients with diastolic blood pressure averaging 115 through 129 mm Hg. J. Amer. med. Ass. **202**, 1028—1034 (1967).
FREIS, E. D.: Veterans administration cooperative study group on antihypertensive agents. Effect of treatment on morbidity in hypertension. II. Results in patients with diastolic blood pressure averaging 90 through 114 mm Hg. J. Amer. med. Ass. **213**, 1143—1152 (1970).
FREIS, E. D.: Modification of hypertension by antihypertensive drug treatment in spontaneously hypertensive rats. In: OKAMOTO, K. (Ed.): Spontaneous Hypertension, pp. 231—237. Tokyo: Igaku Shoin Ltd. 1972.
FREIS, E. D., ROSE, J. C., HIGGINS, T. F., FINNERTY, F. A., JR., KELLY, R. T., PARTMOPE, E. A.: The hemodynamic effects of hypotensive drugs in man. IV. 1-hydrazinophthalazine. Circulation 8, 199—204 (1953).
FRIEDMAN, H., HEINE, W. J.: Demonstration of antihydralazine antibody in hydralazine induced lupus erythematosus. Experientia (Basel) **19**, 10—11 (1963).
GAMSKI, M.: Binazin, ein neues Phthalazinderivat. Z. ges. inn. Med. **28**, 234—235 (1973).
GARDNER, D. L.: The response of the dog to oral 1-hydrazinophthalazine (hydralazine). Brit. J. exp. Path. **38**, 227—235 (1957).

Gardner, D. L., Brooks, P. W.: Prevention of vascular necrosis in rats with adrenal regeneration hypertension by incomplete control of raised blood pressure. Brit. J. exp. Path. **43**, 276—287 (1962).

Gaunt, R., Renzi, A.: Apresoline (1-Hydrazinophthalazine) in the experimental Eclampsia-like syndrome and related aspects of water metabolism. Amer. J. Physiol. **175**, 313—318 (1953).

Gertner, S. B., Romano, A.: The effect of hydralazine on ganglionic transmission. J. Pharmacol. exp. Ther. **138**, 309—314 (1962).

Gottlieb, T. B., Katz, F. H., Chidsey, C. H.: Continued therapy with vasodilator drugs and beta-adrenergic blockade in hypertension. A comparative study of minoxidil and hydralazine. Circulation **45**, 571—582 (1972).

Grimson, K. S., Chittum, J. R., Metcalf, B. H.: Actions of 1-hydrazinophthalazines (C 5968) on vasomotor reflexes and hypertension in dog and man. Fed. Proc. **9**, 279 (1950).

Grimson, K. S., Orgain, E. J., Rowe, C. R., Jr., Sieber, H. A.: Caution with regard to use of hexamethonium and "apresoline". J. Amer. med. Ass. **149**, 215—220 (1952).

Gross, F.: Drug therapy of hypertension: What we have, what we need, what we expect. Amer. J. Cardiol. **34**, 471—475 (1974).

Gross, F.: Summary of round-table discussion on antihypertensive treatment. In: Sambhi M. P. (Ed.): Systemic Effects of Antihypertensive Agents, pp. 585—589. New York: Stratton Intercontinental Medical Book Corporation 1976.

Gross, F., Druey, J., Meier, R.: Eine neue Gruppe blutdrucksenkender Substanzen von besonderem Wirkungscharakter. Experientia (Basel) **6**, 11—12 (1950).

Gross, F., Schuler, W., Tripod, J., Meier, R.: Hemmung der Diaminoxydase (Histaminase) durch Phthalazinderivate. Experientia (Basel) **8**, 229—230 (1952).

Gross, F., Noelpp, B., Sulser, F., Doebelin, R., Kündig, H.: Vergleichende Untersuchungen über die medikamentöse Beeinflussung verschiedener Formen von experimenteller Hypertension. Klin. Wschr. **33**, 372—378 (1955).

Gupta, K. P., Bhargava, K. P.: Mechanism of tachycardia induced by intracerebroventricular injection of hydralazine (1-hydrazinophthalazine). Arch. int. Pharmacodyn. **155**, 84—89 (1965).

Hahn, B. H., Sharp, G. C., Irvin, W. S., Kantor, D. S., Gardner, C. A., Bagby, M. K., Perry, H. M., Jr., Osterland, C. K.: Immune responses to hydralazine and nuclear antigens in hydralazine-induced lupus erythematosis. Ann. intern. Med. **76**, 365—374 (1972).

Heine, W. J., Friedman, H.: Hydralazine lupus syndrome associated with a possible anti-hydralazine antibody. J. Amer. med. Ass. **182**, 726—729 (1962).

Henn, M. J., Perkins, T. W., Hargraves, M. M., Odel, H. M.: Acute systemic lupus erythematosus syndrome from hydralazine hydrochloride. Arch. intern. Med. **95**, 857—862 (1955).

Hildreth, E. A., Biso, C. E., McCrewy, T. A.: Persistence of the "hydralazine syndrome". J. Amer. med. Ass. **173**, 657—660 (1960).

Hoobler, S. W., Dontas, A. S.: Drug treatment of hypertension. Pharmacol. Rev. **5**, 135—174 (1953).

Hoobler, S. W., Blaquier, P.: Therapeutic use of hydralazine (Apresoline) and Rauwolfia compounds in hypertension. In: Moyer, J. (Ed.): Hypertension. The First Hahnemann Symposium on Hypertensive Disease, pp. 384—390. Philadelphia-London: W. B. Saunders Company 1959.

Hughes, W. M., Dennis, E., Moyer, J. H.: Treatment of hypertension with oral reserpine alone and in combination with hydralazine or hexamethonium. Amer. J. med. Sci. **229**, 121—134 (1955).

Ingenito, A. J., Barrett, J. P., Procita, L.: Centrally mediated peripheral hypotensive effects of reserpine and hydralazine when perfused through the isolated in situ cat brain. J. Pharmacol. exp. Ther. **170**, 210—220 (1969).

Johnson, R. L., Freis, E. D., Schnaper, H. W.: Clinical evaluation of 1-hydrazinophthalazine (C 5968) in hypertension with special reference to alternating treatment with hexamethonium. Circulation **5**, 833—841 (1952).

Jounela, A. J., Pasanen, M., Mattila, M. J.: Acetylator phenotype and the antihypertensive response to hydralazine. Acta med. scand. **197**, 303—306 (1975).

Judson, W. E., Hollander, W., Wilkins, R. W.: The effects of intravenous apresoline (hydralazine) on cardiovascular and renal function in patients with and without congestive heart failure. Circulation **13**, 664—674 (1956).

Katila, M., Frick, M. H.: Continued dihydralazine and propranolol in the treatment of hypertension. Int. J. clin. Pharmacol. **4**, 111—114 (1970).

Kaufman, M.: Pancytopenia following use of hydralazine ("apresoline"). J. Amer. med. Ass. **151**, 1488—1490 (1953).

KEBERLE, H., FAIGLE, J. W., HEDWALL, P., RIESS, W., WAGNER, J.: Plasma concentrations and pharmacological response in animals. In: DAVIES, D. S., PRICHARD, B. N. C. (Eds.): Biological Effects of Drugs in Realition to Their Plasma Concentrations. pp. 13—24. London: Macmillan 1973.

KIRKENDALL, W. M., PAGE, E. B.: Polyneuritis occurring during hydralazine therapy. J. Amer. med. Ass. **167**, 427—432 (1958).

KIRPEKAR, S. M., LEWIS, J. J.: Pharmacological properties of hydralazine, dihydralazine and some related compounds. J. pharm. Pharmacol. **9**, 877—887 (1957).

KIRPEKAR, S. M., LEWIS, J. J.: Effects of reserpine and hydralazine on isolated strips of carotid arteries. J. pharm. Pharmacol. **10**, 255—259 (1958a).

KIRPEKAR, S. M., LEWIS, J. J.: Antagonism to the actions of hydralazine, reserpine, potassium cyanide, sodium azide and anoxia on arterial smooth muscle. J. pharm. Pharmacol. **10**, 307—314 (1958b).

KIRPEKAR, S. M., LEWIS, J. J.: Some effects of reserpine and hydralazine upon tissue respiration and the concentration of adenosine nucleotides in certain tissues. Brit. J. Pharmacol. **14**, 40—45 (1959a).

KIRPEKAR, S. M., LEWIS, J. J.: Some effects of hydralazine on blood iron and an iron-containing enzyme system. J. pharm. Pharmacol. **11**, Suppl., 203T (1959b).

KOCH-WESER, J.: Vasodilation for vasospastic hypertension. New Engl. J. Med. **289**, 213—214 (1973).

KOCH-WESER, J.: Vasodilator drugs in the treatment of hypertension. Arch. intern. Med. **133**, 1017—1027 (1974).

LECLERC, G., WERMUTH, C.-G., MILSCH, F., SCHWARTZ, J.: Synthèses et corrélations de Hansch dans une série d'hydrazinopyridazines hypotensives. Europ. J. med. Chem. Chim. Ther. **11**, 107—113 (1976).

LEE, R. E., SELIGMAN, A. M., GARBEL, D., FULTON, L. A., CLARK, M. A.: Reserpine-hydralazine combination therapy of hypertensive disease, with hydralazine in doses perorally below the toxic range. Ann. intern. Med. **44**, 456—465 (1956).

LEE, S. L., SIEGEL, M.: Drug induced systemic lupus erythematosus. In: MEYLER, L., PECK, H. M. (Eds.): Drug Induced Diseases. Amsterdam: Excerpta Medica Foundation pp. 239—248. 1968.

LESSER, J. M., ISRAILI, Z. H., DAVIS, E., DAYTON, P. G.: Fate of hydralazine ^{14}C in man and dog. Clin. Pharmacol. Ther. **14**, 140 (1973).

LESSER, J. M., ISRAILI, H., DAVIS, C., DAYTON, P. G.: Metabolism and disposition of hydralazine ^{14}C in man and dog. Drug Metab. Dispos. **2**, 351—360, 1974.

LEWIS, R., SCHWARTZ, R., HENRY, W. B., JR.: Canine systemic lupus erythematosus. Blood **25**, 143—160 (1965).

LIM, R. K. S., MOFFITT, R. L., GLASS, H. G.: Observations on the mechanism of central hypertension. J. Pharmacol. **113**, 33—34 (1955).

LINÉT, O., VAN ZWIETEN, P. A., HERTTING, G.: Effect of hydrazinophthalazines on catecholamines in rats. Europ. J. Pharmacol. **6**, 121—124 (1969).

LIU, TSAN Z., SHEN, JEN-TA, LOKEN, H. F.: Inhibition of dopamine-β-hydroxylase by hydralazine. Proc. Soc. exp. Biol. (N. Y.) **145**, 294—297 (1974).

MARKS, P. A., REYNELL, P. C., BRADLEY, S. E.: Hemodynamic effects of L-hydrazinophthalazine in the dog, with special reference to circulating splanchnic blood volume. Amer. J. Physiol. **183**, 144—148 (1955).

MCCOY, F. W., LEACH, W. J.: Experimental attempt to produce the L-E syndrome (arthritis) in swine with hydrazinophthalazine. Proc. Soc. exp. Biol. (N. Y.) **101**, 183—186 (1959).

MCISAAC, W. M., KANDA, M.: The metabolism of 1-hydrazinophthalazine. J. Pharmacol. exp. Ther. **143**, 7—13 (1964).

MCNICOL, M. W., HUTCHISON, H. E.: Severe toxic reaction to hydralazine. Lancet **1956 II**, 1288.

MEIER, M., HEDWALL, P. R., BRUNNER, H.: Beeinflussung der Wirkungen von Hydralazin durch Beta-Blockade. Naunyn-Schmiedebergs Arch. exp. Path. Pharmak. **251**, 131—132 (1965a).

MEIER, M., HEDWALL, P. R., BRUNNER, H.: Wirkungen von Hydralazin und Propranolol auf Coronardurchblutung und Sauerstoffverbrauch des Myokard. Helv. physiol. Acta **23**, C36—C38 (1965b).

MEIER, R., TRIPOD, J., BRÜNL, C.: Änderung der blutdrucksenkenden Wirkung von Apresolin und Nepresol durch Reaktion mit Serumbestandteilen. Naunyn-Schmiedebergs Arch. exp. Path. Pharmak. **223**, 338—341 (1954).

MEIER, R., GROSS, F., TRIPOD, J., TURRIAN, H.: Pharmakologische Charakterisierung von synthetischem Hypertensin. Experientia (Basel) **13**, 361—362 (1957).

MEIER, R., TRIPOD, J., WIRZ, E.: Classification d'une série d'antagonistes de la serotonine et analyse de ses points d'attaque vasculaires périphériques. Arch. int. Pharmacodyn. **117**, 185—196 (1958).

Mellander, S., Johansson, B.: Control of resistance, exchange, and capacitance functions in the peripheral circulation. Pharmacol. Rev. **20**, 117—196 (1968).
Merrill, D. H., Kenyon, K.: 1-Hydrazinophthalazine (Apresoline) in the treatment of hypertensive disease: a clinical trial with a control group. Amer. J. med. Sci. **226**, 623—631 (1953).
Miller, A. J., Abrams, D. L., Kaplan, B. M.: Persistent reversal of severe systemic hypertension after prolonged toxic reaction to hydralazine. Cardiology **60**, 251—256 (1975).
Möllerberg, H.: Attempts to produce the "hydralazine syndrome" in the albino rat. Acta med. scand. **161**, 443—445 (1958).
Monier, J. C.: Collagenose posthydralazinique chez le rat. Algerie Med. **64**, 421 (1960).
Moore-Jones, D., Perry, H. M., Jr.: Radioautographic localization of hydralazine-1-C^{14} in arterial walls. Proc. Soc. exp. Biol. (N. Y.) **122**, 576—579 (1966).
Morrow, J. D., Schroeder, H. A., Perry, H. M., Jr.: Studies on the control of hypertension by Hyphex. II Toxic reactions and side effects. Circulation **8**, 829—839 (1953).
Moyer, J. H.: Hydralazine (Apresoline) hydrochloride: pharmacological observations and clinical results in the therapy of hypertension. Arch. intern. Med. **91**, 419—439 (1953).
Moyer, J. H., Brest, A. N.: Hydralazine in the treatment of hypertension. Med. Clin. N. Amer. **45**, 375 (1961).
Moyer, J. H., Handley, C. A., Huggins, R. A.: Some pharmacodynamic effects of 1-hydrazinophthalazine (C 5968) with particular reference to renal function and cardiovascular response. J. Pharmacol. exp. Ther. **103**, 368—376 (1951).
Moyer, J. H., Huggins, R. A., Handley, C. A.: Further cardiovascular and renal hemodynamic studies following the administration of hydralazine (1-hydrazinophthalazine) and the effect of ganglionic blockade with hexamethonium on these responses. J. Pharmacol. exp. Ther. **109**, 175—182 (1953).
Muller, J. C., Rast, C. L., Jr., Pryor, W. W., Orgain, E. S.: Late systemic complications of hydralazine (apresoline) therapy. J. Amer. med. Ass. **157**, 894—899 (1955).
Nagaoka, A., Kikuchi, K., Aramaki, Y.: Depressor responses to the spontaneously hypertensive rats to the antihypertensive agents. Jap. J. Pharmacol. **19**, 401 (1969).
Page, I. H.: Treatment of essential and malignant hypertension. J. Amer. med. Ass. **147**, 1311—1318 (1951).
Page, J. H., McCubbin, J. W.: Renal vascular and systemic arterial pressure responses to nervous and chemical stimulation of the kidney. Amer. J. Physiol. **173**, 411—420 (1953).
Page, I. H., Dustan, H. P.: Editorial. Persistence of normal blood pressure after discontinuing treatment in hypertensive patients. Circulation **25**, 433—436 (1962).
Paz, M. A., Seifter, S.: Immunological studies of collagens modified by reaction with hydralazine. Amer. J. med. Sci. **263**, 281—290 (1972).
Perry, H. M., Jr.: Method of quantitating 1-hydrazinophthalazine in body fluids. J. Lab. clin. Med. **41**, 566—573 (1953).
Perry, H. M.: Late toxicity to hydralazine resembling systemic lupus erythematosus or rheumatoid arthritis. Amer. J. Med. **54**, 58—72 (1973).
Perry, H. M., Camel, G. H.: Guanethidine: Some pharmacologic and clinical observations. In: Symposium on Guanethidine (Ismelin), Ciba, Basel. Sponsored by the University of Tennessee, Memphis, 1960, pp. 69—74.
Perry, H. M., Jr., Schroeder, H. A.: A syndrome simulating collagen disease caused by 1-hydrazinophthalazine (apresoline). J. Amer. med. Ass. **154**, 670—673 (1954).
Perry, H. M., Schroeder, H. A.: Studies on the control of hypertension. VI. Some evidence for the reversal of the process during hexamethonium and hydralazine therapy. Circulation **13**, 528—536 (1956).
Perry, H. M., Jr., Schroeder, H. A., Morrow, J. D.: Studies on the control of hypertension by Hyphex. IV. Levels of the agents in urine and blood. Amer. med. Sci. **228**, 405—416 (1954).
Perry, H. M., Jr., Comen, P., Yunice, A.: Distribution of hydralazine-1-C^{14} after injection into normal mice. J. Lab. clin. Med. **59**, 456—461 (1962).
Perry, H. M., Jr., Schroeder, H. A., Latanzaro, F. J., Moore-Jones, D., Camel, G. H.: Studies on the control of hypertension. VIII. Mortality, morbidity, and remissions during twelve years of intensive therapy. Circulation **33**, 958—972 (1966).
Pifferi, G., Parravicini, F., Carpi, C., Dorigotti, L.: Synthesis and antihypertensive properties of new 3-hydrazinopyridazines. J. med. Chem. **18**, 741—746 (1975).
Pigeon, G., Genest, J.: Prolonged hydralazine hydrochloride administration in 132 hypertensive patients—study of toxicity. Canad. med. Ass. J. **83**, 743—746 (1960).
Raskin, N. H., Fishman, R. A.: Pyridoxine-deficiency neuropathy due to hydralazine. New Engl. J. Med. **273**, 1182—1185 (1965).
Reidenberg, M. M., Drayer, D., DeMano, A. L., Bello, C. T.: Hydralazine elimination in man. Clin. Pharmacol. Ther. **14**, 970—977 (1973).
Reinhardt, D. J., Waldun, J. M.: Lupus erythematosus-like syndrome complicating hydralazine (apresoline) therapy. J. Amer. med. Ass. **155**, 1491—1492 (1954).

REIS, M. E., VAN ZWIETEN, P. A.: Hypotensive effect of hydralazine, injected into the vertebral artery of the cat. Arch. int. Pharmacodyn. **169**, 494—499 (1967).
REUBI, F. C.: Renal hyperemia induced in man by a new phthalazine derivative. Proc. Soc. exp. Biol. (N. Y.) **73**, 102—103 (1950a).
REUBI, F. C.: Le flux sanguin rénal. Aspects physiopathologiques, cliniques et thérapeutiques. Helv. med. Acta **17**, Suppl. 26, 9—108 (1950b).
REUTTER, F.: Die Behandlung der akuten Blutdruckkrise. Ther. Umsch. **22**, 49—53 (1965).
REYNOLDS, H., CALDWELL, J. R.: Hydralazine syndrome, hypersensitivity or toxicity? Its significance in understanding of collagen disease. J. Amer. med. Ass. **165**, 1823—1826 (1957).
REZA, M. J., DORNFELD, L., GOLDBERG, L. S.: Hydralazine therapy in hypertensive patients with idiopathic systemic lupus erythematosus. Arthr. Rheum. **18**, 335—338 (1975).
ROWE, G. G., HUSTON, J. H., MAXWELL, G. M., CROSLEY, A. P., JR., CRUMPTON, C. W.: Hemodynamic effects of 1-hydrazinophthalazine in patients with arterial hypertension. J. clin. Invest. **34**, 115—120 (1955).
SANNERSTEDT, R., STENBERG, J., JOHNSSON, G., WERKÖ, L.: Hemodynamic interference of alprenolol with dihydralazine in normal and hypertensive man. Amer. J. Cardiol. **28**, 316—320 (1971).
SANNERSTEDT, R., STENBERG, J., VEDIN, A., WILHELMSSON, C., WERKÖ, L.: Chronic beta adrenergic blockade in arterial hypertension. Hemodynamic influences of dihydralazine and dynamic exercise and clinical effects of combined treatment. Amer. J. Cardiol. **29**, 718—723 (1972).
SANO, J., TANIGUCHI, K., GAMO, T., TAKESADA, M., KAKIMOTO, Y.: Die Katechinamine im Zentralnervensystem. Klin. Wschr. **38**, 57—62 (1960).
SARDI, A., CARAVAGGI, A. M., BALDONI, E.: Hemodynamic activity of L 6150. Systemic and coronary circulation. Naunyn-Schmiedebergs Arch. Pharmacol. **279**, 301—312 (1973).
SCHAPER, W. K. A., JAGENEAU, A. H. M.: Der Einfluß blutdrucksenkender Substanzen auf Elektrocardiogramm, Blutdruck und Herzfrequenz nicht narkotisierter Hunde. Arzneimittel-Forsch. **11**, 1102—1106 (1961).
SCHAUB, F., NAGER, F., SCHRITHIN, W., VÖLLM, K., HANY, A.: Der heutige Stand der Hypertoniebehandlung. Schweiz. med. Wschr. **94**, 769—775, 803—810 (1964).
SCHMID, A., KELLNER, H.: Kreislaufveränderungen unter Apresolin und ihre Bedeutung für die Frage der Blutdruckregulation. Cardiologia (Basel) **23**, 349—358 (1953).
SCHMITT, H., GICQUEL, J.: Action de l'hydrazinophthalazine (C 5968) et de la dihydrazino-1,4-phthalazine (C 7448) sur les centres vasomoteurs. Arch. int. Pharmacodyn. **105**, 269—278 (1956).
SCHROEDER, H. A.: Effects on hypertension of sulfhydryl and hydrazine compounds. J. clin. Invest. **30**, 672—673 (1951).
SCHROEDER, H. A.: The effect of 1-hydrazinophthalazine in hypertension. Circulation **5**, 28—37 (1952a).
SCHROEDER, H. A.: Control of hypertension by hexamethonium and 1-hydrazino-phthalazine (apresoline) in hypertensive subjects: preliminary observations. Arch. intern. Med. **89**, 523—540 (1952b).
SCHROEDER, H. A.: Hypertensive Disease. Cause and Control, p. 474. Philadelphia: Lea and Febiger 1953.
SCHROEDER, H. A.: Mechanism of Hypertension, p. 122. Springfield, Ill.: Charles C. Thomas 1957.
SCHROEDER, H. A.: The pharmacology of hydralazine. In: MOYER, H. (Ed.): Hypertension. The First Hahnemann Symposium on Hypertensive Disease, pp. 332—344. Philadelphia-London: Saunders 1959.
SCHROEDER, H. A., PERRY, H. M., JR.: Survival rates in severe hypertension intensively treated with hydralazine and ganglionic blockade. In: BOCK, K. D., COTTIER, P. (Eds.): Essential Hypertension, pp. 307—316. Berlin-Göttingen-Heidelberg: Springer 1960.
SCHROEDER, H. A., MORROW, J. D., PERRY, H. M., JR.: Studies on the control of hypertension by hyphex. I. Effects on blood pressure. Circulation **8**, 672—680 (1953).
SCHULER, W., MEIER, R.: Vergleich der aminooxydasehemmenden und der blutdrucksenkenden Wirkung von Hydrazinophthalazine. Helv. physiol. Acta **13**, 106—112 (1955).
SCHULER, W., WYSS, E.: Specificity of the in vitro action of antihypertensive hydralazine derivatives antagonistic to reserpine on the enzyme and metal catalysis of biogenous amines. Arch. int. Pharmacodyn. **128**, 431—468 (1960).
SCHULERT, A. R.: Physiological disposition of hydralazine (1-hydrazinophthalazine) and a method for its determination in biological fluids. Arch. int. Pharmacodyn. **132**, 1—15 (1961).
SHACKMAN, N. H., SWILLER, A. I., MORRISON, M.: Syndrome simulating acute disseminated lupus erythematosus. Appearance after hydralazine ((apresoline) therapy. J. Amer. med. Ass. **155**, 1492—1494 (1954).

SIEGEL, M., LEE, S. L., PERESS, N. S.: The epidemiology of drug-induced systemic lupus erythematosus. Arthr. Rheum. **10**, 407—415 (1967).

SIGUIER, F., BÉTOURNÉ, C., BONNET DE LA TOUR, J.: Le lupus érythémateux hydralazinique. Sem. Hôp. Paris **34**, 773—784 (1958).

SLONIM, N. B.: Arthralgia, headache, prostration and fever during hydralazine therapy. J. Amer. med. Ass. **154**, 1419 (1954).

STEIN, D. H., HECHT, H. H.: Cardiovascular and renal responses to the combination of hexamethonium and 1-hydrazinophthalazine ((apresoline) in hypertensive patients. J. clin. Invest. **34**, 867—874 (1955).

STUNKARD, A., WERTHEIMER, L., REDISH, W.: Studies on hydralazine, evidence for a peripheral site of action. J. clin. Invest. **33**, 1047—1053 (1954).

TANGRI, K. K., BHARGAVA, K. P.: The central hypotensive action of 1-hydrazinophthalazine (C 5968). Arch. int. Pharmacodyn. **125**, 331—342 (1960).

TAYLOR, R. D., DUSTAN, H. P., LORCORAN, A. C., PAGE, I. H.: Evaluation of 1-hydrazinophthalazine (apresoline) in treatment of hypertensive disease. Arch. intern. Med. **90**, 734—749 (1952).

TRIPOD, J., MEIER, R.: Détermination et classification pharmacodynamique de l'action vasculaire périphérique de l'Apresoline, du Nepresol et du Serpasil. Arch. int. Pharmacodyn. **99**, 104—125 (1954).

TRIPOD, J., MEIER, R.: Charakterisierung des pharmakodynamischen Wirkungsspektrums blutdrucksenkender Stoffe. Naunyn-Schmiedebergs Arch. exp. Path. Pharmak. **232**, 470—480 (1958).

UEDA, H., YAGI, S., KANEKO, Y.: Hydralazine and plasma renin activity. Arch. intern. Med. **122**, 387—391 (1968).

WAGNER, J.: Pharmacokinetics and metabolism of hydralazine: Specific affinity for blood vessels. Experientia (Basel) **29**, 767 (1973).

WAGNER, J., HEDWALL, P.: Correlation between the pharmacokinetics and the hypotensive action of hydralazine in the rat. Naunyn Schmiedebergs Arch. Pharmacol. **274**, R 122 (1972).

WAGNER, J., HEDWALL, P.: Pharmacokinetics and pharmacological action of vasodilators. International Symposium on Hypertension, Monte Carlo 1975, MILLIEZ, P., SAFAR, M. (Eds.), Vol. 2, pp. 331—342.

WALKER, H. A., WILSON, S., ATKINS, E. C., GARRETT, H. E., RICHARDSON, A. P.: The effect of 1-hydrazinophthalazine (C 5968) and related compounds on the cardiovascular system of dogs. J. Pharmacol. exp. Ther. **101**, 368—378 (1951).

WERKÖ, L.: The place of β-adrenergic blocking drugs in the treatment of mild to moderate arterial hypertension. In: BERGLUND, G., HANSSON, L., WERKÖ, L (Eds.): Pathophysiology and Management of Arterial Hypertension, pp. 228—233. Göteborg: Astra 1975.

WERLE, E., SCHAUER, A., HARTUNG, G.: Einfluß von Hydrazin- und Guanylhydrazinderivaten auf die Aktivität der Monaminoxydase, Diaminoxydase, Dopadecarboxylase und Histidindecarboxylase. Klin. Wschr. **33**, 562—567 (1955).

WESTER, A., ZAAL, G. A., DELEEUW, P. W., BIRKENHÄGER, W. H.: Haemodynamic and endocrinological changes during antihypertensive treatment with a new vasodilator substance (L6150) and propranolol. Clin. Sci. Molec. Med. **51**, Suppl. 3, 605s—607s, 1976.

WESTER, P. O.: The urinary excretion of trace elements before and during treatment with hydralazine. Acta med. scand. **197**, 307—309 (1975).

WILKINSON, E. L., BACKMAN, H., HECHT, H. H.: Cardiovascular and renal adjustments to a hypotensive agent (1-hydrazinophthalazine: Ciba Ba 5968, apresoline). J. clin. Invest. **31**, 872—879 (1952).

YONKMAN, F. F., FREIS, E. D.: Rational elimination of side reactions and/or tolerance in the development of potentially valuable drugs. Angiology **3**, 36—41 (1952).

ZACEST, R., KOCH-WESER, J.: Relation of hydralazine plasma concentration to dosage and hypotensive action. Clin. pharmacol. Ther. **13**, 420—425 (1972).

ZACEST, R., STANLEY, P. E.: The influence of acetylation phenotype on plasma hydralazine levels in man following oral and intravenous administration. Recent Advances in Hypertension, pp. 343—350 (1975). MILLIEZ, P., SAFAR, M., (Eds.): Boehringer Ingelheim

ZACEST, R., GILMORE, E., KOCH-WESER, J.: Treatment of essential hypertension with combined vasodilation and beta-adrenergic blockade. New Engl. J. Med. **286**, 617—622 (1972).

ZAK, S. B., GILLERAN, T. G., KARLINER, J., LUKAS, G.: Identification of two new metabolites of hydralazine from human urine. J. med. Chem. **17**, 381—382 (1974a).

ZAK, S. B., BARTLETT, M. F., WAGNER, W. E., GILLERAN, T. G., LUKAS, G.: Disposition of hydralazine in man and a specific method for its determination in biological fluids. J. pharm. Sci. **63**, 225—229 (1974b).

ZAK, S. B., LUKAS, G., GILLERAN, T. G.: Plasma levels of real and "apparent" hydralazine in man and rat. Drug Metab. Dispos. **5**, 116—121, 1977.

ZBINDEN, G.: Progress in Toxicology. Special Topics. Vol. 2, p. 80. Berlin-Heidelberg-New York: Springer 1976.
ZIMMER, H., MCMANUS, J., NOVINSON, T., HESS, E. V., LITWIN, A. H.: A major metabolite of 1-hydrazinophthalazine. Arzneimittel-Forsch. **20**, 1586—1587 (1970).
ZIMMER, H., KOKOSA, J., GARTRIZ, D. A.: Identification of 3-methyl-s-triazolo[3,4-a]phthalazine, a human hydralazine metabolite, by gas chromatography—mass spectrometry. Arzneumittel-Forsch. **23**, 1028—1029 (1973).
ZIMMER, H., GLASER, R., KOKOSA, J.: 3-hydroxymethyl-s-triazolo [3,4-a]phthalazine, a novel urinary hydralazine metabolite in man. J. med. Chem. **18**, 1031—1033 (1975).
ZWIETEN, A. VAN: Pharmakologische und biochemische Wirkungen von Hydralazin und Dihydralazin. Arzneimittel-Forsch. **18**, 79—84 (1968).

Section III Nitroprusside

ADAMS, A. P., CLARKE, T. N. S., EDMONDS-SEAL, J., FÖEX, P., PRYS-ROBERTS, C., ROBERTS, J.: Effects of sodium nitroprusside on myocardial contractility and haemodynamics. Brit. J. Anaesth. **45**, 120 (1973).
ADAMS, A. P., CLARKE, T. N. S., EDMONDS-SEAL, J., FÖEX, P., PRYS-ROBERTS, C., ROBERTS, J. G.: The effects of sodium nitroprusside on myocardial contractility and haemodynamics. Brit. J. Anaesth. **46**, 807—817 (1974).
AHEARN, D. J., GRIM, C. E.: Treatment of malignant hypertension with sodium nitroprusside. Arch. intern. Med. **133**, 187—191 (1974).
AMA Committee on Hypertension: The treatment of malignant hypertension and hypertensive emergencies. J. Amer. med. Ass. **228**, 1673—1679 (1974).
AMARANATH, L., KELLERMEYER, W. F.: Tachyphylaxis to sodium nitroprusside. Anesthesiology **44**, 345—348 (1976).
ANDERSON, R. A., RAE, W.: Stability of sodium nitroprusside solutions. Aust. J. pharm. Sci. NS **1**, 45—46 (1972).
BARON, G., KREYE, V. A. W.: Effects of drugs on ^{45}Ca uptake by isolated vascular smooth muscle membranes. Pflügers Arch. **343**, R54 (1973).
BASTRON, R. D., KALOYANIDES, G. J.: Effect of sodium nitroprusside on function in the isolated intact dog kidney. J. Pharmacol. exp. Ther. **181**, 244—249 (1972).
BHATIA, S. K., FROHLICH, E. D.: Hemodynamic comparison of agents useful in hypertensive emergencies. Amer. Heart J. **85**, 367—373 (1973).
BLEIFELD, W., HANRATH, P.: Die hämodynamische Basis der Therapie des akuten Myokardinfarktes. Dtsch. med. Wschr. **100**, 1345—1350 (1975).
BOEV, K., GOLENHOFEN, K., LUKANOW, J.: Selective suppression of phasic and tonic activation mechanisms in stomach smooth muscle. In: BÜLBRING, E., SHUBA, F. (Eds.): Physiology of Smooth Muscle, pp. 203—208. New York: Raven Press 1976.
BOWER, P. J., PETERSON, J. N.: Methemoglobinemia after sodium nitroprusside therapy. New Engl. J. Med. **293**, 865 (1975).
BREEMEN, C. VAN: Transmembrane calcium transport. Second Int. Symposium on Vascular Neuroeffector Mechanisms, Odense, Denmark, 1975. Abstract in: Blood Vessels **12**/6, Nr. 4, 1975.
BURKE, D. H., MANN, D. E.: Influence of several autonomic drugs on sodium nitroprusside and oxotremorine-induced hypothermia in immature and mature mice. J. pharm. Sci. **59**, 1814—1818 (1970).
CARLINER, N. H., DENUNE, D. P., FINCH, C. S., JR., GOLDBERG, L. I.: Sodium nitroprusside treatment of ergotamine-induced peripheral ischemia. J. Amer. med. Ass. **227**, 308—309 (1974).
CASINELLI, C. M.: La accion hipotensora del nitroprusiato aplicaciones terapéuticas. An. Fac. Med. (Lima) **39**, 1330—1331 (1956).
CAUJOLLE, F., PHAM HUU CHANH, LECONTE, P.: Pharmacologie du nitrosopentacyanoferrate-III de cobalt. Arch. int. Pharmacodyn. **172**, 487—495 (1968).
CHATTERJEE, K., PARMLEY, W. W., GANZ, W., FORRESTER, J., WALINSKY, P., CREXELLS, C., SWAN, H. J. C.: Hemodynamic and metabolic responses to vasodilator therapy in acute myocardial infarction. Circulation **48**, 1183—1193 (1973).
COHN, J. N., FRANCIOSA, J. A., NOTARGIACOMO, V. A.: Nitroprusside and dobutamine effect on myocardial oxygen supply/demand in experimental myocardial infarction. Circulation, Suppl. to **49/50**, III-103 (1974).
DAVIDSOHN, K.: Versuche über die Wirkung des Nitroprussidnatriums. Diss., Albertus-Universität, Königsberg, Prussia, 1887.
DAVIES, D. W., KADAR, D., STEWARD, D. J., MUNRO, I. R.: A sudden death associated with the use of sodium nitroprusside for induction of hypotension during anaesthesia. Canad. Anaesth. Soc. J. **22**, 547—552 (1975a).

DAVIES, D. W., GREISS, L., KADAR, D., STEWARD, D. J.: Sodium nitroprusside in children: observations on metabolism during normal and abnormal responses. Canad. Anaesth. Soc. J. **22**, 553—560 (1975b).
EPPENS, H.: Sodium nitroprusside in hypotensive anaesthesia. Brit. J. Anaesth. **45**, 124 (1973).
FORRESTER, J. S., CHATTERJEE, K., SWAN, J. C.: Hemodynamic monitoring in patients with acute myocardial infarction. J. Amer. med. Ass. **226**, 60—61 (1973).
FRANCIOSA, J. A., GUIHA, N. H., LIMAS, C. J., RODRIGUERA, E., COHN, J. N.: Improved left ventricular function during nitroprusside infusion in acute myocardial infarction. Lancet **1972 I**, 650—654.
FRANCIOSA, J. A., AKHTAR, N., NOTARGIACOMO, A., COHN, J. N.: Hemodynamic and metabolic response to nitroprusside infusion in experimental acute myocardial infarction. Circulation, Suppl. to VII and VIII, IV-169 (1973).
GIFFORD, R. W., JR.: Treatment of hypertensive emergencies associated with essential hypertension. In: MOYER, J. (Ed.): Hypertension. The First Hahnemann Symposium on Hypertensive Disease, pp. 615—622. Philadelphia: W. B. Saunders Comp. 1959.
GIFFORD, R. W., JR.: Hypertensive emergencies and their treatment. Med. clin. N. Amer. **45**, 441—452 (1961).
GLUSA, E., MARKWARDT, F., STUERZEBECHER, J.: Effects of sodium nitroprusside and other pentacyanonitrosyl complexes on platelet aggregation. Haemostasis **3**, 249—256 (1974).
GOLDSTEIN, F., RIEDERS, F.: Conversion of thiocyanate to cyanide by an erythrocytic enzyme. Amer. J. Physiol. **173**, 287—290 (1953).
GOLENHOFEN, K.: Theory of P and T systems for calcium activation in smooth muscle. In: BÜLBRING, E., SHUBA, F. (Eds.): Physiology of Smooth Muscle, pp. 197—202. New York: Raven Press 1976.
GRIFFITHS, D. P. G., CUMMINS, B. H., GREENBAUM, R., GRIFFITH, H. B., STADDON, G. E., WILKINS, D. G., ZORAB, J. S. M.: Cerebral blood flow and metabolism during hypotension induced with sodium nitroprusside. Brit. J. Anaesth. **46**, 671 (1974).
GUIHA, N. H., LIMAS, C. J., FRANCIOSA, J. A., COHN, J. N.: Treatment of refractory heart failure with sodium nitroprusside. Circulation **46**, Suppl. II, 105 (1972).
HÄUSLER, G.: The effects of sodium nitroprusside (SNP) on vascular smooth muscle. Experientia (Basel) **31**, 729 (1975).
HÄUSLER, G., THORENS, S.: Pharmacology of vasoactive antihypertensives. In: BEVAN, J. A., BURNSTOCK, G., JOHANSSON, B., MAXWELL, R. A., NEDERGAARD, O. A. (Eds.): Vascular Neuroeffector Mechanims, pp. 232—241. Basel: Karger 1976.
HERMANN, L.: Über die Wirkung des Nitroprussidnatriums. Pflügers Arch. ges. Physiol. **39**, 419 (1886).
HILL, H. E.: A contribution to the toxicology of sodium nitroprusside. 1. The decomposition and determination of sodium nitroprusside. Aust. chem. Inst. J. Proc. **9**, 89 (1942).
HILTON, J. G.: Effects of sodium nitroprusside on blood pressure responses to epinephrine. Amer. J. Physiol. **196**, 738—740 (1959).
HILTON, J. G., TUMLINSON, W. B.: Effect of sodium nitroprusside on blood pressure responses to histamine. Amer. J. Physiol. **199**, 325—327 (1960).
HÖBEL, M., RAITHELHUBER, A.: Separation of sodium nitroprusside metabolites by thin-layer chromatography (TLC). Naunyn Schmiedebergs Arch. Pharmacol., Suppl. to **282**, R 33 (1974).
HÖBEL, M., RAITHELHUBER, A.: Untersuchungen über den Stoffwechsel und die Organverteilung von ^{14}C-markiertem Natrium-Nitroprussid an Ratten. Arzneimittel-Forsch. **26**, 11, 2015—2019, (1976).
HÖBEL, M., ANWEILER, J., RAITHELHUBER, A.: Sodium nitroprusside: Degradation in ox and human blood, distribution in rat organs and excretion in urine and feces of the rat. Naunyn Schmiedebergs Arch. Pharmacol., Suppl. to **287**, R 81 (1975).
JACK, R. D.: Toxicity of sodium nitroprusside. Brit. J. Anaesth. **46**, 952 (1974).
JOHNSON, C. C.: The actions and toxicity of sodium nitroprusside. Arch. int. Pharmacodyn. **35**, 480—496 (1929).
JUNG, F., PETSCH, G.: Über die hypotensive Wirkung von Pentacyanoferraten, insbesondere von Nitroprussid-Natrium. Acta biol. med. germ. **19**, 781—783 (1967).
KANEKO, Y., IKEDA, T., TAKEDA, T., UEDA, H.: Renin release during acute reduction of arterial pressure in normotensive subjects and patients with renovascular hypertension. J. clin. Invest. **46**, 705—716 (1967).
KATZ, R. L., WOLF, C. E.: Sodium nitroprusside for controlled hypotension and hypertensive emergencies. In: MARK, L. C., NGAI, S. H. (Eds.): Highlights of Clinical Anesthesiology, pp. 48—54. New York: Harper & Row 1971.
KOMAREK, J., MANSFELD, C.: Der Einfluß von Natriumnitroprussid auf das Kreislaufsystem, myokardiale Dynamik, Kontraktilität und Sauerstoffverbrauch des linken Ventrikels beim Hund. Herz/Kreisl. 8, 15—21 (1976).
KREYE, V. A. W.: The action of sodium nitroprusside on isolated smooth muscle. Fifth Int. Congress on Pharmacology, San Francisco, 1972. Abstracts of Volunteer Papers, p. 130.

Kreye, V. A. W.: Untersuchungen zum zellulären Wirkungsmechanismus vasodilatorischer Pharmaka unter besonderer Berücksichtigung von Natrium-Nitroprussid. Thesis, University of Heidelberg, 1974.
Kreye, V. A. W.: Inhibition of nitroprusside-induced relaxation of isolated vascular smooth muscle by cyanide. Cause of clinical tachyphylaxis? Naunyn Schmiedebergs Arch. Pharmacol. **297**, Suppl. II, R30 (1977a).
Kreye, V. A. W.: Organic nitrates, sodium nitroprusside and vasodilation. In: Vanhoutte, P. M., Leusen, I. (Eds.) Mechanisms of vasodilatation. Basel, S. Karger, 1977b, in press:
Kreye, V. A. W., Lüth, J. B.: Effect of sodium nitroprusside, temperature, and calcium withdrawal on the relaxation speed of vascular smooth muscle. In: Betz, E. (Ed.) Ionic actions on vascular smooth muscle. Berlin-Heidelberg-New York, pp. 145—149, Springer, 1976.
Kreye, V. A. W., Baron, G. D., Lüth, J. B., Schmidt-Gayk, H.: Mode of action of sodium nitroprusside on vascular smooth muscle. Naunyn Schmiedebergs Arch. Pharmacol. **288**, 381—402 (1975).
Kreye, V. A. W., Raithelhuber, A., Höbel, M.: Sodium nitroprusside toxicity and antidotes. Naunyn Schmiedebergs Arch. Pharmacol., Suppl. to **293**, R264 (1976).
Kyncl, J.: Circulatory effects of sodium nitroprusside. Naunyn Schmiedebergs Arch. Pharmacol. **269**, 390—391 (1971).
Lang, K.: Die Rhodanbildung im Tierkörper. Biochem. Z. **259**, 243 (1933).
Lowson, J. A.: Correspondence. Sodium nitroprusside in hypotensive anaesthesia. Brit. J. Anaesth. **44**, 908 (1972).
Luka, N. L., Kumazawa, T., Merin, R.: Myocardial hemodynamic and metabolic response to sodium nitroprusside. Circulation, Suppl. to **49/50**, III-189 (1974).
Da Luz, P. L., Forrester, J. S., Wyatt, H. L., Tyberg, J. V., Chagrasulis, R., Parmley, W. W., Swan, H. J. C.: Simultaneous improvement in ischemic function and metabolism by nitroprusside. Circulation, Suppl. to **49/50**, III—102 (1974).
MacRae, W. R.: Induced hypotension for middle ear surgery. Proc. roy. Soc. Med. **64**, 1223—1224 (1971).
Mani, M. K.: Nitroprusside revisited. Brit. med. J. **1971 III**, 107—108.
McDowall, D. G., Keaney, N. P., Turner, J. M., Lane, J. R., Okuda, Y.: The toxicity of sodium nitroprusside. Brit. J. Anaesth. **46**, 327—332 (1974).
Merrifield, A. L., Blundell, M. D.: Toxicity of nitroprusside. Brit. J. Anaesth. **46**, 324 (1974).
Miller, F. N., Van Maanen, E. F.: Cardiovascular effects of sodium nitroprusside in the dog. Pharmacologist **10**, 156 (1968).
Moraca, P. P., Bitte, E. M., Hale, D. E., Wasmuth, C. E., Poutasse, E. F.: Clinical evaluation of sodium nitroprusside as a hypotensive agent. Anesthesiology **23**, 193—199 (1962).
Mueller, H., Evans, R., Religa, A., Farmelant, M., Ayres, S.: Nitroprusside effect on cardiac perfusion and metabolism in myocardial infarction. Circulation, Suppl. to **49/50** III-194 (1974a).
Mueller, H., Religa, A., Evans, R., Ayres, S.: Metabolic changes in ischemic myocardium by nitroprusside. Amer. J. Cardiol. **33**, 158 (1974b).
Mukherjee, D., Feldman, M. S., Helfant, R. H.: Nitroprusside therapy. Treatment of hypertensive patients with recurrent resting chest pain, ST-segment elevation, and ventricular arrhythmias. J. Amer. med. Ass. **235**, 2406—2409 (1976).
Nourok, D. S., Gwinup, G., Hamwi, G. J.: Phentolamine-resistant pheochromocytoma treated with sodiumnitro prusside. J. Amer. med. Ass. **183**, 841—844 (1963).
Nourok, D. S., Glassock, R. J., Solomon, D. H., Maxwell, M. H.: Hypothyroidism following prolonged sodium nitroprusside therapy. Amer. J. med. Sci. **248**, 129 (1964).
Page, I. H., Corcoran, A. C., Dustan, H. P., Koppanyi, T.: Cardiovascular actions of sodium nitroprusside in animals and hypertensive patients. Circulation **11**, 188—198 (1955).
Palmer, R. F., Lasseter, K. C.: Medical intelligence/drug therapy/sodium nitroprusside. New Engl. J. Med. **292**, 294—297 (1975).
Parade, D.: Die Behandlung der hypertonen Krise mit Natriumnitroprussid. Med. Welt **23**, 373—375 (1972).
Parmley, W. W., Chatterjee, K., Charuzi, Y., Swan, H. J. C.: Hemodynamic effects of noninvasive systolic unloading (nitroprusside) and diastolic augementation (external counterpulsation) in patients with acute myocardial infarction. Amer. J. Cardiol. **33**, 819—825 (1974).
Playfair, L.: On the Nitroprussides: A New Class of Salts. London: RJE Taylor 1849.
Posner, M. A., Rodkey, F. L. Tobey, R. E.: Nitroprusside-induced cyanide poisoning: Antidotal effect of hydroxocobalamine. Anesthesiology **44**, 330—335 (1976).
Raithelhuber, A., Höbel, M.: Sodium nitroprusside: Metabolism, distribution and excretion in rats. Naunyn Schmiedebergs Arch. Pharmacol. **293**, Suppl. R54 (1976).
Reske, S. N.: Untersuchung zur Pharmakokinetik von Natrium-Nitroprussid. Dissertation, Heidelberg, 1976.

Robie, N. W., McNay, J. L.: Comparative regional blood flow effects of minoxidil and nitroprusside. Pharmacology **33**, 583 (1974).
Ross, G., Cole, P. V.: Some cardiovascular actions of sodium nitroprusside in the dog. Brit. J. Anaesth. **45**, 120 (1973a).
Ross, G., Cole, P. V.: Cardiovascular actions of sodium nitroprusside in dogs. Anaesthesia **28**, 400—406 (1973b).
Rowe, G. G., Henderson, R. H.: Systemic and coronary hemodynamic effects of sodium nitroprusside. Amer. Heart J. **87**, 83—87 (1974).
Schiffmann, H., Fuchs, P.: Controlled hypotension effected by sodium nitroprusside. Acta anaesth. scand. **23**, Suppl., 704—709 (1966).
Schlant, R. C., Tsagaris, T. S., Robertson, R. J., Jr.: Studies on the acute cardiovascular effects of intravenous sodium nitroprusside. Amer. J. Cardiol. **9**, 51—59 (1962).
Sheps, S. G.: Hypertensive crisis. Postgrad. med. **49**, 95—99 (1971).
Siegel, P., Moraca, P. P., Green, J. R.: Sodium nitroprusside in the surgical treatment of cerebral aneurysms and arteriovenous malformations. Brit. J. Anaesth. **43**, 790 (1971).
Smith, R. P., Kruszyna, H.: Nitroprusside produces cyanide poisoning via a reaction with hemoglobin. J. Pharmacol. exp. Ther. **191**, 557—563 (1974).
Stinson, E. B., Holloway, E. L., Derby, G. R. N., Oyer, P. E., Hollingsworth, J., Griepp, R. B., Harrison, D. C.: Comparative hemodynamic responses to chlorpromazine, nitroprusside, nitroglycerin, and trimethaphan immediately after open-heart operations. Circulation, Suppl. I to **51/52**, 26—33 (1975).
Styles, M., Coleman, A. J., Leary, W. P.: The hemodynamic effects of sodium nitroprusside. Anesthesiology **38**, 173—176 (1973).
Taylor, T. H., Styles, M., Lamming, A. J.: Sodium nitroprusside as a hypotensive agent in general anaesthesia. Brit. J. Anaesth. **42**, 859—864 (1970).
Thienes, C. H.: Altered responses of smooth muscle to autonomic drugs produced by physical and chemical changes. Arch. int. Pharmacodyn. **31**, 447—500 (1926).
Tountas, C. J., Georgopoulos, A. J., Kyriakou, K. V., Marselos, A. A.: The effect of sodium nitroprusside on coronary circulation. J. cardiovasc. Surg. **6**, 100—103 (1965).
Tuzel, I.: Sodium nitroprusside: A review of its clinical effectiveness as a hypotensive agent. J. clin. Pharmacol. **14**, 494—503 (1974).
Verhaege, R. H., Shepherd, J. T.: Effect of nitroprusside on smooth muscle and adrenergic neurotransmission in isolated blood vessels. Circulation **51/52**, Suppl. II, 58 (1975).
Vesey, C. J., Cole, P. V., Linnell, J. C., Wilson, J.: Some metabolic effects of sodium nitroprusside in man. Brit. med. J. **1974 II**, 140—142.
Vorburger, C.: Die hypertensive Krise: Ther. Umsch. **24**, 190—195 (1967).
Wilbrandt, R., Piehl, W., Neuhaus, G., Freylan, M. D., Freund, H. W., Göhring, H. J., Behrenbeck, D. W., Fritz, K.: Die Behandlung hypertoner Krisen mit Natriumnitroprussid. Dtsch. med. Wschr. **95**, 1822—1827 (1970).
Wildsmith, J. A. W., Marshall, R. L., Jenkinson, J. L., MacRae, W. R., Scott, D. B.: Haemodynamic effects of sodium nitroprusside during nitrous oxide/halothane anaesthesia. Brit. J. Anaesth. **45**, 71—74 (1973).

Section IV Diazoxide

Review article: Diazoxide: a review of its pharmacological properties and therapeutic use in hypertensive crises. Drugs **2**, 78—137 (1971).
Baer, L., Goodwin, F. J., Laragh, J. H.: Diazoxide-induced renin release in man: dissociation from plasma and extracellulai fluid volume changes. J. clin. Endocr. Metab. **29**, 1107—1109 (1969).
Balsam, M. J., Baker, L., Kaye, R.: Hyperosmolar nonketotic coma associated with diazoxide therapy for hypoglycemia. J. Paediat. **78**, 523—525 (1971).
Bartorelli, C., Gargano, N., Leonetti, G., Zanchetti, A.: Hypotensive and renal effects of diazoxide, a sodium retaining benzothiadiazine compound. Circulation **27**, 895—903 (1963).
Beamer, V. L., McDonald, R. H., Jr.: Failure of repeated diazoxide injections to modify the course of severe hypertension. Amer. Heart J. **79**, 742—751 (1970).
Bhatia, S. K., Frohlich, E. D.: Hemodynamic comparison of agents useful in hypertensive emergencies. Amer. Heart J. **85**, 367—373 (1973).
Blackard, W. G., Aprill, C. N.: Mechanism of action of diazoxide. J. Lab. clin. Med. **69**, 960—967 (1967).
Boyarsky, S., Labay, P.: The effect of diazoxide, an antidiuretic thiazide in ureteral peristalsis. Clin. Res. **16**, 474 (1968).
Calesnik, B., Katchen, B., Black, J.: Importance of dissolution rates in producing effective diazoxide blood levels in man. J. pharm. Sci. **54**, 1277—1280 (1965).
Charles, M. A., Danforth, E., Jr.: Nonketoacidotic hyperglycemia and coma during intravenous diazoxide therapy in uremia. Diabetes **20**, 501—503 (1971).

Conway, J., Keitzer, F., Miller, J.D.: Hemodynamic effects of a sodium retaining thiazide derivative: preliminary observations. J. Lab. clin. Med. **58**, 809 (1961).
Crout, J.R., Andreasen, F.V.V., Parks, R.I., Heimbach, D.M.: Intravenous Diazoxide in Hypertension. Clin. Res. **18**, 337 (1970).
Davidov, M.E., Mroczek, W.J., Gavrilovich, L., Finnerty, F.A.: Outpatient therapy of resistant hypertension. Clin. Res. **22**, 4A (1974).
DeBroe, M., Mussche, M., Ringoir, S., Bosteels, V.: Oral diazoxide for malignant hypertension. Lancet **1972I**, 1397.
Dollery, C.T., Pentecort, B.L., Samaan, N.A.: Drug induced diabetes. Lancet **1962II**, 735—737.
Ehrlich, E.N.: Cortisol responses to diazoxide in man and their possible relationship to effective blood volume. Metabolism **19**, 469—479 (1970).
Fajans, S.S., Floyd, J.C., Knopf, R.F., Rall, J., Guntsche, E.M., Conn, J.W.: Benzothiadiazine suppression of insulin release from normal and abnormal islet tissue in man. J. clin. Invest. **45**, 481—491 (1966).
Finnerty, F.A., Jr.: Treatment of acute hypertension in pregnancy. Obstet. Gynec. Dig. **12**, 30—37 (1970).
Finnerty, F.A., Jr.: Relationship of extracellular fluid volume to the development of drug resistance in the hypertensive patient. Amer. Heart J. **81**, 563—566 (1971).
Finnerty, F.A., Jr.: Hypertensive crisis. J. Amer. med. Ass. **229**, 1479—1480 (1974).
Finnerty, F.A., Jr., Kakaviatos, N., Tuckman, J., Magill, J.: Clinical evaluation of diazoxide; a new treatment for acute hypertension. Circulation **28**, 203—208 (1963).
Finnerty, F.A., Jr., Davidov, M., Kakaviatos, N.: Hypertensive vascular disease. The long-term effect of rapid repeated reductions of arterial pressure with diazoxide. Amer. J. Cardiol. **19**, 377—384 (1967).
Finnerty, F.A., Jr., Kakaviatos, N., Davidov, M.: The long-term effect of repeated acute reductions of arterial pressure with diazoxide in patients with severe hypertension. Ann. N. Y. Acad. Sci. **150**, 461—463 (1968).
Finnerty, F.A., Jr., Davidov, M., Mroczek, W.J., Gavrilovich, L.: Influence of extracellular fluid volume on response to antihypertensive drugs. Circulat. Res. **27**, Suppl. I, 71—82 (1970).
Frerichs, H., Gerber, R., Creutzfeldt, W.: Insulinsekretion in vitro: Hemmung der glucose-induzierten Insulinabgabe durch Diazoxide. Diabetologica **2**, 269—276 (1966).
Frerichs, H., Creutzfeldt, C., Creutzfeldt, W.: Klinische Beobachtungen und experimentelle Befunde bei der Behandlung des Hyperinsulinismus mit Diazoxide. Verh. dtsch. Ges. inn. Med., 73. Kongreß, 1086—1091 (1967).
Frerichs, H., Creutzfeldt, C., Creutzfeldt, W.: Wirkungsmechanismus und Ergebnisse der Diazoxid-Therapie bei B-Zelltumoren. 14. Symposium Dtsche. Ges. Endokrinol. S. 146—154. Berlin-Heidelberg-New York: Springer 1968.
Gifford, R.W., Jr.: Management of hypertension complicated by cerebrovascular disease. Drug Ther. **1**, 22—25, 30—31, 34—38 (1971).
Gilmore, E., Weil, J., Chidsey, C.: Treatment of essential hypertension with a new vasodilator in combination with β-adrenergic blockade. New Engl. J. Med. **282**, 521—527 (1970).
Graber, A.L., Porte, D., Jr., Williams, R.H.: Clinical use of diazoxide and mechanism for its hyperglycaemic effects. Diabetes **15**, 143 (1966).
Green, O.C., Berger, J.: The clinical use of diazoxide in leucine-sensitive hypoglycaemia. Ann. N Y. Acad. Sci. **150**, 356—366 (1968).
Greene, J.A.: Effects of diazoxide on renal function in the dog. Proc. Soc. exp. Biol. (N. Y.) **125**, 375—379 (1967).
Guedon, J., Buisson, C., Bursaux, E.: Les résistances périfériques totales dans l'hypertension artérielle humaine. Effects hémodynamiques du diazoxide. Rev. europ. Etud. clin. biol. **17**, 212—218 (1972).
Hamby, W.M., Jankowski, G.J., Pouget, J.M., Dunea, G., Gantt, C.L.: Intravenous use of diazoxide in the treatment of severe hypertension. Circulation **37**, 169—174 (1968).
Henrich, W.L., Cronin, R., Miller, P.D., Anderson, R.J.: Hypotensive Sequelae of Diazoxide and Hydralazine Therapy. J. Amer. med. Ass. **237**, 264—265, (1977).
Hofbauer, K.G., Bauereiss, K., Schwarz, K., Gross, F.: Comparative studies on isoproterenol and diazoxide in the isolated perfused rat kidney. Naunyn Schmiedebergs Arch. Pharmacol. **293**, Suppl., R37 (1976).
Hutcheon, D.E., Barthalmus, K.S.: Antihypertensive action of diazoxide: A new benzothiadiazine with antidiuretic properties. Brit. med. J. **1962II**, 159—161.
Janes, R.G., Roelf, R.J., Wilson, W.R.: Effect of guanethidine and adrenal demedullation in hyperglycaemia responses to diazoxide in rats. Proc. Soc. exp. Biol. (N. Y.) **117**, 572—575 (1964).
Janis, R., Triggle, D.: Effect of diazoxide on aortic reactivity to calcium in spontaneously hypertensive rats. Canad. J. Physiol. Pharmacol. **51**, 621—626 (1973).

Johnson, B.: Renal actions of diazoxide in hypertensives. Clin. Res. **16**, 386 (1968).
Johnson, B. F.: Diazoxide and renal function in man. Clin. Pharmacol. Ther. **12**, 815—824 (1971).
Just, H., Stein, J.: Studies on the effect of diazoxide, a new hypotensive drug, on the systemic and pulmonary circulation in hypertensive subjects. Z. Kreisl.-Forsch. **58**, 925—936 (1969).
Kakaviatos, N., Finnerty, F. A.: Preliminary observations on the value of diazoxide administered intravenously in man. Angiology **13**, 541—544 (1962).
Kakaviatos, N., Tuchman, J., Finnerty, F. A.: An antihypertensive agent which reduces peripheral resistance. Clin. Res. **10**, 174 (1962).
Kakaviatos, N., Davidov, M., Gavrilovich, L., Finnerty, F. A.: Diazoxide and furosemide in hypertension. Lancet **1967 II**, 725
Kakaviatos, N., Davidov, M., Finnerty, F. A., Jr.: Acute reduction of arterial pressure associated with an increase in effective renal plasma flow. Clin. Res. **16**, 62 (1968).
Kincaid-Smith, P., Fang, P., Laver, M. C.: A new look at the treatment of severe hypertension. Clin. Sci. molec. Med. **45**, 75s—87s (1973).
Koblenzer, P. J., Baker, L.: Hypertrichosis lamyoginosa associated with diazoxide therapy in prepubertal children: a clinico-pathologic study. Ann. N.Y. Acad. Sci. **150**, 373—382 (1968).
Koch-Weser, J.: Vasodilator drugs in the treatment of hypertension. Arch. intern. Med. **133**, 1017—1027 (1974).
Koch-Weser, J.: Diazoxide. New Engl. J. Med. **294**, 1271—1274 (1976).
Kuchel, O., Fishman, L. M., Liddle, G. W., Michelakis, A.: Effect of diazoxide on plasma renin activity in hypertensive patients. Ann. intern. Med. **67**, 791—799 (1967).
Kumar, G. K., Dastoor, F. C., Robayo, J. R., Razzaque, M. A.: Side effects of diazoxide. J. Amer. med. Ass. **236**, 275—276 (1976).
Landesman, K., Wilson, K. H.: The relaxant effect of diazoxide on isolated gravid and nongravid human myometrium. Amer. J. Obstet. Gynec. **161**, 120—125 (1968).
Landesman, K., Coutinho, E. M., Wilson, K. H., Lopes, A. C. V.: The relaxant effect of diazoxide on nongravid human myometrium. Amer. J. Obstet. Gynec. **102**, 1080—1084 (1968).
Landesman, R., de Souza, J. A., Coutinho, E. M., Wilson, K. H., de Souza, M. B.: The inhibitory effect of diazoxide in normal term labor. Amer. J. Obstet. Gynec. **103**, 430—433 (1969).
Langdon, R. G., Wolff, F. W.: Diabetogenic action of diazoxide. Brit. med. J. 1962/II, 926.
Lee Won Ro, Mroczek, W. J., Davidov, M. E., Finnerty, F. A. Jr.: Nonemergency use of slow infusions of diazoxide. Clin. Pharmacol. Ther. **18**, 154—157 (1975a).
Lee Won Ro, Finnerty, F. A. Jr., Davidov, M. E., Mroczek, W. J.: The effect of β-adrenergic blockade on diazoxide induced tachycardia. Clin. Res. **23**, 191 A (1975b).
Leonetti, G., Grazi, S., Ligresti, A., Romano, S., Zanchetti, A.: Autonomic and renal effects of intravenous diazoxide. A study of the mechanisms of its hypotensive action in man. Pharmacol. clin. **2**, 206—215 (1970).
Levy, J. V.: Verapamil and Dizoxide Antagonism of agonist-induced contractions of aortic strips from normal and spontaneously hypertensive rats (SHR). Res. Commun. chem. Path. Pharmacol. **11**, 387—401 (1975).
Limas, C. J., Freis, E. D.: Minoxidil in severe hypertension with renal failure: effect of its addition to conventional antihypertensive drugs. Amer. J. Cardiol. **31**, 355—361 (1973).
Lockwood, C. H., Nicholls, D. M., Troop, V. L., Lewis, J. A.: Diazoxide therapy in hypertension. Amer. J. Med. Sci. **246**, 312—318 (1963).
Loubatières, A., Mariani, M. M., Atric, R.: The action of diazoxide on insulin reaction, medullo-adrenal secretion, and the liberation of catecholamines. Ann. N.Y. Acad. Sci. **150**, 226 (1968).
Malaisse, W., Malaisse-Lagae, F.: Effects of glycodiazin and glibenclamide upon insulin secretion *in vitro*. Europ. J. Pharmacol. **9**, 93—98 (1970).
Mathew, T. H., Kincaid-Smith, P.: The use of diazoxide in hypertensive crises with particular reference to the control of hypertension in severe renal failure. Drugs **2**, 73—77 (1971).
McLaine, P. N., Drummond, K. N.: Intravenous diazoxide for severe hypertension in childhood. J. Pediat. **79**, 829—832 (1971).
McNeill, J. H., Barnes, R. V., Davis, R. S., Hook, J. B.: The effect of vasodilator drugs on noradrenaline constrictor response in the isolated mesenteric artery. Canad. J. Physiol. Pharmacol. **47**, 663—669 (1969).
Miller, W. E., Gifford, R. W. Jr., Humphrey, D. C., Vidt, D. G.: Management of severe hypertension with intravenous injections of diazoxide. Amer. J. Cardiol. **24**, 870—875 (1969).
Milton, R. M., Taylor, R. M.: Further studies on the renal pharmacology of diazoxide. Fed. Proc. **21**, 432 (1962).
Moore, P. F.: The effects of diazoxide and benzothiadiazine diuretics upon phosphodiesterase. Ann. N.Y. Acad. Sci. **150**, 256—260 (1968).
Mroczek, W. J., Davidov, M., Gavrilovich, L., Finnerty, F. A. Jr.: The value of agressive therapy in the hypertensive patients with azotemia. Circulation **40**, 893—904 (1969).

MROCZEK, W. J., LEIBEL, B. A., DAVIDOV, R. N. M., FINNERTY, F. A. JR.: The importance of the rapid administration of diazoxide in accelerated hypertension. New Engl. J. Med. **285**, 603—606 (1971).
MROCZEK, W. J., LEE, W. R., DAVIDOV, M. E., FINNERTY, F. A. JR.: Vasodilator administration in the presence of β-adrenergic blockade. Circulation **53**, 985—988 (1976).
MULLER, S. A.: Hirsutism. Amer. J. Med. **46**, 803—817 (1969).
NAYLER, W. G., MCINNES, I., SWANN, J. B., RACE, D., CARSON, V., LOWE, T. E.: Some effects of the hypotensive drug diazoxide on the cardiovascular system. Amer. Heart J. **75**, 223—232 (1968).
NEARY, D., THURSTON, H., POHL, J. E. F.: Development of extrapyramidal symptoms in hypertensive patients treated with diazoxide. Brit. med. J. **1973 III**, 474—475.
O'BRIEN, K. P., GRIGOR, R. R., TAYLOR, P. M.: Intravenous diazoxide in treatment of hypertension associated with recent myocardial infarction. Brit. med. J. **1975 IV**, 74—77.
OKUN, R., RUSSEL PATTERSON, R., WILSON, W. R.: Use of diazoxide with trichlormethiazide for hypertension. Arch. intern. Med. **112**, 882—888 (1963).
PENNINGTON, J. C., PICKER, R. H.: Diazoxide and the treatment of the acute hypertensive emergency in obstetrics. Med. J. Aust. **59/II**, 1051—1054 (1972).
POHL, J. E. F., THURSTON, H.: Use of diazoxide in hypertension with renal failure. Brit. med-J. **1971 IV**, 142—145.
POHL, J. E. F., THURSTON, H., SWALES, J. D.: The antidiuretic action of diazoxide. Clin. Sci. **42**, 145—152 (1972a).
POHL, J. E. F., THURSTON, H., DAVIS, D., MORGAN, M. Y.: Successful use of oral diazoxide in the treatment of severe toxaemia of pregnancy. Brit. med. J. **1972 II**, 568—570 b.
POWELL, W. J. JR., GREEN, R. M., WHITING, R. B., SANDERS, C. A.: Action of diazoxide on skeletal muscle vascular resistance. Circulat. Res. **28**, 167—178 (1971).
PRUITT, A. W., DAYTON, P. G., PATTERSON, J. H.: Studies of diazoxide in children. Pharmacologist **13**, 196 (1971).
PRUITT, A. W., DAYTON, P. G., PATTERSON, J. H.: Disposition of diazoxide in children. Clin. Pharmacol. Ther. **14**, 73—82 (1973).
RAMASWAMY, D., RICHARDSON, D. W.: Mechanism of circulatory effects of intravenous diazoxide. Circulation **38**, Suppl. 6, 160 (1968).
ROWE, G. G., LEICHL, T. R., BOAKE, W. C., KYLE, J. C., CRUMPTON, C. W.: The systemic and coronary hemodynamic effects of diazoxide. Amer. Heart J. **66**, 636—643 (1963).
RUBIN, A. A., ROTH, F. E., WINBURY, M. M.: A nondiuretic benzothiadiazine with antihypertensive properties. Nature (Lond.) **192**, 176—177 (1961).
RUBIN, A. A., ROTH, F. E., TAYLOR, R. M., ROSENKILDE, H.: Pharmacology of Diazoxide, an antihypertensive, nondiuretic benzothiadiazine. J. Pharmacol. exp. Ther. **136**, 344—352 (1962).
RUBIN, A. A., ZITOWITZ, L., HAUSLER, L.: Acute circulatory effects of diazoxide and sodium nitrite. J. Pharmacol. exp. Ther. **140**, 46—51 (1963).
SAUBAR, S. S., MITCHELL, S. A., LOCKEY, R. F., VLCEK, E. A., GREENE, J. A. JR.: Metabolic effects of hypotension induced by hemorrhage and by hypotensive drugs. Clin. Res. **15**, 410 (1967).
SCHMITT, H., SCHMITT, H., LAUBIE, M.: Actions du diazoxide sur le système cardiovasculaire, sur le métabolisme du myocarde et sur les décharges sympathiques. Arch. int. Pharmacodyn. **171**, 339—355 (1968).
SCOTT, J. C., COWLEY, A. W.: The effect of diazoxide on coronary blood flow. Amer. J. Cardiol. **24**, 865—869 (1969).
SELLERS, E. M., KOCH-WESER, J.: Protein-binding and vascular activity of diazoxide. New Engl. J. Med. **281**, 1141—1145 (1969).
SELLERS, E. M., KOCH-WESER, J.: Displacement of warfarin from human albumin by diaz-oxide and ethacrynic, mefenamic, and nalidixic acids. Clin. Pharmacol. Ther. **11**, 524—529 (1970).
SELLERS, E. M., KOCH-WESER, J.: Influence of intravenous injection rate on protein binding and vascular activity of diazoxide. Ann. N.Y. Acad. Sci. **226**, 319—332 (1973).
SPITZER, J. J., SCOTT, J. C.: Effects of diazoxide on myocardial free fatty acid metabolism and hemodynamics in the dog. Arch. int. Pharmacodyn. **184**, 405—414 (1970).
SPONER, G., SCHELLING, P., GROSS, F.: Differential effect of propranolol on the cardiovascular and diabetogenic actions of diazoxide. Naunyn Schmiedeberg's Arch. Pharmacol. **294**, R 20, 77 (1976).
STANTON, H., WHITE, J.: Hypotensive actions of drugs on unanaesthetized normotensive and "metacorticoid" hypertensive rats determined by a direct recording technique. Arch. int. Pharmacodyn. **154**, 351—363 (1973).
STAQUET, M., YABO, R., VICTORA, J., WOLFF, F. W.: An adrenergic mechanism for hyperglycemia induced by diazoxide. Metabolism **14**, 1000—1009 (1965).
STEINKE, J., SOELDNER, J. S.: Metabolic effects of diazoxide in normal subjects, patients with diabetes mellitus, and patients with organic hypoglycemia. Ann. N.Y. Acad. Sci. **150**, 326—336 (1968).

Suzuki, T.: Studies on the renin-angiotensin-aldosterone system: Effect of the antihypertensive agent diazoxide on plasma renin activity and its clinical application especially in screening primary aldosteronism and its similar disorders. Jap. Circulat. J. **34**, 187—197 (1967).
Swales, J. D., Thurston, H., Pohl, J. E. F.: Sodium conservation in chronic renal failure. Studies using oral diazoxide. Clin. Sci. **43**, 771—778 (1972).
Symchowicz, S., Winston, L., Black, J., Smith, M., Calesnick, B., Tabachnik, I. I. A.: Diazoxide blood levels in man. J. pharm. Sci. **56**, 912—914 (1967).
Tabachnik, I. I. A., Gulbenkian, A.: Mechanism of diazoxide hyperglycemia in animals. Ann. N.Y. Acad. Sci. **150**, 204—218 (1968).
Tabachnik, I. I. A., Gulbenkian, A., Seidman, F.: The effect of a benzothiadiazine, diazoxide on carbohydrate metabolism. Diabetes **13**, 408—418 (1964).
Tabachnik, I. I. A., Gulbenkian, A., Seidman, F.: Further studies on the metabolic effects of diazoxide. J. Pharmacol. exp. Ther. **150**, 455—462 (1965).
Taylor, J., Green, R. D.: Evidence for an antagonistic action of diazoxide at alpha-adrenergic receptors in rabbit aorta. Europ. J. Pharmacol. **12**, 385—387 (1970).
Taylor, R. M.: Renal aspects of certain antihypertensive agents. Angiology **14**, 79—83 (1963).
Taylor, R. M., Rubin, A. A.: Studies on the renal pharmacology of diazoxide, an antidiuretic benzothiadiazine. J. Pharmacol. exp. Ther. **144**, 284—292 (1964).
Thirwell, M. P., Zsotér, T. T.: The effect of diazoxide on the veins. Amer. Heart J. **83**, 512—517 (1972).
Thomson, A. E., Nickerson, M., Gaskell, P., Grahame, G. R.: Clinical observations on an antihypertensive chlorothiazide analogue devoid of diuretic activity. Canad. med. Ass. J. **87**, 1306—1310 (1962).
Thomson, G. R., Anderson, R. W., Ballantyne, L. M.: The effects of intravenous diazoxide, a non-diuretic thiazide, upon blood pressure, electrolyte and uric acid excretion. Mich. Med. **65**, 17—21 (1966).
Thurston, H., Pohl, J. E. F., Swales, J. D.: The effect of oral diazoxide on hypertension and sodium secretion in chronic renal failure. Clin. Sci. molec. Med. **45**, 175s—179s (1973).
Topliss, J. G., Yudis, M. D.: Correlation of antihypertensive activity with structure in a series of 2H-1,2,4-Benzothiadiazine 1,1-Dioxides, using the substituent constant approach. J. med. Chem. **15**, 394—400 (1972).
Updike, S. J., Harrington, A. R.: Acute diabetic ketoacidosis: A complication of intravenous diazoxide treatment for refractory hypertension. New Engl. J. Med. **280**, 768 (1969).
Wales, J. K., Wolff, F. W.: Haematological side effects of diazoxide. Lancet **1967 I**, 53—54.
Wales, J. K., Grant, A. M., Wolff, F. W.: Reversal of diazoxide effects by tolbutamide. Lancet **1967 I**, 1137—1138.
Walfish, P. G., Natale, R., Chang, C.: Beta-adrenergic receptor mechanisms in the metabolic effects of diazoxide in fasted rats. Diabetes **19**, 228—233 (1970).
Wegienka, L. C., Simpson, R. G., Karam, J. H., Forsham, P. H.: Clinical experience with diazoxide. Ann. N.Y. Acad. Sci. **150**, 383—394 (1968).
Weller, J. M., Borondy, P. E.: Effects of benzothiadiazine drugs on carbohydrate metabolism. Metabolism **14**, 708—714 (1965).
Wilkenfeld, B. E., Levy, B.: The effects of theophylline, diazoxide and imidazole on isoproterenol-induced inhibition of the rabbit ileum. J. Pharmacol. exp. Ther. **169**, 61—67 (1969).
Wilson, W. R., Okun, R.: Acute hemodynamic effects of diazoxide in man. Circulation **28**, 89—93 (1963).
Wilson, W. R., Kirkendall, W. M.: Effects of intravenous diazoxide in treatment of severe hypertension. Clin. Res. **12**, 196 (1964).
Wohl, A. J.: Electronic Molecular Pharmacology: The Benzothiadiazine Antihypertensive Agents. I. Pharmacological aspects of Tautomerism and Conformation. Molec. Pharmacol. **6**, 189—194 (1970a).
Wohl, A. J.: Electronic Molecular Pharmacology: The Benzothiadiazine Antihypertensive Agents. II. Multiple regression analyses relating biological potency and electronic structure. Molec. Pharmacol. **6**, 195—205 (1970b).
Wohl, A. J., Hausler, L. M., Roth, F. E.: Studies on the mechanism of antihypertensive action of diazoxide *in vitro* vascular pharmacodynamics. J. Pharmacol. exp. Ther. **158**, 531—539 (1967).
Wohl, A. J., Hausler, L. M., Roth, F. E.: Mechanism of the antihypertensive effect of diazoxide: *in vitro* vascular studies in the hypertensive rat. J. Pharmacol. exp. Ther. **162**, 109—114 (1968).
Wolff, F.: Diazoxide hyperglycemia and its continued relief by tolbutamide. Lancet 1964/I, 309—310.
Zarday, Z., Victora, J., Wolff, F. W.: The effect of diazoxide on catecholamines. Metabolism **15**, 257—261 (1966).
Zitowitz, L., Rubin, A. A.: Some acute cardiovascular actions of diazoxide (SRG-95213), a non-diuretic antihypertensive benzothiadiazine. Fed. Proc. **21**, 114 (1962).

Section V Minoxidil

BONACCORSI, A., FRANCO, R., GARATTINI, S., CHIDSEY, C.: Mechanism of vasodilator activity of the antihypertensive minoxidil. Circulation 48, Suppl. IV, 45 (1973).
BRYAN, R.K., HOOBLER, S.W., ROSENZWEIG, J., WELLER, J.M.: Effect of minoxidil on blood pressure and hemodynamics in severe hypertension. Amer. J. Cardiol. **39**, 786—801, 1977
CARLSON, R.G., FEENSTRA, E.S.: Toxicologic studies with the hypotensive agent minoxidil. Toxicol. appl. Pharmacol. **39**, 1—11, 1977.
CHIDSEY, C.A.: Clinical and pharmacokinetic studies of minoxidil, a new antihypertensive agent. Clin. Sci. molec. Med. **45**, 171s—173s (1973).
DORMOIS, J.C., YOUNG, J.L., NIES, A.S.: Minoxidil in severe hypertension: Value when conventional drugs have failed. Amer. Heart J. **90**, 360—368 (1975).
DUCHARME, D.W., FREYBURGER, W.A., GRAHAM, B.E., CARLSON, R.G.: Pharmacologic properties of minoxidil: a new hypotensive agent. J. Pharmacol. exp. Ther. **184**, 662—670 (1973).
EDITORIAL: New vasodilator drugs for hypertension. Brit. med. J. **1973 IV**, 185—186.
FREYBURGER, W.A., WEEKS, J.R., DUCHARME, D.W.: Cardiovascular actions of the hypotensive agent, N,N-diallyl-melamine (U 7720). Naunyn Schmiedebergs Arch. Pharmacol. **251**, 39—47 (1965).
GIBALDI, M.: Pharmacokinetic and pharmacodynamic studies of bethanidine and minoxidil in man. In: MILLIEZ, P., SAFAR, M. (Eds.): Recent Advances in Hypertension, pp. 307—315. Ingelheim: Boehringer 1975.
GILMORE, E., WEIL, J., CHIDSEY, C.: Treatment of essential hypertension with a new vasodilator in combination with β-adrenergic blockade. New Engl. J. Med. **282**, 521—527 (1970).
GOTTLIEB, T.B., KATZ, F.H., CHIDSEY, C.A.: Combined therapy with vasodilator drugs and β-adrenergic blockade in hypertension: a comparative study of minoxidil and hydralazine. Circulation **45**, 571—582 (1972a).
GOTTLIEB, T.B., THOMAS, R.C., CHIDSEY, C.A.: Pharmacokinetic studies of minoxidil. Clin. Pharmacol. Ther. **13**, 436—441 (1972b).
HARTNETT, M.N., BENNETT, W.M., McDONALD, W., HARNER, M.H., PORTER, G.A.: Minoxidil therapy for severe hypertension. Clin. Res. **23**, 466A (1975).
HUMPHREY, S.J., WILLIAMS, J.E., ZINS, G.R.: Renal tubular site of enhanced sodium reabsorption in dogs treated with direct peripheral vasodilators. Fed. Proc. **30**, 607 (1971).
HUMPHREY, S.J., WILSON, E., ZINS, G.R.: Whole body tissue blood flow in conscious dogs treated with minoxidil. Fed. Proc. **33**, 583 (1974).
KINCAID-SMITH, P.S.: The treatment of resistant hypertension. Drugs **11**, Suppl. 1, 78—86 (1976).
KOBLENZER, P.J., BAKER, L.: Hypertrichosis lamyoginosa associated with diazoxide therapy in prepubertal children: a clinico-pathologic study. Ann. N.Y. Acad. Sci. **150**, 373—382 (1968).
LIEBAU, G., HAYDUK, K., BUNDSCHU, H.D., MENZ, H.P.: Klinische Erfahrungen mit Minoxidil, einem neuen Antihypertonikum. Verh. dtsch. Ges. inn. Med. **80**, 277—279 (1974).
LIMAS, C.J., FREIS, E.D.: Minoxidil in severe hypertension with renal failure: effect of its addition to conventional antihypertensive drugs. Amer. J. Cardiol. **31**, 355—361 (1973).
LIMAS, C., GUIHA, N.H., FREIS, E.D.: Treatment of severe resistant hypertension with minoxidil. Clin. Pharmacol. Ther. **13**, 145 (1972).
MARTIN, W.B., ZINS, G.R., FREYBURGER, W.A.: The use of minoxidil, an experimental arteriolar dilator, in 510 patients with refractory hypertension. Clin. Sci. molec. Med. **48**, 189s—190s (1975).
MEHTA, P.K., MAMDANI, B., SHANSKY, R.M., MAHURKAR, S.D., DUNEA, G.: Severe hypertension. Treatment with minoxidil. J. Amer. med. Ass. **233**, 249—252 (1975).
MROCZEK, W.J., SAHETA, N.P., Won Ro LEE, DAVIDOV, M.E., FINNERTY, F.A. JR.: Minoxidil in patients with severe hypertension. Clin. Res. **23**, 198A (1975).
MULLER, S.A.: Hirsutism. Amer. J. Med. **46**, 803—817 (1969).
MUTTERPERL, R.E., FRAYDA, D.O., DIAMOND, R.N., LOWENTHAL, D.T.: Long-term effects of minoxidil in the treatment of malignant hypertension in chronic renal failure. J. clin. Pharmac. **16**, 498—509, 1976.
O'MALLEY, K., McNAY, J.L.: Technique for rapid control of hypertension with oral minoxidil. Clin. Sci. molec. Med. **48**, 185s—187s (1975).
O'MALLEY, K., VELASCO, M., McNAY, J.L.: Adrenergic mechanism of minoxidil-induced increase in plasma renin activity. Clin. Res. **21**, 953 (1973).
O'MALLEY, K., VELASCO, M., WELLS, J., McNAY, J.L.: Control plasma renin activity and changes in sympathetic tone as determinants of minoxidil-induced increase in plasma renin activity. J. clin. Invest. **55**, 230—325 (1975a).
O'MALLEY, K., VELASCO, M., WELLS, J., McNAY, J.L.: Mechanisms of the hypotensive effect of propranolol in minoxidil-treated hypertensive patients. Clin. Res. **23**, 200A (1975b).
PERRY, H.M., JR., COMEN, P., YUNICE, A.: Distribution of hydralazine-1-C^{14} after injection into normal mice. J. Lab. clin. Med. **59**, 456—461 (1962).

Pettinger, W. A., Keeton, K.: Altered renin release and synergistic antihypertensive activity of vasodilating drugs and propranolol. Clin. Res. **21**, 472 (1973).
Pettinger, W. A., Mitchell, H. C.: Minoxidil—an alternative to nephrectomy for refractory hypertension. New Engl. J. Med. **289**, 167—171 (1973).
Pettinger, W. A., Campbell, W. B., Keeton, K.: The adrenergic component of renin release induced by vasodilating antihypertensive drugs in the rat. Circulat. Res. (in press).
Pluss, R. G., Orcutt, J., Chidsey, C. A.: Tissue distribution and hypotensive effects of minoxidil in normotensive rats. J. Lab. clin. Med. **79**, 639—647 (1972).
Redmond, D. P., Traub, Y. M., McDonald, R. H., Jr., Shapiro, A. P.: Minoxidil and the management of severe hypertension. A relationship to renal function. Clin. Pharmacol. Ther. **15**, 217 (1974).
Sannerstedt, R., Bronson, L., Berglund, G., Werkö, L.: Minoxidil—haemodynamic and clinical experiences with a new peripheral vasodilator. Acta med. scand. **197**, 409—414 (1975).
Shen, D., O'Malley, K., Gibaldi, M., McNay, J. L.: Pharmacodynamics of minoxidil as a guide for individualizing dosage regimens in hypertension. Clin. Pharmacol. Ther. **17**, 593—598 (1975).
Velasco, M., O'Malley, K., Robie, N. W., Wells, J., Israili, Z. H., McNay, J. L.: Differential effects of propranolol on heart rate and plasma renin activity treated with minoxidil. Clin. Pharmacol. Ther. **16**, 1031—1038 (1974).
Wagner, J.: Pharmacokinetics and metabolism of hydralazine: Specific affinity for blood vessels. Experientia (Basel) **29**, 767 (1973).
Wagner, J., Hedwall, P.: Correlation between the pharmacokinetics and the hypotensive action of hydralazine in the rat. Naunyn Schmiedebergs Arch. Pharmacol. **274**, Suppl. R 122 (1972).
Wagner, J., Hedwall, P.: Pharmacokinetics and pharmacological actions of vasodilators. Int. Symposium on Hypertension, pp. 331—342. Milliez, P., Safar, M., (Eds.). Monte Carlo: 1975.
Werner, K., Heimsoth, V. H., Bock, K. D.: Klinisch experimentelle Untersuchungen mit dem Piperidinopyrimidin-Derivat Minoxidil. Verh. dtsch. Ges. inn. Med. **80**, 275—277 (1974).
Wilburn, R. L., Blaufuss, A., Bennett, C. M.: Long-term treatment of severe hypertension with minoxidil, propranolol, and furosemide. Circulation **52**, 706—713 (1975).
Youngdale, G. A., Anger, D. G., Anthony, W. Z., Da Vanzo, J. P., Greig, M. E., Heinschman, R. V., Kearting, H. H., Szmuszkovicz, J.: Synthesis and pharmacological activity of 3-12-pynolidinyl) indoles. J. med. Chem. **7**, 415—427 (1964).
Zacest, R., Frewin, D. B., Robinson, M. A., Wilson, L. L., Lawrence, J. R., Clarkson, A. R., Jackson, B.: Clinical and hemodynamic effects of minoxidil in refractory hypertension. Drugs **11**, Suppl. 1, 177—184 (1976).
Zins, G. R.: The *in vivo* production of a potent long-acting hypotensive metabolite from diallyl-melamine. J. Pharm. exp. Ther. **150**, 109—117 (1965).
Zins, G. R., Emmert, D. E., Walk, R. A.: Hypotensive metabolite production and sequential metabolism of N,N-diallylmelanine in rats, dogs, and man. J. Pharm. exp. Ther. **159**, 194—205 (1968).

Section VI Guancydine

Clark, D. W., Goldberg, L. I.: Guancydine: A new antihypertensive agent. Use with quinethazone and guanethidine or propranolol. Ann. intern. Med. **76**, 579—585 (1972).
Cummings, J. R., Grace, J. L., Jr.: Loss of guancydine's angiotensin inhibitory action in nephrectomized rats and reestablishment of blockade by cross circulation. Pharmacologist **11**, 270 (1969).
Cummings, J. R., Welter, A. N., Grace, J. L., Jr., Lipchuk, L. M.: Cardiovascular actions of guancydine in normotensive and hypertensive animals. J. Pharmacol. exp. Ther. **161**, 88—97 (1968).
Cummings, J. R., Welter, A. N., Grace, J. L., Jr., Gray, W. D.: Angiotensin blocking actions of guancydine. J. Pharmacol. exp. Ther. **170**, 334—346 (1969).
Druey, J., Tripod, J.: Hydralazines. In: Schlittler, E. (Ed.): Antihypertensive Agents, pp. 223—262. New York-London: Academic Press 1967.
Ellenbogen, L., Chan, P. S., Cummings, J. R.: Effect of guancydine on catecholamine synthesis, storage, and catabolism. Fed. Proc. **31**, 522 (1972).
Ellenbogen, L., Chan, P. S., Cummings, J. R.: Effects of guancydine on catecholamine synthesis, storage and catabolism. Arch. int. Pharmacodyn. **207**, 170—179 (1974).
Freis, E. D., Hammer, J.: Guancydine, a new type of antihypertensive agent: a preliminary communication. Med. Ann. D.C. **38**, 69—72 (1969).
Gadekar, S. M., Nibi, S., Cohen, E.: Hypotensive activity of some cyanoguanidines. J. med. Chem. **11**, 811—814 (1968).
Gussin, R. Z., Cummings, J. R., Stokey, E. H., Ronsberg, M. A., Malone, L. C.: The effect of guancydine, a new antihypertensive, on fluid and electrolyte excretion. Proc. Amer. Soc. Nephrol. **3**, 25 (1969).

GUSSIN, R. Z., STOKEY, E. H., RONSBERG, M. A., MALONE, L. C., CUMMINGS, J. R.: Mechanisms of antihypertensive-induced fluid retention. Clin. Res. 18, 500 (1970).
GUSSIN, R. Z., STOKEY, E. H., RONSBERG, M. A., MALONE, L. C., CUMMINGS, J. R.: The effect of guancydine on fluid and electrolyte excretion: a comparison with hydralazine and reserpine. Arch. int. Pharmacodyn. **192**, 135—151 (1971).
HAMMER, J., ULRYCH, M., FREIS, E. D.: Hemodynamic and therapeutic effects of guancydine in hypertension. Clin. Pharmacol. Ther. **12**, 78—90 (1971).
KOCH-WESER, J.: Vasodilator drugs in the treatment of hypertension. Arch. intern. Med. Med. **133**, 1017—1027 (1974).
RUSSO, C., MENDLOWITZ, M.: The effect of guancydine on blood pressure, vascular reactivity, and norepinephrine uptake in essential hypertension. Clin. Pharmacol. Ther. **13**, 875—878 (1972).
RUSSO, C., SUCK, A., MENDLOWITZ, M., GITLOW, S., WOLF, R. L., BERTINI, L. M.: The effect of guancydine in hypertensive patients. Fed. Proc. **29**, 447 (1970).
STENBERG, J., SANNERSTEDT, R., WERKÖ, L.: Haemodynamic studies on the antihypertensive effect of guancydine. Europ. J. clin. Pharmacol. **3**, 63—67 (1971).
VILLARREAL, H., ARCILA, H., RAMIREZ, M. A., SIERRA, P.: Effects of guancydine on systemic and renal hemodynamics in arterial hypertension. Clin. Pharmacol. Ther. **12**, 838—842 (1971).
WELTER, A. N., GRACE, J. L., JR.: Angiotensin antagonism by guancydine (1 cyano-3-t-amyl guanidine). Fed. Proc. **26**, 460 (1967).
WERKÖ, L.: New treatment for hypertension. Europ. J. clin. Pharmacol. **3**, 61—62 (1971).
WERNING, C., SCHWEIKERT, H. V., STIEL, D.: Erste Erfahrungen in der Langzeitbehandlung mit dem Antihypertensivum Guancydine. Dtsch. med. Wschr. **95**, 1756—1761 (1970).
WORCEL, M., PAPADIMITRIOU, A., MEYER, P.: Blockade of the effects of angiotensin, oxytocin, norepinephrine, 5-hydroxytryptamine, and acetylcholine by guancydine. J. Pharmacol. exp. Ther. **179**, 42—46 (1971).

Section VII Prazosin

ADRIAENSEN, H., VRYENS, R.: Prazosin in the treatment of hypertension. Practitioner **214**, 268—273 (1975).
ALTHUIS, T. H., HESS, H.-J.: Synthesis and identification of the major metabolites of prazosin formed in dog and rat. J. Med. Chem. **20**, 146—149, 1977.
AMERY, A., VERHIEST, W., CROONENBERGHS, J., FAGARD, R.: Double Blind Cross Over Study With a New Vasodilator— Prazosin— in the Treatment of Mild Hypertension, pp. 100—110. Amsterdam: Excerpta Medica 1974.
BENDALL, M. J., BALOCH, K. H., WILSON, P. R.: Side effects due to treatment of hypertension with prazosin. Brit. med. J. **1975 II**, 727—728.
BLOOM, D. S., ROSENDORF, C., KRAMER, R.: Clinical evaluation of prazosin as the sole agent for the treatment of hypertension: A double blind cross-over study with methyldopa. Curr. ther. Res. **18**, 144—150 (1975).
BOLLI, P., SIMPSON, F. O.: New vasodilator drugs for hypertension. Brit. med. J. **1974 I**, 637.
BOLLI, P., WOOD, A. J., PHELAN, E. L., LEE, D. R., SIMPSON, F. O.: Prazosin: Preliminary clinical and pharmacological observations. Clin. Sci. molec. Med. **48**, 177s—179s (1975).
CAIRNS, S. A., JORDAN, S. C.: Prazosin treatment complicated by acute febrile polyarthritis. Brit. Med. J. 1976 II, 1425—25.
CAMBRIDGE, D., DAVEY, M. J., MASSINGHAM, R.: Prazosin, a selective antagonist of post-synaptic α-adrenoceptors. Brit. J. Pharmac. **59**, 514 P—515 P, 1977.
CAVERO, I.: Cardiovascular effects of prazosin in dogs. Clin. Sc. Mol. Med. **51**, 6095—612s, 1976.
COHEN, B. M.: Prazosin hydrochloride (CP-12299-1) an oral antihypertensive agent. J. clin. Pharmacol. **10**, 408—417 (1970).
CONSTANTINE, J. W.: Analysis of the hypotensive action of prazosin. In: COTTON, D. W. K. (Ed.): Prazosin: Evaluation of a New Anti-Hypertensive Agent, pp. 16—36. Amsterdam: Excerpta Medica 1974.
CONSTANTINE, J. W., MCSHANE, W. K., SCRIABINE, A., HESS, H.-J.: Analysis of the hypotensive action of prazosin. In: ONESTI, G., KIM, K. E., MOYER, J. H. (Eds.): Hypertension, Mechanisms and Management, Chapter 6, pp. 429—444. Baltimore- Grune and Stratton Inc. 1973.
CURTIS, J. R.: Prazosin in patients with chronic renal failure. Brit. med. J. **1974 III**, 742—743.
CURTIS, J. R., BATEMAN, F. J. A.: Use of prazosin in management of hypertension in patients with chronic renal failure and in renal transplant recipients. Brit. med. J. **1975 IV**, 432—434.
FERNANDES, M., SMITH, SANFORD, I., WEDER, A., KIM, K. E., GOULD, A. B., BUSBY, P., SWARTZ, C., ONESTI, G.: Prazosin in the treatment of hypertension. Clin. Sci. molec. Med. **48**, Suppl. 2, 181s—184s (1975).

Gabriel, R., Meek, D., Gosh, B. C.: Collapse after prazosin hydrochloride. Lancet **1975 I**, 1095, a.
Gabriel, R, Meek, D., Mamtora, H.: Adverse reactions to prazosin. Brit. med. J. **1975 IV**, 41, b.
Graham, R. M., Thornell, J. R., Gain, J. M., Bagnoli, C., Oates, H. F. and Stohes, G. S.: Prazosin: The first dose phenomenon. Brit. Med. J. 1976/IV, 1293—94.
Hayes, J. M., Graham, R. M., O'Connell, B. P.: Prazosin in hypertension. Brit. med. J. **1974 IV**, 108.
Hess, H. J.: Biochemistry and structure-activity studies with prazosin. Excerpta med. (Amst.) 3—15 (1974).
Hua, A., Macdonald, J. M., Myers, J. B., Kincaid-Smith, P.: Studies with prazosin—a new hypotensive agent I. Open clinical study of prazosin in combination with other antihypertensive agents. Med. J. Aust. **63**, 559—561 (1976).
Kellaway, G. S. M.: Adverse drug reactions during treatment of hypertension. Drugs **11**, Suppl. 1, 91—99 (1976).
Kincaid-Smith, P., Hua, A.: Prazosin and hydralazine in the treatment of hypertension. Brit. med. J. 1974/**III**, 804—805.
Kincaid-Smith, P., Fang, P., Laver, M. C.: A new look at the treatment of severe hypertension. Clin. Sci. molec. Med. **45**, 75s—87s (1973).
Küchel, O., Fishman, L. M., Liddle, G. W., Michelakis, A.: Effect of diazoxide on plasma renin activity in hypertensive patients. Ann. intern. Med. **67**, 791—799 (1967).
Lund-Johansen, P.: Hemodynamic changes at rest and during exercise in long-term prazosin therapy of essential hypertension. In: Prazosin, Evaluation of a New Anti-Hypertensive Agent, pp. 43—51. Amsterdam: Excerpta Medica 1974.
Masoni, A., Tommasi, A. M., Baggioni, F., Bagni, B.: Hemodynamic Study in Man of Medium-term Treatment With a new Amino-quinazoline Antihypertensive Agent, pp. 54—63. Amsterdam: Excerpta med. 1974.
Massingham, R., Hayden, M. L.: A comparison of the effects of prazosin and hydralazine on blood pressure, heart rate and plasma renin activity in conscious renal hypertensive dogs. Europ. J. Pharmacol. **30**, 121—124 (1975).
Mroczek, W. J., Potin, S., Davidov, M. E., Finnerty, F. A., Jr.: Prazosin in hypertension: a double blind evaluation with methyldopa and placebo. Curr. ther. Res. **16**, 769—777, 1974.
Okun, R.: Dosage schedule routine for prazosin: Two cross-over trials comparing t.i.d. with q.i.d. administration and t.i.d. with l.i.d. administration, pp. 82—91. Amsterdam: Excerpta med. 1974.
Onesti, G., Fernandes, M. A., Kim, K. E., Swartz, C. D.: Prazosin in the treatment of hypertension. Clin. Pharmacol. Ther. **15**, 216, 1974.
Paul, R. R., Sharma, P. L., Wahi, P. L.: A phase II study of prazosin hydrochloride in hypertensive subjects. Int. J. clin. Pharmacol. **14**, 271—74, 1976.
Pettinger, W. A., Keeton, K.: Altered renin release and synergistic antihypertensive activity of vasodilating drugs and propranolol. Clin. Res. **21**, 472, 1973.
Pitts, N. E.: The clinical evaluation of prazosin hydrochloride, a new antihypertensive agent, pp. 149—163. Amsterdam: Excerpta med. 1974.
Richardson, D. W., Ramaswamy, D., Ramirez, A.: Effect of furazosin on arterial pressure and cardiac output in human hypertension. Circulation **38**, Suppl. VI., 164 (1968).
Rosendorff, C.: Prazosin: severe side effects are dose-dependent. Brit. med. J. **1976 III**, 508.
Safar, M. E., Weiss, Y. A., London, G. L., Milliez, P. L.: Short-term hemodynamic studies with prazosin, pp. 64—69. Amsterdam: Excerpta med. 1974.
Schirger, A., Sheps, S. G.: Prazosin—New antihypertensive agent J. Amer. med. Ass. **237**, 989—991, 1977.
Scriabine, A., Constantine, J. W., Hess, H. J., McShane, W. K.: Pharmacological studies with some new antihypertensive aminoquinazolines. Experientia (Basel) **24**, 1150—1151 (1968).
Stokes, G. S., Weber, M. A.: Prazosin: Preliminary report and comparative studies with other antihypertensive agents. Brit. med. J. **1974 II**, 298—300.
Stokes, G. S., Graham, R. M., Gain, J. M., Davis, P. R.: Influence of dosage and dietary sodium on the first dose effect of prazosin. Brit. Med. J. 1977, I, 1507—1508.
Thulin, T., Saetre, H., Vikesdahl, O., Warmenius, S., Persson, G., Scherstin, B.: Multicenter study of the antihypertensive effect of prazosin hydrochloride (prazosin) on mild and moderate hypertension, pp. 126—137. Amsterdam: Excerpta med. 1974.
Venables, T. A., Duff, R. S.: A comparative trial of prazosin and methyldopa, pp. 111—117. Amsterdam: Excerpta med. 1974.
Wohl, A. J.: Electronic molecular pharmacology: the benzothiadiazine antihypertensive agents. I. Pharmacological aspects of tautomerism and conformation. Molec. Pharmacol. **6**, 189—194 (1970).
Woods, A. J., Phelan, E. L., Simpson, F. O.: Cardiovascular effects of prazosin in normotensive and genetically hypertensive rats. Clin. Exp. Pharm. Physiol. **2**, 297—304, 1975.

Chapter 9

Antihypertensive Effect of Diuretics

J. CONWAY

With 5 Figures

I. Introduction

Since the introduction of the long acting benzothiadiazine diuretics by NOVELLO and SPRAGUE in 1957 and the demonstration of their blood pressure lowering actions (HOLLANDER and WILKINS, 1957; FREIS et al., 1958), a vast literature has developed attesting to this effect, though considerable controversy has surrounded the mode of action. The fall in blood pressure, however, is quite modest, approximately 20/12 mmHg in the recumbent and standing positions.

The antihypertensive effect of diuretics had in fact been noted earlier with mercurial diuretics (VIERSMA, 1946) and this was later confirmed by others (HOLLANDER et al., 1959; McQUEEN and MORRISON, 1960). It has also been demonstrated for compounds related indirectly to the thiazides, such as chlorthalidone (KAKAVIATOS and FINNERTY, 1962; HUTCHEON et al., 1965) and furosemide (DAVIDOV et al., 1967), and to such chemically unrelated compounds as ethacrynic acid (DOLLERY et al., 1964; CONWAY and LEONETTI 1965) and spironolactone (HOLLANDER et al., 1959; HOLLANDER, 1961; CRANSTON and JUEL-JENSEN, 1962).

The diuretic and non-renal actions of diuretics have been the subject of a comprehensive review by PETERS and ROCH-RAMEL in an earlier edition of this Handbook (1969). The present article therefore is limited to a discussion of the antihypertensive action of diuretics with emphasis on the mode of action on the cardiovascular system in man. No attention is given to the practical aspects of use of drugs for the treatment of hypertension or to their side effects.

II. Acute Haemodynamic Response to Diuretics (1-7 Days)

The diuretic response to the thiazide compounds demonstrates a rather flat dose response curve, the maximal diuretic dose of hydrochlorothiazide being 50 to 100 mg. This also corresponds to the optimal hypotensive dose. The duration of the effect of a single dose is approximately 8 h. When an adequate dose is given twice daily a cumulative loss of about 300 mEq. of sodium occurs in 2 to 3 days (HOLLANDER et al., 1959; FREIS et al., 1960; VENNING et al., 1962; HUTCHEON et al., 1965) and this is accompanied by weight loss (Fig. 1). Plasma volume falls by approximately 10% (WILSON and FREIS, 1959; DUSTAN et al., 1959; HANSEN, 1968), end-diastolic pressure falls and consequently cardiac output is reduced (CROSLEY et al., 1958; ALEKSANDROW et al., 1959a; VILLARREAL et al., 1962a).

As cardiac output falls, total peripheral resistance rises due to the activity of homeostatic reflexes (Dustan et al., 1959; Seriu, 1965). Glomerular filtration rate also declines, as a result of reflex action and partly as a consequence of the direct effect of the diuretic on the kidney (Castle et al., 1959; Crosley et al., 1960; Villarreal et al., 1962b). Plasma renin and angiotensin II levels increase in response to the sodium loss (Veyrat et al., 1964; Castenfors, 1967; Bourgoignie et al., 1968; Werning et al., 1969; Catt et al., 1970, 1971).

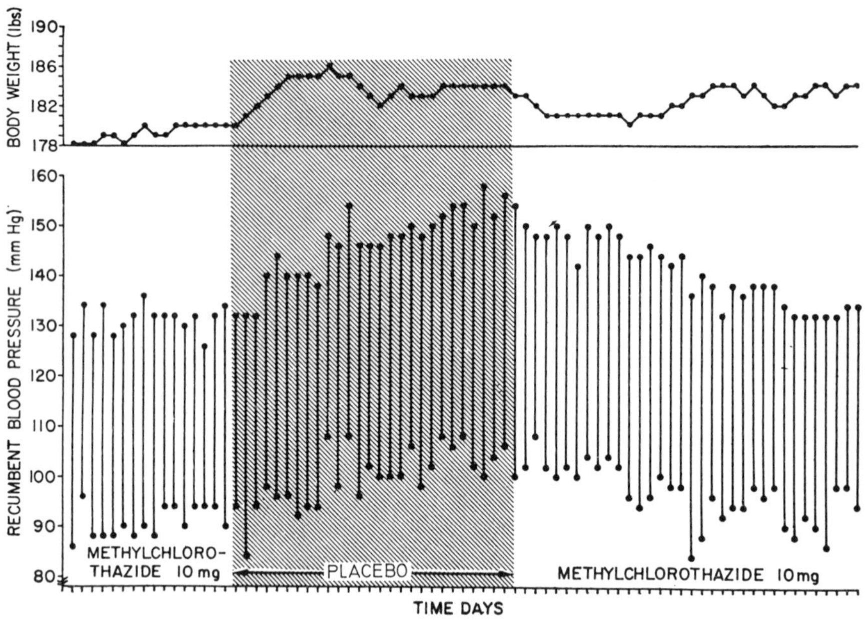

Fig. 1. Timing of the changes in body weight and blood pressure in a patient going off and then on thiazide therapy

The potent diuretics, furosemide and ethacrynic acid, produce a more dramatic loss of sodium. The fall in arterial pressure then becomes more evident and the response of the renin-aldosterone system is more obvious. These diuretics have therefore been extensively used in the analysis of the acute hypotensive effects of the diuretics. Thus it has been shown that reduction in plasma volume does not fully account for the fall in pressure. After a diuretic, plasma volume can be restored without returning blood pressure to the control level (Varnauskas, 1961; Winer, 1961a, b; Finnerty, Davidov, and Kakaviatos, 1968). There is, however, some divergence of opinion on this point (Wilson and Freis, 1959, Dustan et al., 1959; McQueen and Morrison, 1960). Replacement of the excreted water with isotonic dextrose solution results in restoration of pressure without correction of the plasma volume deficit (Davidov et al., 1969). The fall in pressure therefore appears to result from the reduction in extracellular fluid volume rather than sodium loss, *per se*, or decline in plasma volume.

The diminished pressor response to intravenously injected noradrenaline had been noted in the earlier studies on diuretics (Aleksandrow et al., 1959b; Hollander et al., 1959; Freis et al., 1960; Winer, 1968). This can apparently be restored by the dextrose infusions, but not by restoration of plasma volume with dextran solution (FINNERTY et al., 1968; DAVIDOV et al., 1969). The diminished response to pressor agents does not therefore appear to be specifically induced by sodium depletion.

From the evidence available it appears that the fall in blood pressure which occurs immediately with diuretic therapy is directly related to excretion of sodium and water and this is reflected in a fall in plasma volume, extracellular fluid volume and cardiac output. The fall in plasma volume alone, however, is not adequate to explain the hypotensive effect, since there is a residual effect which results from the reduced extracellular fluid volume.

It is perhaps unfortunate that the full haemodynamic picture has not been examined when plasma volume or extracellular fluid volume are restored after diuretic therapy, since it would be more satisfactory to know the levels of both cardiac output and blood pressure after these manoeuvres. Hence there is a little uncertainty about a possible effect of diuretics on blood vessels at even this stage of their hypotensive action.

III. Chronic Haemodynamic Response

The hypotensive effect of the diuretics is maintained undiminished for as long as the drug therapy is continued. It has also been shown that during continuous treatment cardiac output is restored and total peripheral resistance is reduced (CONWAY and LAUWERS, 1960; VILLARREAL et al., 1962a; LUND-JOHANSEN, 1970). Diuretic therapy apparently produces an effect on the vascular tree and this will be discussed more fully below.

There is a divergence of opinion as to whether plasma volume, extracellular fluid volume, or indeed the initial sodium loss, is maintained. Balance studies reveal that sodium loss is limited to 2 to 3 days and thereafter subjects regain some of the deficit (HOLLANDER et al., 1959; VENNING et al., 1962; HITZENBERGER et al., 1968). Balance studies are, however, accurate only over short periods. Thus the retention of sodium observed towards the end of the first week of therapy may merely represent an oscillation or overshoot of the regulating mechanisms and the state of sodium balance after a period of weeks cannot be detected by them. Unfortunately measurements of exchangeable sodium values are also difficult to interpret. While the initial loss of sodium is reflected in a fall in exchangeable sodium, the level after several weeks of continued treatment is restored to near control levels (LAUWERS and CONWAY, 1960; CONWAY and LEONETTI, 1965; GIFFORD et al., 1961). HANSEN (1968) showed however that the initial reduction of 218 mEq. in exchangeable sodium was only partially restored after 3 months of therapy (to 132 mEq below control). The figure agrees quite well with the value found for chlorthalidone (HEALY et al., 1970). Restoration of measured exchangeable sodium after chronic diuretic therapy, however, may not indicate an actual retention of the ion, since a normal value could equally result from activation of the large, previously nonexchangeable sodium pool. Hence the state of sodium balance after chronic diuretic therapy must remain unknown until suitable methods become available.

Measurements of extracellular fluid volume have generally shown a fall of about 10% as diuretic therapy was initiated (WILSON and FREIS, 1959; MCQUEEN and MORRISON, 1960; BARTORELLI et al., 1966; LETH, 1970) but levels returned to a value closer to control after some weeks or months of treatment (WILSON and FREIS, 1959; LAUWERS and CONWAY, 1960; CRANSTON et al., 1963; BARTORELLI et al., 1966; LETH, 1970). It is uncertain whether there is complete or partial restoration in extracellular fluid volume with time (see also TARAZI et al., 1970).

Plasma volume measurements after chronic diuretic therapy have also given conflicting results. While some have found that the initial reduction of about 10% in volume was not maintained (WILSON and FREIS, 1959; CONWAY and LAUWERS, 1960; GIFFORD et al., 1961), others have reported a persistent reduction of about 7% (WINER, 1961; HANSEN, 1968, TARAZI et al., 1970; LUND-JOHANSEN, 1970; LETH, 1970). All these studies on extracellular fluid and plasma volumes have unfortunately been made on limited numbers of subjects, and take no account of seasonal or temperature variations. Upon the evidence it is difficult therefore to determine the true position.

An assumption surrounding this point needs examination. It is implied that if the reduction in plasma volume persists, the mechanism responsible for the fall in blood pressure must be the same on long term diuretic therapy as it was initially. This of course may be so, but the evidence does not support it. A fall in peripheral resistance on long-term therapy has been demonstrated by the 3 groups who have looked for it; and it should be noted that one of them, LUND-JOHANSEN (1970), found a reduced resistance in spite of a persistent reduction in plasma volume.

The position of potassium balance after chronic treatment with diuretics is also confused. While TALSO and CARBALLO (1960) could detect no change in exchangeable potassium on thiazide therapy, REMENCHIK et al., (1966) demonstrated a reduction of exchangeable potassium and naturally occurring K^{40}, by whole body counting, in 9 non-oedematous subjects who were given hydrochlorothiazide (100 mg/day) for 4 weeks.

ANDERSON et al., (1971) however could detect no such change in total body potassium (K^{40}). With chlorthalidone and furosemide respectively. HEALY et al. (1970) demonstrated reductions of exchangeable potassium of 317 mEq and 247 mEq. Although these changes were significant, they form a small proportion of the body potassium pool. The hypokalemia commonly observed is partly a reflection of the accompanying alkalosis (TALSO and CARBALLO, 1960; SCHWARTZ, 1966).

The loss of electrolytes which occurs as treatment starts, is complete within 2 to 3 days; but as this occurs, regulating mechanisms which tend to conserve sodium are activated so that a balance is eventually struck. The point at which equilibrium is achieved will depend upon the potency and duration of activity of the diuretic, the sodium intake, and the strength of the mechanisms concerned with sodium retention. For this reason results from various groups studying fluid and electrolyte shifts tend to differ.

The behaviour of the renin-angiotensin-aldosterone system after diuretic therapy illustrates further the balance of forces at play. Plasma renin activity, or angiotensin II levels, rise over the course of approximately a week and then decline (Fig. 2). Even after long term therapy some observers have found elevated levels (TARAZI et al., 1970; OVERTURF et al., 1972), while others have not (BOURGOIGNE, 1968; WERNING et al., 1969; CATT et al., 1970, 1971 [Fig. 3]).

In rats receiving chlorothiazide an increase in the granularity of the juxtaglomerular apparatus is, in addition, anatomical evidence for the increased activity of the renin-angiotensin system (TOBIAN et al., 1962).

Since sodium loss diminishes gradually over a few days of continued treatment, it is sometimes stated that "escape" from the influence of the diuretic has occured. Although a true "escape" of tubular cells from the action of thiazides can be demonstrated (PETERS, 1966), it does not apply to chronic treatment in man. The apparent waning of the diuretic effect is due to the operation of complex sodium retaining mechanisms, leading to the balance between the two opposing forces.

Wherever the point of equilibrium may be between these forces, the persistence of the diuretic activity during long-term therapy can be seen when the drug is withdrawn. A large increase in weight then ensues (Fig. 1), and sometimes oedema develops. Plasma volume and extracellular fluid volume increase and overshoot above normal (WILSON and FREIS, 1959; TARAZI et al., 1970) and then decline slowly. The return takes a surprisingly long time and in the work of TARAZI et al. the process of readjustment is seen to persist for 4 weeks.

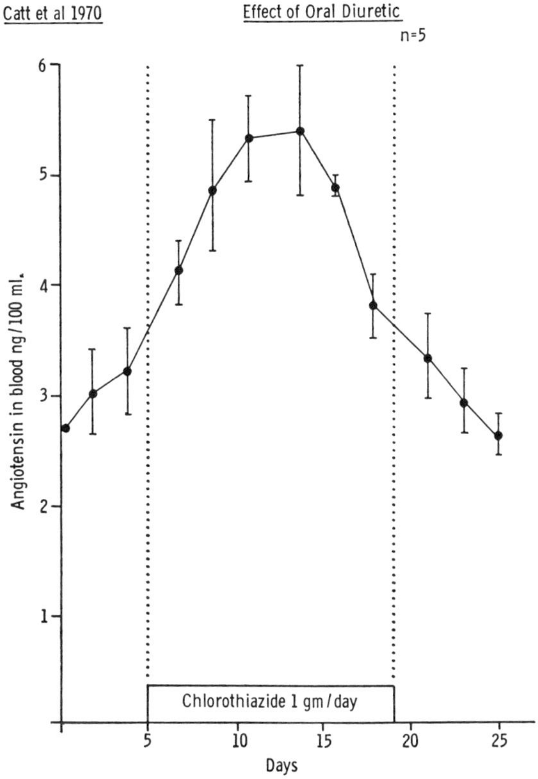

Fig. 2. The effect of chlorothiazide on the angiotensin II levels in the blood. From CATT et al., Circulation Research 1970, with permission

Some of the differences of opinion regarding the status of sodium and water balance during long-term diuretic therapy, stem from the fact that the changes are relatively small in relation to the control measurements and their repeatability. This applies even more forcibly when the tissue electrolyte changes are considered. From studies in rats, WELLER and HAIGHT (1963) and TALSO et al. (1966) found no change in skeletal muscle electrolytes, but others have found some evidence for an increase in tissue sodium and loss of potassium (TOBIAN et al., 1962; WOLF and GESSLER, 1964). In one study, hydrochlorothiazide was reported to reduce total muscle and intracellular water, sodium and potassium content in man (VILLAMIL et al., 1963). In passing it should be noted that thiazides are without effect on tissue ions in nephrectomized animals (ORBISON, 1962). Furthermore no changes have been reported in the sodium and potassium content of vascular tissues in rats treated with hydrochlorothiazide (Tobian et al., 1962; Daniel, 1962; Weller and Haight, 1963).

In conclusion therefore the composition of tissue electrolytes and the disposition of fluid within the body during continued duiretic therapy rests upon an equilibrium between the continued action of the duiretic and the homeostatic mechanisms opposing the sodium and water loss. The resulting balance appears to be so close to normal as to make estimates of the actual status difficult. It is likely however that some deficit in extracellular fluid, and plasma volume, persists at some intermediate level between the control value and the fall produced as diuretic therapy is started.

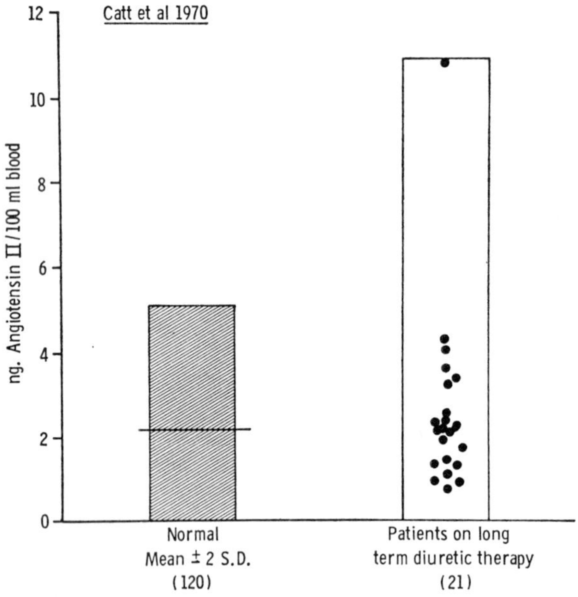

Fig. 3. The effect of chronic therapy with chlorothiazide on angiotensin II levels. From Catt et al., Circulation Research 1970, with permission

IV. Characteristics of the Hypotensive Response

Although a fall in blood pressure can be seen soon after an adequate diuresis has been established, and the diuretic effect is fully achieved within 3 to 4 days, it is not generally appreciated that the effect on blood pressure takes about 3 weeks to become fully manifest (Hall and Owen, 1959; Conway and Palmero, 1963). After the diuretic is withdrawn the reverse is observed, weight rises over a few days, overshoots, and the settles at a higher level, at which time pressure itself rises slowly over a period of 3 weeks. This is illustrated in Fig. 1 and it is a point of importance since it demonstrates that the hypotensive effect of the diuretic is not a direct ar immediate result of the loss of extracellular fluid. A delay of similar has been noted in the hypotensive response to spironolactone in patients with primary aldosteronism (Brown et al., 1972). The timing of this is reminiscent of the changes which occur in the opposite direction as pressure rises when patients are placed upon a sodium retaining substance (Borst and Geus, 1963). The fall in pressure with diuretics must therefore depend, in part at least, upon a gradual change, perhaps in electrolyte distribution, which ensues after the acute loss of electrolytes and water with the initiation of therapy.

The mean fall in blood pressure with diuretics is modest, and is only slightly affected by increasing the dose (BORHANI, 1960; CRANSTON et al., 1963), in spite of the demonstration of a increase in blood level when this is done (MCLEOD et al., 1970). Larger doses, however, lead to augmented hypokalemia, hyperuricemia and nitrogen retention.

The hypotensive effect is variable from one patient to another and, as shown in Fig. 4, it is related to the initial, or control blood pressure level (CRANSTON et al.,

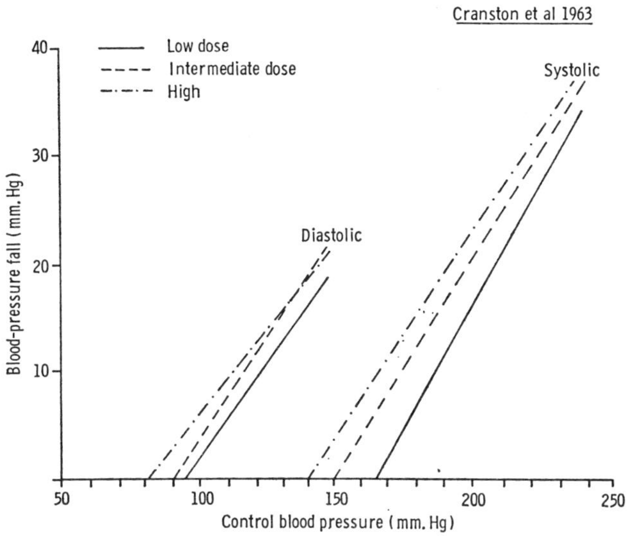

Fig. 4. Regression lines of blood-pressure fall on control blood pressure at low, intermediate and high doses of diuretics. From CRANSTON et al., Lancet **1963**, with permission

1963, ANDERSON et al., 1971). This point is of some importance since it has been reported that blood pressure is not reduced in normotensive subjects (FREIS and WILSON, 1959). Diuretics are therefore regarded as having an "antihypertensive" effect rather than a "hypotensive" one. Since the change in blood pressure is small and the response is related to blood pressure level, the response in normal subjects may be difficult to detect and it will be necessary to examine this point more rigorously.

Providing that an adequate dose is given, all diuretics achieve the same hypotensive effects. Spironolactone appears to be as effective as hydrochlorothiazide and chlorthalidone (HOLLANDER, 1961; CRANSTON and JUEL-JENSEN, 1962; DARRACOTT VAUGHAN et al., 1973), but triamterene is less effective (CRANSTON et al., 1965), and the same may apply to amiloride (KAMPFF-MEYER et al., 1968; PATERSON et al., 1968). These are weaker diuretics but they will reverse the hypokalemia produced by thiazides and give a small additional fall in pressure when they are administered concurrently.

Paradoxically furosemide, one of the most potent diuretics, in a dose of 40 mg twice daily, is less effective in reducing pressure than hydrochlorothiazide at a dose of 50 mg twice daily (ANDERSON et al., 1971). This probably results from the shorter duration of action of furosemide. When sodium intake is restricted, a potent diuretic, ethacrynic acid, can be added to thiazide treatment to achieve further reduction in blood pressure (CONWAY and LEONETTI, 1965), but hypokalemia and hyperuricemia then become a problem. The combination can be useful as a temporary measure in patients who are resistant to hypotensive therapy, providing renal function is good.

The fall in blood pressure produced by diuretics affects the recumbent and standing pressures equally and the effect is maintained during exercise (VARNAUSKAS et al., 1961; LUND-JOHANSEN, 1970). The work of LUND-JOHANSEN on the haemodynamic effect of longterm thiazide therapy illustrates that cardiac output remains normal, whilst the hypotensive effect is maintained. This applies both at rest and during exercise. Peripheral resistance is, therefore, reduced (Fig. 5).

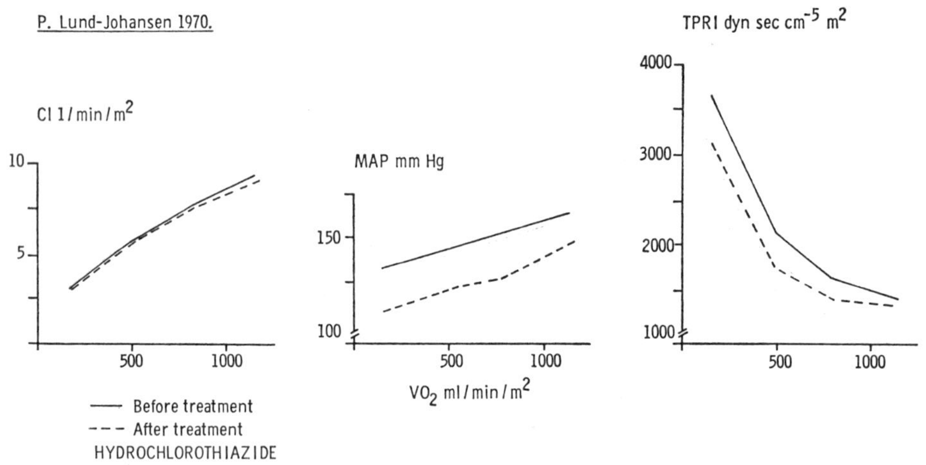

Fig. 5. The effect of long-term therapy with hydrochlorothiazide on cardiac index (CI) mean arterial pressure (MAP) and total peripheral resistance (TPRI) at rest and during exercise. The level of exercise is indicated by the oxygen consumption (VO_2). From LUND-JOHANSEN, Acta med. Scand. 1970, with permission

Hence, the haemodynamic response to diuretics is a physiologically satisfactory one. In this regard it should be mentioned in passing that a question hangs over the response to chlorthalidone. This compound appeared to produce some of its hypotensive action by reduction of cardiac output. The numbers of subjects involved however were small (nine in all) and the blood pressure responses were greater than those found in the subjects treated with hydrochlorothiazide, thereby making comparison of the haemodynamic effects difficult (LUND-JOHANSEN, 1970).

V. Interaction Between Diuretics and Other Antihypertensive Drugs

In addition to their hypotensive effects the diuretics have the important property of enhancing the response of other agents which lower blood pressure. In the initial studies on chlorothiazide it was noted that the mild hypotensive agents, reserpine and hydralazine, were rendered more effective when a diuretic was added and patients who had previously undergone a sympathectomy had an unusually large fall in pressure (HOLLANDER and WILKINS, 1957; FREIS et al., 1958).

This was confirmed by many others for ganglionic blocking agents (TAPIA et al., 1957; HALL and OWEN, 1959; DUSTAN et al., 1959; RØNNOV-JESSEN, 1955; FREIS et al., 1960; WINER, 1961b), reserpine (SMITH et al., 1964), methyldopa (WILSON et al., 1963; COLWIL et al., 1964; SMITH et al., 1966), guanethidine (LEISHMAN et al., 1961; RØNNOV-JESSEN and HANSEN, 1969), vasodilators (TAYLOR et al., 1952; SMITH et al., 1964; GILMORE et al., 1970) and clonidine (JUNGLING, 1968; ONESTI et al., 1969).

Diuretic therapy, therefore, interacts with a variety of agents differing in pharmacological action. Several possibilities exist for this interaction.

First, antonomic blocking agents interfere with the reflex responses to the fall in blood pressure (DUSTAN et al., 1959; SERIU, 1965), and hence to some extent hinder the increase in peripheral resistance which accompanies the fall in cardiac output produced by the diuretics. Blocking agents also interfere with the renin response to sodium depletion (KANEKO et al., 1965; MOHAMMED et al., 1969).

It is more usual however to think of the diuretics interacting in the opposite manner with antihypertensive agents; that is with the sodium retention which occurs as blood pressure is reduced. It has been amply shown, for example, that thiazides reverse this sodium retention (RØNNOV-JESSEN and HANSEN 1969). The precise mechanism for sodium retention with hypotensive drugs has not been fully elucidated. Certainly a reduction in glomerular filtration plays a part (SMITH, 1965) but sodium retention occurs without a fall in filtration rate. BIRKENHAGER et al. (1962) noted that retention was more pronounced in subjects with marked diurnal excretory rhythm and suggested that the nocturnal loss of sodium was inadequate. LAULER et al. (1963) suggested that the hypotensive agents accentuated the normal retention of sodium which occurs on standing. SMITH (1965) suggested that sympathetic blocking agents stimulate active tubular reabsorption of sodium and this has also been proposed as the mechanism for the sodium retention which occurs with diazoxide (POHL et al., 1972).

Sodium retention, produced by so many hypotensive agents, is one of the most important mechanisms by which hypertensive patients develop resistance to hypotensive agents (FINNERTY, 1971). Recently DUSTAN et al., (1972) have also made the interesting observation that, when sympathetic nervous function is reduced, blood pressure level becomes directly related to plasma volume. These facts demonstrate the practical importance of maintaining concurrent diuretic therapy when autonomic blocking agents are being administered for the control of hypertension.

Finally, it has been shown that chlorothiazide interferes with the excretion of mecamylamine (HARINGTON and KINCAID-SMITH, 1958) but there are unfortunately no other studies of the manner in which diuretics may interfere with the pharmacokinetics of other agents.

VI. Mode of Antihypertensive Action

The description of the status of the individual on long term diuretic therapy leaves many uncertainties and differences of opinion. However, it is agreed, as noted earlier, that peripheral resistance is reduced. The mechanism whereby this comes about is unknown. It is even open to doubt that the fall in resistance is necessarily an effect of the drug at all. It could be argued that the diuresis causes a fall in cardiac output, and with time this could result, by some undefined means, in a fall in peripheral resistance. Something similar to this has in fact been reported after propranolol therapy (TARAZI et al., 1972) and there is also some evidence that it occurs with long-term treatment with guanethidine (VILLARREAL et al., 1964, CHAMBERLAIN and HOWARD, 1964).

That vague constellation of ideas which surrounds "resetting of baroreceptors" should be mentioned here, although the term has been debased beyond any useful meaning. Nevertheless it is possible that the fall in vascular resistance could come about as a result of a failure of the regulative reflexes which were set off when cardiac output falls. With these two explanations, however, it would be a little difficult to explain the fact that cardiac output returns to normal. These possibilities remain, however, and should not be forgotten.

The suggestion has been made that thiazides reduce resistance by virtue of a direct dilator effect on blood vessels. This came to prominence when a non diuretic analogue, diazoxide, was discovered (Rubin, 1961). Such a direct action can be dismissed for a variety of reasons. As noted in the introduction, diuretics of extremely diverse chemical structure lower blood pressure with equal effectiveness. For example, for a given diuretic effect, a mercurial gives the same hypotensive response as a thiazide (Hall and Owen, 1959). Generally the change in blood pressure is related to the change in extracellular fluid volume (Freis and Wilson, 1959; Hall and Owen, 1959). Even amongst the benothiadiazines there is a wide range of dosage, yet the antihypertensive action is related to the diuretic effect and increasing the dose above that which achieved an adequate diuresis causes no greater fall in pressure. Most damaging, perhaps, to the theory of a direct dilator action is the fact that withdrawal of the compound does not lead to an immediate rise in pressure (Fig. 1), in spite of the fact that the thiazides are known to leave the body within 48 h. Furthermore, Hollander et al. (1959) have shown that blood pressure does not rise when thiazides are withdrawn if sodium intake is restricted. Finally, the thiazides do not affect the tone of excised vascular tissue in animals (Daniel and Nash, 1965).

The antihypertensive action, therefore, depends upon the diuretic action, even though the reduction in vascular resistance is not an immediate consequence of the diuresis. This is supported by the fact that in individual hypertensive patients the fall in blood pressure produced by diuretics is related to the fall produced by moderate sodium restriction (Parijs et al., 1973).

A reduction in plasma volume could not account for the reduction in peripheral resistance, but nothing is know of the vascular effect of a sustained reduced extracellular fluid volume. This could affect the vessel wall by changing the volume of fluid between individual vascular cells, reducing wall stiffness (Zelis et al., 1968) or reducing tissue pressure on the outside of minute vessels. It is of interest in passing to note that several diuretics, albeit at high dosage, influence the rate of flow of lymph into the thoracic duct. This action persists in nephrectomized animals (Szwed et al., 1972). It could be important because it demonstrates a non-renal action of a wide variety of diuretics on the mobility of extracellular fluid. This could influence the distribution of body fluids and perhaps vascular function.

A change in the sodium gradient between the interior of the cell and its environment has been suggested as a possible mechanism of action of diuretics producing vasodilatation (Friedman et al., 1960). This is difficult to demonstrate and the finding has been disputed (Daniel, 1962; Villamil et al., 1963).

Continued sodium loss could result in a diminished response of vascular tissue to naturally occuring pressor substances and a diminished reactivity to noradrenaline has been proposed (Bock u. Sun, 1960; Preziosi et al., 1959; Gillenwater et al., 1962).

Although there is no universal agreement on this point (Daniel and Nash, 1965), a similar reduction in responsiveness of the forearm vasculature has been observed in normal subjects after one week of chlorothiazide therapy (Feisal et al., 1961). A similar effect was observed in dogs after the same duration of therapy.

The response to sympathetic nerve stimulation is also reduced by chlorothiazide treatment (AOKI and BRODY, 1965) and the catecholamine content of variuos organs is reduced after hydrochlorothiazide therapy (PREZIOSI et al., 1961; HOLLANDER et al., 1959). These effects have all been elicited after short-term treatments with diuretics but FREIS et al. (1960) and ECKSTEIN et al. (1964) have shown a reduction in the response to noradrenaline after long-term therapy. Long-term thiazide therapy in rabbits and dogs also results in a reduction in the sensitivity of blood vessels to noradrenaline, but not to other vasoactive compounds (ZSOTÉR et al., 1970).

Clearly the mode of action of the diuretics in lowering blood pressure remains speculative. Work in this area is hindered by the fact that the change in blood pressure is quite small and generally the animal models for hypertension respond irregularly, if at all, to diuretic therapy (WELLER and HAIGHT, 1963; FREGLEY, 1961; TOBIAN and COFFEE, 1964; STANTON and WHITE, 1965; NICHOLAS, 1971).

Present evidence therefore points to the fall in pressure as an indirect and delayed effect of the diuretic action. This could be due to a change in extracellular fluid volume within the vessel wall or its immediate surroundings. Alternatively vascular smooth muscle contraction may be affected by a change in electrolyte distribution. There is some evidence that vascular responses to vasoconstrictor agents, particularly noradrenaline, are affected. This might not be of sufficient degree to produce postural hypotension but, whatever the effect on blood vessels, it is clear that the regulation of blood pressure with changes in posture and with exercise remains normal. For this reason diuretic therapy remains the most satisfactory regimen for hypertension. One could only wish that it were more potent.

VII. An Abnormality of Sodium Regulation in Hypertension?

There is an additional possibility that, within the disease complex known as essential hypertension, there is a subgroup in which sodium handling is abnormal, and this group might respond exceptionally well to diuretic therapy. An examination of such subjects could reveal that the mode of action of diuretics is to interfere with this derangement.

When diuretics emerged as useful antihypertensive agents it was indeed hoped that their use might reveal important information about the relationship between sodium metabolism and hypertension. That hope has not been realized, but there is an increasing body of information which points to an abnormality in the regulation of sodium distribution in quite a large proportion of hypertensive subjects.

The demonstration that some 25% of hypertensive patients, without primary aldosteronism, have low levels of plasma renin or have a blunted response to sodium depletion, to thiazide diuretics and to other stimuli, is of interest (HELMER and JUDSON, 1968; CREDITOR and LOSCHKY, 1968; WOODS et al., 1969; CHANNICK, ALDIN and MARKS, 1969; JOSE et al., 1970; OELKERS et al., 1970; JERUM and DOYLE, 1969; MOLZAHN, 1972; COGHLAN et al., 1972). These subjects have a greater pool of exchangeable sodium (JOSÉ et al., 1970; WOODS et al., 1969) and suffer a greater loss of sodium than usual when they pass from a high to a low sodium diet (WEINBERGER et al., 1968; BROWN et al., 1971). The fall in pressure was also greater on a low sodium diet in these subjects compared with hypertensives with normal exchangeable sodium levels (BROWN et al., 1971).

The patient with a low plasma renin activity behave as if they have an expanded extracellular fluid volume, which may be due to an adaptation to prolonged ingestion of a high sodium diet, or the presence of an unidentified sodium retaining hormone. Alternatively there may be a defect in the sympathetic nervous system governing the release of renin (Kaneko et al., 1965). These patients respond to blockade of steroid synthesis by aminoglutethimide with a fall in blood pressure (Woods et al., 1969). They also respond to spironolactone and other diuretics whereas hypertensives with normal plasma renin activity do not. (Spark and Melby, 1971; Carey, Douglas, and Liddle, 1972; Darracott Vaughan et al., 1973). This, taken with the fact others have shown that the response to thiazides in hypertensives generally is correlated with their response to spironolactone (Cranston and Juel-Jensen, 1962; Conway and Palermo, 1963; Darracott Vaughan et al., 1973), suggests that the response to diuretics may be related to an abnormality in sodium metabolism.

VIII. Summary and Conclusions

The acute hypotensive effect of diuretics is almost certainly the direct result of the fall in extracellular fluid and plasma volume, with a consequent reduction in cardiac output. At this stage peripheral resistance rises, due to reflex action, but it is inadequate to compensate fully for the reduced output and blood pressure falls.

On present evidence, the fall in extracellular fluid volume appears to exert an effect which is independant of the coincident fall in plasma volume. Whether this influences cardiac output or peripheral resistance is unknown.

As diuretic therapy is maintained over longer periods, a balance is achieved between the opposing forces of the continued action of the diuretic on the kidney and a variety of neurogenic and hormonal mechanisms concerned with sodium retention. After several weeks of treatment, therefore, the status of the fluid and electrolyte balance in the various compartments of the body is difficult to assess. It is probable that extracellular fluid and plasma volume continue to be marginally reduced and there is a small reduction in total body sodium and potassium. The antihypertensive action of diuretics, which takes about 3 weeks to be fully manifest, is maintained by a fall in peripheral resistance.

The mechanism responsible for the sustained fall in pressure and vascular resistance has not been elucidated but there is ample evidence to support the idea that the hypotensive effect results from the diuretic action, rather than a direct dilator action of the thiazides on blood vessels.

Four possible mechanisms for the hypotensive effect of diuretics present themselves:

1) There may be a gradual decline in the activity of the neurogenic and hormonal reflex activity which attempts to maintain blood pressure in the face of the reduced cardiac output produced acutely by the diuretic.

2) A reduction in extracellular fluid volume could influence the diameter of resistance vessels or reduce tissue pressure.

3) Sodium loss and an alteration in ionic distribution in vascular muscle could reduce the tone of blood vessels or influence their response to normally circulating vasoconstrictor substances, notably noradrenaline.

4) Reduction in vasomotor tone may result from enhanced storage and binding of noradrenaline which ocurs with sodium depletion. There may also be a substantial proportion of hypertensive subjects with an abnormality in the regulation of sodium distribution. These are, or behave as though they are, retaining excessive amounts of sodium and diuretic therapy could interfere with this abnormality.

Evidence for and against each of these can be gathered from the literature. The fact that the hypotensive action of diuretics has been with us for more than a decade should not deflect us from research into their mode of action.

References

ALEKSANDROW, D., WYSZNACKA W., GAJEWSKI, J.: Studies on the mechanism of hypotensive action of chlorothiazide. New Engl. J. Med. **260**, 51—55 (1959a).

ALEKSANDROW, D., WYSZNACKA, W., GAJEWSKI, J.: Influence of chlorothiazide upon arterial responsiveness to nor-epinephrine in hypertensive subjects. New Engl. J. Med **261**, 1052—1055 (1959b).

ANDERSON, J., GODFREY, B. E., HILL, D. M., MUNRO-FAURE, A. D., SHELDON, J.: A comparison of the effects of hydrochlorothiazide and Frusemide in the treatment of hypertensive patients. Quart. J. Med. NS **40**, 541—560 (1971).

AOKI, V. S., BRODY, M. J.: Effect of thiazides on the sympathetic nervous system. Pharmacologist **7**, 145 (1965) (Abstract).

BARTORELLI, C., GARGANO, N., LEONETTI, G.: Potassium loss and potassium replacement during long-term diuretic treatment in hypertension. In: Antihypertensive Therapy. An International Symposium. F. Gross (Ed.). Berlin-Heidelberg-New York: Springer 1966.

BIRKENHAGER, W. H., STATIUS VAN EPS, L. W., VRIES, L. A. DE: Reversal of rhythmic water and sodium excretion patterns during ganglionic or adrenergic block. Acta med. scand. **172**, 105—115 (1962).

BORHANI, N. O.: Chlorothiazide and hydrochlorothiazide. A comparative study of their hypotensive, saluretic and hyperuricemic action. Ann. intern. Med. **53**, 342—358 (1960).

BORST, J. G. G., GEUS, A. B.: Hypertension explained by Starling's theory of circulatory homeostasis. Lancet **1963** I, 677—682.

BOURGOIGNIE, J. J., CATANZARO, F. J., PERRY, H. M.: Renin-Angiotensin Aldosterone System during chronic thiazide therapy of benign hypertension. Circulation **37**, 27—35 (1968).

BRAVO, E. L., TARAZI, R. C., DUSTAN, H. P.: Beta-adrenergic blockade in diuretic-treated patients with essential hypertension. N. Engl. J. Med., **292**, 66—70 (1975).

BROWN, J. J., DAVIS, D. L., FERRISS, J. B., FRASER, R., HAYWOOD, E., LEVER, A. F., ROBERTSON, J. I. S.: Comparison of surgery and prolonged spironolactone therapy in patients with hypertension, aldosterone excess and low plasma renin. Brit. med. J. **1972**, II, 729—734.

BROWN, J. J., DAVIES, D. L., LEVER, A. F., ROBERTSON, J. I. S.: Plasma renin concentration in human hypertension. Brit. med. J. **1966**, II, 267—272.

BROWN, W. J., BROWN, F. K., KRISHNAN, I.: Exchangeable sodium and blood volume in normotensive and hypertensive humans on high and low sodium intake. Circulation **43**, 508—519 (1971).

BÜHLER, F. R., BURKART, F., LÜTOLD, B. E., KÜNG, M., MARBET, G., PFISTERER, M.: Antihypertensive beta-blocking action as related to renin and age: A pharmacologic tool to identify pathogenetic mechanisms in essential hypertension. Amer. J. Cardiol., **36**, 653—669 (1975).

BÜHLER, F. R., LARAGH, J. H., SEALEY. J. E., BRUNNER, H. R.: Plasma aldosterone-renin interrelationship in various forms of essential hypertension. Amer. J. Cardiol. **32**, 554—561 (1973).

CAREY, R. M., DOUGLAS, J. G., LIDDLE, G. W.: Spironolactone in patients with essential hypertension and suppressed plasma renin activity. Clin. Res. **20**, 72 (1972) (abstract).

CASTENFORS, J.: Effect of ethacrynic acid on plasma renin activity during supine exercise in normal subjects. Acta physiol. scand. **70**, 215—220 (1967).

CASTLE, C. H., CONRAD, J. K., HECHT, H. H.: Observations on the diuretic effect of chlorothiazide. Arch. intern. Med. **103**, 415—420 (1959).

CATT, K. J., CAIN, M. D., COGHLAN, J. P., ZIMMET, P. Z., CRAIN, E., BEST, J. B.: Metabolism and blood levels of Angiotensin II in normal subjects, Renal Disease and essential hypertension. Circulation Res. **26** and**27**, Suppl. II, 177—193 (1970).

CATT, K. J., ZIMMET, P. Z., CAIN, M. D., CRAN, E., BEST, J. B., COGHLAN, J. P.: Angiotensin II blood-levels in human hypertension. Lancet **1971 I**, 459—469.

CHAMBERLAIN, D. A., HOWARD, J.: Guanethidine and methyldopa: a haemodynamic study. Brit. Heart. J. **26**, 528—536 (1964).

CHANNICK, B. J., ALDIN, E. V., MARKS, A. D.: Suppressed plasma renin activity in hypertension Ann. intern. Med. **123**, 131—140 (1969).

COGHLAN, J. P., DOYLE, A. E., JERUMS, J., SCOGGINS, B. A.: The effects of sodium loading and deprevation on plasma renin and plasma and urinary aldesterone in hypertension. Clin. Sci. **42**, 15—23 (1972).

COLWILL, J. M., DUTTON, A. M., MORRISSEY, J., YU, P. N.: Alpha-methyldopa and hydrochlorothiazide. New Engl. J. Med. **271**, 696—703 (1964).

CONWAY, J., LAUWERS, P.: Hemodynamic and hypotensive effects of long-term therapy with chlorothiazide. Circulation **21**, 21—27 (1960).

CONWAY, J., LEONETTI, G.: Hypotensive effect of ethacrynic acid. Circulation **31**, 661–664 (1965).
CONWAY, J., PALMERO, H.: The vascular effect on the thiazide diuretics. Arch. intern. Med. **111**, 203—207 (1963).
CRANSTON, W. I., JUEL-JENSEN, B. E.: The effects of spironolactone and chlorthalidone on arterial pressure. Lancet **1962 I**, 1161—1164.
CRANSTON, W. I., JUEL-JENSEN, B, E, SEMMENCE, A, M, JONES, R. P. C. H., FORBES, J. A., MUTCH, L. M. M.: Effect of oral diuretis on raised arterial pressure. Lancet **1963 II**, 966—970.
CRANSTON, W. I., SEMMENCE, A. M., RICHARDSON, D. W., BARNETT, C. F.: Effect of triamterene (Dyrenium) on elevated arterial blood pressure. Amer. Heart. J. **70**, 455—460 (1965).
CREDITOR, N. C., LOSCHKY, U. K.: Incidence of suppressed renin activity and of normo-kalemic primary aldosteronism in hypertensive negro patients. Circulation **37**, 1027—1035 (1968).
CROSLEY, A. P., JR., COSTELLO, C., FREEMAN, J. D., WHITE, D. H., JR., ROWE, G. C.: The acute effects of carbonic anhydrase inhibitors on systemic hemodynamics. J. clin. Invest. **37**, 887 (1958) (abstract).
CROSLEY, A. P., JR., CULLEN, R. C., WHITE, D., FREEMAN, J. J., CASTILLO, C. A., ROWE, G. C.: Studies on the mechanism of action of chlorothiazide in cardiac and renal diseases. I. Acute effects on renal and systemic hemodynamics and metabolism. J. Lab. clin. Med. **55**, 191—202 (1960).
DANIEL, E. E.: On the mechanism of antihypertensive action of hydrochlorothiazide in rats. Circulation Res. **11**, 941—954 (1962).
DANIEL, E. E., NASH, C. W.: The effect of diuretic and non-diuretic benzothiadiazines and of structurally related diuretic drugs on active ion transport and contractility in smooth muscles. Arch. Int. Pharmacodyn. **158**, 139—154 (1965).
DARRACOTT VAUGHAN, E., LARAGH, J. H., GAVRAS, I., BUHLER, F. R., HARALAMBOS, G., BRUNNER, H. R., BAER, J.: Volume factor in low and normal renin essential hypertension. Amer. J. Cardiol. **32**, 523—532 (1973).
DAVIDOV, M., GAVRILOVICH, L., MROCZEK, W., FINNERTY, F. A., JR.: Relation of extracellular fluid volume to arterial pressure during drug-induced saluresis. Circulation **40**, 349—355 (1969).
DAVIDOV, M., KAKAVIATOS, N., FINNERTY, F. A., JR.: Antihypertensive properties of furosemide. Circulation **34**, 125—135 (1967).
DAVIES, D. L., WILSON, G. M.: Diuretics: Mechanism of action and clinical application. Drugs **9**, 178—226 (1975).
DOLLERY, C. T., PARRY, E. H. O., YOUNG, D. S.: Diuretic and hypotensive properties of ethacrynic acid: A comparison with hydrochlorothiazide. Lancet **1964 I**, 947—952.
DUSTAN, H. P., CUMMING, G. R., CORCORAN, A. C., PAGE, I. H.: A mechanism of chlorothiazide enhanced effectiveness of antihypertensive, ganglioplegic drugs. Circulation **19**, 360—365 (1959).
DUSTAN, H. P., TARAZI, R. C., BRAVO, E. L.: Dependence of arterial pressure on intravascular volume in treated hypertensive patients. New Engl. J. Med. **286**, 816—866 (1972).
ECKSTEIN, J. W., WNEDLING, M. G.: Effect of prolonged treatment with chlorothiazide on cardiovascular responses to norepinephrine, J. Lab. clin. Med. **64**, 853—854 (1964
FEISAL, K. A., ECKSTEIN, J. W., HORSLEY, A. W., KEASLIGH, H. H.: Effects of chlorothiazide on forearm vascular responses. J. appl. Physiol. **16**, 549—552 (1961).
FINNERTY, A., JR.: Relationship of extracellular fluid volume to the development of drug resistance in the hypertensive patient. Amer. Heart J. **81**, 563—565 (1971).
FINNERTY, F. A., JR., DAVIDOV, M., KAKAVIATOS, N.: Relation of sodium balance to arterial pressure during drug-induced saluresis. Circulation **37**, 175—183 (1968).
FREGLEY, M. J.: Effect of chlorothiazide and hydrochlorothiazide on blood pressure and thyroid activity of hypertensive rats. Amer. J. Cardiol. **8**, 890—898 (1961).
FREIS, E. D., WANKO, A., SCHNAPER, H. W., FROHLICH, E. D.: Mechanism of the altered blood pressure responsiveness produced by chlorothiazide. J. clin. Invest. **39**, 1277—1281 (1960).
FREIS, E. D., WANKO, A., WILSON, I. M., PARRISH, A. E.: Treatment of essential hypertension with chlorothiazide (Diuril). J. Amer. med. Ass. **166**, 137—140 (1958).
FRIEDMAN, S. M., NAKASHIMA, M., FRIEDMAN, C. L.: Relation of saluretic and hypotensive effects of hydrochlorothiazide. Amer. J. Physiol. **198**, 148—152 (1960).
GESSLER, U., NEUHAUS, M.: Experimentelle Untersuchungen intra- und extracellularer Elektrolyt- und Wassergehaltsveränderungen nach Chlorthalidonbehandlung. Arch. exp. Path. Pharmakol. **244**, 63—70 (1962).
GIFFORD, R. W., MATTOX, V. R., ORVIS, A. L., SONES, D. A., ROSEVEAR, J. W.: Effect of thiazide diuretics on plasma volume, body electrolytes, and excretion of aldosterone in hypertension. Circulation **24**, 1197—1205 (1961).
GILLENWATER, J. Y., SCOTT, J. B., FRÖHLICH, E. D.: Effect of chlorothiazide on response of renal vascular bed to vasoactive substances. Circulation Res. **11**, 283—286 (1962).

GILMORE, E., WEIL, J., CHIDSEY, C.: Treatment of essential hypertension with a new vasodilator in combination with betaadrenergic blockade. New Engl. J. Med. **282**, 521—527 (1970).

HALL, R., OWEN, S. G.: The hypotensive effect of chlorothiazide. Lancet **1959 I**, 129—130.

HANSEN, J.: Hydrochlorothiazide in the treatment of hypertension. Acta med. scand. **183**, 317—321 (1968).

HARINGTON, M., KINCAID-SMITH, P.: Effect of chlorothiazide on the hypotensive action of mecamylamine and on its urinary excretion. Lancet **1958 I**, 403—404.

HEALY, J. J., MCKENNA, T. J., CANNING, B. St., JR., BRIEN, T. G., DUFFY, G. J., MULDOWNEY, F. P.: Body composition changes in hypertensive subjects on long-term oral diuretic therapy. Brit. med. J. **1**, 716—719 (1970).

HEIDER, C., DENNIS, E., MOYER, J. H.: Chlorothiazide potentiation and ganglionic blockade in patients with hypertension. Ann. N. Y. Acad. Sci. **71**, 456—464 (1958).

HELMER, O. M., JUDSON, W. E.: Metabolic studies on hypertensive patients with suppressed plasma renin activity not due to hyperaldosteronism. Circulation **28**, 965—976 (1968).

HITZENBERGER, G., KAMPFFMEYER, H., CONWAY, J.: The diuretic effect of desmethyl-pipazurolguanidine (MK-870) in man. J. clin. Pharm. Therap. **9**, 71—79 (1968).

HOLLANDER, W.: The antihypertensive activity of aldosterone antagonists. In: Brest, A. N., Moyer, J. H. (Eds.): Hypertension recent advances, pp. 269—274. Lea and Febiger 1961.

HOLLANDER, W., CHOBANIAN, A. V., WILKINS, R. W.: Relationship between diuretic and antihypertensive effects of chlorthiazide and mercurial diuretics. Circulation **19**, 827—838 (1959).

HOLLANDER, W., WILKINS, R.: Chlorothiazide: A new type of drug for the treatment of arterial hypertension. Boston Med. Quart. **8**, 69—73 (1957).

HOLLANDER, W., YAGI, S., KRAMSCH, D. M.: *In vitro* effects of vasopressor agents on the metabolism of the vascular wall. Circulation **30** (Supp. II), 1—10 (1964).

HUTCHEON, D. E., LEONARD, G. B., SCHWARTZ, M. L.: The antihypertensive action of chlorthalidone. J. med. Soc. N. J. **62**, 172—175 (1965).

JERUMS, G., DOYLE, A. E.: Renal sodium handling and responsiveness of plasma renin levels in hypertension. Clin. Sci. **37**, 79—90 (1969).

JOSE, A., CROUT, J. R., KAPLAN, N. M.: Suppressed plasma renin activity in essential hypertension. Ann. intern. Med. **72**, 9—16 (1970).

JUNGLING, K.: Klinische Untersuchungen mit dem neuen Antihypertonikum, Catapresan. Med. Welt **39**, 2105—2112 (1968).

KAKAVIATOS, N., FINNERTY, F. A.: Comparison of chlorthalidone, a long-acting antihypertensive and diuretic agent with chlorothiazide. Amer. J. Cardiol. **101**, 570—574 (1962).

KAMPFFMEYER, H., CONWAY, J.: The antihypertensive and diuretic effects of amiloride (N-amidino-3,5-diamino-6-chlorophrazine-carboxamide hydrochloride alone and in combination with hydrochlorothiazide. J. Clin. Pharm. Therap. **9**, 350—354 (1968).

KANEKO, Y., TAKEDA, T., IKEDA, T., TAGAWA, H., ISHI, M., TAKABATAKE, Y., UEDA, H.: Effect of ganglion-blocking agents on renin release in hypertensive patients. Circulation Res. **27**, 97—103 (1970).

LARAGH, J. H.: Symposium on hypertension: Mechanisms and Management. Vacocontriction Volume analysis for understanding and treating hypertension: The use of renin and aldosterone profiles. Amer. J. Med. **55**, 261—274 (1973).

LAULER, D. P., VAGNUCCI, A. I., HICKLER, R. B., THORN, G. W.: Clinical features of sodium retention induced by antihypertensive therapy. Circulation **28**, 754—756 (1963).

LAUWERS, P., CONWAY, J.: Effect of long-term treatment with chlorothiazide on body fluids, serum electrolytes and exchangeable sodium in hypertensive patients. J. Lab. clin. Med. **56**, 401—406 (1960).

LEBEL, M., SCHALEKAMP, M. A., BEEVERS, D. G., BROWN, J. J., DAVIES, D. L., FRASER, R., KREMER, D., LEVER, A. F., MORTON, J. J., ROBERTSON, J. I. S., TREE, M., WILSON, A.: Sodium and the renin-angiotensin system in essential hypertension and mineralocorticoid excess. Lancet **1974 II**, 308—310.

LEISHMAN, A. W. D., MATHEWS, H. L., SMITH, A. J.: Guanethidine Hypotensive drugs with long action. Lancet **1961 II**, 1044—1048.

LETH, A.: Changes in plasma and extracellular fluid volumes in patients with essential hypertension during long-term treatment with hydrochlorothiazide. Circulation **42**, 479—485 (1970).

LETH, A., IBSEN, H., SEDERBERG-OLSEN, P.: The effect of triamterene on plasma and extracellular fluid volume and blood pressure in ten thiazide-treated hypolkalemic patients with essential hypertension. Scand. J. clin. Lab. Invest. **30**, 437—440 (1972).

LUND-JOHANSEN, P.: Hemodynamic changes in long term diuretic therapy of essential hypertension. Acta med. scand. **187**, 509—518 (1970).

MCLEOD, P. J., OGILVIE, R. I., RUEDY, J.: Effects of large and small doses of hydrochlorothiazide in hypertensive patients. J. clin. Pharm. Therap. **11**, 733—739 (1970).

McQueen, E. G., Morrison, R. B. I.: The hypotensive action of diuretic agents. Lancet **1960 I** 1209—1212.

Mohammed, S., Fasola, A, F., Privitera, P. J., Lipicky, R. J., Martz, B. L., Gaffney, T. E.: Effect of methyldopa on plasma renin activity in man. Circulation Res. **25**, 543—547 (1969).

Molzahn, M., Pressmann, T. H., Halim, S., Lohmann, F. W., Oelkers, W.: Orthostatic changes of haemodynamics, renal function, plasma catecholamine and plasma renin concentration in normal and hypertensive man. Clin. Sci. **42**, 209—222 (1972).

Nicholas, T. E.: Responses of mean arterial pressure to pressor agents and diuretics in renal hypertensive and salt hypertensive rats. Brit. J. Pharmacol. **42**, 179—192 (1971).

Novello, F. C., Sprague, J. M.: Benzothiadiazine dioxides as novel diuretics. J. Amer. cxem. Soc. **79**, 2028—2029 (1957).

Oelkers, W., Magnus, R., Samwer, K. F.: Das Verhalten der Plasmareninkonzentration nach akuter Natriurese und nach Orthostase bei Gesunden und Hypertonikern. Klin. Wschr. **48**, 598—607 (1970).

Onesti, G., Schwartz, A. B., Kim, K. E., Swartz, C., Brest, A. N.: Pharmacodynamic effects of a new, antihypertensive Drug, Catapres (ST-155). Circulation **39**, 219—228 (1969).

Orbison, J. L.: Failure of chlorothiazide to influence tissue electrolytes in hypertensive and non-hypertensive nephrectomized dogs. Proc. Sec. Exp. biol. Med. **110**, 161—164 (1962).

Overturf, M., Fritz, A., McBride, J.: Renin activity, sodium and potassium in hypertensive patients. J. Chron. Dis. **25**, 621—634 (1972).

Parijs, J., Joossens, J. V., van der Linden, Versteken, G., Amery, A. K. P. C.: Moderate sodium restriction and diuretics in the treatment of hypertension. Amer. Heart J. **85**, 22—34 (1973).

Paterson, J. W., Dollery, C. T., Haslam, R. M.: Amiloride hydrochloride in hypertensive patients. Brit. med. J. **1**, 422—423 (1968).

Peters, G.: Pharmacology of diuretics. In: Gross, F. (Ed.): Antihypertensive Therapy. An International Symposium. Berlin-Heidelberg-New York: Springer 1966.

Peters, G., Roch-Ramel, F.: Handbook of experimental pharmacology. Herken, H. (Ed.). Vol. 24, p. 257—435. Heffter and Heubner 1969.

Pohl, J. E. F., Thurston, H., Swales, J. D.: The antidiuretic action of diazoxide. Clin. Sci. **42**, 145—152 (1972).

Preziosi, E., Bianchi, A., Loscalzo, B., Schaepdryver, de, D. F.: On the pharmacology of chlorothiazide. Arch. int. Pharmacodyn. **118**, 467—495 (1959).

Preziosi, E., Shaepdryver, A. F., de, Marmo, E., Miele, E.: On the mechanism of the antihypertensive effect of hydrochlorothiazide. Arch. int. Pharmacodyn. **131**, 209—229 (1961).

Remenchik, A. P., Miller, C., Talso, P. J., Willoughby, E. O.: Depletion of body potassium by diuretics. Circulation **33**, 796—801 (1966).

Rønnov-Jessen, V.: Heart failure from retention of salt and water caused by treatment with pentolinium. Lancet **1955 I**, 122—124.

Rønnov-Jessen, V., Hansen, J.: Blood volume and exchangeable sodium during treatment of hypertension with guanethidine and hydrochlorothiazide. Acta med. scand. **186**, 155—163 (1969).

Rubin, A. A., Roth, F. E., Winbury, M. M.: A non-diuretic benzothiadiazine with antihypertensive properties. Nature (Lond.) **192**, 176—177 (1961).

Safar, M., Milliez, P.: Le traitement médical de l'hypertension artérielle: étude hémodynamique. Rev. Europ. Etudes Clin. Biol. **16**, 334—342 (1971).

Saito, I., Misumi, J., Kondo, K., Saruta, T., Matsuki, S.: Effects of furosemide and chlorothiazide on blood pressure and plasma renin activity. Cardio. Res. **10**, 149—152 (1976).

Schwartz, W. B.: Pathogenesis and replacement of diuretic-induced potassium and chloride loss. Ann. N. Y. Acad. Sci. **139**, 506—510 (1966).

Seriu, Y.: A clinical study of the role of catecholamine in blood pressure. Jap. Circulation J. **29**, 433—488 (1965).

Shalekamp, M. A., Ledel, M., Beevers, D. G., Fraser, R., Kolsters, G., Birkenhäger, W. H.: Body fluid volume in low-renin hypertension. Lancet **1974 II**, 310—311.

Smith, A. J.: Fluid retention produced by guanethedine. Circulation, **31**, 490—496 (1965).

Smith, W. M., Bachman, B., Galante, J. G., Hanowell, E. G., Johnson, W. P., Koch, C. E., Jr., Korfmacher, S. D., Thurm, R. H., Bromer, L.: Co-operative Clinical Trial of aplhamethyldopa. Ann intern. Med. **65**, 657, 671 (1966).

Smith, W. M., Damato, A. M., Galluzzi, N. J., Garfield, C. F., Hanowell, E. G., Stimson, W. H., Thurm, R. H., Walsh, J. J., Bromer, L.: The evaluation of antihypertensive therapy co-operative clinical trial method I. Double-blind control comparison od chlorothiazide, rauwolfia serpentina, and hydralazine. Ann. intern. Med. **61**, 829—846 (1964).

Spark, R. F., Melby, J. C.: Hypertension and low renin activity: presumptive evidence for mineralocorticoid excess. Am. J. intern. Med. **75**, 831 (1971).

STANTON, H. C., WHITE, J. B., JR.: Hypotensive actions of drug on unanaesthetized normotensive and "metacorticoid" hypertensive rats, determined by a direct recording technique. Arch. int. Pharmacodyn. **154**, 351—363 (1965).
SWALES, J. D.: Sodium Metabolism in Disease. Lloyd-Luke 1975.
SZWED, J. J., KLEIT, S. A., HAMBURGER, R. J.: Effect of furosemide and chlorothiazide on the thoracic duct lymph flow in the dog. J. Lab. clin. med. **79**, 693—700 (1972).
TALSO, P. J., CARBALLO, A. J.: Effects of benzothiadiazines on serum and total body electrolytes. Ann. N.Y. Acad. Sci. **88**, 822—840 (1960).
TALSO, P. J., REMENCHICK, A.P., CUTILLETTA, A.F.: Effects of diuretic agents on serum and tissue electrolytes in rats. Proc. Soc. exp. Biol. (N.Y.) **122**, 78—81 (1966).
TAPIA, F. A., DUSTAN, H. P., SCHNECKLOTH, R. A., CORCORAN, A. C., PAGE, I. H.: Enhanced effectiveness of ganglion-blocking agents in hypertensive patients during the administration of a saluretic agent (chlorothiazide). Lancet **II**, 1831—1833. (1957)
TARAZI, R. C., DUSTAN, H. P.: Beta adrenergic blockade in hypertension. Amer. J. Cardiol. **29** 633—640 (1972).
TARAZI, R. C., DUSTAN, H. P., FRÖHLICH, E. D.: Long-term thiazide therapy in essential hypertension. Circulation **41**, 709—717 (1970).
TAYLOR, R. D., DUSTAN, H. P., CORCORAN, A. C., PAGE, I. H.: Evaluation of 1-hydrazinophlhalazine (Apresoline) in treatment of hypertensive disease. Arch. intern. Med. **90**, 734—749 (1952).
TOBIAN, L., COFFEE, K.: Effect of thiazide drugs on renovascular hypertension in contrast to their effect in essential hypertension. Proc. Soc. exp. Biol. **119**, 196—198 (1964).
TOBIAN, L., JANECEK, J., FOKER, J., FERREIRA, D.: Effect of chlorothiazide on renal juxtaglomerular cells and tissue electrolytes. Amer. J. Physiol. **202**, 905—908 (1962).
VARNAUSKAS, E., CRAMER, G., MALMCRONA, R., WERKO, L.: Effect of chlorothiazide on blood pressure and blood flow at rest and on exercise in patients with arterial hypertension. Clin. Sci., **20**, 407—416 (1961).
VENNING, E. H., DYRENFURTH, I., DOSSETOR, J., B. BECK, J. C.: Effect of chlorothiazide upon, aldosterone excretion an Na and K balance in essential hypertension. J. Lab. clin. Med. **60**, 79—85 (1962).
VEYRAT, R., DE CHAMPLAIN, BOUCHER, R., GENEST, J.: Measurement of human arterial renin activity in some physiological and pathological states. Canad. med. Ass. J. **90**, 215—219 (1964).
VIERSMA, H. J.: De behandeling van hypertensie met zoutloos diet en met uidrijving van keukenzout. Amsterdam: N. V. Noord-Hollandsche Uitgevers Maatschappij 1946.
VILLAMIL, M. F., YEYATI, N., ENERO, M. A., RUBIANES, S., TAQUINI, A. G.: Effect of long term treatment with hydrochlorothiazide on water and electrolytes. Amer. Heart J. **65**, 194—207 (1963).
VILLARREAL, J., EXAIRE, J. E., REVOLLO, A., SONI, J.: Effects of chlorothiazide on systemic hemodynamics in essential hypertension. Circulation **26**, 405—408 (1962a).
VILLARREAL, H., EXAIRE, J. E., RUBIO, V., DAVILA, H.: Effect of guanethidine and bretylium tosylate on systemic and renal hemodynamics in essential hypertension. Amer. J. Cardiol. **14**, 633—643 (1964).
VILLARREAL, H., REVOLLO, A., EXAIRE, J. E., LARRONDON, F.: Effects of chlorothiazide on renal hemodynamisc. Circulation **26**, 409—412 (1962b).
WEINBERGER, H., DOWDY, A. J., NOKEZ, G. W., LEUTSCHER, J. A.: Plasma renin activity and aldosterone secretion in hypertensive patients during high and low sodium intake and administration of diuretic. J. clin. Endocr. **28**, 357—371 (1968).
WELLER, J. M., HAIGHT, A. S.: Effect of chlorothiazide on blood pressure and electrolytes of normotensive and hypertensive rats. Proc. Soc. exp. Biol. **112**, 820—825 (1963).
WERNING, C., BAUMANN, K., SCHÖNBECK, M., GYSLING, E., WEIDMANN, P., SIEGENTHALER, W.: Die Wirkung länger dauernder Hydrochlorothiazid-Gaben auf die Plasma-Renin-Aktivität und die Aldosteronexkretionsrate bei Normalpersonen. Klin. Wschr. **47**, 318—324 (1969).
WILSON, I. M. and FREIS, E. D.: Relationship between plasma and extracellular fluid volume depletion and the antihypertensive effect of chlorothiazide. Circulation **20**, 1028—1036 (1959).
WILSON, W. R., OKUN, R., TETREAULT, L., FALLIS, N.: Methyldopa and hydrochlorothiazide in primary hypertension. J. Amer. med. An. **185**, 819—825 (1963).
WINER, B. M.: The antihypertensive action of benzothiadiazines. Circulation **23**, 211—218 (1961a).
WINER, B. M.: The antihypertensive mechanisms of salt depletion induced by hydrochlorothiazide. Circulation **24**, 788—796 (1961b).
WINER, B. M., LUBBE, W. F., COLTON, T.: Antihypertensive actions of diuretics. J. Amer. med. Ass. **204**, 775—779 (1968).

Wolf, K., Gessler, U.: Experimentelle Untersuchungen zum Elektrolytstoffwechsel nach Chlorthalidonbehandlung. Arch. exp. Path. Parmakol. **247**, 136—143 (1964).

Woods, J. W., Liddle, G. W., Stant, E. G., Michelakis, A. M., Brill, B. B.: Effect of an adrenal inhibitor in hypertensive patients with suppressed renin. Arch. intern. Med. **123**, 366—370 (1969).

Zelis, R., Mason, D. T., Brauwald, E.: A comparison of the effects of vasodilator stimuli on peripheral resistance in vessels in normal subjects and in patients with congestive heart failure. J. clin. Invest. **47**, 960—970 (1968).

Zsoter, T. T., Hart, F., Radde, I. C.: Mechanism of antihypertensive action of prolonged administration of hydrochlorothiazide in rabbit and dog. Circulation Res. **27**, 717—725 (1970).

Chapter 10

The Pathophysiology of Adrenal Inhibitors with Respect to their Antihypertensive Activity

R. GAUNT and J. C. MELBY

With 18 Figures

I. Introduction

The corticosteroids are essential for the maintenance of normal blood pressure. Adrenal insufficiency is characterized by hypotension. In susceptible species excesses of all known corticosteroids can cause hypertension. The adrenal cortex is to some degree a "permissive" sustaining factor in many types of hypertension as first established in renal hypertension by GOLDBLATT (1934). Adrenal dysfunction is the apparent primary cause of some uncertain but significant fraction of hypertensive disease in man. It follows, therefore, that "chemical adrenalectomy" by the use of drugs or competitive antagonists of adrenal steroids could have a role in the therapeutic management of high blood pressure. This is indeed the case but that this role of the adrenal cortical inhibitors is at present a relatively minor one is due to a combination of (a) etiologic uncertainties concerning conditions logically calling for their use, (b) lack of highly specific drugs for such use, and (c) the metabolic ingenuity of the adrenal in thwarting attempts to alter its complex secretory functions in accordance with man-made concepts of desirable ends.

II. Adrenocortical-Related Hypertension (Mineralocorticoid Hypertensive Syndromes)

Three known mineralocorticoid hormones are secreted by the human adrenal cortex: aldosterone, deoxycorticosterone (DOC) and 18–OH–11-deoxycorticosterone (18–OH–DOC) (Figs. 1–3). Since the discovery of DOC by STEIGER and REICHSTEIN in 1937 and aldosterone by SIMPSON et al. (1953), several extensive reviews have appeared on the regulation of biosynthesis of these steroids (MUELLER, 1971) and the activity of these substances on the regulation of electrolyte metabolism (GAUNT, 1971). The discovery of 18–OH–DOC as an endogenous secretory product of the rat adrenal by BIRMINGHAM and WARD in 1961 and of the human adrenal by MELBY et al. (1971) has been followed by studies on the mineralocorticoid activity of this steroid as discussed in this chapter. Aldosterone is a product of the zona glomerulosa, and its secretion is activated by a complicated interplay of ACTH, angiotensin II and potassium ion. DOC and 18–OH–DOC are largely secreted by the zona fasciculata, under the influence of ACTH. Aldosterone's mineralocorticoid activity in terms of stimulation of active sodium transport approximates 50 times that of 18–OH–DOC and 25 times that of DOC. In view of the amounts generally secreted, alrosterone is the pre-eminent steroid

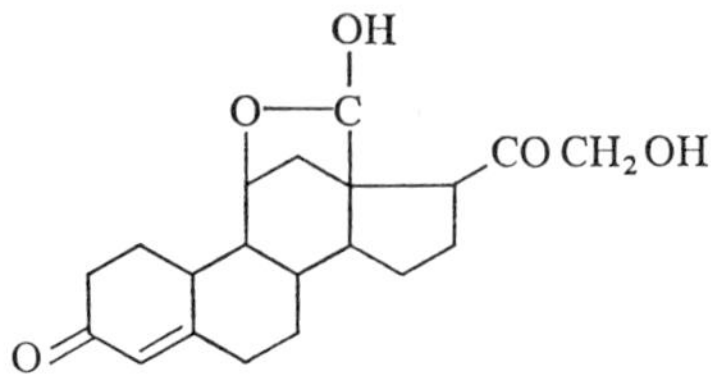

Fig. 1. Aldosterone

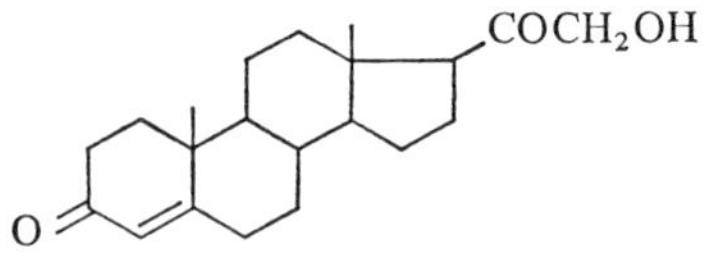

Fig. 2. 11-deoxycorticosterone

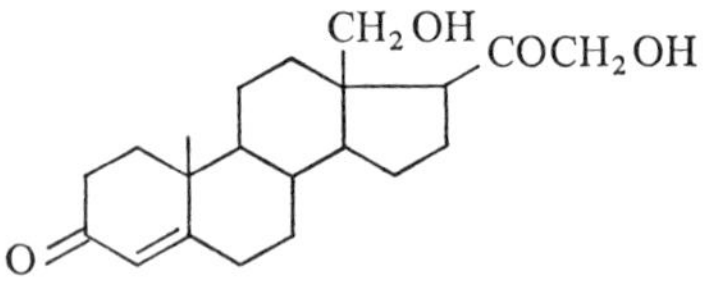

Fig. 3. 18-OH-DOC

hormone influencing sodium metabolism in man. These mineralocorticoids administered in quantity to experimental animals induce sodium retention, expansion of the extracellular fluid volume and ultimately hypertension. Hypertension has long been observed in man, apparently resulting from the hypersecretion of each of these mineralocorticoids. Aldosterone excess generally occurs alone in those hypertensive disorders in which it is involved, 18–OH–DOC and DOC excess may occur independently or together, as in Cushing's syndrome. The development of drugs for the treatment of steroid-related hypertension can now be greatly aided by progress in the identification of the bewildering array of abnormalities in steroid biosynthesis apparently causing some 20% of the cases of hypertension otherwise diagnosed as "essential". The mineralocorticoid-hypertensive syndromes as now recognized are classified below, and in most cases the type of drug needed in their management, although ones not necessarily available, is at least suggested by the etiologic factors involved:

I. Aldosterone Excess

A. Aldosterone-producing adenoma or (rarely) carcinoma – primary aldosteronism (Conn's syndrome) (CONN, 1955).

B. Bilateral adrenocortical nodular hyperplasia – idiopathic hyperaldosteronism (MELBY, 1968).

C. Hereditary glucocorticoid suppressible aldosteronism (SUTHERLAND et al., 1966).

D. Congenital hyperaldosteronism with bilateral zona glomerulose hyperplasia (MORAN et al., 1960).

II. *Isolated Deoxycorticosterone Excess*

A. DOC-producing adenoma.

B. Idiopathic (ACTH-independent) hypersecretion of DOC (BROWN et al., 1972).

C. 11β-Hydroxylase deficiency – congenital virilizing adrenocortical hyperplasia (EBERLEIN and BONGIOVANNI, 1956).

III. *Isolated 18–OH-11-Deoxycorticosterone Excess*

A. Idiopathic hypersecretion of 18–OH–DOC (MELBY et al., 1971).

B. 18–OH–DOC-producing adenoma (ROVNER et al., 1971).

IV. *Concurrent 18–OH–DOC and DOC Secretory Excess*

A. 17α-Hydroxylase deficiency – (Biglieri's syndrome) (BIGLIERI et al., 1966).

B. Cushing's syndrome with excessive secretion of ACTH (BIGLIERI et al., 1968; MELBY et al., 1972).

V. *Unidentified Mineralocorticoid Secretory Excess*

A. Hyporeninemic hypertension (low-renin essential hypertension) (WOODS et al., 1969; SPARK and MELBY, 1971).

B. Cordisol-producing adrenocortical carcinomas and adenomas.

In the discussion to follow, the format will follow the above classification. However, Cushing's syndrome will be treated separately as will hyporeninemic hypertension (low-renin essential hypertension).

A. Hyperaldosteronism

The hypertensive disorders due to excessive secretion of aldosterone might be considered "primary" since the hypersecretion of aldosterone is not stimulated via the renin-angiotensin system. Characteristically, all of the hypertensive disorders in which aldosterone hypersecretion is "primary" exhibit a reduced plasma renin activity, hyporesponsiveness to physiologic stimuli normally causing renin secretion by the kidney, hypertension and hypokalemia. This discussion specifically excludes those hypertensive disorders in which aldosterone secretory excess is associated with elevated plasma renin activity due either to a renin-producing tumor of the kidney or to renal effects of accelerated hypertension. Estimates of hypertension, due to aldosterone excess, in the hypertensive population vary from 0.5 to 7.5%. Agents which selectively inhibit aldosterone biosynthesis in the absence of increased deoxycorticosteroid production, and agents which competitively inhibit the action of aldosterone, are effective in reversing all of the manifestations of primary aldosteronism.

1. Aldosterone-Producing Adenoma

In nearly 70% of patients exhibiting primary aldosterone secretory excess, solitary aldosterone-producing adenomas are found. In but a tiny fraction of these patients is the adrenal tumor malignant. Disapparance of hypertension occurs only in two-thirds of patients having solitary adenomas removed by unilateral adrenalectomy; obviously various other causal factors may co-exist.

2. Idiopathic Hyperaldosteronism — with Bilateral Nodular Adrenocortical Hyperplasia

Nearly one-third of patients with primary aldosterone secretory excess have marked nodular hypertrophy of the zona glomerulosa of the adrenal cortices. Bilateral total adrenalectomy relieves hypertension completely in only about two-thirds of these patients, but with suitable replacement therapy it corrects the metabolic abnormalities in the remainder. Possible dependence of idiopathic hyperaldosteronism on the anterior pituitary is suggested by the observation that dexamethasone induces a significant reduction in aldosterone secretion.

3. Glucocorticoid-Suppressible Aldosteronism

In a related observation Sutherland et al. (1966) have described a rare form of hyperaldosteronism occurring in families in which suppressive doses of dexamethasone reduce aldosterone secretion and blood pressure.

4. Congenital or Juvenile Aldosteronism

This rare condition begins in childhood, producing hypertension and potassium depletion (Moran et al., 1960). The adrenal cortices show a markedly hyperplastic adrenal glomerulosa with diffuse involvement. Sub-total adrenalectomy may relieve hypertension and the metabolic disturbances.

B. Excessive DOC Secretion

Hypertension may be associated with excessive secretion of DOC, but severe alterations in potassium metabolism, as possibly predictable from animal work (Gross, 1956; Hall and Hall, 1967), are said to be less frequently observed than in patients with hyperaldosteronism. DOC is secreted largely by the zona fasciculata of the adrenal and is usually ACTH dependent. Adenomas secreting exclusively DOC are very rare.

1. Idiopathic Hypersecretion of DOC

Brown et al. (1972) have reported the occurrence of persistently raised plasma DOC levels in 35% (six) of 21 hypertensive patients who exhibited suppressed plasma renin activity. In these patients markedly elevated plasma levels of DOC was the sole steroid abnormality observed. Since DOC secretion is ordinarily ACTH dependent, it was unexpected that in a few patients so treated dexametha-

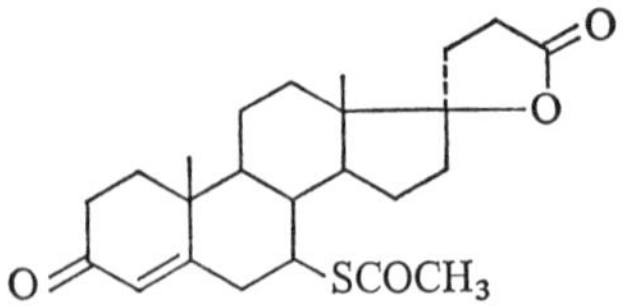

Fig. 4. Sprioneolactone

sone failed to reduce blood pressure. The competitive inhibitor of mineralocorticoid action, spironolactone (Fig. 4), however, reduced blood pressure into the normal range. It is conceivable that the isolated DOC excess in these patients was due to a DOC-producing adrenocortical adenoma. However, pathologic evidence was not available.

2. 11α-Hydroxylase Deficiency — an Inborn Error of Corticosteroid Biosynthesis Associated with Virilizing Hyperplasia of the Adrenal Cortex

The hypertension in this rare form of virilizing hyperplasia of the adrenal cortex was described by EBERLEIN and BONGIOVANNI (1956). It is due to the excessive production of DOC by the zona fasciculata resulting compensatorially from the inadequate biosynthesis of corticosterone (Fig. 5) and cortisol with

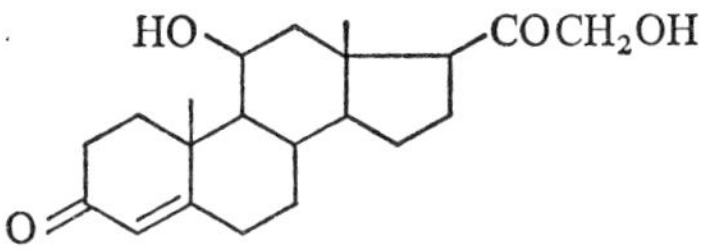

Fig. 5. Corticosterone

consequent uninhibited ACTH secretion. The administration of cortisol or one of its synthetic analogs activates long loop negative feedback inhibition of pituitary ACTH secretion and DOC production diminishes as does the blood pressure.

C. 18=OH=DOC Hypersecretion

MELBY et al. (1971) described the association of hypersecretion of 18–OH–DOC, suppressed plasma renin activity and restoration of normal blood pressure when pituitary suppression was induced by dexamethasone. Idiopathic isolated 18–OH–DOC excess has been noted in patients subsequently shown to have bilateral adenomatous hyperplasia of the adrenal cortices. A single patient having a solitary adrenal adenoma, excess secretion of 18–OH–DOC and hypertension has been described by ROVNER et al. (1971).

D. Concurrent Hypersecretion of DOC and 18-OH-DOC

1. 17α-Hydroxylase Deficiency

BIGLIERI et al. (1966) described a syndrome in which patients lacked secondary sex characteristics and were otherwise characterized by hypertension, hypokalemia, low urinary 17-ketosteroids and 17-hydroxycorticosteroids, and elevated tetrahydro-DOC and metabolites of corticosterone. In these patients there was also an increased excretion of 18–OH–DOC (MELBY et al., 1972). In fact they produce 8 to 20 times as much 18–OH–DOC as is normally secreted and 10 to 20 times as much DOC. The resulting hypertension and hypokalemia is readily understandable. The excessive steroid production and the hypertension can be abolished by the administration of ACTH-suppressive doses of dexamethasone.

2. 18=OH=DOC and DOC Secretory Excess in Cushing's Syndrome

18–OH–DOC secretory excess was seen in all of 13 patients with Cushing's syndrome due to abnormal regulation of ACTH secretion by the hypothalamus and pituitary, *i.e.*, Cushing's disease (MELBY et al., 1972). This was also true in patients with ectopic ACTH production by extra adrenal neoplasm. While DOC hypersecretion was demonstrated frequently in patients with other varieties of Cushing's disease, it was invariable in patients with neoplastic sites of ectopic ACTH secretion. Neither DOC nor 18–OH–DOC excess could be found in patients with primary adrenocortical tumors. In most patients with marked increments in 18–OH–DOC secretion, plasma renin activity was suppressed, and hypertension and hypokalemia invariably were present. Such increments in DOC secretion had been shown previously by BIGLIERI et al. (1968) in patients with ectopic ACTH secretion from non-endocrine tumors. It is reasonable to assume that the enormous quantities of 18–OH–DOC and DOC secreted in the ectopic (ACTH) form of Cushing's syndrome is the sole or primary cause of the concomitant hypertension and hypokalemic alkalosis. This is also likely true, although the excess mineralocorticoid production is less (roughly three-fold), in patients with Cushing's syndrome of pituitary origin. It is pertinent that the hypertension-inducing properties of DOC in animals are well-known and those of 18–OH–DOC have recently been demonstrated (RAPP et al., 1973; BIRMINGHAM et al., 1973; GOTSHALL and DAVIS, 1973).

The more florid aspects of Cushing's syndrome are presumably due to glucocorticoid excess, and its possible role in the accompanying hypertension has to be considered. The incidence of hypertension in patients without endocrine disease, treated with synthetic cortisol analogs, is only 16% (SAVAGE et al., 1962); in patients treated with ACTH, on the other hand, it is nearly twice as great. CHRISTY (1966) previously had proposed that the difference observed in response to glucocorticosteroids vs. ACTH in terms of hypertension could be explained by mineralocorticoid secretion stimulated by ACTH, an idea entirely compatible with observations cited above.

The observed occurrence of hypokalemic alkalosis and hypertension in patients with Cushing's syndrome due to a primary adrenocortical tumor secreting largely cortisol leaves open the role of cortisol itself. Cortisol (Fig. 6) can cause mild

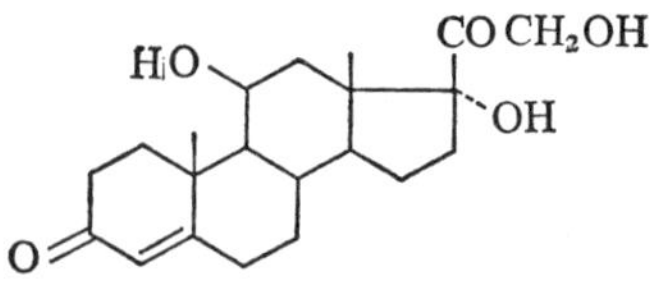

Fig. 6. Cortisol

hypertension in susceptible animals (GAUNT et al., 1959), an experimental syndrome differing markedly from that caused by mineralocorticoids, and this steroid could be a contributory cause of hypertensive disease in human Cushing's syndrome. BAGSHAWE (1960) has reported a patient with adrenocortical carcinoma producing excessive aldosterone and cortisol, a combination since noted by others. The potential complexity of causal relations in such cases is illustrated by the fact that cortisol can antagonize the natriuretic action of aldosterone, an effect in turn blocked by prolactin (HORROBIN et al., 1973). Also, the possibility that as yet unidentified mineralocorticoids may be involved in the hypertension induced by cortisol-secreting adrenocortical carcinomas has to be considered.

E. The Problem of Hyporeninemic Hypertension (Low-Renin Essential Hypertension) — Mineralocorticoid Syndrome

It has been estimated that approximately 20% of patients with essential hypertension exhibit suppressed plasma renin activity (*e.g.*, HELMER et al., 1968; WOOD et al., 1969). As stated above, hyporeninemic hypertension is also observed in patients with demonstrable mineralocorticoid excess. The known mineralocorticoid-hypertension syndromes account for some 25% of patients with hyporeninemic hypertension and somewhat more than five per cent of the entire hypertensive population. The large number of patients with hyporeninemic hypertension without demonstrable cause exhibit many of the same features found in patients with demonstrable mineralocorticoid hypertension. They contrast sharply with patients who have normally responsive plasma renin activity and essential hypertension. Patients with hyporeninemic hypertension can have expanded blood volume, reduced aldosterone secretion and plasma aldosterone levels which cannot be stimulated by salt depletion and erect posture; they become normotensive when treated with inhibitors of steroid biogenesis and competitive inhibitors of mineralocorticoid activity. By contrast, patients with essential hypertension and normally responsive plasma renin activity tend to have contracted blood volume, normally responsive aldosterone secretion and plasma aldosterone levels which rise briskly in response to sodium deprivation and erect posture. In such cases treatment with the known adrenal inhibitors generally fails to reduce blood pressure (SPARK and MELBY, 1971). The recent observations implicating 18–OH–DOC and DOC secretory excess in the genesis of hyporeninemic hypertension in some patients have intensified an as yet unsuccessful search for unidentified mineralocorticoids in remaining patients where such potential factors are not recognized.

The development in the last two decades of pharmacologic agents to palliate hypertensive disease has been one of great practical utility, although for the most part such drugs are used empirically and selected on a trial-and-error basis. In steroid-related hypertension, it is now clear that the way is open to develop and select drugs with highly specific sites of action which should meet individual needs based on sophisticated differential diagnostic considerations. The limited successes and potential leads in this direction are discussed below.

III. Inhibitors of Steroid Secretion

A. In vitro Studies

KAHNT and NEHER (1972) have extended their already broad survey of the *in vitro* effect of a large number of chemical entities on steroidogenesis in beef adrenal homogenates. While the *in vivo* effects of no compound can be established with certainty from *in vitro* systems, the procedures used by these authors have produced results generally correlating well with the quality of action of compounds known to be effective in modifying adrenal function in intact animals and man. As yet, however, their work points mainly to potentialities for future developments. For instance, in extension of previous work showing the variable effect of drugs (KAHNT and NEHER, 1966), an inhibition of aldosterone synthesis being one of the most common effects, they have recently used a group of 3- and 4-pyridine derivatives to modify the biosynthesis of corticosterone and cortisol selectively to achieve the following: corticosterone stimulation; cortisol stimulation; total stimulation; total inhibition; cortisol inhibition; corticosterone inhibition. To carry such work into human pharmacology is of self-evident importance but also a task of prodigious magnitude.

B. Metyrapone (Metopirone) (Fig. 7)

This drug, synthesized by BENCZE and ALLEN (1959), was first shown by CHART et al. (1958) to inhibit corticosteroidgenesis in the dog. In massive intravenous doses it can apparently completely inhibit adrenal steroid secretion. In moderate and chronically tolerable amounts, however, it acts primarily (although not exclusively) as an 11 β-hydroxylase inhibitor (LIDDLE et al., 1958; JENKINS and THORN, 1958), causing in dog and man an inhibited output of cortisol and particularly aldosterone (TUCCI et al., 1967). This is followed, as a result of the release from cortisol inhibition, by an enhanced ACTH output. With normal pathways of steroidogenesis blocked, the effect of ACTH is to increase the output of two normally minor 11-deoxy steroids: 11-deoxycortisol and 11-deoxycorticosterone (GAUNT et al., 1965).

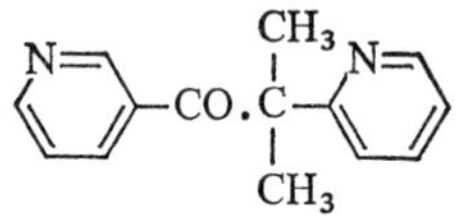

Fig. 7. Metyrapone

This pattern of effect is the basis of the widespread use of metyrapone as a diagnostic test for pituitary ACTH reserve. If pituitary function is normal, the drug causes a compensatory rise of ACTH secretion, resulting in a marked increase in total 17-OH corticosteroid secretion, due principally to 11-deoxycortisol.

Both 11-deoxycortisol and particularly 11-deoxycorticosterone are salt-retaining, hypertension-invoking steroids. Hence, the findings seem logical that the chronic administration of metyrapone in dogs (ADLIN and CHANNIK, 1966; MARKS et al., 1971) and in hypertension-prone rats with regenerating adrenals (COLBY et al., 1970) causes or accelerates hypertensive disease. In the case of the dog, although not the rat, this finding was somewhat enigmatic because the dog is unusually resistant to the pressor effects of exogenous DOC.

Nevertheless, as an example of the fact that the subtleties of applied pharmacology are legion, metyrapone, when combined with other drugs which inhibit other aspects of adrenal steroidogenesis, *e.g.*, aminoglutethimide (see below) or dexamethasone (COPPAGE et al., 1959) can have a beneficial role in various types of human disorders including hypertensive disease. The rationale presumably is that aminoglutethimide adds to the adrenal secretory suppressive action of metyrapone and thus prevents the compensatory rise in 11-deoxy steroids usually induced by the latter. JONES et al. (1970) found the combination of metyrapone and aminoglutethimide is particularly useful in Cushing's syndrome of whatever variety. Effects were manifested by reductions in cortisol secretion rates, blood pressure, insulin requirements, Cushingoid appearance, and enhancement of general well-being.

C. Aminoglutethimide (Elipten) — A-G (Fig. 8)

This drug was first used as an anticonvulsive agent, and some years after its introduction both laboratory and clinical work unexpectedly established that it inhibited adrenal steroidogensis (Rev: GAUNT et al., 1968; HUGHES and BURLEY, 1970; TOUITOU et al., 1973a, b). Primarily it acts to inhibit at an early stage the conversion of pregnenolone to progesterone by inhibition of the desmolase system and as a consequence dampens the output of all major corticosteroids; aldosterone secretion is particularla susceptible to its action. A compensatory increase in ACTH output results in adrenal hypertrophy and, presumably due to an inhibition of its metabolic use, to an accumulation of adrenal cholesterol. As would be expected A–G can also affect gonadal steroidsgenesis with resulting alterations in reproductive functions – a problem now being extensively investigated. The adrenal, however, is apparently more sensitive to the action of A–G than the gonads; hence in human therapeutic dosage gonadal dysfunction is not an important or limiting factor in its use.

MANCHENO-RICE et al. (1973) and others (cf. TOUITOU et al., 1973) consider the adrenal glomerulosa to be more sensitive to A–G inhibition than the fasciculata

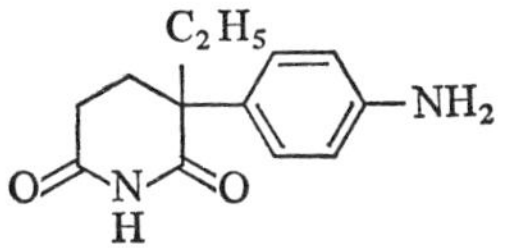

Fig. 8. Aminoglutethimide

in normal men, with the result that its suppression of aldosterone secretion is profound and continuous, whereas the fasciculata-based secretion of DOC and 18–OH–DOC may be unaffected or actually increased. Presumably this is the result of a compensatory increment of ACTH secretion due to a loss of cortisol inhibition since it in turn could be inhibited by dexamethasone. These findings give support to those of others (see below) that A–G plus an ACTH-suppressant therapy would be useful in cases of mineralocorticoid excess.

The remarkable specificity of action of A–G is shown by the fact that chemically it differs from the widely used hypnotic, glutethimide (DORIDEN) only by the presence of an amino group. Glutethimide, however, unlike aminoglutethimide, has no effect of practical importance on adrenal function (CHART, 1969).

Effects in Hypertension[1]. Aminoglutethimide has been little studied in the animal models of experimental hypertension. In one instance, however, CHART et al. (1969) found it unequivocally effective in ameliorating adrenal regeneration hypertension in rats, a syndrome in which spironolactone is also markedly active. The rationale of this result has since become probably apparent. There is growing evidence that the pressor influence of regenerating adrenals is due to an early high production of DOC followed by a relatively high output of 18–OH–DOC (GAUNT et al., 1974). Despite questions raised by the above-mentioned observations in *normal* human subjects, one suspects that in this case (in which high endogenous output of ACTH results from the operation) that A–G suppresses 11-deoxy steroid output.

Adrenal regeneration hypertension, since its discovery by SKELTON (1955), has been much studied as an experimental oddity without demonstrable relevance to any particular human condition. It may turn out to be the best experimental model available for the screening of drugs particularly suited to that large population of human hypertensives characterized by low or normal aldosterone secretion and low plasma renin values.

WOODS, LIDDLE, MICHELAKIS, and BRILL (1969) were the first to note that A–G was effective in a certain type of human hypertension. Patients with the now well-recognized syndrome of hypertension occurring without aldosterone or DOC excess, with low plasma renin and high exchangeable sodium values responded to A–G (0.75 gm/day) with a prolonged and significant reduction in blood

[1] Despite its apparent utility in treating diseases characterized by adrenal dysfunction as well as in certain malignancies, A-G is not at present commercially available anywhere in the world. It is distributed, under the limitations of research use, by various national Pharmaceutical Divisions of the CIBA-Geigy Corporation.

pressure. Compensatory elevations of identifiable steroid secretion were prevented by the use of 7.5 mg of prednisolone per day.

MELBY and co-workers (unpublished) have confirmed these findings in patients with primary aldosteronism and those with low-renin hypertension. Doses of 1 to 2 g/day of A–G produced results equivalent to those of 400 mg/day of spironolactone in terms of weight loss and return of blood pressure to normal or near-normal levels. Other evidence of the similarity of response of low-renin hypertension to A–G and spironolactone and the non-responsiveness of other forms of essential hypertension have been presented (SPARK and MELBY, 1971; CAREY et al., 1972).

In secondary hypoaldosteronism (congestive heart failure, hepatic cirrhosis and idiopathic edema), A–G caused reduced aldosterone excretion, sodium diuresis, and a rise in plasma renin activity in 32 of 37 patients (KÜCHEL et al., 1970). These authors thought tne drug was useful particularly in those patients resistant to more conventional therapies.

3 β-Hydroxysteroid Dehydrogenase Inhibitors

A series of steroidal compounds has been synthesized in the Sterling-Winthrop Research Institute during the last decade which acts as inhibitors of 3 β-hydroxysteroid dehydrogenase: steroid Δ isomerase enzyme systems. These have been of interest and use as laboratory tools and some are now available of potential use in man (NEUMANN et al., 1970).

The first of these extensively studied was cyanotrimethylandrostenolone (Fig. 9), whose adrenal-inhibiting properties were first noted by BURNHAM et al. (1963). GOLDMAN and associates (GOLDMAN, 1970) found that this and related compounds, acting as analogs of 3 β-hydroxysteroid dehydrogenase and isomerase

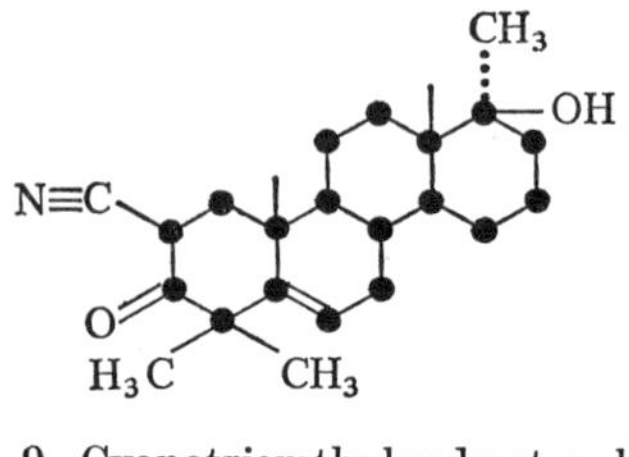

Fig. 9. Cyanotriemthylandrostenolone

substrates, act with great potency and remarkable irreversibility to block steroid biosynthesis in the adrenal, testis and ovary. Using these inhibitors as tools, they have produced in animals experimental models of developmental defects in man presumably due to genetic steroidogenic enzyme deficiencies. Such compounds could not be used in man in part because of the months-long persistence of their effects.

More recently, however, new compounds, particularly Win-24540 (Fig. 10), have shown selective reversible effects on the adrenal without comparable gonadal involvement (NEUMAN et al., 1970; POTTS, personal communication). In animals Win-24540 seems to block or inhibit the secretion of all major corticosteroids, permitting accumulation in adrenal vein blood of pregnenetriol, 17-hydroxypregnenolone and pregnenolone. The compound is tolerable and potentially useful in man (MELBY, unpublished) as made evident by inhibited secretion, obviously in all zones of the adrenal, of cortisol, aldosterone, DOC, 18–OH–DOC and corticosterone. A compensatory response to the expected concomitant hypersecretion of ACTH is an increased output of the C-19 steroids. dehydroepiandrosterone and its sulfate ester. Win-24540 in doses up to 1 g daily reduced cortisol secretion to a normal range in two patients with Cushing's syndrome without causing signs of clinical hypoadrenalism. It also reduced excessive aldosterone

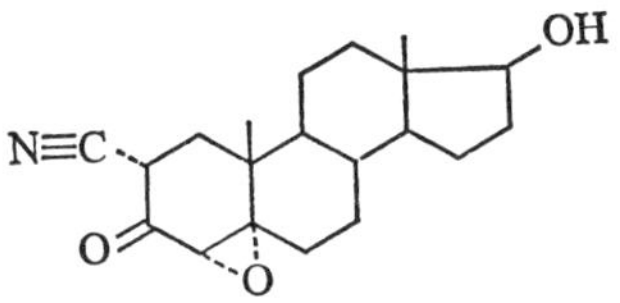

Fig. 10. 4-α,4-Epoxy-17β-hydroxy-3-oxo-5α-androstane-2α-carbonitrile (Win-24540)

secretion in patients with primary aldosteronism without unacceptable reductions in cortisol output. Its possible effects in hyporeninemic hypertension are awaited with interest.

IV. Inhibitors of Corticosteroid Secretion of Potential Interest in Hypertension

A number of compounds are listed below (a larger list is more extensively discussed elsewhere – GAUNT et al., 1965), which, because of their mode of action, could potentially have some use in selected cases of hypertensive disease. With the exception of o,p′-DDD (mitotane), however, which has other demonstrated uses, these compounds have served largely as experimental tools in animal experimentation; clinical study has been either lacking or scanty.

A. o,p′-DDD (Fig. 11)

The first pharmacological inhibitor of the adrenal cortex discovered was the insecticide DDD (WOODWARD and NELSON, 1949). In the dog it was shown, as has since been widely confirmed, to cause cytotoxic atrophy of the inner layers of the adrenal, the zona glomerulosa largely escaping its effects. Later work showed that these morphological aspects of the drug's action were associated in man with secretory deficiencies, particularly of the glucocorticoids.

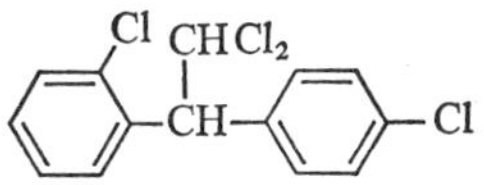

Fig. 11. Mitotane (o,p′-DDD)

Commercial DDD is made up of a mixture of isomers, and the initial work of NICHOLS and HENNIGAR (1957) as well as CUETO and BROWN (1958) showed that the most active and toxicologically tolerable of these isomers was o,p′-DDD. Hence this compound has been used in most recent studies. The adrenal-inhibiting response of the DDDs has a marked species specificity, the rat being largely unresponsive to it.

The adrenal atrophy which occurs in responsive species after administration of the DDD isomers is reversible and resembles that of ACTH deficiency; the drug causes loss of steroidogenic, but not hyperemic, responsiveness of the adrenal to ACTH. Its mechanism of action is unknown.

The main use of o′p'-DDD in man has been in cases with adrenal tumors or Cushing's syndrome in which frequently excess glucocorticoid production and/or the progress of metastatic disease can be inhibited. Since it affects mainly the adrenal fasiculata, its effects on aldosterone are slight, if any (TEMPLE et al., 1969); it lacks demonstrated potentialities for the therapy of hypertensive disease, but being primarily an inhibitor of cortisol secretion, could be of limited use insofar as cortisol may be involved in such diseases. Whathever the mechanism may be, o,p′-DDD reduced blood pressure in renal hypertensive rats (FREGLY, 1968).

B. Heparinoids

Heparin and the semi-synthetic polysaccharide, Ro-1-8307, have been shown by the original extensive work of MAJOOR and collaborators (MAJOOR, 1968) and later work of numerous others (*e.g.* ABBOT et al., 1966; CONN et al., 1966) to be fairly specific inhibitors of aldosterone secretion. The functional effect of such drugs is associated with morphological manifestations of adrenal glomerular inhibition (CHREMOS et al., 1969; LEVINE et al., 1972). *In vitro*, at least, they inhibit angiotensin (SEALEY et al., 1967) although this suggested mechanism of action is not confirmed in man (FORD and BAILEY, 1966).

The heparinoids affect electrolyte metabolism in a manner consistent with and expected from their induction of aldosterone deficiency. The clinical use of such preparations would presumably be limited by their anticoagulant action, albeit that is less with Ro-1-8307 than with heparin.

C. GPA-2282 (Fig. 12)

GPA-2282 [3-methyl-2-(3-pyridyl) indole methansulfonate] in dogs and man has shown the unusual pattern of reducing the secretion rate of 18−OH-corticosterone and aldosterone (to about 30% of control levels), increasing that of DOC and corticosterone without markedly affecting the secretion of cortisol or 18−OH−DOC (MELBY et al., 1972). It could not be used in hyperaldosteronism or hypertensive disease because of the self-defeating property of increasing DOC secretion (MELBY, unpublished).

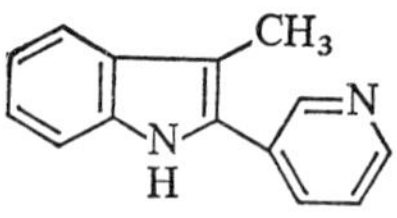

Fig. 12. GPA-2282

D. SU-9055 and Related Compounds

There are several known compounds, none of demonstrated clinical utility, which in intact animals act primarily as 17α-hydroxylation inhibitors, among which are those designated as Su-9055 (Fig. 13), Su-8000 and Su-10603. One aspect of their acute effects is inhibition of the secretion of cortiscol and compensatory hypersecretion of corticosterone and deoxycorticosterone (CHART et al., 1962). When given with an 11β-hydroxylase inhibitor, the results are predictable as a summation of the effects of each compound separately.

In vitro studies show that again complete specificity is lacking and other enzyme systems may be inhibited as well as those involving 17 α-hydroxylation. It is also apparently true in the *in vitro* systems of KAHNT and NEHER (1962) that each such compound may have its own individualistic profile as regards its effectiveness in modifying various steroidogenic steps.

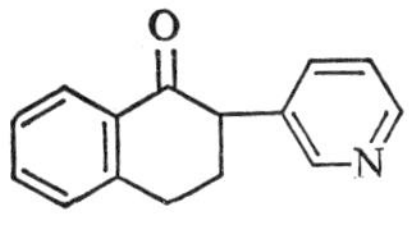

Fig. 13. Su-9055

Inhibition of 17 α-hydroxylation *in vivo* is a property of a rather wide range of drugs, including one of the monoamine oxidase inhibitors mentioned below and some thiosemicarbazones (GAUNT et al., 1965). In the one human trial of such compounds, Su-9055's clearest effect was to inhibit 18-oxidation and thus reduce aldosterone secretion (BLEDSOE et al., 1964).

Effects in hypertensive disease have not been studied.

E. SKF-12185 2(p-aminophenyl)-2-phenylethylamine (SKF-12185) (Fig. 14)

SAUNDERS and COLLEAGUES (1966) first reported that this compound inhibited adrenal function in rats and guinea pigs. It also had unequivocal effects on corticosteroid secretion in man, as various workers have seen (TUCCI et al., 1966; GABRILOVE, 1967, 1968). It inhibits the secretion of cortisol and aldosterone, which results in a metyrapone-like compensatory elevation of ACTH and 11-deoxycortisol secretion. Most available data point to an inhibition of 11 α-hydroxylation as the primary effect of the compound in man. Complete specificity in that respect, however, would be unusual. The compound may have potentially useful effects in states of hypercorticoidism, but, if so, that is yet to be demonstated.

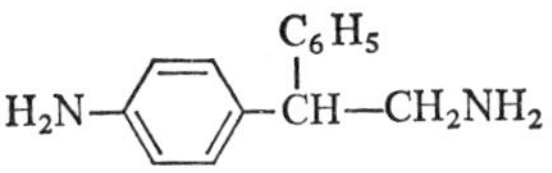

Fig. 14. SKF-12185

F. Monamine Oxidase Inhibitors

At least three monamine oxidase inhibitors, nialamide (Fig. 15), α-ethyltryptamine (Monase; Fig. 16), and tranylcypromine (Parnate; Fig. 17), have some sort of adrenal-inhibiting effects. The fact that they inhibit monamine oxidase seems to be only coindicental and not causal. This can be inferred from (a) the fact that numerous monamine oxidase inhibitors are not adrenal inhibitors, including, in our experience, the most potent known of such compounds (Su-11739; N-methyl-N-(2-propynyl)-1-indanamine HCl) (Fig. 18) and (b) the fact that the known adrenal inhibitors of this group act at different sites.

GOLD and COLLEAGUES (1960) showed that *nialamide*, along with several other drugs which were pharmacologically but not chemically related, inhibited the rise of 17-deoxysteroids normally induced in man by metyrapone. Apparently this was due to an effect on the pituitary in which the expected hypersecretion of ACTH was prevented. This interpretation was consistent with the observation that nialamide reduced adrenal weight and adrenal plasma corticosterone in rats (JASMIN and RICHER, 1966).

TULLNER and HERTZ (1964) showed that in dogs α-ethyltryptamine, given intravenously, sharply reduced corticosteroid secretion for one to two hours and

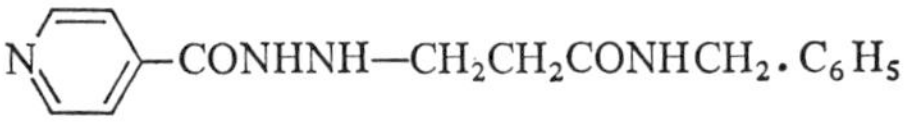

Fig. 15. Nialamide

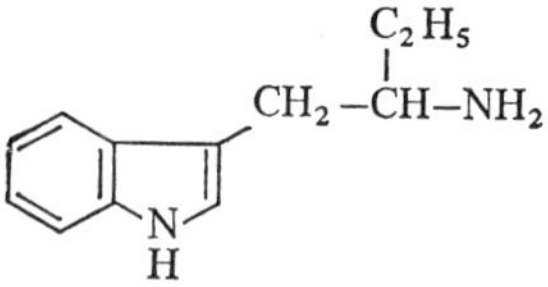

Fig. 16. α-ethyltryptamine

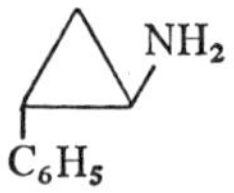

Fig. 17. Tranylcypromine

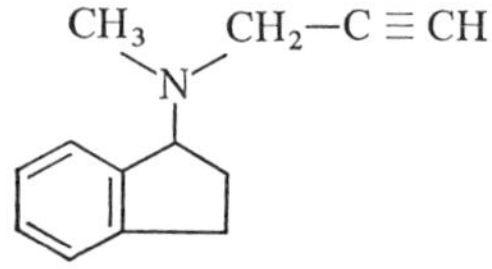

Fig. 18. (N-Methyl-N(2-Propinyl)I-indanamine, Su 11.739

that this was due also to inhibition of ACTH secretion. These facts, including opinion as to site of action, were verified by LORENZEN and GANONG (1967), who found the effect, however curiously related to its pressor action.

In contrast, in dogs, *tranylcypromine* acts apparently directly on the adrenal to block 17α-hydroxylation. This manifests itself by a reduction in the output of cortisol and 11-deoxycortisol and a rise in corticosterone and aldosterone (JOHNSON et al., 1965). In this respect it resembles, but only in part, the17α-hydroxylation inhibitors discussed above. It differs also from α-ethyltryptamine in that its adrenal-inhibiting effect cannot be overcome with either ACTH or angiotensin. The doses of trancylcypromine necessary to achieve adrenal inhibition in dogs were distinctly higher than those used in clinical practice. Effects, if any, of the compound on adrenal function in man are apparently not recorded.

V. Competitive Inhibitors of Mineralocorticoids

For many years private investigators and the pharmaceutical industry poured enormous effort into the theoretically promising search for steroidal compounds which would inhibit the end organ response to steroid hormones, *i.e.*, competitive inhibitors. This search in general was without notable success. An exception, however, concerned competitive antagonists to the mineralocorticoids.

LANDAU noted a natriuretic action of progesterone in human subjects, an effect apparently due to inhibition of aldosterone effects (LANDAU and LUGIBIHL, 1958). In the laboratories of Searle and Co. a series of steroidal lactones were then synthesized which were clearly shown to block the renal salt-retaining action of mineralocorticoids in animals (KAGAWA et al., 1957) and man (LIDDLE, 1957). From this work there evolved the compound spironolactone (Aldactone; Fig. 6), which is extensively used as a diuretic, antihypertensive and diagnostic agent.

While the renal site of action of spironolactone is perhaps the one of major importance, the drug, in addition, antagonizes the effect of mineralocorticoids, mainly aldosterone, at all sites at which such steroids affect electrolyte transport. These include the salivary glands, sewat glands, gastro-intestinal tract, epithelium of toad bladder, amphibian skin, etc. It is also a weak anti-androgen (STEELMAN et al., 1969).

The drug apparently acts by displacing aldosterone from its effective receptor sites (SWANECK et al., 1970), for which purpose, however, the requisite molar excess of spironolactone is in the order of 10,000 times the aldosterone involved (FANESTIL, 1968).

Spironolactone is much the most widely used clinically of all the drugs known to inhibit the action of or suppress the secretion of adrenal steroids, because aside from its world-wide commercial availability, of its unequivocal effectiveness in selected patients as a diuretic and antihypertensive agent. It also has relatively low toxicity. It has the advantage, relative to the thiazide diuretics, that by its antagonism of the kaliuretic as well as the anti-natriuretic action of the corticosteroids, it can be used to deplede body sodium without loss of potassium. It is, however, a weak drug relative to the strong diuretics now available. Hence it is frequently used in combination with thiazides, in which case the natriuretic and antihypertensive effects of the two are approximately additive, while the thiazide-promoted potassium loss is circumvented.

The antihypertensive activity of spironolactone is best observed when spironolactone is administered in adequate doess to patients with the mineralocorticoid-hypertensive syndromes. Spironolactone in a dose of 400 mg/day, given for a period of from three to five weeks, to patients with primary aldosteronism resulted in a 2 to 3 kg loss in body weight occurring from the seventh to the tenth day of therapy. This was followed by a significant reduction of blood pressure, which in most patients reached normal range by the third week of therapy (MELBY, 1968). This work was extended by SPARK and MELBY (1969) who studied 20 patients with solitary aldosterone-producing adenomas and contrasted them with 20 patients with accelerated hypertension, raised plasma renin activity and secondary aldosteronism. The expected response (reduction in both body weight and blood pressure) occurred in patients with primary aldosteronism, but patients with secondary aldosteronism were less affected. One of the authors (J. C. M.) has extended these studies to a large number of patients with various disorders of which hypertension was the common feature. Results are shown in Table 1. Patients with primary aldosteronism due to solitary adenomas were most responsive; those with bilateral hyperplasia were somewhat less so. Only seven of

24 patients with secondary aldosteronism responded at all and these exhibited only a negligible reduction in body weight.

Response to therapy of essential hypertension with spironolactone was dependent on the status of plasma renin activity. As previously noted, approximately 70 to 75% of patients with essential hypertension exhibit plasma renin activity which can be stimulated by erect posture or sodium depletion; the remainder show suppressed or hyporesponsive plasma renin activity. The first of several studies (*e.g.* ESCH and PLACHETA, 1973) demonstrating the specificity of the spironolactone response for patients with low-renin hypertension was that of SPARK and MELBY (1971), here extended in Table 1. Eighty per cent of patients

Table 1. *Effect of spironolactone in high dosage on various types of hypertension (400 mg/day for 3—5 weeks)*

	No. of patients	No. responding	Mean reduction in blood pressure (mm Hg)	Mean reduction in diastolic blood pressure	Weight loss (kg)
Primary aldosteronism					
Solitary adrenal adenoma	46	46	—46/28	26%	—2.6
Bilateral adrenal nodular hyperplasia	19	19	—34/22	20%	—2.2
Secondary aldosteronism					
With accelerated hypertension	24	7	(16/10)[a]	(8%)[a]	(—0.6)[a]
Essential hypertension					
Normal plasma renin activity	43	9	(—28/20)[b]	(16%)[b]	(—0.8)[b]
Essential hypertension					
Low plasma renin activity	32	32	—38/26	25%	—2.7

[a] Figures from 7 (30%) cases showing any hypotensive response.
[b]. Figures from 9 (20%) cases showing any hypotensive response.

with essential hypertension and normally responsive plasma renin activity did not respond with a measurable reduction in blood pressure or body weight to large doses of spironolactone. In contrast all patients with suppressed plasma renin activity and essential hypertension were responsive, *i.e.*, reminiscent of cases of primary aldosteronism. This characteristic response of patients with hyporeninemic hypertension to spironolactone, as well as to aminoglutethimide (WOODS et al., 1969), has been viewed as indirect evidence for the existence of an as yet unidentified mineralocorticoid as the cause of this syndrome. In any case, the presence or absence of responsiveness to spironolactone in essential hypertension permits segregation of a large fraction of such patients in which etiology of the disease must have distinctive features and in which appropriate therapy can be rationally devised. Unfortunately when the large doses of spironolactone shown in Table 1 are used, increased side effects may intervene. These include impotence and gynecomastia in males and irregular menses in females (SPARK and MELBY, 1968; CLARK, 1965; LEVITT, 1970). Obviously spironolactone is not completely devoid of sex hormone-like effects. Also, in practical therapy it is of interest that effects of spironolactone can be antagonized by aspirin (TWEEDALE and OGILVIE, 1973).

It is of pharmacologic interest that, from much more limited experience, it appears that the specific potential indications for aminoglutethimide are the same as those for spironolactone, namely, in hypertension associated with demonstrable hypercorticoidism and/or hyporenism. With A–G the results are apparently obtained by an inhibition of steroid secretion while spironolactone blocked steroid action.

VI. Reserpine and Pharmacologically Related Drugs

The effect of reserpine, chlorpromazine and pharmacologically related drugs on adrenal cortical function has been extensively studied and comprehensively reviewed (GAUNT et al., 1965). The data are enormously confusing and generalizations necessarily guarded. It is certain that an initial large dose of such drugs causes an outpouring of ACTH and corticosteroids, generally followed with continued drug administration by a period of relative non-responsiveness to stimuli normally expected to cause ACTH release. This refractoriness may be due either to an insulation of the hypothalamic-pituitary system from stimuli which normally impinge upon it or more likely to drug-induced depletion of stores of pituitary ACTH. Whatever may be the complex pharmacology involved, no evidence exists that corticoadrenal influences are significantly involved in the antihypertensive actions of drugs such as reserpine.

VII. Concluding Remarks

The subject matter of this chapter involves much experimental and relatively little applied pharmacology. Eventual wider application seems certain as the present prototype drugs are improved and new ones found. It is a field *par excellance* for application of the at times disdained but still highly productive art of molecular manipulation. Past history and current inferrence make it all but certain that new drugs with greater selectivity and specificity of action can be found or synthesized and that they can be used with fine discrimination to alter the numerous endocrine metabolic aberrations which may lead to hypertension.

Aside from the development of better drugs, the major evident problem in this field is to the cause of hypertension in that large sub-group of "essential" hypertensives which can now be segregated on the basis of definable criteria. They approximate 20% of the hypertensive population and are characterized by (a) low plasma renin velues, which are unresponsive to stimuli normally expected to elevate renin; (b) high levels of total body exchangeable sodium; (c) have no demonstrable excess output of any known steroid; and, (d) respond particularly well to the antihypertensive effects of drugs blocking some aspect of adrenal cortical function. In other words, such patients act as if they had mineralocorticoid hypertension. Unless alternative causes become manifest, a search must continue in these cases for a possible mineralocorticoid-like humor which could be a specific target of pharmacological attack.

Addendum I

On the Use of Aminoglutethimide (A-G) as an Adrenal Inhibitor

It has generally been found that the adrenal "escapes" from some of the inhibiting effects of A–G, given in tolerable doses, due to compensatory hypersecretion of ACTH. Usually dexamethasone is given concomitantly to suppress such hypersecretion.

SANFORD et al.[2] found, however, that A–G stimulated the metabolic degredation

[2] SANFORD, E. J., DRAGO, J. H., ROHNER, T, H., Jr., SANTEN, R., LIPTON, A.: "Aminoglutethimide Medical Adrenalectomy for Advanced Prostatic Carcinoma" J. of Urol. **115**, 170—174 (1976).

of dexamethasone so that increasing and monitored doses of the latter had to be used to maintain adrenal suppression. If instead of dexamethasone, cortisol was used its metabolism was uninfluenced by A–G. Hence rather constant and predictable doses of both drugs, as established in each patient, could be given for long periods. They applied such therapy in mammary and prostatic cancer with encouraging results. Presumably then a combination of A–G and cortisol would be the regimen of choise when A–G is used in cardiovascular diseases.

Addendum II

Further Observations in Selective Inhibition of Adrenal 3β-Hydroxysteroid Dehydrogenase:Δ 5 Isomerase Activity byTrilostane (4α, 5-Epoxy-17β-hydroxy-3-oxo-5α-androstane-2α Carbonitrile)

Trilostane has been demonstrated to completely inhibit ACTH induced rises in corticosterone and cortisol secretion by rats and guinea pigs respectively (POTT, G. O., RYAN, W. T., HARDING, H. R.: Selective inhibitor of adrenal 3β-hydroxysteroid dehydrogenase: Δ5 isomerase. Presented at the 57th Annual Meeting of The Endocrine Society, New York City, June 18–20, 1975). KOMANICKY et al. (KOMANICKY, P., SPARK, R. F., MELBY, J. C.: Treatment of Cushing's syndrome with inhibitor of adrenal steroidogenesis. Presented at the 58th Annual Meeting of The Endocrine Society, San Francisco, California, June 23–25, 1976) administered Trilostane in 7 patients with Cushing's syndrome from one to thirty-two weeks in a dose of 200–500 mg/day. All patients treated with Trilostane exhibited both biochemical and clinical improvement in their disease. The average cortisol secretion rate diminished from 71 mg/24 hr. to 37 mg/24 hr. shortly after introduction of therapy. Urinary 17-hydroxycorticosteroids and urinary free cortisol excretion were reduced by fifty percent as were plasma cortisol levels. Reciprocal rise of urinary dehydroepiandrosterone sulfate from 1.3 mg/24 hr. to 5.7 mg/24 hr. was noted. Urinary 17-ketosteroids also increased from 18 mg/24 hr. to 43 mg/24 hr. thus confirming the site of action of Trilostane at 3β-hydroxysteroid dehydrogenase: Δ5,4 isomerase level. Urinary tetrahydroaldosterone excretion fell from 31 µg/24 hr. to 11µg/24 hr. as did urinary 18-hydroxy tetrahydroDOC and urinary tetrahydro DOC. The reduction in both glomerulosa and fasiculata mineralocorticoid was associated with a rise in plasma renin activity which may have partially overcome the block. Interestingly, there was no alteration in plasma testosterone levels. Plasma dehydroepiandrosterone levels did not rise in parallel with plasma dehydroepiandrosterone sulfate levels. This observation requires further explanation. Plasma potassium levels increased, plasma glucose levels diminished and mean arterial blood pressure fell from hypertensive levels into the normotensive range. Patients with Cushing's syndrome on long-term Trilostane therapy exhibited no side effects from this medication. In patients with primary aldosteronism, we have also observed marked reduction in aldosterone secretion rate following administration of Trilostane with incomplete remission of the clinical manifestations of primary aldosteronism. HOLLIFIELD et al. (HOLLIFIELD, J. W., MCKENNA, T. J., WOLLFF, J. M., CHICK, W. T., LIDDLE, G. W.: Inhibition of adrenal biosynthesis in the treatment of steroid excess states. Presented at the 57th Annual Meeting of The Endocrine Society, New York City, June 18–20, 1975) and BAER et al. (BAER, L., POTTS, G., LITTLE, F., LARAGH, J. H.: Aldosterone suppression with a new adrenal inhibitor: Exposure of its role in hypertension. Presented at the 57th Annual Meeting of The Endocrine Society, New York City, June 18–20, 1975) demonstrated inhibition of aldosterone secretion in patients with primary aldosteronism but failed to observe complete clinical remission in some of their patients. All patients exhibited increments in plasma potassium levels but not all patients exhibited reduction in elevated blood pressure. Aldosterone secretion and excretion rates were diminished by more than sixty percent in patients treated with Trilostane. Similarly, both of these groups also failed to observe a uniform effect on blood pressure by Trilostane in patients with low-renin essential hypertension. HOLLIFIELD et al. observed significant reduction in mean arterial blood pressure in 4 of 7 patients whereas BAER et al. observed no reduction in mean arterial pressure in any of 7 patients with low-renin hypertension studied. The curious inconsistency in treatment of patients with low-renin hypertension by Trilostane may have to do with patients selection. It is possible that the mineralocorticoid-hypertensive syndrome may not be influenced by adrenal inhibitors and the block in mineralocorticoid biosynthesis is less than complete. Furthermore, it is not at all certain that low-renin hypertension is due to mineralocorticoid excess in a majority of cases. Trilostane is currently being used to inhibit the development of secondary aldosteronism induced by diuretic therapy in treatment of hypertensive patients. Diuretic induced secondary hyperaldosteronism does not supervene in patients receiving modest doses of Trilostane.

References

ABBOTT, E. C., GORNALL, A. G., SUTHERLAND, D. J. A., STIEFEL, M., LAIDLAW, J. C.: The influence of a heparin-like compound on hypertension, electrolytes and aldosterone in man. Canad. med. Ass. J. **94**, 1155 (1966).

ADLIN, E. V., CHANNICK, B. J.: Effects of prolonged inhibition of 11 β-hydroxylase in the dog. Endocrinology **78**, 511 (1966).

BAGSHAWE, K. D.: Hypokalemia ,carcinoma and Cushing's syndrome. Lancet **1960 II**, 284.

BENCZE, W. L., ALLEN, M. J.: Chemistry and structure-activity relationships of amphenone analogues. J. Med. Pharm. Chem. **1**, 395 (1959).

BIGLIERI, E. G., HENON, M. A., BRUST, W.: 17-Hydroxylation deficiency in man. J. Clin. Invest. **45**, 1946 (1966).

BIGLIERI, E. G., SLATON, P. E., SCHAMBELAN, M., KRONFIELD, S. J.: Mineralocorticoid hypertension. Amer. J. Med. **45**, 170 (1968).

BIRMINGHAM, M. K., OLIVER, J. T., LI, M., CHAN, T. H., BARTOVA, A., STEWART, P. B.: Hypertensive action of 18-Hydroxydeoxycorticosterone (18—OH—DOC). Fed. Proc. **32**, 352 (Abst. 762) (1973).

BIRMINGHAM, M. K., WARD, P. J.: Identification of the Porter-silber chromagen secreted by the rat adrenal. J. biol. Chem. **236**, 1661 (1961).

BLEDSOE, T., ISLAND, D. P., RIONDEL, A. M., LIDDLE, G. W.: Modification of aldosterone secretion and electrolyte excretion in man by a chemical inhibitor of 18-oxidation. J. clin. Endocr. **24**, 740 (1964).

BROWN, J. J., FERRISS, J. B., FRASER, R., LEVER, A. F., LOVE, D. R., ROBERTSON, J. I. S., WILSON, A.: Apparently isolated excess deoxycorticosterone in hypertension. Lancet **1972 II**, 243.

BURNHAM, D. F., BEYLER, A. L., POTTS, G. O.: Adrenal blocking action of a new steroid, cyanotrimethylandrostenolone. Fed. Proc. **22**, 270 (1963).

CAREY, R. M., DOUGLAS, J. G., SCHWEIKERT, J., R., LIDDLE, G. W.: The syndrome of essential hypertension and suppressed plasma renin activity. Arch. intern. Med. **130**, 849 (1972).

CHART, J. J.: The effect of aminoglutethimide and realted compounds on steroid secretion. Progress in Endocrinology ICS 184, Excerpta Med. Found. 809 (1969).

CHART, J. J., GISOLDI, E., GAUNT, R.: Effect of aminogluthetimide in adrenal regeneration hypertension. Proc. Soc. exp. Biol. & Med. **132**, 202 (1969).

CHART, J. J., SHEPPARD, H., ALLEN, M. J., BRNCZE, W. L., GAUNT, R.: New amphenone analogs as adrenocortical inhibitors. Experientia (Basel) **14**, 151 (1958).

CHART, J. J., SHEPPARD, H., MOWLES, T., HOWIE, N.: Inhibitors of adrenal corticosteroid 17 α-hydroxylation. Endocrinology **71**, 479 (1962).

CHREMOS, A. N., LAIDLAW, J. C., RUSE, J. L.: Effect of a sulfated mucopolysaccharide (Ro 1-8307) on the zona glomerulosa of regenerating rat adrenal glands and of intact glands in sodiumdeprived rats. Endrocinology **85**, 337 (1969).

Christy, N. P.: Adrenal cortical steroids in various types of hypertension. In: Manger, W. M. (Ed.): Hormones and hypertension, p. 169. Springfield/Ill.: Thomas 1966.

Clark, Eugene: Spironolactone therapy and gynecomastia: J. Amer. med. Ass. **193**, 163 (1965).

Colby, H. D., Skelton, F. R., Brownie, A. C.: Metopirone-induced hypertension in the rat. Endocrinology **86**, 620 (1970).

Conn, J. W.: Primary aldosteronism, a new clinical syndrome. J. Lab. clin. Med. **45**, 3 (1955).

Conn, J. W., Rovner, D. R., Cohen, E. L., Anderson, J. E., Jr.: Inhibition by heparinoid of aldosterone biosynthesis in man. J. clin. Endocr. **26**, 527 (1966).

Coppage, W. S., Jr., Island, S., Smith, M., Liddle, C. W.: Inhibition of aldosterone secretion and modification of electrolyte excretion in man by a chemical inhibitor of 11 β-hydroxylation. J. clin. Invest. **38**, 2101 (1959).

Cueto, C., Brown, J. H. U.: The chemical fractionation of an adrenocorticolytic drug. Endocrinology **62**, 326 (1958).

Eberlein, W. R., Bongiovanni, A. M.: Plasma and urinary corticosteroids in the hypertensive form of congenital adrenal hyperplasia. J. biol. Chem. **223**, 85 (1956).

Esch, I., Placheta, P.: Treatment of essential hypertension with spironolactone with reference to the plasma renin activity. Wien. klin. Wschr. **85**, 413 (1973).

Fanestil, D. D.: Mode of spirolactone action: competitive inhibition of aldosterone binding to Kidney mineralocorticoid receptors. Biochem. Pharm. **17**, 2240 (1968).

Ford, H. C., Bailey, R. E.: The effect of heparin on aldosterone secretion and metabolism in primary aldosteronism. Steroids **7**, 30 (1966).

Fregly, M. J.: Effect of o,p′-DDD and metyrapone (Su-4885) on development of renal hypertension in rats. Tox. Appl. Pharmacol. **12**, 548 (1968).

Gabrilove, J. L., Nicolis, G. L., Gallagher, T. F.: Effect of SK and F (dl-2(p-aminophenyl)-2-phenylethylamine) on adrenocortical function in primary aldosteronism. J. clin. Endocr. **27**, 1337 (1967).

Gabrilove, J. J., Nicolis, G. L., Gallagher, T. F.: The effect of d-2(p-aminophenyl)-2-phenylethylamine (SK and F-12185) in Cushing's syndrome associated with adrenocortical carcinoma. Metabolism. **17**, 936 (1968).

Gaunt, R.: Steroid action on electrolyte and water metabolism. In: Christy, N. P. (Ed.): The Human Adrenal Cortex, 301. New York: Harper and Row 1971.

Gaunt, R., Chart, J. J., Renzi, A. A.: Inhibitors of adrenal cortical function. Ergebn. Physiol. **56**, 114 (1965).

Gaunt, R., Gross, F., Renzi, A. A., Chart, J. J.: The adrenal cortex in hypertension (with particular reference to adrenal regeneration hypertension). In: Moyer, J. (Ed.): Hypertension, The First Hahnemann Symposium on Hypertensive Disease, p. 219. Philadelphia: W. B. Saunders Company.

Gaunt, R., Melby, J. C., Dale, S. L., Grekin, R. J., Brown, R. D.: Adrenal regeneration hypertension. Endocrinology, Proc. IV, Intl. Cong., Washington, D. C., June 18—24, 1972 Excerpta Med., Amsterdam 740 (1974).

Gaunt, R., Steinetz, B. G., Chart, J. J.: Pharmacologic alteration of steroid hormone function. Clin. Pharmacol. **9**, 657 (1968).

Gold, E. M., DiRaimondo, V. C., Kent, J. R., Forsham, P. H.: Comparative effects of certain non-narcotic central nervous system analgesics and muscle relaxants on the pituitary adrenocortical system. Ann. N. Y. Acad. Sci. **86**, 178 (1960).

Goldblatt, H., Lynch, J., Hanzal, R. F., Summerville, W. W.: I. The production of persistent elevation of systolic blood pressure by means or renal ischemia. J. exp. Med. **59**, 347 (1934).

Goldman, A. A.: Animal Models of Inborn Errors of Steroidogenesis and Steroid Action. In: 21. Colloquium der Gesellschaft für Biologische Chemie, Mosbach/Baden, p. 389. Berlin-Heidelberg-New York: Springer 1970.

Gotshall, R. W., Davis, J. O.: Mineralocorticoid activity of 18-hydroxy-deoxycorticosterone in the dog. Amer. J. Physiol. **224**, 1116 (1973).

Gross, F.: Experimental analysis of the effects of aldosterone and other corticosteroids. Rev. ibér. Endocr. **3**, 603 (1956).

Hall, C. E., Hall, O.: The comparative hypertensive activities of the acetates of d-aldosterone and deoxycorticosterone. Acta Endocr. **54**, 399 (1967).

Helmer, O. M., Judson, W. E.: Metabolic studies on hypertensive patients with suppressed plasma renin activity not due to hyperaldosteronism. Circulation **38**, 965 (1968).

Horrobin, D. F., Manku, M. S., Burstyn, P. G.: Saluretic action of aldosterone in the presence of excess cortisol: restoration of salt-retaining action by prolactin. J. Endocr. **56**, 343 (1973).

HUGHES, S. W. M., BURLEY, D. M.: Aminoglutethimide: a "side-effect". Turned to therapeutic advantage. Postgrad. med. J. **46**, 409 (1970).
JASMIN, G., RICHER, G. L.: Effect of Nialamide on Plasma and Adrenal Corticosterone in Rats. In: Program of the Forty-Third Meeting of the Endocrine Society, New York City, June 1961, 70 (1966).
JENKINS, J. S., THORN, G. W.: Inhibition of adrenal steroid 11-oxygenation in the dog. Science **128**, 478 (1958).
JOHNSON, P. C., LORENZEN, L. C., BIGLIERI, E. G., GANONG, W. F.: The effect of the monoamine oxidase inhibitor. tranylcypromine on adrenocortical secretion in dogs Amer. Zool. **5**, 689 (Abst. 290) (1965).
JONES, J. E., VAITUKAITIS, J. L., MELBY, J. C.: The pharmacological control of Cushing's syndrome. Program, the endocrine society. St. Louis, Mo., Abst. 66, p. 69, June 10—12, 1970.
KAGAWA, C. M., CELLA, J. A., VAN ARMAN, C. G.: Action of new steroids in blocking effects of aldosterone and deoxycorticosterone on salt. Science **126**, 1015 (1957).
KAHNT, F. W., NEHER, R.: On the specific inhibition of adrenal steroid biosynthesis. Experientia (Basel) **18**, 499 (1962).
KAHNT, F. W., NEHER, R.: Über die Adrenale Steroid-Biosynthese *in vitro*: III. Selective Hemmung der Nebennierenenden-Funktion. Helvet. chim. Acta **49**, 725 (1966).
KAHNT, F. W., NEHER, R.: On adrenocortical steroid biosynthesis *in vitro*. Part V. Activators and inhibitors — evidence for the presence of substrate-specific 21-hydroxylase. Acta Endocr. **70**, 315 (1972).
KÜCHEL, O., HORKY, K., GREGOROVA, I.: The treatment of secondary hyperaldosteronism with oedema by amino-glutethimide. Pharm. Clin. **2**, 138 (1970).
LANDAU, R. L., LUGIBIHL, K.: Inhibition of the sodium-retaining influence of aldosterone by progesterone. J. clin. Endocr. **18**, 1237 (1958).
LEVINE, J. H., LAIDLAW, J. C., RUSE, J. L.: Effects of a sulfated mucopolysaccharide (RO 1-8307) on zona glomerulosa width and steroid production by the rat adrenal cortex. Canad. J. Physiol. Pharm. **50**, 270 (1972).
LEVITT, J. I.: Spironolactone therypy and amenorrhea. JAMA **211**, 2014 (1970).
LIDDLE, G. W.: Sodium diuresis induced by steroidal antagonists of aldosterone. Science **126**, 1016 (1957).
LIDDLE, G. W., LANCE, E. M., HARRIS, A. P.: Alteration in adrenal steroid patterns in man resulting from treatment with a chemical inhibitor of 11 β-hydroxylation. J. clin. Endocr. **18**, 906—(1958).
LORENZEN, L. C., GANONG, W. F.: Effect of drugs related to α-ethyltryptamine on stress-induced ACTH secretion in the dog. Endocrinology **80**, 889 (1967).
MAJOOR, C. L. H.: Aldosterone suppression by heparin. New Engl. J. Med. **279**, 1172 (1968).
MANCHENO-RICE, E., KUCHEL, O., WOWACZYNSKI, W., SETH, K. J., SASAKI, C., DAWSON, K., GENEST, J.: A dissociated effect of amino-gluethimide on the mineralocorticoid secretion in man. Metabolism **22**, 123 (1973).
MARKS, A. D., ADLIN, E. V., CHANNICK, B. J.: Effect of metyrapone on plasma renin activity in dogs. Amer. J. Physiol. **221**, 1604 (1971).
MELBY, J. C.: Aldosterone Inhibitors (Adrenal Cortex, Chapter 5), p. 477. In: ASTWOOD, E. B., CASSIDY, C. E. (Ed.): Clinical Endocrinology II. New York: Grune and Stratton 1968.
MELBY, J. C., DALE, S. L., GREKIN, R. J., GAUNT, R., WILSON, T. E.: 18-Hydroxy-11-deoxy-corticosterone (18—OH—DOC) secretion in experimental and human hypertension. Rec. Progr. Hormone Res. **28**, 287 (1972).
MELBY, J. C., DALE, S. L., WILSON, T. E.: 11-Hydroxy-deoxycorticosterone in human hypertension. Circulat Res. **28**, (Suppl.) 2 II-143 (1971).
MORAN, W., GOETZ, F. C., KENNEDY, B. J., MELBY, J. C., ZIMMERMAN, B.: Primary hyperaldosteronism without adrenal tumor. Amer. J. Med. **28**, 638 (1960).
MÜLLER, J.: Regulation of aldosterone biosynthesis. Monographs on endocrinology, Vol. 5. Berlin-Heidelberg-New York: Springer 1971.
NELSON, A. A., WOODARD, G.: Severe adrenal cortical atrophy (cytotoxic) and hepatic damage produced in dogs by feeding 2,2-*bis* (parachlorophenyl)-1,1-dichloroethane (DDD or TDE). Arch. Path. **48**, 387 (1949).
NEUMANN, H. C., POTTS, G. O., RYAN, W. T., STONER, S. W.: Steroidal heterocycles XIII. J. med. Chem. **13**, 948 (1970).
NICHOLS, J., HENNIGAR, G.: Studies on DDD, 2-2,*bis*(parachlorophenyl)-1,1-dichloroethane. Exp. Med. Surg. **15**, 310 (1957).
RAPP, J. M., KNUDSEN, K. D., IWAI, J., DAHL, L. K.: Genetic control of blood pressure and corticosteroid production in rats. Circulation Res. **32**, (Suppl. 1) I-139 (1973).

ROVNER, D. R., CONN, J. W., VADER, S. D.: Rapid production of 18-OH-11-deoxycorticosterone (18—OH—DOC) by a non-functioning adrenal adenoma. Endocrinology **88**, (Supplement, p. A-94, Abstr. 104) (1971).

SAUNDERS, H. L., STECIW, B., KOSTOS, V., TOMOSZEWSKI, J.: Adrenal inhibition in the rat and guinea pig by 2-(p-Aminophenyl)-2-phenylethylamine (SKF-12185). Steroids **7**, 513 (1966).

SAVAGE, O., COPEMAN, W. S. C., CHAPMAN, L., WELLS, M. V., TREADWELL, B. L. J.: Pituitary and adrenal hormones in rheumatoid arthritis. Lancet **1962 I**, 232.

SEALEY, J. E., GERTEN, J. N., LEDINGHAM, J. G. G., LARAGH, J. H.: Inhibition of renin by heparin. J. clin. Endocr. **27**, 699 (1967).

SIMPSON, S. A., TAIT, J. F., WETTSTEIN, A., NEHER, R., VAN EUW, J., REICHSTEIN, R.: Isolierung eines neuen kristallisierten Hormons aus Nebennieren mit besonders hoher Wirksamkeit auf den Mineralstoffwechsel. Experientia (Basel) **9**, 333 (1953).

SKELTON, F. R.: Development of hypertension and cardiovascular-renal lesions during adrenal regeneration in the rat. Proc. Soc. exp. Biol. **90**, 342 (1955).

SPARK, R. F., DALE, S. L., KAHN, P. C., MELBY, J. C.: Activation of aldosterone secretion in primary aldosteronism. J. clin. Invest. **48**, 96 (1969).

SPARK, R. F., MELBY, J. C.: Aldosteronism in hypertension: the response to spironolactone. Ann. intern. Med. **69** (4), 685 (1968).

SPARK, R. F., MELBY, J. C.: Hypertension and low plasma renin activity: presumptive evidence for mineralocorticoid excess. Ann. intern. Med. **75**, 831 (1971).

STEELMAN, S. L., BROOKS, J. R., MORGAN, E. R.: Antiandrogenic activity of spironolactone. Steroids **14**, (4) 449 (1969).

STEIGER, M., REICHSTEIN, T.: Desoxy-corticosterone (21-oxyprogesterone). Aus Δ-3-Oxo-Etio-Cholensäure. Helv. chim. Acta **20**, 1164 (1937).

SUTHERLAND, D. J., RUSE, J. L., LAIDLAW, J. C.: Hypertension, increased aldosterone secretion and low plasma renin activity relieved by dexamethasone. Canad. med. Ass. J. **95**, 1109 (1966).

SWANECK, G. E., CHU, L. L. H., EDELMAN, I. S.: Stereospecific binding of aldosterone to renal chromatin. J. biol. Chem. **245**, 5382 (1970).

TEMPLE, T. E., JONES, D. J., LIDDLE, G. W., DEXTER, R. N.: Treatment of Cushing's disease. Correction of hypercortisolism by o,p'-DDD without induction of aldosterone deficiency. New Engl. J. Med. **281** 801 (1969).

TOUITOU, Y., LEGRAND, J. C., DESGREZ, P.: Adrenocortical steroidogenesis and aminoglutethimide. I. Biochemical studies. Biomedicine **18**, 185 (1973).

TOUITOU, Y., LEGRAND, J. C., DESGREZ, P.: Adrenocortical steroidogenesis and aminoglathemide (A.G.). **II.** Cytochemical and ultrastructural changes. Practical and theoretical values. Biomedicine 18, 272 (1973b).

TUCCI, J. R., ESPINER, E. A., JAGGER, P. I., LAULER, D. P.: The effect of metyrapone on aldosterone secretion in man. Acta Endocr. **56**, 376 (1967).

TUCCI, R. R., ESPINER, E. A., JAGGER, P. I., LAULER, D. P., THORN, G. W.: Effect of new adrenal blocking agent in Cushing's syndrome and primary aldosteronism. Clin. Res. **14**, 478 (1966).

TULLNER, W. W., HERTZ, R.: Suppression of corticosteroid production in the dog by monase. Proc. Soc. exp. Biol. **116**, 837 (1964).

TWEEDDALE, M. B., OGILVIE, R. I.: Antagonism of spironolactone-induced natriuresis by aspirin in man. New Engl. J. Med. **289**, 198 (1973).

WOODS, J. W., HILL, C., LIDDLE, G. W., STANT, E. G., MICHELAKIS, A. M., BRILL, A. B.: Effect of an adrenal inhibitor in hypertensive patients with suppressed renin. Arch. intern. Med. **123**, 366 (1969).

Chapter 11

Interferences with the Renin-Angiotensin System and Their Effects on High Blood Pressure

D. GANTEN and F. GROSS

With 6 Figures

Originally, a chapter on the renin-angiotensin system (RAS) was not planned for inclusion in this volume on antihypertensive agents. However, in view of the recent development of various competitive antagonists to angiotensin II, as well

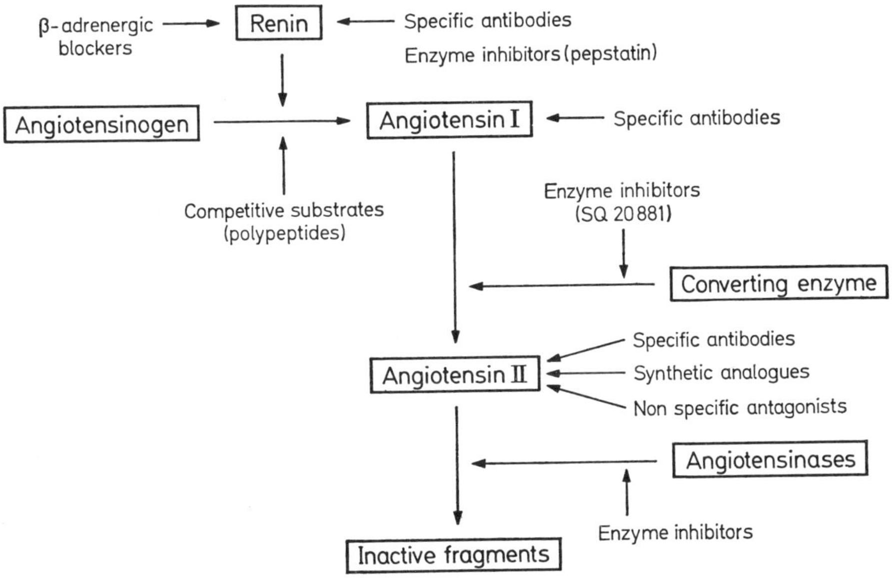

Fig. 1. The renin-angiotensin system and possible interference of various substances

---

Abbreviations Used

RAS = renin-angiotensin system (kidney, plasma)
iso-RAS = iso-renin-angiotensin system (extrarenal tissue)
AI = angiotensin I, decapeptide
AII = angiotensin II, octapeptide
PRA = plasma renin activity
CE = AI converting enzyme
CEI = AI–CE inhibitor
saralasin = 1-sarcosine-8-alanine-AII analogue, P 113
SHR = spontaneously hypertensive rats

as of other drugs which interfere with the activity of the RAS, it was necessary to refer to the possibilities of lowering blood pressure in cases in which hypertension is renin dependent. To improve understanding this chapter gives a short review of the biochemistry and pathophysiology of the RAS (Fig. 1). The discussion is limited to those aspects necessary for the understanding of mechanisms underlying the pathogenesis of renin-dependent forms of high blood pressure and to drugs that may interfere at various levels with the RAS. The inhibitory effect of β-adrenergic blockers on the release of renin from the kidney is discussed in Chapter 13, p. 602. Only a limited number of the recent references and reviews on that topic are quoted in this context.

I. Components of the RAS

A. Renin (EC 3.4.99.19)[1]

Renin from human kidneys has been purified and characterized by several groups of workers (HAAS et al., 1953, 1965; HAAS and GOLDBLATT, 1967; SKEGGS et al., 1976). The methodology for purification has been improved by the application of affinity chromatography techniques and by using renin inhibitors such as pepstatin and other peptides as ligands (CORVOL et al., 1973; MURAKAMI et al., 1973; MAJSTRORAVICH, 1974; MURAKAMI and INAGAMI, 1975; POULSEN et al., 1975). The most highly purified renin has been prepared by MURAKAMI and INAGAMI (1975), who obtained a 180000-fold purified enzyme with a molecular weight of 40000. This is in good agreement with earlier data (PEART et al., 1966 [m. w.40000]; RUBIN, 1972 [m.w. 43000]; BOYD, 1974 [m.w. 40000]). Several authors have described various forms of renal renin (HAAS et al., 1953; COHEN et al., 1972; SKEGGS et al., 1974, 1976). These differences may be attributed either to the presence of isoenzymes or to partial proteolysis of renin during the purification procedure; other investigators have found only one form (MURAKAMI and INAGAMI, 1975).

Several authors have described inactive precursors of renin with molecular weights of about 60000 (BOYD, 1974) in the rabbit (LECKIE and MCCONNELL, 1975), dog (JAMES and HALL, 1974), pig (RUBIN, 1972; BOYD, 1974), and in man (MORRIS and LUMBERS, 1972; DAY et al., 1975; SKINNER et al., 1975). These inactive forms may be activated by acidification, by enzymes, or by cold storage (MORRIS and LUMBERS, 1972; OSMOND et al., 1973; DAY et al., 1975; LECKIE and MCCONNELL, 1975; SEALEY and LARAGH, 1975; SKINNER et al., 1975). The terms "pro-renin," "big-renin", and "big-big-renin" have been coined for these inactive precursors, but in accordance with the terminology for other enzymes the term reninogen is more appropriate.

Relatively pure and angiotensinase-free enzymes that are similar to kidney renin have also been isolated from various extrarenal tissues. In order to distinguish them from kidney renin these enzymes are called isorenins. A more appropriate group name for renin and isorenins would be angiotensinogen hydrolases (angiotensin-I-forming) (GANTEN et al., 1976a, b). The submaxillary gland (WERLE

[1] Enzyme Nomenclature, New York: Elsevier Publishing Company, 1972.

et al., 1957; OLIVER and GROSS, 1966; BING and POULSEN, 1971), the female genital tract (GROSS et al., 1964; ANDERSON et al., 1968; SYMONDS et al., 1968; CARRETERO, 1971a; ESKILDSEN, 1973; SKINNER et al., 1975), the adrenal gland (RYAN, 1972; GANTEN et al., 1976b), neural tissue (FISCHER-FERRARO et al., 1971; DAUL et al., 1975; GANTEN et al., 1976a, b), and the arterial wall (DENGLER, 1956; GANTEN et al., 1976b) are of particular interest in this respect. In some species, enzyme concentrations in extrarenal tissues exceed those in the kidney, and the AII formed may exert metabolic effects at or near the site of its production. Both the renal and extrarenal enzymes are (probably) glycoproteins, have neither serin in the active center nor metal-containing prosthetic groups, and have specific substrate requirements. They are not dialysable, can be precipitated by ammonium sulfate, are heat=labile, relatively stable in acid milieú, and produce in most species a sustained blood pressure increase, which is specially pronounced after bilateral nephrectomy (for review see: PAGE and MCCUBBIN, 1968; LEE, 1969; GROSS, 1971; GANTEN et al., 1976a, b; SKEGGS et al., 1976).

B. Angiotensinogen (Renin Substrate)

Numerous efforts have been made to purify and characterize angiotensinogen (for review see SKEGGS et al., 1976). Estimations of its molecular weight range from 40000 (MÉNARD et al., 1974), 57000 (SKEGGS et al., 1976), to 110000 (EGGENA et al., 1976). In electrophoresis studies, rat angiotensinogen migrated with the prealbumin-albumin fraction (NASJLETTI et al., 1971), whereas MÉNARD et al. (1974) found it in the albumin and postalbumin region. GREEN and BUMPUS (1954), and SEN et al. (1972) observed that the major fractions migrated with the α_1- and α_2-globulin fractions. These discrepancies may be due to multiple forms of substrates occurring in plasma (SKEGGS et al., 1976), but they may also be caused by alterations of the molecule during the purification procedure.

Angiotensinogen is a glycoprotein. The amino acid compositions of all forms described so far are essentially identical, while differences have been attributed mainly to variations in the glucosamine, sialic acid or the neutral hexose carbohydrate moieties.

Treatment of renin substrate with trypsin yielded a tetradecapeptide among other peptide fragments. The purified tetradecapeptide which was later synthesized served as renin substrate and upon incubation with renin yielded the decapeptide angiotensin I (AI) and the tetrapeptide Leu-Val-Tyr-Ser (Table 1). It was found that renin specifically hydrolyses the bond between the two leucines in Positions 10 and 11 of the tetradecapeptide (POULSEN, 1973; SKEGGS et al., 1976). The source of plasma angiotensinogen is the liver (NASJLETTI and MASSON, 1973) but angiotensinogen has also been found in the lymph (HORKY et al., 1971), in the kidney (JOHNSTON et al., 1973) and in high concentrations in brain tissue and in CSF (GANTEN et al., 1971, 1976a, b; MALAYAN and REID, 1976; REID and DAY, 1977). In plasma (POULSEN, 1973) and in brain tissue (HOFFMAN et al., 1976) angiotensinogen concentrations may be a rate-limiting factor for the formation of angiotensin I.

Table 1. *Synthetic peptides that inhibit the renin-angiotensinogen reaction* (oMe, *methyl ester;* oEt, *ethyl ester*; ol, *deoxidized form*; *α-bromoisocaproic acid* BIC)

↓ Trypsin

Renin substrate (angiotensinogen) glycoprotein (nol. wt. 58000)														
Asp 1	Arg 2	Val 3	Tyr 4	Ileu (Val) 5	His 6	Pro 7	Phe 8	His 9	Leu 10	Leu 11	Val 12	Tyr 13	Ser 14	Synthetic tetradecapeptide renin substrate SKEGGS et al. (1957, 1968)
									Leu	Leu	Val	Tyr	oMe	KOKUBU et al. (1973)
									Leu	Leu	Val	Tyr	oEt	
									Leu	Leu	Val	Phe	oMe	
									Leu	Leu	Val	Phe	oEt	
									Leu	Leu	Leu	Tyr	oMe	
									Leu	Leu	Val	Tyr	ol	
									Leu	Leu	Val	Phe	ol	
									His	Leu	Leu	Val	Tyr oEt	
					His	Pro	Phe	His	Leu	Leu	Val	Tyr		
					D-His	Pro	Phe	His	Leu	Leu	Val	Tyr		
					D-His	Pro	Phe	His	Leu	Leu	Val	Phe		
					D-His	Pro	Phe	His	D-Leu	Leu	Val	Tyr		POULSEN et al. (1973)
					D-His	Pro	Phe	His	Leu	D-Leu	Val	Tyr		BURTON et al. (1975)
					D-His	Pro	Phe	His	Ile	Leu	Val	Tyr		
				Pro	His	Pro	Phe	His	Leu	Phe	Val	Tyr		
										BIC	Val	Tyr	Ser OH	
									BIC	Leu	Val	Tyr	Ser OH	SUKETA and INAGAMI (1975)
										BIC	Val	Tyr	NH_2	

C. Angiotensin-I-Converting Enzyme (CE) (E.C. 3.4.15.1)

CE is a peptidyl-dipeptide hydrolase which cleaves the dipeptide leucine-histidine from the carboxyl-end of the decapeptide AI, resulting in the formation of the octapeptide angiotensin II (AII). It was originally discovered by SKEGGS et al. (1954) in plasma. NG and VANE (1967) showed that the principal site of conversion was the lung. This observation has been confirmed by several investigators (for review see VANE, 1974; ERDÖS, 1976). Converting enzyme activity has been demonstrated in a number of tissues including the kidney, vascular tissue, brain and others (ROTH et al., 1969; CUSHMAN and CHEUNG, 1971; YANG and NEFF, 1972; POTH et al., 1975; GANTEN et al., 1976a, b). The degree to which these tissues contribute to the conversion of plasma AI to AII (KREYE and GROSS, 1971) is difficult to measure because of tissue-binding of the peptides and tissue angiotensinase activity. In aortic blood plasma, AI levels are about 10 to 20 times higher than AII levels and it may be that local tissue conversion of the decapeptide contributes to the effective AII concentration at the receptor site. In the adrenal gland tissue of rats and dogs no measurable converting enzyme activity was found.

Purified converting enzyme has a large carbohydrate moiety, contains zinc, and requires chloride for its action. Estimates of the molecular weight of the purified enzyme range from 140000 to 480000 (UEDA et al., 1971; DORER et al., 1972; SOFFER et al., 1974). NAKAJIMA et al. (1973) reported a molecular weight of 206000 with subunits of 70000. The β-CE ("tonin") described by BOUCHER et al. (1974) is probably a different enzyme, as it forms AII directly from renin substrate (SCHILLER et al., 1976). So far, its biologic significance is unknown.

D. Structure of AII

The first pure preparation of angiotensin was isolated by SKEGGS et al. (1954, 1955) and its amino acid sequence was determined by ELLIOT and PEART (1957) which was subsequently confirmed by the synthesis of the octa- and decapeptides (BUMPUS et al., 1957; SCHWYZER et al., 1957). It was found that angiotensin of various species had the same amino acid sequence with the exception of Position 5 which is isoleucine or valine, depending on the species (for review see PAGE and McCUBBIN, 1968; GROSS, 1971; KHOSLA et al., 1974; REGOLI et al., 1974). By replacing various amino acids the activity of AII is reduced or changed.

Position 1: Since angiotensinase activity in plasma depends mainly on aminopeptidase activity, asparagin in Position 1 contributes primarily to the duration of action of angiotensin (RINIKER et al., 1962). It also affects the binding affinity of the peptide for the receptor (REGOLI et al., 1974). The heptapeptide Des-Asp-angiotensin II has also been called angiotensin III and retains biologic activity. It is not known whether the heptapeptide is of physiologic significance.

Position 2: Arginine in this position is protonated at physiologic pH (PRINTZ et al., 1972) and plays a role in binding the peptide to the receptor site (electrostatic interaction, hydrogen bonding). The D-isomer of arginine increased the activity of the heptapeptide, but decreased the activity of the octapeptide.

Position 3: Valine appears to participate in intramolecular hydrogen bonding and thus determines the three-dimensional conformation of AII to the gamma turn model of PRINTZ et al. (1972) or the beta turn model of FERMANDJIAN et al. (1971).

Position 4: Ionization of the phenol group of tyrosine in this position influences affinity to AII receptors, which may be concluded from the fact that the pK is 10 in the natural peptide, 8 in the monoiodinated, and 6 in the diiodinated form of

AII. The iodinated derivatives are much less biologically active than the non-iodinated form (LIN et al., 1970), indicating that the free hydroxyl group is essential for receptor binding.

Position 5 is taken by valine in sheep (CAIN et al., 1970) and beef, while isoleucine occurs in the human (ARAKAWA and NAKAMURA, 1967), horse, rat, and pig. Both peptides are equally active biologically.

Position 6: Histidine can act as a proton donor or acceptor at physiologic pH. The five-membered imidazole ring is of crucial significance for the biologic activity and for the three dimensional conformation of AII (PRINTZ et al., 1972).

Position 7: The bond of proline in this position with the 6-histidine is reported to be toward a "cis" conformation, which determines the secondary structure and provides the orientation for 8-phenylalanine (WEINKAM and JÖRGENSEN, 1971).

Position 8: Phenylalanine is essential for the biologic activity of AII, the heptapeptide 1 to 7 being completely inactive. If the phenyl ring is eliminated, the 8-alanine or other analogs retain the binding capacity to the receptor but lose most of the biologic activity. The binding capacity, on the other hand, depends on the free carboxylic group since the methyl and amide derivatives of 8-phenylalanine have very low affinity to the receptors (KHOSLA et al., 1974; REGOLI et al., 1974).

E. Angiotensinases

All peptidases in plasma and tissue that inactivate AI or AII are called angiotensinases, but it is not known whether specific angiotensinases exist. Enzymes such as aminopeptidases, carboxypeptidases, chymotrypsin, trypsin, pepsin, and papain inactivate angiotensin (CROXATTO and CROXATTO, 1942; CROXATTO et al., 1965; KHAIRALLAH and PAGE, 1967). However, these peptidases have some substrate specificity and therefore have different affinity to various analogs of angiotensin (BUMPUS et al., 1964; for review see LEDINGHAM, 1974).

II. Pathophysiological Significance of the RAS

Since the discovery by GOLDBLATT (1934) that experimental renal artery stenosis in dogs and other species may cause sustained hypertension, the RAS was considered mainly as a pathogenetic mechanism, until GROSS in 1958 established the physiologic significance of renin and angiotensin in the regulation of sodium balance. It is now evident that in most forms of high blood pressure the RAS is not primarily involved in the pathogenesis, but it may be secondarily stimulated, mostly by a negative sodium balance induced by high blood pressure. Although renin-dependent forms of hypertension can be produced experimentally in animals and also exist in man, they account for only a small fraction of experimental and clinical forms of high blood pressure. Nevertheless, the measuring of the activity of the RAS and the analysis of the factors which may influence it, is of significance for the understanding of the pathophysiology of both the renin-dependent and the non-renin-dependent forms of hypertension (for literature see PAGE and McCUBBIN, 1968; GROSS, 1971; LARAGH, 1973; OPARIL and HABER, 1974; SAMBHI, 1976).

A. Experimental Hypertension in Animals

1. Renal Hypertension

The RAS is stimulated following reduction of renal perfusion pressure (for review see: DAVIS and FREEMAN, 1976). This can be achieved by placing silver clips on one or both renal arteries or by other procedures such as cellophane wrapping or by placing a figure-of-eight ligature around the kidney. The increased secretion of renin results in elevated AII levels in plasma. Circulating AII will then 1) increase peripheral resistance by its direct vasoconstrictor effect (GROSS et al., 1963; GROSS, 1971), 2) stimulate aldosterone secretion, thereby inducing sodium and water retention (GROSS, 1958; GENEST et al., 1976), 3) lead to increased sympathetic tone by its effect on the CNS (SEVERS and DANIELS-SEVERS, 1973), 4) stimulate the release of antidiuretic hormone (HUTCHINSON et al., 1976), and 5) stimulate water uptake (FITZSIMONS, 1972). These effects contribute to a rise in arterial blood pressure.

In several models of renal hypertension, however, the RAS is not activated at all and may even be suppressed (DIETZ et al., 1977). Various authors have stated that the RAS may be activated in the initial stages of renal hypertension and then return to normal levels while blood pressure remains high (LEDINGHAM, 1971; SWALES et al., 1972; KRAMER and OCHWADT, 1972). In the acute malignant phase of hypertension the RAS may be stimulated secondary to natriuresis and diuresis induced by high blood pressure and nephrosclerosis (LIARD, 1973; GROSS et al., 1975; MÖHRING et al., 1975). Present knowledge can be summarized as follows: 1) In those types of renal hypertension in which salt and water loss occur (e.g. one renal artery clamped and the contralateral kidney untouched) the RAS is stimulated in order to maintain homoiostasis by increasing mineralocorticoid secretion. The feedback mechanism may secondarily then be overridden by pressure-induced natriuresis and diuresis. 2) In those types of renal hypertension in which salt and water is retained (e.g. both renal arteries clamped or contralateral kidney removed) the RAS will only initially be slightly stimulated and then suppressed (GUYTON et al., 1972; DIETZ et al., 1977).

2. Spontaneous (Genetic) Hypertension

Spontaneously hypertensive (SH) rats are considered the animal model most closely related to human essential hypertension. Most authors agree that there is a slight activation of the plasma RAS at the age of 5 to 8 weeks in SH rats as compared to controls (SEN et al., 1972; SINAIKO and MIRKIN, 1974). In contrast, CZYZEWZKI and PETTINGER (1973), and FORMAN and MULROW (1974) found no change in plasma renin activity (PRA), while LEE (1973) even observed a progressive decrease of PRA. Differences in methodology (BAGBY et al., 1976) and strains of SH rats may in part account for the discrepancies of results. However, it is generally accepted that once high blood pressure is established in SH rats it is independent of an activated RAS. Recent studies indicate that the Iso-RAS in the brain (GANTEN et al., 1976a, b) is activated in certain strains of SH rats. This activation is reflected by an increased level of AII-like material in CSF of SH rats of the New Zealand strain (GANTEN et al., 1976a, b) and by an increased isorenin concentration in certain brain areas of the Kyoto "stroke-prone strain" of SH rats (HOFFMAN et al., 1977).

B. Hypertension in Man

1. Essential Hypertension

Patients with essential hypertension have been classified into three different major subpopulations: 20% to 30% have subnormal PRA, the majority of patients (50% to 80%) have normal values and some 10% to 15% have high renin values (BRUNNER et al., 1972b; CRANE et al., 1972; OPARIL and HABER, 1974).

It was postulated (BRUNNER et al., 1972b) that elevated PRA constituted a risk factor in essential hypertension and that plasma renin levels may be useful for the prognosis of the disease and also for the selection of antihypertensive therapy. However, most investigators found no evidence for such claims (GENEST et al., 1973; for review see OPARIL and HABER, 1974). On the basis of the available data it can be stated that the RAS is not of pathophysiologic significance in essential hypertension, nor can direct conclusions be drawn from the PRA levels on either prognosis or therapy. PRA in essential hypertension is indicative of the state of sodium balance.

2. Renal Hypertension

Sclerosis of the renal arteries associated with stenosis is a common finding in patients over age 50, but many of them are normotensive. For the diagnosis of renovascular hypertension it is necessary to measure renal function and to determine the pressure gradient over the stenosis. Among others, the assay of PRA in renal venous blood is a useful diagnostic tool for estimating the degree of the stenosis (GROSS et al., 1965; GENEST et al., 1966; HUSSAIN et al., 1973). If PRA is elevated in the venous blood from the affected kidney before or after a stimulating manoeuver such as tilting, salt deprivation, administration of diuretics or vasodilators, and if other findings favor the diagnosis of renal hypertension, the chances of improvement by surgery will be approximately 80% to 95% (AMSTERDAM et al., 1969; HUNT and STRONG, 1973). However, PRA in the peripheral venous blod can be in the normal range also in patients who respond to surgical intervention (COHEN et al., 1966; AMSTERDAM et al., 1969; HUSSAIN et al., 1973). Strict control of sodium balance, multiple sites of blood sampling and calculation of renin secretion from both kidneys before and after stimulation of the RAS (BROWN et al., 1965; WOODS and MICHELAKIS, 1968) will improve the significance of PRA measurement to predict the success of surgical interventions (FOSTER et al., 1973; HUNT and STRONG, 1973).

3. Renin-Secreting Tumors

The most typical but rare form of renin-dependent hypertension is the renin-secreting tumor which can occur in the kidney ("primary reninism") (CONN et al., 1972) as well as in extrarenal tissue ("ectopic primary reninism") (GANTEN et al., 1976b). Two histologic types have been described in the kidney: the hemangiopericytoma or juxtaglomerular cell tumor (KIHARA et al., 1968; EDDY and SANCHEZ, 1971; BONNIN et al., 1972; CONN et al., 1972; SCHAMBELAN and BIGLIERI, 1972; BROWN et al., 1973; GHERARDI et al., 1974) and the nephroblastoma or Wilms' tumor (VOÛTE et al., 1971; GANGULY et al., 1973; DAY et al., 1975). Ectopic primary reninism was observed in tumors of the lung (HAUGER-KLEVENE, 1970; GENEST et al., 1975) and in the orbital region (YOKOYAMA, 1976). These tumors contained large amounts of renin and induced hypertension which was cured after removal of the tumors.

III. Interference with the RAS

A. The Renin-Substrate Reaction

1. Peptide Inhibitors

Systemic studies with various synthetic renin substrates have indicated that the C-terminal tetrapeptide sequence Leu-Leu-Val-Tyr is the specific determinant for the binding of the active site of renin (SKEGGS et al., 1974, 1976; KOKUBU et al., 1973; POULSEN, 1973; INAGAMI et al., 1974). Various peptides have therefore been synthesized which may compete with the natural substrate for the active site of renin and in this way prevent the formation of AI (Table 1). On the basis of their studies, KOKUBU et al. (1973) claimed the following structural requirements for an antirenin activity: a) a Leu-Leu bond with L-Leu at the *N*-terminal, b) at the *C*-terminal the aromatic amino acids tyrosine and phenylalanine are essential, and c) replacement of valine by leucine does not reduce antirenin activity. The methyl- or ethylesters of oligopeptides with such an amino acid sequence acted as competitive inhibitors of the renin-substrate reaction *in vitro* and *in vivo*.

While KOKUBU et al. (1973) synthesized mainly tetrapeptides containing the amino acid sequence 10 to 13, PARIKH and CUATRECASAS (1973) obtained a potent inhibitor by replacing L-Leu in Positions 10 and 11 by D-Leu in the complete tetradecapeptide substrate. POULSEN et al. (1976) synthesized octapeptides containing the sequence 6 to 13 of the tetradecapeptide. These peptides were true competitive inhibitors of the enzyme-substrate reaction. Peptides in which D-Leu was substituted for L-Leu on either side of the leucyl-leucine bond, were not cleaved by renin. However, at physiologic pH, the inhibitory constants of these peptides increased and the solubility decreased to an extent that no inhibition could be demonstrated *in vivo*. These peptides were later modified (BURTON et al., 1975; POULSEN et al., 1976) in order to increase solubility. In the most effective inhibitor, phenylalanine replaced leucine in Position 11 and solubility was increased by substituting proline to the terminal amino group (POULSEN et al., 1976).

SUKETA and INAGAMI (1975) used L-α-isocaproic acid (BIC) which has a hydrocarbon side chain identical to that of leucine and may function as a leucine substitute. They synthesized renin inactivators of the general structure α-bromoisocaproyl-oligopeptide (BIC-oligopeptide), which were directed toward the active site of renin. The activity of these oligopeptides was tested against pure isorenin from mouse submaxillary gland. The most potent inactivators of enzyme activity are shown in Table 1. SUKETA and INAGAMI found "pH-dependent" and "pH-independent" inactivators, the latter of which had blocked *C*-terminal groups. This finding is of theoretical interest with respect to interactions of substrate binding to the active site of the enzyme at different degrees of electric charge and ionization (SUKETA and INAGAMI, 1975). Studies with various inhibitors and enzymes from kidneys of primates and nonprimates have also suggested that during evolution the specific substrate site has been preserved, whereas the enzyme site for human renin differs from that of renin from nonprimates (POULSEN et al., 1976).

At present the competitive renin substrates that prevent the formation of AI have been used mainly to elucidate the biochemistry and kinetics of the renin-angiotensinogen interactions and have served as a tool for the purification of the enzyme by means of affinity chromatography (PARIKH and CUATRECASAS, 1973; MAJSTRORAVICH et al., 1974; POULSEN et al., 1975). Provided these peptides are sufficiently soluble, they may become useful for further studies of renin-dependent forms of hypertension.

2. Pepstatin

A pentapeptide (Fig. 2) produced by some actinomycetes strains had originally been found to interfere with the reaction of pepsin with its substrate and was therefore called pepstatin (MORISHIMA et al., 1970; UMEZAWA et al., 1970; AOYAGI et al., 1971). Its structure is shown in Figure 2. This peptide also inhibits the action of renin with its substrate *in vitro* (GROSS et al., 1972) and *in vivo* (MILLER et al., 1972). In view of the similarities between the acid proteases pepsin and renin it was not surprising that both enzymes were affected by the same substance. Pepstatin also inhibits tissue isorenins and cathepsin D. The kinetics of enzyme inhibition by pepstatin have been studied in detail by ORTH et al. (1974) and McKOWN et al. (1974) and correspond to a noncompetitive type of inhibition. A competitive inhibitory mechanism has been claimed by MILLER et al. (1972) and CORVOL et al. (1973).

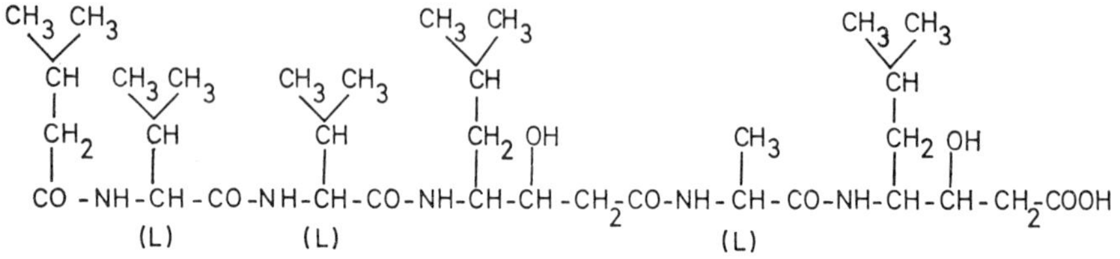

P E P S T A T I N

Fig. 2. Structure of the acid protease and renin inhibitor pepstatin (UMEZAWA et al., 1970)

In renin-dependent forms of experimental hypertension, pepstatin produces a short-term fall in blood pressure. The poor solubility of pepstatin in water as well as the short duration of its action prevent its use in diagnosis of renin-dependent forms of hypertension. However, pepstatin has been used as a ligand for the purification of acid proteases by affinity chromatography (CORVOL et al., 1973; MURAKAMI et al., 1973; MURAKAMI and INAGAMI, 1975).

3. Other Inhibitors of Renin

Besides heparin, bile acids (KOKUBU et al., 1973), PGs (KOTCHEN et al., 1974; ZAHN and GANTEN, 1976), antitrypsin (SCHARPE et al., 1976) and hemoglobin (WORKMAN et al., 1974), further inhibitors of the renin substrate reaction have been described. Lysophosphoglycerides resulting from the action of phospholipase A on parent phosphoglycerides and various analogues of lysophosphatidyl ethanolamine are renin inhibitors *in vitro* and cause a reduction of blood pressure *in vivo* as well as a reduction of PRA in renal hypertensiverats. They are without diagnostic or therapeutic significance (for review see TURCOTTE et al., 1975; SCHARPE et al., 1976).

B. Immunological Interferences

Among the possible interferences with the RAS, pharmacologic and immunologic approaches may be differentiated. In principle, antibodies may be produced against any component of the RAS, e.g., against the enzyme in the form of an antirenin and against the substrate in the form of angiotensinogen antibodies, provided these proteins are available in a form sufficiently pure to produce specific antibodies (HAAS et al., 1965; MICHELAKIS et al., 1974; EGGENA et al., 1976).

Antibodies against synthetic AI and AII have been prepared by coupling the hapten angiotensin with large molecules such as albumin and γ-globulin or by adsorption to charcoal (see reviews: FREEDLENDER et al., 1974; VALLOTON, 1974). A number of experiments with active or passive immunization have been carried out to characterize renin dependence of blood pressure in experimental renal hypertension (CHRISTLIEB et al., 1969; EIDE et al., 1973; JOHNSTON et al., 1973; CHRISTLIEB and HICKLER, 1972; HEDWALL, 1968; BRUNNER et al., 1971, 1972a, b; CARRETERO et al., 1971a, b). In certain renin-dependent forms of experimental renal hypertension the administration of antibodies was followed by a fall in blood pressure (BRUNNER et al., 1971, 1972a; CARRETERO et al., 1971b). However, the increase in blood pressure induced by a clip on one renal artery in the presence of an untouched contralateral kidney was not prevented in rats immunized against angiotensin (JOHNSTON et al., 1973; EIDE et al., 1973). The failure of active immunization to inhibit experimental renal hypertension could be caused either by inaccessibility of angiotensin at the receptors to circulating antibodies or by the fact that the RAS is not of pathogenic significance for that type of hypertension. The former assumption is supported by the observations that pharmacologic inhibitors of renin or angiotensin lower blood pressure in renin-dependent forms of hypertension in cases in which active immunization is ineffective (DAVIS et al., 1974).

The interpretation of results obtained by immunologic techniques is further complicatec by the fact that active and passive immunization and the subsequent binding of AII to circulating antibodies may induce an increase in PRA and plasma concentration of AII. In rabbits, the latter may increase from 100 pg/ml before immunization to more than 100 ng/ml after immunization (OSTER et al., 1975). The effectiveness of blockade of the RAS by antibodies against AII depends 1) on the specificity and affinity of the antibody, 2) on the levels of free AII not bound to antibodies, 3) on AII receptor occupancy and affinity, 4) on the feedback control of renin secretion by AII, and 5) on the distribution volume and half-life of the AII antibodies. These parameters have not been controlled in most *in vivo* studies. Hence, results using the immunologic approach of blocking the RAS have to be interpreted with caution.

In vitro, antibodies to renin (HAAS et al., 1965), to extrarenal isorenins (MICHELAKIS et al., 1974), to angiotensinogen (EGGENA et al., 1976), and to angiotensin have been used to characterize, inhibit, or measure the respective antigens (for review see BOYD and PEART, 1974; FREEDLENDER et al., 1974; VALLOTON, 1974).

C. Inhibitors of Angiotensin-I-Converting Enzyme (CEI)

1. Experimental Results

Non-peptide inhibitors of CE have been reviewed by BAKHLE (1974), and only peptides will be discussed here. Certain peptides behave as competitive or non-competitive inhibitors of the enzyme, others inhibit CE through product inhibition (e.g., bradykinin, methionine-kallidin, AII, 1-Sar-8-Ala-AII (saralasin) and insulin (SANDER et al., 1971; BING et al., 1974; DORER et al., 1974; CHIU et al., 1976). A number of peptides have been isolated from the venom of the snake *Bothrops jararaca*. Originally, these peptides were characterized as inhibitors of kininases, which enhance the action of kinins (bradykinin potentiating factor). At the same time many of these peptides are potent inhibitors of CE and block the conversion of AI to AII, preventing in this way the formation of AII and accumulating AI (FERREIRA et al., 1970; CHEUNG and CUSHMAN, 1973; BAKHLE, 1974). Various of these peptides have been synthesized by ONDETTI et al. (1971) and the non-apeptide Glu-Tryp-Pro-Arg-Pro-Gln-Ileu-Pro-Pro (SQ 20881) has attracted the most attention. The *C*-terminal Pro-Pro makes this peptide resistant to hydrolysis for CE, which results in a potent inhibition of the enzyme *in vivo* and *in vitro* (BAKHLE, 1972, 1974; CUSHMAN and CHEUNG, 1972). The nonapeptide SQ 20881 is preferable to the other peptide inhibitors from *B. jararaca* because of its longer duration of action *in vivo*, which is about 30 to 90 min (DAVIS et al., 1974; BING and POULSEN, 1975; CASE et al., 1976b). An advantage over some AII antagonist is that SQ 20881 has no agonistic (vasoconstrictor) activities (CASE et al., 1976b; SAMUELS et al., 1976).

The question whether CE itself plays a rate-limiting and regulatory role in hypertension or salt and volume imbalance is not yet settled, and further investigations in to the heterogenity of CE in different species and tissues are required. The CEI SQ 20881 has been used in order to demonstrate the presence of CE in various organs, such as the kidney (HOFBAUER et al., 1973), the brain (FITZSIMONS, 1972; GANTEN et al., 1976a, b; HOFFMAN et al., 1976), and the arteries (MALIK and NASJLETTI, 1976) and has been used experimentally and clinically (KRIEGER et al., 1971; ENGEL et al., 1972; KEIM et al., 1972; MILLER et al., 1972; BING and NIELSEN, 1973; GAVRAS et al., 1974; CASE et al., 1976b; SAMUELS et al., 1976; SANCHO et al., 1976) to investigate renin dependence of high blood pressure. Using the CEI SQ 20881 in various experimental models the following results have been obtained: In the normal, sodium-replete animal, administration of CEI has no effect on blood pressure. If the sodium balance is negative, the RAS increasingly contributes to the maintenance of blood pressure, which is indicated by the hypotensive effect the CEI exerts under such conditions. Also in volume depletion induced by hemorrhage, CEI may induce a decrease in blood pressure. Experimental renal hypertension can be prevented when administration of CEI is started at the same time as the stenosis is applied to the renal artery. In the early phase of congestive heart failure, when PRA and aldosterone are elevated, CEI induced marked hypotension. With increasing retention of salt and water PRA decreased and CEI has less effect on blood pressure (JOHNSON and DAUIS, 1973a, b; JOHNSON et al., 1974; SAMUELS et al., 1976). Subsequent to adrenalectomy, pretreatment with hypotensive drugs, or anaesthesia, the inhibition of CE activity may results in a decrease in blood pressure (DAVIS et al., 1974; BING and POULSEN, 1975; SAMUELS et al., 1976).

Administration of SQ 20881 stimulates the activity of the RAS and PRA increases. This effect is probably not the result of blood pressure decrease or reflex β-adrenergic stimulation, but is caused by the removal of the negative feedback which AII has on renin release from the kidney (BING, 1973; PETTINGER et al., 1973; McDONALD et al., 1975; SAMUELS et al., 1976).

2. Clinical Results

In man the CEI (SQ 20881) was first shown by COLLIER et al. (1973) to reduce the rate of AII formation. CEI alone has little or no effect on blood pressure in normal supine human subjects. Following the administration of CEI, sodium-replete subjects maintained blood pressure during 30 min of tilting. Although PRA rose significantly, plasma aldosterone remained unchanged, demonstrating the lack of AII formation and the dependence of aldosterone secretion on AII. In subjects submitted to mild sodium depletion, CEI lowered blood pressure in the recumbent position, but a dramatic fall in blood pressure occurred, accompanied by fainting when they were tilted (SAMUELS et al., 1976). GAVRAS et al. (1974) demonstrated the antihypertensive effect of CEI in renovascular hypertension, malignant hypertension, certain types of essential hypertension, and in patients maintained on a low sodium intake. Subsequent studies have confirmed that CEI is a suitable agent to estimate the participation of the RAS in the hypertensive state.

The effective doses of the CEI SQ 20881 are between 0.25 and 4.0 mg/kg (GAVRAS et al., 1974; CASE et al., 1976b; SANCHO et al., 1976). Since the peptide has no effect on blood pressure by its own it can be administered as slow intravenous bolus injection, or as an infusion of 10 to 100 μg/kg/min (CASE et al., 1976b; SANCHO et al., 1976). It has been suspected that SQ 20881 by inhibition of kininases might cause kinin accumulation which in turn could participate in the hypotensive response (GREEN et al., 1972; SANCHO et al., 1976). This question needs further investigation. The following results, however, indicate that the blood pressure lowering effect of SQ 20881 is the consequence of an inhibition of AII formation: 1) The CEI does not affect blood pressure in anephric patients, 2) good correlations have been found between the depressor effects of CEI and the PRA before administration of the drug, 3) in those patients or experimental conditions, in whom SQ 20881 was effective in lowering blood pressure, angiotensin blockade resulted in quantitatively and qualitatively similar depressor responses.

Since completion of this chapter, ONDETTI et al. (1977) have synthesized a new class of potent CEI. These compounds are mercaptoalkanoyl or carboxyalkanoyl derivatives of proline. Similarly to SQ 20881, they inhibit the conversion of AI to AII *in vitro* and *in vivo*, and they augment the response to bradykinin. Contrary to all other compounds, however, they are active when administered by mouth and have been shown to lower blood pressure in rats with renal hypertension after oral administration.

One of these CEI (D-2-methyl-3-mercaptopropranoyl-L-proline, SQ 14,225) has been tested in man by FERGUSON et al. (1977). SQ 14,225 effectively blocked conversion of AI to AII within 15 min after oral administration, the degree and duration of the inhibition being dose related. Doses 1 to 20 mg given by mouth to subjects of 63 to 73 kg body wt. effectively inhibited the pressor responses to AI and had no effect on pressor responses to AII. A 20 mg oral dose resulted in complete blockade of intravenously administered AI for more than 2 h and in partial inhibition for over 4 h. SQ 14,225 represents an advance in the development of inhibitors of the RAS, the main advantage being its oral efficacy and the lack of angiotensin-like pressor activity. Since this compound also inhibits kinin inactivation, the contribution of the kininogenase system to its biologic effects needs to be studied.

D. AII Antagonists at the Receptor Site

1. Experimental Results

The actions of angiotensin in the various target organs (GOODFRIEND et al., 1974; GANTEN et al., 1976a) are antagonized by a number of drugs that interfere with the sympathetic or parasympathetic nervous system, or by compounds such as ouabain, kinins, vasodilators, prostaglandins, or diuretics. These effects may be indirect, non-specific, or limited to certain tissues (for review see TÜRKER et al., 1974).

After many fruitless attempts the progress made in peptide chemistry has allowed the synthesis of numerous analogs of angiotensin (BUMPUS et al., 1957; SCHWYZER et al., 1957) but only recently various octapeptides which may be considered as specific competitive antagonists of AII have been prepared (MARSHALL et al., 1970; PALS et al., 1971a, b; KHOSLA et al., 1972 to 1974; NEEDLEMAN et al., 1972; SEN et al., 1974; WISSMANN et al., 1974; for review see KHOSLA et al., 1974; REGOLI et al., 1974; TÜRKER et al., 1974; STOKES and EDWARDS, 1976).

This review will mention only those analogs that are of experimental significance and may be used clinically in the diagnosis and perhaps also in the treatment of renin-dependent forms of hypertension (Table 2).

Angiotensin is believed to act on specific receptors in target tissues such as vascular smooth muscle, adrenal glands, brain, and other organs (SWANSON et al., 1973; GLOSSMANN et al., 1974; SAKAI et al., 1974; MCLEAN et al., 1975; BENNET and SNYDER, 1976; DEVYNCK and MEYER, 1976; GANTEN et al., 1976a, b; SALT-

Table 2. *Amino acid sequence of angiotensin* II *and angiotensin* II *analogs that have been used to block angiotensin* II *effects at the receptor* (– *indicates identical amino acid as in angiotensin* II)

1 Asp-	2 Arg-	3 Val-	4 Tyr-	5 Ileu-Val	6 His-	7 Pro-	8 Phe	Angiotensin II
Sar-	—	—	—	—	—	—	Ala	(PALS et al., 1971)
Sar-	—	—	—	—	—	—	Ileu	(KHOSLA et al., 1972, 1974)
N-methyl Ileu	—	—	—	—	—	—	Ileu	(SEN et al., 1974)
Sar	—	—	—	—	—	—	Threo	(SEN et al., 1976)
—	—	—	—	—	—	—	Gly	(WISSMANN et al., 1974)
—	—	—	Phe	—	—	—	Tyr	(MARSHALL et al., 1970)

MAN et al., 1976; THURSTON, 1976). These receptors fulfil the criteria of specificity, high affinity, reversibility of binding, and saturation. From the conformation of the AII molecule it is evident that the binding itself is influenced by the sequence of amino acids and by the tertiary structure of AII. The biologic activity appears to depend almost exclusively on the phenylalanine in Positon 8. Therefore, 8-substituted analogs of AII have proved to be the most potent competitive inhibitors of the natural peptide. The first angiotensin analog to be effective *in vivo* was phenylalanine-4-tyrosine-8-AII, which produced a dose-dependent parallel shift in the pressor dose-responsiveness to exogenous AII (MARSHALL et al., 1970). This AII antagonist exhibited a high degree of specificity and did not alter the uterine dose-response curves for bradykinin, oxytocin, vasopressin, or serotonin (MARSHALL, 1976; NEEDLEMAN et al., 1976). Although the substance represented a useful prototype of AII antagonists, it had marked agonistic AII-like activity and was less potent than subsequently synthesized octapeptides (TÜRKER et al., 1971; NEEDLEMAN et al., 1972; REGOLI and PARK, 1972; SWEET et al., 1973; REGOLI et al., 1974). Today, the most widely used AII analog is saralasin, in which asparagin in Position 1 is replaced by sarcosine, and phenylalanine in Position 8 by alanine. 1-Sar-8-Ala-AII antagonist (saralasin, P 113), which however, has less AII-like activity than most other AII analogs. Saralasin has been used almost exclusively to antagonize AII effects, and data on pharmacodynamics and pharmacokinetics are scarce. The replacement of asparagine in Position 1 by sarcosine has prolonged the biologic half-life of this analog in plasma because it is more resistant to aminopeptidases (PALS et al., 1971a, b; PALS and MASUCCI, 1973; HALL et al., 1974). While the biologic half-life of AII is less than 1 min, that for saralasin is between 3 and 8 min (PETTINGER et al., 1974). An infusion period of less than 20 min is required to achieve effective stable plasma concentrations *in vivo* (PETTINGER et al., 1974).

The 8-Ileu-AII has also been reported to be a potent antagonist of AII (TÜRKER et al., 1972; YAMAMOTO et al., 1972) but it has more pronounced agonistic activity (BUMPUS et al., 1973). Several 8-substituted derivatives of AII cause release of catecholamines from the adrenal medulla (MUNOZ-RAMIREZ et al., 1975), which makes them less useful for clinical studies. SEN et al. (1976) reported that the 1-Sar-8-Threo-AII antagonist had no agonistic effect on blood pressure under the conditions studied and does not stimulate catecholamine release from the adrenal gland.

Experimental studies with AII antagonists have helped to define more precisely the role of the RAS under various pathophysiologic conditions, especially in hypertension (for review see DAVIS et al., 1974), and were also useful in the identification of angiotensin receptors in various tissues (GANTEN et al., 1976a, b).

It has been suggested that AII receptors differ from each other depending upon the target organs of AII (DEVYNCK and MEYER, 1976). The characteristics of AII receptors have been most intensively studied in vascular smooth muscle, in the adrenal gland, and in the brain. The 1-sarcosine-substituted analogs of angiotensin, which are relatively resistant to aminopeptidase degradation, are more potent inhibitors of angiotensin effects on vascular smooth muscle than on the steroidogenic response in the adrenal cortex (PEACH and CHIU, 1974; STEELE and LOWENSTEIN, 1974). The *N*-terminal asparagine appears to participate in the mediation of the myotropic effect of AII since the heptapeptide Des-Asp-AII (angiotensin III) retains only 50% of the vasoconstrictor effect of AII. In contrast, Des-Asp-AII is fully active on adrenal gland receptors mediating steroid hormone release (BLAIR-WEST et al., 1971; GOODFRIEND and PEACH, 1975). Correspondingly, the effect of AII on adrenal receptors is blocked by the heptapeptide inhibitor Des-Asp-8-Ileu-AII, while this compound has no inhibitory effect on vascular smooth muscle receptors (BRAVO et al., 1975). The concept of different AII receptors in the vascular smooth muscle and the adrenal cortex is also supported by the observations of WILLIAMS et al. (1974), that saralasin antagonized AII in rabbit aortic strips as well as in rat glomerulosa cells, while 4-Phe-8-Tyr-AII antagonized AII only in the rabbit aorta, but was inactive on adrenal gland receptors. Although further work is needed to fully characterize angiotensin receptors, it can be presumed that differences of receptors also exist in other target tissues of AII. Hence, it may be possible to selectively block AII effects on vascular smooth muscle, on adrenal cortex, on the kidney, on the brain, and on other tissues by various antagonists which are specific with respect to the tissue receptors.

In vivo, saralasin and 1-Sar-8-Ileu-AII as well as other inhibitors administered either by bolus injection or by infusion have been shown invariably to antagonize the pressor effect of exogenous AII in animals and man. Acute and chronic renal hypertension induced by unilateral renal artery stenosis in the presence of a contralateral untouched kidney was transitorily reversed by saralasin (Fig. 3). Saralasin was, however, ineffective, in hypertension induced by bilateral renal artery stenosis or by stenosis of the renal artery after preceding unilateral nephrectomy. Only when the animals were subjected to severe sodium restriction which resulted in an increase in plasma AII concentration did saralasin lower blood pressure. Saralasin was not effective in animals made hypertensive by the infusion of norepinephrine, tyramine, or vasopressin (BRUNNER et al., 1971, 1972a, 1973, 1974; GAVRAS et al., 1973; SWEET et al., 1973; NEEDLEMAN et al., 1976). In hypertension caused by overdosage of mineralocorticoid hormones such as desoxycorticosterone or positive sodium balance with suppressed PRA, a marked pressor effect of angiotensin antagonists was noted even at low doses, which indicates the partial agonistic activity of these compounds at the vascular smooth muscle receptor (GLESS et al., 1977; KEIM et al., 1976; MACGREGOR and DAWES, 1976; DIETZ et al., 1977).

The effects of AII concentrations in plasma or in brain on central mechanisms of blood pressure and volume regulation have been more precisely defined by means of AII analogs (FISCHER-FERRARO et al., 1971; GANTEN et al., 1971, 1976a, b). Injection of saralasin into the ventricular system of the brain in SH rats of the New Zealand strain (GANTEN et al., 1976a, b), of the Kyoto strain (PHILLIPS et al., 1975), and of the Kyoto stroke-prone substrain (MANN et al., 1976) resulted in a significant fall in arterial blood pressure, whereas no such effect was seen in normotensive control rats after either intraventricular or intravenous injection (Fig. 4). The blood pressure decrease due to central administration of AII antagonists persisted after nephrectomy, which indicates that AII produced in the brain is antagonized. Similar results were reported by SCHÖLKENS (1976), but other investigators could not confirm these observations (ELGHOZI et al., 1976). FUXE et al. (1976) and PHILLIPS and FELIX (1976) have suggested that AII plays a role in the CNS. On the basis of the results available it can be concluded that brain AII receptors are stimulated by AII in the circulating blood and by AII generated inside the blood-brain barrier. Both receptor sites may participate in the regulation of blood pressure. The degree of stimulation of the receptors inside or outside the blood-brain barrier depends on the levels of circulating plasma AII and local brain AII and varies in different models of hypertension (Severs and Daniels-Severs, 1973; Ganten et al., 1976a, b).

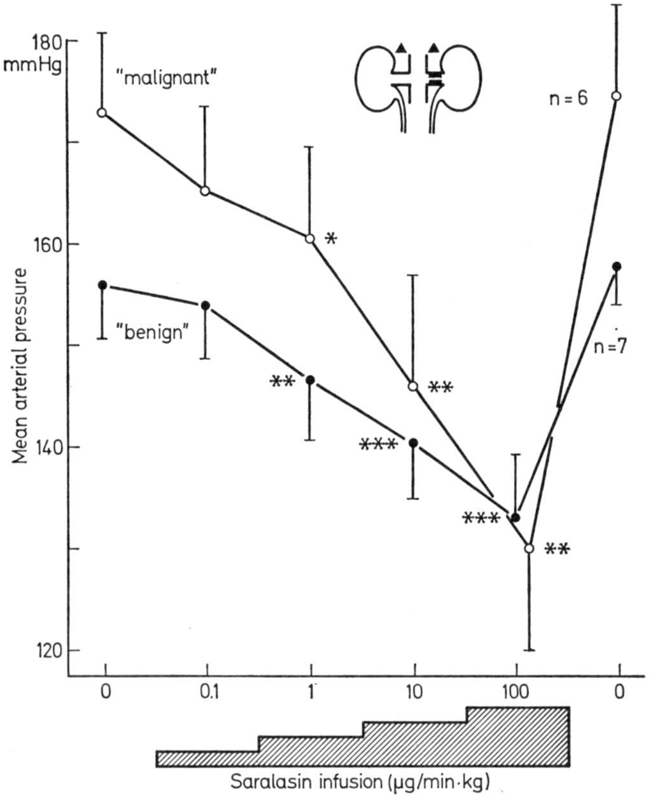

Fig. 3. Effects of cumulative intravenous infusions of saralasin on mean arterial blood pressure *(ordinate)* of renal hypertensive rats (one kidney clamped, the contralateral kidney untouched). "Malignant" hypertensive rats had negative sodium balance, higher plasma renin activity and more pronounced nephrosclerosis as compared with "benign" renal hypertensive rats. Saralasin was given as continuous infusion of increasing cumulative doses as indicated on the abscissa (from Mann et al., 1976)

AII antagonists have also been used in pathophysiologic situations other than hypertension. In those circumstances AII may act at the cellular level (e.g., in the transfer of electrolytes across membranes, ATPase activity, nucleic acid synthesis, protein synthesis, and cell proliferation) or on regulatory systems not directly involved in blood pressure regulation (e.g., water intake, release of antidiuretic hormone, regulation of peripheral vascular resistance in different organs) (for review see Goodfriend et al., 1974; Ganten et al., 1976a, b).

Some experimental data refer to the effects of AII antagonists in hemorrhagic shock (Needleman et al., 1976). The renal vasculature is especially sensitive to vasoconstriction, and the activity of the PRA is stimulated by blood loss.

AII is a potent renal vasoconstrictor and in addition may also enhance adrenergic tone. During hemorrhagic shock AII antagonists have been shown to decrease the overall peripheral resistance, to reverse the renal cortical vasoconstriction, and to prolong survival time in dogs after severe hemorrhage. The hypothesis that by antagonizing AII the perfusion of the kidney in hemorrhagic shock may be improved is attractive, but further studies are needed before it can be accepted.

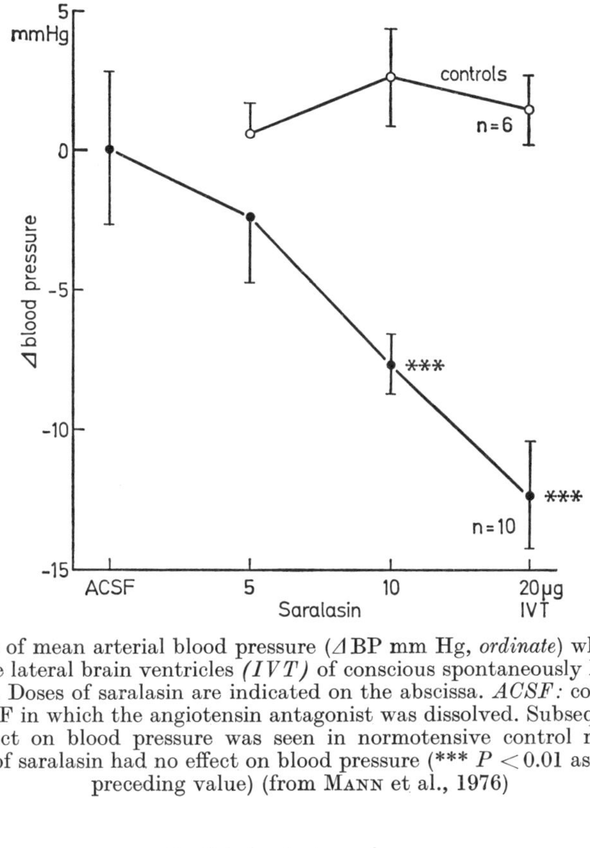

Fig. 4. Decrease of mean arterial blood pressure (ΔBP mm Hg, *ordinate*) when saralasin was injected into the lateral brain ventricles *(IVT)* of conscious spontaneously hypertensive rats (age: 20 weeks). Doses of saralasin are indicated on the abscissa. *ACSF:* control injection of 2 µl artificial CSF in which the angiotensin antagonist was dissolved. Subsequent to saralasin infusion no effect on blood pressure was seen in normotensive control rats. Intravenous administration of saralasin had no effect on blood pressure (*** $P < 0.01$ as compared to the preceding value) (from MANN et al., 1976)

2. Clinical Experience

In recent years many groups have undertaken clinical studies to investigate whether AII antagonists can be used for the diagnosis or treatment of renin-dependent forms of hypertension (for review see: CASE et al., 1976a; GANTEN and GROSS, 1976; STREETEN et al., 1976. Recent articles: DONKER and LEENEN, 1974; LARAGH, 1975; MARKS et al., 1975; SREETEN et al., 1975a, b; BECKERHOFF et al., 1976; GEYSKES et al., 1976). Saralasin has been mainly used in these investigations and, despite its mild vasopressor effect, is the most widely applied AII antagonist. The blood pressure decreasing effect of saralasin correlates well (diastolic pressure better than systolic pressure) with PRA or plasma concentration of AII (CASE et al., 1976a; STREETEN et al., 1976). Because PRA in man is primarily influenced by sodium balance, the degree of the saralasin response is also determined by the sodium intake. Normotensive subjects who did not respond to saralasin infusions could be converted into saralasin responders by sodium depletion, indicating that during sodium depletion AII contributes to the maintenance of blood pressure. In sodium-depleted patients pretreated with diuretics or vasodilating drugs, severe hypotensive effects and fainting can be induced by the administration of AII antagonists. In contrast, when the same individuals were sodium loaded, the effect of saralasin was reversed, inducing a pressor response (MACGREGOR and DAWES, 1976; GLESS et al., 1977) (Fig. 5). Pressor effects of saralasin have also been

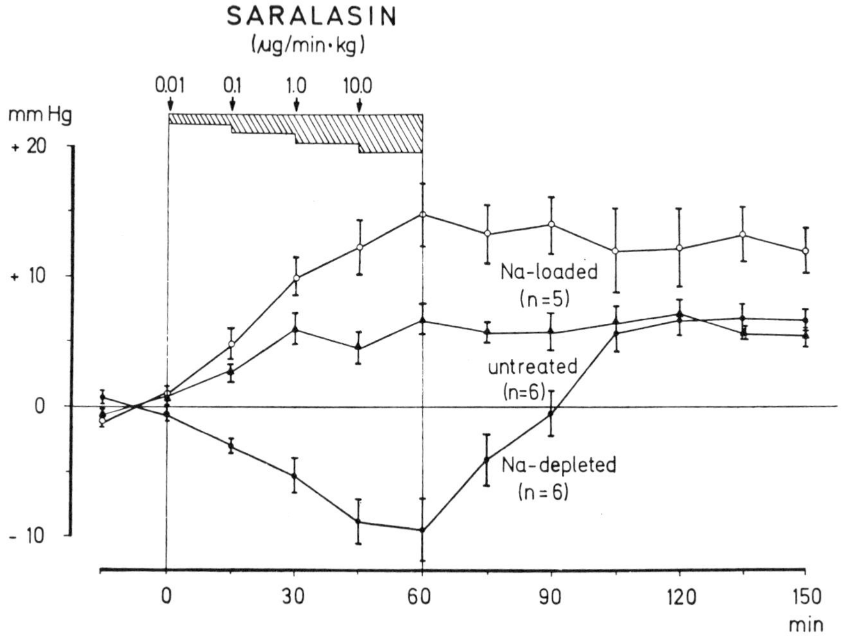

Fig. 5. Effect of cumulative doses of saralasin on diastolic blood pressure in normotensive patients *(ordinate)*. Doses of saralasin were continuously infused over 15 min for each dose. They are indicated between the 30- and 90-min period of the test *(abscissa)*. Patientsiwere tested on a control diet (▲—▲, untreated); no significant changes in blood pressure could be observed (nonresponders). Following pretreatment with chlorthalidone (●—●, Na-depleted), a significant decrease in blood pressure in the same patients was observed (responders); an agonistic response to saralasin occurred after sodium loading (○—○, Na-loaded). PRA was increased in Na-depleted patients, normal in untreated and suppressed in Na-loaded patients. The data demonstrate that according to the state of sodium balance blood pressure can become renin dependent or indepependent (from GLESS et al., 1977)

observed in patients with "low renin" essential hypertension (CASE et al., 1976a; KEIM et al., 1976). Pharmacodynamic studies comparing agonistic effects of saralasin with AII in various states of salt balance have not been reported in the literature.

Pretreatment of patients with diuretics, tilting, or other procedures which stimulate the activity of the RAS may therefore convert non-responders into saralasin responders. Thus the number of (false) positive responders may be increased when saralasin is used as a screening agent for renin-dependent hypertension.

Pharmacokinetic studies were facilitated by the availability of a radioimmunoassay for saralasin. Plasma concentrations of saralasin were correlated to the antagonistic effect on vascular smooth muscle, to renin release from the kidney and to aldosterone secretion. The half-life in man was 3.2 min, and an infusion period of 12 to 15 min was necessary to obtain a steady-state plasma level. Three to 10 min were needed to demonstrate the antagonistic effect on the vasoconstrictor action while 30 to 60 min were required to obtain an effect of saralasin on the secretion of aldosterone (PETTINGER and MITCHELL, 1976).

Saralasin has been given as bolus injections of 1 to 100 µg/kg (MARKS et al., 1975) but mostly in the form of infusions of between 0.01 and 20 µg/kg/min. After bolus injections, and also after the infusion of high doses in patients with low renin, severe increases in blood pressure have been observed. Such a hypertensive response may not occur until several hours after drug administration (KEIM et al., 1976). Severe hypotensive responses have been observed in patients with high PRA and angiotensin-dependent blood pressure levels (PETTINGER and MITCHELL, 1975). The hypertensive as well as the acute hypotensive episodes (CASE et al., 1976a) may be dangerous, and blood pressure of patients should be monitored for several hours after the administration of saralasin. If saralasin is given in cumulative doses (MACGREGOR and DAWES, 1976; GLESS et al., 1977), starting at low levels of 0.01 µg/kg/min and increasing the doses to 0.1, 1.0, and 10 µg/kg/min, each doses being infused over a period of 15 to 20 min, unwanted blood pressure responses can be discovered early and dangerous adverse reactions avoided. The plasma levels of saralasin during the infusion of the antagonist are extremely high (Fig. 6). Saralasin concentrations in plasma (1000 ng/ml) are higher than

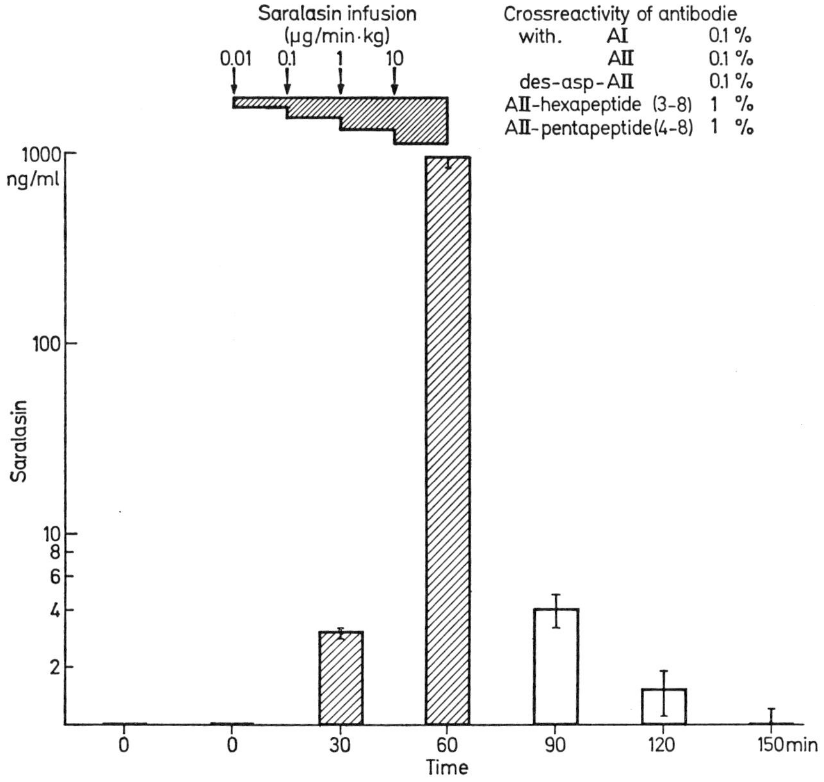

Fig. 6. Plasma concentrations of 1-sarcosine-8-alanine-angiotensin II antagonist (Saralasin) in normotensive patients. Saralasin was infused intravenously at increasing doses of 0.01, 0.1, 1.0, and 10.0 µg/kg body weight and min over 15 min for each dose. Plasma concentrations of saralasin were determined at 30 min intervals by radioimmunoassay before, during, and after termination of the infusion. (The antibody against saralasin was kindly provided by Dr. Bickerton, Norwich Pharmacal Company, New York)

those needed for the inhibition of circulating AII. Concentrations of AII in plasma of normal human subjects rarely exceed 100 pg/ml and, when the RAS is stimulated, remain in most cases below 1000 pg/ml. Hence it is possible to demonstrate angiotensin-dependency of blood pressure with doses of saralasin lower than those used by most authors. Plasma concentrations of saralasin under these conditions are shown in Figure 6. In order to increase the sensitivity to saralasin, activation of the RAS by various stimuli ("priming"), such as pretreatment with diuretics, restriction of sodium intake, tilting, and upright posture, prior to the administration of the drug has been suggested. However, false positive responses and untoward reactions may occur, and it is preferable to administer cumulative doses as already described.

It can be concluded that the RAS participates in the maintenance of blood pressure in those patients who respond with a blood pressure decrease to saralasin. Surgical correction of renal artery stenosis may be successful if saralasin infusion lowers blood pressure, even if the PRA is in the normal range. In this respect the use of saralasin as a screening method may be superior to the assay of PRA or the measurement of plasma AII concentrations, and may even be of equal diagnostic value to renin determinations in both renal veins.

E. Conclusions and Outlook

The RAS offers various possibilities for selective interference with its activity. Inhibitors of renin may be naturally ocurring substances (pepstatin) or the more specific renin substrate analogs. Such substances have not been extensively used *in vivo* so far, but rapid progress is being made in the synthesis of water-soluble derivatives. CE can be blocked by peptides isolated from snake venom. CEI leads to accumulation of AI and reduced formation of AII. In clinical use, CEI has the advantage of a longer duration of action than have the presently available AII antagonists and has no agonistic effect on blood pressure. Analogs of AI, AII, and AIII have been used in a wide variety of *in vitro* and *in vivo* systems. They are receptor specific and block the action of the effector peptides at the target organ. Tissue-specific receptor antagonists may be available in the future. The activity of the RAS is increased following the administration of CEI and angiotensin antagonists.

The development of substances that interfere with the RAS has resulted in a more rational approach to the pathophysiology, diagnosis, and perhaps treatment of certain pathologic conditions characterized by a high activity of the RAS such as some forms of hypertension, congestive heart failure, hypovolemic shock, and others. Interference with the RAS at various levels by means of a variety of inhibitors has already been demonstrated to be more informative than the use of a single inhibitor. It should be possible not only to sort out, but also to influence selectively by drugs individual effects of AII in the various target organs.

At present, drugs which interfere with the RAS are mainly of experimental or diagnostic interest. The practical use of these peptides is limited by the short duration of their action and the need for parenteral administration. Orally effective angiotensin antagonists with a long duration of action need to be developed, but even if such drugs were available their use would still be restricted to the small percentage of patients with hypertension in which the RAS plays a significant role in the maintenance of high blood pressure, and to conditions in which high renin initiates a vicious circle by the stimulation of, e.g., adrenergic activity in hemorrhagic shock.

References

AMSTERDAM, E. A., COUCH, N. P., CHRISTLIEB, R., HARRISON, J. H., CRANE, C., DOBRZINSKY, S. J., HICKLER, R. B.: Renal vein renin activity in the prognosis of surgery for renovascular hypertension. Amer. J. Med. **47**, 860—868 (1969).

ANDERSON, R. C., HERBERT, P. N., MULROW, P. J.: A comparison of properties of renin obtained from the kidney and uterus of the rabbit. Amer. J. Physiol. **215**, 774—778 (1968).

AOYAGI, T., KUNIMOTO, S., MORISHIMA, H., TAKEUCHI, T., UMEZAWA, H.: Effect of pepstatin on acid proteases. J. Antibiot. (Tokyo) **24**, 687—694 (1971).

ARAKAWA, K., NAKAMURA, M.: Studies on human angiotensin. Circulat. Res. **20/21**, (Suppl. 2), 101—207 (1967).

BAGBY, S. P., MCDONALD, W. J., PORTER, G. A.: Optimal renin methodology in spontaneously hypertensive and Wistar Kyoto rats. Clin. Res. **24**, 124A (1976).

BAKHLE, Y. S.: Inhibition of converting enzyme by venom peptides. In: GENEST, J., KOIW, E. (Eds.): Hypertension, pp. 541—547. Berlin-Heidelberg-New York: Springer 1972.

BAKHLE, Y. S.: Converting enzyme *in vitro* measurement and properties. In: PAGE, I. H., BUMPUS, F. M. (Eds.): Angiotensin. Handbook of Experimental Pharmacology, Vol. 37, pp. 41—80. Berlin-Heidelberg-New York: Springer 1974.

BECKERHOFF, R., VETTER, W., FURRER, J., NUSSBERGER, J., SCHMIED, U., SIEGENTHALER, W.: Angiotensin blockade with saralasin. Effect on normal blood pressure and on renovascular hypertension. Dtsch. med. Wschr. **101**, 398—401 (1976).

BENNET, J. B., SNYDER, S. H.: Angiotensin II binding to mammalian brain membranes. J. biol. Chem. **251**, 7423—7430 (1976).

BING, J.: Rapid marked increase in plasma renin in rats treated with inhibitors of the renin system. Acta path. microbiol. scand. A **81**, 254—262 (1973).

BING, J., NIELSEN, K.: Role of the renin system in normo- and hypertension. Acta path. microbiol. scand. A **81**, 3, 254—262 (1973).

BING, J., POULSEN, K.: The renin system in mice. Acta path. microbiol. scand. A **79**, 134—138 (1971).

BING, J., POULSEN, K.: Time course of changes in the plasma renin after blockade of the renin system. Acta path. microbiol. scand. A **83**, 454—466 (1975).

BING, J., POULSEN, K., MARKUSSEN, J.: The ability of various insulins and insulin fragments to inhibit the angiotensin I converting enzyme. Acta path. microbiol. scand. A **82**, 777—782 (1974).

BLAIR-WEST, J. R., COGHLAN, J. P., DENTON, D. A., FUNDER, J. W., SCOGGINS, B. A., WRIGHT, R. D.: The effect of the heptapeptide (2—8) and hexapeptide (3—8) fragments of angiotensin II on aldosterone secretion. J. clin. Endocr. **32**, 575—578 (1971).

BONNIN, J. M., HODGE, R. L., LUMBERS, E. R.: A renin-secreting renal tumor associated with hypertension. Aust. N.Z. J. Med. **2**, 178—181 (1972).

BOUCHER, R., ASSELIN, J., GENEST, J.: A new enzyme leading to the direct formation of angiotensin I. Circulat. Res. **34**, (Suppl. 1), 203—209 (1974).

BOYD, G. W.: A protein bound form of porcine renal renin. Circulat. Res. **35**, 426—438 (1974).

BOYD, G. W., PEART, W. S.: Angiotensin immunoassay. In: PAGE, I. H., BUMPUS, F. M. (Eds.): Angiotensin. Handbook of Experimental Pharmacology, Vol. 38, pp. 211—223. Berlin-Heidelberg-New York: Springer 1974.

BRAVO, E. L., KHOSLA, M. C., BUMPUS, F. M.: Action of [1-des (aspartic acid), 8-isoleucine] angiotensin II upon the pressor and steroidogenic activity of angiotensin II. J. clin. Endocr. **40**, 530—533 (1975).

BROWN, J. J., DAVIES, D. L., LEVER, A. F., ROBERTSON, J. I. S.: Relationship between sodium balance, renin, and aldosterone in physiological and pathological situations in man. In: TCHERDAKOFF, P. (Ed.): CIHTA symposium on hypertension, pp. 141—157. Paris: Expansion Scientifique 1965.

BROWN, J. J., FRASER, R., LEVER, A. F., MORTON, J. J., ROBERTSON, J. I. S.: Primary excess and deficiency of renin: two contrasting cases. In: EISENBACH, G. M. (Ed.): Proceedings in the First Symposium on Nephrology, pp. 235—256. Hannover 1973.

BRUNNER, H. R., KIRSHMAN, J. D., SEALEY, J. E., LARAGH, J. H.: Hypertension of renal origin: evidence for two different mechanisms. Science **174**, 1344—1346 (1971).

BRUNNER, H. R., CHANG, P., WALLACH, R., SEALEY, J. E., LARAGH, J. H.: Angiotensin vascular receptors: their avidity in relationship to sodium balance, the autonomic nervous system, and hypertension. J. clin. Invest. **51**, 58—67 (1972a).

BRUNNER, H. R., LARAGH, J. H., BAER, L., NEWTON, M. A., GOODWIN, F. T., KRAKOFF, L. R., BARD, R. H., BÜHLER, F. R.: Essential hypertension: renin and aldosterone, heart attack and stroke. New Engl. J. Med. **286**, 441—449 (1972b).

BRUNNER, H.R., GAVRAS, H., LARAGH, J.H., KEENAN, R.: Angiotensin-II blockade in man by sar'-ala'-angiotensin II for understanding and treatment of high blood pressure. Lancet **1973 II**, 1045—1048.

BRUNNER, H.R., GAVRAS, H., LARAGH, J.H., KEENAN, R.: Hypertension in man. Exposure of the renin and sodium components using angiotensin II blockade. Circulat. Res. **34** (Suppl. 1), 35—43 (1974).

BUMPUS, F.M., SCHWARZ, H., PAGE, I.H.: Synthesis and pharmacology of the octapeptide angiotensin. Science **125**, 886—887 (1957).

BUMPUS, F.M., SMEBY, P.R., PAGE, I.H., KHAIRALLAH, P.A.: Distribution and metabolic fate of antiotensin II and various derivatives. Canad. med. Ass. J. **90**, 190—193 (1964).

BUMPUS, F.M., SEN, S., SMEBY, R.R., SWEET, C., FERRARIO, C.M., KHOSLA, M.D.: Use of angiotensin II antagonists in experimental hypertension. Circulat. Res. **32/33** (Suppl. 1), 150—158 (1973).

BURTON, J., POULSEN, K., HABER, E.: Competitive inhibitors of renin. Inhibitors effective at physiological pH. Biochemistry **14**, 3892—3898 (1975).

CAIN, M.D., CATT, K.J., COGHLAN, J.P., BLAIR-WEST, J.R.: Evaluation of angiotensin II metabolism in sheep by radioimmunoassay. Endocrinology **86**, 955—964 (1970).

CARRETERO, O.A., BUJAK, B., HOULE, J.A.: Renin isozymes of extrarenal origin. Amer. J. Physiol. **220**, 1468—1472 (1971a).

CARRETERO, O., KUK, P., PIWONSKA, S., HOULE, J., MARIN-GREZ, M.: Role of the renin-angiotensin system in the pathogenesis of severe hypertension in rats. Circulat. Res. **29**, 654—663 (1971b).

CASE, D.B., WALLACE, J.M., KEIM, H.J., SEALEY, J.E., LARAGH, J.H.: Usefulness and limitations of saralasin, a partial competitive agonist of angiotensin II, for evaluating the renin and sodium factors in hypertensive patients. Amer. J. Med. **60**, 825—836 (1976a).

CASE, D.B., WALLACE, J.M., KEIM, H.J., WEBER, M.A., DRAYER, J.I.M., WHITE, R.P., SEALEY, J.E., LARAGH, J.H.: Estimating renin participation in hypertension: Superiority of converting enzyme inhibitor over saralasin. Amer. J. Med. **61**, 790—796 (1976b).

CHEUNG, H.S., CUSHMAN, D.W.: Inhibition of homogenous angiotensin-converting enzyme of rabbit lung by synthetic venom peptides of *Bothrops jararaca*. Biochim. Biophys. Acta **293**, 451—463 (1973).

CHIU, A.T., RYAN, J.W., STEWART, J.M., DORER, F.: Formation of angiotensin III by angiotensin-converting enzyme. Biochem. J. **155**, 189—192 (1976).

CHRISTLIEB, A.R., HICKLER, R.B.: Blood pressure response and antibody formation in spontaneously hypertensive rats and normal albino rats after immunization against angiotensin II. Endocrinology **91**, 1064—1070 (1972).

CHRISTLIEB, A.R., BIEBER, T.U.L., HICKLER, R.B.: Studies on the role of angiotensin in experimental renovascular hypertension: An immunological approach. J. clin. Invest. **48**, 1506—1518 (1969).

COHEN, E.L., ROVNER, D.R., CONN, J.W.: Postural augmentation of plasma renin activity: importance in diagnosis of renovascular hypertension. J. Amer. med. Ass. **197**, 973—978 (1966).

COHEN, S., TAYLOR, J.M., MURAKAMI, K., MICHELAKIS, A.M., INAGAMI, T.: Isolation and characterization of renin-like enzymes from mouse submaxillary glands. Biochemistry **11**, 4286—4293 (1972).

COLLIER, J.G., ROBINSON, B.F., VANE, J.R.: Reduction of pressor effects of angiotensin I in man by synthetic nonapeptide which inhibits converting enzyme. Lancet **1973 I**, 72—74.

CONN, J.W., COHEN, E.L., LUCAS, C.P., MCDONALD, W.J., MAYOR, G.H., BLOUGH, W.M. JR., EVELAND, W.C., BOOKSTEIN, J.J., LAPIDES, J.: Primary reninism. Hypertension, hyperreninemia, and secondary aldosteronism due to renin-producing juxtaglomerular cell tumors. Arch. intern. Med. **130**, 682—696 (1972).

CORVOL, P., DEVAUX, C., MÉNARD, J.: Pepstatin, an inhibitor for renin purification by affinity chromatography. FEBS Letters **34**, 189—192 (1973).

CRANE, M.G., HARRIS, J.J., JOHNS, V.J. JR.: Hyporeninemic hypertension. Amer. J. Med. **52**, 457—466 (1972).

CROXATTO, R., CROXATTO, H.: Destruction of hypertension and pepsitensin by an aminopeptidase obtained from yeast. Science **96**, 519—520 (1942).

CROXATTO, H., CROXATTO, R., ILLANES, G., SALVESTINI, H.: Action de la quimotrepsinia y de la tripsina sobre la Hypertensina y los principios presor y ocitocico de la post hypotisio Rev. Med. Aliment. (Santiago) **5**, 300—302 (1965).

CUSHMAN, D.W., CHEUNG, H.S.: Concentrations of angiotensin-converting enzyme in tissues of the rat. Biochim. biophys. Acta (Amst.) **250**, 261—265 (1971).

CUSHMAN, D.W., CHEUNG, H.S.: Studies *in vitro* of angiotensin-converting enzyme of lung and other tissues. In: GENEST, J., KOIW, E. (Eds.): Hypertension, pp. 532—541. Berlin-Heidelberg-New York: Springer 1972.

CZYZEWSKI, L. B., PETTINGER, W. A.: Failure of feedback suppression of renin release in the spontaneously hypertensive rat. Amer. J. Physiol. **225**, 234—239 (1973).
DAUL, C. B., HEATH, R. G., GAREY, R. E.: Angiotensin-forming enzyme in human brain. Neuropharmacology **14**, 75—80 (1975).
DAVIS, J. O., FREEMAN, R. H.: Mechanisms regulating renin release. Physiol. Rev. **56**, 1—56 (1976).
DAVIS, J. O., FREEMAN, R. H., JOHNSON, J. A., SPIELMAN, W. S.: Agents which block the action of the renin-angiotensin system. Circulat. Res. **34**, 3, 279—285 (1974).
DAY, R. P., LUETSCHER, J. A., GONZALES, C. M.: Occurrence of big renin in human plasma, amniotic fluid, and kidney extracts. J. clin. Endocr. **40**, 1078—1084 (1975).
DENGLER, H.: Über einen reninartigen Wirkstoff in Arterienextrakten. Naunyn-Schmiedebergs Arch. exp. Path. Pharmak. **227**, 481—487 (1956).
DEVYNCK, M. A., MEYER, P.: Angiotensin receptors in vascular tissue. Amer. J. Med. **61**, 758—767 (1976).
DIETZ, R., LÜTH, B., MANN, J. F. E., GROSS, F.: Ist eine Stimulation des Renin-Angiotensin-Systems (RAS) notwendig für den Druckanstieg nach Nierenarterienstenose? Therapiewoche **46**, 7568 (1977).
DONKER, A. J. M., LEENEN, F. H. H.: Infusion of angiotensin II analogue in two patients with unilateral renovascular hypertension. Lancet **1974 II**, 1535—1537.
DORER, F. E., KAHN, J. R., LENTZ, K. E., LEVINE, M., SKEGGS, L. T.: Purification and properties of angiotensin-converting enzyme from hog lung. Circulat. Res. **31**, 356—366 (1972).
DORER, F. E., KAHN, J. R., LENTZ, K. E., LEVINE, M., SKEGGS, L. T.: Hydrolysis of bradykinin by angiotensin-converting enzyme. Circulat. Res. **34**, 824—827 (1974).
EDDY, R. L., SANCHEZ, S. A.: Rein-secreting renal neoplasm and hypertension with hypokalemia. Ann. intern. Med. **75**, 725—729 (1971).
EGGENA, P., CHU, C. L., BARRET, J. D., SAMBHI, M. P.: Purification and partical characterization of human angiotensinogen. Biochim. biophys. Acta (Amst.) **427**, 208—217 (1976).
EIDE, J., LÖYNING, E., AARS, H., AKRE, S.: Autoregulation of renal blood flow in rabbits immunized with angiotensin II. Scand. J. clin. Lab. Invest. **31**, 123—127 (1973).
ELGHOZI, J. L., ALTMAN, J., DEVYNCK, M. A., LIARD, J. F., GRÜNFELD, J. P., MEYER, P.: Lack of hypotensive effect on central injection of angiotensin inhibitors in spontaneously hypertensive (SH) and normotensive rats. Clin. Sci. Mol. Med. **51**, 385s—389s (1976).
ELLIOT, D. F., PEART, W. S.: The amino acid sequence in a hypertensin. Biochem. J. **65**, 246—254 (1957).
ENGEL, S. L., SCHAEFFER, T. R., GOLD, B. I., RUBIN, B.: Inhibition of pressor effects of angiotensin I and augmentation of depressor effects of bradykinin by synthetic peptides. Proc. Soc. exp. Biol. (N. Y.) **140**, 240—244 (1972).
ERDÖS, E. G.: Conversion of angiotensin I to angiotensin II. Amer. J. Med. **60**, 749—759 (1976).
ESKILDSEN, P. C.: Renin in different tissues, amniotic fluid and plasma of pregnant and non-pregnant rabbits. Acta path. microbiol. scand. A **81**, 263—268 (1973).
FERGUSON, R. K., TURINI, G. A., BRUNNER, H. R., GAVRAS, H. and MCKINSTRY, D. N.: A specific orally active inhibitor of angiotensin-converting enzyme in man. Lancet **1977/II**, 775—778.
FERMANDJIAN, S., MORGAT, J. L., FROMAGEOT, P.: Studies of angiotensin II conformations by circular dichroism. Europ. J. Biochem. **24**, 252—258 (1971).
FERREIRA, S. H., BARTELT, D. C., GREENE, L. J.: Isolation of bradykinin-potentiating peptides from Bothrops jararaca venom. Biochemistry **9**, 2583—2593 (1970).
FISCHER-FERRARO, C., NAHMOD, V. E., GOLDSTEIN, D. J., FINKIELMAN, S.: Angiotensin and renin in rat and dog brain. J. exp. Med. **133**, 353—361 (1971).
FITZSIMONS, J. T.: Thirst. Physiol. Rev. **52**, 468—561 (1972).
FORMAN, B. H., MULROW, P. J.: Effect of propranolol on blood pressure and plasma renin activity in the spontaneously hypertensive rat. Circulat. Res. **35**, 215—221 (1974).
FOSTER, J. H., DEAN, R. H., PINKERTON, J. A., KHAMY, R. K.: Ten years experience with the surgical management of reno-vascular hypertension. Ann. Surg. **177**, 755—766 (1973).
FREEDLENDER, A. F., FYHRQUIST, F., HOLLEMANS, H. J. G.: Renin and the angiotensins. In: JAFFE, B. M., BEHRMAN, H. R. (Eds.): Methods of hormone radioimmunoassay, pp. 455—467. New York-London: Academic Press, Inc. 1974.
FUXE, K., GANTEN, D., HÖKFELT, T., BOLME, P.: Immunohistochemical evidence for the existence of angiotensin II containing nerve terminals in the brain and spinal cord of the rat. Neurosc. Letters **2**, 229—234 (1976).
GANGULY, A., GRIBBLE, J., TUNE, B., KEMPSON, R. L., LUETSCHER, J. A.: Renin-secreting Wilm's tumor with severe hypertension. Ann. intern. med. **79**, 835—837 (1973).
GANTEN, D., GROSS, F.: Angiotensin Antagonisten zur Diagnostik und Behandlung des renin-abhängigen Hochdrucks. Med. Klin. **71**, 2043—2050 (1976).

GANTEN, D., MARQUEZ-JULIO, A., GRANGER, P., HAYDUK, K., KARSUNKY, K. P., BOUCHER, R., GENEST, J.: Renin in dog brain. Amer. J. Physiol. **221**, 1733—1737 (1971).

GANTEN, D., HUTCHINSON, J. S., SCHELLING, P., GANTEN, U., FISCHER, H.: The iso-renin angiotensin systems in extrarenal tissue. Clin. exp. Pharmacol. Physiol. **3**, 103—126 (1976a).

GANTEN, D., SCHELLING, P., VECSEI, P., GANTEN, U.: Iso-renin of extrarenal origin. The tissue angiotensinogenase systems. Amer. J. Med. **60**, 760—772 (1976b).

GAVRAS, H., BRUNNER, H. R., VAUGHAN, E. D., LARAGH, J. H.: Angiotensin-sodium interaction in blood pressure maintenance of renal hypertensive and normotensive rats. Science **180**, 1369—1372 (1973).

GAVRAS, H., BRUNNER, H. R., LARAGH, J. H., SEALEY, J. E., GAVRAS, I., VUKOVICH, R. A.: An angiotensin converting-enzyme inhibitor to identify and treat vasoconstrictor and volume factors in hypertensive patients. New Engl. J. Med. **291**, 817—821 (1974).

GENEST, J., TREMBLAY, G. Y., BOUCHER, R., DE CHAMPLAIN, J., ROJO-ORTEGA, J. M., LEFEBVRE, R., RAY, P., CARTIER, P.: Diagnostic significance of humoral factors in renovascular hypertension. In: GROSS, F. (Ed.): Antihypertensive therapy, pp. 518—540. Berlin-Heidelberg-New York: Springer 1966.

GENEST, J., BOUCHER, R., KUCHEL, O.: Renin in hypertension: how important as a risk factor? Canad. med. Ass. J. **109**, 475—478 (1973).

GENEST, J., ROJO-ORTEGA, J. M., KUCHEL, O., BOUCHER, R., NOWACZYNSKI, W., LEFEBVRE, R., CHRÉTIEN, M., CANTIN, J., GRANGER, P.: Malignant hypertension with hypokalemia in a patient with renin producing pulmonary carcinoma. Trans. Ass. Amer. Phycns. **88**, 192—201 (1975).

GENEST, J., NOWACZYNSKI, W., KUCHEL, O., BOUCHER, R., ROJO-ORTEGA, J. M., CONSTANTOPOULOS, G., GANTEN, D., MESSERLI, F.: The adrenal cortex and essential hypertension. In: Recent progress in hormone research, Vol. 37, pp. 377—427. New York: Academic Press 1976.

GEYSKES, G. G., VOS, J., BOER, P., MEES, E. J. D.: Renin dependency of blood pressure. Analysis by angiotensin II antagonist P 113 in hypertensive patients treated with salt depletion and propranolol. Lancet **1976 I**, 1049—1051.

GHERARDI, G. J., ARYA, S., HICKLER, R. B.: Juxtaglomerular body tumor: a rare occult but curable cause of lethal hypertension. Hum. Pathol. **5**, 236—240 (1974).

GLESS, H., GRAM, B., MANN, H., SCHELLING, P., GANTEN, D.: Effect of salt loading and salt restriction on agonistic and antagonistic effects of saralasin (in press) (1977).

GLOSSMANN, H., BAUKAL, A. J., CATT, K. J.: Properties of angiotensin II receptors in the bovine and rat adrenal cortex. J. biol. Chem. **3**, 825—834 (1974).

GOLDBLATT, H., LYNCH, J., HANZAL, R. F., SUMMERVILLE, W. W.: Studies on experimental hypertension I. The production of persistent elevation of systolic blood pressure by means of renal ischemia. J. exp. Med. **59**, 347—379 (1934).

GOODFRIEND, T. L., PEACH, M. J.: Angiotensin III: (des-aspartic acid-1)-angiotensin II. Circulat. Res. **36** (Suppl. 1), 38—48 (1975).

GOODFRIEND, T. L., FYHRQUIST, F., ALLMANN, D.: Biochemical effects of angiotensin. In: PAGE, I. H., BUMPUS, F. M. (Eds.): Handbook of Experimental Pharmacology, pp. 511—517. Berlin-Heidelberg-New York: Springer 1974.

GREEN, A. A., BUMPUS, F. M.: The purification of hog renin substrate. J. biol. Chem. **210**, 281—287 (1954).

GREEN, L. J., CAMARGO, A. C. M., KRIEGER, E. M., STEWARD, J. M., FERREIRA, S. H.: Inhibition of the conversion of angiotensin I to II and potentiation of bradykinin by small peptides present in Bothrops jararaca venom. Circulat. Res. **30/31** (Suppl. 2), 62—70 (1972).

GROSS, F.: Renin und Hypertensin, physiologische oder pathologische Wirkstoffe? Klin. Wschr. **36**, 693—706 (1958).

GROSS, F.: Pharmacology of naturally occurring polypeptides and lipid-soluble acids. In: WALKER, J. M. (Ed.): Encyclopedia of Pharmacology and Therapeutics, pp. 73—286. Oxford: Pergamon Press 1971.

GROSS, F., REGOLI, D., SCHAECHTELIN, G.: Renal content and blood concentration of renin. In: WILLIAMS, P. C. (Ed.): Hormones and the kidney, pp. 293—300. London-New York: Academic Press 1963.

GROSS, F., SCHAECHTELIN, G., ZIEGLER, M., BERGER, M.: A renin-like substance in the placenta and uterus of the rabbit. Lancet **1964 I**, 914—916.

GROSS, F., BRUNNER, H., ZIEGLER, M.: Renin-angiotensin-system, aldosterone and sodium balance. Rec. Prog. Hormone Res. **21**, 119—177 (1965).

GROSS, F., LAZAR, J., ORTH, H.: Inhibition of the renin-angiotensinogen reaction by pepstatin. Science **175**, 656 (1972).

GROSS, F., DIETZ, R., MAST, G. J., SZOKOL, M.: Salt loss as a possible mechanism eliciting an acute malignant phase in renal hypertensive rats. Clin. exp. Pharmacol. Physiol. 2, 323—333 (1975).

GUYTON, A.C., COLEMAN, T.G., GRANGER, H.J.: Circulation: Overall regulation. Ann. Rev. Physiol. **34**, 13—46 (1972).
HAAS, E., GOLDBLATT, H.: Kinetic constants of the human renin and human angiotensinogen reaction. Circulat. Res. **20**, 45—55 (1967).
HAAS, E., LAMFROM, H., GOLDBLATT, H.: Ultraviolet spectroscopy of renin. Arch. Biochem. **44**, 79—94 (1953).
HAAS, E., GOLDBLATT, H., GIPSON, E.C.: Extraction, purification, and acetylation of human renin and the production of antirenin to human renin. Arch. Biochem. **110**, 534—539 (1965).
HALL, M.M., KHOSLA, M.C., KHAIRALLAH, P.A., BUMPUS, F.M.: Angiotensin analogs: The influence of sarcosine substituted in position 1. J. Pharmacol. exp. Ther. **188**, 222—228 (1974).
HAUGER-KLEVENE, J.H.: High plasma renin activity in oat cell carcinoma: A renin-secreting carcinoma? Cancer (Philad.) **26**, 1112—1114 (1970).
HEDWALL, P.R.: Effect of rabbit antibodies against angiotensin II on the pressure response to angiotensin II and renal hypertension in the rat. Brit. J. Pharmacol. **31**, 623—629 (1968).
HOFBAUER, K.G., ZSCHIEDRICH, H., RAUH, W., ORTH, H., GROSS, F.: Reaction of endogenous renin with exogenous renin substrate within the isolated perfused rat kidney. Proc. Soc. exp. Biol. (N. Y.) **142**, 796—799 (1973).
HOFFMAN, W.E., SCHELLING, P., PHILLIPS, M.I., GANTEN, D.: Evidence for local angiotensin formation in brain of nephrectomized rats. Neurosci. Letters **3**, 299—303 (1976).
HOFFMAN, W.E., GANTEN, D., SCHELLING, P., HAEBARA, H., PHILLIPS, M.I., MANN, J.F.E.: Brain iso-renin: possible physiological role in thirst and blood pressure regulation. Pathologie et Biologie (in press) (1977).
HORKY, K., ROJO-ORTEGA, J.M., RODRIGUEZ, J., BOUCHER, R., GENEST, J.: Renin, renin substrate, and angiotensin I-converting enzyme in the lymph of rats. Amer. J. Physiol. **220**, 307—311 (1971).
HUNT, J.C., STRONG, C.G.: Renovascular hypertension. Mechanisms, natural history and treatment. In: LARAGH, J.H. (Ed.): Hypertension manual, pp. 509—536. New York: Yorke Medical Books, Dun-Donnelly 1973.
HUSSAIN, R.A., GIFFORD, R.W. JR., STEWART, B.H., MEANEY, T.F., MCCORMACK, L.J., VIDT, D.G., HUMPHREY, D.C.: Differential renal venous renin activity in diagnosis of renovascular hypertension: review of 29 cases. Amer. J. Cardiol. **32**, 707—715 (1973).
HUTCHINSON, J.S., SCHELLING, P., MÖHRING, J., GANTEN, D.: Pressor action of centrally perfused angiotensin II in rats with hereditary diabetes insipidus. Endocinology **99**, 819—823 (1976).
INAGAMI, T., MISONO, K., MICHELAKIS, A.M.: Definitive evidence for similarity in the active site of renin and acidic protease. Biochem. Biophys. Res. Commun. **2**, 503—509 (1974).
JAMES, S.K., HALL, R.C.: The nature of renin released in the dog following hemorrhage and frusemide. Pflügers Arch. ges. Physiol. **347**, 323—328 (1974).
JOHNSON, J.A., DAVIS, J.O.: Angiotensin II: important role in the maintenance of arterial blood pressure. Science **179**, 906—907 (1973a).
JOHNSON, J.A., DAVIS, J.O.: Effects of a specific competitive antagonist of angiotensin II on arterial pressure and adrenal steroid secretion in dogs. Circulat. Res. **32/33** (Suppl. 1), 159—168 (1973b).
JOHNSON, J.A., DAVIS, J.O., SPIELMAN, W.S., FREEMAN, R.H.: The role of the renin-angiotensin system in experimental renal hypertension in dogs. Proc. Soc. exp. Biol. (N. Y.) **147**, 387—391 (1974).
JOHNSTON, C.J., MENDELSOHN, F.A.O., HUTCHINSON, J.H., MORRIS, B.: Composition of juxtaglomerular granules isolated from rat kidney cortex: In: SAMBHI, M.P. (Ed.): Mechanisms of hypertension, pp. 238—248. Amsterdam: Exerpta Medica 1973.
KEIM, G.R. JR., KIRPAN, J., PETERSON, A.E., MURPHY, D.F.: Inhibition of angiotensin I-initiated hemodynamic changes in anesthetized dogs by a synthetic nonapeptide. Proc. Soc. exp. Biol. (N. Y.) **140**, 149—152 (1972).
KEIM, H.J., DRAYER, J.I., CASE, D.B., LOPEZ-OVEJERO, J., WALLACE, J.M., WEBER, M.A., LARAGH, J.H.: A role for renin in rebound hypertension and encepholapathy after infusion of saralasin acetate (Sar-1-Ala-8-Angiotensin II). New Engl. J. Med. **295**, 1175—1177 (1976).
KHAIRALLAH, P.A., PAGE, I.H.: Plasma angiotensinases. Biochem. Med. **1**, 1—8 (1967).
KHOSLA, M.C., LEESE, R.A., MALOY, W.L., FERREIRA, A.T., SMEBY, R.R., BUMPUS, F.M.: Synthesis of some analogs of angiotensin II as specific antagonists of the parent hormone. J. med. Chem. **15**, 792—795 (1972).
KHOSLA, M.C., HALL, M.M., SMEBY, R.R., BUMPUS, F.M.: Factors that influence the antagonistic properties of angiotensin II antagonists. J. med. Chem. **16**, 829—832 (1973).

Khosla, M.C., Smeby, R.R., Bumpus, F.M.: Structure-activity relationship in angiotensin II analogs. In: Page, I.H., Bumpus, F.M. (Eds.): Angiotensin. Handbook of Experimental Pharmacology, pp. 126—167. Berlin-Heidelberg-New York: Springer 1974.
Kihara, I., Kitamura, S., Hoshino, T., Seida, H., Watanabe, T.: A hitherto unreported vascular tumor of the kidney: a proposal of "juxtaglomerular cell tumor". Acta path. jap. **18**, 197—206 (1968).
Kokubu, T., Hiwada, K., Ito, T., Ueda, E., Yamamura, Y., Mizoguchi, T., Shigezane, K.: Peptide inhibitors of renin angiotensinogen reaction system. Biochem. Pharmacol. **22**, 3217—3223 (1973).
Kotchen, T.A., Hedrick, J.L., Miller, M.C., Talwalkar, R.T.: Effect of prostaglandins on the velocity of the reaction between human renin and homologous renin substrate. J. clin. Endocrinol. **39**, 530—535 (1974).
Kramer, P., Ochwadt, B.: Wasserhaushalt und Elektrolytstoffwechsel bei Ratten mit experimentellem und spontanem Hochdruck. Pflügers Arch. ges. Physiol. **332**, 56—72 (1972).
Kreye, V.A.W., Gross, F.: Conversion of angiotensin I to angiotensin II in peripheral vascular beds of the rat. Amer. J. Physiol. **220**, 1294—1296 (1971).
Krieger, E.M., Salgado, H.C., Assan, C.J.: Greene, L.L.J., Ferreira, S.H.: Potential screening test for detection of overactivity of renin-angiotensin system. Lancet **1971 I**, 269—271.
Laragh, J.H.: Hypertension manual. New York: Yorke Medical Books, Dun-Donnelly 1973.
Laragh, J.H.: Angiotensin blockade: New pharmacologic tools for understanding and treating hypertension. New Engl. J. Med. **292**, 695—696 (1975).
Leckie, B.J., McConnell, A.: A renin inhibitor from rabbit kidney. Conversion of a large inactive renin to a smaller active enzyme. Circulat. Res. **36**, 513—517 (1975).
Ledingham, J.G.: Mechanisms in renal hypertension. Proc. roy. Soc. Med. **64**, 409—418 (1971).
Ledingham, J.G.: Catabolism of angiotensin II. In: Page, I.H., Bumpus, F.M. (Eds.): Angiotensin. Handbook of Experimental Pharmacology, pp. 111—125. Berlin-Heidelberg-New York: Springer 1974.
Lee, D.R.: Plasma renin activity in genetically hypertensive rats measured by a radioimmunoassay of angiotensin I. Proc. Univ. Otago med. Sch. **51**, 34—35 (1973).
Lee, M.R.: Renin and Hypertension. London: Lloyd-Luke 1969.
Liard, J.F.: Sodium retention versus renin-angiotensin system in experimental renal hypertension. Canad. J. Physiol. Pharmacol. **51**, 238—241 (1973).
Lin, S.Y., Ellis, H., Weisblum, B., Goodfriend, T.L.: Preparation and properties of iodinated angiotensins. Biochem. Pharmacol. **19**, 651—662 (1970).
MacGregor, G.A., Dawes, M.: Agonist and antagonist effects of sar-1-ala-8-angiotensin II in salt loaded and salt depleted normal man. Brit. J. clin. Pharmacol. **3**, 483—487 (1976).
Majstroravich, J., Ontjes, D.A., Roberts, J.C.: Affinity chromatography of renin using inhibitory renin substrate analogs. Proc. Soc. exp. Biol. (N.Y.) **146**, 674—679 (1974).
Malayan, S.A., Reid, I.A.: Antidiuresis produced by injection of renin into the third cerebral ventricle of the dog. Endocrinology **98**, 329—335 (1976).
Malik, K.U., Nasjletti, A.: Facilitation of adrenergic transmission by locally generated angiotensin II in rat mesenteric arteries. Circulat. Res. **38**, 26—30 (1976).
Mann, J.F.E., Phillips, M.I., Haebara, H., Lüth, B., Dietz, R., Ganten, D.: Wirkung von intraventrikulär und intravenös injiziertem Saralasin auf den Blutdruck renal und spontan hypertoner Ratten. Therapiewoche **46**, 7553 (1976).
Marks, L.S., Maxwell, M.H., Kaufmann, J.J.: Saralasin bolus test. Rapid screening procedure for renin mediated hypertension. Lancet **1975 IV**, 784—787.
Marshall, G.R.: Structure-activity relations of antagonists of the renin-angiotensin system. Fed. Proc. **35**, 2491—2501 (1976).
Marshall, G.R., Vine, W., Needleman, P.: A specific competitive inhibitor of angiotensin II. Proc. nat. Acad. Sci. (Wash.) **67**, 1624—1630 (1970).
McDonald, K.M., Traher, S., Aisenbrey, G., deTorrente, A., Schrier, R.W.: Effect of angiotensin II and an angiotensin II inhibitor on renin secretion in the dog. Amer. J. Physiol. **228**, 1562—1567 (1975).
McKown, M.M., Workman, R.J., Gregerman, R.I.: Pepstatin inhibition of human renin. Kinetic studies and estimation of enzyme purity. J. biol. Chem. **748**, 7770—7774 (1974).
McLean, A.S., Sirett, N.E., Bray, J.J., Hubbard, J.I.: Regional distribution of angiotensin II receptors in the rat brain. Proc. Univ. Otago med. Sch. **53**, 19—20 (1975).
Ménard, J., Breminer, J., Corvol, P.: Physicochemical properties of plasma renin substrate in normal, binephrectomized and estrogen-treated rats. Amer. J. Physiol. **226**, 1434—1437 (1974).
Michelakis, A.M., Yoshida, H., Menzie, J., Murakami, K., Inagami, T.: A radioimmunoassay for the direct measurement of renin in mice and its application to submaxillary gland and kidney studies. Endocrinology **94**, 1101—1105 (1974).

MILLER, E. D., SAMUELS, A. J., HABER, E., BARGER, A. C.: Inhibition of angiotensin conversion in experimental renovascular hypertension. Science **177**, 1108—1109 (1972).

MILLER, R. P., POPER, C. J., WILSON, C. W., DE VITO, E.: Renin inhibition by pepstatin. Biochem. Pharmacol. **21**, 2941—2944 (1972).

MÖHRING, J., MÖHRING, B., NÄUMANN, H. J., PHILIPPI, A., HOMSY, E., ORTH, H., DAUDA, G., KAZDA, S., GROSS, F.: Salt and water balance and renin activity in renal hypertension of rats. Amer. J. Physiol. **228**, 1847—1855 (1975).

MORISHIMA, H., TAKITA, T., AOYAGI, T., TAKEUCHI, T., UMEZAWA, H.: The structure of pepstatin. J. Antibiot. (Tokyo) **23**, 263—265 (1970).

MORRIS, B. J., LUMBERS, E. R.: The activation of renin in human amniotic fluid by proteolytic enzymes. Biochim. biophys. Acta (Amst.) **289**, 385—391 (1972).

MUNOZ-RAMIREZ, H., KHOSLA, M. C., BUMPUS, F. M., KHAIRALLAH, P. A.: Influence of the adrenal gland on the pressor effect and antagonistic potency of angiotensin II analogs. Europ. J. Pharmacol. **31**, 122—135 (1975).

MURAKAMI, K., INAGAMI, T.: Isolation of pure and stable renin from hog kidney. Biochem. Biophys. Res. Commun. **3**, 757—763 (1975).

MURAKAMI, K., INAGAMI, T., MICHELAKIS, A. M., COHEN, S.: An affinity column for renin. Biochem. Biophys. Res. Cummun. **2**, 482—487 (1973).

NAKAJIMA, T., OSHIMA, G., YEH, H. S. J., IGIC, R., ERDÖS, E. G.: Purification of the angiotensin I converting enzyme of the lung. Biochim. biophys. Acta (Amst.) **315**, 430—438 (1973).

NASJLETTI, A., MASSON, G. M. C.: Stimulation of angiotensinogen formation by renin and angiotensin I. Proc. Soc. exp. Biol. (N. Y.) **142**, 307—310 (1973).

NASJLETTI, A., LEWIS, L. A., MASSON, G. M. C.: Electrophoretic studies on renin substrate from various species. Amer. J. Physiol. **220**, 804—807 (1971).

NEEDLEMAN, P., JOHNSON, E. M. JR., VINE, W., FLANIGAN, E., MARSHALL, G. R.: Pharmacology of antagonists of angiotensin I and II. Circulat. Res. **31**, 862—867 (1972).

NEEDLEMAN, P., DOUGLAS, J. R. JR., JAKSCHIK, B. A., BLUMBERG, A. L., ISAKSON, P. C., MARSHALL, G. R.: Angiotensin antagonists as pharmacological tools. Fed. Proc. **35**, 2488—2493 (1976).

NG, K. K. F., VANE, J. R.: Conversion of angiotensin I to angiotensin II. Nature (Lond.) **216**, 762—766 (1967).

OLIVER, W. J., GROSS, F.: Verhalten des Renin-ähnlichen Prinzips in der Speicheldrüse der weißen Maus unter verschiedenen Bedingungen. Naunyn-Schmiedebergs Arch. exp. Path. Pharmak. **255**, 55—56 (1966).

ONDETTI, E. C., WILLIAMS, N. J., SABO, E. F., PLUSCEG, J., WEAVER, E. R., KOCY, O.: Angiotensin converting enzyme inhibitors from the venom of Bothrops jararaca. Isolation, elucidation of structure, and synthesis. Biochemistry **19**, 4033—4039 (1971).

ONDETTI, M. A., RUBIN, B. CUSHMAN, D. W.: Design of specific inhibitors of angiotensin-converting enzyme: A new class of orally active antihypertensive agents. Science **196**, 441—444, 1977.

OPARIL, S., HABER, E.: The renin angiotensin system. New Engl. J. Med. **291**, 389—401 and 446—457 (1974).

ORTH, H., HACKENTHAL, E., LAZAR, J., MIKSCHE, U., GROSS, F.: Kinetics of the inhibitory effect of pepstatin on the reaction of hog renin with rat plasma substrate. Circulat. Res. **35**, 52—55 (1974).

OSMOND, D. H., ROSS, L. J., SCIAFF, K. D.: Increased renin activity after cold storage of human plasma. Canad. J. Physiol. Pharmacol. **51**, 705—708 (1973).

OSTER, P., BAUKNECHT, H., HACKENTHAL, E.: Active and passive immunization against angiotensin II in the rat and rabbit. Circulat. Res. **37**, 607—614 (1975).

PAGE, I. H., MCCUBBIN, J. W.: Renal Hypertension. Chicago: Year Book Medical Publishers 1968.

PALS, D. T., MASUCCI, F. D.: Plasma renin and the antihypertensive effect of 1-Sar-8-Ala-Angiotensin II. Europ. J. Pharmacol. **23**, 115—119 (1973).

PALS, D. T., MASUCCI, F. D., DENNING, G. S., SIPOS, F., FESSLER, D. C.: Role of the pressor action of angiotensin II in experimental hypertension. Circulat. Res. **29**, 673—681 (1971a).

PALS, D. T., MASUCCI, F. D., SIPOS, F., DENNING, G. S. JR.: A specific competitive antagonist of the vascular action of angiotensin II. Circulat. Res. **29**, 664—672 (1971b).

PARIKH, I., CUATRECASAS, P.: Substrate analog competitive inhibitors of human renin. Biochem. Biophys. Res. Commun. **54**, 1356—1361 (1973).

PEACH, M. J., CHIU, A. T.: Stimulation and inhibition of aldosterone synthesis in vitro on angiotensin II and analogues. Clin. Res. Proc. **34/35** (Suppl. 1), 7—13 (1974).

PEART, W. S., LLOYD, A. M., THATCHER, G. N., LEVER, A. F., PAYNE, N., STONE, N.: Purification of pig renin. Biochem. J. **99**, 708—716 (1966).

PETTINGER, W. A., MITCHELL, H. C.: Renin release, saralasin, and the vasodilator-β-blocker drug interaction in man. New Engl. J. Med. **292**, 1214—1217 (1975).

Pettinger, W. A., Mitchell, H. C.: Clinical pharmacology of angiotensin antagonists. Fed. Proc. **35**, 2521—2525 (1976).

Pettinger, W. A., Campbell, W., Keeton, D., Tanaka, K.: The use of P 113, a selective angiotensin antagonist, in studying cardiovascular and endocrine effects of altered renin release. Pharmacologist **15**, 241 (1973).

Pettinger, W. A., Keeton, K., Tanaka, K.: Radioimmunoassay and pharmacokinetics of saralasin in the rat and hypertensive patients. Clin. Pharmacol. Ther. **17**, 146—158 (1974).

Phillips, M. I., Felix, D.: Specific angiotensin II receptive neurons in the cat subfornical organ. Brain Res. **109**, 531—540 (1976).

Phillips, M. I., Phipps, J., Hoffman, W. E., Leavitt, M.: Reduction of blood pressure by intracranial injection of angiotensin blocker in spontaneously hypertensive rats. Physiologist **18**, 350 (1975).

Poth, M. M., Heath, R. G., Ward, M.: Angiotensin-converting enzyme in human brain. J. Neurochem. **25**, 83—85 (1975).

Poulsen, K.: Kinetics of the renin system. The basis for determination of the different components of the system. Scand. J. clin. Lab. Invest. **31** (Suppl. 132) (1973).

Poulsen, K., Burton, J., Haber, E.: Purification of hog renin by affinity chromatography using the synthetic competitive inhibitor D-Leu-6-octapeptide. Biochim. biophys. Acta (Amst.) **400**, 258—262 (1975).

Poulsen, K., Haber, E., Burton, J.: On the specificity of human renin: studies with peptide inhibitors. Biochim. biophys. Acta (Amst.) **452**, 533—537 (1976).

Printz, M. P., Nemethy, G., Bleich, H.: Proposed models for angiotensin II in aqueous solution and conclusions about receptor topography. Nature (Lond.) New Biol. **237**, 135—140 (1972).

Regoli, D., Park, W. K.: Pressor and myotropic effect and antagonist properties of several analogs of angiotensin II. Canad. Physiol. J. Pharmacol. **50**, 99—112 (1972).

Regoli, D., Park, W. K., Rioux, F.: Pharmacology of angiotensin. Pharmacol. Rev. **26**, 69—123 (1974).

Reid, I. A., Day, R. P.: Interactions and properties of same components of the renin-angiotensin system in brain. In: Buckley, J. P., Ferrario, C. (Eds.): Central Actions of Angiotensin and Related Hormones. New York: Pergamon Press 1977. pp. 267—282

Riniker, B., Brunner, H., Schwyzer, R.: β-Asp-1-Val-5-hypertensin II, ein Hypertensin-Analoges mit besonders hoher biologischer Aktivität. Angew. Chem. **74**, 469—475 (1962).

Roth, M., Weitzmann, A. F., Piquilloud, Y.: Converting enzyme content of different tissues of the rat. Experientia (Basel) **25**, 1247 (1969).

Rubin, I.: Purification of hog renin. Properties of purified hog renin. Scand. J. clin. Lab. Invest. **29**, 51—58 (1972).

Ryan, J. W.: Distribution of a renin-like enzyme in the bovine adrenal gland. Experientia (Basel) **29**, 407—408 (1972).

Sakai, K. K., Marks, B. H., George, J., Koestner, A.: Specific angiotensin II receptors in organ-cultured canine supra-optic nucleus cells. Life Sci. **14**, 1337—1344 (1974).

Saltman, S., Fredlund, P., Catt, K.: Actions of angiotensin II antagonists upon aldosterone production by isolated adrenal glomerulosa cells. Endocrinology **98**, 894—903 (1976).

Sambhi, M. P. (Ed.): Systemic Effects of Antihypertensive Agents. Proceedings of the Pennwalt Symposium. New York: Stratton Intercontinental Book Corp. 1976.

Samuels, A. J., Miller, E. D., Fray, J. S., Haber, E., Barger, A. C.: Renin-angiotensin antagonists and the regulation of blood pressure. Fed. Proc. **35**, 2512—2520 (1976).

Sancho, J., Re, R., Burton, J., Barger, A. C., Haber, E.: The role of the renin angiotensin aldosterone system in cardiovascular homeostasis in normal human subjects. Circulation **53**, 400—405 (1976).

Sander, G. E., West, D. W., Huggins, C. G.: Peptide inhibitors of pulmonary angiotensin I converting enzyme. Biochim. biophys. Acta (Amst.) **242**, 662—667 (1971).

Schambelan, M., Biglieri, E. G.: Regulation and secretion of hyper-reninemia from renin-secreting tumor (RST). Clin. Res. Proc. **20**, 439 (1972).

Scharpe, S., Eid, M., Cooreman, W., Lauwers, A.: α-1-antitrypsin, an inhibitor of renin. Biochem. J. **153**, 505—507 (1976).

Schiller, P. W., Demassieux, S., Boucher, R.: Substrate specificity of tonin from rat submaxillary gland. Circulat. Res. **39**, 629—632 (1976).

Schölkens, B. A.: Blutdruckverhalten experimentell hypertoner Ratten nach zentraler Gabe 1,8-disubstituierter Angiotensin-II-Analoga. Therapiewoche **26**, 7550 (1976).

Schwyzer, R., Iselin, B., Kappeler, H., Rinker, B., Rittel, W., Zuber, H.: Synthese von Hypertensin-peptiden. Chimia (Aarau) **11**, 335—336 (1957).

Sealey, J. E., Laragh, J. H.: "Prorenin" in human plasma? Methodological and physiological implications. Circulat. Res. **36** (Suppl. 1), 10—16 (1975).

SEN, S., SMEBY, R. R., BUMPUS, F. M.: Effect of mercuric chloride on plasma renin substrate level in rats. Amer. J. Physiol. **22**, 38—44 (1972).

SEN, S., SMEBY, R. R., BUMPUS, F. M.: Angiotensin antagonist and possible release of catecholamine. Proc. Soc. exp. Biol. (N. Y.) **147**, 847—849 (1974).

SEN, S., BUMPUS, F. M., TARAZI, R. C., KHAIRALLAH, P. A., ZACHARIAH, N. Y.: Effect of chronic administration of angiotensin antagonists in rats. Fourth Meeting of the International Society of Hypertension, Sydney, 1976, Abstract 44.

SEVERS, W. B., DANIELS-SEVERS, A. E.: Effects of angiotensin on the central nervous system. Pharmacol. Rev. **25**, 415—449 (1973).

SINAIKO, A., MIRKIN, B. L.: Ontogenesis of the renin-angiotensin system in spontaneously hypertensive and normal Wistar rats. Circulat. Res. **34**, 693—696 (1974).

SKEGGS, L. T. JR., MARCH, W. H., KAHN, J. R., SHUMWAY, N. P.: The purification of hypertensin I. J. exp. Med. **100**, 363—370 (1954).

SKEGGS, L. T. JR., MARSH, W. H., KAHN, J. R., SHUMWAY, N. P.: Amino acid composition and electrophoretic properties of hypertensin I. J. exp. Med. **102**, 435—440 (1955).

SKEGGS, L. T., DORER, F. E., KAHN, J. R., LENTZ, K. E., LEVINE, M.: The biological production of angiotensin. In: PAGE, J. H., BUMPUS, F. M. (Eds.): Handbook of ExperimentalPharmacology, pp. 1—16. Berlin-Heidelberg-New York: Springer 1974.

SKEGGS, L. T., DORER, F. E., KAHN, J. R., LENTZ, K. E., LEVINE, M.: The biochemistry of the renin-angiotensin system and its role in hypertension. Amer. J. Med. **60**, 737—748 (1976).

SKINNER, S. L., CRAN, E. J., GIBSON, R., TAYLOR, R., WALTERS, W. A. W., CATT, K. J.: Angiotensins I and II, active and inactive renin, renin substrate, renin activity, and angiotensinase in human liquor amnii and plasma. Amer. J. Obstet. Gynec. **121**, 626—630 (1975).

SOFFER, R. L., REZA, R., CALDWELL, P. R. B.: Angiotensin-converting enzyme from rabbit pulmonary particles. Proc. nat. Acad. Sci. (Wash.) **71**, 1720—1724 (1974).

STEELE, J. M. JR., LOWENSTEIN, J.: Differential effects of an angiotensin II analogue on pressor and adrenal receptors in the rabbit. Circulat. Res. **35**, 592—600 (1974).

STOKES, G. S., EDWARDS, K. D. G.: Drugs affecting the renin-angiotensin-aldosterone system. Use of angiotensin inhibitors. In: Progress in Biochemical Pharmacology. Series editor R. Paoletti, S. Karger, Basel, München, Paris, London, New York, Sydney, 1976.

STREETEN, D. H. P., FREIBERG, J. M., ANDERSON, G. H., DALAKOS, T. G.: Identification of angiotensinogenic hypertension in man using 1-sar-8-ala-angiotensin II (saralasin, P 113). Circulat. Res. **36** (Suppl. 1), 125—132 (1975a).

STREETEN, D. H. P., ANDERSON, G. H., FREIBERG, J. M., DALAKOS, T. G.: Use of an angiotensin II antagonist (saralasin) in the recognition of "angiotensinogenic" hypertension. New Engl. J. Med. **292**, 657—662 (1975b).

STREETEN, D. H. P., ANDERSON, G. H., DALAKOS, T. G.: Angiotensin blockade: Its clinical significance. Amer. J. Med. **60**, 817—824 (1976).

SUKETA, Y., INAGAMI, T.: Actuve site directed inactivators of mouse submaxillary renin. Biochemistry **14**, 3188—3194 (1975).

SYMONDS, E. M., STANLEY, M. A., SKINNER, S. L.: Production of renin by *in vitro* cultures of human chorion and uterine muscle. Nature (Lond.) **217**, 1152—1153 (1968).

SWALES, J. D., THURSTON, H., QUEIROZ, F. P., MEDINA, A.: Sodium balance during the development of experimental hypertension. J. Lab. clin. Med. **80**, 539—547 (1972).

SWANSON, L. W., MARSHALL, G. R., NEEDLEMAN, P., SHARPE, L. G.: Characterization of central angiotensin II receptors involved in the elicitation of drinking in the rat. Brain Res. **49**. 441—446 (1973).

SWEET, C. S., FERRARIO, C. M., KHOSLA, M. C., BUMPUS, F. M.: Antagonism of peripheral and central effects of angiotensin II by [1-sarcosine, 8-isoleucine] angiotensin II. J. Pharmacol. exp. Ther. **185**, 35—41 (1973).

THURSTON, H.: Vascular angiotensin receptors and their role in blood pressure control. Amer. J. Med. **61**, 768—778 (1976).

TURCOTTE, J. G., YU, C., LEE, H., PAVANARAM, S. K., SEN, S., SMEBY, R.: Synthesis of lysophosphatidylethanolamine analogs that inhibit renin activity. J. med. Chm. **18**, 1184—1190 (1975).

TURKER, R. K., YAMAMOTO, M., KHAIRALLAH, P. A., BUMPUS, F. M.: Competitive antagonism of 8-ala-angiotensin II to angiotensin I and II on the isolated rabbit aorta and rat ascending colon. Europ. J. Pharmacol. **15**, 285—291 (1971).

TURKER, R. K., HALL, M. M., YAMAMOTO, M., SWEET, C. S., BUMPUS, F. M.: A new, long lasting competitive inhibitor of angiotensin. Science **177**, 1203—1205 (1972).

TURKER, R. K., PAGE, I. H., BUMPUS, F. M.: Antagonists of angiotensin. In: PAGE, I. H., BUMPUS, F. M. (Eds.): Angiotensin. Handbook of Experimental Pharmacology, pp. 162—169. Berlin-Heidelberg-New York: Springer 1974.

UEDA, E., AKUTSHU, H., YAMAMURA, Y.: Partial purification and properties of angiotensin I converting enzyme from rabbit plasma. Jap. Circulat. J. **35**, 801—806 (1971).
UMEZAWA, H., AOYAGI, T., MORISHIMA, H., MATSUZAKI, M., HAMADA, M., TAKEUCHI, T.: Pepstatin, a new pepsin inhibitor produced by actinomycetes. J. Antibiot. (Tokyo) **23**, 259—262 (1970).
VALLOTON, M.B.: Immunogenicity and antigenicity of angiotensin I and II. In: PAGE, I.H., BUMPUS, F.M. (Eds.): Angiotensin. Handbook of Experimental Pharmacology, pp. 185—200. Berlin-Heidelberg-New York: Springer 1974.
VANE, J.R.: The fate of angiotensin I. In: PAGE, I.H., BUMPUS, F.M. (Eds.): Angiotensin. Handbook of Experimental Pharmacology, pp. 17—40. Berlin-Heidelberg-New York: Springer 1974.
VOÛTE, P.A.JR., VAN DER MEER, J., STANGAARD-KLOOSTERZIEL, W.: Plasma renin activity in Wilms' tumor. Acta Endocr. (Kbh.) **67**, 197—202 (1971).
WEINKAM, R., JORGENSEN, E.C.: Angiotensin II analogs. IX. Conformation studies of angiotensin II by proton magnetic resonance. J. Amer. chem. Soc. **93**, 7038—7044 (1971).
WERLE, E., VOGEL, R., GÖLDEL, L.T.: Über ein blutdrucksteigerndes Prinzip in Extrakten aus der Glandula submaxillaris der weißen Maus. Naunyn-Schmiedebergs Arch. exp. Path. Pharmak. **230**, 236—264 (1957).
WILLIAMS, G.H., McDONNELL, L.M., RAUX, M.C., HOLLENBERG, N.K.: Evidence for different angiotensin II receptors in rat adrenal glomerulosa and rabbit vascular smooth muscle cells. Circulat. Res. **34**, 384—390 (1974).
WISSMANN, H., SCHOELKENS, B., LINDNER, E., GEIGER, R.: Chemie und Wirkungsweise neuer Angiotensin-II-Antagonisten: 8-C-Phenylglycin-Analoga des [5-Isoleucin]-Angiotensins II. Hoppe-Seylers Z. physiol. Chem. **355**, 1083—1096 (1974).
WOODS, J.W., MICHELAKIS, A.M.: Renal vein renin in renovascular hypertension. Arch. intern. Med. **122**, 392—393 (1968).
WORKMAN, R., McKOWN, M.M., GREGERMAN, R.I.: Renin: inhibition by proteins and peptides. Biochemistry **13**, 3029—3035 (1974).
YAMAMOTO, M., TÜRKER, R.K., KHAIRALLAH, P.A., BUMPUS, F.M.: A potent competitive antagonist of angiotensin II. Europ. J. Pharmacol. **18**, 316—322 (1972).
YANG, H.-Y.T., NEFF, N.H.: Distribution and properties of angiotensin converting enzyme of rat brain. J. Neurochem. **19**, 2443—2450 (1972).
YOKOYAMA, H.: Studies on the simultaneous measurement of plasma renin activity and plasma aldosterone concentration in patients with various endocrine, hypertensive, edematous diseases; its clinical evaluation and significance. Folia endocr. jap. **52**, 729—750 (1976).
ZAHN, P., GANTEN, D.: Influence of $^{+}$H-ion concentrations and of prostaglandins on the activity of extrarenal angiotensinogenases. Naunyn Schiedebergs Arch. Pharmacol. **293** (Suppl.), R36 (1976).

Chapter 12

Veratrum Alkaloids with Antihypertensive Activity

O. Krayer and E. Meilman

With 6 Figures

I. Introduction

The rational use of certain Veratrum alkaloids in the treatment of hypertension has its scientific origin and pharmacological basis in the observation of von Bezold and Hirt (1867) that, in the mammalian circulation, veratrine, a mixture of alkaloids from Sabadilla seeds, causes a decrease in blood pressure. Von Bezold[1] assumed this to be due to reflex activity originating in the heart. Already in 1862, in the course of studies on the innervation of the heart (von Bezold, 1863) he had arrived at the conclusion that there are sensory vagal fibers in the heart. His idea that stimulation of these fibers had a vasodepressor effect antedated the discovery of the depressor nerves by Cyon and Ludwig (1866).

Von Bezold assumed the sensory nerve endings for the reflex arc to be spread out under the inner surface of the heart and their stimulation to lead to inhibition of the vasomotor center thus causing vasodilatation. Von Bezold and Hirt did not clearly decide on the relative importance of the vagal fibers versus the true depressor fibers in the effect of veratrine, nor did they advance conclusive proof that sensory vagal fibers from the lungs, or from the abdominal area, were not responsible for the effect. However, von Bezold thought of, and rejected, both possibilities.

In 1887, Lissauer, using cevadine, one of the constituent alkaloids of veratrine, did not accept von Bezold's interpretation of the mechanism of its vasodepressor action. On the other hand, Watts Eden (1892) considered it possible to ascribe the vasodepressor effect of small doses of protoveratrine, an alkaloid obtained by Salzberger (1890) from *Veratrum album*, to the reflex inhibition of the vasomotor center caused by stimulation of the depressor nerves[2].

In 1915, Cramer, working with an extract from *Veratrum viride*, confirmed von Bezold's concept of a reflex decrease in blood pressure due to vasodilatation. He observed that this effect was obtainable with small doses and, as a rule, was

[1] For details concerning the life and work of A. von Bezold see Herrlinger and Krupp, 1964.

[2] Ludwig assumed that the depressor nerves originate in the heart. This was challenged by later authors, especially Köster and Tschermack (1902), who traced their origin to the aorta.

accompanied by a reflex decrease in heart rate and by a slowing or stoppage of the respiration. All these changes were dependent upon the integrity of the vagus nerves. Probably under the influence of the studies of Brodie (1900) and Brodie and Russell (1900), Cramer ascribed the effect to a selective action of the *Veratrum viride* alkaloids upon the endings of afferent vagal fibers in the lungs.

In his review on veratrine and protoveratrine, Boehm (1920), in whose laboratory Lissauer and Watts Eden had done their work, did not resolve the controversy between the earlier authors. However, he concisely stated von Bezold's concept: „Der primäre Abfall des Blutdruckes wird durch die Reizung von (sensiblen) Herznerven erklärt, die, im Stamm des Vagus verlaufend, depressorisch wirken und die Wirkung des eigentlichen N. depressor nach Ansicht von von Bezold noch übertreffen können"[3].

In 1935, Jarisch and Henze (1937) began studies on the circulatory action of the European mistletoe, *Viscum album*. They provided evidence that the observed vasodepressor and cardiodecelerator actions were due to a reflex originating in the heart. The afferent impulses were carried by vagal fibers. The reflex was similar, in general, to the depressor reflex and carotid sinus reflex but independent of both. Corroborative evidence for the reflex nature of the phenomenon was advanced showing that a reciprocal inhibition of accelerans activity accompanied the reflex bradycardia, and an increase in organ volume, especially of the liver, accompanied the reflex decrease in blood pressure.

Searching for other substances with similar pharmacological properties, Jarisch and his associates became aware of the Veratrum alkaloids through the review of Boehm, mentioned above. Thereupon, they carried out extensive studies on the anatomy and physiology of the cardiac nerves and on the action of veratrine and substantiated von Bezold's concept (Jarisch and Richter, 1939a, b; for further lit. see Krayer, 1961).

According to Jarisch's definition, the apparatus of the cardiovascular and cardiocardiac reflex revealed by veratrine consists of: a) the reflexogenous zone in the heart, predominantly in the muscles of the ventricles; b) the afferent pathway in the vagus nerves; and c) the efferent pathway. As with every depressor reflex, the efferent pathway has two divisions, one in the sympathetic outflow of the autonomic nervous system to the vessels and to the heart where decrease in discharge leads to vasodilatation in the vascular bed and to reduction in the rate of the heart, and the other in the parasympathetic (vagal) outflow to the heart where increase in discharge causes a decrease in heart rate. It is this reflex which, in the strict sense, is now correctly referred to as the Bezold-Jarisch Effect (Strughold and Benzinger, 1942; Krayer, 1961).

The unequivocal experimental proof for the existence of the Bezold-Jarisch Effect rests on studies with direct application of Veratrum alkaloids into the coronary circulation and on electrophysiological studies recording alteration of impulse discharge caused by Veratrum alkaloids in afferent (vagal) fibers from mechanoreceptors in the heart.

The Veratrum alkaloids can also cause reflex vasodepressor and cardiodecelerator effects which originate from areas of the circulatory system outside the heart, i.e., the aorta, the carotid sinus area, the pulmonary vascular bed. On the other hand, no direct effect upon the central nervous system is involved in this action.

[3] The primary fall in blood pressure is explained as being due to the stimulation of (sensory) depressor cardiac nerves which are carried in the stem of the vagus and whose effect, according to von Bezold, may even surpass that of the true N. depressor (translation by Krayer from Boehm, 1920, p. 271, lines 32—35).

Even when used in the small doses required for their reflex hypotensive effect, the Veratrum alkaloids may find access to such targets as, e.g., stretch receptors in the lungs, receptors for sensations of temperature and of taste, receptors for the elicitation of nausea and vomiting. Hence, action upon some or all of such additional reflexogenous zones may contribute, in man, to the overall effect of therapeutic doses of the Veratrum alkaloids.

II. Botanical Origin and Chemistry[4]

The Veratrum alkaloids with hypotensive activity are found in various genera, e.g., Veratrum, Schoenocaulon, Zygadenus, of the tribe Veratreae of the plant family Liliaceae. Of the genus Veratrum, the two species *Veratrum album* and *Veratrum viride* are the most important because, in the past, they have been the source of the therapeutically useful alkaloids. Of the genus Schoenocaulon, the species *Schoenocaulon officinale*, often referred to as Sabadilla, has attracted scientific interest for a century and a half. The Sabadilla seeds were the source of veratrine, a mixture of alkaloids first isolated in 1818 by MEISSNER. Several species of Zygadenus, e.g., *Zygadenus venenosus* and *Zygadenus paniculatus*, have long been recognized in North America as livestock poisons (KRAYER et al., 1953).

The modern chemistry of the Veratrum alkaloids started with the work of POETHKE (1937a, b) and JACOBS and CRAIG (CRAIG and JACOBS, 1942; JACOBS and CRAIG, 1943). In the subsequent broad efforts to clarify the structure of these compounds, the extensive and thorough work of KUPCHAN and his coworkers (KUPCHAN and BY, 1968) must rank as the most important contribution.

All hypotensive Veratrum alkaloids belong to the ceveratrum[5] group. The important substances are ester derivatives of the alkamines protoverine, germine, zygadenine, and veracevine. These alkamines contain the modified steroid cevane nucleus with its nitrogen in the tertiary configuration. They have as a common feature an α-ketol hemiketal system in rings A and B. The ceveratrum alkamines are highly hydroxylic containing 7 to 9 atoms of oxygen. In the plants they occur mostly in the esterified state. The hypotensive activity resides in the ester alkaloids, the alkamines themselves are devoid of this pharmacological property. A list of some of the ceveratrum alkaloids is given in Table 1.

For therapeutic purposes as antihypertensive agents, only the polyacyl compounds of protoverine, i.e., protoveratrine A and protoveratrine B, and of germine, i.e., germitetrine, germitrine, and neogermitrine, have proved to be useful. When mixtures of alkaloids of *Veratrum viride* were successfully employed, e.g., Veratrone, Veriloid, the active principles were polyacyl germine derivatives. The protoveratrines are illustrative of the group.

As already mentioned, protoveratrine was first isolated by SALZBERGER (1890) from *Veratrum album*. POETHKE (1937a, b, 1938) improved the extraction methods. He assumed protoveratrine to be a triacyl ester of protoverine. Protoveratrine was later found also in *Veratrum viride*. Almost simultaneously (1952—1953) various authors (for references see KUPCHAN and AYRES, 1960) succeeded in demonstrating that protoveratrine extracted from its plant source consists of two closely related

[4] For a detailed study of the alkaloids in the plants of the tribe Veratreae, the botanical taxonomy of the tribe, and the relation of occurrence and structure of the alkaloids to the taxonomy, see KUPCHAN, ZIMMERMAN, and AFONSO (1961).

[5] The name *ceveratrum* alkaloids was introduced by FIESER and FIESER (1959) to distinguish this group from the *jerveratrum* alkaloids (see KUPCHAN and BY, 1968) which have different chemical, pharmacological, and toxicological properties.

Table 1. *Ceveratrum alkaloids*[a]

	Formula	Acyl groups at				Plant source
		C_3	C_6	C_7	C_{15}	
Protoverine	$C_{27}H_{43}NO_9$					
Esters of Protoverine						
Protoveratrine A	$C_{41}H_{63}NO_{14}$	HMB	Ac	Ac	MB	VA VV
Protoveratrine B	$C_{41}H_{63}NO_{15}$	t-DMB	Ac	Ac	MB	VA VV
Germine	$C_{27}H_{43}NO_8$					
Esters of Germine						
Germitetrine	$C_{41}H_{63}NO_{14}$	HMAB		Ac	MB	VA
Germitrine	$C_{39}H_{61}NO_{12}$	MB		Ac	HMB	VA VV
Neogermitrine	$C_{36}H_{55}NO_{11}$	Ac		Ac	MB	VA VV ZV
Germerine	$C_{37}H_{59}NO_{11}$	MB			HMB	VA VV
Germidine	$C_{34}H_{53}NO_{10}$	Ac			MB	VV ZV
Neogermidine	$C_{34}H_{53}NO_{10}$			Ac	MB	VV ZV
Zygadenine	$C_{27}H_{43}NO_7$					
Esters of Zygadenine						
Veratroylzygadenine	$C_{36}H_{52}NO_{10}$	Ve				VA VV ZV
Vanilloylzygadenine	$C_{35}H_{49}NO_{10}$	Va				ZV
Veracevine	$C_{27}H_{43}NO_8$					
Esters of Veracevine						
Cevadine	$C_{32}H_{49}NO_9$	An				SO
Veratridine	$C_{36}H_{51}NO_{11}$	Ve				SO

Ac = acetyl; An = angeloyl; HMAB = erythro-2-hydroxy-2-methyl-3-acetoxybutyryl; HMB = (*d*)-2-hydroxy-2-methylbutyryl; MB = (*l*)-2-methylbutyryl; t-DMB = (*d*)-threo-2,3-dihydroxy-2-methylbutyryl; Va = vanilloyl; Ve = veratroyl; VA = *Veratrum album*; VV = *Veratrum viride*; ZV = *Zygadenus venenosus*; SO = *Schoenocaulon officinale*.

[a] The data assembled in this table were taken in part from KUPCHAN and FLACKE (1967) and in part from BENFORADO (1967).

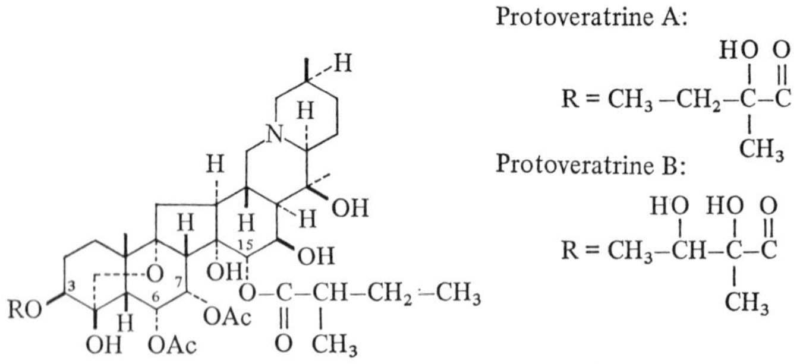

Fig. 1. The protoveratrines

compounds, protoveratrine A and protoveratrine B, and that the protoveratrines are tetra-esters of protoverine. The elucidation of the complete structures of protoveratrine A and protoveratrine B (Fig. 1) was reported by KUPCHAN and AYRES (1960)

III. Pharmacological Actions of Small Doses of the Hypotensive Ceveratrum Alkaloids

A. Circulation

1. Hypotensive Action

It was CRAMER (1915) who first stressed the important fact that the hypotensive effect of his *Veratrum viride* extract could be reliably observed only if small doses were used. This remains true for the therapeutically useful hypotensive action of the individual alkaloids.

All the naturally occurring ester alkaloids of Table 1 cause a transient decrease in blood pressure in the mammalian circulation (rabbit, cat, dog, man). The polyacyl alkaloids, i.e., protoveratrine A, protoveratrine B, germitetrine, germitrine, neogermitrine, are more potent than the mono-esters and most of the di-esters. Within the active dosage range for an individual animal, e.g., 0.5 to 5 μg/kg of protoveratrine[6] given intravenously in the anesthetized dog, the fall in blood pressure is proportional to the dose. The same has been shown for protoveratrine on intravenous administration in man (MEILMAN and KRAYER, 1950, 1952). The Veratrum ester alkaloids also differ in regard to the onset and duration of action after single intravenous doses, as shown by a comparison of veratridine and protoveratrine. In the dog, the intravenous injection of veratridine close to the heart is followed by a latency period of a few seconds after which the blood pressure falls abruptly, reaching the lowest level within 30 sec, and within 2 to 3 min returns to the level of the control period or slightly below. With a dose of protoveratrine causing the same maximal fall in blood pressure, the decrease is less abrupt. The minimum is reached in 1 to 3 min, and the return to a steady level, usually below the control level, requires 10 to 30 min. Similar differences between the two alkaloids have been observed in man (MEILMAN and KRAYER, 1950). Like protoveratrine, the germine esters germitetrine, germitrine, and neogermitrine have a greater potency than veratridine (KUPCHAN and FLACKE, 1967), and germitetrine also has a longer duration of action (BENFORADO et al., 1960).

The decrease in blood pressure, as a rule, is accompanied by a decrease in heart rate [Fig. 2 (man) see also Fig. 3 (dog)]. Unless it is intense, the cardiodecelerator effect per se is unlikely to contribute to the blood pressure fall.

A decrease in arterial resistance in various vascular beds of the circulation occurs during the hypotensive response to the Veratrum ester alkaloids. Quantitative measurements in the femoral arteries of anesthetized dogs showed a marked absolute increase in blood flow during the blood pressure fall caused by intravenous administration of protoveratrine (see Fig. 3), various germine esters, or veratridine. The vasodilatation is not brought about by a direct action upon the motor elements of the vessel wall but is transmitted by the nervous system, as was demonstrated in perfusion experiments using the hindlegs in the dog (MOE et al., 1944; KRAYER et al., 1944; BENFORADO et al., 1960). Atropine had no influence upon the vasodi-

[6] Whenever the term "protoveratrine" is used in this and subsequent sections of the present chapter, it refers to mixtures of protoveratrine A and protoveratrine B containing from one third to approximately one half protoveratrine B. On parenteral administration, the hypotensive activity of protoveratrine B may be slightly less than that of protoveratrine A. When protoveratrine A was compared quantitatively with mixtures of the protoveratrines containing 53% A and 47% B (ABREU et al., 1954), or two thirds A and one third B (ROTHLIN and CERLETTI, 1954), no significant difference in hypotensive potency could be detected.

latation, showing that cholinergic vasodilator pathways (UVNÄS, 1954) are not involved (BENFORADO et al., 1960).

The time courses of the vasodilatation in the femoral vascular bed and of the decrease in blood pressure are not parallel (BENFORADO et al., 1960). FLACKE et al. (1960) adduced evidence, in the dog, to show that a decrease in cardiac output, as a rule, participates in the hypotensive response. The relative contribution of decrease in resistance in various parts of the circulatory system and of decrease in cardiac output was found to be dependent upon the level of vascular

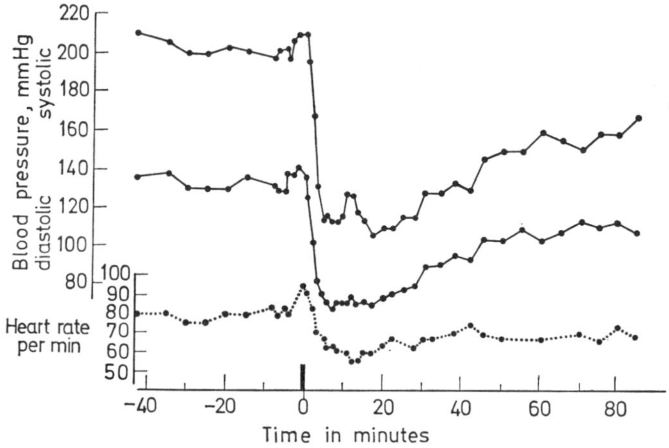

Fig. 2. The effect of protoveratrine A upon blood pressure and heart rate of a 36-year old woman with essential hypertension. At the signal, 0.09 mg (1.8 μg/kg) of protoveratrine A was administered intravenously. The blood pressure was measured in the recumbent position with a sphygmomanometer (MEILMAN and KRAYER, from KRAYER, 1958)

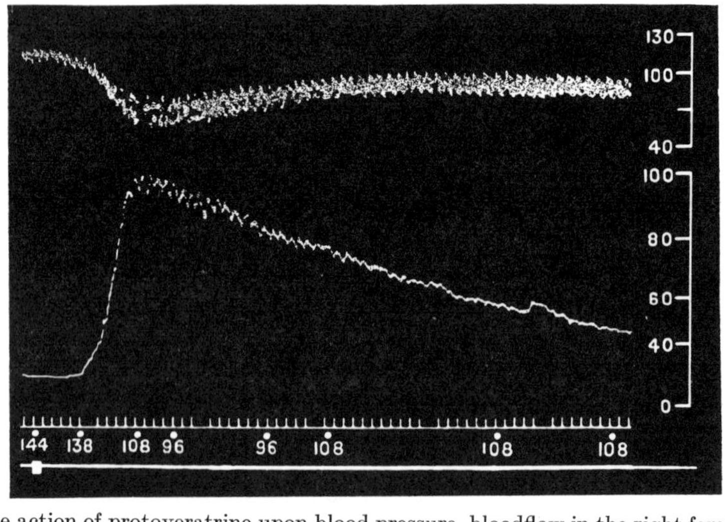

Fig. 3. The action of protoveratrine upon blood pressure, bloodflow in the right femoral artery and heart rate. Dog 15.5 kg (June 11, 1943). Anesthesia with sodium pentobarbital. From top to bottom: blood pressure, in mm Hg; bloodflow (with differential manometer) in cm³/min; time in 5 sec; horizontal row of figures: heart rate/min. At the signal, intravenous injection of 20 μg (1.3 μg/kg) of protoveratrine (60% A + 40% B) (KRAYER, 1950)

tone and cardiac output existing prior to the injection of the alkaloids. Decrease in cardiac output may, in part, be due to a decrease in venous return resulting from an increase in capacitance on the venous side. Because the atrial pressures were increased in two thirds of the hypotensive responses to Veratrum ester alkaloids, FLACKE et al. (1960) considered it possible that, in these cases, neurogenically induced decrease in myocardial contractility, due to a decrease in sympathetic discharge to the cardiac ventricles, played a role in the overall effect upon cardiac output.

It is now an established fact that the hypotensive effect of small doses of Veratrum ester alkaloids is reflex in nature, and that it is caused by their action upon receptor areas in the heart itself especially in the ventricles, in the aorta and carotid sinuses, and in the pulmonary vascular bed. ABREU et al. (1954) showed, in the dog, that protoveratrine A caused a hypotensive effect after severing the vagus nerves as long as the carotid sinus nerves were intact, and after carotid sinus denervation provided the vagus nerves were functioning. After cutting both, carotid sinus and vagus nerves, the administration of protoveratrine A led to blood pressure increase. Similar results with protoveratrine A were obtained in the cat (FERNANDEZ and CERLETTI, 1955). Likewise, BENFORADO et al. (1960) were able to produce the characteristic hypotensive effect, in the dog, as long as one of the receptor areas, either in the chest or in the carotid sinus, was in nervous connection with the central nervous system. Denervation of both these main receptor areas abolished the hypotensive effect of all alkaloids they examined, i.e., veratridine, and the di- and tri-esters of germine; instead, hypertension and cardioacceleration were uniformly produced by all alkaloids.

Some of the difficulties in the interpretation of the reflex effects of the Veratrum ester alkaloids upon the circulation result from the necessity to conduct the animal experiments under anesthesia. For example, in the cat, too deep a level of anesthesia with barbituric acid derivatives obscures the reflex effects of protoveratrine A which are clearly demonstrable under *light* barbiturate anesthesia, or under chloralose-urethane anesthesia (FERNÁNDEZ and CERLETTI, 1955). While a direct effect upon the central nervous system is not involved in the hypotensive action of small doses of protoveratrine, or therapeutically useful germine esters (FERNÁNDEZ and CERLETTI, 1955; WANG et al., 1955), nevertheless, the central regulatory areas must be in an appropriate state of excitability for unimpeded reflex action to occur (GELLHORN, 1958; KUPCHAN and FLACKE, 1967).

The receptor areas in the heart were first unequivocally demonstrated by DAWES (1947) who injected veratridine, cevadine, and protoveratrine directly into the coronary arteries, or into segments thereof. The most striking effects were obtained from injections into the circumflex branch of the left coronary artery which mainly supplies the left ventricle (Fig. 4 A and B). To elicit the hypotensive response it was sufficient, for intracoronary injection, to use 1/10 to 1/20 of the minimal dose effective when administered into the cavity of the left ventricle. These experiments showed clearly also the difference in the time course between the effect of the mono-ester veratridine and that of protoveratrine with its two constituent tetra-esters. Corroborative evidence for the observations of DAWES was provided, e.g., by AVIADO et al. (1949, 1951) and ROTHLIN and CERLETTI (1954); see also DAWES and COMROE (1954).

Following the lead of AMANN and SCHAEFER (1943) numerous attempts have been made to demonstrate the changes in the activity of the mechanoreceptors of the heart under the influence of the Veratrum ester alkaloids by recording the action potentials of afferent nerve fibers (PAINTAL, 1963). Of particular interest in this regard are the ventricular pressure receptors which, unlike other cardiovascular mechanoreceptors, are stimulated by relatively small doses of Veratrum ester alkaloids, i.e., doses required to elicit the Bezold-Jarisch Effect (Jarisch and Zotterman, 1948; Schaefer, 1950, 1960; Paintal, 1955, 1963; Kramer, 1959; Doutheil and Kramer, 1959; Neil, 1960; Neil and Joels, 1961).

There is a markedly increased electrical activity in the afferent fibers of these ventricular pressure receptors which sets in after a latency period ranging from 5 to 15 sec depending on the type of alkaloid injected into the right atrium

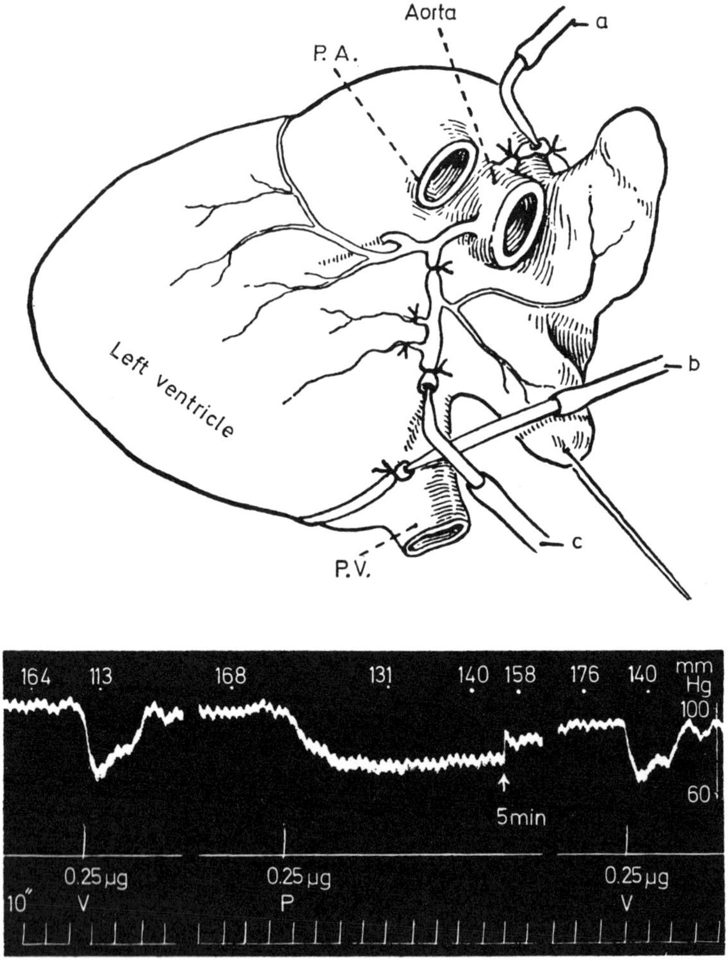

A

B

Fig. 4. A Left lateral diagram of preparation for simultaneous perfusion of the coronary arteries of the dog. Cannulae are shown in the right coronary artery (a); the peripheral end of the left circumflex (b); and the central end of the left circumflex (c) which now feeds only the left superior atrial coronary artery. The aorta, pulmonary artery (P.A.) and pulmonary veins (P.V.) have been divided (Dawes, 1947). B Direct injection of protoveratrine and veratridine into the coronary circulation. Dog 7.8 kg. Pentobarbital sodium. Record of heart rate (beats per minute) above and blood pressure below. At arrow, above 5 min, recording was stopped for five minutes. Injection of 0.25 µg protoveratrine (P) into the left circumflex coronary artery causes a more prolonged fall of blood pressure and heart rate than 0.25 µg veratridine (V). Time in 10-second intervals (Protoveratrine: 60% A + 40% B) (Dawes, 1947)

(PAINTAL, 1955). The duration of stimulation also depends upon the nature of the alkaloids and may vary from 1 to 18 sec in the case of the mono-ester veratridine, to 1 to 15 min in the case of Veriloid, a mixture of alkaloids containing various germine di- and poly-esters. The main effect is the production of a continuous discharge which may attain high frequency and which overshadows the phasic discharge resulting from the cardiac rhythm (PAINTAL, 1963).

Increased activity in afferent fibers from left atrial mechanoreceptors under the influence of Veratrum ester alkaloids was reported by PAINTAL (1955, 1957) and NEIL and JOELS (1961); afferent fibers from right atrial receptors require higher doses of the alkaloids (PAINTAL, 1957; NEIL and JOELS, 1961).

Veratrine (JARISCH et al., 1952; WITZLEB, 1952) and protoveratrine (DONTAS, 1955) also increase the impulse frequency in afferent fibers of carotid sinus and aortic baroreceptors.

A study of DONTAS (1955) has given us some insight into the complexity of the interaction of the diverse impulse discharge reaching the vasomotor center from various receptor areas under the influence of protoveratrine. It also has provided information on the resulting change in efferent vasomotor impulse discharge leading to the hypotensive effect. The experiments were conducted in cats under light chloralose-urethane anesthesia, neuromuscular blockade with decamethonium or tubocurarine, and artificial respiration. The participation of the carotid and aortic afferents and the resulting alteration in the splanchnic discharge was studied during protoveratrine-induced hypotension.

DONTAS concludes that the complete hypotensive response to intravenous protoveratrine requires access of the drug to the cardiac receptor areas with afferent fibers running in the vagus *and* to the receptor areas in the aortic arch and in the carotid sinus area whose afferent fibers run, respectively, in the depressor and in the carotid sinus nerves. If all these areas are denervated, as mentioned above, protoveratrine causes an increase in blood pressure.

There are two phases in the hypotensive response: a relatively brief early and a longer lasting late phase. The early phase, seen in the normal animal, is not modified by severing the carotid sinus nerves but is prevented by vagotomy. The late hypotensive phase, seen in the normal animal, is a composite effect. Receptor areas served by afferent vagal, mainly cardiac, fibers contribute to it, because it is not prevented by severing the aortic and carotid sinus nerves; receptor areas of the carotid sinus contribute to it, because, in the vagotomized animal, the late hypotensive phase remains.

The early hypotensive phase is characterized by strong participation of afferent impulses carried by the vagus and coming from the heart (and probably the lungs). According to DONTAS, stimulation of baroreceptors of the aorta and the carotid sinus does not contribute to this phase, because baroreceptor activity in the aortic arch and in the carotid sinus *decreases* during this phase. On the efferent side, in the preganglionic splanchnic fibers, there is profound inhibition of discharge. At the same time, there is complete *refractoriness* of the splanchnic discharge to chemoreceptor stimulation in the carotid body. In fact, stimulation by anoxia and by drugs (cyanide, acetylchloline, lobeline) now intensifies the protoveratrine-induced bradycardia instead of producing the expected increase in heart rate.

The late hypotensive phase is characterized by participation of afferent impulses from areas served by the vagus (heart and lungs). It is associated with baroreceptor activation in the aortic arch and in the carotid sinus. Inhibition of splanchnic discharge is no longer complete. However, there is low grade continuous activity instead of the highly synchronized normal pattern of discharge, and this leads to decreased effectiveness of vasoconstrictor outflow. During the late phase, splanchnic activity can again be increased by chemoreceptor stimulation in the carotid body by anoxia and by drugs.

DONTAS' observations on the alteration of chemoreceptor activity in the carotid body and on the difference of the time course of the mechanoreceptor activity in different receptor areas indicate that the hypotensive activity of the Veratrum ester alkaloids, or at least of protoveratrine, is not in a simple way related to alteration in the mechanoreceptor activity of the pressor-homeostatic mechanism of the mammalian circulatory system. This is emphasized also by the important observation (RICHARDSON et al., 1952; RUBIN and BURKE, 1952) that the rise in arterial blood pressure, normally elicited in the vagotomized animal by simultaneously clamping both carotid arteries, is reduced, or absent, during the hypotensive action of the Veratrum ester alkaloids. Despite further investigation, this phenomenon has not, as yet, been adequately explained (ABREU et al., 1954; GOTH and HARRISON, 1954; WANG et al., 1955; BORISON et al., 1955).

At the cellular level, the Veratrum ester alkaloids cause their stimulating (and simultaneously desensitizing) effect probably by an action upon the regenerative region of the receptor, rather than the generator region or the nerve fiber central to the regenerative region (PAINTAL, 1957, 1964, 1971). In medullated nerve fibers, Veratrum ester alkaloids are known to induce a negative afterpotential on which repetitive afterdischarge may be superimposed; at higher concentrations depolarization occurs (see ULBRICHT, 1969). Similarly, repetitive afterdischarge induced by Veratrum ester alkaloids in the receptor might explain the high frequency firing observed when the receptor is excited by its natural stimulus; and depolarization of the regenerative region might lead to receptor discharge in the absence of a natural stimulus as is also observed with Veratrum ester alkaloids (PAINTAL, 1964).

2. The Cardiac Action

The hypotensive Veratrum ester alkaloids have a direct cardiac action which resembles that of the cardiac glycosides (KRAYER and ACHESON, 1946). This could be clearly demonstrated in the heart-lung preparation (HLP) of the dog with the heart in a state of failure (KRAYER and MENDEZ, 1942; MOE and KRAYER, 1943; KRAYER et al., 1944, 1953). The minimal effective therapeutic dose of protoveratrine in the failing heart (HLP) was smaller than that of veratridine. However, maximal therapeutic effect could be reached with veratridine, but not with protoveratrine, before toxic effects intervened (KRAYER et al., 1944). In a comprehensive study, BENFORADO (1957) using the method of FARAH and MARESH (1948) examined the therapeutic, irregularity, and lethal doses of several pure Veratrum ester alkaloids (protoveratrine A, protoveratrine B, germitetrine, neogermitrine, germidine, vanilloyl and veratroyl zygadenine, veratridine, and cevadine) in the HLP of the dog. As with the cardiac glycosides, on continuous infusion of the minimal lethal dose, the therapeutic effect manifested itself by decrease in right atrial pressure; this was followed by the onset of cardiac irregularities and eventually by ventricular fibrillation. For protoveratrine the minimal cardiac irregularity dose in the HLP was approximately two to five times the dose required in the intact dog to produce a 25% to 40% decrease in blood pressure. This makes it entirely improbable that any direct deleterious cardiac effect is involved in the hypotensive response. The therapeutic ranges of the Veratrum ester alkaloids in the HLP of the dog lack the remarkable uniformity of those of the cardiac glycosides. Instead, the relative therapeutic and irregularity doses of the Veratrum ester alkaloids vary from substance to substance and with the same substance the variability is high (BENFORADO, 1957).

Attempts to analyze the positive inotropic action of veratridine and cevadine were made by REITER (1963) using the isometrically contracting, isolated guinea-pig papillary muscle. As with the cardioactive steroids of the digitalis type, the effect of the Veratrum ester alkaloids was found to depend on the outside sodium concentration, indicating that sodium ions play a key role in the cellular mechanism in contrast to what is known about the inotropic effect of the catecholamines.

The increase in force of contraction is the consequence of an acceleration of force development as shown by the increase in the steepness of the ascending limb of the isometric contraction curve. In this regard, the inotropic effect resembles that of the cardiac glycosides, catecholamines, increase in Ca^{++} concentration, or increase in contraction frequency. However, in contrast to these inotropic interventions, cevadine and veratridine cause a marked retardation of relaxation, so that total contraction time is prolonged. Similar observations were already made by STRAUB (1903) who studied the effect of veratrine upon the isolated heart of *Aplysia limacina*. Simultaneous recording of isometric contraction curves and transmembrane action potentials of guinea-pig papillary muscles (REITER, 1963) revealed a prolongation of the action potentials concomitant with the characteristic alteration of the relaxation process caused by cevadine and veratridine.

The investigation of the inotropic effect was extended by KOCH-WESER (1966) to protoveratrine A, protoveratrine B, germitrine, germerine, and germidine. In guinea-pig atrial strips and kitten papillary muscles, the 50% effective concentration was lowest for the tetra-esters, protoveratrine A and protoveratrine B, and highest for the mono-esters, cevadine and veratridine. The inotropic effect was not inhibited by a β-adrenoceptor-blocking agent, propranolol.

With doses used therapeutically, in man, for their hypotensive effect, it is improbable that the positive inotropic cardiac action of the Veratrum ester alkaloids will become manifest. However, in patients with heart failure treated with full doses of cardiac glycosides, protoveratrine may have additive effects on the heart (see below).

B. Respiration

With doses of the Veratrum ester alkaloids of the order required for hypotensive therapeutic action, respiratory effects usually are inconspicuous, except for a tachypnea with inspiratory emphasis which has been observed under experimental conditions (MOE et al., 1944; ZIPF and MARQUARDT, 1966). Higher doses cause respiratory depression and apnea; e.g., in the guinea pig, doses of 1 to 15 µg/kg protoveratrine A led to tachypnea while apnea occurred at the dosage level of 20 µg/kg or above (ZIPF and MARQUARDT, 1966).

Reflex effects probably originating in the stretch receptors of the lungs with afferent pathways in the vagi are mainly responsible for the respiratory changes (KRAYER and ACHESON, 1946; DAWES, 1947; AVIADO et al., 1949, 1951; KRAYER et al., 1953; PAINTAL, 1957), weak excitation of the receptors leading to tachypnea, strong excitation to apnea. For the overall respiratory action of large doses of Veratrum ester alkaloids additional sites, peripheral as well as central, have been implicated (for lit. see BENFORADO, 1967).

The action upon the stretch receptors of the lungs can be elicited by the polyesters protoveratrine A, protoveratrine B, and germitetrine with smaller doses than those needed of the mono-esters, e.g., veratridine, or cevadine. Moreover, the effect of these polyesters develops more slowly and lasts longer than that of the mono-esters, which calls to mind the differences between the hypotensive effects of the two types of alkaloids.

C. Emetic Action

In the mammals which possess a vomiting mechanism, all hypotensive Veratrum ester alkaloids have an emetic effect on enteral as well as on parenteral administration. Local effects upon the mucosal membranes of the gastrointestinal tract (SWISS, 1952), or on specific sensory receptors in the gastrointestinal tract with afferent fibers in the vagus nerves are not involved. The receptor areas of the lungs, the heart, and the large vessels, with afferent fibers in the vagi and the carotid sinus nerves, so important for the hypotensive effect, are of no importance for the emetic response (BORISON et al., 1955). The denervation of the heart in the monkey, for example, does not influence the emetic effect of protoveratrine (PENG and WANG, 1962).

The systematic analysis of the site of action in the cat (BORISON and FAIRBANKS, 1952; BORISON et al., 1955; BORISON and SAMPSON, 1961) indicates that there is no direct effect upon the vomiting center in the lateral reticular formation of the medulla oblongata. The chemoreceptor trigger zone, which plays an important role in the emetic effect of apomorphine and the cardiac glycosides, is not involved. This was also established for the action of protoveratrine in the monkey (PENG and WANG, 1962). While the emetic response remains after severing the vagus nerves below the nodose ganglia, emesis no longer occurs after cutting the vagi cephalad to them. The available evidence suggests that the emetic action of the hypotensive Veratrum ester alkaloids is a reflex phenomenon, and that the receptors of the afferent pathways are located in the nodose ganglia of the vagus nerves or in close proximity to them.

If equihypotensive doses of different Veratrum ester alkaloids are compared, no difference in the hypotensive/emetic activity ratio can be observed in animals on intravenous or other parenteral administration (SWISS, 1952; ABREU et al., 1954). After the complete elucidation of the chemical structures of protoveratrine A, and protoveratrine B (KUPCHAN and AYRES, 1960) and after differences between the hypotensive/emetic activity ratio of protoveratrine A and that of protoveratrine B had been observed in man (WINER, 1956 a,b, 1957, 1960), a large series of related protoverine derivatives was prepared by partial synthesis (KUPCHAN et al., 1962). An extensive pharmacological study which employed many of these compounds, administered intravenously in the unanesthetized dog, did not show conclusively that substances had been found with a significantly greater margin between hypotensive and emetic doses than that of protoveratrine A (WEAVER et al., 1962).

IV. Therapeutic Use

The use of protoveratrine in the treatment of human hypertension was first proposed by KRAYER because it combined the advantage of a well-characterized therapeutic agent with two features of its hypotensive activity which made it preferable to the pharmacologically better known alkaloid veratridine, i.e., on intravenous injection, the hypotensive action of protoveratrine developed more slowly and it lasted longer than that of veratridine. Moreover, clinical trials with veratridine soon showed that its hypotensive dose and its toxic emetic dose were essentially the same (MEILMAN and KRAYER, 1950). The first human experiments and clinical trials with protoveratrine were carried out by MEILMAN at the Beth Israel Hospital in Boston. As protoveratrine, and later protoveratrine A, became commercially available, interest in their clinical and experimental use spread in the USA and subsequently in Europe and elsewhere.

A. Circulatory Action

The antihypertensive effect of protoveratrine appears to be independent of the etiology of the hypertensive disease. There is a considerable variability in the effect, so that the optimal dose leading to an adequate decrease in blood pressure must be established for the individual patient (MEILMAN and KRAYER, 1952; WILBRANDT, 1954; WINER, 1960). Using protoveratrine by intravenous administration in a group of 51 hypertensives, MEILMAN and KRAYER (1952) determined the dose which decreased the blood pressure to 150 mm Hg systolic and 90 mm Hg diastolic or less (Fig. 5). The majority required 1.5 to 1.9 μg/kg body weight; in seven it was between 1.1 and 1.5 μg/kg, and in thirteen between 1.9 and 3.0 μg/kg. In the experience of MEILMAN, this individual optimal intravenous dose, once

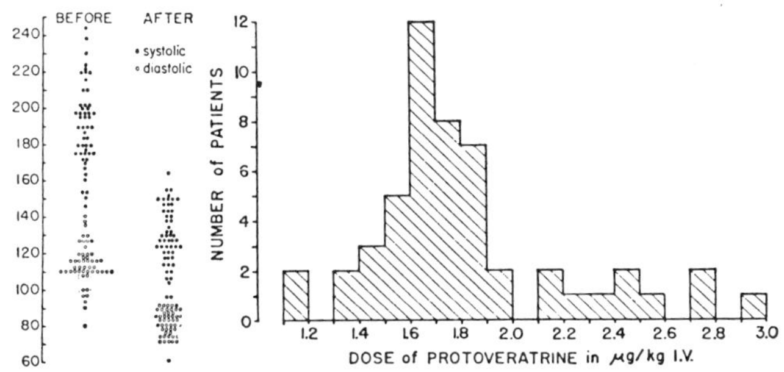

Fig. 5. The optimal intravenous dose of protoveratrine as determined in 51 adult hypertensive patients. The dose in μg/kg body weight which lowers blood pressure to or below 150 mm Hg systolic and to or below 90 mm Hg diastolic (regardless of initial blood-pressure level) is plotted against the number of patients giving the same response. The actual blood-pressure readings before and after protoveratrine are given on the left (Protoveratrine: 60% A + 40% B) (MEILMAN and KRAYER, 1952)

established, induces a reproducible fall in systolic and diastolic blood pressure on repeated use and, in most patients, is free of significant adverse effects.

In a comparative study on ten hypertensive patients, WINER (1960) found protoveratrine B slightly less potent on intravenous administration than protoveratrine A. Employing criteria similar to those of MEILMAN and KRAYER (1952), he also determined the optimal intravenous dose of protoveratrine B. In a total number of thirty-four hypertensives, it was 1.8 to 3.0 μg/kg in twenty-eight; between 1.2 and 1.8 μg/kg in two; and between 3.0 and 3.7 μg/kg in four.

Because the therapeutic range is narrow, great care is needed in establishing the individual optimal dose. On intravenous administration in man, the full blood pressure-decreasing effect of protoveratrine (and of protoveratrine A, or protoveratrine B as well) requires 10 to 15 min (see Fig. 2) (MEILMAN and KRAYER, 1952; WINER, 1960). Hence, in order to find the optimal dose in patients whose antihypertensive response to an initial test dose of 1.0 to 1.5 μg/kg was inadequate, additional doses of 20 μg (total) may be given at 10-min to 15-min intervals.

A valuable method for achieving and maintaining an adequate hypotensive effect is the continuous intravenous infusion of protoveratrine (MEILMAN and

KRAYER, 1952; MEILMAN, 1953a; KÄSER, 1954; CURRENS et al., 1956; SIKKEL and WOLFF, 1959). It permits controlled lowering of the blood pressure to levels which are not excessive; and it appears to reduce the incidence and severity of adverse effects such as nausea and vomiting.

The antihypertensive effect of the intravenous infusion of protoveratrine is illustrated in Fig. 6 by the results obtained in a case of malignant hypertension.

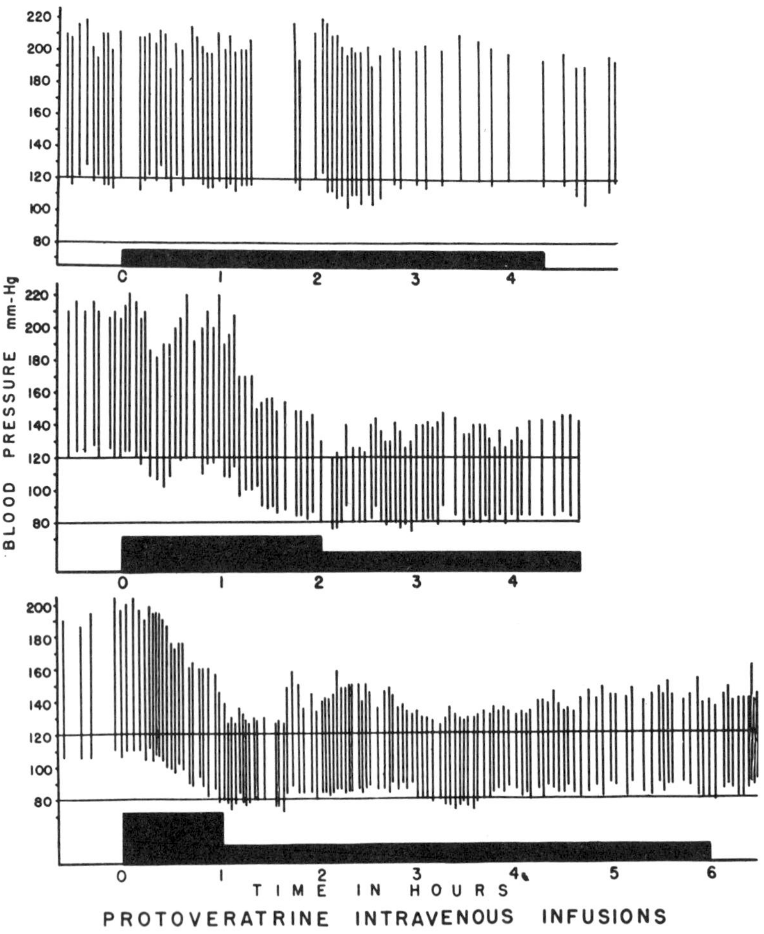

Fig. 6. A. M., 37 year old woman, body weight 60 kg. Malignant hypertension. Response of the blood pressure to continuous infusion of protoveratrine. Ordinates, blood pressure in mm Hg, measured with sphygmomanometer in the recumbent position. Abscissae, time in hours. Black bars, time of infusion. Rates of infusion are per total body weight (not per kg!); *top*: 1 μg/min; *middle*: 2 μg/min for 2 hours then reduced to 1.1 μg/min; *bottom*: 3 μg/min for 1 h then reduced to 1.1 μg/min. For further explanation see text (Protoveratrine: 60% A + 40% B) (MEILMAN and KRAYER, 1952)

In this patient, the infusion rate of 1.0 μg/min protoveratrine did not lower the blood pressure. A gradual fall in blood pressure could be induced by continuous infusion at priming rates of 2 μg/min, or 3 μg/min (for the patient as a whole) leading to adequate blood pressure levels within two hours, or one hour, respectively. Thereafter, the blood pressure could be maintained at the reduced level by the continuous infusion of 1.1 μg of protoveratrine per minute.

The rate of intravenous infusion of a drug capable of maintaining a steady blood pressure, reduced from its hypertensive level to the normal range, must be equal to the rate of elimination of the drug by the human body as a whole. Hence this rate of elimination of protoveratrine could be determined for hypertensive patients by experiments of the above kind. In twenty hypertensives, the values ranged between 0.6 μg/min and 2.0 μg/min; for fifteen of the twenty, it was of the order of 1.0 μg/min (MEILMAN and KRAYER, 1952).

When protoveratrine is administered by intramuscular (or subcutaneous) injection (MEILMAN and KRAYER, 1952; KÄSER, 1954; KRAYER, 1958) two to three times the intravenous dose is required, i.e., 4 to 6 μg/kg body weight. The administration is rendered painless by the use of a local anesthetic such as procaine hydrochloride (KÄSER, 1954). Variability in response is greater than on intravenous administration. Maximal hypotensive action is reached in about thirty minutes. The blood pressure returns gradually to the starting level within four to six hours; but occasionally it takes as long as twelve hours. Cumulative effects usually become apparent when the optimal dose is administered at intervals shorter than eight hours. There is no conclusive evidence that tolerance to the antihypertensive effect of protoveratrine develops on prolonged administration. After one to two weeks of treatment, the incidence of vomiting appears to increase in the experience of some authors (MEILMAN and KRAYER, 1952; DOYLE and SMIRK, 1953).

Oral administration of protoveratrine (MEILMAN and KRAYER, 1952; HOOBLER et al., 1952; CURRENS et al., 1953; LEHR, 1957; ALIMURUNG and GRAJO, 1958) made it possible to treat effectively only about one out of four or five patients without more than occasional side effects. It is of interest in this connection, that protoveratrine A and protoveratrine B differ only slightly in their antihypertensive activity when administered intravenously (WINER, 1960). On oral administration, however, protoveratrine B is much less potent than protoveratrine A (WINER, 1956a, b; WYSS and SPÜHLER, 1956; GRAY and HAMER, 1957) presumably as a result of poor absorption, or degradation during the course of absorption. The advent of agents more reliable in their effect when given by the oral route has left no place for the *oral* use of protoveratrine A, protoveratrine B, or other Veratrum ester alkaloids in the prolonged treatment of hypertension.

The slowing of the pulse which accompanies the antihypertensive effect of protoveratrine, or other Veratrum ester alkaloids, is usually due to a sinus bradycardia, but sometimes to other bradyarrhythmias, such as varying degrees of heart block, nodal rhythm, or sinus arrest. These alterations of rate and rhythm can be promptly overcome by the administration of atropine (atropine sulfate 0.4 to 1.0 mg, i.v.) without, as a rule, influencing the effect on the blood pressure. In some instances, the antihypertensive effect is diminished, or even abolished, when atropine causes the bradycardia to be replaced by a tachycardia (MEILMAN and KRAYER, 1950, 1952; HOOBLER and CORLEY, 1950; CURRENS et al., 1953; WINER, 1960). There is suggestive evidence that patients with congestive heart failure, treated with cardiac glycosides, are more sensitive than others to the bradyarrhythmia-producing effect of the Veratrum ester alkaloids, and also more readily develop premature ventricular beats (MEILMAN and KRAYER, 1952; MARGOLIN et al., 1956).

The electrocardiogram may show not only bradycardia, but first or second degree heart block. The acute fall in blood pressure caused by protoveratrine may result in prompt elevation of inverted T in lead 1, or elevation of depressed S-T segment in leads V-4, 5, 6. Some patients exhibit transient T-wave changes, usually inversion, sharply localized to V-3 and V-4. Presumably, these are not ischemic changes because they are readily reversed by administration of atropine but not oxygen (MEILMAN, 1956). In patients with angina pectoris, protoveratrine does not induce electrocardiographic changes indicative of ischemia.

As in experimental animals, protoveratrine produces the fall in blood pressure in the hypertensive patient mainly by decreasing total peripheral resistance (DURAND et al., 1957). Decrease in cardiac output may be a contributing factor (MYERS et al., 1951, 1952; HOOBLER et al., 1955). Resistance to bloodflow was found to be decreased in the vascular bed of the brain (CRUMPTON et al., 1951), arm and leg (HOOBLER et al., 1955; CURRENS et al., 1955) and kidney (MEILMAN, 1953a).

In a variety of cardiac conditions, DURAND et al. (1957) found that pulmonary arterial resistance, as well as peripheral arterial resistance, was lowered by protoveratrine in their hypertensive patients. In patients with congestive heart failure without hypertension, the decrease in pulmonary arterial resistance, due to administration of protoveratrine, was especially striking in that pulmonary arterial pressure fell despite an increase in cardiac output. These studies may explain the improvement of pulmonary congestion and relief of dyspnea in hypertensive patients suffering from congestive heart failure when the blood pressure is reduced by protoveratrine or other Veratrum ester alkaloids (BLACK and LYONS, 1954).

During the action of therapeutic doses of protoveratrine in human hypertension, in conformity with the experimental results reported above, the autonomic regulation of the vascular system is fully operative except for setting a new equilibrium at a lower level of blood pressure (DURAND et al., 1957). Hence the pressor response to cold remains unimpeded and postural hypotension does not occur. Likewise, the pressure response to the Valsalva maneuver is not impaired. This is contrary to the action of the ganglioplegic substances which completely disrupts the regulatory mechanism. Because the motor elements of the effector system at the vascular site are fully functioning, vasoconstriction can be readily induced by substances such as ephedrine or norepinephrine when an undesirable fall in blood pressure occurs following the administration of Veratrum ester alkaloids.

B. Action on Renal Function

Administered intravenously in a single optimal dose to hypertensive patients (see Fig. 5), protoveratrine induces a fall in glomerular filtration rate (GFR; inulin) of about 22% during the initial relatively fast fall of blood pressure. When the lowered level of blood pressure is maintained, the GFR rises but not quite to the control values. On the other hand, the effective renal plasma flow (ERPF; p-aminohippurate extraction) falls only 8% during the initial phase of the blood pressure fall. Subsequently, ERPF returns, in 60 to 90 min, to or occasionally above control values during the prolonged level of reduced blood pressure. If the decrease in blood pressure is gradually induced over a period of one hour by continuous infusion of protoveratrine, ERPF does not fall at all. These findings are consistent with renal vasodilatation (MEILMAN, 1953a).

Acute falls in blood pressure lead to transient oliguria probably as a result of the decrease in GFR (MEILMAN, 1952, 1953a). However, there is no evidence of prolonged water retention when blood pressure is maintained at low levels with protoveratrine.

C. Side Effects and Toxic Actions

Protoveratrine and other Veratrum ester alkaloids owe their therapeutic usefulness and effectiveness to gaining access in a selective way to sensory nerve endings in the circulatory system. However, there are other sensory nerve endings not involved in the hypotensive effect which equally lack barriers to the penetration of the low concentrations of protoveratrine and other Veratrum ester alkaloids used therapeutically. As a result, various side effects are encountered.

The experimental, or therapeutic, use of Veratrum ester alkaloids, in man, usually is accompanied initially by sensations of prickling and tingling, and by gustatory and thermal sensations. Intravenous doses of protoveratrine, or protoveratrine A, for example, give rise to the appearance of paresthesia of the lips and of the tongue, and to a sensation of warmth in the face, mouth, throat, hands, epigastrium, perineum, and feet. Intensity, spread, and duration of the sensation of warmth are proportional to the dose. It precedes the fall of blood pressure and may last as long as twenty-five minutes. There is no reddening of the skin but, with larger doses, sweating may occur in the neck, chest, and hands. Occasionally, salivation and rhinorrhea are noticed.

Nausea and vomiting are more discomforting than the symptoms and signs just described and may militate against the therapeutic use of the Veratrum ester alkaloids. It is to be kept in mind that the incidence of nausea and vomiting can be reduced and their intensity diminished by the technique of administration, at least on intravenous administration. Rapid injection, e.g., of the optimal dose of protoveratrine, may precipitate nausea and vomiting, while slow injection and, especially, continuous infusion, leading to the same decrease in blood pressure, are usually devoid of adverse effects.

All Veratrum ester alkaloids so far available as antihypertensive therapeutic agents are capable of causing nausea and vomiting. As was pointed out above in connection with experimental studies in mammals, no substances have as yet been found which, on parenteral administration, clearly differ in their hypotensive/emetic activity ratio if equihypotensive doses are compared. However, WINER (1957, 1960), on intravenous administration to patients with hypertensive disease, observed a significantly wider margin between the hypotensive and emetic doses of protoveratrine B than that between the hypotensive and emetic doses of protoveratrine A. Germitetrine was similar to protoveratrine A in regard to its hypotensive/emetic activity ratio (WINER, 1957).

Nausea and vomiting are disagreeable and uncomfortable but not dangerous side effects of the therapy with Veratrum ester alkaloids. Nausea, with a severe oppressive feeling in the chest, and vomiting might suggest coronary insufficiency. However, this chest discomfort is said by patients with true angina pectoris to be different from their anginal pain. In patients with coronary artery disease and angina, protoveratrine administration does not induce an attack of angina pectoris.

Despite the long, and fairly widespread therapeutic use of Veratrum ester alkaloids in the form of mixtures or as pure substances, no fatal poisoning has become known. With excessively large doses of protoveratrine, relaxation, lethargy, weakness, giddiness, and collapse may occur, due to the severe hypotension. A patient with poor blood supply to the brain might suffer transient cerebral ischemia during such an episode (CURRENS et al., 1953). In a patient under treatment with digitoxin, an accidental overdose of $2^1/_2$ times the effective oral dose of protoveratrine caused severe hypotension, A-V dissociation, and ectopic beats but was not fatal (BLACK and LYONS, 1954). Even 50 mg of protoveratrine by mouth, i.e., 75 times the usual dose, had no serious sequelae in a patient with hypertensive disease (Currens et al., 1953). Neuromuscular effects of a myotonic nature were observed only after the oral administration of large doses of protoveratrine B to hypertensive patients (Winer, 1956a, b; 1957).

D. Indications

Protoveratrine by parenteral administration remains a useful remedy for acute hypertensive states, or encephalopathy which may occur in the course of all types of hypertension, including malignant hypertension, eclampsia, acute nephritis, and steroid-induced hypertension. Pulmonary edema secondary to hypertension also responds promptly (Currens et al., 1953; Meilman, 1956).

Hydralazine would be contraindicated in acute hypertensive states where cardiac failure is a hazard.

Rauwolfia alkaloids of the reserpine type are not suitable for the treatment of a hypertensive crisis because several hours are required for the antihypertensive effect to develop. The same is true of alpha-methyldopa. In addition to their antihypertensive activity, reserpine and alpha-methyldopa have a sedative effect. The latter will obscure the return of mental alertness, which, therefore, cannot serve as an indicator of the recovery of a patient from hypertensive encephalopathy. Protoveratrine, administered to a comatose patient, will lower the blood pressure reliably and in a short time and, in fact, may "awaken" the patient.

Some of the most favorable reports on the use of mixtures of Veratrum ester alkaloids, or of protoveratrine, concern toxemia of pregnancy[7] especially when seizures occur (Bryant and Fleming, 1940; Finnerty and Fuchs, 1953; Käser, 1954; Currens et al., 1956; Krupp et al., 1956; Sikkel and Wolff, 1959). For an illness of reasonably limited time such as eclampsia, characterized by generalized arteriolar and capillary vasoconstriction, protoveratrine is an important therapeutic agent (Meilman, 1953b; Käser, 1954; Winkler and Cangello, 1958; Reid, 1962). Indeed, it has definite advantages. Its arteriolar action reduces vasospasm. Like hydralazine, protoveratrine – by intravenous administration – permits a controllable, graded lowering of the blood pressure. However, hydralazine causes tachycardia and increased cardiac output in these patients who may be on the verge of pulmonary edema. Hence protoveratrine is preferable.

Despite a 25% failure rate with respect to blood pressure reduction, magnesium sulfate is still used in the treatment of toxemia of pregnancy. Depression of reflexes is a hazard, especially when oliguria is present. Finnerty and Fuchs (1953) consider Veratrum ester alkaloids more effective and producing less adverse effects than magnesium sulfate. According to Käser (1954) and Reid (1962) treatment of severe pre-eclampsia and eclampsia with protoveratrine is superior to the use of the classical methods.

When used as an antihypertensive agent in pregnancy, reserpine should be discontinued for several days prior to delivery, in order to obviate the threat of respiratory obstruction in the newborn due to salivation and nasal congestion (Aaron, 1972; Reid, 1972, personal communication). Protoveratrine has no such effect.

[7] The therapeutic use of Veratrum ester alkaloids in pregnancy became questionable when Binns et al. (1963, 1968) recognized that cyclopia and related cephalic malformations in lambs, long known to North American sheep rangers, occur when the ewes feed on Veratrum plants (*Veratrum californicum*, Durand) during a critical period (the 14th day) of gestation. The available evidence indicates that this teratogenic activity is *not* a property of protoveratrine, or other ceveratrum ester alkaloids (Keeler and Binns, 1966). The teratogenic agents are some of the jerveratrum alkaloids, i.e., jervine, cyclopamine, and cycloposine (Keeler, 1970).

V. Summary

Hypotensive Veratrum ester alkaloids continue to have their main therapeutic usefulness in the treatment of acute hypertensive states, such as eclampsia, malignant hypertension, hypertensive pulmonary edema, and hypertensive encephalopathy. In all these conditions further disturbance of consciousness should be avoided and drugs which increase cardiac output are contraindicated. For these therapeutic indications the Veratrum ester alkaloids should be administered by the intravenous or intramuscular route, and in the form of well characterized preparations, such as protoveratrine A, protoveratrine B, or a known mixture of the two.

Acknowledgements

The authors are indebted to Drs. J. M. Benforado, W. E. Flacke, P. Honerjäger, D. E. Reid, and M. Reiter for reading the manuscript and suggesting improvements. During the writing of this review the senior author served as Visiting Professor in the Institut für Pharmakologie und Toxikologie der Technischen Universität München, West Germany. The hospitality of its Director, Professor Dr. Melchior Reiter, and the expert technical help of its secretarial staff and its photographer greatly facilitated the literary work.

References

Aaron, H. (Ed.): Drugs in pregnancy. The Medical Letter **14**, 94—96 (1972).

Alimurung, M. M., Grajo, M. Z.: Oral protoveratrine in the treatment of hypertension. Amer. J. Cardiol. **2**, 361—371 (1958).

Abreu, B. E., Richards, A. B., Alexander, W. M., Weaver, L. C.: Cardiovascular, emetic and pharmacodynamic properties of certain Veratrum alkaloids. J. Pharmacol. exp. Ther. **112**, 73—79 (1954).

Amann, A., Schaefer, H.: Über sensible Impulse im Herznerven. Pflügers Arch. ges. Physiol. **246**, 757—789 (1943).

Aviado, D. M., Li, T. H., Kalow, W., Schmidt, C. F., Turnbull, G. L., Peskin, G. W., Hess, M. E., Weiss, A. J.: Respiratory and circulatory reflexes from the pertused heart and pulmonary circulation of the dog. Amer. J. Physiol. **165**, 261—277 (1951).

Aviado, D. M., Pontius, R. G., Schmidt, C. F.: The reflex respiratory and circulatory actions of veratridine on pulmonary, cardiac and carotid receptors. J. Pharmacol. exp. Ther. **97**, 420—431 (1949).

Benforado, J. M.: Studies on Veratrum alkaloids. XXVI. Comparison of the cardiac action of various tertiary amine ester alkaloids. J. Pharmacol. exp. Ther. **120**, 412—425 (1957).

Benforado, J. M.: The Veratrum Alkaloids. In: Root, W. S., Hofmann, F. G. (Eds.): Physiological Pharmacology, Vol. 4, p. 331—398. New York: Academic Press 1967.

Benforado, J. M., Flacke, W., Swaine, C. R., Mosimann, W.: Studies on Veratrum alkaloids. XXIX. The action of some germine esters and of veratridine upon blood pressure, heart rate and femoral blood flow in the dog. J. Pharmacol. exp. Ther. **130**, 311—320 (1960).

Bezold, A. v.: Untersuchungen über die Innervation des Herzens. 2 Bände, Leipzig: Engelmann 1863.

Bezold, A. von, Hirt, L.: Über die physiologischen Wirkungen des essigsauren Veratrins. Untersuch. a. d. physiol. Laborat. in Würzburg. Leipzig 1867.

Binns, W., James, L. F., Shupe, J. L., Everett, G.: A congenital cyclopiantype malformation in lambs induced by maternal ingestion of a range plant, *Veratrum californicum*. Amer. J. Vet. Res. **24**, 1164—1175 (1963).

Binns, W., Shupe, J. L., Keeler, R. F., James, L. F.: Chronologic evaluation of teratogenicity in sheep fed Veratrum californicum. J. Amer. Vet. med. Ass. **147**, 839—842 (1968).

BLACK, M. M., LYONS, R. H.: Prolonged depression of atrioventricular conduction caused by large dosages of protoveratrine. Amer. Heart J. **48**, 266—269 (1954).

BOEHM, R.: Veratrin und Protoveratrin. In: Heffters Handbuch d. exper. Pharmakologie. Bd. 2, Teil 1, S. 249—282. Berlin: Springer 1920.

BORISON, H. L., FAIRBANKS, V. F.: Mechanism of Veratrum-induced emesis in the cat. J. Pharmacol. exp. Ther. **105**, 317—325 (1952).

BORISON, H. L., FAIRBANKS, V. F., WHITE, C. A.: Afferent reflex factors in Veriloid-induced hypotension. Arch. internat Pharmacodyn. **101**, 189—199 (1955).

BORISON, H. L., SAMPSON, S. R.: The vagal body: receptor site for emetic action of Veratrum alkaloids? Fed. Proc. **20**, 169 (1961).

BRODIE, T. G.: The immediate action of an intravenous injection of blood serum. J. Physiol. (Lond.) **26**, 48—71 (1900).

BRODIE, T. G., RUSSELL, A. E.: On reflex cardiac inhibition. J. Physiol. (Lond.) **26**, 92—106 (1900).

BRYANT, R. D., FLEMING, J. G.: Veratrum viride in the treatment of eclampsia: II. J. Amer. med. Ass. **115**, 1333—1339 (1940).

CRAIG, L. C., JACOBS, W. A.: The veratrine alkaloids. XIII. The dehydrogenation of protoveratrine. J. biol. Chem. **143**, 427—432 (1942).

CRAMER, W.: On the action of Veratrum viride. With some remarks on the interrelationship of the medullary centers. J. Pharmacol. exp. Ther. **7**, 63—82 (1915).

CRUMPTON, C. W., FRIEDLAND, C. K., KUO, P. T., SCHNABEL, T. G., JR., FOLTZ, E. L., PAGE, R. G., ALANIS, J., HAFKENSCHIEL, J. H.: The hemodynamic actions of protoveratrine in essential hypertension. J. clin. Invest. **30**, 634 (1951).

CURRENS, J. H., MCGINTY, J. F., KHAMBATTA, R. B., GORDON, I.: The effect of intravenous protoveratrine on digital pulse volume and digital skin temperature in hypertensive patients. Circulation **11**, 440—446 (1955).

CURRENS, J. H., MYERS, G. S., WHITE, P. D.: The use of protoveratrine in the treatment of hypertensive vascular disease. Amer. Heart J. **46**, 576—592 (1953).

CURRENS, J. H., REID, D. E., NEWELL, J. L.: Hypertension associated with pregnancy; incidence and treatment with particular reference to protoveratrine. J. Amer. med. Ass. **161**, 1232—1239 (1956).

CYON, E., LUDWIG, C.: Die Reflexe eines der sensiblen Nerven des Herzens auf die motorischen der Blutgefäße. Ber. üb. d. Verh. d. Königl. sächs. Ges. d. Wiss. zu Leipzig **18**, 307—328 (1866).

DAWES, G. S.: Studies on Veratrum alkaloids. VII. Receptor areas in the coronary arteries and elsewhere as revealed by the use of veratridine. J. Pharmacol. exp. Ther. **89**, 325—342 (1947).

DAWES, G. S., COMROE, J. H.: Chemoreflexes from the heart and lungs. Physiol. Rev. **34**, 167—201 (1954).

DONTAS, A. S.: Effects of protoveratrine, serotonin and ATP on afferent and splanchnic nerve activity. Circulation Res. **3**, 363—373 (1955).

DOUTHEIL, U., KRAMER, K.: Über die Differenzierung kreislaufregulierender Reflexe aus dem linken Herzen. Pflügers Arch. ges. Physiol. **269**, 114—129 (1959).

DOYLE, A. E., SMIRK, F. H.: The use of the pure Veratrum alkaloids neogermitrine and protoveratrine in hypertension. Brit. Heart J. **15**, 439—449 (1953).

DURAND, J., VORIDIS, E., SCÉBAT, L.: Action de la protovératrine sur l'hémodynamique circulatoire. Rev. franç. Ètud. clin. Biol. **2**, 1005—1012 (1957).

FARAH, A., MARESH, G.: Determination of the therapeutic, irregularity, and lethal doses of cardiac glycosides in the heart lung preparation of the dog. J. Pharmacol. exp. Ther. **92**, 32—42 (1948).

FERNÁNDEZ, E., CERLETTI, A.: Studies on the hypotensive mechanism of protoveratrine. Arch. internat. Pharmacodyn. **100**, 425—435 (1955).

FIESER, L. E., FIESER, M.: Steroids, p. 867—895. New York: Reinhold 1959.

FINNERTY, F. A., JR., FUCHS, G. J.: Veratrum treatment of toxemia of pregnancy: controlled study. Amer. J. Obstet. Gyn. **66**, 830—841 (1953).

FLACKE, W., BENFORADO, J. M., SWAINE, C. R., MOSIMANN, W.: Studies on Veratrum alkaloids. XXX. The action of some esters of germine on cardiac output and vascular tone with some observations on drug-induced decrease of positive inotropic sympathetic tone. J. Pharmacol. exp. Ther. **130**, 321—327 (1960).

GELLHORN, E.: Dependence of protoveratrine-induced hypotension on the hypothalamus. Proc. Soc. exp. Biol. (N. Y.) **97**, 400—402 (1958).

GOTH, A., HARRISON, F.: Influence of protoveratrine on effect of vasoactive drugs. Proc. Soc. exp. Biol. (N.Y.) **87**, 437—439 (1954).

GRAY, I. R., HAMER, N. A.: Protoveratrine A in treatment of hypertension. Brit. med. J. **5045**, 609—612 (1957).

HERRLINGER, R., KRUPP, J.: Albert von Bezold 1836—1868, ein Pionier der Kardiologie. Stuttgart: G. Fischer 1964.

HOOBLER, S. W., CORLEY, R. W.: The hypotensive action of protoveratrine. Univ. Michigan med. Bull. **16**, 362—368 (1950).

HOOBLER, S. W., CORLEY, R. W., KABZA, T. G., LOYKE, H. F.: Treatment of hypertension with oral protoveratrine. Ann. intern. Med. **37**, 465—481 (1952).

HOOBLER, S. W., KABZA, T. G., CORLEY, R. W.: The effect of protoveratrine on the cardiac output and on some regional circulations in man. J. clin. Invest. **34**, 559—564 (1955).

JACOBS, W. A., CRAIG, L. C.: The veratrine alkaloids. XIX. On protoveratrine and its alkamine protoverine. J. biol. Chem. **149**, 271—279 (1943).

JARISCH, A.: Vom Herzen ausgehende sensible Erregungen. Schriften der deutschen Akademie der Luftfahrtforschung **7**, 61—68 (1943).

JARISCH, A., HENZE, C.: Über Blutdrucksenkung durch chemische Erregung depressorischer Nerven. Naunyn-Schmiedebergs Arch. exp. Path. Pharmak. **187**, 706—730 (1937).

JARISCH, A., LANDGREN, S., NEIL, E., ZOTTERMAN, Y.: Impulse activity in the carotid sinus nerve following intra-carotid injection of potassium chloride, veratrine, sodium citrate, adenosin-triphosphate and dinitrophenol. Acta physiol. scand. **25**, 195—211 (1952).

JARISCH, A., RICHTER, H.: Die Kreislaufwirkung des Veratrins. Naunyn-Schmiedebergs Arch. exp. Path. Pharmak. **193**, 347—354 (1939a).

JARISCH, A., RICHTER, H.: Die afferenten Bahnen des Veratrineffektes in den Herznerven. Naunyn-Schmiedebergs Arch. exp. Path. Pharmak. **193**, 355—371 (1939b).

JARISCH, A., ZOTTERMAN, Y.: Depressor reflexes from the heart. Acta physiol. scand. **16**, 31—51 (1948).

KÄSER, O.: Die Behandlung der hypertensiven Spättoxikosen mit gefäßerweiternden Mitteln, insbesondere mit Protoveratrin. Schweiz. med. Wschr. **84**, 171—180 (1954).

KEELER, R. F.: Teratogenic compounds in Veratrum californicum (Durand). IX. Structure-activity relation. Teratology **3**, 169—174 (1970).

KEELER, R. F., BINNS, W.: Teratogenic compounds of Veratrum californicum (Durand). II. Production of ovine fetal cyclopia by fractions and alkaloid preparations. Canad. J. Biochem. **44**, 829—838 (1966).

KOCH-WESER, J.: Myocardial action of Veratrum alkaloids. Abstracts Internat. Pharmacol. Congress S. Paulo, Brazil 1966 No. 505.

KÖSTER, G., TSCHERMACK, A.: Über Ursprung und Endigung des N. depressor und N. laryngeus superior beim Kaninchen. Arch. Anat. u. Entwicklungsgesch. Suppl. 225—294 incl. Taf. I-XI (1902).

KRAMER, K.: Die afferente Innervation und die Reflexe von Herz und venösem System. Verhandl. Deutsch. Ges. Kreisl.-Forsch. 25. Tagung, p. 142—163. Darmstadt: Steinkopff 1959.

KRAYER, O.: Untersuchungen über die Kreislaufwirkung der Veratrumalkaloide. Naunyn-Schmiedebergs Arch. exp. Path. Pharmak. **209**, 405—420 (1950).

KRAYER, O.: Veratrum Alkaloids. In: DRILL, V. A. (Ed.): Pharmacology in Medicine. 2nd Ed. Chapter 34, 515—524. New York: McGraw-Hill 1958.

KRAYER, O.: The history of the Bezold-Jarisch Effekt. Naunyn-Schmiedebergs Arch. exp. Path. Pharmak. **240**, 361—368 (1961).

KRAYER, O., ACHESON, G. H.: The pharmacology of the Veratrum alkaloids. Physiol. Rev. **26**, 383—446 (1946).

KRAYER, O., KUPCHAN, S. M., DELIWALA, C. V., ROGERS, B. H.: Untersuchungen über die Veratrumalkaloide. XVIII. Die chemischen und pharmakologischen Beziehungen zwischen den Zygadenusalkaloiden und den Veratrumalkaloiden. Naunyn-Schmiedebergs Arch. exp. Path. Pharmak. **219**, 371—385 (1953).

KRAYER, O., MENDEZ, R.: Studies on Veratrum alkaloids. I. The action of veratrine upon the isolated mammalian heart. J. Pharmacol. exp. Ther. **74**, 350—364 (1942).

KRAYER, O., MOE, G.K., MENDEZ, R.: Studies on Veratrum alkaloids. VI. Protoveratrine: Its comparative toxicity and its circulatory action. J. Pharmacol. exp. Ther. **82**, 167—186 (1944).

KRUPP, R.J., PIERCE, C., FARRIS, C., JACOBS, A.: Protoveratrine in the treatment of toxemia of pregnancy. Amer. J. Obstet. **71**, 247—254 (1956).

KUPCHAN, S.M., AYRES, C.I.: Veratrum alkaloids. XXXIX. The structures of protoveratrine A and Protoveratrine B. J. Amer. Chem. Soc. **82**, 2252—2258 (1960).

KUPCHAN, S.M., BY, A.W.: Steroid Alkaloids: The Veratrum Group. In: MANSKE, R.H.F. (Ed.): Alkaloids. Vol. 10, p. 193—285. New York: Academic Press 1968.

KUPCHAN, S.M., FLACKE, W.E.: Hypotensive Veratrum Alkaloids. In: SCHLITTLER, E. (Ed.): Antihypertensive Agents. Vol. 7, p. 429—458. New York: Academic Press 1967.

KUPCHAN, S.M., FUJITA, E., GRIVAS, J.C., WEAVER, L.C.: Veratrum alkaloids. L. Structure-activity relationships in a series of synthetic hypotensive analogs of protoveratrine. J. Pharm. Sci. **51**, 1140—1144 (1962).

KUPCHAN, S.M., ZIMMERMAN, J.H., AFONSO, A.: The alkaloids and taxonomy of Veratrum and related genera. Lloydia **24**, 1—26 (1961).

LEHR, P.: Die Behandlung der Hypertonie mit Protoveratrin. Dtsch. Arch. klin. Med. **203**, 630—646 (1957).

LISSAUER, H.: Untersuchungen über die Wirkungen der Veratrumalkaloide. Naunyn-Schmiedebergs Arch. exp. Path. Pharmak. **23**, 36—76 (1887).

MARGOLIN, E.G., LEVINE, H.D., MERRILL, J.P.: Cardiac arrhythmias associated with protoveratrine. Amer. Heart J. **52**, 257—268 (1956).

MEILMAN, E.: The mechanism of protoveratrine-induced oliguria. J. clin. Invest. **31**, 649 (1952).

MEILMAN, E.: Clinical studies on Veratrum alkaloids. III. The effect of protoveratrine on renal function in man. J. clin. Invest. **32**, 80—89 (1953a).

MEILMAN, E.: Clinical studies on Veratrum alkaloids. IV. Use of protoveratrine in toxemia of pregnancy. J. Amer. med. Ass. **153**, 540—545 (1953b).

MEILMAN, E.: The management of hypertensive cardiovascular disease. Circulation **8**, 596—607 (1956).

MEILMAN, E., KRAYER, O.: Clinical studies on Veratrum alkaloids. I. The action of protoveratrine and veratridine in hypertension. Circulation **1**, 204—213 (1950).

MEILMAN, E., KRAYER, O.: Clinical studies on Veratrum alkaloids. II. The dose-response relations of protoveratrine in hypertension. Circulation **6**, 212—221 (1952).

MOE, G.K., BASSETT, D.L., KRAYER, O.: Studies on Veratrum alkaloids. V. The effect of veratridine and cevine upon the circulation in anesthetized dogs, with particular reference to femoral arterial flow. J. Pharmacol. exp. Ther. **80**, 272—284 (1944).

MOE, G.K., KRAYER, O.: Studies on Veratrum alkaloids. II. The action of veratridine and cevine upon the isolated mammalian heart. J. Pharmacol. exp. Ther. **77**, 220—228 (1943).

MYERS, G.S., FRIEDLICH, A.L., SCANNELL, J.G., O'NEILL, J.R., MCGINTY, J.F., CURRENS, J.H.: The hemodynamic effects of protoveratrine in hypertensive patients with congestive failure. Proc. New Engl. Cardiovasc. Soc. 4—7 (1951—1952).

NEIL, E.: Afferent impulse activity in cardiovascular receptor fibers. Physiol. Rev. **40**, Suppl. 4, 201—208 (1960).

NEIL, E., JOELS, N.: The impulse activity in cardiac afferent vagal fibres. Naunyn-Schmiedebergs Arch. exp. Path. Pharmak. **240**, 453—460 (1961).

PAINTAL, A.S.: A study of ventricular pressure receptors and their role in the Bezold reflex. Quarterly J. exp. Physiol. **40**, 348—363 (1955).

PAINTAL, A.S.: The influence of certain chemical substances on the initiation of sensory discharges in pulmonary and gastric stretch receptors and atrial receptors. J. Physiol. (Lond.) **135**, 486—510 (1957).

PAINTAL, A.S.: Vagal afferent fibres. Ergeb. Physiol. **52**, 74—156 (1963).

PAINTAL, A.S.: Effects of drugs on vertebrate mechanoreceptors. Pharmacol. Rev. **16**, 341—380 (1964).

PAINTAL, A.S.: Action of drugs on sensory nerve endings. Ann. Rev. Pharmacol. **11**, 231—240 (1971).

PENG, M. T., WANG, S. C.: Emetic responses of monkeys to apomorphine, hydergine, deslanoside and protoveratrine. Proc. Soc. exp. Biol. (N.Y.) **110**, 211—215 (1962).

POETHKE, W.: Die Alkaloide von Veratrum album. 1. Mitteilung: Darstellung der Alkaloide und ihre Verteilung in Rhizomen, Wurzeln und Blattbasen. — Germerin, ein neues Alkaloid von Veratrum album. Arch. Pharmazie **275**, 357—379 (1937a).

POETHKE, W.: Die Alkaloide von Veratrum album. 2. Mitteilung: Die einzelnen Alkaloide und ihre Beziehungen zueinander. Protoveratridin, Germerin, Protoveratrin. Arch. Pharmazie **275**, 571—599 (1937b).

POETHKE, W.: Die Alkaloide von Veratrum album. 3. Mitteilung: Jervin, Pseudojervin, Rubijervin. Einteilung der Alkaloide. Arch. Pharmazie **276**, 170—181 (1938).

REID, D.E.: Hypertensive (toxemic) pregnancy. In: A Textbook of Obstetrics, p. 785—791. Philadelphia, London: W.B. Saunders 1962.

REITER, M.: Über die inotrope Wirkung von Veratridin und Cevadin auf den Herzmuskel. Naunyn-Schmiedebergs Arch. exp. Path. Pharmak. **246**, 45 (1963).

RICHARDSON, A. P., WALKER, H. A., FARRAR, C. B., GRIFFITH, W., POUND, E., DAVIDSON, J. R.: The mechanism of the hypotensive action of Veratrum alkaloids. Proc. Soc. exp. Biol. (N.Y.) **79**, 79—85 (1952).

ROTHLIN, E., CERLETTI, A.: Pharmakologische Grundlagen der Therapie mit Veratrum-alkaloiden. Schweiz. med. Wschr. **84**, 137—142 (1954).

RUBIN, B., BURKE, J. C.: Bioassay of Veratrum viride. I. Effect of vergitryl on carotid sinus pressor reflex. J. Pharmacol. exp. Ther. **105**, 409—420 (1952).

SALZBERGER, G.: Über die Alkaloide der weißen Nieswurz (Veratrum album). Arch. Pharmazie **228**, 462—483 (1890).

SCHAEFER, H.: Central control of cardiac function. Physiol. Rev. **40**, Suppl. **4**, 213—231 (1960).

SCHAEFER, H.: Elektrophysiologie der Herznerven. Ergeb. Physiol. **46**, 71—125 (1950).

SIKKEL, A., WOLFF, J.: The use of protoveratrine in toxaemia of pregnancy. Gynaecologia (Basel) **147**, 42—62 (1959).

STRAUB, W.: Quantitative Untersuchung des Eindringens von Alkaloiden in lebende Zellen. Pflügers Arch. ges. Physiol. **98**, 233—240 (1903).

STRUGHOLD, Benzinger: See Jarisch, A. (1943), discussion.

SWISS, E. D.: The emetic properties of Veratrum derivatives. J. Pharmacol. exp. Ther. **104**, 76—86 (1952).

ULBRICHT, W.: The effect of veratridine on excitable membranes of nerve and muscle. Ergeb. Physiol. **61**, 18—71 (1969).

UVNÄS, B.: Sympathetic vasodilator outflow. Physiol. Rev. **34**, 608—618 (1954).

WANG, S. C., NGAI, S. H., GROSSMAN, R. G.: Mechanism of vasomotor action of Veratrum alkaloids: extravagal sites of action of Veriloid, protoveratrine, germitrine, neogermitrine, germerine, veratridine, and veratramine. J. Pharmacol. exp. Ther. **113**, 100—114 (1955).

WATTS EDEN, T.: Untersuchungen über die Wirkungen der Veratrumalkaloide. II. Über die Wirkungen des Protoveratrins. Naunyn-Schmiedebergs Arch. exp. Path. Pharmak. **29**, 440—472 (1892).

WEAVER, L. C., JONES, W. R., KUPCHAN, S. M.: Veratrum alkaloids. LI. Hypotensive-emetic relationships in the unanesthetized dog among analogs of protoveratrines. J. Pharm. Sci. **51**, 1144—1148 (1962).

WILBRANDT, R.: Behandlung der Hypertonie mit Protoveratrin. Schweiz. med. Wschr. **84**, 142—146 (1954).

WINER, B. M.: A comparison between protoveratrine A and protoveratrine B orally in arterial hypertension, a therapeutically important difference in activity. New Engl. J. Med. **255**, 1173—1179 (1956a).

WINER, B. M.: Studies of two pure Veratrum alkaloids, Protoveratrine A and Protoveratrine B. Circulation **14**, 1019 (1956b).

WINER, B. M.: Studies of pure Veratrum alkaloids, Protoveratrine A, Protoveratrine B, and Germitetrine B. Circulation **16**, 953 (1957).

WINER, B. M.: Comparative studies of protoveratrine A and protoveratrine B intravenously in hypertensive man. Circulation **22**, 1074—1082 (1960).

WINKLER, E. G., CANGELLO, V. W.: Protoveratrine in toxemia of pregnancy. Amer. J. Obstet. Gyn. **75**, 433—443 (1956).

Witzleb, E: Über die Wirkung des Veratrins auf die chemo- und pressoreceptorischen Aktionspotentiale im Carotissinusnerven. Pflügers Arch. ges. Physiol. **256**, 234—241 (1952).

Wyss, St., Spühler, O.: Protoveratrin in der Behandlung der Hypertonien. Acta med. scand. **153**, 221—236 (1956).

Zipf, H. F., Marquardt, H.: Zur Differenzierung der Wirkung verschiedener Veratrum-Alkaloide auf die Lungendehnungsreceptoren und auf die Atemtätigkeit. Naunyn-Schmiedebergs Arch. Pharmak. exp. Path. **254**, 287—300 (1966).

Chapter 13

The Clinical Pharmacology of Antihypertensive Drugs

J. A. OATES, M. E. CONOLLY, B. N. C. PRICHARD, D. G. SHAND, and G. SCHAPEL

I. Introduction

J. A. OATES and M. E. CONOLLY

The current drugs and strategy for treating hypertension are the result of truly remarkable advances during the past 20 years. The pathways to discovery of new antihypertensive drugs have been varied. The vasodilators were developed largely as a result of systematic searches for compounds that lower blood pressure in experimental animals. By contrast, there was no evidence from investigations in animals that the beta-adrenergic blockers, methyldopa, clonidine, or the oral diuretics could lower blood pressure. Importantly, each of these drugs had been developed for the purpose of affecting a biological system of sufficient importance to merit their investigation in man. Only after they were introduced into clinical investigation was their antihypertensive action discovered.

Parallelled with pharmacologic advances, there have been small but significant improvements in the understanding of the nature of essential hypertension. Important differences have emerged within the population labeled as "essential hypertension". Although the fundamental abnormalities in hypertension are far from clear, it is now possible to characterize subsets of the hypertensive population that respond differently to various classes of drugs, thus improving the rationale for selecting specific therapy for an individual patient.

For many patients, the optimal control of hypertension is dependent on the use of available agents in concert. By employing rational combinations of drugs that lower pressure by differing mechanisms, it is possible to achieve greater antihypertensive action with fewer side effects than with a single drug.

With an improved understanding of the pharmacokinetics and fate of antihypertensive drugs in man, it is possible to predict more precisely their accumulation, to establish a rationale for loading doses when needed, and to anticipate the expected differences in plasma levels achieved within the hypertensive population. Furthermore, knowledge of drug interactions that result in loss of blood pressure control can prevent patients from being unnecessarily deprived of needed reductions in blood pressure. The relationship between interindividual differences in metabolic pathways of drugs and susceptibility to toxicity provides a basis for safer selection of therapy in the future.

With the range of useful agents available and with present information to aid in selecting and combining drugs, the physician can offer patients an excellent prospect for preventing the cardiovascular complications of hypertension with minimal adverse effect on the quality of their lives.

II. The Guanidinium Adrenergic Neuron Blocking Drugs

J. A. OATES and M. E. CONOLLY

The prototype drug for this class is guanethidine. Following its successful employment in the treatment of hypertension, bethanidine, debrisoquin, and a number of other ring-substituted guanidiniums have been developed, all of which share the ability to lower blood pressure in man by inhibition of peripheral adrenergic transmission.

A. The Fate of these Drugs in Relation to their Use in Therapy

The highly selective effect of guanethidine and related drugs on adrenergic neurons results from the fact that these ring-substituted bases are substrates for the norepinephrine pump (MITCHELL and OATES, 1970). This energy requiring membrane transport system uniquely concentrates them at their site of action. Inhibition of the norepinephrine pump will prevent the uptake of these guanidiniums into the adrenergic neuron (BRODIE et al., 1965; MITCHELL and OATES, 1970), and thereby prevent their pharmacologic effect (STONE et al., 1964; LEISHMAN et al., 1963; MITCHELL et al., 1970). The concentration of these drugs within the adrenergic neuron is key to the kinetics of their distribution and disposition in man.

1. Distribution: Relation to Regimens for Drug Administration and Interaction with Other Drugs

a) Kinetics of Neuronal Storage in Man

Following its intravenous administration, guanethidine's elimination from the body is that of a multicompartmental distribution, (OATES et al., 1971 and KAUFMANN et al., to be published). There is an initial rapid phase of disposition dominated by removal of the drug from the plasma compartment, and two subsequent phases determined primarily by the rates of uptake into and release from extravascular pools. The late phase of disposition has a half-life of approximately 5 days and represents the phase when the other body pools have come into equilibrium with a pool that has the slowest net rate of removal. The half-life of the "late-phase pool" corresponds with the long duration of guanethidine's clinical action. Administration of protriptyline, which inhibits uptake of guanethidine into the neuronal pool, will substantially decrease the amount of drug eliminated during the late phase of disposition. Furthermore, amphetamine, known to release guanethidine from the adrenergic neuron (CHANG et al., 1965; SHAND et al., 1973), releases the drug from the late-phase pool. All of this evidence supports the concept that the late-phase pool represents primarily guanethidine stored in the adrenergic neuron and is therefore the pool that determines the kinetics of the drugs' pharmacologic effect in man.

The late phase of bethanidine's elimination has a half-life of approximately 12 h. This is considerably shorter than that of guanethidine, consistent with its shorter duration of clinical effect. The amount of bethanidine eliminated during the late phase also is decreased by protripytline (KAUFMANN et al., to be published).

b) Methods for Administration of Guanethidine to Patients, Based on the Kinetics of the Neuronal Pool

Because of the long half-life of the late-phase pool of guanethidine, repeated administration of the same daily dose will lead to accumulation in the late-phase pool to a much greater extent than other pools, and that pool will dominate the kinetics of the drug during maintenance therapy. If the pool with a half-life of 5 days were to totally dominate the kinetics of the pharmacologic effect, then initiation of therapy with a given daily maintenance dose should lead to slow accumulation of the drug in the late phase pool such that 90% of maximal pharmacologic effect would not be apparent for about 17 days, a lag period that approximates the delay in maximal antihypertensive effect seen when therapy is initiated with a given daily maintenance dose. With this type of accumulation kinetics, it was predicted that blood pressure reduction in patients with severe hypertension could be achieved more rapidly with guanethidine by a regimen for loading the drug to the desired level of effect prior to initiation of maintenance therapy at a much lower daily dose. Accordingly, a method has been devised for loading guanethidine in hospitalized patients urgently requiring reduction of blood pressure (Shand et al., 1975). The loading regimen recognizes that the nearly maximal effect from a single oral dose is not apparent for at least 6 h and that patients will differ in the amount of drug required during the load to satisfactorily reduce blood pressure. To design the load, it was necessary to predict a ratio of loading to maintenance doses. If the late phase pool with a half-life of 5 days were to totally dominate the kinetics at steady state, resembling a 1 compartment model, the loss of one-eighth of the drug in that pool daily would require its replacement with a maintenance dose of one-eighth of that in the body each day. Assuming that the actual kinetics would closely approximate this one compartment model, a fraction of one-seventh of the load lost daily was tested, and was found to be a practical prediction of daily loss, with the realization that accumulation in this multicompartmental system is far more complex than the one compartment model and that such a fraction is only a very useful clinical approximation.

Based on these assumptions, the guanethidine load is begun with a single dose of 75 mg, as this is equivalent to a maintenance dose of 10 mg; excessive reduction of blood pressure was not expected from this single dose and has not been observed. After the initial dose, the load is continued with subsequent doses of 25 to 30% of the total drug previously loaded, given at 6 hourly intervals during the day but omitting the dose that would fall in the middle of the night. The maximal single dose given during the load has been 150 mg. When blood pressure begins to fall, longer intervals between doses and smaller percentage increments are in order, and the determination of when the load is complete is based on the reduction of standing blood pressure to the desired level. When the load is completed, the amount in the body is approximated by estimating a loss of one-seventh of the drug present in the body each day. The maintenance dose is then calculated to be one-seventh of the amount in the body at the end of the load. The total amount of drug loaded to bring about reduction of blood pressure over a 2 to 3 day period has been 125 to 525 mg (uncorrected for elimination). A typical loading program would be as follows: Day 1 — 75 mg at 6 a.m., 25 mg at 12 m, 35 mg at 6 p.m.; Day 2 — 45 mg at 6 a.m., 60 mg at 12 m (noon), and discontinuation of the load when the standing blood pressure has fallen to desired levels by 6 p.m. A maintenance dose of 30 mg daily would be initiated about 1 day later. The clinical application of this loading regimen has extended the use of guanethidine to patients requiring reduction of blood pressure over a 1 to 3 day period and for those whose treatment is initiated by rapidly acting antihypertensives with the aim of discontinuing them as soon as adrenergic neuron blockade is achieved with guanethidine, which can then be continued for long term therapy.

c) *Drug Interactions in Man, Based on Altered Distribution to the Adrenergic Neuron*

a. Drugs that inhibit the norepinephrine pump in peripheral adrenergic neurons will antagonize the antihypertensive effects of the guanidinium adrenergic neuron blockers. The tricyclic antidepressants are competitive inhibitors of the norepinephrine pump, and it has been demonstrated in controlled studies that the antihypertensive effects of guanethidine, bethanidine, and debrisoquin in man are almost totally abolished by concomitant administration of tricyclic antidepressants such as desipramine (MITCHELL et al., 1970). The effect of bethanidine can be prevented for a week following the administration of as little as 50 mg of desipramine. Inhibition of the action of the guanidinium antihypertensives is produced also by imipramine (LEISHMAN et al., 1963), amitriptyline (MEYER et al., 1970), and even the least potent of the tricyclics, doxepin, when given in doses of more than 100 mg daily (FANN et al., 1971a). In patients with severe hypertension, the loss of control of blood pressure resulting from this drug interaction can lead to serious clinical complications such as the initiation of the malignant phase of hypertension.

Chlorpromazine is less potent as an inhibitor of the norepinephrine pump, but in the doses employed in psychiatric therapy, it too will antagonize the antihypertensive effects of guanethidine (FANN et al., 1971b). As chlorpromazine is a much less potent competitive inhibitor, its antagonism can be partially overcome by increasing the dose of guanethidine.

Drugs identified in animal studies as inhibitors of the norepinephrine pump must be evaluated in man to determine whether their potency and bioavailability combine to produce significant inhibition of the norepinephrine pump in patients in the doses used clinically. Inhibition of this transport mechanism in man may be evaluated in several ways. Significant blockade of the norepinephrine pump will antagonize the pressor response to the indirectly acting amine, tyramine, which must be transported into the adrenergic neuron in order to release norepinephrine. Thus, a rightward shift of partial dose-response curves to tyramine in man results from administration of desipramine, protriptyline, amitriptyline (MITCHELL et al., 1970), and doxepin (FANN et al., 1971a). The pressor response to norepinephrine itself must be measured concomitantly in order to exclude receptor blockade as a cause for reduced pressor sensitivity to tyramine. Inhibition of the norepinephrine pump can also be assessed by measuring the effect of drugs on the late-phase storage pool of guanethidine (OATES et al., 1971). The effect of plasma from patients receiving potential inhibitors of the norepinephrine pump on amine uptake into the rat iris, brain slices, or other tissues rich in adrenergic neurons can be used as an *in vitro* bioassay (BORGÅ et al., 1970). For evaluating directly the antagonism of the guanidinium antihypertensives, bethanidine is an optimal test drug; because of its more rapid turnover in the human adrenergic neuron, antagonism of its antihypertensive effect is seen more abruptly following blockade of the norepinephrine pump. Many of the drugs that inhibit the norepinephrine pump will also block amine uptake into platelets and cause a reduced level of the platelet serotonin after serotonin uptake in the platelets has been inhibited for a week or more (FANN et al., 1971). Whether the order of potency as inhibitors of the platelet amine pump corresponds with that for the norepinephrine pump in adrenergic neurons however, remains to be determined.

b. Amphetamine will release guanethidine from its storage sites in adrenergic neurons. Guanethidine levels in adrenergically innervated tissues are reduced by amphetamine administration (CHANG et al., 1965). Blockade of sympathetic nerves, such as that to the cat spleen, can be reversed by amphetamine (DAY and RAND,

1962), and the antihypertensive effect of guanethidine in man is antagonized within hours by administration of dextroamphetamine 10 mg (GULATI et al., 1966). We have shown that considerable release of guanethidine from the cat spleen by amphetamine is associated with a rapid antagonism of guanethidine's action on the splenic nerve (SHAND et al., 1973). Furthermore, the administration of amphetamine 10 mg, 3 times daily to patients will cause release of ^{3}H-guanethidine from the body in the late-phase of its elimination (OATES et al., 1971). This release, presumably from the neuronal pool, is associated with clinical antagonism of guanethidine's antihypertensive effect.

Antagonism of the effect of guanethidine by ephedrine probably results from release of guanethidine from the neuron terminal together with inhibition of its uptake into the neuron.

2. Delivery of the Adrenergic Neuron Blockers into the Systemic Circulation after Oral Administration

The delivery of orally administered guanethidine into the systemic circulation is incomplete. When administered as a powder and gelatin capsules, only about 50% of guanethidine is absorbed from the intestinal tract (RAHN and GOLDBERG, 1969). After absorption, metabolism during the first pass through the liver inactivates a significant fraction of the drug (MCMARTIN et al., 1970) but the amount removed by first pass metabolism has not been precisely quantified. Thus, a combination of incomplete absorbtion and appreciable first pass metabolism combine to yield only a fraction of orally administered guanethidine to the systemic circulation. Further studies to define precisely that fraction and its relation to dose and dosage form would be useful.

The absorbtion of orally administered bethanidine is nearly complete; following oral administration of ^{14}C bethandine, virtually all of the administered radioactivity is excreted in the urine in patients with normal renal function. Transformation of the drug during first pass metabolism has not been examined directly, but in light of evidence (see below) that metabolic clearance of this drug is low, it is unlikely that first pass metabolism causes any appreciable reduction in the amount of drug available to the systemic circulation. Thus, nearly all of orally administered bethandine reaches the systemic circulation as unchanged drug.

3. Disposition of the Guanidinium Adrenergic Neuron Blocking Drugs

a) *Guanethidine*

Our studies with intravenously administered guanethidine (KAUFMANN et al., to be published), and those of MCMARTIN et al. (1970) indicate that once guanethidine reaches the systemic circulation, approximately half of it is eliminated by renal excretion of the unchanged drug and half by metabolism. In the few patients where this has been measured, renal clearance of guanethidine has been found to be in the range of 200 to 400 ml/min suggesting that tubular secretion of the drug augments removal by glomerular filtration. Two major metabolites of guanethidine are excreted in the urine, guanethidine N-oxide and 2-(6-carboxyhexylamino) ethylguanidine (MCMARTIN et al., 1970).

b) *Bethanidine*

Following its intravenous administration, bethanidine is eliminated into the urine almost entirely as the unchanged molecule (KAUFMANN et al., to be published), indicating that renal excretion is the principal pathway of bethanidine elimination. Thus, renal failure is likely to prolong the effect and enhance the accumulation of bethanidine (DOYLE and MORLEY, 1965).

B. The Effects of Guanethidine on Sympathetic Reflexes and Cardiovascular Control in Man

Inhibition of sympathetic reflexes by guanethidine in man has been demonstrated by its blockade of the Valsalva overshoot (COHN et al., 1963). Interestingly, the increase in venous capacity produced by guanethidine does not occur as quickly after an intravenous dose as does blockade of the Valsalva reflex; on chronic therapy most but not all patients with blocked Valsalva reflexes exhibited blockade of the venoconstrictor reflexes as well. Associated with the inhibition of sympathetic reflexes is a slight drop in peripheral vascular resistance (COHN et al., 1963; RICHARDSON, 1960) which is remarkable in light of the rise in peripheral vascular resistance seen when blood pressure is lowered without inhibiting sympathetic reflexes.

In hypertensive patients without cardiac failure, the cardiac output is decreased acutely following intravenously administered guanethidine (COHN et al., 1963), an effect associated with a decrease in the filling pressure of the right heart which reflects the increase in venous capacitance. During chronic therapy, there is a reduction in the resting output that results from a diminished cardiac rate; stroke volume is not decreased (KAHLER et al., 1962; RICHARDSON et al., 1960).

Plasma volume is expanded by guanethidine treatment (MULHEIMS, 1962). Guanethidine may worsen cardiac failure in patients with cardiac disease (GAFFNEY and BRAUNWALD, 1964), and some hypertensive patients receiving guanethidine will retain sodium (SMITH, 1965), even to the point of developing cardiac failure (LEISHMAN et al., 1961). In addition, we have found that the acute reduction of elevated arterial pressure with bethanidine may be associated with profound sodium retention. The extent to which this results from removal of the sympathetic inotropic drive to the heart versus a decrease in glomerular filtration rate (RICHARDSON, 1960) is not clear. In normal subjects, however, the increase in plasma volume produced by guanethidine is not due to sodium retention; it is postulated that with the increased venous capacitance, blood moves from the extravascular compartment into the venous system as a result of lower capillary pressure produced by a decrease in postcapillary resistance (WEIL and CHIDSEY, 1968).

An additional consequence of the expanded plasma volume produced by guanethidine is the development of tolerance to the antihypertensive effect of guanethidine (LEISHMAN et al., 1961). Once sympathetic reflexes are inhibited, blood pressure becomes a direct function of blood volume (DUSTAN et al., 1972) Accordingly, the reduction of the intravascular volume by diuretics, low sodium diet, or both will augment the antihypertensive effect of guanethidine substantially.

C. The Spectrum of Clinical Effects

Selective distribution of these drugs to adrenergic neurons leads to a constellation of clinical effects that is highly targeted. Thus, interference with peripheral adrenergic transmission is the basis for most of its pharmacologic effects in man.

Consistent with the impaired peripheral adrenergic transmission and resultant blockade of the baroreceptor reflex, the greatest hypotensive effect is seen in the standing position. There is much less reduction of pressure in the supine position, and therefore guanethidine produces more orthostatic hypertension relative to any given reduction in supine pressure than does methyldopa (OATES et al., 1965) which interferes with sympathetic function by a different mechanism. Accordingly, when compared with methyldopa, guanethidine produces far more symptoms related to orthostatic hypotension and this is its most disagreeable effect for patients. Bethanidine resembles guanethidine in this regard (PRICHARD et al., 1968).

After exercise, arterial pressure often falls even lower than the standing pressure at rest. Severe hypotension may result. Exercise-related hypotension results primarily from the failure of peripheral resistance to rise reflexly during and after exercise (KHATRI and COHN, 1970). This inability to increase resistance is particularly likely to lead to hypotension immediately after upright leg exercise when dependent venous pooling leads to a decreased cardiac output.

As sexual ejaculation in the male is a sympathetic function, the guanidinium adrenergic blockers frequently prevent or delay ejaculation. This disturbing drug effect is much less of a problem with methyldopa (OATES et al., 1965). Diarrhea is commonly associated with the use of guanethidine, but occurs infrequently with effective doses of bethanidine (PRICHARD et al., 1968). Thus, guanethidine-induced diarrhea cannot be readily attributed to adrenergic neuron blockade. Sedation and fatigue, common unpleasant effects during treatment with methyldopa, are less troublesome with guanethidine and bethanidine; this probably results from the relatively poor distribution of guanethidine and bethanidine into the central nervous system. Furthermore, the remarkable concentration and persistence of the guanidinium adrenergic neuron blockers in peripheral adrenergic neurons achieves a pharmacologic effect with minimal exposure of other body tissues to the drugs. Therefore, specific organ toxicity and immunologic reactions are exceedingly rare.

III. Methyldopa

M. E. CONOLLY and J. A. OATES

A. Introduction

Methyldopa (α-methyl-dihydroxyphenylalanine, Aldomet) is one of the most widely used antihypertensive drugs. Its introduction into therapeutics followed the unexpected discovery of its hypotensive property made during a systematic study of aromatic amino L-acid decarboxylase-inhibitors in man (OATES et al., 1960). Following early studies indicating that blood pressure reduction was not the result of decarboxylase inhibition, more recent evidence localizes the hypotensive action to the central nervous system, mediated by α-methyl-norepinephrine, a false neurotransmitter resulting from biotransformation of methyldopa. An important feature of this drug is that the pressure reduction is almost as effective in the recumbent as in the standing position, and there is little further fall after exercise. The drug is generally well-tolerated; the most frequent side effects are related to its pharmacologic effects on the central nervous system.

B. Pharmacokinetics

1. Oral Administration

Absorption is rapid, incomplete, and variable, both from subject to subject and in the same subject on different days. In radiolabeled studies, renal elimination, which was essentially complete within 24 h, accounted for about 30 to 70% of the administered radioactivity (SJOERDSMA et al., 1963; BUHS et al., 1964; PRESCOTT et al., 1966; AU et al., 1972). Absorption, while influenced by numerous physiochemical factors within the lumen of the gut, may finally be effected by a stereospecific transport system (LIN et al., 1962) since AU et al. found only 8 to 13% of the administered ^{14}C to appear in the urine after administration of radiolabeled D-α-methyldopa. There are no data on biliary excretion of methyldopa in man, but the finding that all the fecal radioactivity is as unchanged methyldopa is compatible with this being entirely unabsorbed drug. Biliary excretion is known to be trivial in the rat (PORTER and TITUS, 1963).

After oral administration, peak plasma levels of methyldopa occur within 2 to 6 h. Doses of 0.5 to 1.0 G produced levels of 2 to 4 μg methyldopa/ml (SJOERDSMA et al., 1963; SAAVEDRA et al., 1974), the plasma content of ^{14}C being estimated as 2.5% of the dose at 2 h (PRESCOTT et al., 1966). There is no relationship between the plasma level of unchanged drug and its effect, nor does the time course of its effect (maximal at 3 to 8 h and lasting up to 24 h) reflect its short (1 to 1.5 h) plasma half-life. These findings are consistent with its action via an active metabolite.

Once absorbed, methyldopa is widely distributed throughout the body. Animal studies show that it is taken up and stored in peripheral adrenergic neurons (MUSCHOLL and MAITRE, 1963) and it also enters the central nervous system (CARLSSON and LINDQVIST, 1962). It undergoes biotransformation to α-methylnoradrenaline both centrally and peripherally. The observed depletion of tissue levels of noradrenaline is not due to inhibition of dopa decarboxylase (DAY and RAND, 1964) but to its stoichiometric displacement by α-methylnoradrenaline (CARLSSON and LINDQVIST, 1962). This compound accumulates in the storage granules, from which it may be displaced by nerve stimulation (MUSCHOLL and MAITRE, 1963; DAY and RAND, 1964) or by reserpine (AU et al., 1972).

L-α-methyldopa is extensively but variably metabolized in man (BUHS et al., 1964; PRESCOTT et al., 1966; AU et al., 1972). Following oral administration of labeled methyldopa, about one-third of the plasma radioactivity is as the sulphate conjugate of methyldopa, and this compound is also a major urinary metabolite. It accounts for 20 to 80% of the urinary radioactivity and a similar fraction is accounted for by unchanged methyldopa. Free and conjugated 3-0-methyl methyldopa make up to 0 to 15% of the urinary radioactivity. Decarboxylation gives rise to α-methyldopamine, which, with its 3-0-methylated derivative, accounts for up to 20% of urine radioactivity. Small amounts of 3-4-dihydroxyphenyl acetone have been detected. The active metabolite, α-methyl noradrenaline has also been found in the urine in quantities comparable to those of noradrenaline (MUSCHOLL and RAHN, 1966, 1968), and its continuing urinary excretion for several days after a single dose of methyldopa is consistent with the hypothesis that it is responsible for the hypotensive action that persists long after methyldopa itself has been eliminated.

2. Parenteral Administration

Few human studies are available. SJOERDSMA et al. (1963) found peak plasma levels after intravenous administration to be 5 to 8 times higher than after oral administration of the same dose. The plasma half-life of the unchanged drug was 1.4 to 1.8 h. GILLESPIE et al. (1962) gave intravenous infusions of up to 1000 mg, and consistently observed that the peak hypotensive effect occurred 6 to 8 h after administration.

The metabolic fate of methyldopa varies according to the route of administration. Following intravenous infusion of methyldopa, 86 to 94% of the drug was recovered unchanged in the urine. Less than 2% of the recovered drug was as α-methyldopamine. In contrast, following oral administration as noted previously, conjugation with sulphuric acid produces one of the major metabolites. These findings indicate that sulphate conjugation occurs primarily during the passage of methyldopa from the gut into the systemic circulation. This pattern of metabolism has been observed with another catechol, isoprenaline, which is conjugated with sulphuric acid during absorption, and this takes place primarily in the gut wall (CONOLLY et al., 1972b).

The foregoing observations on the metabolic fate of methyldopa have recently been confirmed and extended to compare the fate of parenteral methyldopa with that of the injected ethyl ester, α methyldopate (SAAVEDRA et al., 1974). Following oral dosing, the sulphate conjugate of methyldopa was found in large quantities in both plasma and urine. There was a considerable variation in the ability of different subjects to effect conjugation. Once again no correlation was noted between metabolic fate and pharmacologic effect.

Given parenterally, the esterified form of methyldopa was less effective than i.v. methyldopa in lowering the blood pressure, apparently because it fails to hydrolyse completely. Consequently only low levels of methyldopa are achieved. Physicians using this form of methyldopa (which is that normally supplied for intravenous use) should be aware of this difference, and adjust the dose accordingly.

C. Mechanism of Action

The current evidence indicates that the hypotensive action of methyldopa is mediated by its active metabolite, α-methylnorepinephrine, which acts within the central nervous system to attenuate efferent sympathetic signals to the resistance vessels. α-Methylnorepinephrine is synthesized from methyldopa within sympathetic neurons of the brain and peripheral nervous system, and is stored in neurosecretory vesicles, replacing norepinephrine on a stochiometric basis (CARLSSON and LINDQVIST, 1962). α-Methyl norepinephrine is released upon nerve stimulation (MUSCHOLL and MAITRE, 1963) and for this reason has been termed a "false-transmitter." In man, following a single dose of methyldopa, there is a reciprocal relationship between α-methylnorepinephrine and norepinephrine excretion in the urine that is consistent with its replacement of norepinephrine in the neurosecretory pool (MUSCHOLL and RAHN, 1968). Furthermore, these studies demonstrated a good correlation between the prolonged hypotensive effect of a single dose of methyldopa and an equivalent long persistence of α-methylnorepinephrine in the body.

There is little evidence that the replacement of norepinephrine by α-methylnorepinephrine in peripheral adrenergic neurons is responsible for the hypotensive effect of methyldopa. The majority of reports indicate that there is little difference between norepinephrine and α-methylnorepinephrine in their potency on adrenergic receptors (MUSCHOLL and MAITRE, 1963; TRINKER, 1971; NIES and SHAND, 1973). In experimental animals FINCH and HAEUSLER (1973) were not able to demonstrate impaired sympathetic nerve function after treatment with methyldopa. In addition, inhibition of the decarboxylase with an inhibitor acting only on the peripheral nervous system does not prevent the hypotensive action of methyldopa even though it blocks the peripheral (but not central) formation of α-methylnorepinephrine (HENNING, 1969).

In contrast, inhibition of either aromatic L-amino acid decarboxylase or dopamine β-oxidase within the central nervous system abolishes the hypotensive action of methyldopa (HENNING, 1969; DAY et al., 1973; FINCH and HAEUSLER, 1973). Furthermore, very small quantities of methyldopa (which would be without effect given systemically) into the central nervous system result in a fall in blood pressure. This has been accomplished either by direct application to the vasomotor centers in the region of the third and fourth ventricles (Heise and Kroneberg, 1972, 1973) or by injection into the vertebrobasilar arterial system (Henning, 1969). The integrity of central adrenergic neurons is a prerequisite for the action of methyldopa. Destruction of these by prior intra-ventricular administration of 6-hydroxydopamine virtually abolishes its hypotensive effect (Haeusler and Finch, 1973). It seems likely that α-methylnorepinephrine is released onto α-adrenergic receptors of the central blood pressure regulating mechanism to exert a depressor action (Heise and Kroneberg, 1972, 1973).

Renin output has been shown to be reduced by methyldopa (Mohammed et al., 1969). It seems certain that this also is centrally mediated. Although this could contribute to the reduction in blood pressure produced by methyldopa, the relationship between therapeutic efficacy and influence on plasma renin levels has not yet been evaluated.

D. Hemodynamic and Renal Effects

Numerous studies have been carried out to investigate the hemodynamic effects of acute oral and intravenous administration of methyldopa (Wilson et al., 1961; Gillespie et al., 1962; Onesti et al., 1964) and of chronic oral administration (Sannerstedt et al., 1962; Sannerstedt et al., 1963; Mohammed et al., 1968; Lund-Johansen, 1972).

Acute studies showed that after oral or intravenous administration of methyldopa (up to 2.5 and 1.25 G respectively) blood pressure fell gradually, reaching its lowest point between 3 to 10 h after the dose, returning to control levels by 24 h. These changes were accompanied by drowsiness and were characterized by a decrease in peripheral vascular resistance. Some laboratories also observed a reduction in heart rate and cardiac output. Cardiovascular reflexes are apparently modified by methyldopa. Thus, in some (but not all) patients the pressure overshoot of the Valsalva maneuver is reduced or abolished (Wilson et al., 1961; Dollery and Harington, 1962). When patients adopt a standing position there may be a further reduction in pressure, and the expected increase in peripheral resistance may not occur (Gillespie et al., 1962; Onesti et al., 1964). However, the orthostatic fall in pressure recorded in any of these studies rarely exceeded 18 mm Hg. Mason and Braunwald (1964) have demonstrated a reduced constrictor response in both arterial and venous beds in response to leg exercise and immersion of the opposite limb in ice cold water. Since there is little, if any, impairment of peripheral adrenergic neuron function in experimental animals during treatment with methyldopa (Finch and Haeusler, 1973), it is most likely that this modification of cardiovascular reflexes is produced by an effect of methyldopa within the central nervous system.

More prolonged studies have provided essentially similar data. Sannerstedt et al. (1962) also showed that the hemodynamic response to exercise was qualitatively normal, and there was no postexercise hypotension (*i.e.* the homeostatic reflexes remained intact). These latter findings were confirmed by Lund-Johansen (1972) although he was unable to demonstrate any consistent alteration of peripheral resistance after 12 months treatment with methyldopa. However, he used relatively low doses (average 896 mg/day) which produced low plasma levels, and only a modest overall reduction in blood pressure was achieved. These workers and others (Oates et al., 1965; Prichard and Gillam, 1969) have shown that during chronic treatment with methyldopa the increased hypotensive effect on standing is much less than that seen with the adrenergic neuron blocking drugs.

Acute and chronic studies (SANNERSTEDT et al., 1963; ONESTI et al., 1964; MOHAMMED et al., 1968) have shown that renal vascular resistance is also reduced so that despite the fall in blood pressure, the renal fraction of the cardiac output is unchanged, or may actually increase. In consequence, renal function is not impaired.

E. Relative Efficacy

Methyldopa has been the subject of a large number of clinical trials during the last 15 years (WILSON et al., 1961; GILLESPIE et al., 1962; ONESTI et al., 1964; OATES et al., 1965; MROCZEK et al., 1972; CONOLLY et al., 1972a). Many of the early studies compared it with other agents then available, whereas more recently methyldopa has been used as the yardstick against which newer agents have been measured.

GILLESPIE et al. (1962) reported 20 patients with initial diastolic pressures in excess of 110 mm Hg in whom the standing diastolic pressure was rapidly lowered to below 100 mm Hg and maintained at that level for up to nine months, using doses of 0.75 to 3.0 G/day. Twelve of these patients also received a diuretic. Two patients were unable to tolerate the required dose of methyldopa because of sedation. No patient developed tolerance to the hypotensive effect, although this has been observed elsewhere (PRESCOTT et al., 1966).

OATES et al. (1965) compared methyldopa with guanethidine and pargyline in 19 patients. An important feature in this trial, all too often neglected in such studies, is that it sought to compare equipotent doses of each drug. These patients had pretreatment diastolic pressure levels of 107 to 145 mm Hg and three had previously had accelerated hypertension. Comparison was based on an eight week period on each drug in a dose large enough to reduce the standing mean arterial pressure by at least 16.7%. On this basis, methyldopa in doses up to 3 G per day, proved as effective as the other two agents in lowering the standing pressure while at the same time producing significantly better control of the supine pressure than either pargyline or guanethidine.

Several recent trials have compared methyldopa with clonidine, since both drugs have in common a predominantly, if not exclusively, central mode of action.

MROCZEK et al. (1972) compared clonidine and methyldopa giving both in combination with chlorthalidone for a period of 12 weeks to 41 moderately or severely hypertensive patients. Methyldopa up to 3 G per day proved as effective in lowering the mean blood pressure in the sitting position as 1.8 mg clonidine.

CONOLLY et al. (1972a) compared clonidine and methyldopa in 13 patients with moderately severe hypertension who were receiving no other drug. In this study no arbitrary limit was placed on the dose to be used. They found methyldopa (average dose 4.15 G per day, range 0.75 to 10.0 G) as effective in lowering the pressure lying, standing, and after exercise, as clonidine (average dose 1.33 mg per day, range 0.33 to 4.2 mg).

F. Side-Effects and Toxicity

Side effects relate to methyldopa's known pharmacology. Their nature is predictable, though their incidence is not, for patients show wide interindividual differences in the dose they can tolerate. Furthermore, patients who prove intolerant to one drug (even to one as similar to methyldopa as clonidine is) may be able to tolerate an alternative (OATES et al., 1965; CONOLLY et al., 1972a). Unwanted effects related to its action on the central nervous system include sedation (which often improves spontaneously as therapy continues) and depression, which may be severe. Dryness of the mouth is more common than is generally realized. By analogy with clonidine (RAND et al., 1969) this may be central in origin. It is a more persistent side effect than sedation (CONOLLY et al., 1972a). Malfunction of the extrapyramidal system may also be induced. Tolerance to the hypotensive action has been described (PRESCOTT et al., 1966) but the mechanism of this loss of effect is unknown.

Unwanted peripheral effects of methyldopa are less common. In patients who depend on a high level of adrenergic tone to maintain myocardial contractility, methyldopa may precipitate cardiac failure. Since the function of peripheral adrenergic nerves is not affected to any degree in most patients, postural hypotension and failure of ejaculation are very rarely encountered. Impotence, which depends on parasympathetic function, cannot occur as a direct effect of methyldopa, but may be a secondary feature of methyldopa-induced depression.

Toxic effects of methyldopa are rarely serious, although there have been occasional fatalities (REHMAN et al., 1973; TOGHILL et al., 1974). Their mechanism is not understood; they are presumed to represent idiosyncratic reactions to the drug.

The most serious form of toxicity relates to hepatic damage. The illness runs a course that is often indistinguishable from viral hepatitis (ELKINGTON et al., 1969) but occasionally massive liver necrosis (SCHWEITZER and PETERS, 1974), sometimes ending fatally (HOYUMPA and CONNELL, 1973; REHMAN et al., 1973) has been encountered. Active chronic hepatitis has also been recorded (GOLDSTEIN et al., 1973). Recently TOGHILL et al. (1974) have described a series of 20 patients in whom there were features of all the above types of liver dysfunction, and also 1 patient presenting as cholestatic jaundice. Obstructive jaundice caused by methyldopa has also been described elsewhere (HOFFBRAND et al., 1974). It is not possible to discern a pattern of dosage or duration of therapy in these cases, but most serious hepatotoxicity could be avoided if liver function tests were performed during the interval of 2 to 4 weeks after starting the drug and at 3 months. In view of the fact that several of the reported fatalities have occurred after a second exposure to methyldopa in patients who had previously developed signs of hepatotoxicity, great care should be taken to avoid ever using methyldopa again in patients with this idiosyncrasy.

An unusual toxic reaction that occurs in about 20% of patients taking methyldopa is the development of a positive direct Coombs' test, which is due to the formation of an immunoglobulin (IgG) specific in most cases for the Rhesus antibody Rh_e (CARSTAIRS et al., 1966). Less than 1% of patients on methyldopa develop a frank hemolytic anemia, although about 5% show a raised reticulocyte count. The explanation for this reaction is not known. However, it has been shown to be a dose-related phenomenon which does not manifest itself until the patient has been taking methyldopa for at least 120 days. This suggests that methyldopa or some metabolite is somehow incorporated into the erythrocyte during hematopoiesis, and that fragments of these cells when broken down by the reticulo-endothelial system possess antigenic properties (WORLLEDGE et al., 1966; CARSTAIRS et al., 1966). Cross matching of blood is not hindered by this problem so long as the hematologist is made aware of its drug-induced origin. Withdrawal of methyldopa causes the Coombs' test to become negative after two to six months in most patients (BRECKENRIDGE et al., 1967).

Development of a positive Coombs' test does not necessarily occur in patients who develop hepatotoxicity, nor is hepatotoxicity usually accompanied by a positive Coombs' reaction.

Equally unrelated to the Coombs' status of these patients is the appearance of antinuclear factor in the serum, which is also related to methyldopa therapy, although it is not dose-related. There is a definite, though less clear cut relationship to duration of therapy (BRECKENRIDGE et al., 1967). These workers found no other evidence of lupus erythematosus, but three cases arising in patients on methyldopa have been reported elsewhere (SHERMAN et al., 1967).

Like most drugs, methyldopa produces occasional febrile reactions and skin rashes. No abnormality of pigment metabolism has been reported, although one patient with retinitis pigmentosa did complain of darkening of vision which cleared when the drug was withdrawn (CONOLLY et al., 1972b).

IV. Clonidine

M. E. CONOLLY and J. A. OATES

Unexpectedphar macologic effects are not always therapeutic disasters, as the history of the imidazoline derivative, clonidine, shows. As a group, the imidazolines have a wide range of pharmacologic activities. Some, such as naphazoline, have α-adrenergic vasoconstrictor effects which have lead to their use as nasal decongestants.

Clonidine (2-(2,6-dichlorophenylamino)-2-imidazoline hydrochloride; Catapres; Catapresan) was originally synthesized with such use in mind, and it caused considerable consternation when, after the nasal instillation of a few drops, the first two volunteers to receive clonidine became very sedated and also hypotensive (GRAUBNER and WOLF, 1966).

This chance finding triggered a larger number of investigations (EHRINGER, 1966; NAYLER et al., 1968; MCRAVEN et al., 1971; ONESTI et al., 1971) which have shown that clonidine is an effective hypotensive agent. It produces pressure control with little orthostatic or exercise-induced hypotension. Although the side-effects are few, some of them are signficiant. A striking feature of this drug is that it achieves its effect when given in only microgram doses.

A. Pharmacokinetics

A gas-chromatograph mass spectrometric assay for clonidine (DRAFFAN et al., 1975) has provided the sensitivity required for assessment of its kinetics in man. The drug is well absorbed, the bioavailable fraction of the dose ranging from 70.6 to 81.5% of an oral dose (DAVIES et al., 1977). The volume of distribution is high, ranging from 3.19 to 5.56 l/kg (DOLLERY et al., 1976). Following oral administration, 33.1 to 41.7% of the dose appears in the urine as unchanged clonidine in the first 24 h. After intravenous dosage 44.7 to 55.4% of the drug is excreted unchanged. In some subjects renal clearance exceeds glomerular filtration rate, suggesting that active renal tubular secretion of the drug takes place.

The metabolism of clonidine in man is still incompletely documented. Parahydroxy-clonidine has been tentatively identified in human urine (REHBINDER, 1970) and some of the excreted radioactivity is in the form of conjugates.

Peak plasma levels occur about 1 h after ingestion, levels of 1.35 ± 0.15 ng/ml being achieved after a single 300 μg dose. Plasma levels following intravenous dosage decline in a biexponential manner with rapid redistribution to the tissues ($t\ 1/2\alpha$ 2.2 to 28.7 min), and a slow elimination phase ($t\ 1/2\beta$ 6.9 to 11.1 h) which corresponds to the plasma half-life after oral dosage (5.2 to 13.0 h). The peak plasma concentrations reported in this study after oral administration were associated with substantial falls of blood pressure in normotensive individuals (−26/−16 mm Hg). Interestingly, with higher plasma levels, achieved after intravenous dosage in one subject, it was observed that no further pressure reduction was achieved with clonidine levels of 2 to 3 ng/ml, while above 3 ng/ml a paradoxical attenuation of the hypotensive effect emerged. This probably represents recruitment of a peripheral α-adrenoreceptor (vasoconstrictor) effect, and may indicate that the optimal hypotensive effect of clonidine may be obtainable only over a very narrow range of plasma concentrations. Consequently, further increases in the dose of clonidine in an attempt to improve pressure control could prove counter-productive.

B. Mechanism of Action

There is now a large body of data which shows that clonidine produces its hypotensive effects through its action on vasomotor centers in the brain stem, possibly via α-adrenergic mechanisms (Bolme and Fuxe, 1971; Schmitt et al., 1971), although it also has peripheral effects which may contribute to the overall response to chronic treatment with clonidine.

Intravenous injections of clonidine produce a brief initial rise in blood pressure which is due to a peripheral α-agonist action, and can be abolished by α-blocking drugs (Constantine and McShane, 1968). The pressor phase is accompanied by a bradycardia which persists throughout the longer hypotensive phase which follows.

It has been shown that hypotension can be produced by injections of very small doses into the cisterna magna (Kobinger, 1967), vertebral artery (Constantine and McShane, 1968), or cerebral ventricle (Sherman et al., 1968). Nayler et al. (1968) were able to prevent the hypotensive effect of clonidine by transection of the upper cervical cord combined with section of vagosympathetic trunks. Schmitt (1970) has shown that intravenous clonidine causes a supression of impulses in the sympathetic nerves, whose time course corresponds to the onset and offset of hypotension. In a recent study, Dollery and Reid (1973) have shown that pretreatment of rabbits with intracisternal 6-hydroxy-dopamine, which causes partial ablation of brain stem and spinal adrenergic neurons, reduces the bradycardia and hypotensive effect of clonidine.

Another effect probably produced by reduction of sympathetic activity at a central level is a fall in renin output, a function known to be influenced by the adrenergic innervation of the kidney.

Peripheral effects which may prove to be of importance in the long term reduction of blood pressure include the reduction of vascular smooth muscle responsiveness to a wide range of compounds including noradrenaline and angiotensin (Zaimis, 1970). Shaw et al. (1971) have shown a peripheral vasodilator effect for clonidine in animals with complete autonomic block.

Recently, clonidine has been shown to inhibit the release of noradrenaline from postganglionic sympathetic nerves when present in concentrations which might reasonably be expected to occur after normal therapeutic doses (Werner et al., 1972). However, since the Valsalva response is not modified by clonidine, the relevance of this observation is doubtful.

C. Hemodynamic Effects in Man

Numerous studies have now demonstrated that clonidine effectively lowers arterial pressure in hypertensive patients. An important feature of its action is that this is achieved without abolishing normal homeostatic mechanisms, so that standing and exercise are not accompanied by troublesome hypotension. A large number of workers, following several different experimental protocols, have provided an interesting picture of the clinical pharmacology of this drug.

1. Acute Intravenous Administration

Intravenous injection of clonidine produces a brief rise in blood pressure, followed by a period of hypotension lasting approximately 4 h. If a large enough dose is given, a fall in heart rate is seen. Cardiac output is reduced. A clear-cut reduction in peripheral resistance may not be seen, but the fact that it remains constant in the face of falling cardiac output and blood pressure indicates an attenuation of the reflex regulation of peripheral resistance.

Barnett and Cantor (1968) gave 150 μg clonidine intravenously to seven supine hypertensive patients. After a brief pressor phase there was a fall in pressure (average −34./−20 mm Hg). Cardiac output fell on average from 6.5 to 5.2 l/min and peripheral resistance increased marginally from a mean of 1791 to 1829 dynes/sec/cm^5.

McRaven et al. (1971) reported a similar study in eight hypertensive patients given two injections of 150 μg each, half an hour apart. Five of these patients showed an initial pressor response to the first injection after which in all eight an average pressure reduction of −26/−16 mm Hg occurred. The second injection reduced the pressure by a further −14/−7 mm Hg. The cardiac index fell from 2.78 to 2.31 and then to 2.10 l/min/m^2 after the two injections. There was a slight but significant reduction of heart rate (81 to 76 beats/min) only after the second injection. There was a significant reduction in left ventricular filling pressure as reflected by the pulmonary artery wedge pressure, and a (statistically non-significant) reduction of mean right atrial pressure. In light of these findings, and of other animal (Nayler et al., 1968) and human studies (Muir et al., 1969), these authors attributed the reduction in cardiac output to a reduction in venous return to the heart, consequent upon redistribution of blood volume to the venous capacitance bed, the latter being caused by the action of clonidine on brainstem vasomotor centers.

The influence of intravenous clonidine on the response to positional change and exercise have been reported by several groups. Barnett and Cantor (1968) in their studies on seven hypertensive patients found that after clonidine-induced hypotension had developed (average pressure reduction of −34/−14 mm Hg), tilting to 60° produced a further average pressure reduction of −26/−7 mm Hg (pretreatment, the mean fall on tilting was −11/0 mm Hg). Cardiac output fell by 1.1 l/min (pretreatment tilting causing a fall of 1.3 l/min) while peripheral resistance (2083 to 2100 dynes/sec/cm^5) was virtually unchanged (in the pretreatment examination there was a modest increase of from 1791 to 2186 dynes/s/cm^5).

In response to exercise in the supine position, blood pressure rose by 26/21 mm Hg (the pretreatment increase was 29/26 mm Hg). Cardiac output rose by 4.6 l/min (the pretreatment increase being 5.5 l/min) and total peripheral resistance fell from 1850 to 1148 dynes/sec/cm^5 (as compared with a fall of 2090 to 1418 dynes/sec/cm^5 before clonidine).

The response to the Valsalva maneuver was not altered by clonidine.

Muir et al. (1969) examined the response to exercise before and after clonidine in eight patients. They found that although the values for the parameters measured (blood pressure, cardiac index, heart rate, stroke volume, and total peripheral resistance) were at all times lower after clonidine, the changes seen on exercise were qualitatively entirely normal. Once again, the response to the Valsalva maneuver remained intact. This group also found evidence, in the form of reduced cardio-pulmonary blood volume, to suggest a redistribution of the total blood volume.

2. Oral Single-Dose Studies

Oral doses are predictably slower to act than intravenous injections, and do not have an initial pressor effect. However, the hemodynamic characteristics of the hypotensive phase are virtually identical.

ONESTI et al. (1971) investigated the effects of 300 to 750 μg of clonidine in seven hypertensive patients. Hypotension began from 30 min after dosing, and some effect persisted for up to 10 h. In the supine position, mean arterial pressure fell from 155 to 128 mm Hg (−17%) while cardiac output decreased from 5.9 to 4.7 l/min (−21%). The heart rate fell from 82 to 74 beats/min, but the calculated peripheral resistance was virtually unchanged (2160 and 2190 dynes/sec/cm^5). When these patients were tilted to 45°, further changes occurred. There was a greater fall in mean arterial pressure, from 151 to 101 mm Hg (−33%), while cardiac output fell from 4.5 to 3.8 l/min (−15%). Heart rate again declined (by 12 beats/min) but peripheral resistance, instead of rising in the pretreatment manner (+27%) actually fell slightly from 2194 to 2147 dynes/sec/cm^5. Renal blood flow was not significantly altered in either the supine or the erect position because the fall in arterial pressure was matched by a reduction of the renal vascular resistance (−15% in the supine studies and −30% in the erect). However, in both positions there was a sharp fall in sodium and chloride excretion, possibly because of changes in renal tubular handling of sodium as a result of the drop in renal perfusion pressure.

3. The Effects of Chronic Oral Therapy

SCHNEIDER (1968) reported a persistent reduction in arterial pressure and peripheral resistance. STENBERG et al. (1968) have indicated that the physiologic-adaptation to exercise is still present after treatment with clonidine for seven days. Similarly, maintenance of renal plasma flow and glomerular filtration rate after prolonged oral therapy has been reported (BOCK et al., 1966).

D. Renin Release and Catechol Amines

Adrenergic mechanisms are of great importance in regulating renin release, and since clonidine has major effects on adrenergic function, it might be anticipated that this drug would modify both catecholamine and renin release. This has been demonstrated by HÖKFELT et al. (1970) and ONESTI et al. (1971).

HÖKFELT and his colleagues have shown that clonidine therapy progressively reduces catecholamine levels in blood and urine of patients with hypertension of varying etiology though not in a patient with a pheochromocytoma, an observation recently confirmed (CONOLLY, unpublished data). Plasma renin and urinary aldosterone secretion rate also fell, taking several days to reach maximal suppression.

ONESTI et al. have also shown that after 4 days treatment with clonidine (400 μg/day) not only was the "supine" plasma renin activity reduced, but the increase normally seen on standing was markedly attenuated.

It seems probable that the reduction of renin and aldosterone are not direct effects of clonidine on renin-producing cells but are produced by the suppression of adrenergic activity, since renin and aldosterone secretion may actually be increased while the patient is receiving clonidine simply by introducing drastic dietary salt restriction. Furthermore, in patients with primary hyperaldosteronism, clonidine does not affect aldosterone output. Finally, ONESTI et al. have shown that clonidine (1 μg/kg) injected into the cisterna magna of the dog reduces renal vein renin markedly, whereas when given into a peripheral vein the same dose is without such effect.

Several groups (HOKFELT et al., 1970; CONOLLY et al., 1972; HUNYOR et al., 1973) have described a pheochromocytoma-like hypertensive crisis, which sometimes follows the abrupt cessation of clonidine therapy. In this situation there is evidence of marked adrenergic over-activity with high plasma and urinary catecholamines. This condition will subside spontaneously over 2 to 3 days, but may be rapidly reversed by reinstitution of clonidine therapy or administration of α-adrenergic blockers. The mechansim is unknown, but if, as has been suggested, clonidine exerts its hypotensive effect by a central α-agonist effect (BOLME and FUXE, 1971) it may be that sudden withdrawal may leave the relevant α-receptors hyposensitive to the endogenous stimulant, thereby permitting "rebound" overactivity.

E. Relative Efficacy

Clonidine has now been widely used in clinical medicine, either alone, or with a diuretic (SMET et al., 1969; ONESTI et al., 1971; MATHEW and PARKER, 1971). In other centers it has been compared with established antihypertensive drugs such as guanethidine (HOOBLER and SAGASTUME, 1970) or methyldopa (AMERY et al., 1970; PUTZEYS and HOOBLER, 1972; MROCZEK et al., 1972; CONOLLY et al., 1972).

The data now available indicate that clonidine is an effective drug in many patients, producing a sustained reduction in blood pressure throughout long periods of treatment. The pressure control is generally free from postural or exercise-induced hypotension. Side-effects, though troublesome in some patients, do not differ from those caused by other drugs (with the exception of the hypertensive crisis following abrupt withdrawal, mentioned above) and may be reduced by giving smaller doses of clonidine in combination with a diuretic.

If rapid reduction of blood pressure is required (*e.g.* in a patient presenting with accelerated hypertension) the use of clonidine by intramuscular injection (starting with a dose of 100 μg) may be considered as an alternative to established drugs such as reserpine, diazoxide, hydralazine, or pentolinium. When given intramuscularly it has no initial pressor effect, whereas, when given by the intravenous route, unless given slowly, this may occur (MROCZEK et al., 1973). Clonidine may be considered preferable to hydralazine or diazoxide in this situation in that its acute effects are not accompanied by an increase in cardiac output, but rather the reverse (BARNETT and CANTOR, 1968; ONESTI et al., 1971).

A clear picture of the efficacy of clonidine and its range of side effects emerges from the titrated-dose crossover comparison between it and methyldopa in 13 patients recently reported by CONOLLY et al. (1972). In this study both drugs were given in equipotent doses without arbitrary upper limits being fixed beforehand. The only indications for not increasing the dose further were the achievement of adequate pressure control or the development of unacceptable side effects. The average doses used were clonidine 1330 μg/day and methyldopa 4.15 G/day. Pretreatment pressures of 196/123 (standing), 201/121 (lying), and 196/109 (after exercise) were respectively reduced to 148/94, 162/97, and 160/91 by clonidine and 146/93, 156/95, and 151/88 by methyldopa. As in other trials sedation (8 on clonidine, 7 on methyldopa) and dry mouth (clonidine 12, methyldopa 8) were the commonest side effects. Not only were these side effects more frequent with clonidine, they were in general also more severe. However, in some cases it was observed that patients unable to tolerate methyldopa fared well on clonidine. There was some diminution of sedation with time, but dryness of the mouth was found to be a persistent symptom. During the trial, one patient became pregnant.

Termination of the pregnancy for reasons unrelated to her hypertension revealed a 10 week fetus with no detectable chromosomal or anatomical abnormality. Clonidine did not cause failure of ejaculation. Evidence of retinal damage during clonidine therapy was sought because of animal toxicity data, but was not found.

In the course of this trial, several patients, despite advice to the contrary, discontinued clonidine therapy abruptly, and in some cases this produced a rebound hypertensive crisis with features of adrenergic overactivity including severe hypertension in excess of pretreatment levels, tachycardia, and high plasma and urinary catecholamines. Considering the well-known problems with continuing compliance with antihypertensive drug regimens, this response to drug discontinuation can be expected to occur frequently. Furthermore, discontinuation of drugs in the context of emergency or elective surgery may cause this situation to arise under circumstances where it may not be recognized. Where clonidine has been continued parenterally throughout the period of surgery, this withdrawal effect has not been seen, and such patients tolerated anesthesia well. Since clonidine is normally well-absorbed from the gut, and presumably not extensively metabolized during first pass through the liver, the necessary parenteral dose was at least 70% of the normal oral dose.

During this trial no toxic effects were detected which could be attributed to clonidine. Hepatic and renal function were unaltered.

Other trials in which clonidine has been used alone (SMET et al., 1969; ONESTI et al., 1971; MATHEW and PARKER, 1971) or in which it has been compared with an established drug such as guanethidine (HOOBLER and SAGASTUME, 1970) or methyldopa (AMERY et al., 1970; PUTZEYS et al., 1972; MROCZEK et al., 1972) have yielded broadly similar results. Direct comparison with the data of CONOLLY et al. is difficult because most of the trials used clonidine in smaller relatively fixed doses, and in the majority of cases a diuretic was administered simultaneously. In the great majority of cases adequate pressure control was achieved by a dose of 1.5 to 3.0 mg per day when concomitant diuretic therapy was used. All studies noted the absence of significant postural and post exercise hypotension, sedation and dry mouth were common and persistent side effects, affecting at least 30% of patients. Tolerance to the hypotensive effect was rarely seen and responded to diuretics. No recognized toxic effects were encountered. Two pregnancies occurring in clonidine treated patients showed no evidence of teratogenicity.

F. Summary

Clonidine is a potent antihypertensive agent. It probably lowers blood pressure by an action on vasomotor centers within the brain, although the exact mechanism remains to be elucidated.

In clinical use it has been found to share with methyldopa the valuable property of lowering both lying and standing blood pressure equally. Also, like methyldopa, it does not produce exercise induced hypotension as it appears to leave homeostatic mechanisms intact.

Side effects are also central in origin. Chiefly they comprise sedation and dry mouth. If clonidine is used alone they may be persistent and troublesome, but if a lower dose of clonidine is combined with a diuretic, results acceptable to both patient and physician may be achieved.

The drug must not be stopped suddenly because of the hypertensive crisis which may result. If emergency situations prevent oral therapy, the intramuscular route may be used instead (not available in the United States). The drug is well-tolerated by patients under general anesthesia.

The scanty human data available suggest that clonidine does not damage the developing fetus.

Though not a drug of first choice in most patients, it is a useful alternative agent in patients in whom other drugs have failed. Despite the similarity of side effects as well as presumed mechanism of action, the patients who cannot tolerate methyldopa are not necessarily the same ones as those who will get severe side effects from clonidine.

V. Beta-Adrenoreceptor Blocking Drugs

B. N. C. PRICHARD, M. E. CONOLLY, D. G. SHAND, and J. A. OATES

A. Introduction

Since the original report of the use of pronethalol in the treatment of hypertension (PRICHARD, 1964) several other β-adrenoceptor blocking drugs have been developed. Most work has been performed with propranolol, first reports also appearing in 1964. Other β-adrenoceptor blocking drugs have subsequently been shown to possess antihypertensive activity and are now becoming generally available, *e.g.* alprenolol, oxprenolol, pindolol, while others are under clinical evaluation.

One feature of antihypertensive therapy with β-adrenergic blocking drugs has been the considerable interindividual variation in the dosage required to achieve a reduction in pressure. The earliest reports emphasize the importance of a flexible dosage regimen (PRICHARD and GILLIAM, 1964, 1966), with relatively high doses required to control the pressure in a subset of the hypertensive population. The several factors found to contribute to this interindividual variation in response will be considered in detail. Identification of groups of hypertensive patients that have responded differently to propranolol has had heuristic value in focusing on the difference in mechanisms whereby high arterial pressure is maintained in essential hypertension.

The weight of evidence indicates that the reduction in arterial pressure is the result of β-adrenergic receptor blockade. A variety of different molecular species that are β-blockers all produce a hypotensive effect, regardless of differences in "membrane stabilizing" activity or other properties. β-blockade in the juxtaglomerular apparatus, heart, and brain have each been postulated as contributors to the hypotensive effect. The current evidence for action via these mechanisms is evaluated, together with an identification of future research directions.

B. Pharmacokinetics and Metabolism

1. Propranolol

The recommended dose of propranolol varies widely, from as little as 10 to as much as 4000 mg daily (PRICHARD et al., 1969). Before such variation can be attributed to differences in sensitivity to the effects of the drug, individual differences in the drug's availability to the receptor must be considered. Propranolol is eliminated by metabolism (BOND, 1967) and is almost completely absorbed from the gut after oral administration (PATERSON et al., 1970). Despite its complete alimentary absorption, less than the administered dose reaches the systemic circulation after oral administration because much of the drug is removed from the portal blood by the liver during its passage from the gut to the systemic circulation. This presystemic (or first pass) effect is very important to the disposition of propranolol and results in different pharmacokinetics according to the route and duration of drug administration. After intravenous administration of therapeutic doses when portal venous drug concentration is relatively low, as much as 90% of the drug is removed during a single passage through the liver. This has been demonstrated directly in the anesthetized dog (SHAND et al., 1971; BRECKENRIDGE et al., 1973), and in the rat (SHAND et al., 1972). Although the hepatic extraction ratio has not been determined directly in man, the data are compatible with essentially complete extraction after intravenous administration (SHAND and RANGNO, 1972; EVANS et al., 1973). As might be predicted, small oral doses are also avidly extracted by the liver and their bioavailability is relatively poor. However, as the dose is increased, this avid extraction process becomes saturated and progressively more drug enters the circulation (SHAND and RANGNO, 1972). Furthermore, during chronic oral administration, the avid extraction process remains saturated during the usual 6 h dosage interval and drug accumulates to give circulating concentrations at steady state which are about two-fold greater than after the first dose (EVANS and SHAND, 1973a). Because the avid hepatic uptake process remains saturated during chronic oral administration, propranolol concentrations are a linear function of dose until with concentrations of 100 to 200 ng/ml at the end of the dosage interval where there is a proportionately greater increase in drug concentrations with dose, presumably due to some saturation of the drug metabolizing enzymes (EVANS and SHAND, 1973a). Despite the reduction in hepatic extraction ratio at steady state, it remains relatively high in absolute terms, indirect estimates of 0.55 to 0.72 being obtained (EVANS and SHAND, 1973b). Consequently, its half-life can be influenced by alterations in hepatic blood flow (NIES et al., 1973a; BRANCH et al., 1973). As a result of these kinetic differences, the half-life of propranolol is shortest after intravenous administration with an average of about 2.5 h (SHAND and RANGNO, 1972; EVANS et al., 1973), longer after a single oral dose, averaging 3.3 h (SHAND and RANGNO, 1972) and longest after discontinuing chronic oral medication when the half-life was about 4.5 h (EVANS and SHAND, 1973b).

The fact that propranolol undergoes considerable presystemic hepatic elimination during its transfer from the gut lumen to the systemic circulation accounts for its low bioavailability. There is also considerable variation in plasma concentrations when the same oral dose is administered to different individuals. Thus, a seven-fold variation in plasma concentrations is found after oral administration in normal subjects compared to only a two-fold difference following intravenous administration (SHAND et al., 1970). Such differences in bioavailability are even more striking in the clinical population, being up to 20-fold (SHAND, 1974). The low and variable oral bioavailability of drugs like propranolol is an unavoidable consequence of their high hepatic extraction ratio and the anatomical arrangement of the liver and its portal circulation (ROWLANDS, 1972; EVANS and SHAND, 1973b).

Interestingly, the two isomers of the drug are eliminated at different rates. In the seven subjects studied after a single oral dose (GEORGE et al., 1972), the *d*-isomer had a shorter half-life than either the racemate or the *l*-isomer. In addition, their data indicated no difference between the half-lives of the racemate and the *l*-isomer (though different doses were used). An explanation for this unusual finding has been provided in studies of the unanesthetized Rhesus monkey. In these experiments *dl*-propranolol reduced liver blood flow as a result of β-blockade while *d*-propranolol, which is devoid of such activity, did not (NIES et al., 1973a). As a result, *dl*-propranolol had a lesser clearance than *d*-propranolol because of the reduced hepatic blood flow (NIES et al., 1973b). The fact that the pharmacologic-effect of the *l*-isomer reduces its own clearance provides a ready explanation of the fact that the half-life of the racemate is not compounded of its two isomers, but is the same as that of the *l*-isomer. It should be mentioned that preliminary data in the anesthetized dog failed to show a significant difference in the steady state intravenous clearance of the two isomers (BRECKENRIDGE et al., 1973). This might be explained by the fact that the expected differences are only of the order of 30%, an effect which might be more difficult to detect in groups of dogs than in the within-animal studies in the monkey.

Another dispositional factor that could influence the response to propranolol is plasma protein binding. The effects of propranolol are reduced by plasma and are a predictable function of free, rather than total drug concentration. Plasma drug binding varies between 90 and 95% in normal subjects and as a consequence free drug concentration varies two-fold (EVANS et al., 1973). Because propranolol's effects as a competitive antagonist are a function of free drug concentration, such plasma binding differences should not produce a gross distortion of the relationship between total plasma concentration and drug efficacy, but could be responsible for the scatter in the data when groups of subjects are studied (COLTART and SHAND, 1970; BODEM et al., 1973). Recent studies indicate that the effects are indeed a function of free drug concentration in plasma and that true receptor sensitivity varies relatively little in normal subjects (SHAND et al., 1975). It should be mentioned, however, that the effects of disease on plasma propranolol binding have yet to be determined. The effects of variations in drug binding in the blood on the pharmacokinetics of this compound are interesting. Because the hepatic extraction ratio greatly exceeds the fraction of free drug in the blood, alterations in binding cannot affect drug clearance nor average steady state total blood concentrations. However, drug binding in the circulation does produce a proportionate reduction in the apparent volume of distribution. In this way drug binding shortens the half-life of the drug and accelerates drug elimination by delivering drug from the tissues to the liver, which can extract both bound and free forms. This is most clearly demonstrated after intravenous administration when drug clearance is relatively constant (EVANS et al., 1973). After oral administration drug half-life is determined by the variation both in plasma drug binding and in hepatic extraction ratio (EVANS and SHAND, 1973b).

The unchanged propranolol which reaches the systemic circulation is widely distributed to the tissues and the apparent volume of distribution is relatively large, of the order of 250 l (EVANS et al., 1973; EVANS and SHAND, 1973b). This is consistent with the finding in animals that the drug is concentrated in the lungs, liver, kidney, and in the brain (HAYES and COOPER, 1971).

The precise pathways of metabolism for propranolol have yet to be elucidated, but at least one active metabolite has been identified (4-hydroxypropranolol) whose formation depends on the route of administration. PATERSON et al. (1970) showed that this metabolite was formed after the administration of single oral doses, but could not be detected after intravenous drug administration. The metabolite 4-hydroxypropranolol is as active a β-blocking agent as propranolol and in addition possesses intrinsic sympathomimetic activity (FITZGERALD and O'DONNELL, 1971). Its presence accounts for the fact that a single oral dose produces a greater degree of β-blockade 2 h after administration for any given plasma propranolol concentration than is seen after intravenous administration when 4-hydroxypropranolol is not formed (COLTART and SHAND, 1970). However, the metabolite has a shorter half-life than the parent compound so that it has no apparent effect at the end of the usual 6-h dosage interval (CLEAVELAND and SHAND, 1972). In addition, these workers showed indirectly that during chronic oral administration most effects of the drug could be attributed to circulating propranolol, suggesting that either less active metabolite is formed, or that it is present in a much smaller proportion to the parent drug than after the single oral dose. This is compatible with the suggestion that 4-hydroxypropranolol is formed as the result of the saturation of its further metabolic conversion or of an alternative pathway (PATERSON et al., 1970) and with the fact that concentrations of propranolol itself accumulate during the attainment of steady state because of the saturation of an avid uptake process for the drug (EVANS and SHAND, 1973a). ZACEST and KOCH-WESER (1972) demonstrated two hypertensive populations with different total plasma level/response curves during chronic drug administration and suggested that the less sensitive group were not producing the active metabolite. While this might be true, such a difference could also be a function of altered plasma drug binding. Unfortunately all these studies are based on inference because technical difficulties prevented the chemical estimation of 4-hydroxypropranolol. While these problems will only be resolved when such methodology is developed, the fact that 4-hydroxypropranolol has a shorter half-life than the parent drug would seem to diminish its clinical importance as it is unlikely to have a significant effect at the end of 6 h. Consequently, the minimum effectiveness of the drug during chronic administration should be largely determined by the circulating concentrations of propranolol present at the end of the dosage interval.

The other major metabolite of propranolol so far identified is naphthoxylactic acid which accounts for 20% of an oral dose and 40% of an intravenous dose (PATERSON et al., 1970). Studies with radiolabeled drug have shown a further large fraction which moves as single peak on electrophoresis. Although mass spectrometry suggested that this might be a conjugate, none of the standard hydrolytic procedures have yielded free propranolol (HAYES and COOPER, 1971). Recently, however, WALLE and colleagues (1972) suggested that 81 to 94% of the circulating metabolites were in the form of a glucuronide conjugate. A number of other metabolites have been found (WALLE and GAFFNEY, 1972) including isopropylamine which possesses tyraminelike activity and propranolol glycol which is said to produce central nervous system depressant effects (SAELENS et al., 1974). The clinical significance of these many metabolites remains to be fully elucidated.

In summary, the disposition of propranolol is very complex, but a salient feature appears to be the large (20-fold) variation in circulating concentrations following the administration of the same oral dose to different individuals. Such variability is likely to contribute, at least in part, to the wide range in clinically effective dose.

2. Alprenolol

Orally administered alprenolol is almost completely absorbed from the gut (JOHANSSON et al., 1971). As with propranolol, a finite proportion of such a dose is extensively metabolized at first pass through the liver, so that doses below 50 mg may give rise to no measurable amounts of unchanged alprenolol in the plasma, while above that dose level, for every two-fold increase in dose, the plasma level of unchanged drug increases four- to six-fold (ABLAD et al., 1972). Extensive hepatic metabolism also explains why 50 mg alprenolol given orally produces no more β-blockade than 5 mg intravenously, and why, after oral administration, the ratio of unchanged drug to metabolites in plasma is so much lower than after intravenous dosing.

Alprenolol is lipid soluble and therefore achieves high concentrations relative to plasma in heart, lung, liver, and skeletal muscles (10 to 50-fold). This is reflected in the high apparent volume of distribution, of approximately 200-l. Peak plasma levels occur about 2 h after ingestion, and decline with a half-life of 1.7 to 2.0 h. Unlike propranolol, there is no significant difference between the half-life after oral and after intravenous administration, though the data available are derived from only a few subjects (JOHANSSON et al., unpublished, quoted by ÅBLAD et al., 1972).

ÅBLAD reported that there was an extremely wide (100-fold) variation in the degree of β-blockade produced by a given plasma level of alprenolol in the five subjects whom they studied. It has not yet been established whether or not there is a wide individual variation in plasma level for a given oral dose as well, but by analogy with propranolol it would seem likely that this would be the case.

3. Oxprenolol

Only one study in four normal subjects following 20 mg is available (RIESS et al., 1970). These data show a short half-life of the order of 2 h with a five-fold variation in the plasma concentrations attained.

4. Pindolol

Approximately 92% of an oral dose of pindolol is absorbed; peak plasma levels occur at 80 min after oral administration of 5 mg and showed a four-fold variation (GUGLER et al., 1974). TURNER and PEEL (1972) found a five-fold variation after 40 mg given as a single dose, but only two-fold variation after prolonged administration of 10 mg q.i.d. Pindolol has a plasma half-life of 3.6 (GUGLER et al., 1974) or 4 h (TURNER and PEEL, 1972) when administered orally, and 3.1 h (GUGLER et al., 1974) or 3.4 h (HICKS et al., 1972) when given intravenously. Less than 40% of the dose is excreted unchanged in the urine, regardless of the routine of administration, indicating extensive metabolism (GUGLER et al., 1974). About 90% of the metabolites are glucuronides and sulphates which are pharmacologically inactive (OHNHAUS et al., 1974). The half-life of pindolol was independent of renal function (OHNHAUS et al., 1974).

C. Relationship of Plasma Concentration to Effect

If plasma concentrations are to be of value in therapeutic management, there must be a definable relationship with the effects of the drug. Because β-adrenergic blocking drugs are competitive antagonists, their efficacy will depend as much on the strength of the stimulus as on the amount of circulating drug, and dosage requirements should be predictably different among patients with different levels of physical activity. As an initial approach COLTART and SHAND (1970) determined the maximally attainable reduction in heart rate with propranolol at various exercise grades in normal subjects. As predicted, the degree of blockade due to a given dose decreased with increasing work loads. Their most significant data were obtained during strenuous exercise, because the effects of vagal withdrawal on the heart rate response are then minimal. After intravenous propranolol administration, it was found that plasma levels of about 100 ng/ml were required to fully antagonize the heart rate response to exercise which produced heart rates of about 170 beats/min following placebo. Considering the shorter half-life and lesser significance of 4-hydroxypropranolol during chronic oral administration (CLEAVE-

LAND and SHAND, 1972), similar plasma levels should confer a very high degree β-blockade at the end of the usual 6-h dosage interval. This appeared also to be the case in the normal population studied by BODEM et al. (1973). As more data have accumulated, however, there appears to be a greater interindividual variation in the plasma level/effect relationship than was originally suggested. Using the isoproterenol dose ratios as an index of β-blockade, (ZACEST and KOCH-WESER, 1972) distinguished two populations of hypertensive patients which were different by about 2.5-fold in the plasma concentration required for a given effect during chronic oral administration. The greatest interindividual variation has been reported by GEORGE et al. (1973) following oral administration of single doses. Despite the fact that 4-hydroxypropranolol production would tend to make propranolol appear more potent, their data suggest that plasma levels greater then 200 to 300 ng/ml might be required for a maximal effect in some subjects. On the basis of these data it can be concluded that there is a good correlation between the effects of propranolol and its plasma concentration in the individual subject, but that there is a significant degree of individual variation, which could result from a number of factors including variable plasma protein binding and production of active metabolites as well as receptor sensitivity. After intravenous administration, variations in plasma binding and receptor sensitivity contributed equally to the differences in the effectiveness of any given total drug concentration (SHAND et al., 1975). Whether such variability is large enough to render total plasma level determinations useless in clinical management is unclear, but seems unlikely. At the present time, it is suggested that plasma concentrations of 100 ng/ml present at the end of a 6-h dosage interval should be associated with a very high degree of β-blockade, although they may not always result in a maximal effect in all patients. Plasma concentrations in the range of 50 to 100 ng/ml are also associated with a reduction in peripheral renin activity (MICHELAKIS and MCALLISTER, 1972). The potential value of plasma level determinations in the hypertensive patient will be discussed later.

Considering the other β-blocking drugs, ÅBLAD et al. (1972) could find no reasonable correlation of the effects of alprenolol with its plasma concentrations. With practolol, FITZGERALD and SCALES (1968) found that the reduction in exercise tachycardia was related to blood levels, the greatest effect being associated with 2 to 3 μg/ml. This was confirmed by BODEM et al. (1973), who found concentrations of 2.5 μg/ml to produce a maximal effect on exercise tachycardia, and by SCHNECK et al. (1972) who showed a significant effect with 2 μg/ml. Recently the β-blocking effects of pindolol have been shown to be a function of plasma concentration, 30 to 100 ng/ml producing a high degree of blockade of exercise heart rate (GUGLER et al., 1975). Obvious individual variation was again noted.

Although the half-lives of the β-blocking drugs are relatively short, their duration of action may be quite prolonged (OLSSON and VARNAUSKAS, 1973; AELLIG and SAMELI, 1973) as this is also dependent on the dose administered. MCDEVITT and SHAND (1975) have recently shown that for propranolol, duration of action after intravenous administration was appropriate for its half-life. If percent reduction of exercise tachycardia was used to measure effectiveness, this declined linearly with time when plasma levels declined exponentially. As a result, 20 mg i.v. would produce effects for 9 h, though the $T^1/_2$ was 3 h. Despite several suggestions to the contrary, there is to date no evidence that the duration of action of this group of drugs is unduly prolonged. It is clear, however, that if a sufficient dose is administered, their effects may last long enough to permit twice daily dosage (BERGLUND et al., 1973).

D. Efficacy in Hypertension

1. Propranolol

Several trials of the effects of propranolol in hypertension have been published. In assessing these data several problems are immediately apparent. There is little uniformity in study design, patient selection, drug dosage used, or the coadministration of diuretics. Considering the highly variable bioavailability of propranolol, it is unfortunate that few of the studies have incorporated plasma concentration determinations. The largest clinical experience comes from the open studies of PRICHARD and GILLAM (1969) and ZACHARIAS et al. (1972). Both of these groups adopted an extremely flexible approach to drug dosage which ranged from as little as 10 mg to as much as 4000 mg. All of the patients studied by ZACHARIAS et al. (1972) and about half of those studied by PRICHARD and GILLAM (1969) were receiving thiazide diuretics, many with potassium supplementation. The experience of these two groups drawn from over 400 patients was very similar; there were few side effects, a distinct advantage over other therapies. These workers considered that over 85% of patients would respond (with diastolic pressure lowering to less than 100 mm Hg) provided the dose was large enough. In this context, 60% of patients studied by ZACHARIAS and co-workers responded to less than 400 mg daily and 20% required more than 600 mg daily. Side effects were not a major problem in their study. Of the total 420 patients only 4 were withdrawn because of heart failure. Symptoms of reduced peripheral blood flow (cold extremities, chillblains, Raynauds disease, or worsening claudication) were experienced by 25 patients. Dizziness was as expected, very rare. Fifteen patients had troublesome dreams, 5 hallucinations, 9 insomnia and 12 complained of fatigue.

Perhaps the most important feature in these studies was the absence of postural and exercise hypotension. The only potent antihypertensive drugs had hitherto been the adrenergic neuron blocking drugs (*e.g.* guanethidine, bethanidine, debrisoquine) and methyldopa. Although there are important differences between them (OATES et al., 1965; PRICHARD et al., 1968; HEFFERNAN et al., 1971), these drugs worked by interfering with important cardiovascular homeostatic reflexes mediated largely by sympathetic vasoconstrictor fibers. The use of these drugs is therefore associated with a further fall in blood pressure on standing, on exercise, or in a hot environment. In contrast, no postural or exercise hypotension was seen in the use of β-adrenergic blockade in the treatment of hypertension (PRICHARD and GILLAM, 1969; or ZACHARIAS et al., 1972); this was confirmed by intraarterial studies. Neither was propranolol associated with an increased postural fall in blood pressure from an increased environmental temperature of 7° C to 30° C as was the case with bethanidine and guanethidine. The rise in blood pressure caused by vasoconstriction during the effort phase of Valsalva's maneuver was not impaired by propranolol in contrast to the reduced rise in pressure seen in the same patients on bethanidine, guanethidine, and methyldopa (PRICHARD et al., 1970). This data indicates that vasoconstrictor reflexes are intact during therapy with β-adrenoceptor blocking drugs.

From their clinical experience ZACHARIAS and COWEN (1970) selected 28 patients who had apparently responded to less than 320 mg daily and showed that the drug was indeed superior to placebo in lowering blood pressure. A smaller, controlled study by WAAL (1966) using doses up to 300 mg daily gave less uniformly successful results, only 30% of the patients being considered to be adequately controlled (as defined by a blood pressure of 140/95 or less).

Several groups have studied the effects of administering propranolol alone. Unfortunately in view of the clinical experience concerning dosage requirement, all of the early, controlled trials employed doses of 320 mg daily or less. PATTERSON and DOLLERY (1966) showed that doses of propranolol that did not exceed 240 mg daily were no better than 50 mg of hydrochlorthiazide in lowering blood pressure. It is interesting to note that these authors found for the most part patients who responded to propranolol did not respond to diuretics and vice versa. HUMPHREYS and DELVIN (1968) performed a double blind crossover comparison between propranolol and placebo in 18 Jamaican Negroes. Utilizing a maximum dose of propranolol of only 360 mg/day, they failed to demonstrate a statistically significant reduction in blood pressure. RICHARDSON et al. (1968) carried out a double blind crossover comparison of propranolol (using a fixed dose of only 120 mg/day) and chlorthalidone (100 mg/day), for five week periods. Two further five week periods were used for combined medication or placebo administration. Nineteen patients completed the trial. The average lying blood pressure during the placebo period was 172/107 mm Hg. This small dose of propranolol reduced the supine pressure by only 9/8 mm Hg and there was no progressive reduction in pressure during the five weeks. Chlorthalidone alone reduced the supine pressure by 23/9 mm Hg, and propranolol and chlorthalidone in combination produced a fall of 33/15 mm Hg. Subsequent studies show propranolol as well as other β-blockers are enhanced by concomitant therapy with a diuretic. In addition, the combination will yield efficacy in a larger fraction of the hypertensive population.

Five additional studies of the effects of propranolol alone are important because the authors have made some attempt to categorize their patient population. These studies (TAZARI et al., 1971; BÜHLER et al., 1972; LYDTIN et al., 1972; HANSSON, 1973; SHAND et al., 1975) will be described later during the discussion of the mechanism of action of propranolol.

2. Alprenolol

Alprenolol has not been as widely used as propranolol, but available data indicate that it is an effective hypotensive agent. FURBERG and MICHAELSON (1969) conducted a 12-week double blind crossover trial in 12 patients of alprenolol up to 400 mg/day, against a placebo. For the group as a whole the supine blood pressure after 12 weeks on placebo was 180/111 mm Hg, and after alprenolol 162/104. Only the reduction in systolic pressure achieved statistical significance. Mean systolic pressure during heavy exercise was also measured. At the end of the placebo period it was 264 mm Hg; it was significantly lower (236 mm Hg) at the end of the alprenolol period. TIBBLIN and ÅBLAD (1969) reported another double blind crossover study in 11 patients, comparing placebo with alprenolol in doses up to 400 mg/day for 8 to 12 weeks. The control lying pressure of 175/111 mm Hg did not differ from the pressure at the end of the placebo (176/110 mm Hg) but a significant reduction to 153/101 mm Hg was produced by alprenolol. The corresponding values in the standing position were 173/121, 171/121, and 152/108 mm Hg – again a significant reduction with alprenolol. Four of the patients studied showed a progressive and continuing fall in blood pressure throughout the alprenolol period, the final reduction in supine pressure being 36/23 mm Hg in this group. Of the 23 patients in these two studies, only 1 withdrew because of side effects. In that patient a marked fall in blood pressure was associated with an exacerbation of anginal pains.

3. Oxprenolol

LEISHMAN et al. (1970) conducted a trial of oxprenolol in 19 patients. Doses of up to 420 mg/day were used. The trial protocol used an open run-in period during which pressure was stabilized, afterward, on an out-patient basis, either oxprenolol or a placebo was given for four-week periods. The mean lying and standing pressures for the two treatment intervals were significantly different, those for the placebo being 173/102 and 165/106 mm Hg and for oxprenolol 160/99 and 151/99 mm Hg. The mean daily dose used was 320 mg/day. No patients suffered from side effects, but five were withdrawn before the double blind part of the trial because of inadequate pressure control, so that those remaining to complete the trial were necessarily preselected. TUCKMAN et al. (1972) reported the effect of oxprenolol in doses of 60 to 600 mg/day (average 374 mg daily) given in open fashion to 17 patients. Their data, reported as mean pressures, confirm that oxprenolol produces pressure reduction without orthostatic hypotension. Control lying and standing pressures were 140 and 139 mm Hg, and both were reduced to 127 mm Hg.

4. Practolol

Significant reduction in pressure by practolol has been demonstrated in double blind studies by LEISHMAN (1970) and PRICHARD (1971) and in a single blind study by ESLER and NESTEL (1973). In the latter study practolol did not reduce plasma renin activity in the supine position, even though the rise on tilting was attenuated. Practolol is no longer recommended for hypertension because of the oculo-mucocutaneous toxicity associated with long-term administration (WRIGHT, 1975 and FELIX et al., 1974). In most countries it has been withdrawn from the market.

It would have been useful to know whether this relatively "cardioselective" β-blocker could produce the same maximal hypotensive response as the more general β-blockers, such as propranolol. Unfortunately, such a dose ranging comparative study has not been done, nor has their relative effect in low-renin hypertension been evaluated. As there was an impression among some investigators that practolol could not achieve the same maximal reduction in blood pressure as propranolol, a comparison of propranolol with another cardioselective β-blocker might yield useful information on the mechanism underlying the hypotensive effect.

5. Pindolol

In a group of hypertensive patients known to respond to β-blocking drugs, pindolol 13 mg daily was approximately equivalent to propranolol 160 mg daily, or oxprenolol 200 mg a day (WAAL-MANNING, 1970), however, LAVER et al. (1974) found a one to five ratio for pindolol and propranolol.

Several subsequent trials have shown pindolol to be an effective hypotensive agent. FELTHAM et al. (1972) in an open study on double blind in 18 patients, used a dosage between 15 and 80 mg a day. In the double blind phase there was evidence of a delay in the maximum hypotensive effect, a lower blood pressure being observed after four weeks active treatment than after two weeks. THORPE (1972) used 15 to 60 mg daily (average 26 mg) in an open study in 20 patients. Subsequently, in a between subject comparison in 14 of the patients blood pressure in placebo ($n = 8$) averaged 182/100 mm Hg after two weeks of active treatment 150/92 mm Hg ($n = 6$) while after eight weeks active treatment 139/86 mm Hg. There was no decline in the blood pressure in the placebo group. MORGAN et al. (1972) obtained a good response in 59% of their series of 86 patients. In these 45 patients who responded, 39 required 30 mg a day or less, the other 10 between 30 and 50 mg, while increasing the dose to 80 mg a day did not effect the remainder. In four patients there was a rise in blood pressure with pindolol, a phenomenon observed by others (COLLINS and KING, 1972).

SIMPSON and WAAL-MANNING (1973) substituted pindolol for other antihypertensive drugs in 43 patients, continuing diuretic unless this was the only treatment used. Blood pressure control was better on pindolol with fewer side effects than in drugs which produced a postural fall in blood pressure. The average dose used was 15 mg a day and the investigators felt that an increase of the dose above 40 to 50 mg daily was not of value.

VAN COLLER (1973) in an open study in 30 patients suggested pindolol at a dosage of 5 mg or 15 mg t.i.d. was more effective than methyldopa 250 mg or 500 mg t.i.d. However these two dose regimes were rather rigid and the order of treatment was not randomized, methyldopa being administered first in all cases, thus no conclusions can be made regarding relatively efficacy. SCHAFFALITZKY DE MUCKADELL and GYNTELBERG (1973) performed a double blind crossover trial in 35 mild and moderately hypertensive patients in a fixed dose comparison used 5 mg b.d. of pindolol with 50 mg b.d. chlorthalidone. The blood pressures at rest on pindolol (157/105 mm Hg) were similar to those on chlorthalidone (157/106 mm Hg), however the systolic pressures on exercise were lower with pindolol (200/113 mm Hg) than on chlorthalidone (219/114 mm Hg). In this study while the dose of chlorthalidone may have been approximately optimum, this was not true for the dose of pindolol used.

LAVER et al. (1974), in a double blind variable dose study in 35 patients, compared pindolol (average dose 57.5 mg daily) with propranolol (average dose 289.3 mg daily) patients who received a diuretic throughout. The blood pressures on both drugs, pindolol supine 138/92 mm Hg, standing 132/90 mm Hg, and propranolol supine 137/90 mm Hg, standing 132/88 mm Hg, were similar. They found less postural effect than on previous treatment, which was methyldopa (average dose, 1160 mg daily) in 26 patients.

E. Combinations with Vasodilators and Other Drugs

In addition to its use alone or with diuretics, propranolol has also been used in combination with hydralazine. In this case the drug is used largely to prevent the reflex sympathetic increase in cardiac output and peripheral renin activity caused by hydralazine. ZACEST et al. (1972) have studied the effects of propranolol and hydralazine in 23 patients who were receiving stable doses of diuretics. They found that 80 to 160 mg of propranolol daily lowered supine and standing blood pressures. Additions of hydralazine produced a further fall in pressure without an increase in heart rate and diastolic pressures of <90 mm Hg were achieved in 17 of the 23 patients. Similar doses of hydralazine alone produced a lesser fall in blood pressure. While it is impossible to decide whether the effects of propranolol and hydralazine or diuretics were synergistic, they were at least additive and propranolol prevented the reflex tachycardia due to hydralazine. Similar results have been found using propranolol in combination with another vasodilator drug minoxidil (GILMORE et al., 1970; PETTINGER and MITCHELL, 1973). It is noteworthy that the doses of propranolol required with vasodilators do not exceed 240 mg daily and in the patients studied by ZACEST et al. (1972) plasma propranolol concentrations did not exceed 100 ng/ml.

There have also been reports of the combination of β-receptor blocking drugs and drugs inhibiting the action of vasoconstrictor nerves, either at the nerve endings or α-adrenoceptor site. DAY and PRICHARD (1971) reported the effects of the combinations of propranolol and methyldopa, and the sympathetic neuron inhibitory drug bethanidine with propranolol. The combination of propranolol with either methyldopa or bethanidine showed at least an additive, possibly a potentiating action. However, the combination of treatment was at the expense of some postural and exercise hypotension, absent on propranolol alone. The combination of the α-adrenoceptor drug phenoybenzamine with propranolol also resulted in a marked fall in blood pressure on assuming the erect posture (BEILIN and JUEL-JENSEN, 1972).

Labetolol is a β-adrenoceptor blocking drug which, in addition, possesses some α-receptor blocking activity, but less than a quarter that of β-blocking action (BOAKES et al., 1971). Our experience with this drug in the long-term treatment of hypertension indicates that many patients can be controlled without postural or exercise hypotension although this may be seen at large doses (PRICHARD and BOAKES, in preparation).

F. Adverse Effects

Unwanted side effects of β-blocking drugs may conveniently be subdivided into two main categories, namely those produced as a result of β-blockade, and those of a nonspecific or idiosyncratic nature. The most serious side effects are related to β-adrenergic blockade and include precipitation of heart failure, bronchospasm, brady-arrhythmia, and heart block. GREENBLATT and KOCH-WESER (1973) reported a 9.3% incidence of adverse reactions to propranolol in an in-patient population. Though no death occurred, one third of these reactions were considered life-threatening and were due to hypotension as a result of heart failure, often associated with profound bradycardia or heart block. Reactions were common in the elderly or in patients with an elevated BUN and tended to occur soon after beginning therapy.

Precipitate hypotension occurs rarely after oral propranolol. It has been reported in patients with cardiomyopathy (BETT, 1968; TAYLOR, 1968). It has occurred after intravenous propranolol (STEPHEN, 1966) and rarely after oral and intravenous practolol (WISEMAN, 1971). Mechanistically, if a patient is dependent on increased adrenergic drive to prevent the appearance of overt heart failure, then clearly β-adrenergic blockade with or without sodium retention may precipitate failure (DORPH and BINDER, 1969). If it be necessary to persist with β-blocking drugs, the failure which they precipitate may often be successfully held at bay with digitalis and diuretics. There is no evidence that any intrinsic sympathomimetic activity which some β-blockers possess is quantitatively of any significance in "making up" for the loss of adrenergic drive produced by their predominant β-blocking effect.

Hcart failure has been reported with β-adrenoreceptor blocking drugs that possess intrinsic sympathomimetic activity, with alprenolol (LUND-LARSEN and SIVERTSSEN, 1969; LYON and NEVINS, 1971), INPEA (DEL BIANCO et al., 1966), oxprenolol (BIANCHI et al., 1969; FORREST, 1972), and pronethalol (APTHORP et al., 1964). There is no any evidence that the direct membrane effect contributes significantly to heart failure.

The response to exercise depends in part on β-adrenergic mechanisms. β-blockade markedly reduces the capacity for an endurance time to heavy exercise, so that patients taking large doses of β-blocking drugs often complain of weakness and exercise intolerance. Intermittent claudication may be made worse.

Asthmatic patients are dependent to a large extent on adrenergic activity to maintain airway patency, and it has been shown that in these patients β-blockade will produce far greater bronchoconstriction than in normal subjects (MCNEILL,

1964). To some extent this problem may be avoided by the use of a selective β_1-blocker, eq. practolol, though the selectivity of this agent is not absolute, and it too may cause bronchoconstriction (WISEMAN, 1971).

Elevation of lowered blood sugar by glycogenolysis is mediated in part by β-receptors in man, and therefore β-blockade could theoretically interfere with this homeostatic mechanism. However, hypoglycemia is very rare but hypoglycemia due to insulin or oral hypoglycemic agents may be exaggerated in diabetics on propranolol. It may also occur in children recovering from anesthesia, and in patients with a partial gastrectomy (DOLLERY et al., 1969). Recently a case has been reported in which ketotic diabetic hyperglycemia was converted to hyperosmolar nonketotic hyperglycemia (PODOLSKY and PATTAVINA, 1973).

Propranolol readily crosses the blood brain barrier, and part of its hypotensive action may depend on this. Side effects of central origin include lack of concentration, loss of ambition, and depression. Confusion, blurring of vision, and visual hallucinations have rarely been reported. Disturbance of sleep patterns, and vivid dreams are not infrequent in patients taking large doses of propranolol. Practolol, despite its apparently much smaller ability to cross the blood brain barrier, has been reported to produce depression, lethargy, and vivid dreams. However, these are rare occurrences.

Nausea, vomiting, colic, and looseness of the bowels have been reported after large doses of propranolol (DOLLERY et al., 1969). Constipation is more common than diarrhea after practolol (WISEMAN, 1971). Skin rashes, purpura (with or without thrombocytopenia), paresthesia, and alopecia have been reported after propranolol.

Recently a number of severe sensitivity reactions have been reported with practolol: a systemic lupus syndrome (RAFTERY and DENMAN, 1973), dry eyes, corneal ulcers, skin lesions – particularly a psoriasiform eruption which may occur from 3 weeks up to 3 years (on average 10 months) after starting practolol (FELIX and DAHL, 1974), and sclerosing peritonitis (BROWN et al., 1974). These reactions mean that practolol should not be used long-term. Data relating to side effects caused by other β-blocking drugs are as yet scanty. In summary, adverse reactions are uncommon except with practolol, especially with correct patient selection (exclusion of heart failure and asthma). They tend to occur soon after initiation of therapy, even with small doses, but once therapy has been instituted, increasing drug dosage is unlikely to be associated with precipitate adverse reactions.

G. Hemodynamic Effects and Mechanism of Action

While it is evident that β-adrenergic blocking drugs can be effective antihypertensive agents, it is by no means clear how this effect is produced. There appears to be a strong case for linking β-blockade and antihypertensive activity. First, many β-blocking drugs are capable of causing some fall in blood pressure, regardless of whether or not they possess membrane stabilizing activity (PRICHARD, 1972; LEISHMAN et al., 1970; FURBERG and MICHAELSON, 1969; TIBBLIN and ABLAD, 1969). Second, PRICHARD (1971) has shown that d-propranolol, which has almost no β-blocking capacity (though retaining the membrane stabilizing activity of the l-isomer), has no hypotensive effect. Several mechanisms have been proposed on the basis of both human and animal studies and include: (1) resetting of the baroreceptors, (2) reduction in cardiac output, (3) reduction in peripheral renin activity, (4) peripheral adrenergic neuron blockade and (5) an effect on the central nervous system. The fact that so many potential mechanisms exist attests to the wide range of effects that these drugs produce and suggests that more than one mechanism might be responsible according to circumstance. The subject is one of more than academic interest since it is becoming evident that the diagnosis of essential hypertension encompasses several distinct pathophysiologic entities, thus raising the real possibility of more specific approaches to treatment.

Any proposed mechanism must explain the fact that β-adrenergic blockade has never been shown to lower the blood pressure acutely after intravenous administration. The many studies of the effects of propranolol during cardiac catherization have all shown an acute reduction of cardiac output and heart rate at rest, with no change in blood pressure and an elevation of total peripheral resistance (SOWTON and HAMER, 1966; WOLFSON et al., 1966; ROBIN et al., 1967; ULRYCH et al., 1968; PARKER et al., 1968; SONNENBLICK et al., 1968). During exercise, propranolol reduces the increase in rate, cardiac output, and blood pressure, but had little effect on peripheral resistance (EPSTEIN et al., 1965; SHINEBOURNE et al., 1967). The acute effects of alprenolol (FORSBERG and JOHNSON, 1967; WASSERMAN, 1970; KERBER et al., 1972) and oxprenolol (GRANDJEAN and RIVIER, 1968; TURNER and PEEL, 1970; TAYLOR et al., 1970) are essentially similar. The cardioselective agent practolol appears to produce a lesser fall in rate and cardiac output and essentially no acute effect on peripheral resistance and blood pressure (BRICK et al., 1968; FINEGAN et al., 1972; SOWTON et al., 1968). GIBSON and COLTART (1972) have suggested that this is due to the way in which cardioselective drugs tend to preserve significant peripheral circulatory β-sympathetic activity.

These acute effects of β-adrenergic blockade are in contrast with those following more prolonged administration. It should be mentioned that the acute drug effects have generally been followed for less than an hour, while the chronic data have generally been obtained after several weeks therapy. Thus, there are few data concerning the precise time course of the antihypertensive effects of these drugs.

PRICHARD and GILLAM (1969) observed that while most of the hypotensive effect of propranolol was seen within two weeks, it may take several weeks for the maximum hypotensive effect to be observed. They contrasted this delayed decline in pressure with its absence on bethanidine, guanethidine, or methyldopa. This later fall may not be seen in mild hypotensive patients. It is not confined to propranolol, it has been observed with pindolol (THORPE, 1972; FELTAM et al., 1972) and sotalol. In a small double blind trial of sotalol, from a group of patients in a larger open study, a significant fall of blood pressure was seen after two weeks active treatment following a period on placebo. However, after six weeks active treatment there was a further significant fall in blood pressure compared to the levels at two weeks (PRICHARD and BOAKES, 1974). Most workers have shown that most of the effect occurs by the next outpatient visit, usually in two weeks, therefore in some cases there were studies in patients with relatively mild hypertension (WAAL, 1966; BUHLER et al., 1972; ZACHARIAS and COHEN, 1970; LYDTIN, 1972). Clearly, further data concerning this point are required.

In patients who have responded to chronic oral administration of propranolol, it is apparent that while cardiac output remains low; the initially (that is following i.v. administration) raised peripheral resistance falls to predrug levels or lower (TARAZI and DUSTAN, 1972; PRICHARD et al., 1970). A series of 48 patients was studied (TARAZI and DUSTAN, 1972) during the administration of modest doses (up to 320 mg daily) for an average of 18 months. Those 26 patients who responded with a pressure reduction showed a fall in peripheral resistance when first studied two to four months after drug administration. The fall in resistance continued until at 18 months when it was an average of 2.2% lower than predrug values. In those patients who did not show a fall in blood pressure, total peripheral resistances remained elevated. These data strongly suggest an adaptive phenomenon underlying the favorable response. A similar study by LYDTIN et al. (1972) reported a somewhat different experience during nine weeks treatment with doses up to 1000 mg daily in 21 patients. These workers concluded that a favorable response could be expected to doses of up to 400 mg daily, but that no further effect would be anticipated by increasing the dosage. Furthermore, the antihypertensive response was well-correlated with the reduction in cardiac output, peripheral resistance being almost uniformly elevated. The discrepancy between these data and those of the Cleveland Clinic may well rest with differences in the populations studied. For example, the mean initial cardiac output of the patients studied by LYDTIN was 4.14 l/m^2, and 3.2 l/m^2 in the patients studied by TAZARI and DUSTAN. In addition, half of the patients studied by LYDTIN et al. (1972) were labile in that their blood pressure fell to below 95 mm Hg during the placebo period. At this time it seems impossible to come to a definitive conclusion concerning the role of a "hyperkinetic circulation" in determining the response of certain patients to apparently modest doses of the drug.

Perhaps the most thought-provoking study of the effects of propranolol in hypertension is that of BUHLER et al. (1972). These workers subdivided their patients according to their peripheral renin activity into high, normal, or low renin groups. All were treated with propranolol up to 540 mg daily and the lowering of blood pressure correlated with their initial plasma renin activity and its subsequent reduction during therapy. The three groups appeared similar regarding age, initial blood pressure, duration of treatment and average dose administered (2 mg/kg/day) Those patients (12) with initially high renin values responded with the greatest average fall in blood pressure and those with normal (23) renin activity with lesser pressure reductions. The 14 patients with initially low renin levels showed only a very small fall in blood pressure or none at all. Furthermore, there was a good correlation in all the patients between the fall in blood pressure and the reduction in circulating plasma renin activity. More recently this series has been expanded (BUHLER et al., 1973) to a total of 74 patients. Taking a diastolic pressure of 95 mm Hg or less as an indication of success, 53% of patients respond (74% in the high renin group, 66% in the normal renin group, and none in the low renin group). It has already been mentioned that with similar doses (up to 540 mg/day) and taking 100 mm Hg as adequate, ZACHARIAS et al. (1972) showed that about 60% of patients responded well. These two figures are not too discrepant when it is considered that the patients of ZACHARIAS et al. were receiving diuretics.

On the basis of their experience, Laragh's group suggested that propranolol constituted a specific therapy for patients with high renin hypertension. This was consistent with the known effects of propranolol in reducing plasma renin activity (WINER et al., 1969; MICHELAKIS and MCALLISTER, 1972), an action which is associated with modest doses. It is well-known that there are adrenergic mechanisms in the kidney which influence renin release (VANDER, 1965), and MICHELAKIS et al. (1969) have demonstrated that adrenaline, noradrenaline, and cyclic AMP can increase renin output from isolated renal cortical cells. Propranolol given intravenously has been shown to block or reduce the release of renin from the kidney when it is subjected to neural stimulation at a peripheral level (VANDER, 1965) or via medullary centers (PASSO et al., 1971). It may be that this effect of propranolol depends entirely upon peripheral (renal) β-receptors. However, other drugs, such as clonidine and possibly methyldopa, appear to lower renin output through their effect on central regulatory mechanisms. Further support for this hypothesis has come from studies of the effects of an antagonist to angiotensin II, which acutely lowered the blood pressure in eight patients with high plasma renin activity but not in four with low or normal renin activity (BRUNNER et al., 1973). A recent study (CASTENFORS et al., 1973) on 17 hypertensive patients treated with chlorthalidone and alprenolol has demonstrated an alprenolol-induced reduction in the erect plasma renin activity which correlated significantly with the additional fall in systolic and diastolic pressure produced by the β-blocking drug. The correlation between supine plasma renin and reduction in blood pressure was significant only for the diastolic values. Practolol has also been found to decrease the elevation in plasma renin in response to tilt (ESLER and NESTEL, 1973). However, there was no effect on supine renin and the antihypertensive effects of the drug were unrelated to the pretreatment renin values.

As noted elsewhere in this section, a delay has been observed between the institution of propranolol therapy and the development of maximum reduction of blood pressure. This delay may add plausibility to the hypothesis that propranolol lowers blood pressure by its effect on the renin-angiotensin-aldosterone system.

Despite the attractiveness of this hypothesis, the greater success rate with propranolol reported by the British workers (PRICHARD and GILLAM, 1969; ZACHARIAS and COGEN, 1972) suggests that even patients with low renin hypertension can respond, but that they might require larger drug doses. Unpublished data in eight of Prichard's patients receiving 400 to 2000 mg daily showed that lack of compliance or low bioavailability was not the cause of their high dosage requirements as plasma concentrations from 125 to 2000 ng/ml were detected at the end of the dosage interval (SHAND and PRICHARD unpublished observations). HANSSON has recently published material concerning the effects of propranolol in a series of 15 patients with normal or low plasma renin activity given no other medication (HANSSON, 1973). When given in doses of 160 or 320 mg daily for four weeks a significant antihypertensive effect was found compared to the initial four week placebo period. Interestingly plasma renin activity was markedly reduced, especially following tilt. However, the reduction in the renin did not correlate with either blood pressure reduction or plasma propranolol levels. By way of comparison, when modest doses were used, only 6 of the 15 patients achieved a diastolic pressure less than 90 mm Hg and 3 did not achieve diastolic pressures less than 100 mm Hg. Plasma propranolol levels were measured and there was a positive correlation between these and the reduction in systolic (though not diastolic pressure). Although individual plasma propranolol concentrations were not reported they were noted to be variable but averaged 123 ng/ml (68 ng/ml in the patients receiving 160 mg/day and 153 with 320 mg/day). The ten hospitalized patients studied by MICHELAKIS and MCALLISTER (1972) had relatively normal peripheral renin, which were lowered by doses up to 320 mg for six days. In only one patient who had the highest renin values was a significant, dose-related fall in blood pressure seen at 160 and 320 mg/day giving peak (2 h) plasma levels of 184 and 574 ng/ml. The other patients with plasma levels up to 200 ng/ml showed only very small blood pressure changes. More recently STOKES et al. (1974) studied nine patients using 240 mg/day propranolol together with a thiazide diuretic and found an adequate and significant antihypertensive response after 3 to 14 months. There was no significant correlation of this response with the reduction of plasma renin activity. Further, when another β-blocker, pindolol was substituted for propranolol, plasma renin levels increased significantly yet the blood pressure remained the same. Unfortunately, the measurements following pindolol substitution were made only 48 h later and it is as yet unclear how long it would take the blood pressure effect (as opposed to that on renin) to recover.

Recent work by VERNIORY et al. (1974) has also failed to show any correlation between plasma renin levels and the antihypertensive effect of sotalol. Moreover,

AMERY et al. (1974) found that atenolol a cardioselective β-adrenoceptor blocking drug without intrinsic sympathomimetic activity (BARRETT et al., 1973; GRAHAM et al., 1973), lowered blood pressure but did not reduce the recumbent plasma renin or affect the increase in plasma renin in response to tilting. Because a reduction in blood pressure is seen in almost all patients when the dose of propranolol is increased sufficiently, it might be speculated that the dose response curve to propranolol was shifted to the right in patients with low plasma renin activity.

The effect that the coadministration of diuretics may have is unclear as it is known that diuretic administration will elevate peripheral renin activity. MICHELAKIS and MCALLISTER (1972) showed that the renin suppressing effects of a given dose of propranolol could be overcome to some extent by sodium restriction. On the other hand, even modest doses of propranolol show an additive effect with diuretics (ZACEST et al., 1972). HOLLANDER (1973) has shown that propranolol (240 mg/day, will attenuate the hyperreninism due to both hydrochlorothiazide and hydralazine.

In this context, TARAZI et al. (1971) measured plasma volume in 14 hypertensive patients free of cardiac failure, whose blood pressure was controlled with 80 to 640 mg propranolol/day, over a period of 3 to 36 months. Out of 12 patients, 9 showed a measurable (greater than 8%) fall in plasma volume after 3 to 9 months, but this persisted for longer than a year in only 5 patients. The importance of this finding is uncertain, since hypertension was controlled in some patients in whom no reduction in plasma volume could be demonstrated. Furthermore, the acute administration of propranolol has been reported to reduce plasma volume without producing any fall in blood pressure (JULIUS et al., 1972). In another study by SEDERBERG-OLSEN and IBSEN (1972), no significant change in plasma volume was found though the extracellular fluid volume increased by 4.8% at the end of four months.

In studies on the effect of propranolol on the renal handling of sodium (EPSTEIN and BRAUNWALD, 1966) β-blockade appeared to alter the kidney's ability to eliminate sodium in the normal subject. The effect was a fall in daytime sodium excretion, with a compensatory increase in nocturnal sodium clearance so that overall, sodium retention did not occur. It was also observed that if, while taking propranolol, normal subjects were given added sodium each day, there was a delay in reestablishing equilibrium, though after a lag of several days, urinary sodium output "caught up" with the increased load. EPSTEIN and his colleagues found that sodium retention with fluid overload was precipitated only in those patients who were dependent on high adrenergic tone to avoid cardiac failure. SINGH et al. (1971) found that oxprenolol up to 240 mg/day would, like propranolol, reverse the day/night sodium excretion ratio, but unlike propranolol, when given four to ten days to patients with moderately severe cardic disease, it did not cause sodium retention. NIES et al. (1971) have suggested, on the basis of a series of experiments in the dog, that the fall in renal blood flow is merely part of the overall systemic adaptation to β-blockade and that the changes in sodium handling mentioned above may result from enhanced sodium reabsorption secondary to reduced peritubular blood flow. Clearly more data are required before judging whether diuretic therapy increases or decreases the number of patients responding to a given dose of propranolol.

There have been several observations in animals that might be taken to suggest a central mode of antihypertensive effect of β-receptor blocking drugs. Intraventricular propranolol in anesthetized cats has a hypotensive effect, an effect also seen with the (+)-isomer (KELLIHER and BUCKLEY, 1970). More recently a fall in blood pressure, preceded by a rise, has been demonstrated in conscious rabbits and in this case the (+)-isomer of propranolol (0.5 mg) produced no fall in pressure (DOLLERY et al., 1973). Intraarterial injection of propranolol (0.1 mg) into the carotid and vertebral vessels gave a more rapid fall of blood pressure than when injected into the femoral artery (STERN et al., 1971). However, the hypotensive action in these experiments was acute, unlike the effect seen in clinical use in man (PRICHARD and GILLAM, 1969). Any hypotensive action in animals shared by the (+)-isomer is unlikely to be of relevance in man as the (+)-isomer is devoid of hypotensive action (WAAL-MANNING, 1970; PRICHARD, 1970). Finally, practolol possesses a definite antihypertensive effect even though studies in the rat show little of the drug crossing the blood brain barrier (SCALES and COSGROVE, 1970).

Propranolol has been found to have adrenergic neuron-blocking properties, comparable to that of guanethidine according to DAY et al. (1968), but 1/6 to 1/20 the action of the guanethidine from the experiments of BARRETT and NUNN (1970). In addition, similar results were obtained with the (+)-isomer. The significance of these findings is uncertain because the concentrations of propranolol required to have an inhibitory effect are higher than those reached in the treatment of hypertension. There are two further reasons why this effect is unlikely to be of relevance in the treatment of hypertension. First the (+)-isomer is inactive as a hypotensive agent. Second the neuron-blocking drugs in the treatment of hypertension are associated with postural and exercise hypotension, and this is not a feature of the use of propranolol. The possibility that propranolol might alter the setting of the baroreceptor (PRICHARD and GILLAM, 1966) by either a peripheral or central mechanism remains, especially since the observation that peripheral resistance tends to return to predrug levels or lower. Experiments in dogs showed that pressor response to carotid occlusion is blunted by chronic propranolol therapy (DUNLOP and SHANKS, 1969). If chronic propranolol administration enhanced baroreceptor sensitivity, an acute reduction in carotid sinus pressure (from carotid occlusion) would leave more inhibitory impulses remaining than in the absence of chronic propranolol administration, and it is possible that with the higher afferent inhibitory traffic that an occulsion would result in a reduced rise in blood pressure. Human data suggest that baroreceptor reflexes in response to pressor effects are blunted in hypertension and that this reflex is enhanced modestly by propranolol in normals (SLEIGHT et al., 1971). However, the fact that atropine abolished the reflex change in the heart rate suggests that the sympathetic component is the lesser, at least in terms of rate changes. It may be noted, however, that preventing the vasopressor outflow by a central mechanism could come within the compass of the term "baroreceptor resetting".

Much of the controversy surrounding the mechanism of action of propranolol centers on the failure of several workers to confirm BUHLER'S original observation on the relationship between renin lowering and antihypertensive efficacy. It should be emphasized however that the conditions of that study have not been reproduced, either because the patients were not categorized as to renin status, a diuretic was added, or different doses were used. A more recent study by HOLLIFIELD et al. (1976) has confirmed that of BUHLER to the extent that modest doses of propranolol (up to 160 mg daily) giving plasma concentrations in the range of 50 to 100 ng/ml lowered the blood pressure only in patients with circulating renin; no antihypertensive effect was seen at these doses in low-renin essential hypertension. In addition, however, these workers investigated a full range of doses in both high- and low-renin patients. In high-renin patients a further lowering of pressure was achieved without a further fall in renin, suggesting a renin-independent effect. This was confirmed in low renin essential hypertensives whose pressure fell moderately with doses up to 960 mg daily giving plasma levels in the range of 170 to 400 ng/ml. Thus, these patients were less sensitive to any given plasma level than those with high renin. On this a dual mechanism of action was postulated: a low dose effect associated with renin-lowering and a high dose effect (possibly involving the central nervous system) independent of peripheral renin status. The effects of low doses on cardiac output might also contribute, especially in labile hypertensives. It was also clear that some overlap between the two dose response curves occurred, such that at doses of 160 to 320 mg daily some effect might be seen irrespective of renin status. This hypothesis at least has the merit of reconciling and explaining much of the conflict in the literature. The final answer will only come when the mechanism of propranolol in low renin essential hypertension is clearly defined.

Patient Selection and Management

There are two important contraindications to be observed in patient selection. Hypertensive patients with asthma should not be given a β-adrenoceptor blocking drug as airway resistance is increased. The use of cardioselective β-adrenoceptor blocking drugs still requires caution as there are not entirely cardiospecific and at higher dosage bronchial smooth muscle is affected. The presence of cardiac insufficiency is the second contraindication as in such instances cardiac output is critically dependent on an increased sympathetic drive to the heart. β-Adrenergic inhibition removes this compensatory mechanism so overt heart failure may be precipitated. This is likely to occur whether or not a β-adrenergic blocking drug possesses intrinsic sympathomimetic activity.

If plasma renin levels are known it would seem reasonable to begin with diuretics in low renin essential hypertensives, as these respond so well. If plasma renin activity is not suppressed, then β-adrenoceptor blocking drugs may be used alone in the first instance.

Many patients obtain an adequate hypotensive response from dosages up to 320 mg a day of propranolol. Nevertheless, a number of patients require much larger doses which lead to higher plasma levels. It is not possible to formulate a rigid dosage schedule; many investigators with various β-adrenoceptor blocking drugs have stressed the variability of the dosage that is required to control the blood pressure, but dosage variation of the same order is seen with other antihypertensive drugs. A diuretic should be added if β-blockers alone do not produce satisfactory control of the blood pressure. On occasions other drugs may be necessary. A variety are available, such as direct vasodilators, sympathetic neuron inhibitory drugs, or methyldopa.

Beta-adrenoceptor blocking drugs represent an important advance in treatment. They offer many advantages, notably lack of postural or exercise hypotension, unlike many other potent drugs. Provided some simple rules of patient selection exclude those in whom adverse affects of β-blockade are predictable, side effects are generally minor.

VI. The Direct Peripheral Vasodilators

G. SCHAPEL and J. A. OATES

These drugs reduce blood pressure by decreasing total peripheral resistance through relaxation of the smooth muscle in the walls of arterioles. Recently the combination of a β-adrenergic receptor-blocking drug with hydralazine, or its more potent analogue, minoxidil, has resulted in improved long-term patient acceptance (MOYER, 1953; HANSSON et al., 1971; ZACEST et al., 1972) and increased antihypertensive effectiveness by preventing the cardiac response and renin release resulting from reflex sympathetic discharge. Furthermore, the two potent parenteral vasodilator drugs, diazoxide and nitroprusside, currently provide the most potent therapeutic agents for dealing with hypertensive emergencies (GIFFORD, 1973; KOCH-WESER, 1974a, b).

1. Hydralazine

Since the discovery of hydralazine (1-hydrazinophthalazine) more than 25 years ago (GROSS et al., 1950), this agent has been the most widely used member of this family of drugs. Reduction in mean arterial pressure corresponds to plasma hydralazine concentration when β-adrenergic reflexes are blocked and sodium and water retention are prevented by diuretic therapy (ZACEST and KOCH-WESER, 1972). Plasma levels of hydralazine have been shown to be related to acetylation phenotype (PRICE et al., 1964; ZACEST and KOCH-WESER, 1972). Thus, the demonstration of higher plasma hydralazine levels in the slow acetylators of this drug appears, at least partly, to explain its variable effect with regard to both hypotensive response (ZACEST and KOCH-WESER, 1972) and the drug-induced lupus-like syndrome (PERRY et al., 1970).

Absorption of hydralazine is rapid and nearly complete, with peak plasma drug levels within 1 to 2 h of oral administration (LESSER et al., 1973 and 1974; ZAK et al., 1974). More than half the oral dose is metabolized presystemicly, suggesting a relatively high hepatic extraction of the drug. Acetylation appears to be a major determinant of the rate of hepatic removal of the drug and therefore its systemic availability (ZACEST and KOCH-WESER, 1972). Rapid acetylation results in a higher hepatic extraction ratio and greater "first-pass "elimination (GIBALDI et al., 1971). Thus, posthepatic plasma drug levels (the area under the plasma level curve) are lower in rapid compared to slow acetylators, despite similar plasma half-life and volume of distribution in both groups (REIDENBERG et al., 1973). The kinetics of distribution and elimination of the drug from the plasma compartment have been incompletely defined, perhaps in part as the result of limitations in the spectrophotometric assay. Measured over short time intervals, plasma half-life of the parent drug has been estimated to vary from 2 to 8 h (REIDENBERG et al., 1973; LESSER et al., 1974; ZAK et al., 1974). Measurements of plasma concentrations of total radioactivity show a disappearance curve with at least two distinct slopes, suggesting the possibility of a "deep pool" for the drug or one of its metabolites (LESSER et al., 1974). This is of interest in light of the extensive and persistent vascular-tissue binding found in the rat (MOORE-JONES and PERRY, 1966).

The clearance of hydralazine from the body is primarily by metabolic transformation. Thus, only a small fraction (3 to 14%) of hydralazine is excreted into the urine unchanged (ZAK et al., 1974). Because of the negligible role of renal elimination, the reports (PERRY et al., 1954; ZACEST and KOCH-WESER, 1972; REIDENBERG et al., 1973) of elevations in the levels of "apparent" hydralazine in renal failure must be viewed in light of the possibility that the relatively nonspecific analytic method for hydralazine could be measuring the accumulation of metabolites when their excretion is impaired. Hopefully improved methodology will resolve this question.

The mechanism by which hydralazine lowers blood pressure consists of direct depression of the myogenic tone of the precapillary resistance vessels, the arterioles (STUNKARD, 1954; ABLAD, 1963), possibly via an increase in arterial cyclic AMP (ANDERSSON, 1973). Results of experiments involving regional and systemic administration of the drug in the presence of interruption of sympathetic vascular innervation (Stunkard, 1954) have generally indicated more pronounced relaxation of the peripheral resistance vessels compared to the postcapillary capacitance vessels, resulting in net egress of filtration fluid into the extravascular space (Ablad, 1963). The increased cardiac index observed during hydralazine administration (Wilkinson et al., 1952; Freis et al., 1953; Rowe et al., 1955; Judson et al., 1956 and 1957) results from sympathetic stimulation of the heart via baroreceptor reflexes that increase stroke volume and heart rate, and probably also from the increased venous return that during chronic therapy may be partly independent of the sympathetic reflex activation. The increase in pulmonary artery pressure and elevated pulmonary vascular resistance seen in certain individuals (Wilkinson et al., 1952; Rowe et al., 1955; Judson et al., 1956 and 1957) may result from the hyperkinetic circulatory state coupled with a normally maintained venous return to the heart. In fact, pulmonary blood volume has been shown to be undiminished after hydralazine compared to that after sodium nitrite (Ablad, 1963).

The sometimes pronounced and frequent increase in renal (Reubi, 1950; Wilkinson et al., 1952; Judson et al., 1956) and hepatic-portal (Freis et al., 1953) blood flow can be explained on the basis of rapid vascular tissue uptake by these vascular beds (Moore-Jones and Perry, 1966; Lesser et al., 1974). This phenomenon, coupled with the bloodflow dependent kinetics of hydralazine, results in reduction of renal and hepatic vascular resistance with preferential distribution of the drug to these more highly vascular organs (Freis et al., 1953; Ablad, 1963).

Investigations on intravenously administered hydralazine in patients with essential hypertension suggest that a sympathetic stimulus is responsible for the increased release of renin by the kidney, since increase of renal venous renin activity was found to correlate with increase in heart rate, rather than the fall in mean arterial pressure, and since hydralazine administration to a renal transplant recipient was not associated with a significant rise of plasma renin activity (Ueda et al., 1970).

Soon after its introduction (Gross et al., 1950) hydralazine was found to be more effective in lowering blood pressure and better tolerated by patients when the chronotropic and inotropic response of the heart to the baroreceptor-mediated increase in sympathetic tone was diminished by surgical (Schroeder, 1951 and 1952) or pharmacologic (Freis et al., 1953; Moyer, 1953; Judson et al., 1956 and 1957) sympathectomy at various levels in the autonomic nervous system. More recently, the use of β-adrenergic blockers in combination with hydralazine (and a diuretic) has optimized its clinical utility (Hansson et al., 1971; Zacest et al., 1972; Berglund, 1973; Hansson and Zweiffler, 1973; Comerford and Pringle, 1974; Pape, 1974). Not only does β-blockade attenuate reflex adrenergic stimulation of the heart, but it also diminishes the adrenergically mediated release of renin with resultant enhancement of antihypertensive efficacy (Pettinger and Keeton, 1975).

Perhaps the main practical advantage of this antihypertensive drug combination is its preference over sympathoplegic drugs by patients (Hansson et al., 1971; Zacest et al., 1972). Because of smoother blood pressure control, with less postural hypotension and lack of sexual or intestinal disturbance, better patient compliance and therefore more effective and prolonged blood pressure lowering should be achieved in the majority of patients receiving this form of antihypertensive therapy.

The major potential adverse effect of hydralazine is a risk of developing a lupus erythymatosus-like syndrome. This is almost never a problem at doses of less than 200 mg daily, and progressively increases with increasing dosage above that amount (PERRY, 1973). The etiology may involve drug-induced altered immunity, or it may involve activation of a latent immune disorder (ALARCON-SEGOVIA, 1967; PERRY, 1973). The end result is certainly associated with abnormal immune responses, as evidenced by the demonstration of circulating antibodies to both hydralazine itself and native deoxyribose nucleic acid. The hydralazine lupus syndrome is rare in blacks. Fast acetylators appear to be at less risk for comparable drug dosage (PERRY, 1973). Acute fever within one to two weeks of exposure may precede more serious clinical toxicity, which is usually associated with the presence of circulating antinuclear antibodies after therapy with hydralazine for 3 to 20 months (PERRY, 1973). Furthermore, increased drug bioavailability associated with slow acetylator phenotype is suggested by the long-term finding of more effective blood pressure control and longer survival in the subset of patients exhibiting toxicity compared to a closely matched group without it (PERRY, 1973).

A somewhat different view has been proposed by investigators (ALARCON-SEGOVIA et al., 1967) who came into contact with this lupus syndrome as a result of referrals based on rheumatologic problems. The past and family history of such patients revealed features consistent with an underlying lupus diathesis in three-quarters of the toxic subset, which comprised 8 to 13% of a hypertensive population receiving large doses of hydralazine (ALARCON-SEGOVIA et al., 1967).

The long range cardiac effects of the hemodynamic changes induced by hydralazine are unknown. Whether cardiac morbidity and mortality are different when hydralazine is used to lower blood pressure as compared with the use of drugs that tend to decrease cardiac contractility is an important therapeutic question.

2. Minoxidil

Recently the orally active peripheral vasodilator, minoxidil, 6-amino-1,2-dihydro-1-hydroxy-2-imino-4-piperidinopyrimidine, has been shown to be a more potent antihypertensive agent than hydralazine in man (GOTTLIEB et al., 1972a). It has also been proposed as "an alternative to nephrectomy for refractory hypertension" (PETTINGER and MITCHELL, 1973). However, minoxidil is still an investigational drug. Currently its administration is restricted to patients whose hypertension fails to respond to maximal doses of conventional antihypertensive therapy, or whose renal function is being jeopardized by accelerating arteriolopathy (LIMAS and FREIS, 1973; PETTINGER and MITCHELL, 1973; DORMOIS et al., in press).

Information about the disposition of minoxidil in the human is limited to reports of studies of plasma, urine, and stool radioactivity following oral administration of ^{14}C-labeled drug to a relatively small number of hypertensive patients (GOTTLIEB et al., 1972b; CHIDSEY, 1973). Absorption was shown to be rapid, taking only one hour to achieve peak plasma levels of radioactivity. The majority of the radioactivity accumulated in the urine within 24 h, implying absorption of a large fraction of the administered dose (GOTTLIEB et al., 1972b). The average half-life for the exponential decline of plasma radioactivity, between 4 and 16 h postdose, was estimated to be slightly in excess of 4 h, in patients whose blood pressure had already been reduced by therapy with nonradioactive drug for 7 to 10 days (GOTTLIEB et al., 1972b). However, the plasma radioactivity was not monitored long enough to exclude a late phase of drug elimination, such as that which would be expected from a "deep pool" in equilibrium with drug in the body. The existence of such a deep vascular tissue pool of isotopically labeled parent compound, or active metabolite, seems likely in light of the demonstration of relative accumulation of radioactivity in the vascular tissue of the rat (PLUSS et al., 1972). It is also suggested by the persistence of the pharmacologic effect of hypotension for days in both the rat (DUCHARME et al., 1973) and man (SHEN et al., 1975), compared to the early plasma half-life measured in hours in both the rat (PLUSS et al., 1972) and man (GOTTLIEB et al., 1972b). A relative persistence of the drug in vascular tissue would explain why an effective therapeutic response with minoxidil can be achieved usually with a twice-daily dosage regimen (LIMAS and FREIS, 1973).

Initial elimination of minoxidil is primarily via metabolism (PLUSS et al., 1972; CHIDSEY, 1973). Although total body clearance has been estimated to approximate hepatic plasma flow (GOTTLIEB et al., 1972b; CHIDSEY, 1973), reliable values for both the clearance and volume of distribution of minoxidil cannot be derived from such data. Only one-tenth of the dose of oral drug could be identified in the urine as parent compound during the first 24-h collection, the remainder comprising a glucuronide and two other incompletely characterized metabolites (GOTTLIEB et al., 1972b; CHIDSEY, 1973). Cumulative urinary excretion of the total radioactivity, administered as ^{14}C-minoxidil, amounted to 95% of the dose over 6 days (GOTTLIEB et al., 1972b). However, further studies are required, involving a specific, chemical method for the identification of minoxidil and its metabolites in plasma, urine, and tissues.

A daily dose of 2 to 40 mg is usually effective in reducing blood pressure significantly to acceptable or normotensive levels, even in association with accelerated or malignant hypertension and significant impairment of creatinine clearance (GOTTLIEB et al., 1972a; LIMAS and FREIS, 1973: PETTINGER and MITCHELL, 1973; DORMOIS et al., in press). The degree of blood pressure reduction by minoxidil has been shown to be dose-related in rats, dogs, and monkeys (DUCHARME et al., 1973). Recently an individualized dosage regimen for minoxidil was proposed as a result of pharmacodynamic observations in man, which revealed that the loading-dose requirement and frequency of daily dosage were proportional to pretreatment mean arterial pressure, whereas the maintenance daily dose was probably unrelated to the severity of the initial hypertension (SHEN et al., 1975).

There was no significant alteration in the glomerular filtration rate of hypertensive patients taking minoxidil for 7 to 14 days, although a small increase in effective renal plasma flow was observed (GOTTLIEB et al., 1972a). This effect on human renal hemodynamic parameters indicates a diminished filtration fraction, consistent with the intrarenal redistribution of blood flow from the outer to the juxtamedullary cortex observed in conscious dogs treated with minoxidil (HUMPHREY et al., 1974). Some clinical investigators have documented markedly diminished urinary sodium excretion with progressive sodium retention, amounting to 20 to 40 mEq daily, and proportional weight gain, even in the absence of renal impairment (GILMORE et al., 1970; GOTTLIEB et al., 1972a), ending in a prompt diuresis on cessation of the drug (GILMORE et al., 1970). The phenomenon is probably caused by excessive sodium reabsorption from the proximal renal tubular fluid. This explanation is supported by the 60 to 80% reduction in fractional volume clearance associated with unaltered fractional free water and sodium clearances in dogs treated with minoxidil or hydralazine, but not in dogs in which similar hypotension was produced by blocking adrenergic reflexes with guanethidine (HUMPHREY et al., 1971). When diuretics are given concomitantly, sodium and fluid retention usually have not been clinically significant problems in patients with relatively normal creatinine clearance (GILMORE et al., 1970; GOTTLIEB et al., 1972a; CHIDSEY, 1973). However, in patients with renal insufficiency, sometimes quite large doses of the more potent loop diuretic, furosemide, have failed to control progressive edema formation and congestive heart failure. Such massive retention of fluid required cessation of minoxidil in two and dialysis in one of 26 patients studied in our unit; this group was characterized by moderate renal failure (half the patients had serum creatinine concentrations greater than 4 mg/dl prior to minoxidil therapy) (DORMOIS et al., in press).

Pulmonary hypertension has been observed in some minoxidil-treated patients (DORMOIS et al., in press). Despite adequate propranolol dosage documented by determination of levels of the drug in blood, these patients exhibited features of high-output, right-sided heart failure and gross fluid overload (DORMOIS et al., in press). It is not yet clear whether such pulmonary hypertension is predominantly due to high cardiac output or to inappropriately high pulmonary vascular resistance. Nor is it evident whether this right-sided cardiac syndrome and some reported instances of pericardial tamponade, while on minoxidil, are etiologically related to the hemorrhagic degenerative lesion observed in the right atrium of dogs on a dose of 20 mg/kg for one month (DUCHARME et al., 1973).

Plasma renin activity has been shown to increase as a result of minoxidil therapy (GOTTLIEB et al., 1972a; VELASCO et al., 1974; PETTINGER and MITCHELL, 1975; DORMOIS et al., in press). Investigation of the effect of renin suppression by propranolol in a minoxidil-treated patient, presenting with accelerated hypertension and a total cervicothoracolumbar sympathectomy one year earlier, suggested that propranolol was contributing to the reduction of blood pressure via renin suppression, rather than solely by blocking sympathetic stimulation of the heart (DORMOIS et al., in press). The differential effect of propranolol on heart rate and plasma renin activity was examined by a controlled study of nine essentially hypertensive patients whose blood pressure had been significantly lowered by minoxidil (VELASCO et al., 1974). Plasma propranolol concentration correlated with degree of bradycardia, whereas it correlated with fractional decrease of plasma renin activity only at plasma drug concentrations of 60 ng/ml or less (VELASCO et al., 1974), corresponding to a daily oral propranolol dose of 80 to 160 mg (MICHELAKIS and MCALLISTER, 1972). Either 60 ng/ml produces maximal suppression of the β-adrenergic stimulus for renin release, or alternatively, the combined and cumulative effects of these two drugs on sodium balance could have introduced an additional variable into their study that obscured the assessment of β-blockade's role in lowering plasma renin activity. The selectively competitive angiotensin antagonist, saralasin, has been shown to potentiate minoxidil-induced renin release in the rat (CAMPBELL et al., 1975). In patients on minoxidil, propranolol has been shown to jointly inhibit the rise in plasma renin activity and to minimize the reduction in mean arterial pressure which occurs in response to saralasin (PETTINGER and MITCHELL, 1975). The implication is that blood pressure reduction by propranolol, in association with a vasodilator, involves suppression of renin release. However, the blood pressure in two of the seven patients studied appeared to depend on a mechanism unrelated to angiotensin since their response to saralasin persisted in the face of progressive inhibition of renin release by propranolol (PETTINGER and MITCHELL, 1975).

Hypertrichosis is a cosmetic problem associated with the higher doses of minoxidil (CHIDSEY, 1973; LIMAS and FREIS, 1973; DORMOIS et al., in press).

3. Diazoxide

(3-methyl-7-chloro-1,2,4 benzothiadiazine-1,1-dioxide)

This des-sulphamoyl analogue of the benzothiadiazine diuretics, bearing a structural similarity to chlorothiazide, was intentionally developed in order to heighten the antihypertensive action, while minimizing the diuretic effect, of this series of compounds (RUBIN et al., 1961a, b, and 1968). Widespread preference for diazoxide in the therapy of life-threatening hypertension is largely explained by its relative ease of administration; likely effectiveness, potency and rapidity of onset of action; and by its relative safety (Drug Ther. Bull., 1971; Gifford, 1973; JAMA Drug Commentary, 1973; The Medical Letter, 1973; Koch-Weser, 1974a, b; Moser, 1974).

A current controversy exists with regard to whether optimal blood pressure reduction is achieved by rapid intravenous injection of a single large bolus, such as 300 mg within 10 sec, versus slow infusion over 10 to 30 min or repeated small doses of 75 to 150 mg every 5 to 15 min. It is difficult to determine from the literature whether this controversy really relates to rate of administration or total dosage, or to both factors.

Average reductions in mean arterial pressure of 25% have been reported with the intravenous administration of 200 to 300 mg of diazoxide, given as two or three divided doses, each within 30 to 40 sec (Kakaviatos and Finnerty, 1962). A number of investigators have subsequently emphasized the need for rapid intravenous injection, over a period of less than 10 to 30 sec, to achieve an optimal magnitude and duration of hypotensive effect (Finnerty et al., 1963; Hamby et al., 1968; Sellers and Koch-Weser, 1969 and 1973; Mroczek et al., 1971). One of the latter studies in adults found that rapid injection appeared to be required for maximal efficacy only in patients with accelerated hypertension and not in those with chronic hypertension (Mroczek et al., 1971). However, recently a crossover study of five pediatric patients at the Vanderbilt Hospital revealed no overall differential blood pressure response to rapid, compared to slow administration, irrespective of the severity of the hypertensive process (Boerth, personal communication). Two crossover studies in adults without malignant hypertension have shown no difference in blood pressure reduction produced by rapid intravenous injection, within 10 and 20 sec, compared to slow infusion within 10 and 30 min (Crout et al., 1970; Johnson and Kapur, 1972).

Although many investigators advocate the administration of a single 300 mg bolus as the initial dose to all patients, adequate hypotensive effectiveness has been demonstrated by administration of a series of smaller boluses of 75 to 150 mg, each given within 15 to 60 sec and repeated every 4 to 5 min until the desired reduction in pressure is obtained (Kakaviatos and Finnerty, 1962; Miller et al., 1969; Jellett et al., unpublished observations; Boerth, personal communication). About 20% of patients will respond to a dose of less than 300 mg, and the infrequent but real adverse effects of excessive blood pressure reduction can be minimized by a dose ranging regimen that recognizes the considerable interindividual variability in response to this drug (Jellett et al., unpublished observations).

Within the therapeutic range for blood levels of diazoxide, 90% of the total drug is said to be reversibly bound to human plasma albumin at one major site "mainly by hydrophobic interaction and to a lesser extent by hydrogen bonding" (Sellers and Koch-Weser, 1969, 1973 and 1974). During the initial intravascular mixing phase, following a rapid intravenous bolus injection, the plasma concentration of diazoxide has been estimated to exceed the plasma protein binding capacity by a critical fraction (Sellers and Koch-Weser, 1969 and 1973). The initially very high blood levels of free drug would thus (according to the theory) be capable of more complete saturation of the pharmacologically active arteriolar receptor sites, resulting in more effective blood pressure reduction. This phenomenon depends on the assumption that the drug-vascular receptor binding process is either irreversible or only very slowly reversible (Sellers and Koch-Weser, 1969 and 1973), considered, at present, to be a somewhat unique pharmacological situation (Crout et al., 1970; Powell et al., 1971; Johnson and Kapur, 1972).

However to date, the results of both experimental and clinical studies mitigate against irreversible diazoxide binding to arteriolar receptors (CROUT et al., 1970; POWELL et al., 1971; JELLETT et al., unpublished observations; BOERTH, personal communication). In a series of intraarterial infusions of diazoxide in the dog, skeletal muscle vascular resistance was found to be acutely reversible, to be related to plasma drug level and independent of plasma albumin concentration (POWELL et al., 1971). Furthermore, some clinical investigators have observed that the degree of hypotension is generally proportional to plasma drug concentration (CROUT et al., 1970) or to the total amount of compound administered (BOERTH, personal communication), although the dose required to reduce blood pressure optimally may vary between individuals (JELLETT et al., unpublished observations). With the sum of information currently available, it does not appear to be firmly established that diazoxide fails to reach an equilibrium between levels of free drug in plasma and vascular receptors, nor is it adequately established that rapid injection yields greater pharmacologic effects at points in time after the early distribution phase.

Following a single intravenous bolus of 300 mg, analysis of drug in plasma reveals a rapidly declining distribution phase, lasting up to 10 min. Subsequent to the distribution phase, plasma levels of about 20 μg/ml are associated with the antihypertensive effect of the initial dose (SELLERS and KOCH-WESER, 1969). The pharmacologic action of diazoxide is relatively brief compared to the average exponential half-life for plasma drug concentration of 24 h (SYMCHOWICZ et al., 1967; SELLERS and KOCH-WESER, 1969 and 1973; MROCZEK et al., 1971). The hypotensive effect in the average patient lasts only 6 to 16 h, although some individuals exhibit duration of response varying from 3 to 72 h (HAMBY et al., 1968; MILLER et al., 1969; SELLERS and KOCH-WESER, 1969 and 1973; MROCZEK et al., 1971). With this plasma half-life, accumulation can be expected when the loading dose (300 mg) is given 8 hourly, resulting in postdistribution levels of 100 μg/ml after 3 days. Interestingly, with repeated administration, higher plasma levels seem to be required to achieve the antihypertensive effect; this may bear on the greater hyperglycemia that occurs with repeated administration of the drug (CHARLES and DANFORTH, 1971).

More than 90% of diazoxide is eliminated in urine, identified either as parent compound or as apparently inactive metabolites (PRUITT et al., 1973a, b, 1974; SELLERS and KOCH-WESER, 1973). Thus prolonged plasma drug half-life, proportional to decreased creatinine clearance, could contribute to greater hyperglycemia seen in patients with renal failure (SELLERS and KOCH-WESER, 1969; UPDIKE and HARRIGTON, 1969; CHARLES and DANFORTH, 1971). The elevation of blood sugar by diazoxide appears to be temporally related to the hypotensive response (BLACKARD and APRILL, 1967; TABACHNICK and GULBENKIAN, 1968; POWELL et al., 1971; JOHNSON and KAPUR, 1972). Reduced rate of insulin secretion is suggested as the principal mechanism of diazoxide-induced hyperglycemia because of the associated low serum immunoreactive insulin levels (TABACHNICK and GULBENKIAN, 1968; CHARLES and DANFORTH, 1971) in patients with impaired glucose tolerance (STEINKE and SOELDNER, 1968).

Diazoxide and nitroprusside both cause peripheral arteriolar dilation. Unlike nitroprusside, however, diazoxide exerts no effect on veins in man or in experimental animals (THIRLWELL and ZSOTER, 1972). The resultant marked fall on total peripheral resistance reduces afterload on the left ventricle, but is followed by sympathetically mediated tachycardia and increased cardiac output, both of which in the dog have been prevented by β-adrenergic sympathetic blockade without affecting the reduction in mean arterial pressure (RAMASWAMY et al., 1968).

Cardiac index is appreciably elevated for approximately 10 min postinjection, despite unaltered stroke index and right atrial pressure (WILSON and OKUN, 1963; MROCZEK et al., 1971). Increased cardiac work may result in excessive myocardial oxygen demand and extension of functional myocardial ischemia (HAMBY et al., 1968; MILLER et al., 1969; JELLETT et al., unpublished observations). Such precipitation or exaggeration of myocardial ischemia occurs, despite reduced cardiac afterload, because of the reflex tachycardia, associated with sustained venous return to the heart and undiminished preload, in contrast to the action of nitroprusside.

Reductions, approaching 30%, in estimated glomerular filtration rate and renal plasma flow have been documented following rapid intravenous injection of therapeutic doses of diazoxide (JOHNSON, 1971; RADO et al., 1973). Antidiuresis and antinatriuresis appear to be related to both renal hemodynamic changes and proximal tubular effects, the latter being reflected by combined reductions of osmolal and free water clearance (JOHNSON, 1971; RADO et al., 1973). Abolition of the antidiuretic effect of diazoxide in hypophysectomized animals (TAYLOR and RUBIN, 1964) has not been confirmed in man. Diazoxide was found capable of reducing urinary volume, free water and osmolal clearance, and sodium excretion in patients with both vasopressin-dependent and nephrogenic diabetes insipidus (POHL et al., 1972; RADO et al., 1973).

A significant increase in plasma renin activity (more than 40 ng/ml/h) has been observed following intravenous diazoxide. Peak values occurred 2 h after administration of 5 mg/kg, given intravenously over 1 min, in renin-responsive hypertensive subjects, comprising 60% of the hypertensive population studied (KUCHEL et al., 1967). Renin response to diazoxide correlated with the responsiveness of plasma renin activity to both upright posture and sodium depletion (KUCHEL et al., 1967). However, diazoxide administration was associated with a significant fall in blood pressure even in renin-unresponsive individuals (KUCHEL et al., 1967; BAER et al., 1969).

4. Nitroprusside

Sodium nitroprusside ($Na_2Fe(CN)_5NO \cdot 2\,H_2O$ or sodium nitrosylpentacyanoferrate) is reported to be the most potent and predictably effective, parenteral agent available for the rapid control of life threatening hypertension "irrespective of etiology" (GIFFORD, 1959, 1961, and 1973; KOCH-WESER, 1974a). Although its toxicology was initially noted in mammals almost 90 years ago (HERMANN, 1886) the unique cardiovascular pharmacology of nitroprusside was not described until some 40 years later (JOHNSON, 1928). A further 27 years elapsed before its pharmacologic properties were applied to the therapy of hypertension (PAGE, 1955). Only recently have sterile dosage forms of this compound become commercially available as Nipride (ROCHE, 1974) or Nitroprus (JAHRE, 1976). As systems for the more precise control of the rate of intravenous administration of this drug have become more generally available, excessive hypotension has become more easily avoidable (PAGE, 1955; AHEARN and GRIM, 1974; TUZEL, 1974).

The onset of the hypotensive effect of nitroprusside is extremely rapid (JOHNSON, 1928 and 1929; PAGE, 1955). This hypotensive action, although much greater for nitroprusside than for the nitrites, is attributed to the nitroso (–NO) grouping possessed by these compounds but not by cyanogen (JOHNSON, 1928 and 1929; PAGE, 1955). Thus, although the toxicity that may result from continuing administration, especially in association with renal impairment, may be related to thiocyanate accumulation (WALD et al., 1939; PAGE, 1955), the hypotensive effect is considered to be due to fall in peripheral vascular resistance caused by arteriolar smooth-muscle relaxation, induced by the nitroprusside radical rather than by its metabolic break-down products (JOHNSON, 1928 and 1929; PAGE, 1955; SCHLANT et al., 1962; STYLES et al., 1973; VESEY et al., 1974).

Nitroprusside is pharmacologically unique in that it is associated with direct peripheral dilatation of both arterioles and veins (JOHNSON, 1929; FRANCIOSA et al., 1972; BHATIA and FROHLICH, 1973). By increasing venous capacitance (JOHNSON, 1929), in contrast to diazoxide (THIRLWELL and ZSOTER, 1972; BHATIA and FROHLICH, 1973), it has the potential to reduce the preload on the heart as well as reducing the afterload (CHATTERJEE et al., 1973; PARMLEY et al., 1974). Thus, the left ventricular end-diastolic pressure is lowered without significantly increasing heart rate (SCHLANT et al., 1962; FRANCIOSA et al., 1972; STYLES et al., 1973). Moreover, in association with a significant fall in heart rate, an improvement in left ventricular performance was noted among patients with refractory heart failure (GUIHA et al., 1974). Furthermore, in contrast to the rapidly, short-acting ganglion-blocking agent, trimethaphan camphorate, which also reduces venous tone (BHATIA and FROHLICH, 1973), nitroprusside does not block autonomic transmission of nerve impulses (JOHNSON, 1929; PAGE, 1955). Hence, its hypotensive effect is not posturally dependent and unwanted effects due to autonomic blockade (GIFFORD, 1973) are not encountered (PALMER and LASSETER, 1975).

Careful intravenous infusion of nitroprusside has proven successful in controlling hypertensive emergencies (MANI, 1971; GIFFORD, 1973; KOCH-WESER, 1974a; TUZEL, 1974; PALMER and LASSETER, 1975). Benefit has also resulted in selected patients who have left ventricular failure associated with acute myocardial infarction and filling pressures greater than 15 mm Hg (FRANCIOSA et al., 1972; CHATTERJEE et al., 1973; PARMLEY et al., 1974). It has been administered to reverse ergotamine toxicity with peripheral limb ischemia (CARLINER et al., 1974). The drug has also been used to achieve controlled hypotension during anesthesia (SCHIFFMANN and FUCHS, 1966; SIEGEL et al., 1971; STYLES et al., 1973; VESEY et al., 1974) and to provide a controlled hypotensive stimulus for renin release in the diagnosis of functionally significant, unilateral renal artery stenosis (KANEKO et al., 1967).

Nitroprusside is converted to both thiocyanate and cyanide in the body (LANG, 1933; PAGE, 1955; AHEARN and GRIM, 1974). Low levels of hydrocyanic acid have been measured in erythrocytes of patients given a single intravenous injection of thiocyanate (GOLDSTEIN and RIEDERS, 1951). Moreover, a four-fold elevation of plasma cyanide was associated with only a slight rise in thiocyanate concentration after intravenous infusion of nitroprusside during anesthesia in man, while accumulation of both cyanide and thiocyanate in blood was documented after prolonged nitroprusside infusion administered for blood pressure control (VESEY et al., 1974). Tracer studies in the rat suggest that equilibrium exists between thiocyanate and cyanide after steady state is achieved (BOXER and RICKARDS, 1952). Renal thiocyanate clearance is quite low, a little more than 2 ml/min, with a half-life of approximately one week in subjects who have normal renal function (WALD et al., 1939; DANZIG and KRINGEL, 1955; PAGE, 1955). A close correlation has also been observed between thiocyanate clearance and total chloride urinary excretion rate in dogs (NICKERSON and THOMAS, 1951), suggesting that chloride balance may influence elimination of thiocyanate from the body.

Immediate, unwanted effects, such as apprehension, diaphoresis, hyperventilation, vomiting, and yawning (GIFFORD, 1961; KANEKO et al., 1967; AHEARN and GRIM, 1974) have been attributed to brain-stem ischemia due to excessive hypotension (JOHNSON, 1929; GIFFORD, 1961). This situation can best be avoided by careful monitoring of blood pressure and appropriate adjustment of infusion rate (GIFFORD, 1961; AHEARN and GRIM, 1974; TUZEL, 1974). Later toxicity, manifested by fatigue, weakness, stupor, psychoneurosis, aphasia, slurred speech, muscle twitching, hyperhidrosis, tinnitus, and hypothyroidism (WALD et al., 1939; PAGE, 1955; NOUROK et al., 1964; AHEARN and GRIM, 1974), appears to be related to accumulation of thiocyanate (DOMZALSKI et al., 1953; PAGE, 1955). Cyanide itself could also contribute to such intoxication after prolonged administration (MOISTER and FREIS, 1949; GOLDSTEIN and RIEDERS, 1951; PINES and CRYMBLE, 1952; VESEY et al., 1974). Nitroprusside administration should be discontinued when plasma thiocyanate levels exceed 10 to 12 mg/dl (PAGE, 1955; GIFFORD, 1961; AHEARN and GRIM, 1974). However, clinical toxicity may develop in association with plasma thiocyanate levels between 5 and 20 mg/dl (PALMER and LASSETER, 1975). Plasma thiocyanate concentration should be monitored when the drug is infused for longer than 36 to 72 h, especially in the setting of impaired renal function (PAGE, 1955; NOUROK et al., 1964; GIFFORD, 1973; AHEARN and GRIM, 1974). Such was the background for the single case-report of nitroprusside-induced hypothyroidism, attributed to blockade of thyroid gland iodide uptake in the presence of thiocyanate accumulation, associated with renal failure and drug infusion for 21 days (NOUROK et al., 1964).

VII. Diuretic Drugs

J. A. OATES and M. E. CONOLLY

Diuretics are used alone or as components of the drug regimen in the majority of patients with hypertension. It is beyond the scope of this chapter, however, to cover the complete clinical pharmacology of the diuretic drugs; this diverse group requires a Handbook of its own. Even so, there are specific points regarding the employment of diuretics in the treatment of hypertension that should be mentioned here.

A. Hypertension Associated with Low Plasma Renin Activity

Approximately 20% of patients with "essential" hypertension have low plasma renin activity and subnormal responsiveness to stimuli that provoke release of renin. They are distinguished from primary aldosteronism by normal or subnormal production of aldosterone. This subset of hypertensive patients is uniquely responsive to spironolactone and diuretic combinations.

A group of patients with "low renin hypertension" can be identified by the failure of plasma renin activity to rise following defined stimuli such as upright posture with or without a low sodium diet (SPARK and MELBY, 1971; and CRANE and HARRIS, 1970); the administration of diazoxide (KUCHEL et al., 1967) or the administration of furosemide (CAREY et al., 1972).

The choice of a renin-stimulation test is determined by its ability to accurately predict patients who are sensitive to spironolactone, and by the ease and safety of the test. An antihypertensive response to spironolactone is almost always seen in patients identified as low renin hypertension by the furosemide stimulation test (CAREY et al., 1972). This test can be carried out with less rigorous control of the sodium in the diet than can sodium deprivation. Earlier studies employed 120 mg of furosemide (40 mg at 6 p.m., 12 midnight, and 6 a.m.) followed by 3 h of upright posture (CAREY et al., 1972). Patients with plasma renin activity of less than 1.67 ng per ml per h (incubation at pH 5.5) are classified as having low renin hypertension. More recently, it has been found that the use of only 80 mg of furosemide (40 mg at 6 p.m. and 6 a.m.) followed by 3 h of upright posture will also provide an adequate stimulus to renin release and will adequately identify those patients who are responsive to spironolactone therapy (HOLLIFIELD and LIDDLE, unpublished data). Care should be taken to avoid excessive orthostatic hypotension that may result from this vigorous diuresis, particularly because of the propensity for cerebral and coronary vascular disease in the hypertensive population.

Spironolactone (400 mg daily) lowered the blood pressure in almost all patients with low renin hypertension in a double blind control study with randomized sequence of administration of drug and placebo (CAREY et a., 1972) as well as in less definitive studies (SPARK and MELBY, 1971; and CRANE and HARRIS, 1970). In contrast, this dose of spironolactone is infrequently effective in reducing arterial pressure in patients with plasma renin activity that responds normally to stimuli. Lesser doses of spironolactone (100 to 200 mg daily) will be adequate to maintain the antihypertensive response in most patients after the initial reduction of blood pressure with 400 mg daily.

In addition to spironolactone, other diuretics and combinations thereof will reduce blood pressure in most patients with low renin hypertension and are more effective in this group than in patients with normal or high stimulated plasma renin activity. The combinations of triamterene-hydrochlorothiazide, spironolactone-hydrochlorothiazide, and hydrochlorothiazide alone (DOUGLAS et al., 1974; and ALDIN et al., 1972) will lower blood pressure in low renin hypertension, but dose-response comparisons with spironolactone have not been carried out. The similar effects of these multiple diuretics suggests that patients with low renin hypertension have hypertension that is uniquely volume dependent. This is consistent with the findings of WOODS et al. (1969), that the exchangeable sodium space is larger in patients with low renin hypertension.

B. Role of Plasma Volume in Determining the Blood Pressure of Patients Receiving Inhibitors of Sympathetic Reflexes

When sympathetic reflexes are inhibited, plasma volume becomes a major determinant of blood pressure. This important principle has particular relevance to patients whose blood pressure is not adequately controlled by the guanidinium adrenergic blockers (*e.g.* guanethidine), methyldopa, reserpine, and the ganglion blockers.

As demonstrated by FRYE and BRAUNWALD (1960), expansion of the blood volume has little effect on blood pressure or cardiac output when sympathetic reflexes are intact, presumably because of a compensating change in sympathetic tone. Following ganglion blockade with trimethaphan, however, blood volume expansion increases blood pressure and cardiac output. The dependence of pressure on volume during sympathetic inhibition is also manifested when volume is reduced. NICKERSON and GOURZIS (1962) found that patients with hypovolemia respond with exaggerated reductions in blood pressure during blockade of α-adrenergic receptors with phenoxybenzamine; in such patients, blood pressure can readily be increased by expanding the blood volume.

The importance of this principle in the treatment of hypertension was demonstrated by DUSTAN et al. (1972). They found a remarkable correlation between plasma volume and blood pressure in patients who were on drugs that inhibit sympathetic reflexes (methyldopa, guanethidine, or a combination of propranolol and hydralazine). One subset of their patients exhibited a poor response to these drugs even though they were receiving some diuretic or combination of diuretics, and this group had a higher plasma volume than patients on similar drugs with adequate blood pressure control. Intensification of diuretic therapy together with moderate limitation of sodium intake resulted in a fall in plasma volume associated with a reduction in blood pressure in these "refractory" patients. Thus, in treated hypertensive patients who have a fixed capacity in their vascular bed due to inhibition of sympathetic reflexes, volume regulation may be key to their successful management.

References

Section II. The Guanidinium Adrenergic Neuron Blocking Drugs

BORGÅ, O., HAMBERGER, B., MALMFORS, T., SJOQUIST, F.: The role of plasma protein binding in the inhibitory effect of nortriptyline on the neuronal uptake of norepinephrine. Clin. Pharmacol. Ther. **11**, 581—588 (1970).

BRODIE, B. B., CHANG, C. C., COSTA, E.: On the mechanism of action of guanethidine. Brit. J. Pharmacol. **25**, 171—178 (1965).

CHANG, C. C., COSTA, E., BRODIE, B. B.: Interaction of guanethidine with adrenergic neurons. J. Pharmacol. exp. Ther. **147**, 303—312 (1965).

COHN, J. N., LIPTAK, T. E., FRIES, S. D.: Hemodynamic effects of guanethidine in man. Circulat. Res. **12**, 298—307 (1963).

DAY, M. D., RAND, M. J.: Antagonism of guanethidine by dexamphetamine and other related sympathomimetic amines. J. Pharm. (Lond.) **14**, 541—549 (1962).

DOYLE, A. E., MORLEY, A.: Studies on the absorption and excretion of ^{14}C bethanidine in man. Brit. J. Pharmacol. **24**, 701—704 (1965).

DUSTAN, H. P., TARAZI, R. C., BRAVO, E. L.: Dependence of arterial pressure on intravascular volume in hypertension. New Engl. J. Med. **286**, 860—861 (1972).

FANN, W. E., KAUFMANN, J. S., GRIFFITH, J. D., DAVIS, J. M., JANOWSKY, D. S., OATES, J. A.: Doxepin: Effects on transport of biogenic amines. Psychopharmacologia (Berl.) **22**, 111—125 (1971).

FANN, W. E., DAVIS, J. M., JANOWSKY, D. S., OATES, J. A.: Chlorpromazine reversal of the antihypertensive action of guanethidine. Lancet **1971 II**, 436—437.

FEAGIN, O. T., KAUFMANN, J. S., OATES, J. A. Unpublished observations.

GAFFNEY, T. E., BRAUNWALD, E.: Importance of the adrenergic nervous system in the support of circulatory function in patients with congestive heart failure. Amer. J. Med. **34**, 320—324 (1963).

GULATI, O. D., DAVE, B. T., GOKHALE, S. D., SHAH, K. M.: Antagonism of adrenergic neuron blockade in hypertensive subjects. Clin. Pharmacol. Ther. **7**, 510—514 (1966).

KAHLER, R. L., GAFFNEY, T. E., BRAUNWALD, E.: The effects of autonomic nervous system inhibition on the circulatory response to vascular exercise. J. clin. Invest. **41**, 1981—1987 (1962).

KAUFMANN, J. S., FEAGIN, O. T., SHAND, D. G., McALLISTER, R. G., PAYNE, N. A., OATES, J. A.: Guanethidine and related agents IV: Kinetic characterization of the pool of drug stored in human adrenergic neurons. To be published.

KHATRI, M., COHN, J. N.: Mechanism of exercise hypotension after sympathetic blockade. Cardiology **25**, 329—338 (1970).

LEISHMAN, A. W. D., MATTHEWS, H. L., SMITH, A. J.: Further experience with guanethidine. Lancet **1961 II**, 4—7.

LEISHMAN, A. W. D., MATTHEWS, H. L., SMITH, A. J.: Antagonism of guanethidine by imipramine. Lancet **1963 I**, 112.

McMARTIN, C., RONDEL, M. B., VINTER, J., ALLAN, B. R., HUMBERSTONE, M. B., LEISHMAN, A. W. D., SANDLER, G., THIRKETTLE, J. L.: The fate of guanethidine in two hypertensive patients. Clin. Pharmacol. Ther. **1970 II**, 423—431.

MEYER, J. F., McALLISTER, C. K., GOLDBERG, L. I.: Insidious and prolonged antagonism of guanethidine by amitriptyline. J. Amer. med. Ass. **213**, 1487—1488 (1970).

MITCHELL, J. R., CAVANAUGH, J. H., ARIAS, L., OATES, J. A.: Guanethidine and related agents III. Antagonism by drugs which inhibit the norepinephrine pump in man. J. clin. Invest. **49**, 1956—1604 (1970).

MITCHELL, J. R., OATES, J. A.: Guanethidine and related agents I. Mechanism of the selective blockade of adrenergic neurons and its antagonism by drugs. J. Pharmacol. exp. Ther. **172**, 100—107 (1970).

MULHEIMS, G. H., BROWN, G. O.: Effect of guanethidine on blood volume in essential hypertension. Proc. Soc. exp. Biol. (N. Y.) **109**, 613—615 (1962).

OATES, J. A., MITCHELL, J. R., FEAGIN, O. T., KAUFMANN, J. S., SHAND, D. G.: Distribution of guanidinium antihypertensives mechanism of their selective action. Ann. N. Y. Acad. Sci. **179**, 302—308 (1971).

OATES, J. A., SELIGMANN, A. W., CLARK, M. A., ROUSSEAU, P., LEE, R. E.: The relative efficacy of guanethidine, methyldopa, and pargyline as antihypertensive agents. N. Engl. J. Med. **273**, 729—734 (1965).
PRICHARD, B. N. C., JOHNSTON, A. W., HILL, I. D., ROSENHEIM, M. E.: Bethanidine, guanethidine and methyldopa in treatment of hypertension: A within-patient comparison. Brit. med. J. **1968 I**, 135—144.
RAHN, K. H., GOLDBERG, L.: Comparison of antihypertensive efficacy, intestinal absorption and excretion of guanethidine in hypertensive patients. Clin. Pharmacol. Ther. **10**, 858—866 (1969).
RICHARDSON, D. W., WYSO, E. M., MAGEE, J. H., CAVELL, G. C.: Circulatory effects of guanethidine. Circulation **22**, 184—190 (1960).
SHAND, D. G., MORGAN, D. H., OATES, J. A.: The release of guanethidine by splenic nerve stimulation: A quantitative evaluation showing dissociation from adrenergic blockade. J. Pharmacol. exp. Ther. **184**, 73—80 (1973).
SHAND, D. G., NIES, A. S., MCALLISTER, R. G., OATES, J. A.: A loadingmaintenance regimen for more rapid initiation of the effect of guanethidine. Clin. Pharmacol. Ther. **18**, 139—144 (1975).
SMITH, A. J.: Fluid retention produced by guanethidine. Circulation **31**, 490—496 (1965).
STONE, C. A., PORTER, C. C., STAVORSKI, J. M., LUDDEN, C. T., TOTARO, J. A.: J. Pharmacol. exp. Ther. **144**, 196—204 (1964).
WEIL, J. V., CHIDSEY, C. A.: Plasma volume expansion resulting from interference with adrenergic function in normal man. Circulation **37**, 54—61 (1968).

Section III. Methyldopa

AU, W. Y. W., DRING, L. G., GRAHAME-SMITH, D. G., ISAAC, P., WILLIAMS, R. T.: The metabolism of ^{14}C-labelled α-methyldopa in normal and hypertensive human subjects. Biochem. J. **129**, 1—10 (1972).
BRECKENRIDGE, A., DOLLERY, C. T., WORLLEDGE, S. M., HOLBOROW, E. J., JOHNSON, G. D.: Positive direct Coombs tests and antinuclear factor in patients treated with methyldopa. Lancet **1967 II**, 1265—1268.
BUHS, R. P., BECK, J. L., SPETH, O. C., SMITH, J. L., TRENNER, N. R., CANNON, P. J., LARAGH, J. H.: The metabolism of methyldopa in hypertensive human subjects. J. Pharm. exp. Ther. **143**, 205—214 (1964).
CARLSSON, A., LINDQVIST, M.: In-vivo decarboxylation of α-methyl metatyrosine. Acta physiol. scand. **54**, 87—94 (1962).
CARSTAIRS, K. C., BRECKENRIDGE, A., DOLLERY, C. T., WORLLEDGE, S. M.: Incidence of a positive direct Coombs' test in patients on α-methyldopa. Lancet **1966 II**, 133—135.
CONOLLY, M. E., BRIANT, R. H., GEORGE, C. F., DOLLERY, C. T.: A crossover comparison of clonidine and methyldopa in hypertension. Europ. J. clin. Pharmacol. **4**, 222—227 (1972a).
CONOLLY, M. E., DAVIES, D. S., DOLLERY, C. T., MORGAN, C. D., PATERSON, J. W., SANDLER, M.: Metabolism of isoprenaline in dog and man. Brit. J. Pharmacol. **46**, 458—472 (1972b).
DAY, M. D., ROACH, A. G., WHITING, R. L.: The mechanism of the antihypertensive action of α-methyldopa in hypertensive rats. Europ. J. Pharmacol. **21**, 271—280 (1973).
DOLLERY, C. T., HARINGTON, M.: Methyldopa in hypertension. Clinical and pharmacological studies. Lancet **1962 I**, 759—763.
ELKINGTON, S. G., SCHREIBER, W. M., CONN, H. O.: Hepatic injury caused by L-Alpha-methyldopa. Circulation **40**, 589—595 (1969).
FINCH, L., HAEUSLER, G.: Further evidence for a central hypotensive action of α-methyldopa in both the rat and the cat. Brit. J. Pharmacol. **47**, 217—228 (1973).
GILLESPIE, L., OATES, J. A., CROUT, R., SJOERDSMA, A.: Clinical and chemical studies with α-methyldopa in patients with hypertension. Circulation **25**, 281—291 (1962).
GOLDSTEIN, G. B., LAM, K. C., MISTILIS, S. P.: Drug induced active chronic hepatitis. Amer. J. dig. Dis. **18**, 177—184 (1973).
HAEUSLER, G., FINCH, L.: On the nature of the central hypotensive effect of clonidine and α-methyldopa. J. Pharmacol. (Paris) **3**, 544—545 (1972).
HEISE, A., KRONEBERG, G.: α sympathetic receptor stimulation in the brain and hypotensive activity of α-methyldopa. Europ. J. Pharmacol. **17**, 315—317 (1972).
HEISE, A., KRONEBERG, G.: Central nervous α-adrenergic receptors and the mode of action of α-methyldopa. Naunyn-Schmeid. Arch. Pharmacol. **279**, 285—300 (1973).
HENNING, M.: Studies on the mode of action of α-methyldopa. Acta physiol. scand. Suppl. 322 (1969).
HOFFBRAND, B. I., FRY, W., BUNTON, G. L.: Cholestatic jaundice due to methyldopa. Brit. med. J. **1974 III**, 559.

Hoyumpa, A. M., Connell, A. M.: Methyldopa hepatitis: report of 3 cases. Amer. J. dig. Dis. **18**, 213—224 (1973).
Lin, E. C. C., Hagihira, H., Wilson, T. H.: Specificity of the transport system for neutral amino acids in the hamster intestine. Amer. J. Physiol. **202**, 919—925 (1962).
Lund-Johansen, P.: Hemodynamic changes in long-term α-methyldopa therapy of essential hypertension. Acta med. scand. **192**, 221—226 (1972).
Mason, D. T., Braunwald, E.: Effect of guanethidine, reserpine and methyldopa on reflex venous and arterial constriction in man. J. clin. Invest. **43**, 1449—1463 (1964).
Mohammed, S., Fasola, A. F., Privitera, P. J., Lipicky, R. J., Martz, B. L., Gaffney, T. E.: Effects of methyldopa on plasma renin activity in man. Circulat. Res. **25**, 543—548 (1969).
Mohammed, S., Hanenson, I. B., Magenheim, H. G., Gaffney, T. E.: Effects of alpha-methyldopa on renal function in hypertensive patients. Amer. Heart. J. **76**, 21—27 (1968).
Mroczek, W. J., Leibel, B. A., Finnerty, F. A.: Comparison of clonidine and methyldopa in hypertensive patients receiving a diuretic — a double-blind crossover study. Amer. J. Cardiol. **29**, 712—717 (1972).
Muscholl, E., Kahn, K. H.: Über den Nachweis und die Bedeutung von α-Methylnoradrenalin im Harn von Hypertoniken bei Verabreichung von α-Methyldopa. Pharmacol. Clin. **I**, 19—29 (1968).
Muscholl, E., Maître, L.: Release by sympathetic stimulation of α-methyl-noradrenaline stored in the heart after administration of α-methyldopa. Experientia (Basel) **19**, 658—659 (1963).
Muscholl, E., Rahn, K. H.: Nachweis von α-Methylnoradrenalin im Harn von Hypertonikern während einer Behandlung mit α-Methyldopa. Klin. Wschr. **44**, 1412—1413 (1966).
Nies, A. S., Shand, D. G.: Hypertensive response to propranolol in a patient treated with methyldopa—a proposed mechanism. Clin. Pharmacol. exp. Ther. **14**, 823—826 (1973).
Oates, J. A., Gillespie, L., Udenfriend, S., Sjoerdsma, A.: Decarboxylase inhibition and blood pressure reduction by α-methyl-3,4-dihydroxy-DL-phenylalanine. Science **131**, 1890—1891 (1960).
Oates, J. A., Seligmann, A. W., Clark, M. A., Rousseau, P., Lee, R. E.: The relative efficacy of guanethidine, methyldopa and pargyline as antihypertensive agents. New Engl. J. Med. **273**, 729—734 (1965).
Onesti, G., Brest, A. N., Novack, P., Kasparian, H., Moyer, J. H.: Pharmacodynamic effects of alpha-methyldopa in hypertensive subjects. Amer. Heart. J. **67**, 32—38 (1964).
Porter, C. C., Titus, D. C.: Distribution and metabolism of methyldopa in the rat. J. Pharmacol. exp. Ther. **139**, 77—87 (1963).
Prescott, L. F., Buhs, R. P., Beattie, J. O., Speth, O. C., Trenner, N. R., Lasagna, L.: Combined clinical and metabolic study of the effects of alpha-methyldopa on hypertensive patients. Circulation **34**, 308—321 (1966).
Prichard, B. N. C., Gillam, P. M. S.: Treatment of hypertension with propranolol. Brit. med. J. **1969I**, 7—16.
Rand, M. J., Rush, M., Wilson, J.: Some observations on the inhibition of salivation by St 155 (2-(2,6-dichlorophenylamine)-2-imidazoline hydrochloride, Catapres, Catapresan. Europ. J. Pharmacol. **5**, 168—172 (1969).
Rehman, O. U., Keith, T. A., Gall, E. A.: Methyldopa induced submassive hepatic necrosis. J. Amer. med. Ass. **224**, 1390—1392 (1973).
Saavedra, J. A., Reid, J. L., Jordan, W., Rawlins, M. D., Dollery, C. T.: Plasma concentration of α-methyldopa and sulphate conjugate after oral and intravenous administration. Europ. J. clin. Pharmacol. (in press) 1974.
Sannerstedt, R., Bojs, G., Varnauskas, E., Werkö, L.: Alpha-methyldopa in arterial hypertension. Acta med. scand. **174**, 53—67 (1963).
Sannerstedt, R., Varnauskas, E., Werkö, L.: Hemodynamic effects of methyldopa (Aldomet) at rest and during exercise in patients with arterial hypertension. Acta med. scand. **171**, 75—82 (1962).
Schweitzer, I. L., Peters, R. L.: Acute submassive hepatic necrosis due to methyldopa. Gastroenterology **66**, 1203—1211 (1974).
Sherman, J. D., Lover, D. E., Harrington, J. F.: Anemia, positive lupus and rheumatoid factors with methyldopa. Arch. intern. Med. **120**, 321—326 (1967).
Sjoerdsma, A., Vendsalu, A., Engelman, K.: Studies on the metabolism and mechanism of action of methyldopa. Circulation **28**, 492—502 (1963).
Stone, C. A., Porter, C. C.: Methyldopa and adrenergic nerve function. Pharmacol. Rev. **18**, 569—575 (1966).
Toghill, P. J., Smith, P. G., Benton, P., Brown, R. C., Matthews, H. L.: Methyldopa liver damage. Brit. med. J. **1974III**, 545—548.

TRINKER, F. R.: The significance of the relative potencies of noradrenaline and α-methylnoradrenaline for the mode of action of α-methyldopa. J. Pharm. (Lond.) **23**, 306—308 (1971).

WILSON, W. R., FISHER, F. D., KIRKENDALL, W. M.: The acute hemodynamic effects of α-methyldopa in man. J. chron. Dis. **15**, 907—913 (1961).

WORLLEDGE, S. M., CARSTAIRS, K. C., DACIE, J. V.: Autoimmune haemolytic anaemia associated with α-methyldopa therapy. Lancet **1966 II**, 135—139.

Section IV. Clonidine

AMERY, A., VERSTRAETE, M., BOSSAERT, H., VERSTREKEN, G.: Hypotensive action and side effects of clonidine-chlorthalidone and methyldopa-chlorthalidone in treatment of hypertension. Brit. med. J. **1970 II**, 392—395.

BARNETT, A. J., CANTOR, S.: Observations on the hypotensive action of Catapres (St-155) in man. Med. J. Aust. **1**, 87—91 (1968).

BOCK, K. D., HEIMSOTH, V. V., MERGUET, P, et al: Klinische und klinische-experimentelle Untersuchungen mit einer neuen blutdrucksenkenden Substanz: Dichlorophenylamino-imidazolin. Dtsch. med. Wschr. **91**, 1761—1770 (1966).

BOLME, P., FUXE, K.: Pharmacological studies on the hypotensive effects of clonidine. Europ. J. Pharmacol. **13**, 168—174 (1971).

CONOLLY, M. E., BRIANT, R. H., GEORGE, C. F., DOLLERY, C. T.: A cross over comparison of clonidine and methyldopa in hypertension. Europ. J. clin. Pharmacol. **4**, 222—227 (1972).

CONSTANTINE, J. W., MCSHANE, W. K.: Analysis of the cardiovascular effects of 2-(2,6-Dichlorophenylamino)-2-imidazoline hydrochloride (Catapres). Europ. J. Pharmacol. **4**, 109—123 (1968).

DAVIES, D. S., WING, L. M. H., REID, J. L., NEILL, E., TIPPETT, P, DOLLERY, C. T.: Pharmacokinetics and concentration-effect relationships of intravenous and oral clonidine. Clin. Pharmacol. Ther. **21** (1977).

DOLLERY, C. T., REID, J. L.: Central noradrenergic neurons and the cardiovascular actions of clonidine in the rabbit. Brit. J. Pharmacol. **47**, 206—216 (1973).

DOLLERY, C. T., DAVIES, D. S., DRAFFAN, G. H., DARGIE, H. J., DEAN, C. R., REID, J. L., CLARE, R. A., MURRAY, S.: Clinical pharmacology and pharmacokinetics of clonidine. Clin. Pharmacol. Ther. **19**, 11—17 (1976).

DRAFFAN, G. H., CLARE, R. A., MURRAY, S., BELLWARD, G. D., DAVIES, D. S., DOLLERY, C. T.: The determination of clonidine in human plasma. Proceedings of the Third International Symposium on Mass Spectrometry in Biochemistry and Medicine, Sardinia, Italy, June 1975.

EHRINGER, H.: Die Wirkung von 2-(2,6-Dichlorophenylamino)-2-imidazolin-hydrochlorid auf die Extremitatendurchblutung, den Blutdruck und die Venenkapazität bei Normotonikern. Arzneimittel-Forsch. **16**, 1165—1169 (1966).

GRAUBNER, W., WOLF, M.: Kritische Betrachtungen zum Wirkungsmechanismus des 2-(2,6-dichlorophenyl-amino)-2-imidazolin-hydrochlorid. Arzneimittel-Forsch. **16**, 1055—1058 (1966).

HANNINGTON, E.: Clonidine hydrochloride (Dixarit) for migraine. Prescriber's J. **12**, 21—22 (1972).

HEILMANN, K.: Untersuchungen über die Wirkung von Catapresan auf den intraokularen Drucker. 1. Mitteilung. Klin. Mbl. Augenheilk. **157**, 182—192 (1970).

HÖKFELT, B., HEDELAND, H., DYMLING, J. F.: Studies on catecholamines, renin and aldosterone following catapresan (2-(2,6-dichloro-phenyl-amine)-2-imidazoline hydrochlori de) in hypertensive patients. Europ. J. Pharmacol. **10**, 389—397 (1970).

HOOBLER, S. W., SAGASTUME, E.: Long term clinical experience with Catapres: Comparison with guanethidine. In: CONOLLY, M. E. (Ed.): Catapres in hypertension—an international symposium, pp. 207—226. London: Butterworths 1970.

HUNYOR, S. N., HANSSON, L., HARRISON, T. S., HOOBLER, S. W.: Effects of clonidine withdrawal: possible mechanisms and suggestions for management. Brit. med. J. **1973 II**, 209—211.

KOBINGER, W.: Über den Wirkungsmechanismus einer neuen antihypertensiven Substanz mit Imidazolinstruktur. Naunyn-Schmiedebergs Arch. Pharmak. exp. Path. **258**, 48—58 (1967).

MATHEW, J. Y., PARKER, M. L.: The use of clonidine (Catapres) in the treatment of hypertension. Med. J. Aust. **2**, 1120—1122 (1971).

MCRAVEN, D. R., KROETZ, F. W., KIOSCHOS, J. M., KIRKENDALL, W. M.: The effect of clonidin on hemodynamics in hypertensive patients. Amer. Heart J. **81**, 482—489 (1971).

MROCZEK, W. J., LEIBEL, B. A., FINNERTY, F. A.: Comparison of clonidine and methyldopa in hypertensive patients receiving a diuretic. Amer. J. Cardiol. **29**, 712—717 (1972).

MUIR, A. L., BURTON, J. L., LAWRIE, D. M.: Circulatory effects at rest and exercise of clonidine, an imidazoline derivative with hypotensive properties. Lancet **1969 II**, 181—185.

NAYLER, W. G., PRICE, J. M., SWANN, J. B., McINNES, I., RACE, D., LOWE, T. E.: Effect of hypotensive drug St-155 (Catapres) on the heart and peripheral circulation. J. Pharmacol. exp. Ther. **164**, 45—59 (1968).
ONESTI, G., SCHWARTZ, A. B., KIM, K. E., PAZ-MARTINEZ, V., SWARTZ, C.: Antihypertensive effect of clonidine. Circulat. Res. **28** (Suppl. II), 53—69 (1971).
PUTZEYS, M. R., HOOBLER, S. W.: Comparison of clonidine and methyldopa on blood pressure and side effects in hypertensive patients. Amer. Heart. J. **83**, 464—468 (1972).
REHBINDER, D.: The metabolism of clonidine (Catapres, St 155). In: CONOLLY, M. E. (Ed.): Catapres in hypertension—an international symposium, pp. 227—236. London: Butterworths 1970.
SCHMITT, H.: Centrally mediated decrease in sympathetic tone induced by 2-(2,6-dichlorophenyl-amino)-2-imidazoline (St 155, Catapres). In: CONOLLY, M. E. (Ed.): Catapres in hypertension—an international symposium, pp. 23—42. London: Butterworths 1970.
SCHMITT, H., SCHMITT, H., FENARD, S.: Evidence for an α sympathomimetic component in the effects of Catapresan on vasomotor centres: antagonism by piperoxan. Europ. J. Pharmacol. **14**, 98—100 (1971).
SCHNEIDER, K. W.: Cardial-Hämodynamik im akuten Versuch, nach chronischer Behandlung und im Belastungstest mit St 155. In: HEILMEYER, L., HOLTMEIER, H. J., PFEIFFER, E. F. (Eds.): Hochdrucktherapie: Symposion über 2-(2,6-dichlorophenylamino)-2-imidazolin-hydrochlorid, pp. 78—83. Stuttgart: Thieme 1968.
SHAFAR, J., TALLETT, E. R., KNOWLSON, P. A.: Evaluation of clonidine in prophylaxis of migraine. Lancet **1972I**, 403—407.
SHAW, J., HUNYOR, S. N., KORNER, P. I.: The peripheral circulatory effects of clonidine and their role in the production of arterial hypotension. Europ. J. Pharmacol. **14**, 101—111 (1971).
SHERMAN, G. P., GREGA, G. I., WOODS, R. J., BUCKLEY, J. R.: Evidence for a central hypotensive mechanism of 2-(2,6-dichlorophenylamino)-2-imidazoline (Catapresan, St 155). Europ. J. Pharmacol. **2**, 326—328 (1968).
SMET, G., HOOBLER, S. W., SANBAR, S., JULIUS, S.: Clinical observations on a new anti-hypertensive drug, 2-(2,6-dichlorophenylamine)-2-imidazoline hydrochloride. Amer. Heart. J. **77**, 473—478 (1969).
STENBERG, J., HOLMBERG, S., NAETS, E., et al: Hemodynamic effects of Catapresan: Central circulation at rest; circulation at rest and under exercise. In: HEILMEYER, L., HOLTMEIER, H. J., PFEIFFER, E. F. (Eds.): Hochdrucktherapie: Symposion über 2-(2,6-Dichlorophenylamino)-2-imidazolin-hydrochlorid, S. 68—75. Stuttgart: Thieme 1968.
VORBURGER, C., BUTIKOFER, E., REUBI, F.: Die akute Wirkung von St 155 auf die cardiale und renale Hämodynamik. In: HEILMEYER, L., HOLTMEIER, H. J., PFEIFFER, E. F. (Eds.): Hochdrucktherapie: Symposion über 2-(2,6-Dichlorophenylamino)-2-imidazolin-hydrochlorid, S. 86—94. Stuttgart: Thieme 1968.
WERNER, U., STARKE, K., SCHÜMAN, H. J.: Actions of clonidine and 2-(2-methyl-6-ethyl-cyclohexylamino)-2-oxazoline on postganglionic autonomic nerves. Arch. int. Pharmacodyn. **195**, 282—290 (1972).
ZAIMIS, E.: On the pharmacology of catapres (St 155). In: CONOLLY, M. E. (Ed.): Catapres in hypertension—an international symposium, pp. 9—22. London: Butterworths 1970.

Section V. Beta-Adrenoreceptor Blocking Drugs

ÅBLAD, B., ERVIK, M., HALLGREN, J., JOHNSSON, G., SOLVELL, L.: Pharmacological effects and serum levels of orally administered alprenolol in man. Europ. J. clin. Pharmacol. **5**, 44—52 (1972).
AELLIG, W. H., PRICHARD, B. N. C., SCALES, B. A.: Blood levels of practolol following intravenous administration. Brit. J. Pharmacol. **40**, 572P (1970).
AELLIG, W. H., SAMELI, K.: Prolonged action of pindolol. Brit. med. J. **1973II**, 365.
AMERY, A., BILLIET, L., FAGARD, R.: Beta receptors and renin release. New Engl. J. Med. **290**, 284 (1974).
BARRETT, A. M., CARTER, J., FITZGERALD, J. D., HULL, R., LE COUNT, D.: A new type of cardioselective adrenoceptive blocking drug. Brit. J. Pharmacol. **48**, 340 (1973).
BEILIN, L. J., JUEL-JENSEN, B. E.: Alpha and beta adrenergic blockade in hypertension. Lancet **1972I**, 979.
BERGLUND, G., ANDERSSON, O., HANSSON, L., OCANDER, R.: Propranolol given twice daily in hypertension. Acta med. scand. **194**, 513 (1973).
BETT, J. H.: Hypotension after oral propranolol. Lancet **1968**I, 302.
BOAKES, A. J., BOEREE, B. H., PRICHARD, B. N. C.: Dose response studies to oxprenolol, pindolol, practolol, propranolol and sotalol on tilt, valsalva and exercise tachycardia. Naunyn-Schmiedeberg's Arch. Pharmacol. **279**, R. 42 (1973).

BOAKES, A. J., KNIGHT, E. J., PRICHARD, B. N. C.: Preliminary studies of the pharmacological effects of 5{1-Hydroxy-2(1-Methyl-3-phenylpropyl)amino-ethyl}Sylicylamide (AH 5158) in man. Clin. Sci. **40**, 18 (1971).

BODEM, G., BRAMMELL, H. L., WEIL, J. V., CHIDSEY, C. A.: Pharmacodynamic studies of beta adrenergic antagonism induced in man by propranolol and practolol. J. clin. Invest. **52**, 747—754 (1973).

BODEM, G., CHIDSEY, C. A.: Pharmacokinetic studies of practolol, a β-adrenergic antagonist, in man. Clin. Pharmacol. Ther. **14**, 26—29 (1973).

BOND, P. A.: Metabolism of propranolol (Inderal); a potent, specific β-adrenergic receptor blocking agent. Nature (Lond.) **213**, 721—723 (1967).

BRANCH, R. A., NIES, A. S., SHAND, D. G.: The disposition of propranolol VIII. General implications of the effect of liver blood flow on elimination from the perfused rat liver. Drug Metab. Disp. **1**, 687—690 (1973).

BRECKENRIDGE, A. M., BURANAPONG, P., DOLLERY, C. T., GEORGE, C. F., MACERLEAN, D., ORME, M. L. E.: Hepatic clearance of propranolol in dogs. Brit. J. Pharmacol. **48**, 336P (1973).

BRICK, I., HUTCHINSON, K. J., McDEVITT, D. G.: Comparison of the effects of ICI 50172 and. propranolol on the cardiovascular responses to alrenaline, isoprenline and exercise. Brit. J. Pharmacol. **34**, 127—140 (1968).

BROWN, J. J., DAVIES, D. L., FERRISS, J. B., FRASER, R., HAYWOOD, E., LEVER, A. F., ROBERTSON, J. I. S.: Comparison of surgery and prolonged spironolactone therapy in patients with hypertension, aldosterone excess and low plasma renin. Brit. J. Pharmacol. **2**, 729—734 (1972).

BROWN, P., BADDELEY, H., READ, A. E., DAVIES, J. D., McGARRY, J.: Sclerosing peritonitis, an unusual reaction to a β-adrenergic blocking drug (Practolol). Lancet **1974 II**, 1477—1481.

BRUNNER, H. R., GAVRAS, H., LARAGH, J. H., KEENAN, R.: Angiotensin II blockase in man by Sar 1—8 angiotensin II for understanding and treatment of high blood pressure. Lancet **1973 II**, 1045—1047.

BUHLER, F. R., LARAGH, J. H., BAER, L., DARRACOTT VAUGHAN, E., BRUNNER, H. R.: Propranolol inhibition of renin secretion. New Engl. J. Med. **287**, 1209—1214 (1972).

BUHLER, F. R., LARAGH, J. H., DARRACOTT VAUGHAN, E., BRUNNER, H. R., GAVRAS, H., BAER, L.: Antihypertensive action of propranolol. Amer. J. Cardiol. **32**, 511—522 (1973).

CASTENFORS, J., JOHNSSON, H., ORO, L.: Effect of alprenolol on blood pressure and plasma renin activity in hypertensive patients. Acta med. scand. **193**, 189—195 (1973).

CLEAVELAND, C. R., SHAND, D. G.: Effect of route of administration on the relationship between β-adrenergic blockase and plasma propranolol level. Clin. Pharmacol. Ther. **13**, 181—195 (1972).

COLLINS, I. S., KING, I. W.: Pindolol (Visken, LB 46). A new treatment for hypertension: Report of a multicentre open study. Curr. ther. Res. **14**, 185 (1972).

COLTART, D. J., GIBSON, D. G., SHAND, D. G.: Plasma propranolol levels associated with suppression of ventricular ectopic beats. Brit. med. J. **1971 I**, 490—491.

COLTART, D. J., SHAND, D. G.: Plasma propranolol levels in the quantitative assessment of β-adrenergic blockade in man. Brit. med. J. **1970 III**, 731—734.

DAY, GILLIAN M., PRICHARD, B. N. C.: Hypotensive action from combination of propranolol and other hypotensive drugs. Brit. J. Pharmacol. **41**, 408 (1971).

DAY, M. D., OWEN, A. A., WARREN, P. R.: An adrenergic neuron blocking action of propranolol in isolated tissues. J. Pharm. (Lond.) **20**, 1305—1345 (1968).

DOLLERY, C. T., PATTERSON, J. W., CONOLLY, M. E.: Clinical pharmacology of β-receptor-blocking drugs. Clin. Pharmacol. Ther. **10**, 765—799 (1969).

DOLLERY, C. T., LEWIS, P. J., MYERS, M. G., REID, J. L.: Central hypotensive effect of propranolol in the rabbit. Brit. J. Pharmacol. **48**, 343P (1973).

DORPH, S., BINDER, C.: Evaluation of the hypotensive effect of beta-adrenergic blockade in hypertension. Acta med. scand. **185**, 443—448 (1969).

DUNLOP, D., SHANKS, R. G.: Inhibition of the carotid sinus reflex by the chronic administration of propranolol. Brit. J. Pharmacol. **36**, 132—143 (1969).

EPSTEIN, S. E., BRAUNWALD, E.: The effect of beta adrenergic blockade on patterns of urinary sodium excretion. Ann. intern. Med. **65**, 20—27 (1966).

EPSTEIN, S. E., ROBINSON, B. F., KAHLER, R. L., BRAUNWALD, E.: Effects of beta adrenergic blockade on the cardiac response to maximal and submaximal exercise in man. J. clin. Invest. **44**, 1745—1753 (1965).

ESLER, M. D., NESTEL, P. J.: Evaluation of practolol in hypertension. Effects on sympathetic nervous system and renin responsiveness. Brit. Heart. J. **35**, 469—474 (1973).

EVANS, G. H., NIES, A. S., SHAND, D. G.: The disposition of propranolol III, decreased half life and volume of distribution as a result of plasma binding in man, monkey, dog and rat. J. Pharmacol. exp. Ther. **186**, 114—122 (1973).

EVANS, G. H., SHAND, D. G.: Disposition of propranolol V. Drug accumulation and steady-state concentrations during chronic oral administration in man. Clin. Pharmacol. Ther. **14**, 487—493 (1973a).

EVANS, G. H., SHAND, D. G.: Disposition of propranolol V. Independent variation in steady state circulating drug concentration and half-life as a result of plasma drug binding in man. Clin. Pharmacol. Ther. **14**, 494—500 (1973b).

FELIX, R. H., IVE, F. A., DAHL, M. G. C.: Cutaneous and ocular reactions to practolol. Brit. med. J. **1974IV**, 321—324.

FELTHAM, P. M., WATSON, O. F., PEEL, J. S., DUNLOP, D. J., TURNER, A. S.: Pindolol in hypertension: A double blind trial. N. Z. Med. **76**, 167 (1972).

FINEGAN, R. E., MARLON, A. M., HARRISON, D. C.: Circulatory effects of practolol. Amer. J. Cardiol. **29**, 315—322 (1972).

FITZGERALD, J. D.: Beta adrenergic blocking drugs. Present position and future. Acta cardiol. (Brux.) **XV**, 199 (1972).

FITZGERALD, J. D., SCALES, B.: Effect of a new adrenergic beta-blocking agent (ICI 50172) on heart rate in relation to its blood levels. Int. J. clin. Pharmacol. **1**, 467—474 (1968).

FITZGERALD, J. D., O'DONNELL, S. R.: Pharmacology of 4-hydroxy-propranolol, a metabolite of propranolol. Brit. J. Pharmacol. **43**, 222—235 (1971).

FORSBERG, S. A., JOHNSSON, G.: Hemodynamic effects of propranolol and H 56/28 in man. A comparative study of two beta adrenergic receptor antagonists Life Sci. **6**, 1147—1154 (1967).

FURBERG, C., MICHAELSON, G.: Effect of Aptin, a β adrenergic blocking agent, in arterial hypertension. Acta med. scand. **186**, 447—450 (1969).

GEORGE, C. F., FENYVESI, T., CONOLLY, M. E., DOLLERY, C. T.: Pharmacokinetics of dextro-, laevo- and racemic propranolol in man. Europ. J. clin. Pharmacol. **4**, 74—76 (1972).

GEORGE, C. F., FENYVEST, T., DOLLERY, C. T.: Pharmacoligical effects of propranolol in relation to plasma levels. In: DAVIES, D. S., PRICHARD, B. N. C. (Eds.): Biological effects of drugs in relation to their plasma concentrations. p. 123: University Park Press 1973.

GIBSON, D. G., COLTART, D. J.: Haemodynamic effects of practolol. Brit. Heart. J. **34**, 95—99 (1972).

GIBSON, D., SOWTON, E.: Effects of ICI 50172 in man during erect exercise. Brit. med. J. **1968I**, 213—215.

GILMORE, E., WEIL, J., CHIDSEY, C.: Treatment of essential hypertension with a new vasodilator in combination with beta-adrenergic blockade. New Engl. J. Med. **282**, 521—527 (1970).

GRAHAM, B. R., LITTLEJOHNS, D. W., PRICHARD, B. N. C., SCALES, B., SOUTHORN, P.: Preliminary observations on the human pharmacology of I.C.I. 66082 in normal volunteers. Brit. J. Pharmacol. **49**, 154 (1973).

GRANDJEAN, T., RIVIER, J. L.: Cardio-circulatory effects of beta-adrenergic blockade in organic heart disease. Brit. Heart J. **30**, 50—59 (1968).

GREENBLATT, D. J., KOCH-WESER, J.: Adverse reactions to propranolol in hospitalized medical patients. Amer. Heart J. **86**, 478—484 (1973).

GUGLER, R., HEROLD, W., DENGLER, H. J.: Pharmacokinetics of pindolol in man. Europ. J. clin. Pharmacol. **7**, 17 (1974).

GUGLER, R., HOBEL, W., BODEN, G., DENGLER, H. J.: The effects of pindolol on exercies induced cardiac acceleration in relation to plasma levels in man. Clin. Pharmacol. Ther. **17**, 127 (1975).

GUYTON, A. C.: Regulation of cardiac output. Anesthesiology **29**, 314—326 (1968).

HOLLANDER, W.: Hypertension, antihypertensive drugs and atherosclerosis. Circulation **48**, 1112—1127 (1973).

HANSSON, L.: Beta-adrenergic blockade in essential hypertension. Acta med. scand. (Suppl.) 550 (1973).

HAYES, A., COOPER, R. G.: Studies on the absorption, distribution and excretion of propranolol in rat, dog and monkey. J. Pharm. exp. Ther. **176**, 302—311 (1971).

HEFFERNAN, A., CARTY, A., O'MALLEY, K., BUGLER, J.: A within-patient comparision of debrisoquine and methyldopa in hypertension. Brit. med. J. **1971I**, 75.

HICKS, D. C., ARBAB, A. G., TURNER, P., MILLS, M.: A comparison of intravenous pindolol and propranolol in normal man. J. clin. Pharmacol. **12**, 212 (1972).

HOLLIFIELD, J. W., SHERMAN, K., VANDERZWAGGR, SHAND, D. G.: Proposed mechanisms of propranol's antihypertensive effect in essential hypertension. New Engl. J. Med. **295**, 68—73 (1976).

HUMPHREYS, G. S., DELVIN, D. G.: Ineffectiveness of propranolol in hypertensive Jamaicans. Brit. med. J. **1968II**, 601—603.

JOHANSSON, R., REGARDH, C. G., SJOGREN, J.: Absorption of alprenolol in man from tablets with different rates of release. Acta pharm. suec. **8**, 59—70 (1971).

JULIUS, S., PASCUAL, P. H., LONDON, R.: Effect of beta-adrenergic blockade on plasma volume in human subjects. Proc. Soc. exp. Biol. (N. Y.) **140**, 982 (1972).
KELLIHER, G. J., BUCKLEY, J. P.: Central hypotensive activity of dl and l-propranolol. J. pharm. Sci. **59**, 1276 (1970).
KERBER, R. E., GOLDMAN, R. H., ALDERMAN, E. L., HARRISON, D. C.: Circulatory responses to beta adrenergic blockade with alprenolol. Amer. J. Cardiol. **29**, 26—32 (1972).
LAVER, M. C., FAND, P., KINCAID SMITH, P.: Double blind comparison of two beta-blocking drugs with previous therapy in the treatment of hypertension. Med. J. Aust. **61**, 174 (1974).
LEISHMAN, A. W. D., THIRKETTLE, J. L., ALLEN, B. R., DIXON, R. A.: Controlled trial of oxprenolol and practolol in hypertension. Brit. med. J. **1970 IV**, 342—344.
LYDTIN, H., KUSUS, T., DANIEL, W., SCHIERL, W., ACKENHEIL, M., KEMPTER, H., LOHMOLLER, G., NIKLAS, M., INGE, W.: Propranolol therapy in essential hypertension. Amer. Heart J. **83**, 589—595 (1972).
McNEILL, R. S.: Effect of a beta-adrenergic blocking agent, propranolol, on asthmatics. Lancet **1964 II**, 1101.
MICHELAKIS, A. M., CAUDLE, J., LIDDLE, G. W.: In vitro stimulation of renin production by epinephrine, norepinephrine and cyclic AMP. Proc. Soc. exp. Biol. (N. Y.) **130**, 748—753 (1969).
MICHELAKIS, A. M., McALLISTER, R. G.: The effect of chronic adrenergic receptor blockade on plasma renin activity in man. J. clin. Endocr. **34**, 386—394 (1972).
MORGAN, T. O., LOUIS, W. J., DAWBORN, J. K., DOYLE, A. E.: The use of pindolol (Visken) in the treatment of hypertension. Med. J. Aust. **2**, 309 (1972).
NIES, A. S., McNELL, J. S., SCHRIER, R. W.: Mechanism of increased sodium reabsorption during propranolol administration. Circulation **44**, 596—604 (1971).
NIES, A. S., EVANS, G. H., SHAND, D. G.: Regional hemodynamic effects of beta-adrenergic blockade with propranolol in the unanesthetized primate. Amer. Heart J. **85**, 97—102 (1973a).
NIES, A. S., EVANS, G. H., SHAND, D. G.: The hemodynamic effects of beta-adrenergic blockade on the flow-dependent hepatic clearance of propranolol. J. Pharmacol. exp. Ther. **184**, 716—720 (1973b).
OATES, J. A., SELIGMANN, A. W., CLARKE, M. A., ROUSSEAU, P., LEE, R. E.: The relative efficiency of guanethidine, methyldopa and pargyline as antihypertensive agents. New Engl. J. Med. **273**, 729 (1965).
OHNHAUS, E. E., NUESCH, E., MEIER, J., KALBERER, F.: Pharmacokinetics of unlabelled and ^{14}C-labelled pindolol in uraemia. Europ. J. clin. Pharmacol. **7**, 25 (1974).
OLLSON, S. B., VARNAUSKAS, E.: Duration of beta-receptor blockade after oral administration of LB 46. Europ. J. clin. Pharmacol. **5**, 214 (1973).
PARKER, J. O., WEST, R. O., DIGIORGI, S.: Hemodynamic effects of propranolol in coronary heart disease. Amer. J. Cardiol. **21**, 11—19 (1968).
PASSO, S. S., ASSAYKEEN, T. A., OTSUKA, K., WISE, B. L., GOLDFIEN, A., GANONG, W. F.: Effects of stimulation of the medulla oblongata on renin secretion in dogs. Neuroendocrinology **7**, 1—10 (1971).
PATERSON, J. W., CONOLLY, M. E., DOLLERY, C. T., HAYES, A., COOPER, R. G.: The pharmacodynamics and metabolism of propranolol in man. Pharmacol. Clin. **2**, 127—133 (1970).
PATTERSON, J. W., DOLLERY, C. T.: Effect of propranolol in mild hypertension. Lancet **1966 II**, 1148—1150.
PETTINGER, W. A., MITCHELL, H. C.: Minoxidil—an alternative to nephrectomy for refractory hypertension. New Engl. J. Med. **289**, 167—171 (1973).
PODOLSKY, S., PATTAVINA, C. G.: Hyperosmolar non-ketotic diabetic coma: a complication of propranolol therapy. Metabolism **22**, 685—693 (1973).
PRICHARD, B. N. C.: Aspects of the evaluation of antihypertensive drugs. In: Proceedings of the International Symposium on Clinical Pharmacology, p. 193. Brussels: Royal Academies of Medicine of Belgium, 1970.
PRICHARD, B. N. C.: Hypotensive action of pronethalol. Brit. med. J. **1964 I**, 1227—1228.
PRICHARD, B. N. C.: Communication—5th International Congress on Pharmacology, San Francisco (1972).
PRICHARD, B. N. C., GILLAM, P. M. S.: The use of propranolol in the treatment of hypertension. Brit. med. J. **1964 II**, 725—727.
PRICHARD, B. N. C., GILLAM, P. M. S.: Treatment of hypertension with propranolol. Brit. med. J. **1969 I**, 7—16.
PRICHARD, B. N. C., JOHNSTON, A. W., HILL, I. L., ROSENHEIM, M. L.: Bethanidine, guanethidine and methyldopa in the treatment of hypertension: a within patient comparison. Brit. med. J. **1968 I**, 135.

PRICHARD, B. N. C., GILLAM, P. M. S., GRAHAM, B. R.: Beta receptor antagonism in hypertension; comparison with the effect of adrenergic neurone inhibition on cardiovascular responses. Int. J. clin. Pharmacol. 4—1, p. 135 (1970a).
PRICHARD, B. N. C., SHINEBOURNE, E., FLEMING, J., HAMER, J.: Haemodynamic studies in hypertensive patients treated by oral propranolol. Brit. Heart J. **32**, 236—240 (1970).
PRICHARD, B. N. C., BOAKES, A. J., DAY, G.: Practolol in the treatment of hypertension. Postgrad. med. J. Suppl. **47**, 84—92 (1971).
RAFTERY, E. B., DENMAN, A. M.: Systemic lupus erythematosus syndrome induced by practolol. Brit. med. J. **1973II**, 452—455.
RICHARDSON, D. W., FREUND, J., GEAR, A. S., MAUCK, H. P., PRESTON, L. W.: Effect of propranolol on elevated arterial pressure. Circulation **37**, 534—542 (1968).
RIESS, W., RAJAGOPALAN, T. G., INHOF, P., SCHMID, K., KEBERLE, H.: Metabolic studies on oxprenolol in animals and man by means of radiotracer techniques and GLC analysis. Postgrad. med. J. **46**, (Suppl.) 32—39 (1970).
ROBIN, E., COWAN, PURI, P., GANGLY, S., DEBOYRIE, E., MARTINEZ, M., STOCK, T., BING, R. J.: A comparative study of nitroglycerine and propranolol. Circulation **36**, 175—186 (1967).
ROWLAND, M.: Influence of route of administration on drug availability. J. pharm. Sci. **61**, 70—74 (1972).
SAELENS, D. A., WALLE, T., PRWITGA, P. J., KNAPP, D. R., GAFFNEY, T.: Central nervous system effects and metabolic disposition of a glycol metabolite of propranolol. J. Pharmacol. exp. Ther. **188**, 86—92 (1974).
SCALES, B., COSGROVE, M. B.: The metabolism and distribution of the selective adrenergic beta blocking agent, practolol. J. Pharmacol. exp. Ther. **175**, 338—347 (1970).
SCHAFFALITZKY DEMUCKADELL, O. B., GYNTELBERG, F.: The antihypertensive effect of a new beta-blocking agent pindolol compared with chlorthalidone. Europ. J. clin. Pharmacol. **5**, 210 (1973).
SCHNECK, D. W., AOKI, V. S., KROETZ, F. W., WILSON, W. R.: Correlation of beta blockade with serum practolol levels after oral administration. Clin. Pharmacol. Ther. **13**, 685—693 (1972).
SEDERBERG-OLSEN, P., IBSEN, H.: Plasma volume and extracellular fluid volume during long-term treatment with propranolol in essential hypertension. Clin. Sci. **43**, 165—170 (1972).
SEEDAT, Y. K., STEWART-WYNNE, E. G., REDDY, J., RANDEREE, M.: Experiences with beta-adrenergic blockade drugs in hypertension. S. Afr. med. J. **47**, 259 (1973).
SHAND, D. G.: Proprandol. Disease-a-Month. October, 1974.
SHAND, D. G., EVANS, G. H., NIES, A. S.: The almost complete hepatic extraction of propranolol during intravenous administration in the dog. Life Sci. **10**, 1417—1421 (1971).
SHAND, D. G., NUCKOLLS, E. M., OATES, J. A.: Plasma propranolol levels in adults with observations in four children. Clin. Pharmacol. Ther. **11**, 112—120 (1970).
SHAND, D. G., RANGNO, R. E.: The disposition of propranolol —1. Elimination during oral absorption in man. Pharmacology **7**, 159—168 (1972).
SHAND, D. G., RANGNO, R. E., EVANS, G. H.: The disposition of propranolol II: Hepatic elimination in the rat. Pharmacology **8**, 344—352 (1972).
SHINEBOURNE, E., FLEMING, J., HAMER, J.: Haemodynamic responses to exercise in hypertension. Place of the sympathetic nervous system evaluated by a new selective beta adrenergic blocking agent ICI 50, 172. Cardiovasc. Res. **2**, 379—383 (1968).
SINGH, B. N., TILL, M. R., KELLY, D. T.: The effects of oxprenolol (Trasicor, Ciba 39089-Ba) on patterns of urinary sodium excretion in man. Amer. J. Cardiol. **27**, 372—375 (1971).
SLEIGHT, P., GOLBBIN, B., PICKERING, T. G.: Baroreflex sensitivity in normal and hypertensive man: The effect of β-adrenergic blockade on reflex sensitivity. Postgrad. med. (Suppl.) **47**, 79—81 (1971).
SONNENBLICK, E. H., ROSS, J., BRAUNWALD, E.: Oxygen consumption of the heart. Newer concepts of its multifactorial determination. Amer. J. Cardiol. **22**, 328—336 (1968).
SOWTON, E., BALCON, R., CROSS, D., FRICK, H.: Haemodynamic effects of ICI 50172 in patients with ischaemic heart disease. Brit. med. J. **1968I**, 215—216.
SOWTON, E., HAMER, J.: Hemodynamic changes after beta adrenergic blockade. Amer. J. Cardiol. **18**, 317—320 (1966).
STEPHEN, S. A.: Unwanted effects of propranolol. Amer. J. Cardiol. **18**, 463—468 (1966).
STERN, S., HOFFMAN, M., BRAUN, K.: Cardiovascular responses to carotid and vertebral artery infusions of propranolol. Cardiovasc. Res. **5**, 425—430 (1971).
STOKES, G. S., WEBER, M. A., THORNELL, I. R.: β-blockers and plasma renin activity in hypertension. Brit. med. J. **1974I**, 60—62.
TARAZI, R. C., FROHLICH, E. D., DUSTAN, H. P.: Plasma volume changes with long-term beta-adrenergic blockade. Amer. Heart J. **82**, 770—776 (1971).
TAYLOR, J. A.: Hypotension after oral propranolol. Lancet **1968I**, 532—533.

TAYLOR, S. H., MAJID, P. A., SAXTON, C., STOKER, J. B.: Comparison of the circulatory effects of oxprenolol and propranolol in hypertensive patients. In: SIMPSON, F. O. (Ed.): Beta adrenergic receptor blocking durgs—an international symposium. Auckland 1970.

TEWARI, S. N., GRANT, R. H. E.: Propranolol in hypertension. Postgrad. med. J. **44**, 509—512 (1968).

THORPE, P.: A controlled study of prindolol (Visken) in hypertension. Med. J. Aust. **2**, 306 (1972).

TIBBLIN, G., ABLAD, B.: Antihypertensive therapy with alprenolol a β-adrenergic receptor antagonist. Acta med. scand. **186**, 451—457 (1969).

TUCKMAN, J., MARTIN, R., HODLER, J.: Hypertensiebehandlung mit hohen Dosen von Oxprenolol, allein oder in Kombination mit dem Vasodilatator Dihydralazin. Helv. med. Acta **36**, 243—244 (1972).

TURNER, A. S., PEEL, J. S.: An evaluation of hypotensive agents. Med. J. Aust. (Suppl. Sept. 16) p. 48 (1972).

TURNER, A. S., PEEL, J. S.: Comparative studies with beta-adrenergic receptor blockade. In: SIMPSON, F. O. (Ed.): Beta adrenergic receptor blocking durgs—an international symposium. Auckland 1970.

ULRYCH, M., FROHLICH, E. D., DUSTAN, H. P., PAGE, I. H.: Immediate hemodynamic effects of beta adrenergic blockade with propranolol in normotensive and hypertensive man. Circulation **37**, 411—416 (1968).

VAN COLLER, P. E.: Clinical experience with Visken (Pindolol) in essential hypertension. Its special comparative action to aldomet (Methyldopa). J. int. med. Res. **1**, 561 (1973).

VANDER, A. J.: Effect of catecholamines and the renal nerves on renin secretion in anesthetized dogs. Amer. J. Physiol. **209**, 659—662 (1965).

VERNIORY, A., STAROUKINE, M., TELERMAN, M., DELWICHE, F.: Effect of sotalol on arterial blood pressure and renin-angiotensin system in hypertensive patients. Experta Medica Symposium on Clinical Advances in beta blocking therapy, in press (1974).

WAAL, H. J.: Hypotensive action of propranolol. Clin. Pharmacol. Ther. **7**, 588—598 (1966).

WAAL-MANNING, H. J.: Comparative studies on the hypotensive effects of beta-adrenergic receptor blockade. In: Simpson Symposium in beta-adrenergic receptor blocking drugs, p. 64. CIBA, Auckland 1970.

WAAL-MANNING, H. J.: Lack of effect of d-propranolol on blood pressure and pulse rate in hypertensive patients. Proc. Univ. Otago med. Sch. **48**, 80 (1970).

WAAL-MANNING, H. J., SIMPSON, F. O.: Comparison of pindolol (Visken) with other antihypertensive drugs. Aust. N. Z. J. Med. **3**, 425 (1973).

WALLE, G., GAFFNEY, T. E.: Propranolol metabolism in man and dog: Mass spectroscopic identification of six new metabolites. J. Pharmacol. exp. Ther. **183**, 83—92 (1972).

WASSERMAN, A. J., PROCTOR, J. D., ALLEN, F. J., KEMP, V. E.: Human cardiovascular effects of alprenolol, a beta-adrenergic blocker: hemodynamic, antiarrhythmic, and antianginal. J. clin. Pharmacol. **10**, 37—49 (1970).

WISEMAN, R. A.: Practolol—accumulated data on unwanted effects. Postgrad. med. J. (Suppl.) Vol. **47**, 68—71 (1971).

WOLFSON, S., HEINLE, R. A., HERMAN, M. V., KEMP, H. G., SULLIVAN, J. M., GORLIN, R.: Propranolol in angina pectoris. Amer. J. Cardiol. **18**, 345—352 (1966).

WRIGHT, P.: Untoward effects associated with practolol administration: Oculomucocutaneous syndrome. Brit. med. J. **1975I**, 595—598.

ZACEST, R., GILMORE, E., KOCH-WESER, J.: Treatment of essential hypertension with combined vasodilation and beta-adrenergic blockage. New Engl. J. Med. **286**, 618—622 (1972).

ZACEST, R., KOCH-WESER, J.: Relation of propranolol plasma level to β-blockade during oral therapy. Pharmacology **7**, 178—184 (1972).

ZACHARIAS, F. J., COWEN, K. J.: Controlled trial of propranolol in hypertension. Brit. med. J. **1970I**, 471.

ZACHARIAS, F. J., COWEN, K. J., PRESST, J., VICKERS, J., WALL, B. G.: Propranolol in hypertension. A study of long-term therapy, 1964—1970. Amer. Heart J. **83**, 755—761 (1972).

Section VI. The Direct Peripheral Vasodilators

ABLAD, B.: A study of the mechanism of the hemodynamic effects of hydralazine in man. Acta pharmacol. (Kbh.) **20**, 1—53 (1963).

AHEARN, D. J., GRIM, C. E.: Treatment of malignant hypertension with sodium nitroprusside. Arch. intern. Med. **133**, 187—191 (1974).

ALARCON-SEGOVIA, D.: Clinical and experimental studies on the hydralazine syndrome and its relationship to systemic lupus erythematosus. Medicine **46**, 1—33 (1967).

Andersson, R.: Cyclic AMP as a mediator of the relaxing action of papaverine, nitroglycerine, diazoxide and hydralazine in intestinal and vascular smooth muscle. Acta pharmacol. (Kbh.) **32**, 321—336 (1973).
Baer, L., Goodwin, F. J., Laragh, J. H.: Diazoxide-induced renin release in man: Dissociation from plasma and extracellular fluid volume changes. J. clin. Endocr. **29**, 1107—1109 (1969).
Bhatia, S. K., Frohlich, E. D.: Hemodynamic comparison of agents useful in hypertensive emergencies. Amer. Heart J. **85**, 367—373 (1973),
Blackard, W. G., Aprill, C. N.: Mechanism of action of diazoxide. J. Lab. clin. Med. **69**, 960—967 (1967).
Berglund, G.: A homogenously investigated, highly selected hypertensive population. Acta med. scand. **194**, 87—91 (1973).
Boerth, R.: Personal communication.
Boxer, G. E., Rickards, J. C.: Studies on the metabolism of the carbon of cyanide and thiocyanate. Arch. Biochem. **39**, 7—26 (1952).
Campbell, W. B., Pettinger, W. A., Keeton, K., Brooks, S. N.: Vasodilating antihypertensive drug-induced aldosterone releasei a study of endogenous angiotensin-mediated aldosterone release in the rat. J. Pharmacol. exp. Ther. **193**, 166—175 (1975).
Carliner, N. H., Denune, D. P., Finch, C. S., Jr., Goldberg, L. I.: Sodium nitroprusside treatment of ergotamine-induced peripheral ischemia. J. Amer. med. Ass. **227**, 308—309 (1974).
Charles, M. A., Danforth, E., Jr.: Nonketoacidotic hyperglycemia and coma during intravenous diazoxide therapy in uremia. Diabetes **20**, 501—503 (1971).
Chatterjee, K., Parmley, W. M., Ganz, W., Forrester, J., Walinsky, P., Crexells, C., Swan, H. J. C.: Hemodynamic and metabolic responses to vasodilator therapy in acute myocardial infarction. Circulation **48**, 1183—1193 (1973).
Chidsey, C. A.: Clinical and pharmacokinetic studies of minoxidil a new antihypertensive agent. Clin. Sci. molec. Med. **45**, Suppl. 1, 171—173 (1973).
Comerford, M. B., Pringle, A.: A long-term study of the antihypertensive effect of alprenolol. Acta med. scand. Suppl. **554**, 15—22 (1974).
Crout, J. R., Andreasen, F. V. V., Parks, R. I., Heimbach, D. M.: Intravenous diazoxide in hypertension. Clin. Res. **18**, 337 (1970).
Danzig, L. E., Kringel, A. J.: Use of the artificial kidney in treatment of thiocyanate psychosis. J. Amer. med. Ass. **158**, 560—563 (1955).
Domzalski, C. A., Kolb, L. C., Hines, E. A.: Delirious reactions secondary to thiocyanate therapy of hypertension. Mayo Clin. Proc. **28**, 272—280 (1953).
Dormois, J. C., Young, J. L., Nies, A. S.: Minoxidil in severe hypertension: Value when conventional drugs have failed. Amer. Heart J. (in press).
Drug Ther. Bull. Emergency reduction of blood pressure. Drug Ther. Bull. **9**, 80 (1971).
Ducharme, D. W., Freyburger, W. A., Graham, B. E., Carlson, R. G.: Pharmacologic properties of minoxidil: a new hypotensive agent. J. Pharmacol. exp. Ther. **184**, 662—670 (1973).
Finnerty, F. A., Jr., Kakaviatos, N., Tuckman, J., McGill, J.: Clinical evaluation of diazoxide: A new treatment for acute hypertension. Circulation **28**, 203—208 (1963).
Franciosa, J. A., Guiha, N. H., Limas, C. J., Rodriguera, E., Cohn, J. N.: Improved left venticular function during nitroprusside infusion in acute myocardial infarction. Lancet **1972 I**, 650—654.
Freis, E. D., Rose, J. C., Higgins, T. F., Finnerty, F. A., Jr., Kelley, R. T., Partenope, E. A.: The hemodynamic effects of hypotensive drugs in man IV. 1-hydrazinophthalazine. Circulation **8**, 199—204 (1953).
Gibaldi, M., Boyes, R. N., Feldman, S.: Influence of firstpass effect on availability of drugs on oral administration. J. pharm. Sci. **60**, 1338—1340 (1971).
Gifford, R. W., Jr.: Treatment of hypertensive emergencies including use of sodium nitroprusside. Mayo Clin. Proc. **34**, 387—394 (1959).
Gifford, R. W., Jr.: Hypertensive emergencies and their treatment. Med. Clin. N. Amer. **45**, 441—452 (1961).
Gifford, R. W.: Treatment of hypertensive emergencies. In: Onesti, G., Kim, K., Moyer, J. (Eds.): Hypertension: Mechanisms management. The XXVI Hahnemann Symposium, pp. 809—817. New York: Grune and Stratton 1973.
Gilmore, E., Weil, J., Chidsey, C.: Treatment of essential hypertension with a new vasodilator in combination with β-adrenergic blockade. New Engl. J. Med. **282**, 521—527 (1970).
Goldstein, F., Rieders, F.: Formation of cyanide in dog and man following administration of thiocyanate. Amer. J. Physiol. **167**, 47—51 (1951).
Gottlieb, T. B., Katz, F. H., Chidsey, C. A.: Combined therapy with vasodilator drugs and beta-adrenergic blockade in hypertension. A comparative study of minoxidil and hydralazine. Circulation **45**, 571—582 (1972a).

GOTTLIEB, T. B., THOMAS, R. C., CHIDSEY, C. A.: Pharmacokinetic studies of minoxidil. Clin. Pharmacol. Ther. **13**, 436—441 (1972b).
GROSS, F., DRUEY, J., MEIER, R.: Eine neue Gruppe blutdrucksenkender Substanzen von besonderem Wirkungscharakter. Experientia (Basel) **6**, 19—21 (1950).
GUIHA, N. H., COHN, J. N., MIKULIC, E., FRANCIOSA, J. A., LIMAS, C. J.: Treatment of refractory heart failure with infusion of nitroprusside. New Engl. J. Med. **291**, 587—592 (1974).
HAMBY, W. M., JANKOWSKI, G. J., POUGET, J. M., DUNEA, G., GANTT, C. L.: Intravenous use of diazoxide in the treatment of severe hypertension. Circulation **37**, 169—174 (1968).
HANSSON, L., OLANDER, R., ABERG, H., MALMCRONA, R., WESTERLUND, A.: Treatment of hypertension with propranolol and hydralazine. Acta med. scand. **190**, 531—534 (1971).
HANSSON, L., ZWEIFLER, A. J.: Combined treatment of hypertension with vasodilatation and beta-adrenergic blockade. Mich. Med. **72**, 695—698 (1973).
HERMANN, L.: Über die Wirkung des Nitroprussidnatriums. In: Pflügers Arch. ges. Physiol. **39**, 419 (1886 Bonn).
HUMPHREY, S. J., WILLIAMS, J. E., ZINS, G. R.: Renal tubular site of enhanced sodium reabsorption in dogs treated with peripheral vasodilators. Fed. Proc. **30**, 607 (1971).
HUMPHREY, S. J., WILSON, E., ZINS, G. R.: Whole body tissue blood flow in conscious dogs treated with minoxidil. Fed. Proc. **33**, 583 (1974).
J.A.M.A. Drug Commentary. Evaluation of diazoxide (Hyperstat I.V.). J. Amer. med. Ass. **224**, 1422—1423 (1973).
JELLETT, L. B., DYE, M. S., MICHELAKIS, A. M., OATES, J. A.: Individualization of antihypertensive therapy with diazoxide, employing a dose-ranging regimen. (Unpublished observations.)
JOHNSON, B. F.: Diazoxide and renal function in man. Clin. Pharmacol. Ther. **12**, 815—824 (1971).
JOHNSON, B. F., KAPUR, M.: The influences of rate of injection upon the effects of diazoxide. Amer. J. med. Sci. **263**, 481—488 (1972).
JOHNSON, C. C.: Mechanism of actions and toxicity of nitroprusside. Proc. Soc. exp. Biol. (N. Y.) **26**, 102—103 (1928).
JOHNSON, C. C.: The actions and toxicity of sodium nitroprusside. Arch. int. Pharmacodyn. **35**, 480—496 (1929).
JUDSON, W. E., HOLLANDER, W., WILKINS, R. W.: The effects of intravenous apresoline (hydralazine) on cardiovascular and renal function in patients with and without congestive heart failure. Circulation **13**, 664—674 (1956).
JUDSON, W. E., HOLLANDER, W., WILKINS, R. W.: The effect of exercise in the supine position on cardiovascular and renal function before and during chronic oral hydralazine therapy. J. Lab. clin. Med. **49**, 672—683 (1957).
KAKAVIATOS, N., FINNERTY, F. A., JR.: Preliminary observations on the value of diazoxide administered intravenously in man. Angiology **13**, 541—544 (1962).
KANEKO, Y., IKEDA, T., TAKEDA, T., UEDA, H.: Renin release during acute reduction of arterial pressure in normotensive subjects and patients with renovascular hypertension. J. clin. Invest. **46**, 705—716 (1967).
KOCH-WESER, J.: Hypertensive emergencies. New Engl. J. Med. **290**, 211—214 (1974a).
KOCH-WESER, J.: Vasodilator drugs in the treatment of hypertension. Arch. intern. Med. **133**, 1017—1027 (1974b).
KUCHEL, O., FISHMAN, L. M., LIDDLE, G. W., MICHELAKIS, A.: Effect of diazoxide on plasma renin activity in hypertensive patients. Ann. intern. Med. **67**, 791—799 (1967).
LANG, K.: Die Rhodanbildung im Tierkörper. Biochem. Z. **259**, 243—256 (1933).
LESSER, J. M., ISRAILI, Z. H., DAVIS, E., DAYTON, P. G.: Fate of hydralazine-^{14}C in man and dog. Clin. Pharmacol. Ther. **14**, 140 (1973).
LESSER, J. M., ISRAILI, Z. H., DAVID, D. C., DAYTON, P. G.: Metabolism and disposition of hydralazine-^{14}C in man and dog. Drug. Metab. Dispos. **2**, 351—360 (1974).
LIMAS, C. J., FREIS, E. D.: Minoxidil in severe hypertension with renal failure. Effect of its addition to conventional antihypertensive drugs. Amer. J. Cardiol. **31**, 355—361 (1973).
MANI, M. K.: Nitroprusside revisited. Brit. med. J. **1971 III**, 407—408.
MICHELAKIS, A. M., MCALLISTER, R. G.: The effect of chronic adrenergic receptor blockade on plasma renin activity in man. J. clin. Endocr. **34**, 386—394 (1972).
MILLER, W. E., GIFFORD, R. W., JR., HUMPHREY, D. C., VIDT, D. G.: Management of severe hypertension with intravenous injections of diazoxide. Amer. J. Cardiol. **24**, 870—875 (1969).
MOORE-JONES, D., PERRY, H. M., JR.: Radioautographic localization of hydralazine-1-C^{14} in arterial walls. Proc. Soc. exp. Biol. (N. Y.) **122**, 576—579 (1966).
MOISTER, F. C., FREIS, E. D.: The metabolism of thiocyanate after prolonged administration in man. Amer. J. med. Sci. **218**, 549—555 (1949).
MOSER, M.: Diazoxide—an effective vasodilator in accelerated hypertension. Amer. Heart J. **87**, 791—795 (1974).

MOYER, J. H.: Hydrallazine (Apresoline) hydrochloride: Pharmacological observations and clinical results in the therapy of hypertension. Arch. intern. Med. **91**, 419—439 (1953).

MROCZEK, W. J., LEIBEL, B. A., DAVIDOV, M., FINNERTY, F. A., JR.: The importance of the rapid administration of diazoxide in accelerated hypertension. New Engl. J. Med. **285**, 603—606 (1971).

NICKERSON, M., THOMAS, J. J.: Renal excretion of thiocyanate. J. Lab. clin. Med. **38**, 194—198 (1951).

NOUROK, D. S., GLASSOCK, R. J., SOLOMON, D. H., MAXWELL, M. H.: Hypothyroidism following prolonged sodium nitroprusside therapy. Amer. J. med. Sci. **248**, 129—138 (1964).

PAGE, I. H.: Cardiovascular actions of sodium nitroprusside in animals and hypertensive patients. Circulation **11**, 188—198 (1955).

PALMER, R. F., LASSETER, K. C.: Sodium nitroprusside. NewEngl. J. Med. **292**, 294—297 (1975).

PAPE, J.: The effect of alprenolol in combination with hydralazine in essential hypertension. A double-blind, crossover study and a long-term follow-up study. Acta med. scand. Suppl. **554**, 55—62 (1974).

PARMLEY, W. W., CHATTERJEE, K., CHARUZI, Y., SWAN, H. J. C.: Hemodynamic effects of noninvasive systolic unloading (nitroprusside) and diastolic augmentation (external counterpulsation) in patients with acute myocardial infarction. Amer. J. Cardiol. **33**, 819—825 (1974).

PERRY, H. M., JR., SCHROEDER, H. A., MORROW, J. D.: Studies on the control of the hypertension by Hyphex. IV. Levels of the agents in urine and blood. Amer. J. med. Sci. **228**, 405—416 (1954).

PERRY, H. M., JR., TAN, E. M., CARMODY, S., SAKOMOTO, A.: Relationship of acetyl transferase activity to antinuclear antibodies and toxic symptoms in hypertensive patients treated with hydralazine. J. Lab. clin. Med. **76**, 114—125 (1970).

PERRY, H. M., JR.: Late toxicity to hydralazine resembling systemic lupus erythematosus or rheumatoid arthritis. Amer. J. Med. **54**, 58—72 (1973).

PETTINGER, W. A., MITCHELL, H. C.: Minoxidil—an alternative to nephrectomy for refractory hypertension. New Engl. J. Med. **289**, 167—171 (1973).

PETTINGER, W. A., KEETON, K.: Altered renin release and propranolol potentiation of vasodilatory drug hypotension. J. clin. Invest. **55**, 236—243 (1975).

PETTINGER, W. A., MITCHELL, H. C.: Renin release, saralasin and the vasodilator-beta-blocker drug interaction in man. New Engl. J. Med. **292**, 1214—1217 (1975).

PINES, K. L., CRYMBLE, M. M.: In vitro conversion of thiocyanate to cyanide in the presence of erythrocytes. Proc. Soc. exp. Biol. (N. Y.) **81**, 160—163 (1952).

PLUSS, R. G., ORCUTT, J., CHIDSEY, C. A.: Tissue distribution and hypotensive effects of minoxidil in normotensive rats. J. Lab. clin. Med. **79**, 639—647 (1972).

POHL, J. E., THURSTON, H., SWALES, J. D.: The antidiuretic action of diazoxide. Clin. Sci. **42**, 145—152 (1972).

POWELL, W. J., JR., GREEN, R. M., WHITING, R. B., SANDERS, C. A.: Action of diazoxide on sketetal muscle vascular resistance. Circulat. Res. **28**, 167—178 (1971).

PRICE EVANS, D. A., WHITE, T. A.: Human acetylation polymorphism. J. Lab. clin. Med. **63**, 394—403 (1964).

PRUITT, A. W., DAYTON, P. G., PATTERSON, J. H.: Disposition of diazoxide in children. Clin. Pharmacol. Ther. **14**, 73—82 (1973a).

PRUITT, A. W., FARAJ, B. A., ISRAILI, Z. H., DAYTON, P. G.: Metabolism of diazoxide. Clin. Res. **21**, 107 (1973b).

PRUITT, A. W., FARAJ, B. A., DAYTON, P. G.: Metabolism of diazoxide in man and experimental animals. J. Pharmacol. exp. Ther. **188**, 248—256 (1974).

RADO, J. P., SZENDE, L., TAKO, J., HALMOS, T.: Effects of intravenous diazoxide and chlorpropamide on renal function in man. Amer. Heart J. **85**, 755—766 (1973).

RAMASWAMY, D., RICHARDSON, D. W.: Mechanism of circulatory effects of intravenous diazoxide. Circulation Suppl. **38**, VI—160 (1968).

REIDENBERG, M. M., DRAYER, D., DEMARCO, A. L., BELLO, C. T.: Hydralazine elimination in man. Clin. Pharmacol. Ther. **14**, 970—977 (1973).

REUBI, F.: Renal hyperemia induced in man by a new phthalazine derivative. Proc. Soc. exp. Biol. (N. Y.) **73**, 102—103 (1950).

Roche: Nipride T. M. (sodium nitroprusside). Nipride package insert. Nutley, New Jersey: Hoffmann-LaRoche Inc. 1974.

ROWE, G. G., HUSTON, J. H., MAXWELL, G. M., CROSLEY, A. P., JR., CRUMPTON, C. W.: Hemodynamic effects of 1-hydrazinophthalazine in patients with arterial hypertension. J. clin. Invest. **34**, 115—120 (1955).

RUBIN, A. A., ROTH, F. E., WINBURY, M. M., TOPLISS, J. G., SHERLOCK, M. H., SPERBER, N., BLACK, J.: New class of antihypertensive agents. Science **133**, 2067 (1961a),

RUBIN, A. A., ROTH, F. E., WINBURY, M. M.: A non-diuretic benzothiadiazine with anti-hypertensive properties. Nature (Lond.) **192**, 176—177 (1961b).

RUBIN, A. A., TAYLOR, R. M., ROTH, F. E.: A brief review of the development of diazoxide as an antihypertensive agent. Ann. N. Y. Acad. Sci. **150**, 457—460 (1968).

SAUNDERS, J. P., HIMWICH, W. A.: Properties of the transsulfurase responsible for conversion of cyanide to thiocyanate. Amer. J. Physiol. **163**, 404—409 (1950).

SCHIFFMANN, H., FUCHS, P.: Controlled hypotension effected by sodium nitroprusside. Acta anaesth. scand. Suppl. **23**, 704—709 (1966).

SCHLANT, R. C., TSAGARIS, T. S., ROBERTSON, R. J., JR.: Studies on the acute cardiovascular effects of intravenous sodium nitroprusside. Amer. J. Cardiol. **9**, 51—59 (1962).

SCHROEDER, H. A.: Effects on hypertension of sulfhydryl and hydrazine compounds. J. clin. Invest. **30**, 672—673 (1951).

SCHROEDER, H. A.: The effect of l-hydrazinophthalazine in hypertension. Circulation **5**, 28—37 (1952).

SELLERS, E. M., KOCH-WESER, J.: Protein binding and vascular activity of diazoxide. New Engl. J. Med. **281**, 1141—1144 (1969).

SELLERS, E. M., KOCH-WESER, J.: Influence of intravenous injection rate on protein binding and vascular activity of diazoxide. Ann. N. Y. Acad. Sci. **226**, 319—332 (1973).

SELLERS, E. M., KOCH-WESER, J.: Binding of diazoxide and other benzothiadiazines to human albumin. Biochem. Pharmacol. **23**, 553—566 (1974).

SHEN, D., O'MALLEY, K., GIBALDI, M., MCNAY, J. L.: Pharmacodynamics of minoxidil as a guide for individualizing dosage regimens in hypertension. Clin. Pharmacol. Ther. **17**, 593—598 (1975).

SIEGEL, P., MORACA, P. P., GREEN, J. R.: Sodium nitroprusside in the surgical treatment of cerebral aneurysms and arteriovenous malformations. Brit. J. Anaesth. **43**, 790—795 (1971).

STEINKE, J., SOELDNER, J. S.: Metabolic effects of diazoxide in normal subjects, patients with diabetes mellitus, and patients with organic hypoglycemia. Ann. N. Y. Acad. Sci. **150**, 326—336 (1968).

STUNKARD, A., WERTHEIMER, L., REDISCH, W.: Studies on hydralazine: Evidence for a peripheral site of action. J. clin. Invest. **33**, 1047—1053 (1954).

STYLES, M., COLEMAN, A. J., LEARY, W. P.: Some hemodynamic effects of sodium nitroprusside. Anesthesiology **38**, 173—176 (1973).

SYMCHOWICZ, S., WINSTON, L., BLACK, J., SMITH, M., CALESNICK, B., TABACHNICK, I. I. A.: Diazoxide blood levels in man. J. pharm. Sci. **56**, 912—914 (1967).

TABACHNICK, I. I. A., GULBENKIAN, A.: Mechanism of diazoxide hyperglycemia in animals. Ann. N. Y. Acad. Sci. **150**, 204—218 (1968).

TAYLOR, R. M., RUBIN, A. A.: Studies on the renal pharmacology of diazoxide, an antidiuretic benzothiadiazine. J. Pharmacol. Ther. **144**, 284—292 (1964).

The Medical Letter. Diazoxide (Hyperstat). Med. Lett. Drug. Ther. **15**, 53—55 (1973).

THIRLWELL, M. P., ZSOTER, T. T.: The effect of diazoxide on the veins. Amer. Heart J. **83**, 512—517 (1972).

TUZEL, I. H.: Sodium nitroprusside: A review of its clinical effectiveness as a hypotensive agent. J. clin. Pharmacol. **14**, 495—503 (1974).

UEDA, H., KANEKO, Y., TAKEDA, T., IKEDA, T., YAGI, S.: Observations on the mechanism of renin release by hydralazine in hypertensive patients. Circulat. Res. **27** (suppl. 2), 201—206 (1970).

UPDIKE, S. J., HARRINGTON, A. H.: Acute diabetic ketoacidosis—a complication of intravenous diazoxide treatment for refractory hypertension. New Engl. J. Med. **280**, 768 (1969).

VELASCO, M., O'MALLEY, K., ROBIE, N. W., WELLS, J., ISRAILI, Z. H., MCNAY, J. L.: Differential effects of propranolol on heart rate and plasma renin activity in patients treated with minoxidil. Clin. Pharmacol. Ther. **16**, 1031—1038 (1974).

VESEY, C. J., COLE, P. V., LINNELL, J. C., WILSON, J.: Some metabolic effects of sodium nitroprusside in man. Brit. med. J. **1974 II**, 140—142.

WALD, M. H., LINDBERG, H. A., BARKER, M. H.: The toxic manifestations of the thiocyanates. J. Amer. med. Ass. **112**, 1120—1124 (1939).

WILKINSON, E. L., BACKMAN, H., HECHT, H. H.: Cardiovascular and renal adjustments to a hypotensive agent (l-hydrazinophthalazine: Ciba BA-5968: Apresoline). J. clin. Invest. **31**, 872—879 (1952).

WILSON, W. R., OKUN, R.: The acute hemodynamic effects of diazoxide in man. Circulation **28**, 89—93 (1963).

ZACEST, R., GILMORE, E., KOCH-WESER, J.: Treatment of essential hypertension with combined vasodilation and beta-adrenergic blockade. New Engl. J. Med. **286**, 617—622 (1972).

ZACEST, R., KOCH-WESER, J.: Relation of hydralazine plasma concentration to dosage and hypotensive action. Clin. Pharmacol. Ther. **13**, 420—425 (1972).
ZAK, S. B., BARTLETT, M. F., WAGNER, W. E., GILLERAN, T. G., LUKAS, G.: Disposition of hydralazine in man and a specific method for its determination in biological fluids. J. Pharm. Sci. **63**, 225—229 (1974).

Section VII. Diuretic Drugs

ALDIN, E. V., MARKS, A. D., CHANNICK, B. J.: Spironolactone and hydrochlorthiazide in essential hypertension—blood pressure response and plasma renin activity. Arch. intern. Med. **130**, 855—858 (1972).
CAREY, R. M., DOUGLAS, J. C., SCHWEIKERT, R., LIDDLE, G. W.: The syndrome of essential hypertension and suppressed plasma renin activity: normalization of blood pressure with spironolactone. Arch. intern. Med. **130**, 849—854 (1972).
CRANE, M. G., HARRIS, J. J.: The effect of spironolactone in hypertensive patients. Amer. J. med. Sci. **260**, 311—329 (1970).
DOUGLAS, J. G., HOLLIFIELD, J. W., LIDDLE, G. W.: The treatment of low—renin essential hypertension—comparison of spironolactone and a hydrochlorothiazide—triamterene combination. J. Amer. med. Ass. **227**, 518—521 (1974).
DUSTAN, H. P., TARAZI, R. C., BRAVO, E. L.: Dependence of arterial pressure on intravascular volumes in treated hypertensive patients. New Engl. J. Med. **286**, 861—866 (1972).
FRYE, R. L., BRAUNWALD, E.: Studies on Starling's Law of the Heart, I. The circulatory response to acute hypervolemia and its modification by ganglionic blockade. J. clin. Invest. **39**, 1043—1050 (1960).
HOLLIFIELD, J. W., LIDDLE, G. W.: (Unpublished data).
KUCHEL, O., FISHMAN, L. M., LIDDLE, G. W., MICHELAKIS, A.: Effect of diazoxide on plasma renin activity in hypertensive patients. Ann. intern. Med. **67**, 791—799 (1967).
NICKERSON, M., GOURZIS, J. T.: Blockade of sympathetic vasoconstriction in the treatment of shock. J. Trauma **2**, 399—411 (1962).
SPARK, R. F., MELBY, J. C.: Hypertension and low plasma renin activity: presumptive evidence for mineralo corticoid excess. Ann. intern. Med. **75**, 831—836 (1971).
WOODS, J. W., LIDDLE, G. W., STANT, E. G., JR., MICHELAKIS, A. M., BRILL, A. B.: Effect of an adrenal inhibitor in hypertensive patients with suppressed renin. Arch. intern. Med. **123**, 366—370 (1969).

Chapter 14

Table of Antihypertensive Drugs

F. Gross and J. B. Lüth

The following tables give information about the most important drugs used today in the treatment of high blood pressure. These lists do not in any way aim for completeness, in particular with respect to brand names, which are much more numerous for several of the mentioned products. The usual forms of administration and average dosages are included, but various other schemes are also recommended for some drugs in some countries.

What is said for the single entities with respect to completeness holds true even more for the fixed combinations, of which only a fraction of those marketed in a number of countries has been included. Some examples of the combinations that make sense to the authors have been mentioned; many have been omitted; however, deletion does not mean in all cases – but it does in some – that the combination is considered useless. If a barbiturate is added to reserpine and a diuretic, it is difficult to ascribe to the new combination an improved effect on the high blood pressure. Quite a few more examples could be given, where the addition of a further ingredient to the basic combination of reserpine and a diuretic is nothing but the mixing in of a special flavor, and not of an antihypertensive component. Some of the readers may also feel that too many drugs and combinations have been listed, and they may never have heard the names of quite a few of them. Despite the incompleteness of the list, it gives an impression of the huge variety of preparations, which will further increase with the growing number of β-adrenergic blockers and their combinations with other drugs.

Rauwolfia Extracts, Reserpine and Derivatives

Generic name	Proprietary name	Formulation	Doses
Deserpidine	Harmonyl	Tabl. 0.25 mg	0.75–1.0 mg for 10–14 days; maintenance dose 0.25 mg daily
Methoserpidine	Decaserpyl	Tabl. 5; 10 mg	Initial dose of 30 mg/day; maintenance dose up to 60 mg daily
Rauwolfia serpentina extracts	Hypercal Hypertane Hypertensan Raudixin Rivadiscin	Tabl. 2 mg Tabl. 2 mg Tabl. 50 mg Tabl. 50 mg Tabl. 150 mg	200 mg/day; maintenance dose 50–300 mg
Alseroxylone fraction	Rauwiloid	Tabl. 2 mg	2–8 mg daily

Rauwolfia Extracts, Reserpine and Derivatives (Continued)

Generic name	Proprietary name	Formulation	Doses
Rescinnamine	Anaprel 500 Moderil	Tabl. 0.5 mg Tabl. 0.25; 0.5 mg	0.5 mg 2–3 times daily
Reserpine	Rau-Sed Sandril Sedaraupin Serpasil	Tabl. 0.25 mg Amp. 2.5 mg/ml; 10 ml Tabl. 0.1 mg Tabl. 0.2 mg Amp. 0.25 (1.0) mg/ml Tabl. 0.25; 0.1; 1 mg Amp. 0.1 mg/ml Drops 0.5 mg/ml	0.05–0.5 mg daily; maintenance dose 0.25–0.5 mg daily
Syrosingopine	Singoserp	Tabl. 1 mg	Initial dose 1–2 mg daily; maintenance dose 0.5 to 3 mg daily

Alpha-methyldopa, Clonidine

Generic name	Proprietary name	Formulation	Doses
Alpha-methyl-dopa	Aldomet, Aldometil Presinol Sembrina	Tabl. 125; 250; 500 mg Tabl. 250 mg Amp. 250 mg/5 ml Sugar-coated tablet 250 mg	0.5–3 g daily
Clonidine	Catapres Catapresan Catapresan 300	Tabl. 0.1 mg Amp. 0.15 mg/ml Tab. 0.15; 0.3 mg	Initial dose 0.075 mg 3 times daily; daily doses of up to 0.9 or 1.2 mg may be necessary; i.v. 0.075 to 0.150 mg

Sympatholytics

Generic name	Proprietary name	Formulation	Doses
Bethanidine	Bethanid Esbatal	Caps. 10 mg Tabl. 10; 50 mg	Initial dose, 10—20 mg daily in divided doses; subsequent doses gradually increased up to 200 mg daily
Debrisoquine	Declinax	Tabl. 10; 20 mg	10 mg twice daily, increasing to 50 mg 3 times daily
Guanethidine	Ismelin	Tabl. 10; 25 mg Amp. 10 mg/ml	10–20 mg daily, initially; subsequent doses increasing at weekly intervals to a maximum of 300 mg daily; maintenance dose 50–75 mg daily
Guanoclor	Vatensol	Tabl. 10; 40 mg	10–20 mg daily
Guanoxan	Envacar	Tabl. 10; 40 mg	Initial, 10 mg daily; subsequent doses gradually increased up to 200 mg daily

Ganglionic Blockers

Generic name	Proprietary name	Formulation	Doses
Chlorisondamine	Ecolid	Tabl. 25 mg Amp. 5 mg/ml	Initial, 10 mg daily; subsequent doses increasing up to 250 mg daily; i.v. 1–2 mg, s.c. 1–15 mg
Hexamethonium	Vegolysen	10% solution for injection, in vials of 25 mg	Initial dose of 5–15 mg s.c., i.m. Administration every 4–6 h is usually necessary
Mecamylamine	Inversine Mekamine Mevasine Revertina Versamine	Tabl. 2.5; 10 mg Tabl. 2.5; 100 mg	Initial dose, 2.5 mg twice daily; subsequent doses gradually increased to a maximum of 60 mg daily
Pempidine	Perolysen Tenormal	Tabl. 1; 5 mg	Initial dose, 2.5 mg every 6h; subsequent doses may be increased gradually to a maximum of 80 mg daily
Pentolinium	Ansolysen Pentilium	Tabl. 10; 40 mg Amp. 0.5% for 10 ml	Initial dose, 1–2.5 mg s.c. every 12 h; subsequent doses increased by 0.5–20 mg; tablets 10–20 mg every 12 h; maintenance dose 100–900 mg
Trimethaphan	Arfonad	Amp. 250 mg/5 ml	Administration by slow i.v. infusion of a freshly prepared solution in sodium chloride, the usual strength of solution being 1 mg/ml. The infusion is started at the rate of 3–4 mg/min and then the rate is adjusted according to the response of the patient

Alpha-adrenergic Blockers

Generic name	Proprietary name	Formulation	Doses
Phenoxybenzamine	Dibenyline, Dibenzyline, Dibenzyran	Caps. 10 mg	10–20 mg initially; subsequent doses increasing up to 240 mg daily
Phentolamine	Regitine, Rogitine	Amp. 10 mg/ml Tabl. 20 mg	5–10 mg i.m./i.v.
Tolazoline	Priscol, Priscoline Toline Tovalad Vasodil Zoline	Tabl. 25 ml Amp. 25 mg/ml Tabl. 25 mg	Up to 200 mg daily in divided doses

Alpha-adrenergic Blocker and Vasodilator

Prazosin	Minipres Hypotens Hypovase	Tabl. 1; 2; 5 mg	0.5–15 mg daily; initially 0.5–1.0 mg daily

Beta-adrenergic Blockers

Generic name	Proprietary name	Formulation	Doses
Alprenolol	Aptin, Gubernal	Tabl. 50 mg Amp. 10 mg/10 ml	100–200 mg daily, increasing up to 400 mg daily in divided doses by mouth; 5–20 mg by i.v. injection at a rate not exceeding 1 mg/min
Atenolol	Tenormin	Tabl. 50; 100 mg	100–300 mg daily
Bupranolol	Betadrenol	Tabl. 40; 100 mg	80–120 mg daily
Bunitrolol	Stresson	Tabl. 10 mg	10-20 mg twice daily
Butidrin	Betabloc, Recetan	Tabl. 50 mg	50–150 mg daily
Metoprolol	Beloc Betaloc Lopresor Seloken	Tabl. 50; 100 mg	100–300 mg daily
Nifenalol	Inpea	Tabl. 50 mg	100–300 mg daily
Oxprenolol	Trasicor slow Trasicor	Tabl. 20; 40; 80 mg Amp. 2 mg 160 mg	1–2 mg i.m., or i.v. 40 to 160 mg daily in divided doses increased to a maximum of 400 mg daily
Pindolol	Visken	Amp. 0.4 mg/2 ml Tabl. 5;15mg; Drops 1 ml = 20 drops = 5 mg	Mean dosage 15 mg daily by mouth; i.v. 0.4–2 mg
Propranolol	Inderal, Dociton	Tabl. 10; 40; 80 mg Amp. 1 mg/1 ml	160–320–2000 mg daily; 3–10 mg by slow i.v. injection
Sotalol	Sotalex, Beta Cardone	Tabl. 160 mg	160–640–1000 mg daily
Timolol	Blocadren, Temserin	Tabl. 5; 10; 15 mg	15–45 mg daily
Toliprolol	Doberol	Tabl. 10; 50 mg	30–150 mg daily

Vasodilators

Generic name	Proprietary name	Formulation	Doses
Dihydralazine	Nepresol	Tabl. 25 mg	25–100 mg daily
Diazoxide	Hyperstat Hypertonalum	Amp. 300 mg/20 ml	Treatment of severe hypertensive crisis: rapid injection of 300 mg i.v. every 4–20 h
Hydralazine	Apresolin Dralzine	Tabl. 25; 50 mg Amp. 20 mg/ml Tabl. 25 mg	50–200 mg daily by mouth; 20–40 mg i.v. or i.m.
Sodium Nitroprusside	Nipride Nipruss	Amp. 50 mg Amp. 60 mg	Infusion of 0.02–0.2 mg per min
Verapamil	Isoptin	Tabl. 40; 80 mg Amp. 5 mg/2 ml	120–240 mg daily by mouth; 5 mg i.v.

Veratrum Alkaloids

Generic name	Proprietary name	Formulation	Doses
Alkavervir	Veriloid	Tabl. 1; 2 mg	9–15 mg daily in three doses at intervals of 6–8 h
Cryptenamine	Unitensen	Tabl. 2 mg Amp. 2 mg	Initial dose, 2 mg twice daily by mouth, for patients in hospital the dose may be increased gradually each day; 1 mg diluted with 20 ml dextrose, i.v. injection may be used at a rate of 1 ml/min. For maintenance therapy of hypertensive crisis, i.m. injections of 1 mg at intervals of 3–6 h
Protoveratrine A + B	Puroverine	Tabl. 0.25 mg Amp. 0.10 mg	0.25–1 mg by mouth every 2–4 h; 0.1–0.4 mg i.m. every 1–6 h

Diuretics

Generic name	Proprietary name	Formulation	Doses
Amiloride	Midamor, Arumil	Tabl. 5 mg	10–40 mg daily
Bendrofluazide, Bendro-flumethiazide	Aprinox Berkozide Bristuric Centyl Naturetin Naturine Pluryl Sinesalin	Tabl. 2.5; 5.0 mg	10 mg daily
Benzthiazide	Aquatag Exasalt Exna NaClex	Tabl. 50 mg	25–50 mg daily
Butizide, Buthiazide	Eunephran Saltucin Ufrix	Tabl. 5.0 mg	10 mg daily
Chlorothiazide	Chlotride Diuril Flumen Miuril Miuzil Salisan Saluren Saluric Yadalan	Tabl. 250; 500 mg	250–500 mg daily
Chlorthalidone	Hygroton Igroton	Tabl. 50; 100 mg	50 mg daily; in severe cases initial doses of 100 mg may be necessary
Clopamide	Adurix Brinaldix	Tabl. 20 mg	20–40 mg twice daily
Clorexolone	Flonatril Nefrolan	Tabl. 10; 25 mg	10 mg twice daily

Diuretics (Continued)

Generic name	Proprietary name	Formulation	Doses
Cyclopenthi-azide	Navidrex Navidrix	Tab. 0.5 mg	Initial dose 1–2 mg daily, increasing up to 4 mg daily
Cyclothiazide	Anhydron Doburil Valmiran	Tabl. 2 mg	2 mg daily
Frusemide, Furosemide	Furantral Furix Lasix	Tabl. 40; 500 mg Amp. 20 mg/2 ml; 250 mg/25 ml	40–400 mg daily
Hydrochloro-thiazide	Aquarius Di-Chlotride Direma Esidrex Esidrix Hydrid Hydro-Aquil Hydro-Diuril Hydro-Saluric Hydrozide Lexxor Oretic	Tabl. 25; 50 mg	25–50 mg twice daily
Hydro-flumethiazide	Diucardin Saluron	Tabl. 50 mg	50–100 mg daily
Indapamid	Natrilix	Coated tab. 2.5 mg	2.5–5 mg once daily
Mefruside	Baycaron	Tabl. 25 mg	50 mg daily in divided doses
Methyclo-thiazide	Aquatensen Duretic Enduron	Tabl. 2.5; 5 mg	2.5–5 mg daily
Metolazone	Zaroxolyn	Tabl. 2.5; 5; 10 mg	2.5–5 mg once daily
Polythiazide	Drenusil Nephril Renese	Tabl. 2 mg Tabl. 1 mg Tabl. 1; 2; 4 mg	1–4 mg daily
Quinethazone	Aquamox Hydromox	Tabl. 50 mg	50 mg twice daily
Spironolactone	Aldactone Osyrol	Coated tabl. 25; 50 mg Coated tabl. 50; 100 mg	100–200 mg daily in divided doses
K-Canrenoate	Aldactone pro injection Osyrol pro injection	Vials 200 mg Vials 200 mg	200–400 mg daily
Triamterene	Diurene Dyrenium Dytac Iatropur Triamteril	Caps. 50 mg	100–250 mg daily in divided doses
Trichlor-methiazide	Esmarin Metahydrin Naqua	Tabl. 2; 4 mg	4–8 mg daily
Xipamid	Aquaphor	Tabl. 40 mg	20–40 mg daily

Combinations of Reserpine, Rauwolfia Extracts and Derivatives With Diuretics

Generic name	Proprietary name	Formulation and content	Doses
Reserpine combined with:			
Bendrofluazide	Albicol Tablets	Reserpine 0.15 mg Bendrofluazide 2.5 mg	Twice daily $^{1}/_{2}$–1 tab.
	Tensanyl	Reserpine 0.1 mg Bendrofluazide 1.25 mg KCl 573 mg	Initial 1 or 2 tab. thrice daily, maintenance 1–3 tab.
Bendroflumethiazide	Raupicin Repicin	Reserpine 0.1 mg Bendroflumethiazide 2 mg KCl 200 mg	1–2 tabl. daily
Benzthiazide	Exna-R	Reserpine 0.125 mg Benzthiazide 50 mg	Dosage individual to the need of the patient
Chlorthalidone	Darebon (mite)	Reserpine 0.25 (0.125) mg Chlorthalidone 50 (25) mg	Initial 1 tabl. daily, maintenance $^{1}/_{2}$ tabl. 3 times weekly
	Hygroton-Reserpin, Regroton	Reserpine 0.25 mg Chlorthalidone 50 mg	1–2 tabl. daily in one dose
Chlorothiazide	Diupres	Reserpine 0.125 mg Chlorothiazide 250 mg	2–3 tabl. daily
Cyclopenthiazide	Navidrex-Serpasil K	Reserpine 0.1 mg Cyclopenthiazide 0.25 mg KCl 600 mg	1–3 tabl. daily
Frusemide, Furosemide	Nortensin	Reserpine 0.4 mg Frusemide 60 mg	Initial dose 1 tabl. daily, maintenance 1 tabl. every 2nd day
	Terbolan	Reserpine 0.1 mg Frusemide 15 mg	3–4 tabl. daily
Hydrochlorothiazide	Hydropres (25; 50)	Reserpine 0.125 mg Hydrochlorothiazide 25; 50 mg	
	Hydrotensin 50	Reserpine 0.125 mg Hydrochlorothiazide 50 mg	
	Salupres	Reserpine 0.625 mg Hydrochlorothiazide 12.5 mg KCl 572 mg	2–3 tabl. daily
	Serpasil-Esidrix	Reserpine 0.1 mg Hydrochlorothiazide 25 mg	
	Serpasil-Esidrex (K)	Reserpine 0.15 mg Hydrochlorothiazide 10 mg KCl 600 mg	1 tabl. 3 times daily
Hydrochlorothiazide and Triamteren	Resaltex	Reserpine 0.125 mg Hydrochlorothiazide 25 mg Triamteren 50 mg	1 tabl. daily
Hydroflumethiazide	Salutensin	Reserpine 0.125 mg Hydroflumethiazide 50 mg	1 tabl. twice daily
Polythiazide	Drenusil-R	Reserpine 0.25 mg Polythiazide 1 mg	1 tabl. daily
	Renese-R Renese-Reserpine	Reserpine 0.25 mg Polythiazide 2 mg	$^{1}/_{2}$–2 tabl. daily

Combinations of Reserpine, Rauwolfia Extracts and Derivatives With Diuretics (Cont'd)

Generic name	Proprietary name	Formulation and content	Doses
Quinethazone	Hydromox-R	Reserpine 0.125 mg Quinethazone 50 mg	1–3 tabl. daily
Trichlormethiazide	Naquival	Reserpine 0.1 mg Trichlormethiazide 4 mg	1–3 tabl. daily
	Metatensin	Reserpine 0.1 mg Trichlormethiazide 2 (4) mg	
Xipamide	Durotan	Reserpine 0.1 mg Xipamide 4 mg	$^1/_2$–2 tabl. daily
Reserpine combined with:			
Rescinnamine Raubasine Butizide	Modenol	Reserpine 0.07 mg Rescinnamine 0.07 mg Raubasine 0.7 mg Butizide 3.3 mg KCl 300 mg	Initial dose 2–3 tabl. daily, maintenance 1 tabl. daily
Deserpidine combined with:			
Hydrochlorothiazide	Oreticyl (25/50)	Deserpidine 0.125 mg Hydrochlorothiazide 25/50 mg	1–2 tabl. daily
Methyclothiazide	Endoronyl, Enduron Harmonyl	Deserpidine 0.25 mg Methyclothiazide 5 mg	Initial dose 1 tabl,. maintenance $^1/_2$–2 tabl.
Methoserpidine combined with:			
Benzthiazide	Decaserpyl Plus	Methoserpidine 10 mg Benzthiazide 20 mg	Initial dose 1 tabl. thrice daily, maintenance 1–5 tabl. daily
Rauwolfia Serpentina extracts combined with:			
Bendroflumethiazide	Rauzide	Rauwolfia Serpentina extract 50 mg Bendroflumethiazide 4 mg	1–4 tabl. daily
Hydroflumethiazide	Rautrax	Rauwolfia Serpentina extract 50 mg KCl 625 mg	Initial dose 1–3 tabl. daily, maintenance 1 tabl.

Combinations of Reserpine With Other Antihypertensive Drugs

Reserpine combined with:			
Methyldopa and Mefruside	Caprinol	Reserpine 0.1 mg Methyldopa 125 mg Mefruside 10 mg	1 tabl. daily

Combination of Reserpine With Vasodilators

Generic name	Proprietary name	Formulation and content	Doses
Reserpine combined with:			
Dihydralazine	Adelphan	Reserpine 0.1 mg Dihydralazine 10 mg	2–3 tabl. daily
	Dralserp	Reserpine 0.1 mg Dihydralazine 25 mg	
Hydralazine	Serpasil-Apresoline	Reserpine 0.2 mg Hydralazine 50 mg	1–2 tabl. daily
Rauwolfia alkaloids and Dihydralazine-Theophylline	Ipharon	Rauwolfia alkaloids 1 mg Dihydralazine-Theophylline 25 mg	1 coated tabl. 2–3 times daily; maintenance dose once or twice daily 1 coated tabl.

Combination of Reserpine With Vasodilators and Diuretics

Generic name	Proprietary name	Formulation and content	Doses
Reserpine combined with:			
Dihydralazine Hydrochlorothiazide	Adelphan-Esidrix Adelphan-Esidrex	Reserpine 0.1 mg Dihydralazine 10 mg Hydrochlorothiazide 10 mg	Initial dose 2–3 tabl. daily, maintenance 1 to 2 tabl daily
	Elfanex	Reserpine 0.1 mg Dihydralazine 10 mg Hydrochlorothiazide 10 mg KCl 300 mg	1–2 tabl. daily
Hydralazine Hydrochlorothiazide	Hydrotensin Plus SER-AP-ES	Reserpine 0.1 mg Hydralazine 25 mg Hydrochlorothiazide 15 mg	1–2 tabl. 3 times daily
Inositolnicotinat Mefruside	Bendigon	Reserpine 0.15 mg Inositolnicotinat 150 mg Mefruside 15 mg	1–3 capsules daily
Dihydroergocristine and Clopamide	Briserin (mite)	Reserpine 0.1 (0.05) mg Dihydroergocristine 0.58 (0.4) mg Clopamide 5 (2.5 mg)	Initial dose 1 tabl. daily, if necessary 2–3 tabl. daily

Combination of Other Antihypertensive Drugs With Diuretics

Generic name	Proprietary name	Formulation and content	Doses
Methyldopa combined with:			
Butizide	Sembrina-Saltucin	Methyldopa 250 mg Butizide 1 mg	2–4 tabl . daily
Chlorothiazide	Aldoclor	Methyldopa 250 mg Chlorothiazide 150 mg	
Hydrochlorothiazide	Aldoril Hydromet	Methyldopa 250 mg Hydrochlorothiazide 15 mg	Initial dose 2–3 tabl. the first 2 days; maintenance: adjusted delating or adding 1 or 2 tablets

Combinatior of Other Anthypertensive Drugs With Diuretics (Continued)

Generic name	Proprietary name	Formulation and content	Doses
Mefruside	Sali-Presinol	Methyldopa 250 mg Mefruside 10 mg	2–3 tabl. daily
Clonidine combined with:			
Chlorthalidone	Combipres	Clonidine 0.1 (0.2) mg Chlorthalidone 15 mg	Initial dose 0.1 mg tabl. once or twice daily, maintenance 0.2 to 0.8 mg daily in divided doses
	Combipresan	Clonidine 0.075 mg Chlorthalidone 15 mg	Initial dose 2 tabl. daily, maintenance 1 tabl. daily
Guanethidine combined with:			
Cyclopenthiazide	Ismelin-Navidrex K	Guanethidine 10 mg Cyclopenthiazide 0.15 mg KCl 400 mg	Initial dose 1 tabl. daily; maintenance dose 1/2 to 4 tabl. daily
Hydrochlorothiazide	Esimil	Guanethidine 10 mg Hydrochlorothiazide 25 mg	Individual dosage to the need of the patient

Combination of Vasodilators and Diuretics

Generic name	Proprietary name	Formulation and content	Doses
Hydralazine Hydrochlorothiazide	Apresoline-Esidrix	Hydralazine 25 mg Hydrochlorothiazide 15 mg	1–2 tabl. 3 times daily

Combination of Two Diuretics

Generic name	Proprietary name	Formulation and content	Doses
Amiloride Hydrochlorothiazide	Moduretic	Amiloride 5 mg Hydrochlorothiazide 50 mg	1–2 tabl. daily
Spironolactone Hydrochlorothiazide	Aldactazide	Spironolactone 25 mg Hydrochlorothiazide 25 mg	2–4 tabl. daily in divided doses
Triamterene Benzthiazide		Triamterene 50 mg Benzthiazide 25 mg	1–2 tabl. daily
Triamterene Hydrochlorathiazide	Dyazide Dytide	Triamterene 50 mg Hydrochlorothiazide 25 mg	1–2 tabl. daily

Combination of Veratrum Alkaloids and Diuretics

Generic name	Proprietary name	Formulation and content	Dose
Cryptenamine Methyclothiazide	Diutensen	Cryptenamine 2 mg Methyclothiazide 2.5 mg	1—4 tabl. daily

Author Index

Page numbers in *italics* refer to the bibliography

6555 Pharma Vol. 39

Subject Index

Handbuch der experimentellen Pharmakologie/ Handbook of Experimental Pharmacology

Heffter-Heubner, New Series

Volume 4:
General Pharmacology

Volume 10:
Die Pharmakologie anorganischer Anionen

Volume 11:
Lobelin und Lobeliaalkaloide

Volume 12:
Morphin und morphinähnlich wirkende Verbindungen

Volume 14: Part 1
The Adrenocortical Hormones I

Part 2
The Adrenocortical Hormones II

Part 3
The Adrenocortical Hormones III

Volume 16:
Erzeugung von Krankheitszuständen durch das Experiment/ Experimental Production of Diseases

Part 1
Blut (In Vorbereitung)

Part 2
Atemwege

Part 3
Heart and Circulation

Part 4
Niere, Nierenbecken, Blase

Part 5
Liver

Part 6
Schilddrüse
(In Vorbereitung)

Part 7
Zentralnervensystem

Part 8
Stütz- und Hartgewebe

Part 9
Infektionen I

Part 10
Infektionen II

Part 11A
Infektionen III

Part 11B
Infektionen IV

Part 12
Tumoren I

Part 13
Tumoren II

Part 14
Tumoren III
(In preparation)

Part 15
Kohlenhydratstoffwechsel, Fieber/ Carbohydrate Metabolism, Fever

Volume 17: Part 1
Ions alcalino-terreux I

Part 2
Ions alcalino-terreux II

Volume 18: Part 1
Histamine

Part 2
Anti-Histaminics

Volume 19:
5-Hydroxytryptamine and Related Indolealkylamines

Volume 20: Part 1
Pharmacology of Fluorides I

Part 2
Pharmacology of Fluorides II

Volume 21:
Beryllium

Volume 22: Part 1
Die Gestagene I

Part 2
Die Gestagene II

Volume 23:
Neurohypophysial Hormones and Similar Polipeptides

Springer-Verlag
Berlin
Heidelberg
New York

Handbuch der experimentellen Pharmakologie/ Handbook of Experimental Pharmacology

Heffter-Heubner, New Series

Volume 24:
Diuretica

Volume 25:
Bradykinin, Kallidin and Kallikrein

Volume 26:
Vergleichende Pharmakologie von Überträgersubstanzen in tiersystematischer Darstellung

Volume 27:
Anticoagulantien

Volume 28: Part 1
Concepts in Biochemical Pharmacology I
Part 3
Concepts in Biochemical Pharmacology III

Volume 29:
Oral wirksame Antidiabetika

Volume 30:
Modern Inhalation Anesthetics

Volume 32: Part 1
Insulin I
Part 2
Insulin II

Volume 34:
Secretin, Cholecystokinin, Pancreozymin and Gastrin

Volume 35: Part 1
Androgene I
Part 2
Androgens II and Antiandrogens/ Androgene II und Antiandrogene

Volume 36:
Uranium – Plutonium – Transplutonic Elements

Volume 37:
Angiotensin

Volume 38: Part 1
Antieoplastic and and Immunosuppressive Agents I
Part 2
Antineoplastic and Immunosuppressive Agents II

Volume 39:
Antihypertensive Agents

Volume 40:
Organic Nitrates

Volume 41:
Hypolipidemic Agents

Volume 42:
Neuromuscular Junction

Volume 43:
Anabolic-Androgenic Steroids

Volume 44:
Haem and Haemoproteins

Volume 45: Part 1
Drug Addiction I
Part 2
Drug Addiction II

Volume 46:
Fibrinolytics and Antifibrinolytics
(In Preparation)

Volume 47:
Kinetics of Drug Action

Volume 48:
Arthropod Venoms

Volume 49:
Gangliomic Transmission (In preparation)

Volume 50:
Inflammation and Antiinflammatory Drugs
(In preparation)

Volume 51:
Ergot Alkaloids and Related Compounds
(In preparation)

Springer-Verlag
Berlin
Heidelberg
New York